Concepts *for* Nursing Practice

Concepts *for* Nursing Practice
CONTENT ORGANIZATION

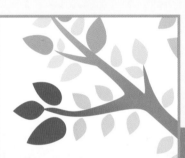

Health Care Recipient Concepts

Health and Illness Concepts

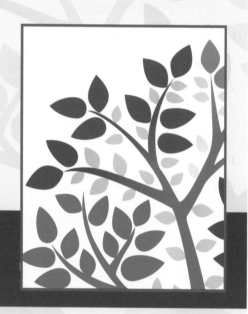

Professional Nursing and Health Care Concepts

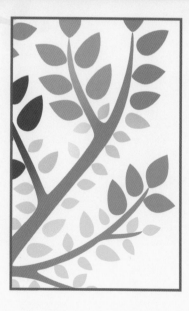

Concepts *for* Nursing Practice

THIRD EDITION

Jean Foret Giddens, PhD, RN, FAAN, ANEF

Dean and Professor
Doris B. Yingling Endowed Chair
School of Nursing
Virginia Commonwealth University
Richmond, Virginia

ELSEVIER

3251 Riverport Lane
St. Louis, Missouri 63043

CONCEPTS FOR NURSING PRACTICE, THIRD EDITION ISBN: 978-0-323-58193-6

Notices

Knowledge and best practice in this field are constantly changing. As new research and experience broaden our understanding, changes in research methods, professional practices, or medical treatment may become necessary.

Practitioners and researchers must always rely on their own experience and knowledge in evaluating and using any information, methods, compounds, or experiments described herein. In using such information or methods they should be mindful of their own safety and the safety of others, including parties for whom they have a professional responsibility.

With respect to any drug or pharmaceutical products identified, readers are advised to check the most current information provided (i) on procedures featured or (ii) by the manufacturer of each product to be administered, to verify the recommended dose or formula, the method and duration of administration, and contraindications. It is the responsibility of practitioners, relying on their own experience and knowledge of their patients, to make diagnoses, to determine dosages and the best treatment for each individual patient, and to take all appropriate safety precautions.

To the fullest extent of the law, neither the Publisher nor the authors, contributors, or editors, assume any liability for any injury and/or damage to persons or property as a matter of products liability, negligence or otherwise, or from any use or operation of any methods, products, instructions, or ideas contained in the material herein.

Previous edition copyrighted 2017, 2013.

Library of Congress Control Number: 2019949909

Executive Content Strategist: Lee Henderson
Senior Content Development Specialist: Heather Bays
Publishing Services Manager: Julie Eddy
Senior Project Manager: Tracey Schriefer
Product Manager: Kathy Withrow
Designer: Renee Duenow

Printed in Canada

Last digit is the print number: 9 8 7 6 5 4

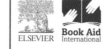

Working together
to grow libraries in
developing countries

www.elsevier.com • www.bookaid.org

ABOUT THE AUTHOR

Dr. Giddens earned a Bachelor of Science in Nursing from the University of Kansas, a Master of Science in Nursing from the University of Texas at El Paso, and a Doctor of Philosophy in Education and Human Resource Studies from Colorado State University. Dr. Giddens has over 30 years' experience in nursing education spanning associate degree, baccalaureate degree, and graduate degree nursing programs in New Mexico, Texas, Colorado, and Virginia. She is an expert in concept-based curriculum development and evaluation, as well as innovative strategies for teaching and learning. Dr. Giddens is the author of multiple journal articles, nursing textbooks, and electronic media and serves as an education consultant to nursing programs throughout the country.

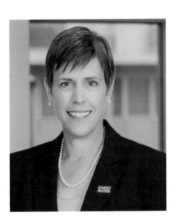

ACKNOWLEDGMENTS

Developing and writing *Concepts for Nursing Practice, Third Edition,* represents an amazing collaboration of educators and clinicians from multiple disciplines across the country. I extend my gratitude and appreciation to the contributors and reviewers for sharing their expertise and wisdom. I also am grateful to my colleagues at Elsevier for their expertise and guidance. Lastly, I extend deep appreciation to my husband Jay—without your friendship, love, and support, I could not accomplish such work.

Gail Elizabeth Armstrong, PhD, DNP, RN
Associate Professor
College of Nursing
University of Colorado
Aurora, Colorado

Debra Bennett-Woods, EdD
Professor Emerita
Health Services Education
Regis University
Denver, Colorado

Janice Bissonnette, PhD, RN, NP
Affiliate Researcher
Epidemiology
Ottawa Hospital Research Institute
Ottawa, Ontario, Canada

Kevin Brigle, PhD, RN, NP
Oncology Nurse Practitioner
Massey Cancer Center
Virginia Commonwealth University
Richmond, Virginia

Lorraine P. Buchanan, MSN, RN
Clinical Assistant Professor
School of Nursing and Health Studies
University of Missouri
Kansas City, Missouri

Lynne Buchanan, PhD, MSN, APRN-NP, BC
Associate Professor
College of Nursing
University of Nebraska Medical Center
Omaha, Nebraska

Susan Caplan, PhD, RN
Assistant Professor
Nursing
Rutgers University
Newark, New Jersey

Barbara M. Carranti, MS, RN
Clinical Associate Professor
Nursing
Le Moyne College
Syracuse, New York

Paul Thomas Clements, PhD, RN, DF-IAFN
Professor in Residence
Director, DNP Program
University of Nevada
Las Vegas, Nevada

Sean P. Convoy, DNP, PMHNP-BC
Assistant Professor
School of Nursing
Duke University
Durham, North Carolina

Patrick Coyne, MSN, RN
Director
Palliative Care
Medical University of South Carolina
Charleston, South Carolina

Constance Dahlin, MSN, AB, ANP-BC, ACHPN, FPCN, FAAN
Director of Professional Practice
Hospice and Palliative Nurses Association
Pittsburgh, Pennsylvania;
Consultant
Center to Advance Palliative Care
New York, New York;
Palliative Nurse Practitioner
North Shore Medical Center
Salem, Massachusetts

Kimberly D. Davis, MS, RN, CNE
Clinical Assistant Professor
Family and Community Health Nursing
School of Nursing
Virginia Commonwealth University
Richmond, Virginia

Jennie De Gagne, PhD, DNP, RN-BC, CNE, ANEF, FAAN
Associate Professor
School of Nursing
Duke University
Durham, North Carolina

Fayron Epps, PhD, RN
Assistant Professor
Byrdine F. Lewis College of Nursing and Health Professions
Georgia State University
Atlanta, Georgia

Sylvia Escott-Stump, MA, RDN, LDN
Clinical Assistant Professor, Ret.
Department of Nutrition Science
East Carolina University
Greenville, North Carolina

Linda Felver, PhD, RN
Associate Professor
School of Nursing
Oregon Health & Science University
Portland, Oregon

Katherine Fletcher, PhD, RN
Clinical Professor
School of Nursing
University of Kansas
Kansas City, Kansas

Nelda Godfrey, PhD, RN, ACNS-BC, FAAN
Associate Dean
Innovative Partnerships and Practice
University of Kansas
Kansas City, Kansas

Sue K. Goebel, MS, RN, WHNP
Associate Professor of Nursing
Department of Health Sciences
Colorado Mesa University;
Women's Health Nurse Practitioner
Integrative Medicine Center
Grand Junction, Colorado

Debra Hagler, PhD, RN, ACNS-BC, CNE, CHSE, ANEF, FAAN
Clinical Professor
College of Nursing and Health Innovation
Arizona State University
Phoenix, Arizona

Ingrid Hendrix, MILS
Nursing Services Librarian
Health Sciences Library and Informatics Center
University of New Mexico
Albuquerque, New Mexico

Kathleen A. Hessler, AA, BA, JD
Director
Compliance & Risk
Simione Healthcare Consultants, LLC
Albuquerque, New Mexico

Nancy Hoffart, PhD, RN
Forsyth Medical Center Distinguished Professor
School of Nursing
University of North Carolina at Greensboro
Greensboro, North Carolina

Beth S. Hopkins, DNP, FNP
Assistant Professor
College of Nursing
Upstate Medical University of the State of New York
Syracuse, New York

Eun-Ok Im, PhD, MPH, FAAN
Professor & Mary T. Champagne Professor
School of Nursing
Duke University
Durham, North Carolina

Nancy Jallo, PhD, RN
Associate Professor
School of Nursing
Virginia Commonwealth University
Richmond, Virginia

Teresa Keller, PhD, RN, MPA
Professor
School of Nursing
New Mexico State University
Las Cruces, New Mexico

Sangmi Kim, PhD, MPH, RN
Postdoctoral Associate
School of Nursing
Duke University
Durham, North Carolina

Kathie Lasater, EdD, RN
Professor Emerita
School of Nursing
Oregon Health & Science University
Portland, Oregon

Mijung Lee, PhD(c), RN
PhD Candidate
School of Nursing
University of Virginia
Charlottesville, Virginia

Judy Liesveld, PhD, PPCNP-BC, CNE
Clinician Educator Professor
Associate Dean of Education and
    Innovation
College of Nursing
University of New Mexico
Albuquerque, New Mexico

Susan Lindner, MSN, RN
Clinical Assistant Professor, Ret.
School of Nursing
Virginia Commonwealth University
Richmond, Virginia

Rebecca S. Miltner, PhD, RN, CNL,
    NEA-BC
Associate Professor
School of Nursing
University of Alabama at Birmingham
Birmingham, Alabama

Ann Nielsen, PhD, RN
Associate Professor of Clinical Nursing
Undergraduate Program
Oregon Health & Science University
Portland, Oregon

Devon Noonan, PhD, MPH
Associate Professor
Nursing
Duke University
Durham, North Carolina

Shelly Orr, PhD, RN, CNE
Assistant Professor
School of Nursing
Virginia Commonwealth University
Richmond, Virginia

Pamela Parsons, PhD, GNP-BC
Associate Professor, Director of Practice and
    Community Engagement
School of Nursing
Virginia Commonwealth University
Richmond, Virginia

Katherine Pereira, DNP, RN
Professor
School of Nursing
Duke University
Durham, North Carolina

Richard A. Pessagno, DNP, CRNP,
    FAANP
Adjunct Instructor
Nursing, DNP Program
Chatham University
Pittsburgh, Pennsylvania;
Psychiatric Nurse Practitioner
Private Practice
Wilmington, Delaware

Elizabeth Reifsnider, PhD, RN, FAAN
College of Nursing and Health Innovation
Center for Health Promotion and Disease
    Prevention
Arizona State University
Phoenix, Arizona

Nancy Ridenour, PhD, APRN, BC, FAAN
Maxine Clark and Bob Fox Dean and
    Professor
Barnes Jewish College;
Adjunct Professor
School of Medicine
Washington University
St. Louis, Missouri

Beth Rodgers, PhD, RN, FAAN
Professor and Chair
Adult Health and Nursing Systems
School of Nursing
Virginia Commonwealth University
Richmond, Virginia

L. Jane Rosati, EdD, RN, ANEF
Professor
School of Nursing
Daytona State College
Daytona Beach, Florida

Carolyn E. Sabo, EdD, RN
Professor
School of Nursing
University of Nevada, Las Vegas
Las Vegas, Nevada

Lana Sargent, PhD, FNP-C, GNP-BC
Assistant Professor
Adult Health & Nursing Systems
Virginia Commonwealth University
Richmond, Virginia

Gwen Sherwood, PhD, RN
Professor Emeritus
School of Nursing
University of North Carolina at Chapel Hill
Chapel Hill, North Carolina

Leigh Ann Simmons, PhD, MFT
Professor and Chair
Department of Human Ecology
University of California, Davis
Davis, California

Leigh Small, PhD, RN, CPNP-PC
Associate Dean of Academic Programs
College of Nursing
University of Colorado
Aurora, Colorado

Debra J. Smith, MSN
Principal Lecturer II
College of Nursing
University of New Mexico
Albuquerque, New Mexico

Angela Renee Starkweather, PhD,
    ACNP-BC, FAAN
Professor & Associate Dean for Academic
    Affairs
School of Nursing
University of Connecticut
Storrs, Connecticut

Amy Szoka, PhD, RN
Chair
School of Nursing
Daytona State College
Daytona Beach, Florida

Ishan C. Williams, PhD
Associate Professor
School of Nursing
University of Virginia
Charlottesville, Virginia

Susan F. Wilson, PhD, RN
Emeritus Associate Professor
Harris College of Health and Health
  Sciences
Texas Christian University
Fort Worth, Texas

Elizabeth Young, MSN, RN
Clinical Instructor
School of Nursing
The University of Kansas;
Clinical Nurse II
Renal and Transplant Progressive Care
The University of Kansas Health System
Kansas City, Kansas

REVIEWERS

Kim Amer, PhD, RN
Associate Professor
School of Nursing
DePaul University
Chicago, Illinois

Joanna V. Bachour, MSN, RN
Assistant Professor Registered Nurse
School of Nursing
Massachusetts College of Pharmacy and
    Health Science University
Worcester, Massachusetts

Joseph Boney, MSN, RN, NEA-BC
Director of Adjunct Faculty Development/
    Nursing Instructor
Second Degree BS in Nursing Program
Rutgers University School of Nursing
Newark, New Jersey

Tiffany M. Caldwell, MSN, RN
INACSL – CAE Healthcare Simulation
    Fellow 2016
Simulation Instructor
School of Nursing Portland Campus
Oregon Health & Science University
Portland, Oregon

Ashley Dru Causey, MSN, RN
OHSU School of Nursing
Undergraduate Program, Portland Campus
Oregon Health and Science University
Portland, Oregon

Tedi Courtney, MSN, RN
Clinical Assistant Professor
School of Nursing
University of Tulsa Oxley College of Health
    Sciences
Tulsa, Oklahoma

Patricia Donovan, MSN, RN
Director of Practical Nursing and
    Curriculum Chair
Practical Nursing Program
The Porter and Chester Institute
Rocky Hill, Connecticut

Kelly Duffy, EdD, MSN, RN
Senior Professor
School of Nursing
RN-BSN program
Daytona State College
Daytona Beach, Florida

Jean C. Farnham, MSN, RN
Nursing Faculty
Health Sciences-Nursing
Santa Rosa Junior College
Santa Rosa, California

Teresa Faykus, DNP, RN, CNE
Professor of Nursing
RN-BSN Coordinator
Nursing
West Liberty University
West Liberty, West Virginia

Linda Felver, PhD, RN
Associate Professor
School of Nursing
Oregon Health & Science University
Portland, Oregon

Rita W. Ferguson, PhD, RN, CHPN, CNE
Clinical Assistant Professor
College of Nursing
The University of Alabama in Huntsville
Huntsville, Alabama

Kari Gali, DNP, RN, PNP-BC
Director of Quality and Population Health
    Design in Distance Health
Cleveland Clinic;
Quality Consultant
American Academy of Pediatrics
Nursing and Medicine;
Adjunct Faculty
Case Western Reserve University
Cleveland, Ohio;
Clinical Preceptor
University of Illinois, Chicago
Chicago, Illinois

Christina N. George, MS, RN, CNE
Assistant Professor of Nursing
Nursing
Tulsa Community College
Tulsa, Oklahoma

Ruth Gliss, MS, RN, CNE
Professor
Nursing
Genesee Community College
Batavia, New York

Pamela Harvey, MSN, RN
Instructor
Medical Assistant Program
Bradford Union Career Technical Center
Starke, Florida

Susan Justice, MSN, RN, CNS
Clinical Assistant Professor
College of Nursing and Health Innovation
University of Texas
Arlington, Texas

Bonny Kehm, PhD, RN
Faculty Program Director
BS & MS Programs in Nursing
School of Nursing
Excelsior College
Albany, New York

Lorraine Kelley, MSN, BSHA/HIS, RN
Faculty
Department of Nursing and Emergency
    Medical Services
Pensacola State College
Pensacola, Florida

Tawnya S. Lawson, MS, RN
Dean
Practical Nursing
Hondros College of Nursing
Westerville, Ohio

Lisa Oken, MSN, RN
Clinical Faculty
VA – Nurse Academic Partnership
Portland VA/Oregon Health Sciences
    University
Portland, Oregon

Barbara J. Pinekenstein, DNP, RN-BC,
    CPHIMS
Clinical Professor
Richard E. Sinaiko Professor in Health Care
    Leadership
School of Nursing
University of Wisconsin, Madison
Madison, Wisconsin

Michele Poradzisz, PhD, RN, CNE, CNL
Professor
School of Nursing
Saint Xavier University
Chicago, Illinois

L. Jane Rosati, EdD, RN, ANEF
Professor
School of Nursing
Daytona State College
Daytona Beach, Florida

Mary Ruiz-Nuve, MSN, RN
Director of Clinical Placement
Practical Nursing
St. Louis College of Health Careers
Fenton, Missouri

Lisa A. Urban, PhD, RN
Professor
School of Graduate and Professional Studies
Stevenson University
Owings Mills, Maryland

Kris B. Weymann, PhD, RN
Assistant Professor
School of Nursing
Oregon Health & Science University
Portland, Oregon

PREFACE

Wisdom means keeping a sense of the fallibility of our views and opinions, and of the uncertainty and instability of the things we most count on.

Gerard Brown

INTRODUCTION TO CONCEPTUAL LEARNING

Conceptual learning is increasingly viewed as a major trend for the future of education—not in nursing alone, but across numerous disciplines. This belief is based on the premise that *concepts* can be used effectively as unifying classifications or principles for framing learning while knowledge increases exponentially.

So, what is a *concept*? Simply stated, a concept is an organizing principle or a classification of information. A concept can be limited or complex in scope and can be useful as a basis for education from preschool through doctoral education. In advanced applications, concepts are considered building blocks or the foundation for theory.

By gaining a deeper understanding of a core set of concepts, a student can recognize and understand similarities and recurring characteristics, which can be applied more effectively than memorized facts. Teaching conceptually turns traditional learning upside down, focusing on generalities (concepts) and then applying this understanding to specifics (exemplars), instead of the traditional educational approach that focuses more heavily on content and facts.

HOW THIS BOOK IS ORGANIZED

The conceptual approach in nursing involves an examination of concepts that link to the delivery of patient care. There are multiple concepts applicable to nursing practice. This book does not attempt to present all nursing concepts, nor does it suggest that the featured concepts chosen are the most important. However, the 57 concepts featured in this book are commonly seen in nursing literature or are representative of important practice phenomena; they are the concepts that apply to the broadest group of patients of various ages and across various health care settings. A simplified concept presentation format using consistent headings is intentionally used so that students will find the approach intuitive; at the same time, an understanding of more formalized conceptual analyses will be fostered. Three overarching groups of concepts, or *units*, are featured:

- **Health Care Recipient Concepts (Unit 1)**—concepts that help us understand the individuals for whom we care
- **Health and Illness Concepts (Unit 2)**—concepts that help us make sense of the multiple health conditions experienced by our patients across the lifespan
- **Professional Nursing and Health Care Concepts (Unit 3)**—concepts that guide our professional practice in the context of health care

These three overarching units are further categorized into *themes,* into which concepts are organized to provide a structured framework. This structured approach promotes a thorough understanding of individual concepts and their important context within related health care concepts.

Each concept provides a full spectrum of information, with separate subheadings for concept definition, risk factors, health assessment, context of the concept to nursing and health care, interrelated concepts, case studies, and examples (exemplars) of concepts in practice. Each piece helps build an understanding of the concept as a whole, which in turn will promote the development of clinical judgment, a key outcome if nursing students are to practice effectively in today's complex health care environment.

FEATURES

Concept discussions include holistic concept diagrams that help visualize conceptual processes, along with *interrelated concepts* diagrams. These illustrations encourage students to build important associations among interrelated concepts. *Case Studies* provide an example of the concept applied in the context of patient care or practice setting.

An extensive list of *exemplars* (boxes at the end of every concept chapter) is based on incidence and prevalence across the lifespan and clinical settings. The *Featured Exemplars* section provides a brief explanation of some of the most important exemplars. Using a custom technology, direct links to selected exemplars have been embedded into a core collection of Elsevier eBooks. This option of linking directly to a curated list of exemplars in a set collection of titles allows for a seamless user experience by uniting concepts to priority exemplars. Although instructors have complete flexibility to choose those concepts and exemplars best suited to their particular institution, these direct links are provided to allow quick access to those exemplars likely to be used in the majority of cases.

Interactive review questions incorporated into a self-assessment student testing engine are provided as an additional feature of this book's Evolve website (http://evolve.elsevier.com/Giddens/concepts). These 250 student questions include multiple-choice and multi-select questions to simulate the NCLEX™ Examination testing experience, along with correct answer options and rationales.

Additional material to support faculty is included on the *Evolve Instructor Resources* site. A number of resources are provided to offer assistance in developing and teaching in a concept-based curriculum. Additionally, TEACH Lesson Plans, PowerPoints, and test banks have all been developed at both the RN and PN level to accommodate all learning needs.

CONCLUSION

Why use a conceptual approach? An exponential generation of new knowledge and information in all areas of our world (including health care and nursing) has made it literally impossible for anyone to know all information within the discipline of nursing. The study of nursing concepts provides the learner with an understanding of essential components associated with nursing practice without becoming saturated and lost in the details for each area of clinical specialty. If concepts are understood deeply, links can be made when these are applied in various areas of nursing practice.

The conceptual approach also fosters future advancement of the nursing discipline. This book serves as a guide to learning about concepts and their application in clinical nursing practice. The conceptual approach provides the foundation for learning, clinical practice, and research efforts needed to continue to build substantive knowledge to the discipline of nursing. The conceptual approach represents a journey that embraces change. Let the journey begin!

Jean Foret Giddens

CONTENTS

Health Care Recipient Concepts

ATTRIBUTES AND RESOURCES

PERSONAL PREFERENCES

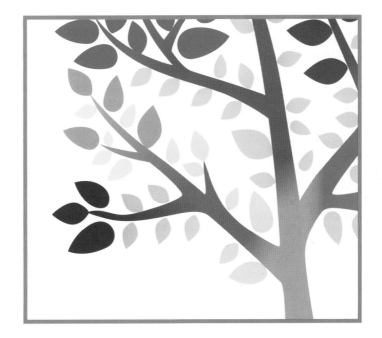

In the not too distant past, health care was delivered in a disease-centered model whereby healthcare providers controlled and directed care with little input from patients regarding their desires or their concerns about the impact of the treatment plan on their lives. Patients were appraised of the plan as opposed to discussing options for disease management.

Health care has moved to a patient-centered model of health care in which patients and their families are active participants in their care.[1] Healthcare services are designed to meet the needs and wishes of the individual. Healthcare professionals counsel and provide advice related to healthcare decisions, based on their clinical expertise and evidence.[1] Fundamental to this is the ability to understand the unique attributes of each and every patient. For the successful delivery of patient-centered care, nurses should understand the concepts presented in this unit. The two themes within this unit are Attributes and Resources and Personal Preferences.

Attributes and Resources includes concepts associated with unique characteristics of the patient: Development, Functional Ability, and Family Dynamics. *Personal Preferences* includes concepts that influence an individual's attitudes and preferences regarding health care: Culture, Spirituality, Adherence, and Self-Management. These concepts are necessary to understand the decision making and behavior of patients, and they inform providers of strategies necessary to reach decisions that are mutually acceptable and agreeable to patients and providers.

---

[1]Institute of Medicine. (2001). *Crossing the quality chasm: A new health system for the 21st century*. Washington, DC: National Academies Press.

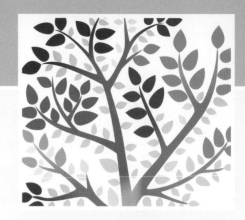

Development

Leigh Small

A basic characteristic of all human life is change. Development is a complex process that involves the integration of an expansive variety of gradual changes that occur across multiple domains and result in an individual's functional abilities. These changes usually increase in complexity according to a dynamic, somewhat predictable sequence that begins at conception and continues over the life span until older age and/or death.[1-4] The individual's state of health, environmental context, and/or life experiences may alter an aspect of an individual's development, causing it to stagnate or regress to an earlier stage. The ability to provide patient-centered, quality care requires nurses to understand and assess the different aspects of an individual's development and appropriately adjust the care they provide. It is also important for nurses to recognize when expected developmental progression in any area is not occurring, so that collaborative interventions can be initiated.

DEFINITION

Development refers to *the sequence of physical, psychosocial, and cognitive developmental changes that take place over the human life span.*[3] Development does not occur as an isolated phenomenon. Rather, it represents the dynamic integration of three aspects of change: growth, differentiation, and maturation. *Physical growth* is a quantitative change in which an increase in cell number and size results in an increase in overall size or weight of the body or any of its parts. *Differentiation* is the process by which initially formed cells and structures become specialized. This is both a quantitative and a qualitative change from simple to complex in which broad global function becomes refined and specific. *Maturation* is the emergence of personal, behavioral, or adultlike physical characteristics or a "ripening." Maturation enables an individual to function in a fully developed and optimal way. Thus maturation increases adaptability and competence for individuals to adjust to new situations.[3] Development, as well as the interrelated processes of growth, differentiation, and adaptation, is significantly impacted by genetics, environmental factors, culture, family values, and personal experiences.[3-6] Therefore the overall concept of development, as defined in this context, affects all aspects of every individual and directs all aspects of nursing care. Times during which development is rapidly occurring (i.e., infancy, childhood, and older adulthood) deserve special attention and in-depth knowledge because nursing care will need to responsively adjust and nurses will need to adapt to the developmental changes of the patient more frequently and on an individual basis.

The unique sets of skills and competencies to be mastered at each developmental stage across the life span for the individual to cope with the environment are called *developmental tasks.*[7] Developmental tasks are broad in scope and are, to a significant degree, determined by culture.[8] The tasks may relate to the individual or to the family. Examples of developmental tasks are stepping up steps unassisted and coping with the loss of a spouse.[9]

The order of developmental task attainment is more important than the chronologic age at which each occurs because, although development is ongoing, its speed varies across individuals. Furthermore, each individual has a unique developmental pace moderated by one's state of health, environment, and social/family context. Rate and level of development are also related to the physiologic maturity of all systems—particularly the neurologic, muscular, and skeletal systems.

SCOPE

The scope of the concept, or extent to which development influences an individual (i.e., expected, delayed, or advanced development; Fig. 1.1), spans the entire life course—from birth to death (Table 1.1). Normal human development is organized and progressive and usually occurs in a predictable sequence. Based on this expected sequence, stages of development have been identified. The traditional stages of development have been identified by general age groups and include embryologic, infant, toddler, preschool, school age, adolescent (teen), young adult, adult, middle age, and older adult. These stages identify characteristics found in the majority of individuals within a stated age range. Although individuals vary in the time of onset of each stage and in the length of time spent in each stage, the sequence itself rarely varies.

Types of Development

Development is a complex and interconnected concept that has been distilled into six overarching categories or domains: physical/physiologic, motoric, social/emotional, cognitive, communication, and adaptive (Fig. 1.2). The accelerated and decelerated paces of development occur somewhat independently within each domain (e.g., physical/physiologic, motor, social, cognitive, and communication). For example, while gross motor skills are changing (i.e., infant walking), language skills may not be developing as quickly. Similarly, an older school-aged child may be demonstrating advanced physical maturation but has not achieved advanced states of emotional maturation. Thus age-related developmental expectancies or norms are always based on an age range—never

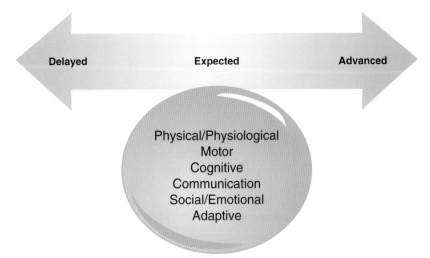

FIGURE 1.1 Scope of Development.

TABLE 1.1	Identified Developmental Age Compared With Chronologic Age
Developmental Age	**Chronological Age**
Birth	Conception through birth
Infant	Birth through 12 months
Toddler	12–36 months
Preschooler	36 months–5 years
School-ager	5–12 years
Adolescent	12–18 years
Young adult	18–35 years
Middle adult	35–65 years
Older adult	
Young-old	65–75 years
Middle-old	75–85 years
Old-old	>85 years

an exact point in time when specific skills will be achieved.[1,3,10] Although the pace of development within each of these domains occurs independently, the progression of skills in the subcategories is also interconnected and reliant on the development in the other domains.

Physical/Physiologic Development

Physical/physiologic development refers to the growth and changes in body tissues and organ systems and the resultant changes in body functions and proportions. Physiologic development includes cellular proliferation, differentiation, and maturation that occurs in each organ and system that allows integrated human functioning necessary for life and health (i.e., infant hematopoietic maturity and secondary sexual characteristic development leading to sexual function). Overall, physical growth and development occur in a bilateral and symmetric way, progressing in a cephalocaudal (head-to-toe) direction (i.e., infants have a disproportionately larger head-to-body ratio compared with that of an adult) and proximodistally (from midline to periphery).

Motoric Development

Motoric development is frequently separated into two major categories: gross and fine motor. Very generally, motoric development progresses from achievement of gross motor to fine motor skills—a process referred to as refinement.[11,12] Gross motor skills involve the use of large muscles to move about in the environment. Examples of gross motor development include the sequential skills of sitting, standing, maintaining balance, cruising, walking, running, walking up stairs without assistance, and more complex physical tasks such as playing soccer. Fine motor skills involve the use of small muscles in an increasingly coordinated and precise manner. Examples of fine motor development include the achievement of the successive skills of batting at an object, reaching and holding an object, transferring an object from hand to hand, holding a pencil in a refined grasp, making marks with a pencil, writing letters, writing words, and the complex skill of creating masterful artwork. Other fine motor skills using the hands and fingers to eat, draw, dress, and play are all required to achieve optimal functioning.[13,14] Fine motor development is contingent upon cognitive and neurologic development.

Social/Emotional Development

Social and emotional development includes the development of self-understanding, understanding others, and understanding social interactions.[1,2,11,12] These different elements of social/emotional development usually occur in this order (e.g., self, others, and social interaction). Knowledge of social/emotional skills is critical because it directs effective communication with an individual(s) and may impact suggested environmental strategies for an individual to attain optimal functioning. For example, young preschool children cannot distinguish between their effort and their ability and are likely to overestimate their competence and abilities. Thus caution should be used regarding self-reported ability(ies), and nurses should seek confirmation (e.g., "Johnnie says that he can swallow pills. Have you seen Johnnie take pills before, or is Johnnie better able to swallow liquid medicine?"). Development of an understanding of others (perspective taking) includes a growing comprehension that other people have emotions and intentions and that objects do not. This understanding is foundational to the development of trust, moral development, and the ability to interact with others. These aspects of development underlie the ability of children to discern the difference between a truth and a lie. A complicating aspect of social/emotional development is emotional regulation, which directly impacts relational interactions (i.e., play, work, and social interactions).[15] This complex aspect of development declines during the aging process in an indeterminable rate, underscoring the need to consider and assess areas of social/emotional development across the life span.

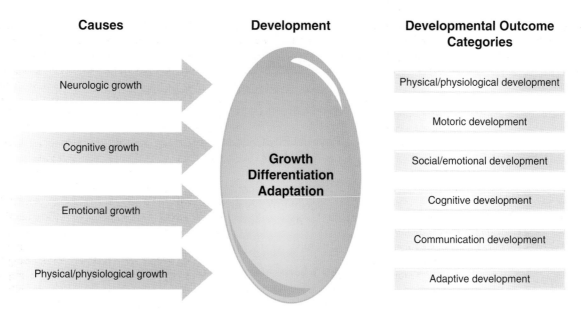

FIGURE 1.2 Development Concept Categories.

Cognitive Development

The cognitive dimension of development relates to working memory capacity, cognitive self-regulation, and the processing and use of information about the environment and objects in the environment. In addition, individuals have an increasing understanding of relationships between self-understanding and information over time. These processes underlie the development of critical thinking skills and executive functioning, which includes learning, forming concepts, understanding, problem solving, reasoning, remembering, and thinking abstractly. Ultimately, these complex aspects of cognitive development, in combination with advanced social/emotional developmental stages, enable moral and spiritual development.[1]

Some have suggested that there are different aspects of intelligence that include analytical, creative, and practical components,[11,12] whereas others have conceptualized intelligence to include many different types of intelligence.[16] Because the brain has reached 90% of its adult weight and has completed the majority of synaptogenesis and myelination by 6 years of age, the individual is deemed to be at an optimal ready state for formal education—a process thought to stimulate cognitive development. In late adulthood, maintenance of cognitive abilities is affected by a decline in the speed of processing, decrements in executive functioning (e.g., attention and memory), and potentially by reduced or limited cognitive stimulation, which leads to continued synaptic pruning and decreased synaptogenesis. Life span cognitive development and "brain science," including the impact of the environment and trauma, have become a primary focus of research recently.

Communication Development

Speech is the spoken expression of language. The three components of speech are (1) articulation, which refers to the pronunciation of sounds; (2) voice, which refers to the production of sound by the vocal cords; and (3) fluency, which refers to the rhythm of speech. Language involves a set of rules shared by a group of people that allows the communication of thoughts, ideas, and emotions. Communication is a process that requires both receptive and expressive skills. Receptive language function is the ability to hear and understand what others say. Expressive language function is the ability to develop and express one's own thoughts, ideas, and emotions.[17] Speech and language development synergistically occurs with cognitive, neurologic, and fine motor development and requires optimal sensory function (e.g., hearing), sensory integration, and interactional relationships to develop and refine.

Simple speech begins with utterances of consonants, increases to include vowels ("ba-ba" and "da-da"), then single words are formed ("no" and "me"), and two- and three-word combinations arise ("me do" and "you up"), leading to the development of meaningful phrases and sentences. This language explosion or "period of exuberance" is an outward demonstration of frontal lobe development and typically occurs in children 18 months to 3 years of age. This is a specific example of a critical developmental time point, meaning that if significant speech and language gains are not made during this time, the delay may have resultant sequelae (i.e., a variety of learning disorders). Speech and language continue to increase in complexity during the life span until older adulthood, a time during which communication and speech may decline or become impaired as a result of health impairment or disease (e.g., expressive aphasia that results from a stroke).

Adaptive Development

Adaptive development refers to the acquisition of a range of skills that enable independence at home and in the community. Adaptive skills are learned and include self-care activities such as dressing/undressing, eating/feeding, toileting, and grooming; management of one's immediate environment; and functional behaviors within the community, such as crossing the street safely, going to the store, and following rules of politeness when interacting with others.[18] Demonstration of skills in this developmental domain requires advanced and complex skills in each of the other developmental domains previously discussed and efficient sensory integration processes. Examples of adaptive development include cooperation; a level of moral and ethical decision making; and abilities to follow social and cultural folkways, mores, taboos, rules, and laws.

ATTRIBUTES AND CRITERIA

Expected Development

A person who is considered to have *normal* development is one who is demonstrating the expected developmental and physical maturation, physiologic function, and/or expected tasks within or across the developmental domains (e.g., physical/physiologic, motor, social, cognitive, and language) that are associated with the individual's chronologic age.

Developmental level refers to an individual's stage of development (e.g., stage of epiphyseal closure in long bone development, Tanner stage of pubertal development, and stage of cognitive development) or ability to independently achieve an outcome (e.g., perspective taking and abstract reasoning).

A *developmental milestone* is an ability or specific skill that most individuals can accomplish in a certain age range.[1,10] The categories of age ranges typically include those individuals who are experiencing rapid developmental change, such as infants, toddlers, preschoolers, school-aged children, and adolescents (teens), with emphasis on the growing child. However, milestone attainment and loss are appreciated across the life span. Common use of the term "developmental milestones" typically refers to changes that involve *motor, social, emotional, cognitive,* and *communication* skills. In the context of this concept presentation, development also includes *physical/physiologic milestones* (Box 1.1). For example, every aspect of physical and physiologic growth and maturation has been carefully mapped and normed to the general population and to several subpopulations (e.g., weight for age, body mass index for age and gender, and kidney and liver growth and development). Classically defined, developmental milestones occur when a confluence of critical changes (i.e., neurologic, cognitive, emotional, and physical) occurs, marking a significant or critical point of maturation. As a result, these milestones provide a basis for developmental assessment and serve as major markers in tracking development.

Abnormal Development

If an individual does not accomplish milestones within a specified age range, or a critical period, he or she may be identified as being *developmentally delayed*, signifying that an essential element of neurologic and/or cognitive maturation has not occurred within an age range and should be investigated. The definition of developmental delay varies, but it usually involves a delay of at least 2.5 standard deviations in one or more areas or subcategories of development. In other words, a

developmental delay would be identified if a developmental change was not found in an individual that can be found in 95% of others of the same chronologic age range. Certain individuals may demonstrate advanced development in one or more developmental domains/categories (see Fig. 1.1). The developmental changes assessed would include physiologic and physical development, motor, cognitive, communication, social/emotional, and adaptive development.[19] Individual delays within a developmental domain may be demonstrated in subtle ways and may not affect overall functioning unless the delays are pronounced and developmental progress continues to lag over time.

An individual who has accomplished a developmental milestone rarely loses this ability unless the individual encounters a significant stressor (e.g., hospitalization or a new disease diagnosis). For example, once a child learns to sit or stand or becomes toilet trained, it is unusual for such skills to be lost without cause. The loss of developmental milestones, or *developmental regression*, is very subtle, and parents often miss this occurring in their own children. Recognizing the loss of a previously attained developmental milestone is as important of an assessment finding as the identification of achieving milestones. When developmental regression has occurred, the underlying cause must be identified with the goal of ameliorating the situation, addressing underlying health conditions impacting development, and restoring developmental gains as soon as possible.

Developmental arrest is the plateau of developmental change in some category and is noted when chronologic age continues to progress but developmental change does not. Developmental arrest can be differentiated from lagging or slowed development because of its significant effects on an individual's functioning. Physical or growth arrest can be the result of underlying health abnormalities or social conditions (e.g., abuse, neglect, or social isolation) that may or may not have been diagnosed. Cessation in physiologic development (organ or system maturation) frequently results in significant functional limitations or chronic health conditions. For example, some believe that developmental arrest that occurs in utero results in a congenital anomaly.[13]

It is estimated that at least 8% of all children from birth to age 6 years have developmental problems and/or delays in one or more areas of neurocognitive development. A *global delay* refers to lag in multiple neurocognitive developmental areas—speech and language, gross and fine motor skills, and personal and social development.[20] Some individuals are identified as having a *pervasive developmental disorder* (PDD), which means that they have a significant developmental delay in many basic milestones and skills that often cross developmental domains. PDD is usually identified by 3 years of age, which is a critical time in an individual's development. Frequently, children with PDD have delays that affect the ability to socialize with others, to communicate, and to use imagination—all skills that usually emerge during this age. Thus children with these conditions often demonstrate confusion in their thinking and generally have problems understanding the world around them—challenges that continue throughout their life. Specific types of developmental delays are presented in the "Clinical Exemplars" section later in this chapter.

There are periods within each of the domains of development that are characterized not only by critical periods (mentioned previously) but also by susceptible or sensitive periods. These are points in the life span when there is greater susceptibility to positive or negative influences (e.g., genetic, environment, culture, family values, and personal experiences), with resulting beneficial or detrimental effects.[7] One example of the latter is the finding that young children with rapidly occurring frontal lobe development, the "period of exuberance," are particularly vulnerable to environmental toxins (e.g., lead intoxication) and exhibit marked detrimental effects from such exposures (e.g., stunted cognitive abilities or learning disabilities).[21]

BOX 1.1 Attributes of Development

Physical/Physiologic Development
- Growth
- Physical characteristic development
- Organ system maturation

Motoric Development
- Fine motor development
- Gross motor development

Cognitive Development
- Critical thinking
- Executive functioning

Communication Development
- Speech
- Language

Social/Emotional Development
- Social skills
- Emotional control

Adaptive Development
- Adaptive skills
- Functional skills
- Environmental Management

THEORETICAL LINKS

Several theories have been developed throughout the years to understand different domains of neurocognitive development and define different developmental levels and/or stages within each domain. Four of the classic theories are presented: Freud's theory of psychosexual development (1930s and 1940s), Erikson's eight stages of psychosocial development (1940s), Piaget's theory of cognitive development (1960s), and Kohlberg's theory of moral development (1980s). Caution should be taken when considering each of these theories because controversy exists regarding their accuracy and applicability.

Freud's Theory of Psychosexual Development

The term *psychosexual*, as used by Freud, refers to any sensual pleasure. Freud believed that at different ages, particular areas of the body provide the chief source of sensual pleasure and that experiences with these pleasure centers significantly impact the development of personality. He outlined five stages of development: oral (birth to 1 year), anal (1 to 3 years), phallic (3 to 6 years), latency (6 to 12 years), and genital (puberty to adulthood). He identified conflicts associated with each stage that must be resolved for development to occur. Under stress, individuals were thought to regress temporarily to an earlier stage. If resolution was not satisfactorily achieved, an individual may become fixated in the stage and personality development would be arrested.[22,23]

The validity and applicability of Freud's theory and associated underlying assumptions are frequently contested because his work was based on adults with mental health diagnoses and their reflections of past life experiences (retrospective data). However, the conceptual view that an individual matures and develops over time in a stagewise process and the environment impacts those changes (i.e., relationships) was novel at the time and proved to be a critical step for the field of psychology. It resulted in other theorists developing and testing hypotheses regarding specific aspects of cognitive and psychological development over the life span (i.e., psychosocial and moral development).

Erikson's Theory of Psychosocial Development

Erikson's theory of development focused on the psychosocial development of an individual across the life span. Erikson was a protégé of Freud, and the theory he developed was an expansion and refinement of Freud's theory specific to psychosocial development. Erikson identified eight stages of psychosocial development thought to occur between birth and death. These stages were identified by the conflict confronting the individual and included trust versus mistrust (birth to 1 year), autonomy versus shame and doubt (1 to 3 years), initiative versus guilt (3 to 6 years), industry versus inferiority (6 to 11 years), identity versus role confusion (11 to 18 years), intimacy versus isolation (18 to 25 years), generativity versus self-absorption and stagnation (25 to 65 years), and integrity versus despair (65 years to death). He also had a stagewise philosophy (every individual moves only in a forward sequential way through each stage or development ceases), in which each stage had a particular task, identified in the form of a conflict, that must be resolved to progress to the next developmental level.[22,24]

Piaget's Theory of Cognitive Development

Piaget's theory of cognitive development sought to explain how children innately organize their world and learn to think.[25] In this theory, cognitive development is viewed as progressing from illogical to logical, from concrete to abstract, and from simple to complex. Underlying assumptions of this theory are that cognitive development is a product of inborn intellectual capacity, nervous system maturation, and perceptual ability, and exposure to new experiences serves as a stimulus for cognitive development. The theory posits that there are four general periods: sensory motor (birth to 2 years), preoperational (2 to 7 years), concrete operational (7 to 11 years), and formal operations (11 years to adulthood). Each period is composed of a number of stages that are age related, sequential, and stepwise forward.[15,26] These pioneering theories resulted in years of debate regarding the influence of nature versus nurture during a person's development; however, more contemporary theories allege that both play an important role.

Kohlberg's Theory of Moral Development

Kohlberg developed a theory that expands on Piaget's cognitive theory to address the development of an individual's moral reasoning across his or her life span.[27] According to Kohlberg, when a conflict in universal values occurs, a moral choice must be made. This choice is based on moral reasoning, which is postulated to develop progressively over three levels: preconventional (18 months to 5 years), conventional (6 to 12 years), and postconventional (12 to 19 years). Each level is composed of two stages. In this theory, development of moral reasoning is dependent on cognitive skills and neurologic maturation, but it is not definitively linked to specific developmental stages.[27] This theory furthered thought regarding other areas that undergo change and development during one's life.

Contemporary Theories

More contemporary scientists and students who study development appraise theories with regard to three main aspects: Does the theory suggest that development is continuous (uninterrupted change over time) or discontinuous (stepwise progression)? Does the theory suggest that there is only one path of development for all children? What is the relative influence of nature and nurture according to the theory being discussed? Careful review and appraisal of those early developmental theories have given rise to many current theories, such as the ecological systems theory, Vygotsky's sociocultural theory, and theories of multiple intelligences.

CONTEXT TO NURSING AND HEALTH CARE

Because of the frequency and intimacy of their patient contact, nurses are uniquely positioned to gain information about (assess) their patients and holistically intervene to improve patient health and functioning. Assessment of all six domains of development is well within a nurse's scope of practice and significantly impacts the care that nurses and other healthcare providers offer. Care modified or directed by a person's development will be most appropriate and more likely to bring patients to optimal well-being and functioning. Therefore it is important to recognize risk factors and age-sensitive time periods during which developmental progress may be threatened.

Risk Recognition

Developmental progress, delay, arrest, advance, or decline occur in all social classes and ethnic groups and across ages. Most frequently, these concepts are discussed in terms of pediatric populations (infancy through adolescence) because change in all categories of development is occurring rapidly.[28,29] Because development in all areas is interdependent, a delay, arrest, or decline during a period of rapid developmental change may place an individual at risk. Several types of risk exist, including the following:

- **Prenatal:** Genetic conditions, congenital infections, and prenatal exposure to environmental toxins, illicit drugs and/or alcohol, or cigarette smoking
- **Birth risk:** Prematurity, low birth weight, birth trauma, and maternal infection

- **Individual risk:** Ill health, malnutrition, physical or mental disabilities, and cognitive impairments
- **Family risk:** Low parental education, poor health of family members, and large family size
- **Situational risk:** Acute life stress, acute mental or physical health crises, acute school/social problems, bullying, interpersonal violence, sexual abuse, and acute conflictual or violent family relationships
- **Social determinants of health:** Poverty, environmental toxins, adverse living conditions, rural or urban living, areas with high prevalence of disease, community with low cohesion, limited access to health-promoting foods and safe physical environments that facilitate healthy activity, and limited access to health care
- **Toxic stress:** Strict or authoritative parenting, child abuse or neglect, exposure to domestic violence, chronic social isolation, and chronic everyday stressors
- **Health status:** Chronic illness (e.g., congenital heart disease, cancer, brain injury, and cystic fibrosis), traumatic or severe injuries, and conditions requiring prolonged bed rest and/or multiple/prolonged hospitalizations[14]

Stressors, as perceived by children, may differ greatly from the stressors that caregivers may sense exist for a child. For example, loss of a pet, a move, integration into a new school, alterations in household members, and/or illness of sibling, family member, teacher, or friend may be extremely stressful for a child. In some cases in which children spend time with different adults in different contexts (e.g., child care and split time with a divorced parent), caregivers may be unaware that their child has experienced these stressors.

Developmental Assessment

Development, as a concept, has implications for all aspects of nursing practice across all populations and healthcare settings. A thorough developmental assessment of all domains and recognition of risk factors that may impact development are essential for early identification of developmental problems. These assessments are also necessary to determine goals for rehabilitation and strategies to compensate and thus optimize function and overall health when limited progression is identified and/or following illness or injury.

Assessment of development should independently occur for every domain of development. These critical assessments require focused attention and intervention, particularly when working with preverbal or young children and older adults with limited abilities to articulate accurate information, in situations with an absent primary caregiver, or in chaotic living situations in which limited historical data are available.

Infants and Children

Gross screening for developmental risks and lags or delays primarily occurs as a part of well-child health visits.[28] These assessments should be completed by healthcare providers with specialized training in child development and require direct observation with planned developmental challenges and parent report of development task accomplishment. Valid and reliable screening instruments are used and frequently involve documentation of specific skills, parent and/or teacher reports, and child reports. A classic tool used to measure developmental status is the Denver Developmental Screening Test II (DDST II). The DDST II is designed for use with children from 1 month to 6 years of age and has been standardized for minority populations. It assesses gross motor, fine motor, language, personal-social skills, and milestones. The two primary limitations to the use of the DDST II involve the limited sensitivity (83%) and specificity (43%) of the tool,[30] leading to a number of referrals for further evaluation of children suspected of being developmentally delayed but who are not truly developmentally delayed. In addition, the use of this tool does not identify children who have other

diagnoses (e.g., cerebral palsy) that may affect the developmental changes anticipated in a child's early years.[3,9,31] Thus the DDST II is recognized as a gross screening tool with inherent error and not a diagnostic tool.

When delay is suspected in any specific area of development, a more in-depth assessment with a valid, reliable, and highly sensitive and specific tool for that particular area is needed for diagnostic purposes. For example, an in-depth language assessment may be needed after a gross screening by the DDST II. Given this situation, a tool such as the Early Language Milestones Scale (ELM Scale-2)[32] may be used to assess auditory visual, auditory receptive, and expressive language in children between the ages of 1 month and 3 years. Assessment of social/emotional development may include the Modified Checklist for Autism in Toddlers–Revised (M-CHAT-R). This tool has been found to be valid and reliable and to have strong sensitivity and specificity.[33] Other examples of developmental screening tools that include parental report are the Ages and Stages Questionnaire (ASQ),[9] the Parents' Evaluation of Developmental Status (PEDS),[34] and the Learn the Signs/Act Early Interactive Milestones Checklist program sponsored by the National Center on Birth Defects and Developmental Disabilities at the Centers for Disease Control and Prevention (CDC).[35]

Detailed information and several assessment tools focused on child development are available from pediatric and developmental textbooks and from reliable websites such as that of the CDC.[35] The Bright Futures website, developed by the American Academy of Pediatrics, includes specific information for healthcare providers.[36] Many internet resources are appropriate for parents and interested care providers (e.g., child care providers), but it should be emphasized that screening tools do not provide a diagnosis. A diagnosis requires a thorough neurodevelopmental history, physical examination, advanced testing and assessment for specific delay, and assessment for potential underlying associated health disturbance.[20]

Adolescents

Routine physical examinations monitor continued development in all areas into the adolescent years. During the adolescent years, teens' major developmental milestones include advanced cognitive thinking and risk-taking behaviors that accompany psychosocial, moral, and sexual development. To assess these areas of development, a HEADSS Adolescent Risk Profile may be used.[37] HEADSS is a screening tool that assesses the teen's *h*ome, *e*ducation, *a*ctivities, *d*rugs, *s*ex, and potential for *s*uicide for the purpose of identifying high-risk adolescents and the need for more in-depth assessment, counseling, and/or anticipatory guidance. Other general adolescent screening tools can be used, including CRAFFT (*C*ar, *R*elax, *A*lone *F*orget, *F*riends, *T*rouble), which is a behavioral health screening tool for use with children younger than age 21 years to assess for behavior health risk, and RAAPS (*R*apid *A*ssessment for *A*dolescent *P*reventive *S*ervices; http://www.possibilitiesforchange.com/raaps),[38] or GAPS (*G*uidelines for *A*dolescent *P*reventive *S*ervices) developed by the American Academy of Pediatrics.[39] It is important to note that teens often develop mental health issues. Some may be the result of the tumultuous social and emotional changes encountered during adolescence, as well as many chronic mental health conditions first manifest during prepubescence or adolescence (e.g., schizophrenia, substance dependence, and bipolar disorder). There are a multitude of specific, high-quality (valid and reliable) assessment tools that can be used with older school-aged children and adolescents to detect the presence and acuity of depression, anxiety, attention-deficit with/without hyperactivity disorder, and other mental health and developmentally associated issues.

Adults

In adulthood, physical examinations and assessments should continue to monitor normal developmental patterns. However, the focus of these interactions frequently involves minor acute or chronic health disturbances. Physical/physiologic, psychological, and cognitive characteristics of individuals are assessed relative to age. For example, older females' reproductive organs are monitored for the normal decline in function. This physiologic change may result in associated symptoms that are disruptive to the individual (e.g., "hot flashes"). In addition, mental health is an aspect of health and wellness that should be assessed in all individuals (e.g., depression). Screening tools designed for use with adults include the Recent Life Changes Questionnaire, the Life Experiences Survey,[15] and the Stress Audit, all of which aim to identify adults in need of supportive interventions and/or services relative to stress and coping.[31]

Older Adults

When adulthood is reached, often there is limited focus on developmental assessment until individuals reach the older adult stage, unless an adult has a serious mental or physical illness or injury or suffers a traumatic event. When this is the case, frequently the focus is on functional assessment (or functional ability)—that is, an assessment of an individual's ability to carry out basic activities of daily living (BADLs) and instrumental activities of daily living (IADLs).[40] BADLs include skills such as hygiene, toileting, eating, and ambulating. IADLs are skills that are needed to function independently and include preparing meals, shopping, taking medications, traveling within the community, and maintaining finances. Functional assessment is described in greater detail in Concept 2, Functional Ability.

Care Delivery

Knowledge of the individual's development in all areas (i.e., physical/physiologic, motoric, social/emotional, cognitive, communication, and adaptive) is critical to nursing care even when no developmental problems exist. It determines appropriate communication strategies, teaching levels and techniques, safety provisions, assistance with activities of daily living, and approaches to therapeutic interventions. An individual's developmental level also determines need for anticipatory guidance, health promotion, and accident or illness prevention interventions. To provide appropriate information on recommended health screenings, immunizations, and chemoprophylaxis, as well as counseling on health topics such as injury prevention, cigarette smoking, alcohol and drug abuse, diet, exercise, and sexual behavior, the developmental level of all areas must be known.

Early identification and intervention are among the most important points when developmental delay(s) is present. In general, regardless of the type of developmental delay, the earlier that intervention occurs, the better the outcome. Management of neurocognitive developmental delay truly requires intradisciplinary collaboration. Early intervention services can include one or more of the following services: nursing, medicine, physical therapy, occupational therapy, psychological intervention, individual and/or family counseling, nutritional consulting, speech and language services, play therapists, audiology services, and assistive technologies. All of these services have as their interprofessional goal to maximally develop a specified area and develop other areas to compensate for an identified disability to optimize future development and functioning (e.g., readiness to learn in a preschool-aged child).

Physical/physiologic developmental limitations and/or challenges are not addressed in this chapter, although the effects of such problems have been suggested and will affect each of the health and illness concepts and thus impact nursing care. For example, glucose regulation of a newborn is affected differently from that of an adult because of the inability of the newborn to feed itself, the limited amount of brown fat for calorie stores, and the differential caloric loss due to temperature instability.[14] Similarly, tissue integrity in an infant is significantly

different than that of a teen, middle-aged adult, or older adult. Premature and young infants have a greater degree of skin barrier dysfunction resulting in a higher transepidermal water loss, increased percutaneous absorption of chemicals, and higher risk for injury and/or bacterial invasion/infection.[14] Therefore the effect of physical/physiologic development should be considered with review of each of the health and illness concepts contained in this text.

INTERRELATED CONCEPTS

Concepts used to describe the human person do not represent isolated phenomena but, rather, phenomena that interrelate with one another. The strength and direction of the impact of one conceptual phenomenon on another vary, given the central concept under consideration. The interrelated concepts are presented in Fig. 1.3. Concepts representing major influencing factors and hence determinants of development include Functional Ability, Nutrition, and Culture with its unique variations in practices and expectations. These appear in green at the top of the diagram, and their influence on development is indicated by the arrow pointing in the direction of the concept. Family Dynamics and the concepts associated with Mood and Cognition have a reciprocal relationship with development, represented by the red ovals with double-headed arrows. The concepts below the influencers (identified in purple at the bottom of the diagram) are the health and illness concepts significantly impacted by development. Note that there are only a few concepts not affected by development. The relationships are indicated by an arrow pointing from development to each of the concepts.

CLINICAL EXEMPLARS

Conditions resulting from problems with development are many and varied; common exemplars are presented in Box 1.2 and can involve any of the developmental domains. Problems may result in a specific problem or deficit affecting one domain, or they may be pervasive or global, affecting many aspects of multiple domains. Causes of developmental problems are similarly complex. A small number of them are clearly identified as genetic or chromosomal problems. However, the causes of the vast majority are unknown, with numerous environmental conditions proposed as probable factors influencing their occurrence. Neurocognitive and physiologic developmental problems may be diagnosed in utero (e.g., Down syndrome diagnosed via amniocentesis, congenital heart disease diagnosed with a sonogram, and kidney development [hydronephrosis] diagnosed by ultrasound). Alternatively, developmental concerns can be diagnosed at birth (e.g., neuromuscular immaturity), or they may become evident with age and ongoing development (e.g., intellectual disability, leg length discrepancies, learning disabilities, and autism).[13] With advances in science and technology, causes of developmental disorders may be more easily identified and understood in the future, resulting in earlier diagnosis with increased accuracy. These advances should improve health outcomes related to developmental disruptions.

Featured Exemplars
Failure to Thrive

One of the most common physical development problems is that of failure to thrive/grow, a condition in which there is a deceleration or loss in weight and subsequent loss of linear growth (height/length). This has many etiologies categorized into three types: endogenous or organic (e.g., diagnosed/undiagnosed disease process, condition of the gastrointestinal tract, and inadequate nutrition), exogenous or nonorganic (e.g., inappropriate or dysfunctional feeding practices), or mixed type.[14] Weight/height loss or deceleration may be the result of emotional

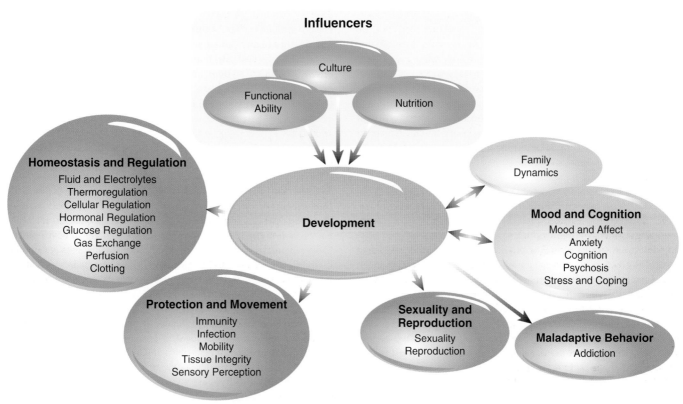

FIGURE 1.3 Development and Interrelated Concepts.

BOX 1.2   EXEMPLARS OF DEVELOPMENTAL DELAY/DISORDERS

Physical/Physiologic Developmental Delay/Disorder
- Angelman syndrome
- Bladder exstrophy
- Hydronephrotic kidney disease
- Cleft lip/palate
- Congenital heart disease
- Cystic fibrosis
- Developmental hip dysplasia
- Down syndrome
- Failure to thrive
- Fragile X syndrome
- Hydrocephaly
- Klinefelter syndrome
- Prader-Willi syndrome
- Spina bifida and other neural tube defects
- Turner syndrome

Motoric Developmental Delay/Disorder
- Cerebral palsy
- Developmental dyspraxia
- Duchenne muscular dystrophy
- Hypertonia
- Hypotonia

Social/Emotional Developmental Delay/Disorder
- Autism spectrum disorder
- Asperger syndrome
- Childhood (pediatric) disintegrative disorder not otherwise specified (PDD-NOS)
- Failure to thrive
- Aggressive/bullying/violent behaviors
- Dysfunctional attachments
- Generalized anxiety disorder
- Obsessive-compulsive disorder
- Reactive attachment disorder
- Separation anxiety disorder

Cognitive Developmental Delay/Disorder
- Attention-deficit disorder
- Attention-deficit/hyperactivity disorder
- Fetal alcohol syndrome
- Rett syndrome

Speech and Communication Developmental Delay/Disorder
- Central auditory processing disorder
- Deafness/conductive hearing loss
- Expressive language disorder
- Receptive language disorder

Adaptive Developmental Delay
- Blindness
- Oppositional defiant disorder
- Traumatic brain injury

 ACCESS EXEMPLAR LINKS IN YOUR GIDDENS EBOOK

stress related to social isolation (e.g., neglect) or mental health difficulties (e.g., depression).

Cleft Lip and Palate

Physiologic developmental problems often have their origins in intrauterine development or embryologic formation and/or cellular division. There may be subtle or overt manifestations that are detected by thorough assessments. One exemplar would be a soft palate abnormality identified through physical examination of the oropharynx. This represents a midline deformity with its beginning in embryologic development. This defect can be demonstrated subtly (e.g., soft palate deformities) or overtly (e.g., cleft lip). It may result in significant functional impairment (inability to suckle from a breast or bottle) and emotional distress (facial deformity), or it may cause little effect on an individual's functioning.

Duchenne Muscular Dystrophy

A classic example of problems with gross and fine motor development identifiable by impaired motoric developmental milestone achievement is Duchenne muscular dystrophy. In this example, a preschool-aged boy may be identified as having difficulty climbing stairs or pedaling/balancing a two-wheeled bicycle. Closer assessment of the young child may identify positive Gower sign, which signifies impaired lower limb motoric development and/or developing weakness. This is a genetic recessive X-linked disorder that involves progressive proximal muscle weakness of the legs and pelvis.

Autism Spectrum Disorder

Perhaps the most commonly occurring impaired social/emotional development problem is autism spectrum disorder (ASD). Children with ASD demonstrate deficits in social communication and interactions across multiple contexts. Associated manifestations include repetitive patterns of behavior, activities, and focused nonhuman interests. These children are most often identified in the toddler or preschool years, and despite intensive interventions, they have symptoms that cause impairment in social, occupational, and interpersonal functioning that persist throughout their life span. Some children suffer mild impairment from their symptoms, whereas others are severely disabled.

Attention-Deficit/Hyperactivity Disorder

Cognitive and intellectual disabilities often evidence themselves in early childhood. One common cognitive disorder is attention-deficit/hyperactivity disorder (ADHD). This is considered to be a minor impairment or learning disability. Symptoms include inattention, impulsivity, and excessive motor activity. Children must demonstrate symptoms prior to age 7 years and have persistent symptoms that cross settings (e.g., school and home) to have this diagnosis. Impairments in executive processing result in disorganized behavior and difficulties with memory, planning, and problem solving.[12] ADHD may also result from injury or disease.

Central Auditory Processing Disorder

Impairments of speech and language are often recognized as learning disabilities. The diagnosis of central auditory processing disorder (CAPD) has become more commonly applied. This disorder affects how the brain receives and processes what is heard. This, like other learning disabilities, is a lifelong problem and often affects an individual's social interactions. Children demonstrate symptoms of this disorder differently based on their age and level of cognitive development. For example, young children may appear to have a speech delay, whereas school-aged children often have difficulty following spoken instructions, do not understand people who speak quickly, and cannot find the right words to say in conversation.

Traumatic Brain Injury

Adaptive development is the result of a complex integration of the multiple skills and abilities easily impacted by injury, illness, substance use, exposure to trauma, or an accumulation of toxic chronic stressors. Traumatic brain injury (TBI) is an example of an adaptive developmental disability defined as an external mechanical force resulting in permanent or temporary brain injury and associated cognitive, physical, or psychosocial dysfunction. Immediate symptoms associated with TBI include deficits in motor coordination, confusion, and irritation. However, persistent symptoms include deficiencies identifying, understanding, processing, and describing emotions; impulsivity; and mood swings. These chronic problems can result in lifelong cognitive and social deficits.

CASE STUDY

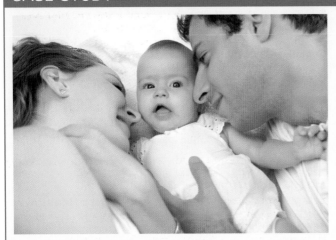

Case Presentation

A first-time mother and father bring their 3-month-old daughter to a clinic appointment. When the nurse asks the parents if they have any concerns about the baby,

the mother responds, "I'm worried because she is still so small. She does lift her head up when she is on her stomach but she doesn't turn over from stomach to side. My neighbor says her grandchild was starting to turn over when she was about 4 months old and my friend's baby who is just about the same age weighs a pound and a half more than mine."

As part of the assessment, the nurse gathers the following information:

- Length at birth: 46 cm (18.4 in.)
- Current length: 57 cm (22.4 in.; increase of 11 cm in 90 days)
- Birth weight: 2786 g (6 lb, 2 oz)
- Current weight: 5100 g (11.2 lb; increase of 2314 g in 90 days, or 25.7 g/day)
- Motor (gross and fine): Kicks when placed on back; holds head up 90 degrees and chest off floor when prone; bears weight on legs when feet placed on solid surface; rudimentary reach/swipe toward objects; pulls objects toward midline
- Reflexes: Moro, tonic neck, and stepping reflexes readily elicited
- Social/emotional behavior: Child attends to faces within 8 to 10 in. away and appears expressive with eye and mouth movements at site of mother or positive expressions of others
- Neurologic/cognitive: Follows a moving object past midline 180 degrees
- Speech and communication: Turns head toward sound; babbles

CASE STUDY—cont'd

Based on knowledge of the different areas of development, the nurse assesses the infant's physical growth by comparing the birth weight and length with the current weight and length. The infant was born at 40 weeks of gestation; therefore the physical growth is determined to be slightly less than the average height and weight for a female infant but with consistent growth acceleration from birth.

Follow-up is needed to review the mother's prenatal and birth history inclusive of intrauterine ultrasound tests, α-fetoprotein test, screens for prenatal infections and immunization titers, and the hospital newborn hearing screening result and newborn screening for inborn errors of metabolism and congenital diseases.

The nurse reviews the assessment findings with the mother and explains that the infant's development falls within the normal ranges at this point. The nurse also explains the different elements of development and the individualized nature of developmental milestones achievement, emphasizing that children normally differ in size, growth, and speed of development. Realizing the importance of providing anticipatory guidance to parents as a way of outlining expected developmental gains over time to decrease unusual expectations and anxiety, and to educate parents regarding abnormal or concerning changes, the nurse provides the parents with a list of developmental milestones for reference and tracking and a list of primitive and postural reflexes with their onset and extinction times. The nurse goes on to explain that even though biologically related, children in the same family normally differ in growth and speed of development.

Case Analysis Questions

1. Consider the length and weight of the infant. At what percentile is the infant for weight and length? Are these findings considered normal?
2. Consider the assessment findings for gross motor, fine motor, social/emotional, neurocognitive, and speech. Which of these milestones are met?

From AndreyPopov/iStock/Thinkstock.

 ACCESS EXEMPLAR LINKS IN YOUR GIDDENS EBOOK

REFERENCES

1. Santrock, J. W. (2014). *Life-span development* (15th ed.). New York: McGraw-Hill.
2. Feldman, R. S. (2015). *Child development* (7th ed.). Englewood Cliffs, NJ: Pearson.
3. Hockenberry, M. J. (2015). Communicating, physical, and developmental assessment. In M. J. Hockenberry & D. Wilson (Eds.), *Wong's nursing care of infants and children* (10th ed.). St Louis: Mosby.
4. Small, L., & Lipman, T. (2018). Children, youth, and families receive care that supports growth and development. In C. L. Betz, M. Krajicek, & M. Craft-Rosenberg (Eds.), *Guidelines for nursing excellence the care of children youth, and families* (2nd ed.). New York: Springer Publishing Company, LLC.
5. Ball, J. W., & Dains, J. E. (2014). *Seidel's guide to physical examination* (8th ed.). St Louis: Mosby.
6. Haith, M., & Benson, J. (2008). *Encyclopedia of infant and early childhood development.* St Louis: Elsevier.
7. Perry, S. E., Hockenberry, M. J., Lowdermilk, D. L., et al. (2014). *Maternal–child nursing care* (5th ed.). St Louis: Elsevier.
8. Trawick-Smith, J. (2013). *Early childhood development: A multicultural perspective* (6th ed.). Upper Saddle River, NJ: Pearson.
9. Wilson, S. F., & Giddens, J. F. (2017). *Health assessment for nursing practice* (6th ed.). St Louis: Elsevier.
10. Sigelman, C. K., & Rider, E. A. (2014). *Lifespan human development* (8th ed.). Belmont, CA: Wadsworth.
11. Berk, L. E. (2018). *Exploring lifespan development* (4th ed.). New York: Pearson.
12. Berk, L. E. (2014). *Development through the lifespan* (6th ed.). New York: Pearson.
13. Chamley, C. A. (2016). *An Introduction to Caring for Children and Young People.* New York: Routledge Taylor and Frances Group.
14. Kliegman, R., Stanton, B. F., Geme, J. W., et al. (2015). *Nelson's textbook of pediatrics* (20th ed.). New York: Elsevier.
15. Sarason, J. G., Johnson, J. H., & Siegal, J. M. (1978). Assessing the impact of life changes: Development of life experiences survey. *Journal of Consulting and Clinical Psychology, 46*(5), 932–946.
16. Gardener, H. (2011). *Frames of mind: The theory of multiple intelligences* (3rd ed.). Philadelphia: Basic Books.
17. Apel, K., & Masterson, J., American Speech-Language-Hearing Association. (2012). *Beyond baby talk* (2nd ed.). New York: Crown Publishing Group.
18. LaBerge, M., & Gale, T. (2006). Adaptive behavior scales for infants and early childhood. *Gale encyclopedia of public health*, Farmington Hills, MI, The Gale Group. Retrieved from http://www.healthofchildren.com/A/Adaptive-Behavior-Scales-for-Infants-and-Early-Childhood.html.
19. Developmental Disabilities Resource Center. (2010). *Glossary of Developmental Disability Terms*, Lakewood, CO, Developmental Disabilities Resource Center. Retrieved from https://ddrcco.com/resources/terms-and-definitions.
20. Tervo, R. (2006). Identifying patterns of developmental delays can help diagnose neurodevelopmental disorders. *Clinical Pediatrics, 45*(6), 509–517.
21. Etzel, R. A. (2010). Developmental milestones in children's environmental health. *Environmental Health Perspectives, 118*(10), A420–A421.
22. Crain, W. (2010). *Theories of development: Concepts and applications* (6th ed.). Englewood Cliffs, NJ: Pearson.
23. Freud, S. (1966). *The ego and the id and other works* (J. Strachy, Trans.) (Vol. 19). London: Hogarth Press and the Institute of Psychoanalysis.
24. Erikson, E. H. (1963). *Childhood and society* (2nd ed.). New York: Norton.
25. Piaget, J. (1969). *The theory of stages in cognitive development.* New York: McGraw-Hill.
26. Singer, D. G., & Revenson, T. A. (1996). *A Piaget primer: How a child thinks.* New York: Penguin Books.
27. Kohlberg, L. (1981). *The philosophy of moral development: Moral stages and the idea of justice.* San Francisco: Harper & Row.
28. Leifer, G. (2015). *Introduction to maternity & pediatric nursing* (7th ed.). St Louis: Saunders.
29. Whitley, P. P. (2004). Developmental, behavioural and somatic factors in pervasive developmental disorders: Preliminary analysis. *Child: Care, Health and Development, 30*(1), 5–11.
30. Glascoe, F. P. 1., Byrne, K. E., Ashford, L. G., et al. (1992). Accuracy of the Denver-II in developmental screening. *Pediatrics, 89*(6 Pt. 2), 1221–1225.
31. Duderstadt, K. (2014). *Pediatric physical examination.* New York: Mosby Inc.
32. Caplan, J., & Gleason, J. R. (2006). Test–retest and interobserver reliability of the Early Language Milestone Scale, ed 2 (ELM Scale-2). *Journal of Pediatric Health Care, 7*(5), 212–219.
33. Robins, D. L., Casagrande, K., Barton, M., et al. (2014). Validation of the Modified Checklist for Autism in Toddlers, Revised with Follow-up (M-CHAT-R/F). *Pediatrics, 133*(1), 37–45.
34. Glasgoe, F. P., & Robertshaw, N. S. (2006). *Parents' Evaluation of Developmental Status: Developmental Milestones* (PEDS:DM). Nashville, Tennessee: Ellsworth & Vandermeer Press.
35. Centers for Disease Control and Prevention. (2014). *Learn the signs. Act early.* Retrieved from https://www.cdc.gov/ncbddd/actearly/index.html.

36. Hagan, J. F., Shaw, J. S., & Duncan, P. (2017). Bright futures: *Guidelines/health supervision of infants, children, & adolescence* (4th ed.). Elk Grove Village, IL: American Academy of Pediatrics.

37. Neinstein, L. S., Gordon, C. M., Katzman, D. K., et al. (2007). *Adolescent health care: A practical guide* (5th ed.). New York: Lippincott Williams & Wilkins.

38. Salerno, J. (2018). *Rapid assessment for adolescent services (RAAPS).* Retrieved from http://www.possibilitiesforchange.com/raaps/.

39. Klein, J. D., Allan, M. J., Elster, A. B., et al. (2001). Improving adolescent health care in community health centers. *Pediatrics, 107*(2), 318–327.

40. Berman, A., Snyder, S. J., & Frandsen, G. (2015). *Kozier & Erb's fundamentals of nursing concepts, process, and practice* (10th ed.). Upper Saddle River, NJ: Pearson.

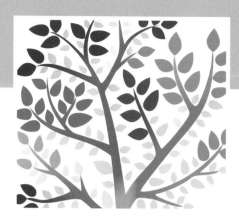

Functional Ability

Lana Sargent

ealth is seen as the level of functional ability for an individual's mind and body. Historically, to be considered in "good health" meant that an individual was free from injury, disability, illness, or pain. A challenge to this view occurred when the World Health Organization (WHO) broadened the definition of health as a "state of complete physical, mental, and social well-being, not merely the absence of disease or infirmity."[1] Expanding and refining the definition of what is considered "good health" or "healthy" is a paradigm shift that is inclusive and more representative of the human population, especially those individuals with disabilities or chronic health conditions. The expanded view of health as it relates to functional ability is supported by one of the four overarching goals of *Healthy People 2030*—to promote healthy development, healthy behaviors, and well-being across all life stages.[2] A key factor in quality of life, and therefore in health, is an individual's ability to function. This view is further supported by the Institute of Medicine report *Crossing the Quality Chasm: A New Health System for the 21st Century*, which emphasizes that a goal of the U.S. healthcare system is "to improve the health and functioning of the people of the United States."[3] Thus the concept of functional ability has implications for collaborative health care across all populations and settings.

DEFINITION

Functional ability refers to the individual's ability to perform the normal daily activities required to meet basic needs; fulfill usual roles in the family, workplace, and community; and maintain health and well-being.[4] Specifically, it reflects the adaptive dimension of development, which is concerned with the acquisition of a range of skills that enable independence in the home and in the community. For the purposes of this concept presentation, functional ability is defined as the *cognitive, social, physical, and emotional ability to carry on the normal activities of life*.[5] Functional ability may differ from functional performance, which refers to the actual daily activities carried out by an individual. Functional impairment and disability refer to varying degrees of an individual's inability to perform the tasks required to complete normal life activities without assistance.

SCOPE

On the broadest and simplest level, the scope of functional ability represents a continuum from full function to disability (Fig. 2.1). This simple linear perspective is useful to acknowledge that a functional ability is a continuum that varies from person to person and within the same person at different points in time. However, the interaction between the health of an individual and disability is a complex process that is influenced by developmental and biologic factors, including current state of health, as well as by psychological, sociocultural, environmental, and politicoeconomic factors. Within the conceptual framework known as the disablement process, the term *function* refers to the positive or neutral interaction between a person's health condition and ability to perform social or physical activities.[6,7] At the other end of the spectrum, *disability* refers to the negative aspects to a person's health condition and social or physical limitation. *Impairment* refers to the physical abnormality that underlies these limitations and is caused by some type of disease process.[7] The scope of conceptualizing function as a complex process that changes based on life span, health, and environment is essential to nursing care and assessment across the entire life course from birth to death.

Life Span Considerations

Functional ability changes across the life span as a function of development (occurring predominantly during the infant, toddler, preschool, school age, adolescent, and young adult developmental stages), although changes in environment, lifestyle, and technology require some continued development of functional skills across the entire life span. In infants and young children, expected development of functional ability is indicated by achievement of developmental milestones. Specialized age-appropriate tests of development are used when indicated to determine developmental delays (see Concept 1, Development). During young and middle adulthood, identification of problems with functional ability requires careful assessment of each developmental milestone. For older adults, functional status ordinarily refers to the safe, effective performance of activities of daily living (ADLs) essential for independent living.[8] For this age group, intentional screening focused on factors known to contribute to a decline in functional ability is essential. A comprehensive, interprofessional assessment, focused on observed functional, social, or cognition changes, should be performed for all individuals not exclusive of environment (institutionalized or community dwelling) or disease state.

ATTRIBUTES AND CRITERIA

Functional ability has two dimensions: attributes and antecedents. Attributes are defining characteristics of functional ability, and

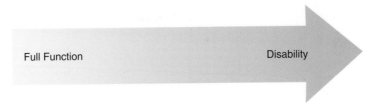

Full Function   Disability

FIGURE 2.1 Scope of Concept Functional Ability Ranges From Full Function to Disability.

antecedents are events that must happen before functional ability can exist. Attributes of functional capacity include the following:

- The capacity to perform specific functional abilities
- The actual or required performance of functional abilities

Antecedents of functional capacity include the following:

- Development of physiologic process: neural, cognitive, endocrine, musculoskeletal, and metabolic
- Acquisition of developmental milestones and skills

At any given time, an individual with the capacity to perform a self-care activity may not complete that activity because of developmental, cultural, environmental, or social factors. Functional ability is further characterized by gradations of capacity or performance. It is not simply a matter of whether the individual *can* or *does* perform the activity but, instead, under what circumstances, with what type and amount of assistance, and in what length of time and with what degree of effort the person *can* or *does* perform the activity. All aspects of this concept presentation are based on these attribute and antecedent principals.

THEORETICAL LINKS

Functional ability is important across the life course because it is a major contributing factor to quality of life. It allows independence and participation in activities that are fulfilling to human nature. Functional ability is also important to healthcare providers and healthcare financers because it can indicate the existence and severity of disease, signal the need for services, monitor success of treatment/disease progression, and facilitate cost-effectiveness in the provision of care.[9] Several theories can be used to translate the complex interaction and dynamic process of functional ability across the life course.

A model of nursing with the concept of functional ability as a cornerstone is the *Roper-Logan-Tierney model of nursing*. According to this model, 12 ADLs are central to human life; these are presented in Box 2.1. This model was developed in Edinburgh and is used throughout Europe and in many other areas of the world to guide nursing education and practice by providing a framework to organize and individualize care. It has a focus on health rather than illness and promotes care directed toward health promotion and wellness. Ongoing patient assessment and facilitation of independence in the patient's normal activities of living are central to the model.[10,11]

The International Classification of Functioning, Disability and Health (ICF) is a framework created by WHO to describe this dynamic (rather than linear) process that occurs between functional ability and disability (Fig. 2.2).[12] The ICF focuses on the changes in functional level; these may be temporary (e.g., recovering from an illness or injury) or long term (e.g., spinal cord injury). The ICF highlights the complex interactions of environment and personal factors and the effect they have on the domains of body function, activity, and the person's ability to participate in hobbies, sports, work, shopping, and driving. This criterion is used in the featured exemplars discussed later to illustrate the complex dynamic process of impairment or limitation in functional ability for certain health conditions.[12]

BOX 2.1   The 12 Activities of Daily Living According to the Roper-Logan-Tierney Model of Nursing

- Maintaining a safe environment
- Breathing
- Communication
- Mobilizing
- Eating and drinking
- Eliminating
- Personal cleansing and dressing
- Maintaining body temperature
- Working and playing
- Sleeping
- Expressing sexuality
- Dying

Data from Roper, N., & Logan, W. W. (2004). *The Roger–Logan–Tierney model of nursing: Based on activities of living*. London: Elsevier/Churchill-Livingstone.

CONTEXT TO NURSING AND HEALTH CARE

Nursing practice has three major dimensions of concern relative to an individual's functional ability: (1) risk recognition, (2) functional assessment, and (3) planning and delivery of individualized care appropriate to level of functional ability. Functional ability is a complex concept that represents the interaction of the physical, psychological, cognitive, and social domains of the human person. Alterations in functional ability occur as primary or secondary problems. Primary problems are those in which the ability to perform a particular function never developed. In contrast, secondary problems occur after functional ability has been attained. Thus secondary problems represent a loss of functional ability.

Two examples of functional ability are the basic activities of daily living (BADLs or ADLs) and the instrumental activities of daily living (IADLs). The BADLs relate to personal care and mobility and include eating as well as hygienic and grooming activities such as bathing, mouth care, dressing, and toileting. IADLs are more complex skills that are essential to living in the community. Examples of IADLs are managing money, grocery shopping, cooking, house cleaning, doing laundry, taking medication, using the telephone, and accessing transportation. BADLs and IADLs are essential to independent living.[13]

Functional ability is a critical consideration in virtually all areas of health care and to all members of the healthcare team representing interprofessional interest. It is a critical element in discharge planning from healthcare facilities. Successful transition is dependent on the functional level in combination with supportive services such as home care services, inpatient or outpatient rehabilitation services, or placement in a long-term care facility. In the rehabilitation setting, the focus is on restoring functional ability and evaluating the functional outcomes of treatment by means of a functional assessment. For long-term care

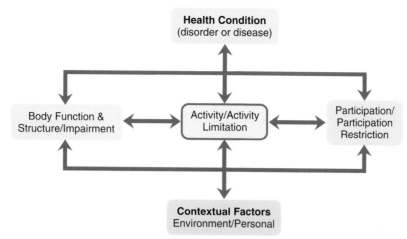

FIGURE 2.2 The International Classification of Functioning, Disability and Health Model (ICF). (Redrawn from World Health Organization [WHO]. [2002]. *Towards a common language for functioning, disability and health.* Geneva: WHO. http://www.who.int/classifications/icf/training/icfbeginnersguide.pdf.)

services, functional impairment—defined as needing assistance with a minimum of two or three ADLs—is a common eligibility criterion.[14]

Risk Recognition

Risk recognition is essential to the early identification of factors that affect function. Actual functional deficiencies lead to subsequent mobilization of resources and support to enhance functional ability. The early identification is critical to the health status of individuals because research has shown that functional deficits are associated with poor health outcomes, whereas good functional ability is associated with positive outcomes. For example, a study of stroke patients revealed that major predictors of independence 5 months after stroke were independent living status and independence in ADLs.[15]

There are multiple risk factors for impaired functional ability because of the numerous variables that impact function, including developmental abnormalities, physical or psychological trauma or disease, social and cultural factors including beliefs and perceptions of health, and physical environment. Research has repeatedly documented age,[15] cognitive function,[16] and level of depression[17] as risk factors for and predictors of functional impairment. Comorbidities and socioeconomic factors have also been implicated. Preclinical disability, defined as task modification without report of difficulty in performing a specific activity, has also been found to be an important predictor of future functional decline and disability in the elderly. In a study of postpartum women, those with postpartum depression (PPD) were 12 times less likely to achieve prepregnancy functional levels than those without PPD. PPD predicted lower personal, household, and social functioning but without deficit in infant care.[18] Sudden onset of functional decline is often indicative of acute illness or worsening of a chronic disease.

Risk reduction should be the focus of care for patients with identified risks. Teaching patient and family about factors associated with maintenance of high-level functional ability is required. These factors include well-balanced nutrition, physical activity, routine health checkups, stress management, regular participation in meaningful activity, and avoidance of tobacco and other substances associated with abuse.[19] In addition, patients need teaching and guidance to develop effective action plans designed to decrease their specific risks. Finally, ongoing assessment of an individual's functional ability can provide continual adjustment of recourses to maximize independence rather than dependence.

Functional Assessment

Comprehensive functional assessment is a time-intensive, interprofessional effort requiring use of multiple assessment tools. Comprehensive functional assessment is indicated under specific circumstances. As discussed for Concept 1, Development, children who are delayed in meeting developmental milestones and accomplishing developmental tasks are referred for assessment across domains of development including that of adaptive behavior, which is analogous to functional ability. Functional abilities are best assessed by observing the function of the child or adult. A comprehensive assessment of functional ability in older adults is indicated when the individual has demonstrated a loss of functional ability, has experienced a change in mental status, has multiple health conditions, or is a frail elderly person living in the community. Screening for functional deficits in older adults should be a part of routine care[19] just as screening for meeting developmental milestones is for children.

An individual's performance of ADLs is basic to functional assessment. ADLs as indicators of functional ability evolved in the late 1950s with the identification of a group of basic physical activities, the performance of which was to be used to evaluate the success of rehabilitation programs. A decade later, IADLs were identified as indicators of ability to live independently in the community. This led to the use of ADLs as a measure of need and eligibility for long-term care and other support services and to the development of an array of assessment tools.

Assessment Tools

The two basic types of assessment tools are self-report and performance based. Self-report tools provide information about the patient's perception of functional ability, whereas performance-based tools involve actual observation of a standardized task, completion of which is judged by objective criteria. Performance-based assessments are preferred because they avoid potential for inaccurate measurement inherent in self-report. They also can measure functional ability with repetition and with consideration of time on task. Potential problems with self-report measures of functional activity stem from the effect of an individual's personal characteristics and preferences as well as environmental factors. Interpretation of what is meant by the question can vary from person to person. Even when vocabulary is correctly understood, the phrasing of the question can lead to an ambiguous response. For example, if a person is asked, "Can you ...?" the answer is based on the person's perception of his or her ability to perform the task, not necessarily on actual ability. Thus overstatements of ability may occur because of a lack of awareness that gradual changes in ability have occurred. Understatements of ability are possible when an individual has not attempted to perform the activity in question because of culture or preference or mistakenly believes that he or she is unable to perform the task. Ability can also be overreported or underreported by individuals based on personal reasons. Pride and the desire to be seen as self-sufficient, fear of losing independence, and fear of long-term care placement are common reasons for overstatement of ability, especially among elders. The 36-Item Short Form (SF-36) remains a "gold standard" as an instrument to measure physical, mental, and social domains in older adults.[20]

Meaningful measurement of functional ability also has to address the areas of dependency and difficulty. Dependency refers to the amount of assistance needed to function, whether it involves the assistance of an adaptive device or another person. *No assistance, partial assistance,* and *total assistance* are examples of common options related to dependency used when scoring functional assessment tools. Common scoring options related to difficulty are *some, a lot,* or *unable to perform.* In addition to functional assessment tools that focus on complex, multidimensional abilities such as ADLs, there are tools designed to assess a specific area of function such as mental status, mobility status, or hand function. There are also tools designed for use with specific populations and age groups.[21-28] The Functional Analysis Screening Tool (FAST) is a 16-titem questionnaire designed to measure social and behavioral functioning validated for assessment of young adults.[29] The FAST measures domains of functioning related to injury (physical or emotional) risk and can provide a verbal report of symptoms. The limitation with behavior function-based scales is that primary behavior and motor stereotypes are maintained with labels. Therefore such tools should simply be a way to gather information during a structured interview that focus on target behaviors.[29]

Table 2.1 presents examples of the wide variety of functional assessment tools. Table 2.2 presents questions and observations associated with functional assessment.

Care Delivery

Knowledge of an individual's functional level in the physical, social/emotional, cognitive, and communication dimensions is essential to planning and implementing effective patient care. Functional level determines the patient's need for assistance and the type and amount of assistance required. It guides the nurse in helping with activities while ensuring use of adaptive equipment and maximizing the patient's independent function. This goal of optimal independent function along with the prevention of functional decline is essential to the improvement of health-related quality of life, which as an outcome of care is an objective for individuals of all ages with chronic illness or disability.[39]

Management of functional activity impairment involves a multidisciplinary effort. Early intervention can include one or more of the following services: nursing, medicine, physical therapy, occupational therapy, psychological intervention, individual and/or family counseling, nutritional consulting, speech and language services, audiology services, home health or homemaker assistance, community services (e.g., day care), support groups, and assistive technologies. When functional activity is impaired, early intervention is critical because generally the earlier the intervention, the better the outcome.[40]

INTERRELATED CONCEPTS

The human person is a complex integrated whole that is greater than the sum of its parts. Therefore it follows that concepts used to describe

TABLE 2.1	Examples of Functional Assessment Tools
Functional Assessment Tool	**Function Assessed/Target Population**
Barthel Index[30]	Activities of daily living
FIM Instrument Functional Independence Measure[31]	Self-care, sphincter control, transfers, locomotion, communication, and social cognition
Dartmouth COOP Functional Health Assessment Charts[32]	Adults: Comprehensive functional and social health
	Adolescents: Comprehensive functional and social health
Now, Growth & Development, Activities of Daily Living, General Health, Environment, and Documentation (NGAGED)[33]	Children ages 2–12 years with physical disabilities: Assesses engagement in life activities—personal, family, social, and school parameters
Functional Activities Questionnaire (FAQ)[34]	Older adults: Assesses IADLs
Folstein Mini-Mental Status Examination (MMSE)[35]	Older adults: Cognitive function
Long-Term Care Minimum Data Set (MDS)[36]	Nursing home residents
36-Item Short Form Survey (SF-36)[20]	Adult patients: Quality-of-life instrument to measure physical, mental, and social domains in older adults
Functional Status Scale (FSS)[26]	Hospitalized children
The Edmonton Functional Assessment Tool[37]	Cancer patients: Functional performance
24-h Functional Ability Questionnaire (24hFAQ)[21]	Outpatient postoperative patients: Functional ability
Geriatric Depression Scale[38]	Older adults: Depression
Inventory of Functional Status after Childbirth[18]	Postpartum women: Functional status

IADLs, Instrumental activities of daily living.

aspects of the human person represent interrelated rather than isolated phenomena. The strength and direction of the impact of one conceptual phenomenon on another vary with the central concept under consideration. Because functional activity depends on the interplay of multiple elements within the physical, psychological, social, and cognitive dimensions and because it allows for purposeful interaction with the environment, a multitude of concepts can be identified as influencing and/or being influenced by it. Fig. 2.3 depicts the most prominent of these interrelationships. Concepts representing major influencing factors and hence determinants of functional ability are **Development, Cognition,** and **Culture,** with its unique variations in practices and expectations. These appear at the top of the diagram, and their influence on functional ability is indicated by the arrow pointing in the direction of this concept. **Family Dynamics** and **Stress and Coping,** as well as the physiologically focused concepts of **Mobility, Nutrition, Sensory Perception, Gas Exchange,** and **Perfusion,** have a clearly reciprocal relationship with functional ability. These concepts surround either side of the concept with double-headed arrows because of their mutual interaction with it. The concepts of **Elimination** and **Sexuality** are shown at the bottom of the figure with arrows pointing from functional ability to them because of the primarily unidirectional relationship of these concepts.

TABLE 2.2   Guide to Functional Assessment Screening

Functional Assessment Component	Sample Questions	Observations/Examinations
Vision	Do you have any difficulty seeing? Do you wear glasses or contact lenses? Do you use any special equipment to help you see, such as a high-intensity light or magnifying glass? When was your last eye exam?	Observe for signs of impaired vision during interaction with patient: turning head to one side in an effort to see better; nonapplicable comments about room seeming dark; feeling for items. Have patient hold a magazine or newspaper and read a line of print. Have patient read a wall clock or sign at a distance.
Hearing	Do you have difficulty hearing? Does anyone tell you that you are hard of hearing? Do you have to ask people to repeat what they say? Can you hear well in crowds? Can you hear when the area is noisy?	Note patient's apparent hearing during your interaction with him or her. Rub your thumb and forefinger together in front of each of patient's ears; patient should easily hear the sound.
Mobility	Do you have any trouble moving? Do you feel steady when you walk? Do you use anything to help you walk? Do you have trouble getting out of bed? Do you have difficulty sitting down or standing up?	Observe patient's general movements; look for obvious limitation of movement in any body part. Have patient put hands together behind neck and then behind waist to assess external and internal rotation of shoulder. Assess lower extremity function, balance, and gait by asking patient to arise from a straight back chair, stand still, walk across room (approximately 10 feet), turn, walk back, and sit down. Note ability to stand up and sit down; balance when sitting, standing, and walking; gait; and ability to turn.
Fall history	Have you had any falls? Have you had any near falls? Do you take any precautions against falling?	
Continence	Do you ever lose control of your bowels? Do you ever lose control of your urine and wet yourself? Do you wear any type of protective pad or underclothes in case of an accident with urine or bowels?	
Nutrition	Have you gained or lost 10 pounds in the past 6 months without trying? What do you typically eat in a day? Do you have difficulty chewing or swallowing? When was your last dental visit?	Note general appearance as related to nutritional status: well nourished, undernourished, emaciated. Obtain weight and determine body mass index.
Cognition	Do you have any trouble with your memory?	Note patient's ability to respond appropriately to questions and directions. Three-item recall at 1 minute; if patient fails this test, follow with MMSE.
Affect	Do you often feel anxious or overstressed? Do you often feel sad or down?	Note patient's expression and if this matches mood.
Home environment	Who do you live with? What type of house do you have: single home, multiple family, apartment? How many floors does the home have? Are there stairs you must use?	
Social participation	What keeps you busy all day? How often do you go out? How often do you have company?	
Activities of Daily Living (basic and instrumental)	Use a reliable, valid assessment tool to assess function related to grooming, toileting, dressing, eating, walking, shopping, meal preparation, housekeeping, travel/driving, money management.	

MMSE, Mini-Mental Status Examination.
From references 13, 35, 38.

CLINICAL EXEMPLARS

Alterations in functional ability may affect one very specific area of function or may be global and affect widespread function. Impaired functional ability is often complex and may involve an array of environmental and individual factors. Furthermore, similar alterations in function can be the result of very different causes.

There are multiple exemplars of situations that change an individual's functional ability. Examples of specific exemplars are presented in Box 2.2 using two major categories of problems for distinction: primary and secondary. Causes of primary problems of functional ability may be genetic in origin (i.e., the result of a congenital defect) or may be a result of trauma, disease, or negative environmental factors occurring during the early years of development. Often, however, as with many developmental problems, the cause is unclear.

Secondary problems of functional activity are more commonly identifiable as the result of aging, disease, trauma, or negative environmental factors. Sudden onset of functional decline is a sign of acute disease such as pneumonia, urinary tract infection, or fluid and electrolyte imbalance. Alternatively, it can be a sign of worsening chronic disease such as diabetes, chronic obstructive pulmonary disease, or heart failure.[41] Depending on the extent of alteration in functional ability, the problem may be termed an impairment, a disability, or a handicap.

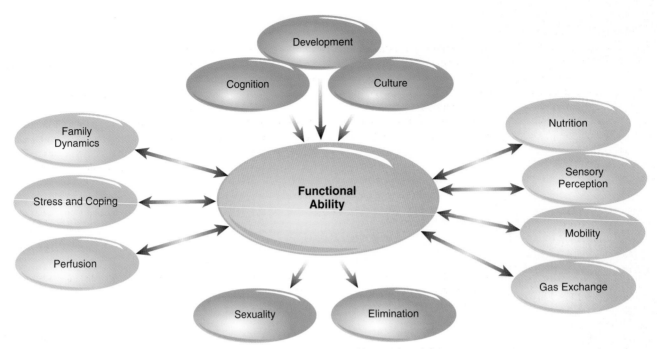

FIGURE 2.3 Functional Ability and Interrelated Concepts.

BOX 2.2   EXEMPLARS OF IMPAIRED FUNCTIONAL ABILITY

Causes of Primary Problems
- Angelman syndrome
- Autism spectrum disorder
- Cerebral palsy
- Down syndrome
- Duchenne muscular dystrophy
- Fetal alcohol syndrome
- Hypoplastic limb
- Malnutrition
- Receptive or expressive language disorder

Causes of Secondary Problems
- Alzheimer disease
- Blindness
- Brain injury
- Cardiovascular disease
- Chronic pain
- Chronic fatigue
- Chronic obstructive pulmonary disease
- Deafness
- Malnutrition
- Multiple sclerosis
- Osteoarthritis
- Parkinson disease
- Rheumatoid arthritis
- Schizophrenia
- Spinal cord injury
- Skeletal fracture
- Stroke

ACCESS EXEMPLAR LINKS IN YOUR GIDDENS EBOOK

Featured Exemplars
Cerebral Palsy

Cerebral palsy (CP) refers to a group of neurologic disorders that affect body movement, posture, and muscle coordination. It is caused by abnormal development or injury to the developing brain in the area responsible for muscle control. This disorder occurs before birth, during the birth process, or within the first years of childhood, and it represents the most common motor disability in childhood. There are four main types of CP (spastic CP, dyskinesic CP, ataxic CP, and mixed CP); thus the severity of symptoms is highly variable. Prevalence estimates of CP range from 1 to 4.5/1000 births.[42]

Autism Spectrum Disorder

Autism spectrum disorder (ASD) refers to a broad category of conditions with a wide range of impairments and disabilities affecting children in early childhood that lasts throughout life. Two general areas of dysfunction are social impairment and repetitive behaviors. Although the cause is not well understood, it is suspected that genetic and environmental factors may be involved. ASD represents a primary problem in functional ability because affected individuals have difficulties meeting BADLs or IADLs. The Centers for Disease Control and Prevention (CDC) estimates that 1 in 68 children have ASD; the rate in males is four or five times higher than in females.[43]

Alzheimer Disease

Alzheimer disease, an irreversible progressive brain disease, is the most common cause of dementia among older adults, affecting an estimated 5 million in the United States.[44] This disorder is characterized by the loss of cognitive functioning (memory, thinking, reasoning, and problem solving) and behavioral changes resulting in a decline of functional ability. The degree of symptoms and functional limitations is directly related to the progression of the disease. Because this occurs in older adults, it is considered a secondary problem in functional ability.

Rheumatoid Arthritis

Rheumatoid arthritis (RA) is a systemic autoimmune condition with genetic predisposition that creates an inflammatory process in the synovial membrane of the joints and other body tissues. Over time, the joint inflammation leads to erosion of the membrane cartilage, causing pain, swelling, and joint deformity; significant impairment in functional ability and mobility results. Affecting less than 1% of the general population, RA is most common among women and individuals older than age 60 years.[45] This is considered a secondary problem in functional ability.

Parkinson Disease

Parkinson disease (PD) is a neurologic disorder caused by a loss of dopamine-producing cells in the brain and resulting in motor disability. Four primary symptoms are tremors, rigidity, bradykinesia, and impaired balance and coordination. This condition most commonly occurs in adults older than age 50 years, with a higher incidence among men than women. Although symptoms are subtle and mild initially, these become more pronounced as the disease progresses and interfere with functional ability.[46] An estimated 1 million Americans have PD, with an estimated 50,000 to 60,000 new cases of PD diagnosed each year.

CASE STUDY

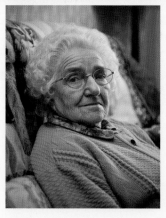

Case Presentation

Mrs. Rose Finney is an 85-year-old woman with ovarian cancer. She presented at the oncology clinic for a scheduled appointment 6 weeks after surgical removal of her ovaries, uterus, a section of large bowel, and as much tumor mass as possible from other areas of her abdomen. The purpose of the visit was a postoperative checkup and planning for chemotherapy. Mrs. Finney was accompanied by a niece with whom she had stayed while recovering from the surgery. The niece lives out of state, and the patient will be returning to her own home after this follow-up appointment.

At this visit, the nurse interviewed the patient to obtain detailed self-report information related to functional ability. The following information was gathered:

- Alert, well-groomed, well-spoken, fiercely independent elderly woman recuperating remarkably well from extensive surgery
- Uncontrolled glaucoma with limited vision in one eye; 20/80 vision with glasses in other eye
- Slightly hard of hearing

- Arthritis in fingers along with lack of strength makes some tasks difficult (e.g., opening jars, using telephone)
- Uncertain walking outdoors, particularly in unfamiliar areas and when ground uneven; no assistive devices
- Medication: Synthroid every morning for 47 years
- Never married, no children
- Lives alone in a single home; bedroom on first floor but laundry facilities and garage are on basement level
- Does not drive
- Only living relatives in addition to the niece are two nephews: One lives out of state and other lives half an hour away
- Telephone contact with closer nephew daily, occasional visits and trips for shopping and other errands
- Three friends in neighborhood, each of whom calls or visits on average every 2 weeks

Case Analysis Questions

1. Based on the information provided, what functional challenges put Mrs. Finney at risk for injury?
2. In addition to managing risk factors within the home, what additional help does she need?
3. What interdisciplinary healthcare team members would be helpful to Mrs. Finney and her family?

From Kirstyokeeffe/iStock/Thinkstock.

  ACCESS EXEMPLAR LINKS IN YOUR GIDDENS EBOOK

REFERENCES

1. National Institutes of Health, World Health Organization. (2011). *Global health and aging*. Retrieved from https://www.nia.nih.gov/research/dbsr/global-aging.
2. U.S. Department of Health and Human Services. (2018). *Healthy People 2030 Framework*. Retrieved from https://www.healthypeople.gov/2020/About-Healthy-People/Development-Healthy-People-2030/Framework.
3. Institute of Medicine, Committee on Quality of Health Care in America. (2001). *Crossing the quality chasm: A new health system for the 21st century*. Washington, DC: National Academies Press.
4. American Thoracic Society. (2007). *Quality of life resource, Functional Status*. Retrieved from http://qol.thoracic.org/sections/key-concepts/functional-status.html.
5. Tappen, R. M. (2011). *Advanced nursing research: From theory to practice*. Sudbury, MA: Jones & Bartlett Learning.
6. Granger, C. V. (1984). A conceptual model for functional assessment. In C. V. Granger & G. E. Gresham (Eds.), *Functional assessment in rehabilitation medicine* (pp. 14–25). Baltimore: Williams & Wilkins.
7. Verbrugge, L. M., Gates, D. M., & Ike, R. W. (1991). Risk factors for disability among US adults with arthritis. *Journal of Clinical Epidemiology*, 44(2), 167–182.
8. Potter, P. A., & Perry, A. G. (2017). *Fundamentals of nursing* (9th ed.). St Louis: Mosby.
9. Min, L. C., Wenger, N. S., Reuben, D. B., et al. (2008). A short functional survey is responsive to changes in functional status in vulnerable older people. *Journal of the American Geriatrics Society*, 56(10), 1932–1936.
10. Roper, N., & Logan, W. W. (2004). *The Roger–Logan–Tierney model of nursing: Based on activities of living*. London: Elsevier/Churchill-Livingstone.
11. Allegoode, M., & Tomey, A. M. (2018). *Nursing theorists and their work* (9th ed.). St Louis: Mosby.
12. World Health Organization (WHO). (2001). *International Classification of Functioning, Disability, and Health*. Geneva: WHO.
13. Goldman, L., & Ausiello, D. (Eds.), (2016). *Cecil medicine* (25th ed.). Philadelphia: Saunders.
14. Geron, S. M. (2002). Functional ability. In *Encyclopedia of aging*. Retrieved from http://www.encyclopedia.com.
15. Hankey, G. J. (2007). *Stroke* (2nd ed.). London: Churchill Livingstone.
16. Royall, D. R., Lauterbach, E. C., & Kaufer, D., the Committee on Research of the American Neuropsychiatric Association. (2007). The cognitive

correlates of functional status: A review from the Committee on Research of the American Neuropsychiatric Association. *Journal of the American Geriatrics Society, 55*, 1705–1711.

17. Van der Weele, G. M., Gussekloo, J., De Waal, M. M., et al. (2009). Co-occurrence of depression and anxiety in elderly subjects aged 90 years and its relationship with functional status, quality of life and mortality. *International Journal of Geriatric Psychiatry, 24*(6), 595–601.

18. Posmontier, B. (2008). Functional status outcomes in mothers with and without postpartum depression. *Journal of Midwifery & Women's Health, 53*(4), 310–318.

19. Bierman, A. S. (2001). Functional status: The sixth vital sign. *Journal of General Internal Medicine, 16*(11), 785–786.

20. Gandek, B., Ware, J. E., Aaronson, N. K., et al. (1998). Tests of data quality, scaling assumptions, and reliability of the SF-36 in eleven countries: Results from the IQOLA Project. International Quality of Life Assessment. *Journal of Clinical Epidemiology, 51*(11), 1149–1158.

21. Hogue, S. L., Reese, P. R., Colopy, M., et al. (2000). Assessing a tool to measure patient functional ability after outpatient surgery. *Anesthesia and Analgesia, 91*(1), 97–106.

22. Hudak, P. L., Amadio, P. C., & Bombardier, C. (1996). Development of an upper extremity outcome measure: The DASH (disabilities of the arm, shoulder and hand) [corrected]. The Upper Extremity Collaborative Group (UECG). *American Journal of Industrial Medicine, 29*(6), 602–608. Erratum in *American Journal of Industrial Medicine, 30*(3), 372, 1996.

23. Leidy, N. K. (1994). Functional status and the forward progress of merry-go-rounds: Toward a coherent analytical framework. *Nursing Research, 43*, 196–202.

24. Pfeffer, R. I., Kurosaki, T. T., Harrah, C. H., Jr., et al. (1982). Measurement of functional activities in older adults in the community. *Journal of Gerontology, 37*(3), 323–329. Reprinted with permission of The Gerontological Society of America, 1030 15th St NW, Suite 250, Washington, DC 20005, via Copyright Clearance. Retrieved from http://www.ncbi.nlm.nih.gov/pubmed/7069156.

25. Center for Functional Assessment Research at SUNY Buffalo. (1993). *Guide for the uniform data set for medical rehabilitation for children* (WeeFIM), Version 4.0. Buffalo, NY, State University of New York at Buffalo.

26. Odetola, F. (2009). Assessing the functional status of children. *Pediatrics, 124*(1), e163–e165.

27. Pollack, M. M., Holubkov, R., Glass, P., et al. Eunice Kennedy Shriver National Institute of Child Health and Human Development Collaborative Pediatric Critical Care Research Network. (2009). Functional status scale: A new pediatric outcome measure. *Pediatrics, 124*(1), e18–e28.

28. Wasson, J. H., Kairys, S. W., Nelson, E. C., et al. (1994). A short survey for assessing health and social problems of adolescents. *The Journal of Family Practice, 38*, 489–494.

29. Iwata, B. A., DeLeon, I. G., & Roscoe, E. M. (2013). Reliability and validity of the functional analysis screening tool. *Journal of Applied Behavior Analysis, 46*(1), 271–284.

30. Neal, L. J. (1998). Current functional assessment tools. *Home Healthcare Nurse, 16*(11), 766–772.

31. Turner-Stokes, T., et al. (1999). The UK FIM+FAM: Development and evaluation. *Clinical Rehabilitation, 13*, 277–287.

32. Nelson, E., Wasson, J., Kirk, J., et al. (1987). Assessment of function in routine clinical practice: Description of the COOP chart method and preliminary findings. *Journal of Chronic Diseases, 40*(Suppl. 1), 55S–63S.

33. Guillet, S. E. (1998). Assessing the child with disabilities. *Home Health Nurse, 16*, 402–409.

34. McDowell, I., & Newell, C. (2006). Functional disability and handicap. In *Measuring health: A guide to rating scales and questionnaires* (3rd ed.). New York: Oxford University Press.

35. Kurlowicz, L., & Wallace, M. (1999). The mini mental status examination (MMSE). *Journal of Gerontological Nursing, 25*(5), 8–9.

36. Centers for Medicare and Medicaid Services. (2010-2016). *Identifiable Data Files-Long Term Care Minimum Data Set(MDS) 3.0.* Retrieved from https://www.resdac.org/cms-data/files/mds-3.0.

37. Kaasa, T., & Wessel, J. (2001). The Edmonton Functional Assessment Tool: Further development and validation for use in palliative care. *Journal of Palliative Care, 17*(1), 5–11.

38. Sheikh, J. I., & Yesavage, J. A. (1986). Geriatric Depression Scale (GDS): Recent evidence and development of a shorter version. In *Clinical gerontology: A guide to assessment and intervention* (pp. 165–173). NY: The Haworth Press.

39. Wilson, I. B., & Cleary, P. D. (1995). Linking clinical variables with health-related quality of life. *JAMA: The Journal of the American Medical Association*, 59–65, 1995.

40. Lubkin, I. M., & Larsen, P. D. (2016). *Chronic illness impact and intervention* (9th ed.). Boston: Jones & Bartlett.

41. Kennedy-Malone, L., Fletcher, K. R., & Martin-Plank, L. (2014). *Advanced practice nursing in the care of older adults*. Philadelphia: FA Davis.

42. Centers for Disease Control and Prevention. (2018). *Basics about cerebral palsy*. Retrieved from http://www.cdc.gov/ncbddd/cp/facts.html.

43. National Institute of Mental Health. (2018). *Autism spectrum disorder*. Retrieved from http://www.nimh.nih.gov/health/topics/autism-spectrum-disorders-asd/index.shtml#part4.

44. National Institute on Aging. (2017). *Alzheimer's disease fact sheet*. Retrieved from https://www.nia.nih.gov/health/alzheimers-disease-fact-sheet.

45. Centers for Disease Control and Prevention. (2018). *Arthritis*. Retrieved from http://www.cdc.gov/arthritis/index.htm.

46. National Institute of Neurologic Disorders and Stroke. (2018). *NINDS Parkinson's disease information page*. Retrieved from https://www.ninds.nih.gov/Disorders/All-Disorders/Parkinsons-Disease-Information-PageB.

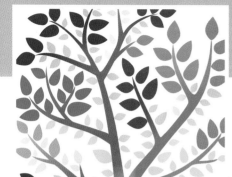

Family Dynamics

Jean Giddens

The *family* has been viewed traditionally as the primary unit of socialization, the basic structural unit within a community. A family is a group of people who are related by heredity, marriage, or living in the same household. Thus a family consists of (1) parents and their children; (2) those related by blood, such as ancestors and descendants; or, in a less restricted definition, (3) any group living together as if they were related by blood. A family is who they say they are.

There are a variety of family configurations: the nuclear family, married-parent families, extended families, married-blended families, cohabiting-parent families, single-parent families, no-parent families, and same-sex families. These are not mutually exclusive classifications. For example, gay couples with children can be represented by the classification of married-parent family, cohabitating-parent family, and married-blended family. For this reason, it is again important to emphasize that a family is who they say they are.

Because families are the foundation of social context and family members act either as a support system or demonstrate a lack of support for members of the family, nurses must understand and appreciate for the ways in which family dynamics influence the delivery of health care to individuals. This concept presentation includes the definition, scope, attributes, theoretical links, and exemplars of concept in the context of professional nursing practice.

DEFINITION

Although *family life* is a universal experience of all people, the term *family* has a different meaning for people because of the varied experiences within families.[1] The wide variability in the configurations of families and the experiences individuals have within families makes it impossible to achieve a universally agreed-upon definition of family. However, the simple definition offered by Kaakinen is helpful: "Family refers to two or more individuals who depend on one another for emotional, physical, and economic support. The members of the family are self-defined."[2, p.5]

Family dynamics is a term that refers to how families interact and behave with one another. For the purposes of this concept presentation, the term family dynamics is defined as *interrelationships between and among individual family members or "the forces at work within a family that produce particular behaviors or symptoms."*[3, p.675] The dynamic is created by the way in which a family lives and interacts with one another. That dynamic—whether positive or negative, supportive or destructive, nurturing or damaging—changes who people are and influences how

they view and interact with the world outside of the family. Influences on family dynamics are many and varied. These include such factors as the family configuration, relationship between the parents, number of children in the family, parental presence or absence, other people living in the home, chronic illness, disability, substance abuse, physical abuse, death, culture, socioeconomic status, unemployment, family values, and parenting practices.

When examining family dynamics, ages within the family should be considered. Young people often have ideas at variance with their parents. Grandparents will likely have views different from those of their grandchildren. The history of the people in the family is important. When a couple marries, they bring with them the culture and norms of their family of origin. This will influence the family dynamics. The role each member plays in the family is significant; it may be important to exchange roles to increase understanding among family members and decrease resentment.

SCOPE

Currently, one emphasis in nursing is providing wellness-oriented family-centered care and empowering families to achieve control over their lives. Wherever nurses practice, they will work with families and observe family dynamics across the life span. Family dynamics occur between couples, with parents and children, and with extended family members. As implied by the word "dynamic," the interactions between family members are fluid and change with growth and development, time, and circumstances. Thus the scope of family dynamics ranges from positive/healthy to negative/dysfunctional (Fig. 3.1) and is shown on a continuum because these dynamics evolve and change over time.

Common traits of families that are positive and healthy include positive and balanced communication and interactions among family members; support, respect, trust, and shared responsibilities; shared rituals, traditions, and religious core; strong sense of right and wrong; sense of play and humor; and shared leisure time.[4] Dysfunctional family dynamics refers to "Family functioning which fails to support the well-being of its members."[5, p.290] Traits associated with dysfunctional family dynamics include behavioral (such as blame, criticizing, enabling, manipulation, power struggles), feelings (such as anger, fear, depression, loneliness, mistrust, rejection), and relationships (such as change/disruption in role, denial, neglect, triangulation).

Multiple variables influence family dynamics. Three key variables include the quality of relationships among family members, the roles

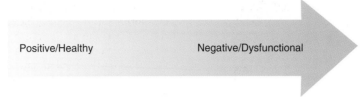

FIGURE 3.1 Scope of Concept on a Continuum from Positive/Healthy to Negative/Dysfunctional.

of family members (and these change over time), and the evolving complexity of the family. These three variables are explored further.

Quality of Relationships

Positive, healthy family dynamics are characterized by relationships that are loving and respectful. Family members support each other, provide nurturance and assistance, and form a unit within society. Family interactions and communications can become negative and dysfunctional as a result of social isolation, perceptions that are inaccurate, and faulty personal interpretations of information.[3] A husband may berate his wife for perceived shortcomings or denigrate a child for having difficulty with school. Siblings may squabble and place blame for incidents. In some instances, a parent and siblings may abuse one child. Observing dysfunctional interactions and communications of parents can lead children to imitate those negative behaviors.

Roles of Family Members

Within the family, individuals assume or are assigned roles: spouse, parent, child, sibling, grandchild, disciplinarian, leader, scapegoat, nurturer, enabler, hero, and so on. Healthy families are able to adapt and adjust to roles that may change over time. For example, as children grow and develop, crises are encountered, illnesses develop, or family members leave home. It may be difficult for family members, especially children, to understand roles, changes in roles, the way changes affect the balance of relationships within the family, and the effects of one family member's actions on the remainder of the family.

Evolving Complexity of the Family

The dynamics change between a married couple when their first child is born. This is because the dynamics in a triad are more complex than those in a dyad (Fig. 3.2); further increases in complexity occur when additional children are born. Extended family relationships add to the complexity, as do divorce, remarriage, and stepchildren. Same-sex families may not be accepted by, or may be estranged from, their families of origin, which precludes receiving support from them. In times of illness and stress, family interactions may change—sometimes for the better and sometimes for the worse. Family members can express concern for the ill member; extended family may gather and provide assistance and support. Old quarrels can be resolved, hurts can be forgiven, love can be expressed, and memories can be shared. At other times, quarrels can arise over past slights, the perceived or real burdens of caregiving, and the strain on family finances. Ill family members can become more demanding, believing they deserve special treatment and care. Death must be faced, burial details settled, and assets divided.

ATTRIBUTES AND CRITERIA

Defining attributes of family dynamics include the following:
- Family, however that is defined, is involved.
- The group of people, the family, have relational obligations.

- Communication, verbal or nonverbal, among family members occurs.
- Interactions among family members are fluid, flexible, and changeable (dynamic).

The family, whether a couple or a multigenerational group, communicates and interacts. The more members involved, the greater the complexity of interaction and communication. Communication and interaction are dynamic and changing and can be positive or negative. Positive interactions and communications are growth producing and produce cohesion. Negative interactions and communications are divisive and disruptive and lead to dysfunction and alienation.

THEORETICAL LINKS

Family Systems Theory

Wright and Leahy describe family systems theory as allowing nurses to "view the family as a unit and thus focus on observing the interaction among family members, and between the family and the illness or problem rather than studying family members individually."[6, p.22] The following are key characteristics of family systems theory: (1) A family system is part of a larger suprasystem and is composed of many subsystems, (2) the family as a whole is greater than the sum of its individual members, (3) a change in one family member affects all family members, (4) the family is able to create a balance between change and stability, and (5) family members' behaviors are best understood from a view of circular rather than linear causality.[6]

Because a change in one family member affects all family members, a change in family dynamics occurs. For example, when Tama, a mother of three children, gives birth to her fourth child, the father and the siblings of the baby experience change and the relationships among the members of the family change. The father, Peter, has to assume additional responsibilities for care of the family while the mother recuperates from the birth. He can prepare meals and do laundry; he can assume some care of the newborn. Siblings must share their mother's love and time with this new member; sibling rivalry may occur. The family attempts to balance this change and restore stability. As the newborn is incorporated into the family, the siblings resume their previous activities.

Because one family member changes, the family changes, and in turn this change affects the member who changed (circular causality). The mother is now the mother of four children, with the additional responsibilities of caring for a newborn and three other children while maintaining her relationship with her partner.

Structural-Functional Theory

The origins of structural-functional theory are in social anthropology.[7,8] In this theory, the family is a social system. Family members have specific roles, such as the father role, mother role, and daughter or son role. Maintaining equilibrium between complementary roles is accomplished through family dynamics. This permits the family to function within the family unit and in society. Some families establish rigid boundaries, and outsiders are kept at a distance. Some families may be isolated and

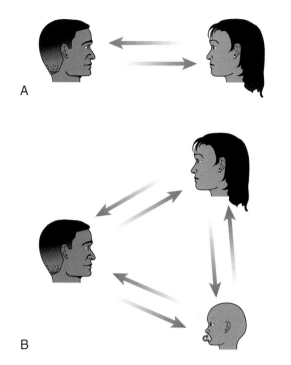

FIGURE 3.2 Complexity of Relationships Within the Family. (A) Dyad. (B) Triad.

may find that in times of crisis their resources are inadequate. Other families maintain open boundaries and give and accept assistance when needed. Some reciprocal relationships within the family can be detrimental, such as designating one member as the family scapegoat or viewing another family member as weak or dependent. Another family member may be identified as the strong or responsible one, and undue expectations may be placed on that member.

Family Stress Theory

The focus of the family stress theory is on the way families react to stress.[9] When faced with a significant stressful event, some families adapt and other families deteriorate; the response is driven by a number of variables, including how the stressor is perceived, other stressors that may also be affecting the family, the resilience of the family as a unit, as well as among individual members, the level of commitment family members have to one another, and availability and accessibility of resources.

Stress of families can also be studied in the contexts in which the family is living, both internal and external. Internal context events are those that the family can change or control (e.g., family structure, psychological defenses, and philosophical values and beliefs). The external context is composed of the time and place in which a family finds itself and over which the family has no control (e.g., culture of the larger society, time in history, economic state of society, maturity of the individuals involved, success of the family in coping with stressors, and genetic inheritance).

Family Life Cycle (Developmental) Theory

Families pass through stages. Relationships among family members move through transitions. Although families have roles and functions, a family's main value is in relationships that are irreplaceable. Developmental changes to the family are part of the life-cycle process, but they also represent adjustments that must be made within the family.[10]

As an example, a couple who goes through stages of dating and then forms a family initially have an exclusive relationship with one another. The relationships change when the family expands and the couple becomes parents to a child. When another child is introduced to the family, the relationships expand. The firstborn child has to relinquish his or her role as an only child and develop a relationship with his sibling. The complexity of relationships increased exponentially as the size of the family increased. Children grow and develop within the family and expand the cycle of their relationships through play groups, school, church, and social club activities. As they mature and change, family relationships will change. As time goes on, the couple grows older and relinquishes their places as primary in the lives of their children. Role reversals may occur as they age; their children as adults may need to care for them and, eventually, deal with their deaths.

CONTEXT TO NURSING AND HEALTH CARE

The family influences and is influenced by other people and institutions. This plays a pivotal role in health care. There are many situations in which the nurse interacts with the family while providing care. Understanding family dynamics and how these dynamics relate to health is important to nurses for the provision of quality nursing care.[11] The family, whether present or absent, influences the patient, either positively or negatively. For nurses to be effective in their care of the family, they must be skilled at conducting a family assessment (including risk recognition) and planning and delivering care appropriate to the situation.

Risk Recognition

During interactions with patients and families, nurses must recognize situations that place families at risk for dysfunction—a number of situations place families at risk. Some of the most common include when the family expands, a situation whereby a family member violates the trust of one or more family members, loss of financial stability, abusive behaviors, substance use and addictions, a severe injury or illness, or death of a family member. A number of disruptions and changes within the family may occur, including changes in roles and relationships of family members, the home and/or living arrangements, finances, priorities, and obligations. These may occur singularly, but in many cases, one issue leads to another or are corelated. As one example, a family member who provides the primary financial support hides a drinking problem from her partner. Due to her addiction, she loses her job and the family is unable to pay outstanding bills. In this scenario, a violation of trust and loss of financial stability occur as a result of the addiction.

Conducting a Family Assessment

A number of culturally sensitive tools have been developed to assess or measure family dynamics (Table 3.1). These and other models are often used in studies of family dynamics. The following example uses the Calgary Family Assessment Model (CFAM) to illustrate a system of family assessment.

The CFAM[6] is widely used by nurses to assess families. Wright and Leahy caution that the nurse must recognize that such an assessment is based on the perspective of the nurse (based on personal and professional life experiences) and interactions with interviewees. The assessment is not "the truth" about the family but is just one perspective at one point in time.

The model is used to ask family members questions about themselves to gain understanding of the structure, development, and function at a point in time. Not all questions within the subcategories are asked at the first interview, and not all questions are appropriate for all families.

TABLE 3.1	Models and Tools to Assess Family Dynamics
Model	**Purpose/Description**
Calgary Family Assessment Model[6]	A multidimensional framework with three major categories: *structural, developmental,* and *functional.* It is embedded in larger worldviews of postmodernism, feminism, and biology of cognition. Theory foundation of model includes systems, cybernetics, communication, and change. Diversity issues are included.
Circumplex Model of Marital & Family Systems[16]	Family model grounded in family systems theory. Includes dimensions of *family cohesion* (emotional bonding that couple and family members have toward one another), *flexibility* (amount of change in its leadership, role relationships, and relationship rules), and *communication* (includes family as a group in relation to listening skills, speaking skills, self-disclosure, clarity, continuity tracking, and respect and regard).
Family Adaptability and Cohesion Evaluation Scales (FACES IV)[17]	Updated version of self-report scale designed to assess full range of cohesion and flexibility dimensions of Circumplex Model.
Dyadic Adjustment Scale[18]	Self-report 32-item questionnaire administered to both members of a couple. Scales include *dyadic consensus, dyadic satisfaction, affectional expression,* and *dyadic cohesion.*
Chinese Family Assessment Instrument (C-FAI)[19]	Self-report measure to assess family functioning in Chinese populations. Contains five dimensions: (1) *mutuality,* (2) *communication and cohesiveness,* (3) *conflict and harmony,* (4) *parental concern,* and (5) *parental control.*
Family Dynamics Measure II (FDM II)[20]	Based on eight bipolar dimensions of Barnhill.[21] First six of dimensions were selected for inclusion: (1) *individuation versus enmeshment,* (2) *mutuality versus isolation,* (3) *flexibility versus rigidity,* (4) *stability versus disorganization,* (5) *clear communication versus unclear or distorted communication,* and (6) *role compatibility versus role conflict.*

Although individuals are interviewed, the focus of a family assessment is on the interaction among the individuals in the family.

The three major categories of the CFAM are structural, developmental, and functional.[6] There are several subcategories for each category. In this brief explanation of the model, only the major categories are addressed.

Structural Assessment

Gaining an understanding regarding the family structure and function is the first step toward understanding the interactions within the family. Assessment of the structure of the family includes determining the members of the family, the relationship among family members in contrast to relationships with those outside the family, and the context of the family. Questions to assess the structure include the following:

- Who is in your family?
- Does anyone else live with you?
- Has anyone moved out recently?
- Is there anyone you think of as family who does not live with you?

Genograms and ecomaps are useful tools to outline the family's internal and external structures. These tools can be hand drawn, or computer programs and apps are available to construct genograms. The ecomap provides a visual depiction of the social and personal relationships of the family members. An example of an ecomap is presented in Fig. 3.3, which shows that the family includes a 35-year-old male (shown as a square in center circle), a 33-year-old female (shown as a circle in center circle), and two children—a boy age 4 and a girl age 2 weeks (shown in center circle). In addition, a number of people with important relationships to members of the exemplar family are shown as purple circles (outside the center circle).

Developmental Assessment

Most nurses are knowledgeable about the stages of child development and adult development, and there is increasing literature about development during senior years. However, family development is more than concurrent development of individuals in a family and is different from family life cycle. Family development considers the vicissitudes of living with both predictable and unpredictable events. Family life cycle describes the typical trajectory followed by most families. The CFAM uses family life cycle to organize the assessment of family development.[6]

Functional Assessment of Family Relationships

Functional assessment addresses how individuals actually behave in relation to one another. The two basic aspects of family functioning are instrumental and expressive. Instrumental aspects include routine activities of daily living, such as preparing meals, eating, sleeping, doing laundry, and changing dressings. Expressive aspects include communication (emotional, verbal, nonverbal, and circular), problem solving, roles, influence and power, beliefs, and alliances and coalitions.[6] The categories are not used to define a family's emotional health; it is the family's judgment of whether they are functioning well that is important.

Care Delivery

Conducting a family assessment and assessing for risks (discussed earlier) are used to determine the current state of a family's function (positive to negative family dynamics). This assessment is used to determine appropriate goals and interventions. Interventions exist to support positive family dynamics and intervene when family dynamics become dysfunctional. Understanding the quality and appropriateness of family dynamics enables nurses to work with families to set goals, create a plan of care, and provide that care while continuing to assess the family. Evaluation of the plan provides the opportunity to make any changes necessary based on observed dynamics of communication and interactions of the family. The nurse's scope of practice, context of the practice setting, the complexity of the issues identified, and experience in family-based care will influence the interventions offered. In some cases, the nurse will identify appropriate referrals; in other cases, the nurse may offer interventions directly. Furthermore, the family's openness to interventions offered by the nurse (or other healthcare providers) is influenced by the relationship and level of trust between the family members and the nurse and other healthcare professionals.

Core Interventions

Core interventions to support families are those that all nurses, regardless of area of practice, should be able to offer. Goals are first determined by the family with the support of the nurse, and then interventions to reach those goals are applied. Core interventions include offering education, facilitating conversation among family members, enhancing understandings, sharing observations, and validating information, perceptions, or feelings (Box 3.1). These may initially seem rather simple;

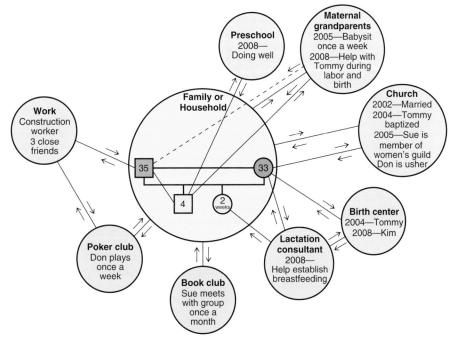

FIGURE 3.3 Example of Ecomap Describing Social Relationships and Depicting Available Supports. (From Lowdermilk, D. L., Perry, S. E., Cashion, K., & Alden, K. R. [2016]. *Maternity and women's health care* [11th ed.]. St Louis: Elsevier.)

however, the complexity becomes clearer when considering that interventions must be tailored to the specific situation and context. Every family and every situation are different, thus the intervention is uniquely applied. In addition, nurses must avoid falling into the trap of thinking "I know what is best for the family." Such an attitude generally does not resonate with families and negatively affects the effectiveness of goals and interactions that could be helpful. Positive rapport and trust must be established and maintained, with an underlying acceptance of the family and their values.

Advanced Interventions

When family dynamics are dysfunctional, significant complexity may exist, making it difficult to determine what is needed and the interventions to offer. In addition to the core interventions (listed earlier), advanced interventions may also be needed. Advanced interventions are carried out by healthcare professionals (nurses, physicians, social workers, psychologists, etc.) with expertise working with families.

Intervening questions. As part of the Calgary Family Intervention Model, interventive questions refer to a systematic approach to introducing questions to the family with the intent to elicit change in three domains of family functioning: cognitive, affective, and behavioral.[6] Two types of interventive questions include linear and circular. *Linear questions* are used to provide the nurse additional information to better understand the problems the family is experiencing; they tend to direct

the conversation for information gathering and tend to focus on cause and effect. As an example, a family consisting of two adults and three children has a young child, Dylan, with a diagnosis of cancer. His prognosis is poor. Since Dylan's diagnosis, the interactions among family members have become dysfunctional. Directed questions might include:

- When did Dylan's illness first affect the family?
- What specific situations following his diagnosis that have been particularly challenging?

Circular questions aim to uncover an explanation of problems and the family's understanding of the problems. These also tend to tease out differences in relationships. Using the same previous scenario, circular questions might include:

- Who in the family is concerned about Dylan's illness and why?
- How have your family routines and interactions changed since Dylan's diagnosis?

There is an art to applying intervening questions. Like most things, it takes time, practice, and experience working with families. Thus the application of interventive questions is most effective among experienced nurses and other healthcare providers who specialize in family nursing.

Other advanced interventions. A number of other interventions are offered for families. These interventions are dependent on situational factors within the family and the underlying issues. Examples include caregiving, family counseling, family therapy, psychiatric care, support groups, palliative care, and hospice. Each of these are interventions beyond the scope of this concept presentation but are addressed throughout this book and from other resources.

INTERRELATED CONCEPTS

The following concepts are related to family dynamics. Fig. 3.4 illustrates how these concepts are related.

Development affects the number and type of interactions within a family and influences the complexity of those interactions. Infants are born; children grow and leave home; marriages occur; parents age and

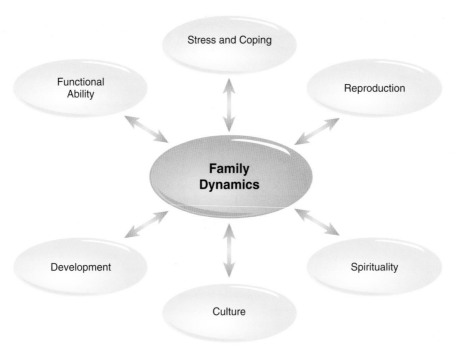

FIGURE 3.4 Family Dynamics and Interrelated Concepts.

die. Families expand and contract as a consequence, and family dynamics change with each of those changes. The presence or absence of the **Functional Ability** of family members affects the self-concept of the family members lacking that ability, and it places stress on the members of the family who are expected to provide assistance. Whether the assistance is offered or not, resentment can occur and lead to dysfunction in the family.

Culture is passed from generation to generation and can affect relationships among family members; for example, the male is always the decision maker; childbirth is the affair of women. Second-generation members of the family may not share the values and customs of first-generation members. Culture has a direct effect on health behaviors. Beliefs, values, and attitudes that are culturally acquired may influence perceptions of illness, healthcare–seeking behavior, and response to treatment.[12] **Spirituality** encompasses a mental or metaphysical belief system, often including belief in a higher being and participation in organized religion. Families often share similar beliefs, but when beliefs diverge, conflicts can occur. Spirituality can bring great comfort in times of stress, illness, and hardship. It can also cause distress when expectations for assistance are not met.

A fundamental purpose of a family is **Reproduction**. The addition of children, whether by birth, adoption, or blending of families, increases the complexity of interactions in a family, introduces stress, and provides the potential for growth and maturation. Infertility creates different stresses through inability to have desired children, through the many tests and procedures undergone to ascertain the cause of the infertility, or through the procedures to try to achieve pregnancy. **Stress and Coping** is a common concept because of the multitude of challenges faced by one or more members of the family. Stress may be from disease onset or sequelae of addictions or substance abuse. It may exist over a period of time such as from an acute infection or for a lifetime, as with a diagnosis of diabetes. Effective coping from within family can provide

a source of support for the family member experiencing stress or, conversely, add to the stress by the family's lack of support.

CLINICAL EXEMPLARS

Positive and negative exemplars of family dynamics provide opportunity to see the wide variety of situations in which family dynamics can be observed (see Box 3.2). The importance of understanding family dynamics when caring for families should lead the nurse to study the factors involved, practice observation of families, and learn appropriate intervention techniques. A detailed discussion of each of these is beyond the scope of this text, but several important exemplars are briefly presented here. Refer to other references for further information about these exemplars and specific interventions for each.

Featured Exemplars
Expanding Family
The family expands by the birth or adoption of a child or by blending families with children through marriage or cohabitation. The family can also expand by incorporating parents or other extended family members. The complexity of communication and interaction is increased in these instances in proportion to the number of individuals involved.

Sibling Rivalry
Sibling rivalry is competition or animosity between and among siblings. It is common with the birth of an infant when the older child competes with the infant for the time and attention of a parent but is usually quickly outgrown. As children grow, the rivalry may be heightened, resulting in arguing and fighting. Sibling rivalry may persist into adulthood. At times, the rivalry is healthy, encouraging the siblings to excel. At other times, lifelong animosity may persist.

BOX 3.2 EXEMPLARS OF FAMILY DYNAMICS

Changes to Family Dynamics
- Expanding family (birth or adoption of an infant; blended family)
- Caregiver role for family member
- Change in socioeconomic status of family
- Chronic illness of family member
- Marriage, divorce/remarriage
- Traumatic injury of family member
- Disability of family member
- Aging of family members
- End-of-life care
- Death of family member

Positive Family Dynamics
- Assistance with child care after birth of new infant
- Respite care for a caregiver
- Support after injury or death of a spouse
- Presence during surgery

- Family reunions
- Celebrations of birthdays and other significant events
- Praying together
- Supportive in-laws
- Sharing care of a dependent family member

Negative/Dysfunctional Family Dynamics
- Child abuse
- Codependency (related to substance abuse by a family member)
- Interfering in-laws
- Intimate partner violence
- Marital infidelity
- Placing blame for birth of a preterm infant or for death of a young child by SIDS
- Sibling rivalry
- Adolescent pregnancy

SIDS, Sudden infant death syndrome.

 ACCESS EXEMPLAR LINKS IN YOUR GIDDENS EBOOK

Intimate Partner Violence

Intimate partner violence is physical, sexual, emotional, or psychological abuse, threatened or actual, by a current or ex-spouse, current or ex-boyfriend or girlfriend, cohabiting partner, or date. Both women and men can be victims. It involves social isolation, emotional distress, and personal safety.[13]

Child Abuse

Child abuse is intentional physical or emotional abuse or neglect, including sexual abuse, of a child, usually by an adult. It is a significant social problem affecting children and can result in disability or death. Child abuse is significantly underreported, so actual incidence is unknown.

Codependency

Codependency is characterized by a relationship in which a person is controlled or manipulated by another who has an illness or addiction. It is a dysfunctional pattern of living and problem solving. It occurs in a setting in which there is addiction, physical or emotional abuse, neglect, or a dysfunction that causes pain and stress.[14,15]

Absent Extended Family

The mobility of contemporary society means that many children move away from their family of origin or retired parents move to a retirement area, often hundreds of miles away. Extended family members often provide child care; help with cooking or cleaning in the event of illness or disability; provide transportation; and, by their presence, have the opportunity to pass on family stories and traditions. When they are absent, there is a void in support and limited opportunity for young children to know their grandparents, aunts and uncles, and other family members.

Aging of Family Members

For many people, healthy aging occurs with retention of their mental and physical capacities. For others, as they age, their capacities and roles may change. Disability and the need for care often come with aging. Hearing and sight may become impaired; mobility may decrease. The aged person may no longer be able to drive. Mental capacity and memory may decline. Adult children may have to provide care for their aging parents.

Death of a Family Member

As part of the cycle of life, family members will die. The death of an infant, child, young parent, middle-aged or older adult, or the aged will have different effects on the family. Tradition, culture, and spiritual beliefs will influence the response to death. Grief may be manifested in a variety of ways and may last a significant length of time.

CASE STUDY

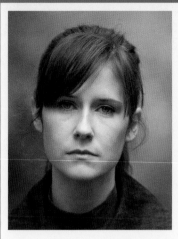

Case Presentation

Erin is a 22-year-old single parent with two children (Stacie, age 5 years, and Monica, age 2 years). Erin dropped out of high school to marry Andrew when she was 17 years old and pregnant. She recently divorced Andrew because of his drinking, affairs, and lack of support of her and the children.

Andrew has a part-time job delivering pizza and spends most of his free time with friends. He only sporadically provides monetary support. Erin and the girls live in a small apartment. Because she has a minimum wage job, Erin relies on food stamps and other types of assistance. Babysitters and rent are major expenses, and Erin continually worries about being able to pay her bills. She would like to earn her GED to get a better job, but she lacks the time and resources to make that happen. Andrew sees the girls only occasionally—usually when Erin asks him to keep the girls so she can work extra shifts. He dislikes spending his time babysitting his daughters and openly verbalizes his frustration with the "whiny girls."

Erin has a strained relationship with her parents. They were angry when she became pregnant, they were against her dropping out of high school to get married, and they consider Andrew a "deadbeat." They do not help Erin financially, citing concerns for their own retirement. Although they live in the same community, they do not babysit the girls very often and have been critical of Erin's parenting style. Erin has always believed that her parents liked her older brother, Dominic, better. He is married and has three children who spend a great deal of time with Erin's and Dominic's parents. Dominic rarely interacts with Erin because they "don't have anything in common."

Recently, after the girls spent time with their father, Erin noticed bruises on the arms and the buttocks of Monica. When she asked the girls what happened, Stacie said, "Daddy got mad when Monica wet her pants and spanked her." A week later, while at a free health clinic getting Stacie immunized for school, Erin shared with the nurse practitioner details of her life and situation: lack of money and support, working too many hours, fear of losing her apartment, and now—Andrew hurting Monica. She said she does not know what to do and began crying.

Case Analysis

1. How would you describe Erin's various families?
2. What findings are indicative of negative or dysfunctional family dynamics?
3. How should the nurse respond to Erin?

From Jupiterimages/Photos.com/Thinkstock.

 ACCESS EXEMPLAR LINKS IN YOUR GIDDENS EBOOK

REFERENCES

1. Galvin, K. M., Braithwaite, D. O., & Bylund, C. L. (2016). *Family communication: Cohesion and change*. New York: Routledge.
2. Kaakinen, J. R. (2018). Family health care nursing. In J. R. Kaakinen, D. P. Coehlo, R. Steele, & M. Robinson (Eds.), *Family health care nursing* (6th ed.). Philadelphia: FA Davis.
3. Mosby. (2013). *Mosby's dictionary of medicine, nursing & health professions* (9th ed.). St Louis: Elsevier.
4. Curran, D. (1984). *Traits of a healthy family*. New York: HarperCollins.
5. NANDA International. (2018). *Nursing diagnoses: Definitions and classification 2018-2020* (11th ed.). New York: Thieme.
6. Wright, L. M., & Leahy, M. (2009). *Nurses and families: A guide to family assessment and intervention* (5th ed.). Philadelphia: Davis.
7. Malinowski, F. (1945). *The dynamics of cultural change*. New Haven, CT: Yale University Press.
8. Radcliffe-Brown, A. (1952). *Structure and function in a primitive society*. New York: Free Press.
9. Boss, P. (2002). *Family stress management* (2nd ed.). Thousand Oaks, CA: Sage.
10. McGoldrick, M., Carter, B., & Garcia-Preto, N. (2010). *The expanded family life cycle: Individual, family and social perspectives* (4th ed.). Englewood Cliffs, NJ: Prentice-Hall.
11. White, M. A., Elder, J. H., Paavilainen, E., et al. (2010). Family dynamics in the United States, Finland and Iceland. *Scandinavian Journal of Caring Sciences*, 24(1), 84–93.
12. Martinez-Campos, R. (2016). Community care: The family and culture. In D. L. Lowdermilk, S. E. Perry, K. Cashion, et al. (Eds.), *Maternity and women's health care* (11th ed.). St Louis: Elsevier.
13. Esposito, N. (2016). Violence against women. In D. L. Lowdermilk, S. E. Perry, K. Cashion, et al. (Eds.), *Maternity and women's health care* (11th ed.). St Louis: Elsevier.
14. All About Counseling. (2018). *Codependency*. Retrieved from http://www.allaboutcounseling.com/codependency.htm.
15. Johnson, R. S. (2018). *Codependency and codependent relationships*. Retrieved from http://bpdfamily.com/content/codependency-codependent-relationships.
16. Olson, D. H., & Gorall, D. M. (2003). Circumplex model of marital and family systems. In F. Walsh (Ed.), *Normal family processes* (3rd ed.). New York: Guilford.
17. Olson, D. H. (2000). Circumplex model of family systems. *Journal of family therapy*, 22(2), 144–167.
18. Spanier, G. (1976). Measuring dyadic adjustment: New scales for assessing the quality of marriage and similar dyads. *Journal of marriage and family*, 38(1), 15–28.
19. Shek, D. T. L. (2002). Assessment of family functioning in Chinese adolescents: The Chinese Family Assessment Instrument. In N. N. Singh, T. Ollendick, & A. N. Singh (Eds.), *International perspectives on child and adolescent mental health* (pp. 297–316). Amsterdam: Elsevier.
20. Lasky, P., Buckwalter, K. C., Whall, A., et al. (1985). Developing an instrument for the assessment of family dynamics. *Western journal of nursing research*, 7(1), 40–57.
21. Barnhill, L. R. (1979). Healthy family systems. *Family Coordinator*, 28(1), 94–100.

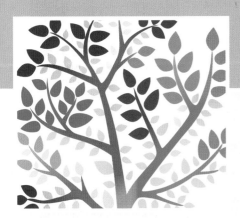

Culture

Susan Caplan

Human beings need to construct meaning from their experiences, and this construction or created reality is known as culture.[1] For most people, culture is defined by its outward manifestations—the foods people eat, the holidays they celebrate, and their countries of origin. However, culture encompasses much more. Culture forms a person's worldview and values, which in turn shapes his or her beliefs about health and illness. The concept of culture is an important aspect of understanding human behavior[2] and, in particular, is a critical part of understanding how to provide person-centered nursing care.

DEFINITION

For the purpose of this concept presentation, culture is defined *a pattern of shared attitudes, beliefs, self-definitions, norms, roles, and values that can occur among those who speak a particular language or live in a defined geographical region.*[2] These dimensions guide such areas as social relationships; expression of thoughts, emotions, and morality; religious beliefs and rituals; and use of technology.

A discussion of culture includes the subconcepts of enculturation, acculturation, assimilation, biculturalism, ethnicity, and ethnic identity. *Enculturation* is the process by which a person learns the norms, values, and behaviors of a culture, similar to socialization. *Acculturation* is the process of acquiring new attitudes, roles, customs, or behaviors as a result of contact with another culture. Both the host culture and the culture of origin are changed as a result of reciprocal influences. Unlike acculturation, *assimilation* is a process by which a person gives up his or her original identity and develops a new cultural identity by becoming absorbed into the more dominant cultural group.[2] Usually, when a minority group or individual assimilates, they do not have a choice about what aspects of the dominant culture they will adopt; rather, the dominant culture's values and practices are imposed upon the less dominant group. In contrast, in the case of *biculturalism*, the individual has a dual pattern of identification and chooses which aspects of the new culture he or she wishes to adopt and which aspects of the individual's original culture he or she wishes to retain.

Ethnicity refers to a common ancestry that leads to shared values and beliefs. It is transmitted over generations by the family and community. Ethnicity is a powerful determinant of one's identity, known as *ethnic identity*. Race is sometimes thought of in biologic terms (for some people, it has a biologic meaning) based on the erroneous belief in the existence of hereditary physical differences among people that

define membership in a particular group.[3] However, there are no genetic characteristics that distinguish one group of people from another, and, in fact, there are more genetic differences among people who are labeled "black" than there are differences between "blacks" and people labeled "white."[3]

SCOPE

The concept of culture is very broad and influences the shared beliefs, values, and behaviors of a group. Cultural norms impact all aspects of life, including everything from interpersonal relationships, family dynamics, and childrearing practices to gender roles, dietary preferences, communication, dress, and religious practices. Cultural norms also significantly influence how people make decisions about treatment preferences, medication adherence, self-care, and perceptions of illness, which in turn affects nursing care and healthcare delivery. The scope of these influences, in the context of health and illness, is illustrated in Fig. 4.1. Kleinman makes the distinction between the Western biomedical model of disease and traditional models of illness.[4] Disease is a response to physiologic causes explained by pathophysiology and manifested by symptoms and signs.[5] In contrast, traditional health beliefs define illness in terms of mind, body, and spiritual and social connections.[5] Therefore all illnesses reflect the influence of the environment, including an individual's cultural experiences.

Causal Beliefs About Illness

Cultural differences can result in different explanations for illness.[5,6] In non-Western cultures, explanatory models of illness might include natural causes (e.g., bacteria, viruses, climate, and environmental irritants), the social world (e.g., punishment for individual behaviors or negative social interactions), or the supernatural world (e.g., ancestral spirits and deities). Western cultures are more likely to endorse solely biomedical causation theories, whereas many non-Western cultures have theories of disease causation that can be characterized as an imbalance with natural, social, or spiritual realms in addition to biomedical causes.[7,8]

Symptoms and Expression of Illness

The manifestation and symptoms of illness can be unique for different cultures. These "culture-bound syndromes or cultural idioms of distress"[6] occur in specific societies and have a constellation of symptoms that are recognized in that culture as a disease entity. For example, *ataque de nervios* is a Latino-Caribbean culture-bound syndrome that usually

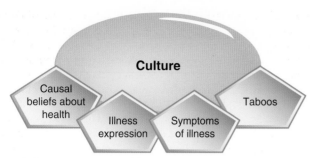

FIGURE 4.1 Scope of Culture Related to Health Care.

occurs in response to a specific stressor and is characterized by disassociation or trancelike states, crying, uncontrollable spasms, trembling, or shouting.[9] *Shenjing shuairuo* or "weakness of nerves" in Chinese culture is described in the *Chinese Classification of Mental Disorders* as a condition caused by a decrease in vital energy that reduces the function of the internal organ systems and lowers resistance to disease.[10] Its symptoms include fatigue, weakness, dizziness, and memory loss. A similar disorder, neurasthenia, has been primarily identified as occurring throughout Asia but can also be found in other cultural groups.[11] The *International Classification of Diseases and Related Disorders* defines this disorder as characterized primarily by extreme fatigue after mental effort and bodily weakness of persistent duration.[12] Neurasthenia is a more socially acceptable illness label in Asia than is depression, which might be considered a mental illness or illness label that is very stigmatizing.[11] Although many Americans would not consider anorexia nervosa or bulimia to be culture-bound syndromes, they may conform to the definition of a culture-bound syndrome[13] because major risk factors for these illnesses are social pressure to be thin and media messages equating beauty and thinness that are more prevalent in Westernized, developed countries.[14]

Taboos

In many cultures, certain illnesses or behaviors that may be characteristic of illnesses are highly stigmatized and are often not revealed to healthcare providers. A patient may deny the existence of socially disapproved symptoms and/or decide not to seek treatment. This is particularly true for mental illnesses (e.g., schizophrenia and depression), suicidal thoughts, behavioral disorders in children (e.g., attention-deficit/hyperactivity disorder [ADHD] and autism spectrum disorders), sexually transmitted infections (e.g., herpes or syphilis), and potentially fatal illnesses (e.g., Ebola and AIDS).[15] In some countries (Malaysia, Singapore, Ghana, Bangladesh, Saudi Arabia, Nigeria) the social stigma of suicide is replicated in the legal sanctions against it. When suicide is outlawed, there is an additional deterrent for an individual contemplating treatment.[16]

ATTRIBUTES AND CRITERIA

The following attributes are related to the concept of culture—that is, conditions common to all cultures: *Culture is learned* through families and other group members; *culture is changeable* and adaptive to new conditions; and cultural values, beliefs, and behaviors are *shared* by all within a group.

Culture Is Learned

Culture may be transmitted to individuals during childhood and adolescence by the process of socialization or enculturation. However, a culture is not limited to members who share the same country of origin or ethnicity and may not be determined solely in childhood; rather, it may encompass any group whose members share certain roles and

values, norms, and attitudes—sometimes referred to as subcultures. Subcultures can include members of racial and ethnic minorities; people of indigenous or aboriginal heritage; professions, such as nursing; people of different socioeconomic levels, such as the "culture of poverty";[17] individuals who are bisexual, gay, lesbian, or transgender; individuals affiliated with particular religious or spiritual groups; age groups, such as teenagers or the elderly; and persons with disabilities. Culture is determined by self-identification, and most people identify with a mix of cultures.

Changing and Adapting

Since the beginning of human history, culture has been constantly changing as people adapt to environmental and technical innovations and in response to globalization and influences of diverse cultural groups. Population migration occurs as a result of regional overpopulation, changes in economic circumstances, the occurrence of catastrophic events (e.g., earthquakes, floods, and famines), and the existence of religious or ethnic conflicts. These migration processes result in ongoing encounters between individuals of different cultures, with subsequent changes and acculturation in both groups.[18]

Shared Beliefs, Values, and Behaviors

Language, rituals, customs (e.g., holiday celebrations), dietary practices, and manner of dress are among the most overt attributes of culture that are readily apparent to non–group members. Some of the less visible attributes of culture, such as values, relationship to authority, social interactions, gender roles, and orientation toward the present or future, are probably the attributes of culture that are most relevant to health care and communication. These kinds of cultural attributes were examined in several landmark studies by Hofstede[19–21] that yielded five dimensions of these attributes. Four of the five dimensions, in addition to religiosity, have particular significance for health care and are presented in the following sections.

Individualism Versus Collectivism

This attribute places value on the degree of closeness and the structure of social relationships, as well as whether loyalties belong to immediate families or to the extended family or clan. The differences in these interpersonal interactions can be thought of as interdependent versus independent and are reflected in the concept of self. Western Europe and the United States are characteristic of individualist societies. Childrearing practices and a "family model of independence" produce a separated or independent sense of self.[21, p.20] The concept of self is distinct and separate from the "non-self," which includes the environment and social worlds.[22] Collectivistic cultures foster development of an interdependent self-concept. People who have an interdependent sense of self consider their social worth in relation to others. The value of collectivism or interdependence in self-concept is most clearly exemplified by Asian cultures, but it also applies to African, Latin American, and some southern European cultures and some minority cultures within the United States.[22,23] Cultural differences in social practices are apparent in the differences in colloquialisms heard in the United States and Japan. For example, in the United States, "the squeaky wheel gets the grease," whereas in Japan, "the nail that stands out gets pounded down."[23, p.224]

Power Distance

Power distance is the acceptance of an unequal distribution of power as legitimate or fair versus illegitimate from the point of view of the less powerful. In cultures that value a more equal distribution of power, people have the expectation that their opinions will be heard and equally valued. People who are less powerful have the right to criticize those in power. In contrast, in cultures in which a greater power distance is observed, people are unlikely to overtly challenge or disagree with people in positions of authority because such power is the result of longstanding formal and hierarchical arrangements. For example, a study of patient/provider communication in respect to HIV adherence revealed that patients were equally divided between preferences for collaborative styles of communication and provider-dominant styles of communication and messages that were delivered using supportive "soft" communication, and tough talk or more demanding kinds of communication.[24]

Masculinity Versus Femininity

Masculinity versus femininity describes how gender roles are conceived and how greatly male and female roles differ. Some societies place greater value on masculine attributes (as defined by Western culture), such as achievement, material success, and recognition, versus more feminine attributes, such as harmonious relationships, modesty, and taking care of others. In some cultures, only men can enact masculine roles, whereas in other cultures gender roles are more flexible. In cultures with more fixed gender roles, women are usually given the role of caretaker for aging relatives and may suffer the stresses of caregiver strain.

Long-Term Versus Short-Term Orientation

Long- versus short-term orientation is the degree to which a culture is oriented to the future and long-term rewards versus the degree to which a culture is oriented to the past or present.[25] Long-term-oriented cultures favor thrift, perseverance, and adapting to changing circumstances. Short-term-oriented cultures are oriented to the present or past and emphasize quick results; they favor respect for tradition and fulfillment of social obligations, although status is not a major issue in relationships and leisure time is important. Among the most long-term-oriented countries are China, Hong Kong, Taiwan, and Japan, whereas the United States, Great Britain, Canada, and the Philippines are among the most short-term-oriented countries.[25]

In a healthcare context, a long-term orientation would be evidenced by the patient who comes in for preventive care visits, receives all of the recommended screening tests and immunizations, and is an active partner in his or her care. A short-term orientation might be evidenced by the individual who seeks treatment for healthcare problems only when the symptoms of an illness become unbearable.

Religiosity

Another cultural dimension is religiosity, which varies according to how much religion permeates one's day-to-day existence and to what degree religious practices can be separated from nonreligious practices. Religion provides a sense of meaning and coherence to help cope with illness and other life adversities.[26] Religion differs from spirituality in that religiosity is an organized and institutionalized practice associated with particular beliefs, whereas spirituality is an individualistic connection to a higher power, which may or may not entail belonging to an organized religion. The majority of people in the United States believe in God (74%), miracles (72%), and heaven (68%), although this has been diminishing over time and with each succeeding generation.[27] Thus religious beliefs are in a state of flux in the United States.

THEORETICAL LINKS

The importance of culture and its influence on human behavior has not always been an accepted theoretical premise. Theories of human behavior have been dominated by the underlying premise of the "psychic unity" of humankind, a theory that states that all human social behavior is derived from evolution.[28] Scientists who believe in these concepts claim that through evolution and natural selection, certain genes in

the species that enhance survival are most likely to be passed down from one generation to the next, and these genes specify cognitive functioning and the manner in which people perceive the world.[29] Therefore thoughts, behaviors, and emotions develop universally and account for such diverse behaviors as favoring relatives (i.e., altruism), creating and following rules, or adopting specific beliefs about religion and warfare.[30] Language, culture, and religion are incidental to or an outgrowth of these genetically determined behavioral processes. Karasz and McKinley[31] refer to "the 'culture-free' approach of traditional health psychology." However, many theorists currently believe that the recognitions of emotions, the social display of emotions, the cognitions and interpretations of emotions and the associated bodily experiences are culturally determined rather than culture free.[32] Relatively recently, behavioral geneticists have shown us how the social environment has a major influence on how genes are expressed. Although there might be inherent biologic factors that produce emotions and behavior, genes interact with the environment to produce differences in emotional responses.[33]

Leininger's Theory of Culture Care Diversity and Universality

Berry and Leininger emphasized the importance of understanding human behavior in the context of culture.[34,35] They applied the concepts of "emic" and "etic," which referred to an approach to understanding behaviors. The term *emic* refers to an approach to understanding culture from within (i.e., the insider's viewpoint), whereas *etic* refers to the application of constructs external to a culture to discover universal characteristics common to all cultures. The assumption of universality can also imply an imposition of an outsider's values, rules, and understanding to another culture or subculture. The concepts of emic and etic are essential aspects of Leininger's theory of culture care diversity and universality.[36]

The central tenet of this theory is that both emic and etic approaches could lead to more responsive approaches to caring, the most important focus of nursing. To provide meaningful and holistic care, social structure factors, such as religion, economics, education, technology, ethnic background, and history, have to be taken into account because these factors have major influences on health, well-being, and illness. This comprehensive approach to nursing formed the basis of Leininger's development of transcultural nursing, the "formal area of humanistic and scientific knowledge and practices focused on holistic culture care … to assist individuals or groups to maintain or regain their health (or well-being)."[36, p.84]

Interprofessional Theory of Social Suffering

The interprofessional theory of social suffering states that relationships and social interactions shape our illness experiences and beliefs about the meaning of suffering. Memories of trauma and suffering exist collectively within a group or culture and are transmitted through shared experiences and learning.[37] All illnesses are a form of social suffering, mediated by cultural and political institutions. Technological advances can treat an individual's disease, but they do not address the root causes of illness, including poverty and the global political economy. Tuberculosis, depression, sexually transmitted infections, substance abuse, domestic violence, posttraumatic stress disorders, and AIDS are not individual problems but, rather, a reflection of social structure and healthcare and political inequities. It is also important to understand the individual's cultural interpretation of illness and suffering. These cultural representations of suffering and the response to it comprise the diversity of human responses to illness and pain. In some cultures, silent endurance is valued, whereas other cultures rail against unjust gods.[37, pp.ix–xiv] Some cultures place a high priority on the well-being and health of their members, whereas other societies are characterized by greater inequities in the health status of their populations.

CONTEXT TO NURSING AND HEALTH CARE

Many nursing students have asked, "Why is there such an emphasis on culture in health care? That's all we keep hearing about." Culture is an essential aspect of health care because of the increasing diversity of the United States. In 2016 the U.S. population was estimated at 323 million. In that year, the non-Hispanic white population of the United States represented 62% of the total population, a drop of five percentage points since 2008.[38] This is due to the aging of the white population and a postrecession decrease in fertility among white women. Currently, children aged 0 to 9 are more likely to be minorities than white.[39] By 2050 the non-Hispanic white population is expected to decrease to 50%, assuming the rate of immigration is constant.[41] Half of the population will be composed of people who identify themselves as belonging to a racial or ethnic minority population, including black, Asian, and Pacific Islander; American Indian, Eskimo, and Aleut; and Hispanic.[40]

In 2016, approximately 12.5% of the U.S. population, or 39 million people, had a disability.[41] Persons with disabilities identify themselves as part of a culture based on shared life experiences; this identification has led to music, publications, and media products unique to that culture, as well as to the disability rights movement to address discrimination in housing, employment, and health care. An estimated 4% of the U.S. population ages 18 to 44 years identified themselves as lesbian, gay, bisexual, or transgender.[42] Persons who are lesbian, gay, bisexual, or transgender experience societal discrimination, societal stigma, and human rights abuses that have led to higher rates of mental illness in addition to higher rates of HIV and sexually transmitted infections.[43,44]

Health Disparities

The increasing cultural diversity in the United States has resulted in the national health objective proposed in *Healthy People 2030:* achieving the highest level of health for all people and communities. Health and well-being is achieved by strengthening physical, social, and economic environments.[45] One of the major goals of *Healthy People 2030* is the elimination of healthcare disparities, and achievement of health equity, which is closely allied with nursing's basic tenet of social justice, which is the belief that all people deserve quality health care and access to care is a basic human right. *Healthy People 2030* emphasizes the need to provide culturally competent healthcare services and to improve health literacy and health education among non-English-speaking populations. This is presented in greater detail as Concept 52, Health Disparities.

Cultural Competency in Nursing

Cultural competence is an expected component of nursing education and professional nursing practice. Culturally competent care means conveying acceptance of the patient's health beliefs while sharing information, encouraging self-efficacy, and strengthening the patient's coping resources. The scope and standards of nursing practice specifically identify cultural competency as it relates to assessment, outcomes identification, planning, and implementation.[46] Cultural competency is currently more of an imperative as we begin to understand that healthcare providers' unconscious biases contribute to disparities in treatment,[47] even though nurses and physicians continue to deny that their own behavior is a factor in healthcare inequalities.[48]

As a nursing student, you might be thinking, "Yes, but we are taught how to communicate with our patients and if I treat everyone with respect and understanding, isn't that sufficient?" By treating everyone the same, we are not providing quality care because we are ignoring

societal factors that contribute to worse health outcomes among vulnerable populations. It is true that communicating respectfully is an essential aspect of communication and every patient is an individual with unique needs. However, failure to recognize the fact that people identify themselves as members of certain groups who have shared experiences of social injustice and who are currently treated differently in health care will result in an inability to understand some of the most essential human experiences of our patients.

Now, you may be saying to yourself, "Yes, I understand cultural competency is important, but really, there are so many other things that we need to learn as nurses."

Rubin defines expert nursing as the ability to recognize qualitative distinctions between patients.[49] The ability to make qualitative distinctions, or to be able to understand differences in the patient's life experiences, requires empathy. Empathy is necessary to understand the individual's self-perceptions of how he or she came to feel that way. Nurses who lack empathy are not practicing evidenced-based care, defined as comprising research-based information, clinical expertise, and patient preferences.[50]

In a cultural sense, this could be illustrated by the description of one nursing student's health assessment and history taking. She writes, "His parents are from India and he practices Hinduism. He goes to Mosques regularly and is a lot like my patient from Sudan, who is also very religious and celebrates Ramadan." This assumption of similarity between Muslim and Hindu practices and the confusion between the two evidence an inability to make qualitative distinctions in a person's history or to really attempt to understand that person's experience of religion. Individualized care or "patient-centered" care is facilitated by cultural competence that respects and acknowledges the patient's values, needs, and preferences.[51]

Developing Cultural Competence

The process of developing cultural competence consists of four interrelated constructs—cultural desire, self-awareness, cultural knowledge, and cultural skill—thus forming the broad components of cultural competency.[52,53]

Cultural Desire

A pivotal construct is *cultural desire*.[52] Cultural desire refers to an interest and intent to understand people who are different from oneself. Cultural desire is a personal choice; this interest is foundational to cultural competence and provides the means for overcoming one's biases and their effect on care. Cultural desire leads to patient-centered care as the nurse becomes more attuned to differences between individuals. Like any other effort to master new skills and knowledge, motivation or cultural desire is a prerequisite.

Self-Awareness

Self-awareness involves identifying and understanding one's own cultural identity. You might think about some aspects of your own cultural identity. Did you grow up with people of the same ethnic background as yourself? Did you gather with extended family and engage in traditional activities? Do members of your family make frequent visits to their country of origin or old neighborhood? Do you participate in ethnic cultural events? Do you speak another language? Do you have pride in your cultural background?

Perhaps you are saying to yourself, "But I grew up in an area where everyone is the same as I am, and we don't have traditions from the countries where my great grandparents came from and we just eat normal American food and celebrate the same holidays as everyone else. *I don't have any cultural identification.*" If you feel that way, ask yourself, "What about the place I grew up? Is it like every other place in the United States? What about the meals I prepare? Does everyone in America celebrate the same holidays? Are all Americans the same? What are my own values and beliefs?"

Perhaps you are saying to yourself, "But I grew up in an area where everyone is from a different culture and I'm very comfortable interacting with other cultures." If you feel that way, ask yourself, "How would I feel living next door to a family with two parents of the same sex or a halfway house for people with chronic severe mental illness? How comfortable do I feel interacting with homeless people? How would I feel if my son or daughter married someone from a religion that I know nothing about? What are my own biases?"

Biases not only are negative stereotypes but also can be any tendency to act, think, or feel in a certain way toward other people. For example, you may believe that Vietnamese people are hardworking, they want their children to do well in school, they expect that their children show respect to their parents, and they stick together. Many nurses believe, "But that really doesn't apply to me, because I know that even if I personally don't like someone or something they've done, I will treat everyone in a professional manner and will treat everyone the same." Nurses grow up with the values and beliefs of their cultures and the society around them. Perhaps you believe that abortion is wrong, that it is immoral to have same-sex relationships, that people with depression could really snap out of it if they wanted to, or that people with substance abuse do not have a mental illness—they make choices. Perhaps you feel angry that some people receive health benefits that are "free" and are paid for by your tax dollars. After all, you work hard to earn money, "Why can't they?" "Why do all of those refugees who have moved into my community get Medicaid and can get medications that I can barely afford?" Is it possible to separate all of these feelings from our practice? Many studies in many fields indicate that those feelings carry over into the care we provide.

Even when one's own values and beliefs are directed against a particular group of people, they may still reflect the biases of the dominant cultural group. For example, nurses from independent cultures will develop nursing objectives based on the cultural value of autonomy—developing one's own potential and maintaining one's independence—and equate "more" of such traits with better health. A patient from a more interdependent, collectivist culture might not share such values. For this patient, it might be expected that he or she is dependent on other family members in times of ill health. Moreover, the family's needs and desires might be valued more highly than obtaining one's own personal goals. The use of the concept of "self-esteem" as part of a nursing diagnosis may reflect the bias that the self is construed similarly in all cultures. As Markus and Kitayama[23] explain, in interdependent cultures, the essence of self is defined by one's relationships to others rather than the inner self. Internal attributes such as desires, abilities, and personality traits are viewed as situation dependent and therefore unreliable. Self is not a constant but, rather, is fluid and changes according to the situation or the relationship. It is important for the nurse to assess the patient's own values and definition of health and to develop mutually agreed upon nursing care plans.[54]

Knowledge

Knowledge as a domain of cultural competency does not imply learning facts about every culture but, rather, exposing one's self to other cultures and being motivated to learn. Knowledge can be acquired by reading journals that represent different groups; visiting ethnic neighborhoods and sampling different foods; learning a foreign language; attending community or professional nursing meetings representing diverse coalitions; speaking with someone from another culture; walking into botánicas, ethnic grocery stores, or herb shops; attending a service at a mosque or synagogue; speaking with a hospital translator; going to a gay pride

---

BOX 4.1 Eight Questions Associated With the RESPECT Model

1. What do you call the problem?
2. What do you think has caused the problem?
3. Why do you think it started when it did?
4. What do you think the sickness does? How does it work?
5. How severe is the sickness? Will it have a long or short course?
6. What kind of treatment do you think you should receive?
7. What are the chief problems the sickness has caused?
8. What do you fear most about the sickness?

From Kleinman, A. (1980). *Patients and healers in the context of culture.* Berkeley, CA: University of California Press.

---

march or Puerto Rican day parade; or reading a novel about someone growing up in another culture.

Skill

Skills are acquired over time by careful attention to the nurse-patient relationship. One element of cultural skill is communication. Collaborative decision making and patient engagement are key aspects of health outcomes, but culturally and linguistically diverse populations require specific strategies to overcome the barriers of language, distrust, low health literacy, and stigma. There are many resources available to learn basic medical terminology on the web, including internet and smartphone applications that serve as translators. There are also assessment questions designed to understand the sociocultural contexts of people's healthcare needs. The RESPECT model of cultural assessment, based on a series of eight questions developed by Kleinman,[55] provides a blueprint to develop skills needed to become culturally competent (Box 4.1).[56] RESPECT is an acronym for *r*espect, *e*xplanatory model, *s*ociocultural context, *p*ower, *e*mpathy, *c*oncerns and fears, and *t*herapeutic alliance/trust.

Respect and *empathy* are attitudes that demonstrate to the patient that his or her concerns are valued and he or she is understood. The nurse can further assess for the patient's *explanatory model*, or understanding of what is the cause of his or her illness, and the *sociocultural context*, which comprises factors in a person's life that may contribute to the current state of health and expectations for treatment, such as poverty, stress, and social support. *Power* refers to the importance of acknowledging that the patient is in a vulnerable position and that there is a difference between patients and healthcare providers in terms of access to resources, knowledge level, and control over outcomes. The loss of power and control that a patient faces can contribute to *concerns and fears* about treatment, illness outcomes, and the future. Bearing in mind the meaning of these concepts in the nursing relationship enhances communication and assessment skills between patient and nurse and creates a *therapeutic alliance and trust*.

Conducting a Cultural Assessment

Assessment has long been recognized as the foundation for competent, patient-centered nursing care. It should be no surprise that cultural assessment is an expected component of nursing care. A cultural assessment helps nurses gain an understanding of the meaning of the illness to the patient, expectations the patient has regarding treatment and care, and the patient's perception about the process. The patient history includes many questions that link to a patient's cultural perspectives and preference. It is most important to apply elements previously described into the history and assessment so these critical data are recognized and understood. Data gained from an interview as it relates to cultural assessment are included in Box 4.2. In addition to data collected as part of an interview, the nurse should observe the patient's behavior (e.g., personal space and eye contact), clothing, and presence of articles as cues for additional or clarifying questions.

INTERRELATED CONCEPTS

Several concepts within this textbook are closely related to the concept of culture and are shown in Fig. 4.2. Health Disparities adversely affect groups of people who have systematically experienced greater obstacles to

---

BOX 4.2   **Data Collected as Part of Cultural Assessment**

Origins and Family
- Where born; if in other country, length of time in United States and circumstances
- Decision making within family
- Cultural group(s) identified with; presence of social network
- Important cultural practices

Communication
- Language spoken at home; skill in speaking, reading, and writing in English
- Preferred methods to communicate with patient and/or family member (how to be addressed, to whom questions are directed, etc.)
- Ways respect is shown to others
- Eye contact, interpersonal space

Personal Beliefs About Health, Illness
- Meaning and belief about cause of illness
- Perception of control over health
- Practices or rituals used to improve health
- Perception of severity of illness
- Expectations for treatment; use of folk remedies, alternative medicine
- Practices that violate beliefs (taboos)
- Concerns or fears about illness or process of treatment

Daily Practices
- Dietary preferences and practices; forbidden foods
- Beliefs about food that pertain to health and illness
- Spiritual beliefs; religious practices
- Special rituals

---

health based on their racial, ethnic, or cultural group; religion; socioeconomic status; gender; age; mental health; cognitive, sensory, or physical disability; sexual orientation or gender identity; geographic location; or other characteristics historically linked to discrimination or exclusion.[57] Culture affects Family Dynamics in many ways, including the manner in which sick family members receive care, beliefs about sharing information with outsiders about a family member's illness, gender roles, and beliefs about appropriate childrearing practices. For example, the dominant practice in America of letting an infant cry himself or herself to sleep to learn how to self-soothe may be construed as a form of neglect, particularly for people of cultures that believe in sharing a bed with an infant.

The concept of Ethics is interrelated because of the different interpretations and values around appropriate behaviors and actions; in some cultures, practices considered appropriate may be considered unethical in others—thus ethics may be nested in cultural context.[58]

Another cultural dimension is Spirituality, which is an individualistic subjective experience of transformation or connection to a higher power. Spirituality may or may not entail belonging to an organized religion. Spirituality is closely interrelated with culture because many spiritual beliefs are embedded within cultural groups.

The concept of Communication is closely related to culture because communication patterns, both verbal and nonverbal, are determined by cultural norms. Degree of eye contact, personal space, and the acceptability of touch all vary by cultures. Culture dictates the nature of relationships and the degree of hierarchy and structure in relationships. In some cultures a high degree of formality and reserve is expected when addressing people of greater social status, whereas in other cultures there is less stratification by age or social standing and it is acceptable to be direct and open with everyone. Similarly, in some cultures, personal revelations or discussion of family problems are taboo, whereas in other cultures there are no such restrictions on communication.

Stress and Coping involve dealing with life's difficulties and are, to a large extent, culturally determined. Cultural belief systems form the basis of a coping strategy by creating a redefinition of negative circumstances.[59] These belief systems may encompass religious beliefs and religiosity, which may have a beneficial effect on health by fostering positive emotions such as hope, gratitude, and reverence.[60] Religiosity may result in decreased symptoms of distress and may help with coping by decreasing loneliness and fostering cultural identity.[61]

The expression and meaning of some symptoms such as Fatigue are influenced by culture. Some cultures seek a biomedical explanation for the medically unexplained symptom of fatigue (such as chronic

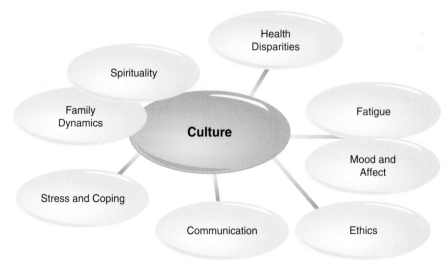

FIGURE 4.2 Culture and Interrelated Concepts.

fatigue syndrome and depression) or a lack of fulfillment, whereas other cultures view fatigue as an imbalance of essential energies.[31] Likewise, Mood and Affect have a strong interrelationship to culture. Depression is the leading cause of nonfatal disease burden and years of life lived with disability worldwide.[62] Rates of depression are highest among the most vulnerable populations—people living in poverty, immigrants, and refugees.[63–65] Experiences of immigration may also contribute to mood disorders because immigrants experience depression from the stress of adjusting to a new culture, loss of family and traditions, loss of social status, and memories of severe deprivation or political violence in their countries of origin.[66] Racial and ethnic minorities are less likely to receive treatment for mood disorders, and when they do receive treatment, it often does not meet the standard of care.[67] Patients have better outcomes when they are culturally and linguistically matched with their mental health provider.[68] Cultural values and beliefs, including the reluctance to share personal problems outside of the family, disclose personal problems, a value on self-sufficiency, recognition of mental health problems, and stigma about mental illness, also create barriers to treatment engagement.[69–72]

CLINICAL EXEMPLARS

There are multiple exemplars of culture in the context of healthcare delivery. These are best presented using the framework of healthcare practices and beliefs, family roles, and patient-provider communication. The most common exemplars of culture as it relates to healthcare and nursing practice are presented in Box 4.3.

Featured Exemplars
Language Preference
An estimated 63 million Americans (21%) speak a language other than English in the home, and 8.5% report that they do not speak English

---

> **BOX 4.3   EXEMPLARS OF CULTURE**
>
> **Health Care Practices/Beliefs**
> - Symptoms of illness
> - Treatment preferences
> - Meaning of illness
> - Control over health and illness
> - Consequences of illness/preventive care
> - Dietary practices
> - Religious healing practices
> - Complimentary alternative or integrative medicine
>
> **Family Roles**
> - Birthrights
> - Childrearing practices
> - Gender roles
> - Family structure
> - Decision making
> - Death and dying
> - Caregiver roles
>
> **Patient-Provider Communication**
> - Language preference
> - Nonverbal communication (eye contact, personal space, touch, body posture)
> - Power distance
> - Taboos
> - Revealing personal information
> - Expression of emotion

 ACCESS EXEMPLAR LINKS IN YOUR GIDDENS EBOOK

---

well (U.S. Census Bureau).[38] Patients with limited English proficiency (LEP) face many healthcare barriers in terms of understanding healthcare information, adherence to treatment plans, and follow-up care due to impaired patient-provider communication. Healthcare providers must ensure that health care is delivered in a manner that takes into account the needs of patients with LEP, often through the use of interpreters. The Agency for Healthcare Research and Quality has a number of tools and guidelines available to help nurses provide quality care to LEP patients.[73]

Decision Making
The values of individualism versus collectivism form cultural differences in the role of the family in determining how people decide to obtain treatments and medical care. For independent cultures, an individual will put himself or herself first in the case of a life-threatening illness, whereas even in such dire situations, members of collectivist cultures may still consult other family members for the best course of action.

Taboo
A taboo is a prohibited or forbidden action or behavior based on moral judgment and/or religious beliefs in the context of one's culture. Taboos are present in all cultures, and what is considered taboo in one culture may not be considered taboo in another. Healthcare providers must maintain awareness that some procedures and treatment practices considered standard of practice may be considered taboo in some cultures. Examples include physical touch of a female patient for an examination without the consent of the husband and administration of blood products.

Power Distance
People from cultures with greater inequality of power distance may be unwilling to disagree with or question the authority of a healthcare provider, whereas people from cultures in which there is an expectation of equality of relationships may not be hesitant in expressing their wishes and needs for their own health care. Therefore when a nurse provides education to the patient who is from a culture that values greater power distance, it might appear that the patient is willing to accept all the nurse's suggestions, when further prompting might elicit additional questions or concerns of the patient.

Symptoms of Illness
The symptoms of an illness may vary depending on how a culture understands and perceives the illness. Thus healthcare providers must consider the possibility that their view of "expected symptoms" associated with certain disorders may be different from that of people from other cultures. For example, in some cultures, it is acceptable to verbalize that one is in pain, whereas in other cultures, the verbalization of pain is seen as a sign of weakness or control. As another example, mental health illnesses are described in bodily terms such as backaches, headaches, and fatigue rather than disturbances in mood and affect.[74]

Beliefs About Illness Control
Beliefs about control one has over health and illness are highly variable depending on one's culture and can impact decisions about health promotion practices or care during times of illness. Individuals who hold a belief that they have control over the course of an illness may "appear" to be more engaged in and actively pursue health screening and treatment options. In some cultures the predominant belief is that what happens is out of one's control, sometimes referred to as fatalism or an external locus of control. In some contexts an external locus of control can be a culturally protective mechanism and serves to preserve a sense of peace and well-being in situations that are out of one's control, such as a terminal illness.

CASE STUDY

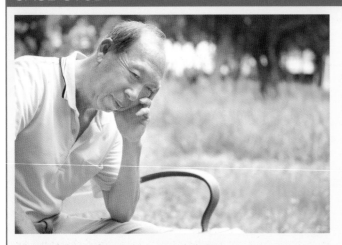

Case Presentation

Mr. Wong is a 78-year-old male from mainland China who has been admitted for rehabilitation following total hip replacement surgery. He has a poor appetite, has experienced weight loss, and has been unable to participate in physical therapy. Thus he is not meeting his goals for rehabilitation. No evidence exists to suggest an underlying disease process.

Ms. Faye, the nurse assigned to care for Mr. Wong, is interested in learning what might be going on with Mr. Wong to better meet his treatment outcomes. Ms. Faye considers the possibility that he does not have adequate pain relief, which could affect his appetite and cause poor participation in physical therapy. She reviews his history to learn more about him. According the health history, Mr. Wong is a widower of 3 years; he has a son and daughter who live in distant cities. Mr. Wong emigrated from China at the age of 38 years and speaks only

Cantonese. He has lived in an ethic neighborhood with other Chinese Americans and has worked as a short-order cook in a Chinese restaurant since arriving in the United States 40 years ago.

Ms. Faye arranges for Mr. Lee, a Cantonese translator who is also Chinese, to help her ask Mr. Wong a few questions. She first asks Mr. Wong if he is in pain. When he responds no, she follows with another question, asking him if he is depressed or anxious. Again, Mr. Wong responds no, that he is fine. During the interaction, Ms. Faye observes that Mr. Wong does not look at her or Mr. Lee, the translator.

After leaving the room, Ms. Faye expresses her frustration to Mr. Lee, mentioning how difficult it will be to help Mr. Wong when he will not communicate. Mr. Lee responds, "Elderly Chinese people believe that they must be stoic about pain and there is a stigma about talking about any mental health problems." This explanation had not occurred to Ms. Faye, who then recognizes her approach may have been offensive and that she had failed to consider the underlying cultural differences beyond language.

Ms. Faye asks Mr. Lee to share more about traditional Chinese beliefs. She then asks Mr. Lee to help her ask Mr. Wong additional questions using a cultural assessment form as a guide. After gathering additional information from Mr. Wong and gaining additional insight from Mr. Lee, Ms. Faye incorporates strategies that include changes to how his food is prepared and served, changes in approaches to pain management, and involving Mr. Wong's son and daughter in his care.

Case Analysis Questions

1. In what way does this case exemplify the concept of culture in the context of health care?
2. Referring to Fig. 4.2, what interrelated concepts are exemplified in this case? What additional concepts apply that are not included in Fig. 4.2?

From Tomwang112/iStock/Thinkstock.

🌿 **ACCESS EXEMPLAR LINKS IN YOUR GIDDENS EBOOK**

REFERENCES

1. Shweder, R. A. (1990). Cultural psychology—What is it? In J. W. Stigler, R. A. Shweder, & G. Herdt (Eds.), *Cultural psychology* (pp. 1–43). Cambridge: Cambridge University Press.
2. Geertz, C. (1973). *The interpretation of cultures.* New York: Basic Books.
3. Cavalli-Sforza, L. (2000). *Genes, peoples, and languages.* Berkley, CA: University of California Press.
4. Kleinman, A. (1988). *Rethinking psychiatry: From cultural category to personal experience.* New York: Free Press.
5. Huff, R. M. (1999). Cross-cultural concepts of health and disease. In R. M. Huff & M. V. Kline (Eds.), *Promoting health in multicultural populations* (pp. 23–39). Thousand Oaks, CA: Sage.
6. American Psychiatric Association. (2013). *Diagnostic and statistical manual of mental disorders* (5th ed.). Washington, DC: Author.
7. Klonoff, E. A., & Landrine, H. (1994). Culture and gender diversity in commonsense beliefs about the causes of six illnesses. *Journal of Behavioral Medicine, 17*(4), 407–418.
8. Opare-Henaku, A., & Utsey, S. O. (2017). Culturally prescribed beliefs about mental illness among the Akan of Ghana. *Transcultural Psychiatry, 54*(4), 502–522.
9. DuraVila, G., & Hodes, M. (2012). Cross-cultural study of idioms of distress among Spanish nationals and Hispanic American migrants: Susto, nervios and ataque de nervios. *Social Psychiatry and Psychiatric Epidemiology, 47*(10), 1627–1637.
10. Chinese Medical Association and Nanjing Medical University. (1995). *Chinese classification of mental disorders* (2nd ed.). Revised (CCMD-2-R). Nanjing: Dong Nan University Press.
11. Molina, K. M., Chen, C., Alegría, M., & Li, H. (2012). Prevalence of neurasthenia, comorbidity, and association with impairment among a nationally representative sample of US adults. *Social Psychiatry and Psychiatric Epidemiology, 47*(11), 1733–1744.
12. World Health Organization. (1992). *International classification of diseases and related disorders (ICD-10).* Geneva: Author.
13. Keel, P. K., & Klump, K. L. (2003). Are eating disorders culture-bound syndromes? implications for conceptualizing their etiology. *Psychological Bulletin, 129*(5), 747–769.
14. Jacobi, C., Hayward, C., de Zwaan, M., et al. (2004). Coming to terms with risk factors for eating disorders: Application of risk terminology and suggestions for a general taxonomy. *Psychological Bulletin, 130*, 19–65.
15. U.S. Department of Health and Human Services. (2001). *Mental health: Culture, race and ethnicity—A supplement to mental health: A report of the Surgeon General.* Rockville, MD: Substance Abuse and Mental Health Services Administration. U.S. Public Health Service No. 01–3613.
16. De Leo, D., & Milner, A. (2010). The Start Study: Promoting suicide prevention for a diverse range of cultural contexts. *Suicide and Life-Threatening Behavior, 40*, 99–106.
17. Moynihan, D. P. (1965). *The Negro family: The case for national action.* Washington, DC: Office of Policy Planning and Research, U.S. Department of Labor. Retrieved from http://www.dol.gov/oasam/programs/history/webid-meynihan.htm.
18. Redfield, R., Linton, R., & Herskovits, M. J. (1936). Memorandum for the study of acculturation. *American Anthropologist, 38*, 149–152.
19. Hofstede, G. (1980). *Culture's consequences: International differences in work-related values.* Beverly Hills, CA: Sage.
20. Hofstede, G. (1991). Empirical models of cultural differences. In N. Bleichrodt & P. Drenth (Eds.), *Contemporary issues in cross-cultural psychology* (pp. 4–20). Lisse, The Netherlands: Swets & Zeitlinger.

21. Kagitcibasi, C. (1997). Individualism and collectivism. In J. W. Berry, M. H. Segall, & C. Kagitcibasi (Eds.), *Handbook of cross-cultural psychology* (2nd ed., Vol. 3). Social behavior and applications. Needham Heights, MA: Allyn & Bacon.

22. Mesquita, B. (2001). Emotions in collectivist and individualist contexts. *Journal of Personality and Social Psychology, 80*(1), 68–74.

23. Markus, H. R., & Kitayama, S. (1991). Culture and the self: Implications for cognition, emotion, and motivation. *Psychological Review, 98,* 224–253.

24. Hurley, E. A., Harvey, S. A., Winch, P. J., et al. (2018). The role of patient-provider communication in engagement and re-engagement in HIV treatment in Bamako, Mali: a qualitative study. *Journal of Health Communication, 23*(2), 129–143.

25. Hofstede, G. (1997). *Culture and organizations: Software of the mind.* New York: McGraw-Hill.

26. Pargament, K. I. (1997). An introduction to the psychology of religion and coping. *The psychology of religion and coping.* New York, NY: Guilford Press.

27. Shannon-Missal, L. (2013). Americans' belief in God, miracles and heaven declines. *The Harris Poll.* Retrieved from http://www.harrisinteractive.com/vault/Harris%20Poll%2097%20-%20Beliefs_12.16.2013.pdf.

28. Matsumoto, D., & Yoo, S. H. (2006). Toward a new generation of cross-cultural research. *Perspectives on Psychological Science: A Journal of the Association for Psychological Science, 1*(3), 234–250.

29. Tooby, J., & Cosmides, L. (1989). Evolutionary psychology and the generation of culture. Part I: Theoretical considerations. *Ethology and Sociobiology, 10,* 29–49.

30. Fukuyama, F. (2011). *The origins of political order: From prehuman times to the French Revolution.* New York: Farrar, Straus & Giroux.

31. Karasz, A., & McKinley, P. S. (2007). Cultural differences in conceptual models of everyday fatigue: A vignette study. *Journal of Health Psychology, 12*(4), 613–626.

32. Hoffman, S. G., & Doan, S. N. (2018). Sociocultural aspects of emotion. In S. G. Hoffman & S. Doan (Eds.), *The social foundations of emotion: developmental, cultural, and clinical dimensions.* Washington, DC: American Psychological Association. Chapter 4.

33. Caspi, A., Moffitt, T. E., Morgan, J., et al. (2004). Maternal expressed emotion predicts children's antisocial behavior problems: Using monozygotic-twin differences to identify environmental effects on behavioral development. *Developmental Psychology, 40*(2), 149–161.

34. Berry, J. W. (1989). Imposed etics–emics–derived etics: The operationalization of a compelling idea. *International Journal of Psychology. Journal International de Psychologie, 24,* 721–735.

35. Leininger, M., & McFarland, M. R. (2002). *Transcultural nursing: Concepts, theories, research and practices* (3rd ed.). New York: McGraw-Hill.

36. Leininger, M. M. (1991). *Culture care diversity and universality, a theory of nursing.* New York: National League for Nursing Press.

37. Kleinman, A., Das, V., & Locke, M. (1997). Introduction. In *Social suffering.* Oakland, CA: University of California Press.

38. U.S. Census Bureau. American FactFinder. *Annual Estimates of the Resident Population 2010 to 2017.* Retrieved from https://factfinder.census.gov/faces.

39. Frey, W. H. (2018). U.S. White population declines and generation 'Z-Plus' is minority white, census shows. *The Avenue.* June 22, The Brookings Institute. Retrieved from https://www.brookings.edu/blog/the-avenue/2018/06/21/us-white-population-declines-and-generation-z-plus-is-minority-white-census-shows/.

40. Ortman, J. M., & Guarneri, C. E. (2009). *United States population projections: 2000 to 2050.* U.S. Census Bureau.

41. U.S. Census Bureau. *American FactFinder, United States: American Community Survey. American Community Survey 1-year estimates, Selected social characteristics in the United States, 2012-2016. Five Year Estimates.* Retrieved from http://factfinder.census.gov.

42. Gates, G. J. *In U.S., More Adults Identifying as LGBT. Gallup. Social and Policy Issues.* 2017. Retrieved from https://news.gallup.com/poll/201731/lgbt-identification-rises.aspx.

43. McLaughlin, K. A., Hatzenbuehler, M. L., & Keyes, K. M. (2010). Responses to discrimination and psychiatric disorders among black, Hispanic, female, and lesbian, gay, and bisexual individuals. *American Journal of Public Health, 100,* 1477–1484.

44. Centers for Disease Control and Prevention (2010). *HIV and AIDS among gay and bisexual men.* Atlanta: Author. Retrieved from http://www.cdc.gov/hiv/risk/gender/msm/facts/index.html.

45. U.S. Department of Health and Human Services, Office of Disease Prevention and Health Promotion. *Healthy People 2030 Framework.* https://www.healthypeople.gov/2020/About-Healthy-People/Development-Healthy-People-2030/Framework.

46. American Nurses Association. (2015). *Nursing scope and standards of practice* (3rd ed.). Silver Spring, MD: Author.

47. Cuellar, N. G. (2017). Unconscious bias: What is yours? *Journal of Transcultural Nursing, 28*(4), 333.

48. Hannah, S. D., & CarpenterSong, E. (2013). Patrolling your blind spots: Introspection and public catharsis in a medical school faculty development course to reduce unconscious bias in medicine. *Culture, Medicine and Psychiatry, 37*(2), 314–339.

49. Rubin, J. (2009). Impediments to the development of clinical knowledge and ethical judgment in critical care nursing. In P. Benner, C. Tanner, & C. Cheslan (Eds.), *Expertise in nursing practice: Caring, clinical judgment, and ethics* (2nd ed., pp. 171–198). New York: Springer.

50. Brown, S. J. (2016). Evidenced-based nursing: *The research–practice connection* (4th ed.). Burlington, MA: Jones & Bartlett.

51. Institute of Medicine. (2003). *Health professions education: A bridge to quality.* Washington, DC: National Academies Press.

52. Campinha-Bacote, J.: *A culturally conscious approach to holistic nursing.* Program and abstracts of the American Holistic Nurses Association 2005 Conference, King of Prussia, PA, June 16–19, 2005.

53. Shen, Z. (2015). Cultural competence models and cultural competence assessment instruments in nursing: A literature review. *Journal of Transcultural Nursing, 26*(3), 308–321.

54. Young, S., & Guo, K. L. (2016). Cultural diversity training: The necessity of cultural competence for health care providers and in nursing practice. *Health Care Management (Philadelphia, Pa.), 35*(2), 94–102.

55. Kleinman, A. (1980). *Patients and healers in the context of culture.* Berkeley, CA: University of California Press.

56. Mostow, C., Crosson, J., Gordon, S., et al. (2010). Treating and precepting with RESPECT: A relational model addressing race, ethnicity, and culture in medical training. *Journal of General Internal Medicine, 25*(Suppl. 2), 146–154.

57. U.S. Department of Health and Human Services. (2011). *HHS action plan to reduce racial and ethnic disparities: a nation free of disparities in health and health care.* Washington, D.C.: U.S. Department of Health and Human Services. Retrieved from http://minorityhealth.hhs.gov/npa/files/Plans/HHS/HHS_Plan_complete.pdf.

58. Ting-Toomey, S., & Chung, L. C. (2012). *Understanding intercultural communication.* New York: Oxford University Press.

59. Folkman, S., & Lazarus, R. S. (1988). The relationship between coping and emotion: Implications for theory and research. *Social Science and Medicine, 26,* 309–317.

60. Emmons, R. A. (2005). Emotion and religion. In R. F. Paloutzian & C. L. Park (Eds.), *Handbook of the psychology of religion and spirituality* (pp. 235–252). New York: Guilford.

61. Rosmarin, D. H., Krumrei, E., & Andersson, G. (2009). Religion as a predictor of psychological distress in two religious communities. *Cognitive Behaviour Therapy, 38,* 54–64.

62. Lopez, A., Mathers, D., Ezzati, C. D., et al. (2006). *Global and regional burden of disease and risk factors, 2001: Systematic analysis of population health data.* London: Onwhyn.

63. Hiott, A., Grzywacz, J. G., Arcury, T. A., et al. (2006). Gender differences in anxiety and depression among immigrant Latinos. *Families, Systems & Health: The Journal of Collaborative Family Healthcare, 24,* 137–146.

64. Huang, F. Y., Chung, H., Kroenke, K., et al. (2006). Racial and ethnic differences in the relationship between depression severity and functional status. *Psychiatric Services, 57,* 498–503.

65. Kessler, R. C., Berglund, P., Demler, O., et al. (2003). The epidemiology of major depressive disorder: Results from the National Comorbidity Survey Replication (NCS-R). *JAMA: The Journal of the American Medical Association, 289*, 3095–3105.

66. Caplan, S. (2007). Latinos, acculturation, and acculturative stress: A dimensional concept analysis. *Policy Politics Nursing Practice, 8*(2), 93–106.

67. Institute of Medicine. (2003). *Unequal treatment: Confronting racial and ethnic disparities in health care.* Washington, DC: National Academy Press.

68. Sue, S. (1988). Psychotherapeutic services for ethnic minorities: Two decades of research findings. *The American Psychologist, 43*, 301–308.

69. Corrigan, P. W., Morris, S., Larson, J. E., et al. (2010). Self-stigma and coming out about one's mental illness. *Journal of Community Psychology, 38*, 1–17.

70. Wang, J., & Lai, D. (2008). The relationship between mental health literacy, personal contacts and personal stigma against depression. *Journal of Affective Disorders, 110*(1), 191–196.

71. Nadeem, E., Lange, H. M., Edge, D., et al. (2007). Does stigma keep poor young immigrant and U.S.-born black and Latina women from seeking mental health care? *Psychiatric Services, 58*, 1547–1554.

72. Caplan, S., & Whittemore, R. (2013). Barriers to treatment engagement for depression among Latinas. *Issues in Mental Health Nursing, 34*, 412–424.

73. Agency for Healthcare Research and Quality. (2012). *Improving patient safety systems for patients with limited English proficiency: A guide for hospitals.* Rockville, MD: Author.

74. Escobar, J. I., Gara, M., Waitzkin, H., et al. (1998). Somatization disorder in primary care. *British Journal of Psychiatry, 173*, 262–267.

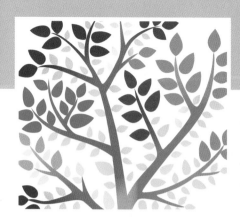

Spirituality

Lorraine P. Buchanan

Spirituality is a concept that has always been present among people. In ancient times there was an awareness that people were more than their bodies, and that that "more," although difficult to describe or quantify, was just as real as the body that could be touched and ministered to. In ancient cultures, there was a sense that people had good and/or bad spirits residing in their bodies, and these spirits influenced the individual's behavior for good or evil. In early Judaism, the care of the sick was a religious obligation, and this obligation continued as Christianity grew and expanded throughout the world.

Spirituality has also long been present in nursing. The earliest hospitals were run by religious orders, and nurses were trained by the Catholic Sisters who ran many of these hospitals. These early "health professionals" did not describe what they did in "spiritual terms," but they believed that the care they provided honored God. As the profession of nursing matured into a unique healthcare discipline, theories and educational methods evolved. Nursing leaders began to examine what made nursing unique and effective. These nurses recognized that nursing involved more than a group of clinical skills—making beds, bathing patients, administering medications, and performing the myriad other tasks that nurses of today still do. What more could nurses provide? One of the concepts identified was the nurse's ability to assess and address the spiritual needs of patients.

In the 1970s and 1980s, the education of nurses moved increasingly into colleges and universities; subsequently, nursing education adopted a scientific approach. With the growing emphasis on evidence-based interventions, spirituality became less visible. However, in 1979 Ruth Stoll published an influential article with guidelines for spiritual assessment in the *American Journal of Nursing*,[1] and in 1989 a book dedicated to spirituality, *Spiritual Dimensions of Nursing Practice*, was published.[2] In more recent years, there has been greater emphasis on spirituality and it is now recognized as an essential component of patient-centered care.[3–5]

DEFINITION

The concept of *spirituality* is an elusive concept to define. Authors who write about spirituality in nursing advocate the position that a patient's quality of life, meaning, purpose, health, and sense of wholeness and connectedness are affected by spirituality, yet the profession of nursing still struggles to clearly define it. Although there a large number of definitions of spirituality, a universal definition does not exist. The lack of clarity in defining spirituality is likely due to the fact that spirituality is unique to each individual, representing a personal experience. Also, spirituality represents "heart" rather than "head" knowledge, and heart knowledge is difficult to encapsulate into words.[2,3]

Definitions of spirituality typically encompass the following ideas: a principle, an experience, attitudes and belief regarding transcendence (God), and the inner person. In the early 1980s O'Brien defined spirituality as "a personal concept, generally understood in terms of an individual's attitudes and belief related to transcendence (God) or to the nonmaterial forces of life and of nature."[6, p.4] O'Brien concluded that most descriptions of spirituality include not only transcendence but also the connection of mind, body, and spirit in addition to love, caring, compassion, and a relationship with the Divine.[6] Individuals can view themselves as being very spiritual—believing that there is a transcendent being—and yet have no association with organized religion.[7] Individuals can also view spirituality in terms of relationships with the environment, with others, or with themselves.[5] Although there is wide variation in the way that spirituality has been defined, for the purposes of this chapter *Spirituality* is defined as "*a dynamic and intrinsic aspect of humanity through which people seek ultimate meaning, purpose, and transcendence and experience relationship to self, family, others, community, society, nature, and the significant or sacred. Spirituality is expressed through beliefs, values, traditions, and practices.*"[8, p.646]

There are other related terms worth mentioning to provide distinction and clarification. *Religion* is defined as beliefs, practices, adopted behaviors, or institutional affiliations guided by a community of faith or specific religious denomination.[5] Religion is the outward expression of a person's spiritual beliefs, such as through attending worship services. It helps people to maintain their faith and spiritual beliefs.[9] A similar term, *religiosity*, is an external expression (public or private) in the form of practicing a belief or faith (whereas spirituality is an internalized spiritual identity or experience). Specifically, religiosity is defined as "the adherence to religious dogma or creed, the expression of moral beliefs, and/or the participation in organized or individual worship, or sacred practices."[10, p.200]

SCOPE

The scope of spirituality is quite broad and complex, encompassing life itself and its meaning as perceived by each individual. Spirituality may be based on religious convictions, teachings, and experiences that provide moral direction and a sense that individuals are part of a larger plan and that each of us belongs to a Higher Being. However, spirituality

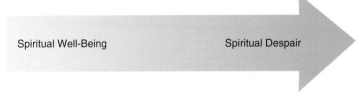

FIGURE 5.1 Scope of Spirituality.

> **BOX 5.1   Attributes of Spirituality**
>
> - Spirituality is universal.
> - Illness impacts spirituality.
> - Patient and/or family must be willing to share and act on spiritual beliefs.
> - Spiritual beliefs and practices are impacted by family and culture.
> - Nurses must be willing to assess and integrate patient beliefs into care.
> - Nurses must be willing to consult with/refer to appropriate spiritual experts.
> - Community-based religious organizations can provide spiritual support/resources.

might have no connection at all to religion and the transcendent but be experienced in the "highs" and "lows" of life with a view that these experiences are viewed as a normal part of living.[11]

What is true is that everyone has a spiritual nature, a sense that there is more than what is experienced day to day, month to month, year to year until death. Spirituality encompasses the mundane activities of life that keep us grounded as well as those magnificent times and experiences when our innermost spirit soars and we may have any number of emotional responses, including exquisite joy, dark and deep sorrow, laughter and fun, and all the emotions in between. Births, deaths, marriages, separations, divorces, terrible diagnoses, joy, and sorrow all possess this ability to touch our spirits in a profound manner. A person may not be the same as he or she was before such an event occurred. Further, the meaning and significance of the event might be experienced only by one individual; others experiencing the same event might be left virtually untouched or unchanged. Regardless, extraordinary events have the power to draw people toward the transcendent or may lead to spiritual distress.[2,11] The scope of spirituality is multidimensional; it is shown in Fig. 5.1 as a continuum ranging from spiritual well-being at one end to spiritual despair at the other.[12]

ATTRIBUTES AND CRITERIA

The attributes of the concept of Spirituality in the context of nursing care are presented in Box 5.1 and described further here:

- Spirituality is universal. All individuals, even those who profess no religious belief, are driven to derive meaning and purpose from life.
- Illness impacts spirituality in a variety of ways. Some patients and families will draw closer to God or however they conceive that higher power to be in an effort to seek support, healing, and comfort. Others may blame and feel anger toward that higher power for any illness and misfortune that may have befallen a loved one or their entire family. Still others will be neutral in their spiritual reactions.
- There has to be willingness on the part of the patient and family to share and act on spiritual beliefs and practices.
- The nurse must be aware that specific spiritual beliefs and practices are affected by family and culture.
- The nurse needs to be willing to assess the concept of spirituality in patients and families and, based on this ongoing assessment, to integrate the spiritual beliefs of patients and families into care.

- The nurse must be willing to refer the patient or family to a spiritual expert (i.e., a minister, priest, rabbi, or imam).
- Community-based religious organizations can provide supportive care to families and patients, and nurses should be aware of these resources.

THEORETICAL LINKS

Puchalski collaborated with many interdisciplinary agencies to create the *Spiritual Care Implementation Model*. It is a relational model that illustrates the process of spiritual care, showing how interdisciplinary healthcare providers should work together to assess and address patients' spiritual needs. The model has two "submodels," one for inpatient settings and another for outpatient settings. The model is also known as the "generalist-specialist model of care." The "generalist" consists of healthcare members who have initial contact with patients and assess for the need of a spiritual care referral. Board-certified chaplains are the "specialist," who would complete a comprehensive spiritual assessment if spiritual distress is noted.[3]

Another theory that closely aligns with spirituality is Atchley's continuity theory of the spiritual self.[13] According to this theory, there is recognition that individuals develop preferences as part of their personalities and that these influence their spiritual self as they grow and age. The continuity theory of the spiritual self is based on the assumption that spirituality sensitizes and guides individuals through a variety of human experiences throughout life. Several key constructs include (1) deep inner silence, (2) insight, (3) compassion, (4) connection with the ground of being, (5) transcendence of the personal self, (6) wonder, and (7) transformation. Furthermore, the continuity theory of the spiritual self proposes a significant role for spiritual beliefs and practices in coping with problems later in life, particularly the experiences of illness, death, and dying. This closely illustrates the notion that spirituality is a lifelong journey.[13]

CONTEXT TO NURSING AND HEALTH CARE

Many healthcare providers recognize assessment and the meeting of spiritual needs as forms of caring. The quality of health care is enhanced by integrating spirituality into patient care. Holistic nursing care focuses on the whole person and addresses all human needs.[4] Spiritual beliefs often contribute to powerful healing and give a sense of peace and positively impacts patients' quality of life, improves health promotion behaviors, and increases activities related to disease prevention.[9]

Professional Mandates to Provide Spiritual Care

The Joint Commission mandates that healthcare facilities provide spiritual care to every patient.[14] As a profession, nursing prides itself on being holistic in its approach to patient care. Nurses tout their ability to conduct thorough assessments of patients' needs, plan nursing interventions to meet all the patients' needs, and provide the necessary care that patients require.

However, nurses shy away from providing spiritual care. The neglect of spirituality is a serious deficit in nursing.[1,3] The American Nurses Association (ANA) Code of Ethics includes a statement regarding nursing's responsibility to address spiritual concerns.[15] In *Nursing Intervention Classification*,[16] two standard nursing interventions are identified that directly relate to spiritual care: Spiritual Support (No. 540) and Spiritual Growth Facilitation (No. 5426). Also, in the *Nursing Outcome Classification*,[17] two spiritual outcomes are identified: Spiritual Health and Personal Health Status. Additionally, the North American Nursing Diagnosis Association International (NANDA-I) includes three specific spiritual nursing diagnoses: "Spiritual Distress," "Risk for Spiritual Distress," and "Readiness for Enhanced Spiritual Well-Being."[18]

The strong emphasis on spirituality within numerous major nursing documents—including statements on ethics, standards for nursing diagnosis, and spiritual intervention classifications—makes it clear that assessing for spiritual needs and addressing spiritual issues is not just an optional duty for nurses but rather a mandate.[9]

Assessment of Spirituality

Providing spiritual care starts with an assessment of a patient's spirituality. The very act of engaging in a conversation about spirituality conveys to the patient and family that nurses are willing to discuss spiritual/religious beliefs and issues. This initial spiritual conversation may very well lead to other opportunities to talk about the impact of spiritual beliefs on the patient's current health issues, such as how the patient will cope, what impact the health crisis will have on the patient's sense of purpose and meaning in life, what adaptations or changes need to be made to accommodate the current health problem, and what difficult choices the patient and family may face. Every one of these issues is spiritual in nature. Nurses may not have the answers, nor is it necessary to have the answers to spiritual issues. It is usually best to listen and encourage the patient and family to talk openly about these issues until they are able to arrive at their own conclusions.[2,19]

Conducting a spiritual assessment is a powerful way to open up the concept of spirituality with a patient and his or her family. Spiritual assessments should be done on every patient initially starting with general questions and following with more thorough questions if spiritual distress is detected.[4,12] The spiritual assessment is done with respect and compassion, ideally at the end of the initial patient assessment.[3–5] A number of spiritual assessment tools that are easy to use are available. The best-known spiritual assessment tool, developed by Puchalski and Romer, uses the acronym FICA for **F**aith and belief, **I**mportance and influence, **C**ommunity, and **A**ddress in care.[20] The questions to ask for each of the four parts of the FICA spiritual assessment tool are presented in Box 5.2.

Nursing Interventions for Spiritual Care

Spiritual care often involves recognizing and honoring the religious beliefs and practices of those in our care. However, spiritual care often does not involve religion. Spiritual care interventions include keeping vigil with a family as a loved one struggles to recover, crying with a family member when their loved one dies, or supporting a newly diagnosed chronically ill patient, redefining the patient's value and life's meaning. Such care can be provided by giving a gentle back rub, speaking soothing words, or reading a prayer or special religious text. Spiritual care cannot be boxed in and narrowly defined. Spiritual care is not limited to those who believe a certain way or who define the transcendent according to a specific doctrine. Spiritual care should be provided to everyone. People may express their spirituality in unique ways, but everyone has a spiritual nature that can be touched through respect, kindness, and compassion. The provision of spiritual care can be viewed through three distinct approaches that include *communication*, *action*, and *presence*.[19]

BOX 5.2   FICA Spiritual History Tool

- **F**aith and belief: "Do you consider yourself spiritual or religious?" or "Is spirituality something important to you" or "Do you have spiritual beliefs that help you cope with stress/difficult times?" (Contextualize to reason for visit if it is not the routine history.) If the patient responds "No," the health care provider might ask, "What gives your life meaning?" Sometimes patients respond with answers such as family, career, or nature. (The question of meaning should also be asked even if people answer yes to spirituality.)
- **I**mportance: What importance does your spirituality have in your life? Has your spirituality influenced how you take care of yourself, your health? Does your spirituality influence you in your healthcare decision making? (e.g., advance directives, treatment, etc.)
- **C**ommunity: Are you part of a spiritual community? Communities such as churches, temples, and mosques, or a group of like-minded friends, family, or yoga, can serve as strong support systems for some patients. Can explore further: "Is this of support to you and how? Is there a group of people you really love or who are important to you?"
- **A**ddress in care: "How would you like me, your healthcare provider, to address these issues in your healthcare?" (With the newer models including diagnosis of spiritual distress, A also refers to the "Assessment and Plan" of patient spiritual distress or issues within a treatment or care plan.)

© C. Puchalski, 1996.
From Puchalski, C., & Romer, A. L. (2000). Taking a spiritual history allows clinicians to understand patients more fully. *Journal of palliative medicine*, 3(1), 129–137.

Communication

Excellent communication involves hearing not just the words being spoken but also understanding nonverbal gestures. The ability to listen is both an art and a learned skill. It requires that the nurse completely attend to the patient with open ears, eyes, and mind. Listening is an active process that requires the nurse's full attention. Nurses must attend to both the auditory and visual stimuli that they receive from the patient, and they must analyze these messages to ascertain the patient's intent. Several barriers may interfere with the nurses' ability to listen actively. Nurses must develop sensitivity to their own internal barriers to active listening as well as to demonstrate great sensitivity to the patient's belief system.

Frequently patients hint at their real concerns and reveal them openly only when nurses consider meanings beyond their words, assess patients' feelings, and inquire about the deeper meaning behind their communications. Likewise, people often do not reveal their most intimate personal thoughts and feelings in a direct manner but rather cloak them and use obscure language. This masking of what represents the true self is a protective measure—arising from the fear that the listener may react in a hurtful way. Thus, rather than exposing their vulnerabilities and accepting the possibility of being hurt, patients may hide what they really feel and allude to their distress only in a roundabout way. This places a burden on the nurse to pick up on and pursue subtle clues that the patient or family member may give.

Several barriers may underlie the nurse's inability to be totally present and communicate effectively with the patient. First, the nurse may be distracted by other things and may not pay attention to the patient. Second, the nurse may miss the meaning of the patient's message because of failure to clarify the meaning of a word, phrase, or facial expression. Third, the nurse may interject personal feelings and reactions into the patient's situation rather than allowing the patient to explore and discuss his or her own feelings and reactions. This last barrier arises when the nurse is busy formulating a response while the patient is still talking. In this instance, the nurse is thinking and cannot hear the patient's message.[19]

Action

The second spiritual intervention, that of taking action, is the implementation of spiritual care. Some spiritual interventions including the following:

- Giving verbal support and encouragement of spiritual beliefs
- Making a referral to a chaplain or pastoral care board-certified professional
- Using religious literature that is meaningful to the patient and the patient's family
- Using prayer with the patient's or family's consent

Underlying these actions, the nurse conveys a powerful message of care, compassion, love, and concern.[2,9,11,19]

Presence

Probably the most important approach to meet patients' spiritual needs is *presence*—the ability to touch another person both physically and spiritually. Presence requires more than just showing up when someone is sick or standing by the bedside, although these actions are important. To fully demonstrate presence, the nurse must be an active listener who can demonstrate empathy, humility, vulnerability, and commitment.

A nurse demonstrates presence through the personal relationship that develops with the patient and the patient's family. This relationship allows the nurse and patient to mutually experience the uniqueness of the other. It is in this relationship that the nurse is able to learn about the patient's spiritual and/or religious needs, wants, hurts, joys, and ambitions. It is through this relationship that the nurse communicates personal spiritual strength and the willingness to care, listen, and be available to the patient. The presence of the nurse touches the patient's distressed spirit, just as a cool hand might soothe a fevered brow.[9,19]

Why Some Nurses Neglect Spiritual Care

Although spirituality should be integrated into the care of all patients, this is, unfortunately, not always the case. There are a number of explanations for the lack of response to spiritual needs. First, the nurse may fail to recognize spiritual needs of the patient and/or family. If a spiritual assessment is not made, the potential to miss a need may occur. There are also times when the nurse recognizes spiritual needs but feels inadequate to meet them. This may be linked to a lack of education, causing poor understanding and absence of needed skills, or low confidence to effectively implement appropriate spiritual care interventions.[3–5] An insufficient focus on spirituality in nursing education may result in nurses feeling inadequate and poorly prepared in this area. Furthermore, some nurses believe that they must be personally "religious" to address and meet the spiritual needs of patients. Another common reason nurses fail to incorporate spirituality into nursing care relates to personal discomfort experienced by the nurse in discussing such a personal and abstract area that does not have concrete answers.[11] Furthermore, religion is sometimes thought of as a private matter and some nurses may be uncomfortable discussing spiritual issues with patients. Many nurses are also uncomfortable or in conflict with their own spirituality.[4]

All of these reasons lead nurses to either avoid spiritual care or, if they recognize a spiritual need, they immediately make a referral to the hospital chaplain. Making a referral to the hospital chaplain and/or a representative from the patient's faith tradition (such as a priest, minister, rabbi, or an imam) is a better response than ignoring the patient's spiritual needs. However, such a response means that the nurse has missed an opportunity to be present to the patient and/or family during the time a spiritual need is expressed.[11] Often, when patients express a spiritual need, it warrants a response from the nurse–even if the response is just to listen and encourage the patient to elaborate on their spiritual concerns. Having a chance to speak about spiritual issues to a willing listener may be all the patient needs. Nurses should be ready to provide support and offer individualized spiritual care when needed.[2,11,19]

INTERRELATED CONCEPTS

Several concepts in this book are closely interrelated with the concept of spirituality and have been mentioned previously. One could make the case that spirituality is interrelated with all concepts presented in this book. Although this may be the case, it is useful to examine those concepts that have the closest links to better understand this concept (Fig. 5.2). One of the closest interrelated concepts is **Culture**. Culture refers to a pattern of shared attitudes, beliefs, and values. Spirituality

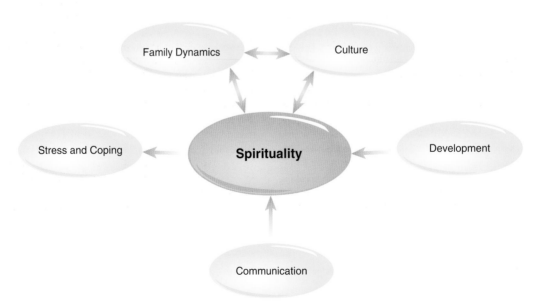

FIGURE 5.2 Spirituality and Interrelated Concepts.

is deeply embedded in an individual's personal belief system and is strongly influenced by the context of that individual's culture. Likewise, spirituality, in itself, can influence culture. When large numbers of individuals share specific spiritual beliefs and/or practices, this can be identified as a religious group with cultural norms. Therefore Fig. 5.2 shows the relationship between spirituality and culture as a bidirectional arrow. Family Dynamics are also closely aligned with spirituality. A person's belief system is strongly influenced within the family unit from early in life. Specific religious practices within a family shape one's view of religion, which closely links with an individual's spirituality. It is also possible that disagreements or changes in one's spiritual beliefs, if different from those held by family members, can lead to changes in relationships. Therefore Fig. 5.2 shows the relationship between spirituality and family dynamics as a bidirectional arrow. A bidirectional arrow is also shown between family dynamics and culture to show that these concepts form a concept cluster. The concept of Development is interrelated because an individual's spirituality is, in part, dependent on his or her developmental stage. Spirituality changes over the course of life, partly based on life experiences and emotional maturity. Spirituality grows as a person ages. Many older adults have strong spiritual beliefs. Another concept linked to spirituality is Stress and Coping. An effective coping strategy for many individuals includes drawing on religion and faith; for this reason the arrow points from Spirituality to Stress and Coping. Finally, the concept of Communication closely aligns with spirituality. Communication is one of the three distinct approaches used to provide spiritual care interventions, as previously discussed. The nurse must be able and willing to actively listen to the patient and notice nonverbal cues as a foundation for understanding the patient's needs, beliefs, and values.[9,19]

CLINICAL EXEMPLARS

There are many exemplars of the concept of Spirituality in the context of health care. It is not expected that nurses will develop expertise in each exemplar. However, nurses should be willing to assess each patient's needs and to confidently and competently discuss and support the patient's spiritual preferences. Common exemplars are presented in Box 5.3.

Featured Exemplars
Faith
Faith, as defined by Dyess, refers to an "evolving pattern of believing, that grounds and guides authentic living and gives meaning in the present moment of inter-relating."[21, p.2728] The term *faith* can refer to a specific religious tradition or belief in something that cannot be touched or seen. Members of an organized religious tradition speak about beliefs and traditions they not only hold dear but also believe are historically trustworthy even though they cannot touch, see, reproduce, or feel the experience. In the context of health care, faith represents a measure of confidence that a force is at work that will lead to a positive outcome (i.e., "God will help me recover"). Faith may also be expressed by patients as confidence in the skill and knowledge of their physicians and nurses.

Hope
Hope refers to beliefs, wishes, and actions taken in situations of uncertainty. Hope is linked to faith and tends to have an emphasis on the

---

BOX 5.3 EXEMPLARS OF SPIRITUALTY

- Faith
- Hope
- Prayer
- Sacraments
- Mindfulness
- Compassion
- Meditation
- Dietary traditions
- Ceremonies
- Rituals
- Grief work
- Religious articles (e.g., candles, oils, rosaries)
- Religious texts (e.g., the Bible, Torah, Qur'an)
- Practice of organized religion:
  - Christian-based faiths
  - Judaism
  - Islam
  - Buddhism
  - Hinduism

ACCESS EXEMPLAR LINKS IN YOUR GIDDENS EBOOK

---

fear of the unknown and of the unseen. For instance, patients may hope for relief from pain even in the face of relentless pain. Nurses must foster hope. When hope for a cure is not possible, nurses can direct patients to reconfigure what they are hopeful about.[9]

Prayer
Prayer is conversation with a higher power, however that higher power is conceived. The conversation may take many forms. Sometimes prayer is asking for something, such as healing for self or others or removal of pain. Prayer can also serve as to give thanks or a way of being in the presence of the transcendent.[9,19]

Sacraments
The term *sacrament* is derived from the Latin *sacramentum,* which means "a sign of the sacred." Sacraments, recognized by Christian faiths, represent special occasions for experiencing God's saving presence. There are variations in the number and meaning of sacraments. For example, the Catholic Church recognizes seven sacraments (Baptism, Holy Communion, Reconciliation, Confirmation, Marriage, Holy Orders, and Anointing of the Sick), whereas most Protestant denominations recognize two sacraments (Baptism and Holy Communion). In the healthcare setting, patients may request Holy Communion or Reconciliation. Baptism may be requested for an infant in an emergency situation.[9]

Mindfulness
Mind, body, and spirit are all interwoven. Mindfulness training helps to strengthen the connection of a person's mind, body, and spirit. Mindfulness helps to reduce anxiety and decrease pain. Other mind-body interventions include relaxation, guided imagery, and music therapy.[9]

CASE STUDY

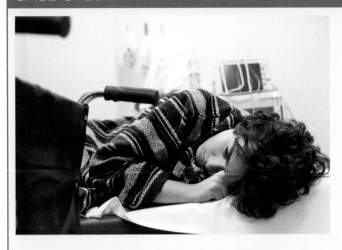

Case Presentation

Robert Klein, a 16-year-old with bilateral amputations below the knee as a result of traumatic injury, was assigned to Mrs. Carlton, a registered nurse on a rehabilitation unit. Mrs. Carlton, who has two teenage sons, found it very difficult to work with Robert. When she was in his room, she felt tearful and was unable to carry on a conversation with him; she also experienced difficulty engaging him in rehabilitation for fear of causing him pain. Her thoughts were on how awful this must be for Robert and what it would be like if this happened to one of her sons. Mrs. Carlton was sympathetic to Robert, but she was ineffective because her close identification with his feelings interfered with her ability to focus on his needs.

One morning, Mrs. Carlton walked into Robert's room and found him crying. Her first response was to leave the room as she thought, "I can't handle this today." But she was able to stop herself, and she went over to Robert and touched his shoulder. He continued to sob and said, "What am I going to do? I wish I were dead. My whole life is sports. I would have qualified for an athletic scholarship if this hadn't happened. I feel like my life is over."

Mrs. Carlton recognized the feelings of despair that Robert was expressing and said to him, "It seems to you like your life is over. You are feeling that this is such an unfair thing to have happened to you. I agree with you, it is, but let's talk about it." Mrs. Carlton responded to Robert in an empathetic manner. She communicated to him that she was present for him, that she understood his feelings, and that she would be with him if he wanted to talk about his situation at greater length. Mrs. Carlton's response did not change Robert's present or his future—her understanding did not change the reality that Robert had experienced bilateral below-the-knee amputations. However, her commitment to be present to Robert, her ability to listen attentively to what he had to say, her encouragement, and her ability to put into words the deep spiritual issue he was facing helped him to open up and draw upon his inner spiritual strength.[19]

Case Analysis Questions

1. What is the first intervention the nurse should include in the nursing plan of care to adequately meet Robert's spiritual needs?
2. Identify three assessment findings of spiritual distress.
3. What are three spiritual care nursing interventions?

From Juanmonino/iStock/Thinkstock.

 ACCESS EXEMPLAR LINKS IN YOUR GIDDENS EBOOK

REFERENCES

1. Stoll, R. (1979). Guidelines for spiritual assessment. *The American Journal of Nursing, 79*(9), 1574–1577.
2. Carson, V. B. (1989). *Spiritual dimensions of nursing practice.* Philadelphia: Saunders.
3. Drury, C., & Hunter, J. (2016). The hole in holistic patient care. *Open Journal of Nursing, 6*(9), 776–792.
4. Puchalski, C. M. (2013). Integrating spirituality into patient care: An essential element of person-centered care. *Polskie Archiwum Medycyny Wewnetrznej, 123*(9), 491–496.
5. Reinert, K. G., & Koenig, H. G. (2013). Re-examining definitions of spirituality in nursing research. *Journal of Advanced Nursing, 69*(12), 2622–2634.
6. O'Brien, M. E. (1982). The need for spiritual integrity. In H. Yura & M. B. Walsh (Eds.), *Human needs and the nursing process.* East Norwalk, CT: Appleton & Lange.
7. Stoll, R. (1989). The essence of spirituality. In V. B. Carson (Ed.), *Spiritual dimensions of nursing practice.* Philadelphia: Saunders.
8. Puchalski, C., Vitillo, R., Hull, S., & Reller, N. (2014). Improving the spiritual dimension of whole person care: Reaching national and international consensus. *Journal of Palliative Medicine, 17*(6), 642–656.
9. Potter, P. A. (2017). Spiritual health. In P. Potter, A. Perry, P. A. Stockert, & A. M. Hall (Eds.), *Fundamentals of Nursing* (9th ed., pp. 773–779). St. Louis: Elsevier.
10. Boswell, G. E., & Boswell-Ford, K. C. (2010). Testing a SEM model of two religious concepts and experiential spirituality. *Journal of Religion and Health, 49*(2), 200–211.
11. Koenig, H. (2013). Why include spirituality? In *Spirituality in patient care: Why, how, when and what* (3rd ed., pp. 6–7). West Conshohocken, PA: Templeton Press.
12. Georgesen, J., & Dungan, J. (1996). Managing spiritual distress in patients with advanced cancer pain. *Cancer Nursing, 19*(5), 376–383.
13. Atchley, R. (2009). *Spirituality and aging.* Baltimore, MD: Johns Hopkins University Press.
14. The Joint Commission (TJC). (2015). *Standards FAQ details.* Retrieved from https://www.jointcommission.org/standards_information/jcfaqdetails.aspx?StandardsFaqId=1492&ProgramId=46.
15. American Nurses Association. (2015). *Code of ethics for nurses with interpretive statements.* Silver Spring, MD: Nursebooks.org.
16. Bulechek, G., Butcher, H., Dochterman, J., & Wagner, C. (Eds.). (2013). *Nursing interventions classification (NIC)* (6th ed.). St Louis: Elsevier.
17. Moorhead, S., Johnson, M., Maas, M., & Swanson, E. (Eds.). (2013). *Nursing outcomes classification (NOC)* (5th ed.). St Louis: Elsevier.
18. NANDA International. (2017). *Nursing diagnoses: Definitions and classifications 2018–2020* (11th ed.). Des Moines, IA: Wiley–Blackwell.
19. Carson, V. B., & Koenig, H. (Eds.). (2008). *Spiritual dimensions of nursing practice* (rev ed.). West Conshohocken, PA: Templeton Press.
20. Puchalski, C., & Romer, A. L. (2000). Taking a spiritual history allows clinicians to understand patients more fully. *Journal of Palliative Medicine, 3*(1), 129–137.
21. Dyess, S. M. (2011). Faith: A concept analysis. *Journal of Advanced Nursing, 67*(12), 2723–2731.

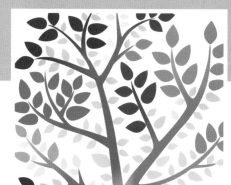

Adherence

Janice Bissonnette

As a healthcare recipient concept representing patient preferences, the term *adherence* has numerous definitions across health care, which has led to contradictory meanings.[1–9] In nursing, the concept of adherence is closely associated with patient-centered care and the nursing expertise required to support a patient's long-term adherence to treatment.[8,9] Nursing plays a major role in supporting patients' acceptance and adjustment to the impact of illness on their lives. Adherence from a patient-centered approach supports the goal of nursing by advocating for what is best in the context of each patient's life. This concept presentation serves as a preliminary step to broadening nurses' appreciation for the complexity of adherence as a patient behavior and represents an integration of what we know about adherence.

DEFINITION

The North American Nursing Diagnosis Association International (NANDA-I) defines "adherence behavior" as a "self-initiated action taken to promote wellness, recovery, and rehabilitation."[10, p.458] Haynes et al. defined adherence as the extent to which patients follow the instructions they are given for prescribed treatments.[11] Christensen offered an alternative definition in keeping with a less paternalistic approach.[12] Adherence in this setting is patient-focused and is the extent to which a person's actions or behaviors coincide with advice or instruction from a healthcare provider intended to prevent, monitor, or ameliorate a disorder.

Cohen, in a concept analysis of adherence related to the nursing practice of patients with cardiovascular disease (CVD), defined adherence as "persistence in the practice and maintenance of desired health behaviors and is the result of active participation and agreement."[13, p.27] Adherence is also associated with terms such as *compliance, concordance, obedience, observance, conformity, acceptance, cooperation, mutuality, persistence,* and *therapeutic alliance.*[14–16]

Before the late 1990s, *compliance* was the more commonly used term to describe a patient's behavior related to following a recommended treatment.[17] The definition of *compliance behavior* as an outcome for nursing diagnostic categories is distinctly different from that for *adherence behavior*. In this context, compliance behavior is "the action taken on the basis of professional advice to promote wellness, recovery, and rehabilitation."[10, p.458] The term *compliance* was the primary descriptor for a patient's obedience to prescribed treatments.[17] Variation and debate exists on how to define *adherence*; how it differs from *compliance* or *concordance*; and how the behavior of adherence relates to patients, healthcare professionals, and system factors.[2,6,7,17–20] The historical transition and change in terminology from *compliance* to *adherence* and *concordance* requires standardization of the taxonomy for *adherence* as a concept for nursing practice.[7,8,21–23] In nursing practice, it is important to determine whether adherence, as a profile of the patient's behavior, is an effective way of characterizing the behavior that individuals demonstrate in response to an agreed upon and informed treatment decision.

SCOPE

The scope of adherence essentially ranges from a total lack of adherence to complete adherence (Fig. 6.1). The degree of adherence within this range includes the patient's intentional or rational decision to stop the medication or change the dose or frequency of the medication.[24] Also included in this range is the patient's unintentional change in medication-taking behavior, which represents a nonpurposeful overlooking of taking the medication.[23,25]

The same applies for health-promotion activities—for example, reducing the amount of recommended exercise, increasing the amount of recommended salt in the diet on weekends, or not attending physicians' appointments. Despite the potential for any degree of nonadherence to influence a patient's disease control or health, it is unclear where, within this range, patients become most at risk for negative outcomes.[21]

The primary situation preceding the evaluation of a patient's adherence behavior is the recommendation or prescription of a treatment by a healthcare professional. Often, the focus is on the patient's adherence to long-term medications or treatments and health-promotion activities in the face of chronic disease.[20] The theme underlying the patient's total or positive adherent behavior suggests that the patient views or believes the professional to be a trusted and knowledgeable source concerning recommended treatment for the disease or health state in question. The action or behavior of adherence assumes some degree of willingness and motivation on the part of the patient to accept all or part of the prescription or recommendation. What is not clear with the behavior of adherence is the degree to which the patient agreed with or was involved in the prescription or recommendation.

Within health care, the consequences of nonadherence fall into three areas: patient-related, health professional–related, and healthcare system–related.[23] Patient-related consequences include increased mortality and morbidity, conflict, attributional uncertainty, embarrassment, and changes in quality of life.[21] Health professional–related consequences include ambivalence, misinterpretation, avoidance, decisional conflict, and lack of empathy.[25–28] Healthcare system–related consequences include increased

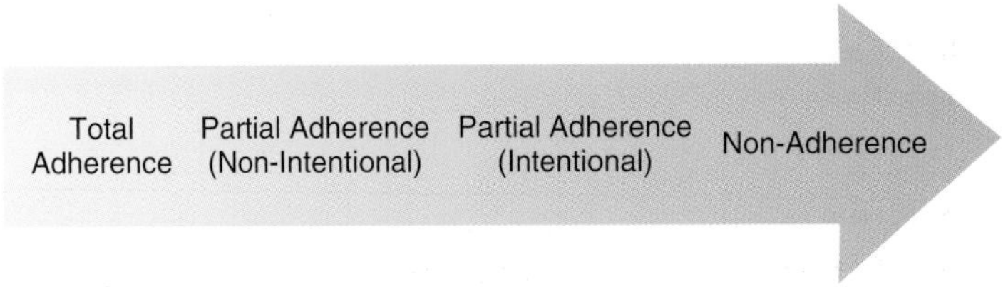

FIGURE 6.1 Scope of Adherence.

BOX 6.1   Attributes of Adherence

- Decisional conflict
- Predictability
- Personal experience
- Power conflict
- Agreement
- Alignment

Data from Christensen, A. J. (2004). *Patient adherence to medical treatment regimens: Bridging the gap between behavioral science and biomedicine.* New Haven, CT: Yale University Press.

costs for and healthcare services.[26,27] Nurses are present in the majority of healthcare settings in which patients receive treatment recommendations. This provides an opportunity to assess motivation and integrate and reinforce treatment adherence strategies with patients.

ATTRIBUTES AND CRITERIA

The attributes of a concept support the identification of situations or behaviors that are best characterized by using the concept of *interest*. A cluster of attributes comprise the real-life definition of a concept as opposed to the dictionary definition.[29] Attributes most commonly associated with adherence include decisional conflict, a patient's personal experience, and agreement (Box 6.1).

In the context of related nursing diagnoses, adherence behavior is the anticipated outcome. For the diagnosis of *Health-Seeking Behaviors*, defined as "the state in which an individual in stable health is actively seeking ways to alter personal health habits, and/or the environment in order to move toward a higher level of health,"[10, p.162] adherence behavior is the outcome. The nursing diagnosis of *Individual Management of Therapeutic Regimen, Effective* is defined as "a pattern of regulating and integrating into daily living a program for treatment of illness and its sequelae that are satisfactory for meeting specific health goals;"[10, p.179] adherence behavior is again considered the expected outcome.

A variable that has significant influence on adherence is motivation. Treatment adherence may not be optimal if an individual is not motivated to do so.[30] Moreover, the degree or source of motivation may influence the extent of adherence. One of the oldest definitions of motivation stems from the psychological use of the term in 1904, which suggests that the term represents an inner or social stimulus for action.[31] Motivation, as with adherence, also runs along a continuum, which varies not only in how much motivation one has but also in the type of motivation. Two major types of motivation are based on the goals that inspire people to act. *Intrinsic motivation* refers to "doing something because it is inherently interesting or enjoyable," and extrinsic motivation refers to "doing something because it leads to a separable outcome."[32, p.55] In an attempt to engage the patient's intrinsic motivation, a patient-centered approach using motivational interviewing (MI) strategies shows some promising results. MI recognizes that patients present at varying stages of motivation and readiness for change. The nurse practicing MI approaches would work collaboratively with patients to prompt conversations about their reasons for change, barriers to change (adherence), and goal setting. A recent systematic review evaluating MI techniques for adolescents and young adults with chronic illness showed improved adherence and symptom reduction in 11 out of the 12 studies included in the review.[33]

THEORETICAL LINKS

Social psychologists have developed many behavioral approaches to guide the assessment of a patient's medication-taking behavior and the overall enhancement of adherence behavior. The social cognition models are the most common theories supporting behavior change associated with adherence or nonadherence.[12,33–35] Common psychological theories include the theory of planned behavior (TPB), the health belief model (HBM), and the self-regulation and self-determination models.[34,35] The primary outcome in each of these models is a specific health behavior based on a deliberate process of decision making. Preexisting intentions, beliefs, motivations, or a patient's degree of confidence in his or her success influences the patient's decision-making process. Interestingly, a recent systematic review suggested that providing feedback guided by measures of adherence significantly improved adherence to treatment in 16 of the 24 studies.[35]

Theory of Planned Behavior

The TPB proposes a model showing how human action is guided.[34] It predicts the occurrence of a specific behavior if that behavior is intentional. As depicted in Fig. 6.2, the model integrates the variables of attitude (e.g., behavioral beliefs), subjective norms (e.g., normative beliefs and motivation), and perceived behavioral control (e.g., confidence and influence on control beliefs), which predict the intention to perform the behavior. In this model, intentions and motivation precede the actual behavior.

The key assumptions of TPB relate to the prediction of whether a person *intends* to do something. The predicators are the patient's attitude or motivation (i.e., if the patient agrees with completing a treatment), the subjective norm (i.e., the amount of social pressure the patient feels to proceed with a treatment), and the perceived behavioral control (i.e., the level of control the patient feels he or she has over the treatment or choice of treatment). By influencing or enhancing these three "predictors," nurses can increase the chance that the individual will intend to proceed with a recommended or prescribed treatment and then actually do it.[34]

For example, a patient presents to a nurse clinician in a diabetes clinic with elevated fasting glucose and hemoglobin A_{1c} (HbA_{1c}) measurements. Will the patient tell the nurse that the elevated measurements are attributable to the fact that he has not been taking his insulin regularly or following his diet? The answer to this question depends on whether the patient *intends* and is motivated to do so. In other words, it is not an automatic, habitual, or thoughtless action. The intention, in turn, depends on the following considerations:

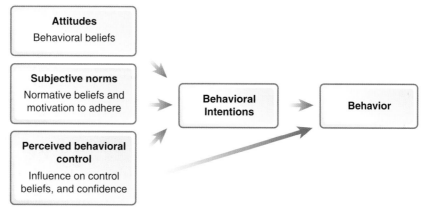

FIGURE 6.2 The Theory of Planned Behavior.

- Whether the patient has a positive or negative *attitude* about revealing his nonadherent behavior.
- To what extent the patient perceives that he experiences social pressure to adhere to healthy lifestyle practices for control of his diabetes and associated health risks, including whether the patient believes the following:
  - The nurse wants to know how he manages his diabetes.
  - Family/friends/significant others would approve of him telling the nurse (normative beliefs).
  - These people's opinions are important to the patient.
  - Whether the patient finds it difficult to discuss his diabetes self-management and adherence with the nurse, resulting in an appropriate treatment plan.

The final behavior is predicted by the degree to which each of the previously mentioned components influences the patient's intention to act.

The Health Belief Model

The HBM first conceptualized beliefs as predictors of preventive health behavior to help explain the lack of initiation of these behaviors by some individuals.[35] The theory hypothesizes that people are more likely to initiate a health-related behavior to the extent that they (1) perceive they could become ill or be susceptible to the problem (e.g., perceived susceptibility), (2) believe that the illness has serious outcomes or will disrupt their daily functioning (e.g., perceived severity), (3) believe that the required recommendation will be effective in reducing symptoms (e.g., perceived benefits), and (4) believe that there are few barriers to initiating the recommendation (e.g., perceived barriers).[36]

For example, using the same scenario previously described, a patient presents to a nurse clinician with elevated fasting glucose and HbA_{1c} measurements. Will the patient tell the nurse the elevation is because he has not been taking his insulin regularly or following his diet? The answer to this question depends on the patient's perceptions of susceptibility, risk, benefits, and barriers. Engaging in a conversation about insulin adherence, in turn, depends on the following factors:
- Whether the patient perceives his diabetes to be severe and his perceptions of susceptibility to the health risks associated with diabetes
- The extent to which the patient perceives that insulin therapy and diet control are beneficial in the control of his diabetes and the reduction of risk factors
- Whether the patient perceives that barriers exist with the use of insulin therapy and diet control

The extent or degree of these perceptions will influence the patient's motivation, engagement, and persistence in the behavior—in this case, whether the patient participates in a conversation about his insulin-taking behavior. The addition of MI strategies in this context may guide the patient to make changes in the interest of his health by eliciting his motivation for change.

CONTEXT TO NURSING AND HEALTH CARE

Dimensions of Adherence

Interactions between patient variables and healthcare provider systems can influence the degree to which a patient follows a prescribed regimen. Some suggest that patients are more likely to adhere when the treatment recommended fits with their expectations.[12] Adherence as a behavior is currently thought to be composed of distinct elements representing adherence to medication, management of adherence, and adherence-related science.[30] Adherence represents three dimensions of thought and attitudes regarding patient behavior associated with recommended treatment and therapies: compliance, persistence, and concordance (Fig. 6.3).

Compliance

Compliance or "obedience" with a prescribed treatment promotes an undertone of blame toward the patient when the patient's behavior does not meet health professionals' expectations.[2] The definition of medication compliance developed by the International Society for Pharmacoeconomics and Outcomes Research group is "the extent to which a patient acts in accordance with the prescribed interval and dose of a dosing regimen."[36, p.46] In this context, compliance is the *behavior of conforming* to treatment for a recommended length of time. The World Health Organization (WHO) attempted to change this by introducing adherence as an alternative to the more paternalistic concept of compliance.[20] Adherence suggests the patient's agreement to prescribed recommendations rather than passive cooperation in obedience to them.[20] Some authors describe the main function of such terms as *compliance* and *adherence* as ideological in that these terms serve as a framework from which healthcare professionals convey their ideas concerning how patients should behave.[37]

Persistence

Another dimension of adherence behavior associated with healthcare therapies is persistence. Persistence appears primarily within the context of chronic disease management therapies.[38] In contrast to compliance, medication persistence is the time from initiation to discontinuation

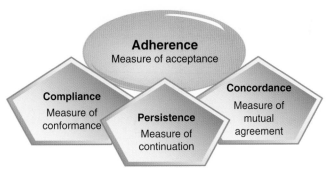

FIGURE 6.3 Dimensions of Adherence.

of a recommended or prescribed treatment and is a *measure of continuation*.[38] In nursing practice, the patient's degree of persistence is of most value when his or her adherence behavior is being assessed. Confirming how often a patient renews or refills his or her prescriptions is a measure of the patient's persistence with continuation of the treatment.

Concordance

Concordance is the most recent term added in an attempt to more accurately reflect the behavior of adherence and suggests that patients and healthcare professionals come to a *mutual agreement* on regimen through a process of negotiation and shared decision making.[18,39] The behavior of concordance reflects the development of an alliance with patients based on realistic expectations.[39]

Interdisciplinary Lens of Adherence

In moving beyond the ideologic and semantic debate, the practical reality of not following a recommended course of treatment, particularly in chronic illness, remains a major cause of poor health outcomes and increased healthcare costs.[35,36] In 2003, the WHO launched a global initiative to improve worldwide rates of adherence to therapies commonly used in treating chronic conditions. Adherence rates with prescribed regimens in chronic illness average 50%, ranging from 0% to 100% depending on the method of measurement.[20]

Adherence is a dynamic concept, influenced in part by the social context of its use. The social or disciplinary context for the purpose of this section is nursing practice, with identification of interrelations between and with other health disciplines. Similar inductive approaches have been applied by nurse researchers for the analysis of such concepts as chronic pain, symptom clusters, conflict in nursing work environments, and adaptive systems.[40] An understanding of the perspectives and uses of adherence within each discipline is fundamental to the clarification of the concept and for the identification of contextual variations.[41,42] The following sections present the major characteristics of adherence emerging from the disciplines of nursing, mental health, general medicine, and pharmacy.

Nursing

In 1973, NANDA accepted noncompliance as a nursing diagnosis. The new diagnostic category reflected little recognition of the impact on nursing practice but resulted more in response to the medically based literature.[41] Kim suggested that the diagnostic taxonomies for nursing appeared to unify communication and documentation between nurses but did not add to the development of nursing science because of the lack of association with an explanatory framework.[40] From 1973 to the present, members of NANDA-I, supported by additional nursing authors, pursued the removal of noncompliance from this diagnostic nomenclature because the term emphasized a paternalistic obligation to follow orders.[41] Interestingly, as discussed previously, the nursing

diagnosis of noncompliance remains in use, with adherence behavior as the expected outcome.

Mental Health

Adherence to therapies is a key component of care in mental health settings.[43] Estimates of medication nonadherence for patients with mental disease are 24% to 90%.[43] One in four patients experiencing psychosis demonstrates nonadherence.[44] Adherence and compliance continue to be described as interchangeable concepts in the mental health literature. An important theme identified from the mental health literature was the association between the patient's nonadherence and his or her feelings of embarrassment when questioned about the nonadherence.[44] Hui et al. reported an underrecognition by mental health clinicians of both the patient's nonadherent behavior and his or her associated feelings of embarrassment.[27] Nonadherence became a symptom of mental illness as opposed to a distinct entity. In more recent publications, various psychosocial interventions have been presented and studied. The key elements of these interventions include psychoeducational strategies, cognitive-behavioral therapy, and MI. Results are promising, and the authors suggest that adherence interventions with an intensive approach and a combination of strategies show results that are more favorable.[42,45]

Medicine

In the general medicine literature, the terms *adherence* and *compliance* are synonymous. Adherence is most frequently associated with efforts to develop a statistically based measurement to predict the presence or risk of adherence and correlation to a health outcome or disease-specific outcomes.[11,12] The chronic disease states most commonly studied for nonadherence rates include asthma, diabetes, HIV/AIDS, transplantation, CVD, hypertension, epilepsy, and cancer.[5,6,13,14,26] Research within these disease states attempts to provide answers to the questions of how to predict, measure, intervene, and treat patients with nonadherent behavior.[11]

Pharmacy

The pharmacy literature mirrors the general medicine literature in nonadherence. Pharmacology research focuses on the development of measurement tools for nonadherence with reference to pharmacist-led interventions to improve patient adherence as a means of achieving therapeutic goals.[19] Some authors describe the general intent of using the term *adherence* to reflect a more active, voluntary, and collaborative relationship between the patient and the healthcare provider but continue to use *compliance* and *adherence* interchangeably.[39]

Power Structure in Health Care

The historical and present-day use of the terms *compliance*, *adherence*, and *concordance* continues to reflect the power structure within the social system of health care. In its ongoing attempt to develop and maintain a power hold, nursing has confronted this power structure without having a clear understanding of its impact on nursing practice. Very few researchers to date have explored the healthcare professional's perceptions and understanding of adherence.

If asked, patients would not label themselves as nonadherent, noncompliant, nonconcordant, or disobedient. When they are confronted with questions regarding nonadherent behavior, patients admit to feeling blamed and accused, stating that very few attempts were being made by nurses or physicians to understand the motivations or basis of decisions to be "nonadherent."[3,12] As with the notion of informed consent, if a patient understands the consequences of nonadherence, do we have the right to make a judgment regarding that individual's choice? After 40 years of studying compliance and adherence, with no clear

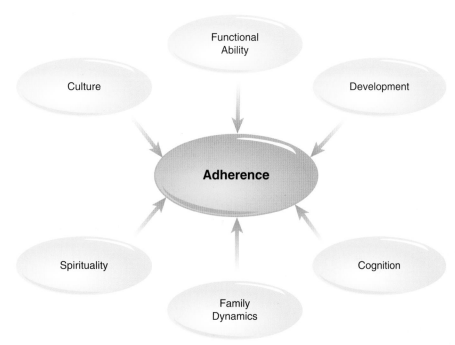

FIGURE 6.4 Adherence and Interrelated Concepts.

development of guidance on how best to intervene, perhaps now is the time to accept this as a phenomenon of human nature with no one solution or one particular investigational approach.

Research attempting to provide an objective measure of adherence reveals variability in identifying a gold standard measure as well as limited success in interventional efforts directed at improving adherence rates.[11,12] There remains an inconsistent definition of adherence as it relates to healthcare recommendations; this has led to the ongoing labeling of patients as nonadherent and unmotivated. Despite the possible replacement of *adherence* with the new language of *persistence* or *concordance*, Russell et al. noted that the understanding of what is best for patients' lives is seldom addressed in the literature.[8]

INTERRELATED CONCEPTS

Several concepts featured in this textbook influence the degree of adherence; those with greatest influence are presented in Fig. 6.4. Understanding how each concept influences nonadherence is a critical part of understanding why the problem occurs and which patients are at highest risk for nonadherence. Sociodemographic characteristics such as Culture, Spirituality, and the stage of Development have been shown to have varying degrees of influence on adherence. Younger patients have consistently demonstrated poorer adherence to prescribed treatment, with adherence again declining in patients above 65 years of age,[12] particularly those with impaired Cognition and those with limited Functional Ability. Similar results have suggested that those with less than 12 years of education and lower household income demonstrate poorer rates of adherence.[12] The quality of Family Dynamics and perceived family support also plays a role in patient adherence, particularly among those with chronic disease.

CLINICAL EXEMPLARS

There are countless clinical exemplars of adherence—so many, in fact, that it would be impossible to explain every situation on the spectrum of nonadherence to adherence. Box 6.2 presents the most common

---

BOX 6.2 EXEMPLARS OF ADHERENCE BEHAVIOR

Medication Management
Short-Term Medication Treatment
- Antibiotics
- Anticoagulants

Long-Term Medication Treatment
- Antihypertensive agents
- Antirejection medications
- Birth control
- Cholesterol-lowering agents
- Insulin

Diet
- Diabetic diet
- Low-cholesterol diet
- Renal diet
- Sodium restrictions

Preventative Health Activities
- Annual influenza vaccination
- Regular exercise
- Smoking cessation
- Use of sunscreen

 ACCESS EXEMPLAR LINKS IN YOUR GIDDENS EBOOK

situations whereby adherence behavior is most often discussed or most important. The three primary categories are medication management, dietary modification, and preventive health activities.

Featured Exemplars
Medication-Taking Behavior

The most common exemplar of adherence is medication-taking behavior, which is associated with short- and long-term medication regimens.

According to the WHO, nonadherence with long-term medications is an ongoing problem that results in serious health risks.[20] The total cost of nonadherence is estimated to be $100 billion annually for the U.S. healthcare system.[42] In their systematic review, Cramer et al. found that adherence and persistence with cardiovascular and glucose-lowering medications were poor.[14] In this review, only 59% of patients took medication for greater than 80% of the expected therapy days.[16]

Dietary Modification

Another common exemplar of adherence behavior is following a diet—either for weight loss or as a specific treatment measure for a medical condition. In the context of chronic illness, such as chronic kidney disease, patients face a long-term commitment to dietary restrictions (e.g., fluid, sodium, and protein) and challenges with ongoing exercise. Nonadherence rates are estimated between 50% and 80% for chronic disease management and lifestyle changes.[20]

Exercise

Exercise is the cornerstone of health-promotion behavior and is a common treatment measure for chronic conditions. If patients do not perceive any benefit from the exercise or if they do not like the activity, sustaining and maintaining the motivation for the change becomes very difficult. Healthcare professionals such as nurses can influence adherence behavior through MI, supporting patients' knowledge development, and using negotiation for realistic and mutually agreed upon goal setting.[46,47]

CASE STUDY

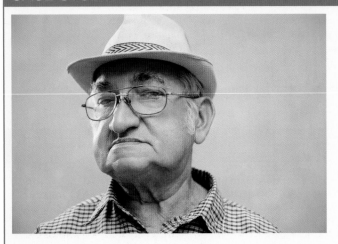

Case Presentation

Martin Herrera is a 65-year-old male admitted to the cardiology unit for a non-ST-elevation myocardial infarction (NSTEMI). It has now been 3 days since Mr. Herrera underwent insertion of a stent; he is preparing for discharge the next day. Prior medical history for Mr. Herrera includes known coronary artery disease, anterior wall myocardial infarction (MI) 2 years earlier, hyperlipidemia, hypertension, and metabolic syndrome. In addition, Mr. Herrera continues to smoke, although he has reduced his smoking to 20 cigarettes per day. In preparing Mr. Herrera for discharge, the nurse reviews his discharge medications, medication-taking behavior before admission, and specific cardiovascular disease (CVD) risk-reduction

strategies (e.g., weight control, exercise, and smoking cessation). Mr. Herrera has admitted to not taking his medications on a regular basis, often missing them 2 or 3 days a week. The most common reason given by Mr. Herrera was forgetfulness and "it won't make a difference anyways."

To begin the assessment of adherence, it is first important to clarify with the patient (1) his beliefs and perceptions about his health risk status, (2) his existing knowledge about CVD risk reduction, (3) any prior experience with healthcare professionals, and (4) his degree of confidence in being able to control his disease. Clarification of these areas reveals the following: (1) Mr. Herrera believes that because he has a very strong family history of CVD, noting that his father died at age 66 years and his brother at age 60 years, nothing he does will change the final outcome; (2) Mr. Herrera states that he saw a video while in the hospital and was given a bunch of pamphlets, but he does not really remember any specifics; in addition, he has never participated in a smoking cessation program; (3) he is seen by a cardiologist every 12 months, but he did not attend his last appointment because he was told that if he did not quit smoking the cardiologist would transfer him for follow-up by his family physician; and (4) Mr. Herrera states that he tried to quit smoking but was only able to go down to 10 cigarettes a day and believes that he is unlikely to be able to smoke any less.

Case Analysis Questions

1. How would you characterize Mr. Herrera's perception regarding his ability to control his health outcomes? Where would he fit on the scope of adherence (see Fig. 6.1)?
2. What areas should the nurse focus on to improve Mr. Herrera's motivation for adherence?

From diego cervo/iStock/Thinkstock.

 ACCESS EXEMPLAR LINKS IN YOUR GIDDENS EBOOK

REFERENCES

1. Akerblad, A., Bengtsson, F., Ekselius, L., et al. (2004). Effects of an educational compliance enhancement programme and therapeutic drug monitoring on treatment adherence in depressed patients managed by general practitioners. *International Clinical Psychopharmacology, 18*(6), 347–354.
2. Bissonnette, J. (2008). A concept analysis: Adherence. *Journal of Advanced Nursing, 63*(6), 634–643.
3. Carpenter, R. (2005). Perceived threat in compliance and adherence research. *Nursing inquiry, 12*(3), 192–199.
4. Dunbar-Jacob, J., & Mortimer-Stephens, M. K. (2001). Treatment adherence in chronic disease. *Journal of Clinical Epidemiology, 54*, S57–S60.
5. De Geest, S., Dobbels, R., Fluri, C., et al. (2005). Adherence to the therapeutic regimen in heart, lung and heart–lung transplant recipients. *The Journal of Cardiovascular Nursing, 20*(55), S85–S95.
6. Gray, R., & Wykes, T. (2002). Cournay K: From compliance to concordance: A review of the literature on interventions to enhance compliance with antipsychotic medication. *Journal of Psychiatric and Mental Health Nursing, 9*, 277–284.
7. Murphy, N., & Canales, M. (2001). A critical analysis of compliance. *Nurs Inquiry, 8*(3), 173–181.
8. Russell, S., Daly, J., Hughes, E., et al. (2003). Nurses and "difficult" patients: Negotiating non-compliance. *Journal of Advanced Nursing, 43*(3), 281–287.

9. Lehane, E., & McCarthy, G. (2009). Medication non-adherence—Exploring the conceptual mire. *International Journal of Nursing Practice*, *15*, 25–31.

10. Johnson, M., Bulechek, G., McCloskey-Dochterman, J., et al. (2001). *Nursing diagnoses, outcomes, & interventions: NANDA, NOC, and NIC linkages*. St Louis: Mosby.

11. Haynes, R. B., Yoa, X., Degani, A., et al. (2005). Interventions to enhance medication adherence [review]. *Cochrane Database Systemat Rev*.

12. Christensen, A. J. (2004). Patient adherence to medical treatment regimens: *Bridging the gap between behavioral science and biomedicine*. New Haven, CT: Yale University Press.

13. Cohen, S. M. (2009). Concept analysis of adherence in the context of cardiovascular risk reduction. *Nursing Forum*, *44*(1), 25–36.

14. Cramer, J. A., Benedict, A., Muszbek, N., et al. (2008). The significance of compliance and persistence in the treatment of diabetes, hypertension and dyslipidaemia: A review. *International Journal of Clinical Practice*, *62*, 76–87.

15. Kyngäs, H., Duffy, M., & Kroll, T. (2000). Concept analysis of compliance. *Journal of Clinical Nursing*, *9*, 5–12.

16. Sackett, D. L., Haynes, R. B., Gibson, E. S., et al. (1975). Randomized clinical trial of strategies for improving medication compliance in primary hypertension. *Lancet*, *1*, 1205–1207.

17. Bissell, P., May, C., & Noyce, P. (2004). From compliance to concordance: Barriers to accomplishing a re-framed model of health care interactions. *Social Science and Medicine*, *58*, 851–862.

18. Farmer, K. (1999). Methods for measuring and monitoring mediations regimen adherence in clinical trials and clinical practice. *Clinical Therapeutics*, *21*(6), 1074–1090.

19. Sabaté, E. (2003). *Adherence to long-term therapies: Evidence for action*. Geneva: World Health Organization.

20. Simpson, S., Eurich, D., Majumdar, S., et al. (2006). A meta-analysis of the association between adherence to drug therapy and mortality. *British Medical Journal*, *333*, 15.

21. Stevenson, F., Cox, K., Britten, N., et al. (2004). A systematic review of the research on communication between patients and health care professionals about medicines: The consequences for concordance. *Health Expectations: An International Journal of Public Participation in Health Care and Health Policy*, *7*, 235–245.

22. Vermeire, E., Hearnshaw, H., Van Royen, P., et al. (2001). Patient adherence to treatment: Three decades of research—A comprehensive review. *Journal of Clinical Pharmacy and Therapeutics*, *26*, 331–342.

23. Crow, J. (2003). Intentional non-adherence. *Pract Nurse*, *26*(6), 12–17.

24. Lehane, E., & McCarthy, G. (2007). Intentional and unintentional medication non-adherence: A comprehensive framework for clinical research and practice? A discussion paper. *International Journal of Nursing Studies*, *44*, 1468–1477.

25. Wilson, H. S., Hutchinson, S. A., & Holzemer, W. L. (2002). Reconciling incompatibilities: A grounded theory of HIV medication adherence and symptom management. *Qualitative Health Research*, *12*(10), 1309–1322.

26. Hui, C., Chen, E., Kan, C., et al. (2006). Anti-psychotics adherence among out-patients with schizophrenia in Hong Kong. *The Keio Journal of Medicine*, *55*(1), 9–14.

27. Hui, C., Chen, E., Kan, C., et al. (2006). Detection of non-adherent behaviour in early psychosis. *Australian and New Zealand journal of psychiatry*, *40*(5), 446–451.

28. Rodgers, B. L. (2000). Concept analysis: An evolutionary view. In B. L. Rogers & K. A. Knafl (Eds.), *Concept development in nursing: Foundations, techniques and applications* (2nd ed., pp. 77–102). Philadelphia: Saunders.

29. Vrijens, B., De Geest, S., Hughes, D. A., et al. (2012). A new taxonomy for describing and defining adherence to medications. *British Journal of Clinical Pharmacology*, *73*, 691–705.

30. American Psychological Association: motivation (n.d.), *Online etymology dictionary*. Retrieved from http://dictionary.reference.com/browse/motivation.

31. Kamali, M., Kelly, B., Clarke, M., et al. (2006). A prospective evaluation of adherence to medication in first episode schizophrenia. *European psychiatry*, *21*(1), 29–33.

32. Pratt, S., Mueser, K., Driscoll, M., et al. (2006). Medication nonadherence in older people with serious mental illness: Prevalence and correlates. *Psychiatric Rehabilitation Journal*, *29*(4), 299–310.

33. Dunbar-Jacob, J. (2007). Models for changing patient behavior. *The American Journal of Nursing*, *107*(6), 20–25.

34. Bandura, A. (2001). Social cognitive theory: An agentic perspective. *Annual Review of Psychology*, *52*, 1–26.

35. Seewoodharry, M. D., Maconachie, G. D., Gillies, C. L., et al. (2017). The Effects of Feedback on Adherence to Treatment: A Systematic Review and Meta-analysis of RCTs. *American Journal of Preventive Medicine*, *53*(2), 232–240.

36. Hamrin, V., Sinclair, V. G., & Gardner, V. (2017). Theoretical approaches to enhancing motivation for adherence to antidepressant medications. *Archives of Psychiatric Nursing*, *31*(2), 223–230.

37. Chisholm, M. A. (2000). Enhancing transplant patients' adherence to medication therapy. *Clinical Transplantation*, *16*(1), 30–38.

38. Cramer, J. A., Burrell, A., Fairchild, C. J., et al. (2008). Medication compliance and persistence: Terminology and definitions. *Value in Health*, *11*(1), 44–47.

39. Fraser, S. (2010). Concordance, compliance, preference or adherence. *Patient Pref Adher*, *4*, 95–96.

40. Kim, H. S., McGuire, D., Tulman, L., et al. (2005). Symptom clusters: Concept analysis and clinical implications for cancer nursing. *Cancer Nursing*, *28*(4), 270–282.

41. Bakker, R. H., Kasterman, M. C., & Dassen, T. W. (1997). Non-compliance and ineffective management of therapeutic regimen: Use in practice and theoretical implications. In M. J. Rant & P. LeMone (Eds.), *Classification of nursing diagnoses: Proceedings of the twelfth conference/North American Nursing Diagnoses Associations* (pp. 196–201). Glendale, CA: CINHAL Information Systems.

42. Kane, J. M., Kishimoto, T., & Correll, C. U. (2013). Non-adherence to medication in patients with psychotic disorders: Epidemiology, contributing factors and management strategies. *World Psychiatry*, *12*(3), 216–226.

43. Sajatovic, M., Valenstein, M., Blow, F. C., et al. (2006). Treatment adherence with antipsychotic medications in bipolar disorder. *Bipolar Disorders*, *8*(3), 232–241.

44. Nose, M., Barbui, C., & Tansella, M. (2003). How often do patients with psychosis fail to adhere to treatment programmes? A systematic review. *Psychological Medicine*, *33*(7), 1149–1160.

45. Akerblad, A., Bengtsson, F., Von Knorring, L., et al. (2006). Response, remission and relapse in relation to adherence in primary care treatment of depression: A 2-year outcome study. *International Clinical Psychopharmacology*, *21*(2), 117–124.

46. Salamon, K. S., Brouwer, A. M., Fox, M. M., et al. (2012). Experiencing type 2 diabetes mellitus: Qualitative analysis of adolescents' concept of illness, adjustment and motivation to engage in self-care behaviors. *The Diabetes Educator*, *38*, 543–551.

47. Copeland, L., McNamara, R., Kelson, M., et al. (2015). Mechanisms of change within motivational interviewing in relation to health behaviors outcomes: A systematic review. *Patient Education and Counseling*, *98*, 401–411.

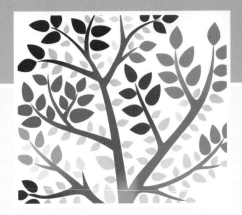

Self-Management

Leigh Ann Simmons and Devon Noonan

Improvements in public health and medical care during the past century have increased people's life expectancy, and now nearly two-thirds of adults living in the United States have one or more chronic diseases, including hypertension, diabetes, and heart disease.[1] As a consequence, a major focus of healthcare services is the ongoing prevention and treatment of chronic diseases that have no cure as opposed to primarily treating acute disease.[2] In fact, data show that approximately 90% of all healthcare expenditures are for the prevention and treatment of chronic disease, with 12% of the population accounting for more than 40% of healthcare spending.[1] This shift toward chronic disease care has required healthcare systems to revamp their approaches to medical treatment. The paternalistic approach, which views the provider as "expert" and the patient as "passive recipient" of medical advice, is largely ineffective at treating chronic diseases that require daily management by patients and their caregivers. Rather, evidence suggests that patient-centered approaches, which emphasize patient–provider partnerships in which patients are active participants in their care, are most effective for addressing chronic disease.[3,4]

Self-management is the primary means by which patients and their caregivers play active roles in their health and medical care. Chronic diseases have significant consequences for patients, including persistent symptoms, daily medication use, changes in health behaviors (e.g., exercise and diet), effects on social and work circumstances, and emotional distress. Patients with chronic disease must continuously and over time engage in healthcare practices and make decisions about health behaviors that influence the course and progression of their disease. These self-management practices reduce risk for complications and comorbid illness and improve long-term prognosis and quality of life.[5] Thus self-management is an essential component of chronic disease care, and providers must teach patients to develop their self-management skills.[2] However, self-management is not limited to controlling chronic disease. Health maintenance also requires individuals to engage in daily health-promoting behaviors that support long-term well-being and reduce chronic disease risk and onset. This chapter presents the concept of self-management within nursing practice.

DEFINITION

There are a number of definitions for self-management in the literature. Clark and colleagues defined self-management as "the day-to-day tasks an individual must undertake to control or reduce the impact of disease on physical health status."[6] Barlow et al. defined self-management as "the individual's ability to manage the symptoms, treatment, physical and psychosocial consequences, and lifestyle changes inherent in living with a chronic condition."[4] For pediatric patients, Modi et al. defined self-management as "the interaction of health behaviors and related processes that patients and families engage in to care for a chronic condition."[7] Although the definitions of self-management vary slightly, some core expectations and skills are consistent across these definitions.[8] First, patients and their caregivers must have sufficient knowledge of the chronic condition and its treatment. Second, they must monitor the condition and respond to information about the current disease state with appropriate cognitive or behavioral responses, all in the context of fluctuating life circumstances (e.g., a patient with diabetes may have to adjust the timing of insulin based on home blood sugar monitoring). Third, they must be able to accurately convey important information about their condition and its management to healthcare providers so that providers can impart the information necessary for patients to develop an effective self-management plan. However, as noted previously, self-management of key health behaviors (e.g., diet, physical activity, sleep, and stress) is also critical for maintaining good health. Given the previously mentioned definitions in concert with the skills necessary to manage both health and chronic disease, the following definition is proposed for purposes of this concept presentation:

Self-management is the ability of individuals and/or their caregivers to engage in the daily tasks required to maintain health and well-being or to respond to the changing physical, psychological, behavioral, and emotional sequelae of a chronic disease based on their knowledge of the condition, its consequences, and the plan of care developed in cooperation with their healthcare team within the context of the daily demands of life.

SCOPE

From a very broad perspective, the scope of self-management as a concept ranges from optimal self-management to a complete absence of self-management. The level or degree of self-care varies from person to person and in different situations across the lifespan. Thus self-management is not a continuous state but rather can be conceptualized on a continuum that can change and is influenced by a number of variables (Fig. 7.1).

Self-management exists within a broad system of collaborative care that includes a partnership among patients, their caregivers, their healthcare providers, and the healthcare system.[9,10] Within this system, each member has an essential role in the partnership. Patients and their

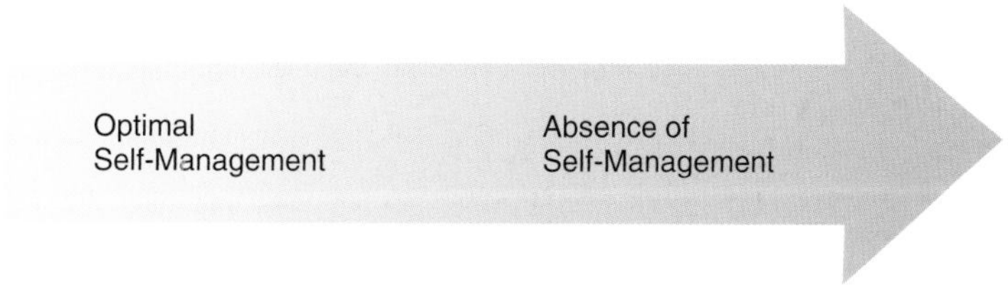

FIGURE 7.1 Scope of Self-Management.

families become the principal caregivers responsible for day-to-day management and accurate reporting of how their health or chronic condition is progressing. Providers become teachers and advisors who are responsible for helping patients and their caregivers to understand health-promoting behaviors. In the case of chronic disease, providers must also help patients and caregivers to understand the condition, acquire necessary management skills, develop an effective management plan, and build confidence in their ability to respond. The healthcare system becomes the care coordinator that organizes and finances the collection of services available to patients for health enhancement and chronic disease prevention as well as management to ensure continuity.[11] Optimal self-management is the by-product of the effective partnership among these members such that health is maximized and the negative consequences of chronic disease—including greater symptomatology, poor disease-related outcomes, reduced quality of life, morbidity, mortality, and excessive healthcare expenditures—are limited.[5]

The scope of self-management can also be characterized in terms of approaches to enhancing the confidence, knowledge, and skills of patients and their caregivers. Self-management education can be provided one-to-one, in groups, or a combination of both. Information may be relayed in person, telephonically, or using self-instruction via mailers, manuals, books, audio- or videotapes, web-based applications, mobile applications, and wearable technology (e.g., accelerometers).[4,5,12] The content of self-management education may include information on guidelines for optimal health-promoting behaviors, the causes and consequences of common chronic diseases, medication management, symptom management, lifestyle behaviors, managing psychosocial effects, social support, and communicating with providers.[4] A variety of entities and individuals may disseminate self-management information and education. These include but are not limited to voluntary healthcare agencies (e.g., the American Heart Association and the American Diabetes Association), state and federal public health systems (e.g., local public health departments and the Centers for Disease Control and Prevention), educational and community-based settings (e.g., schools, worksites, and the Young Men's Christian Association [YMCA]), inpatient institutions (e.g., hospitals and long-term care facilities), ambulatory clinics (e.g., primary and specialty clinics and also ambulatory surgical centers), diverse healthcare providers (e.g., nurses, pharmacists, and physicians), and peers (e.g., others with the same diagnosis who have successfully managed their disease). Most self-management education programs are run separately from clinical patient care but in collaboration with healthcare professionals,[13] although the increased use of technology is allowing for more integration of self-management education and patient monitoring of behaviors into the clinic. For example, wearable technology has been incorporated into (a) cardiac care to monitor abnormal heart rhythms, (b) Parkinson disease management to monitor gait disturbances, (c) neurological monitoring for seizures, and (d) poststroke rehabilitation to monitor exercise goals and physical activity.[14] As these technologies improve in both the types of data collected and ease of patient use, they will increasingly be used in clinical care.

Finally, self-management is essential across the lifespan.[5,11] During the infant, toddler, and school-age years, parents or other caregivers take primary responsibility for self-management skills on behalf of their children. During adolescence, parents and children often share responsibility for these tasks until early adulthood, when now-grown children assume full responsibility from their parents for managing their health or condition. As adults, individuals continue to self-manage their health or chronic condition unless they develop significant disability (e.g., age-associated cognitive decline and accident) that prevents them from handling some or all of the required tasks. In this case, partners, children, or other caregivers assist with or assume management as needed. The provider's role in assisting patients with self-management depends on the life stage and requires the provider to facilitate patients and caregivers to effectively transition roles and responsibilities in self-management strategies. In particular, clinicians should assess the self-management skills of patients and caregivers as well as the social contexts in which these skills are being used (e.g., poverty, neighborhood violence, etc.) to determine the types and levels of supports patients may need to successfully manage their health.[15]

ATTRIBUTES AND CRITERIA

Five key attributes characterize self-management: self-efficacy, patient engagement, health education, patient-provider partnership, and disease management.

Self-Efficacy

Self-efficacy is having the confidence in one's knowledge and abilities to reach a desired outcome.[16] Patients increase self-efficacy through (1) educational experiences that improve knowledge about their health or their chronic condition and its management, (2) ongoing successful performance of the daily tasks required to enhance health or manage their disease and minimize symptoms, (3) engaging in shared decision making and collaborative problem solving with providers and caregivers about their health or disease, and (4) linkages to individual and community-based support services.[5]

Patient Engagement

Patient engagement is linked to self-efficacy and refers to having the knowledge, skills, ability, and willingness to be an active participant in one's health and health care.[17,18] Patients with greater self-efficacy are more likely to be engaged in the process of their care and to develop the necessary partnerships with their healthcare team that enable them to optimize their health or manage their chronic disease.

Health Education

Health education refers to any combination of learning experiences designed to help patients and their caregivers improve health (or a chronic condition) by enhancing their knowledge, skills, and confidence or influencing their attitudes.[19] As a central feature of chronic disease care, patients must frequently be taught about the condition itself as well as how to manage it. This self-management education complements traditional patient education and includes core features such as problem-solving skills, decision making, the utilization of resources, forming a strong patient-provider team relationship, taking action, and self-tailoring.[20]

Patient–Provider Relationship

The *patient–provider relationship*, in which patients take responsibility for their health (or chronic condition) and the "provider," or members of the healthcare team as well as the health system in which care is being provided, serves as the vehicle through which optimal self-management occurs. A strong patient–provider relationship is essential to patient-centered care in which patients' needs, concerns, problems, and values remain at the center of care and self-management approaches are responsive to patients' unique needs and preferences.[11,20]

Disease Management

Disease management is a system of coordinated healthcare interventions and communications for patients with chronic conditions that require significant self-management efforts.[21] The primary goal of disease management programs is to improve population health and reduce healthcare costs by mitigating the future complications of chronic conditions through effective self-care.

THEORETICAL LINKS

Two key theories within the field of psychology underpin self-management and its attributes: social cognitive theory and cognitive-behavioral theory.

Social Cognitive Theory

Social cognitive theory is based on the idea that individuals' expectations influence their behaviors.[22,23] Thus individuals with high self-efficacy, or those who believe they can organize and execute a course of action necessary to produce a desired outcome, are more likely to view difficult tasks as things to be mastered versus avoided. Individuals in good health remain confident that they can maintain their health by practicing positive health behaviors. Among individuals with chronic disease, those with greater self-efficacy—or those who believe they can perform well—will be more likely to successfully manage their condition. Self-management education that helps patients increase self-efficacy by improving their knowledge of the disease and the tasks essential to managing the disease and its symptoms frequently results in better health behaviors and outcomes.

Cognitive-Behavioral Theory

Cognitive-behavioral theory is similar to social cognitive theory in that the theoretic foundation is the notion that thoughts affect behavior. Thus helping people to change the way they think about (1) their health or illness and (2) themselves in relation to their health or illness is necessary to help them self-manage effectively (Fig. 7.2).[24,25] Several features of cognitive-behavioral theory are evident in self-management education and practices. Specifically, cognitive-behavioral theory assumes an active, involved patient who is responsible for engaging in specific actions as part of a plan the patient develops with his or her provider that is responsive to the patient's individual needs and preferences.

CONTEXT OF NURSING AND HEALTH CARE

Nurses help patients and their caregivers with self-management throughout the lifespan in diverse clinical and community-based settings and across the continuum of care from health enhancement/wellness to chronic disease prevention, management of ongoing disease, and recovery

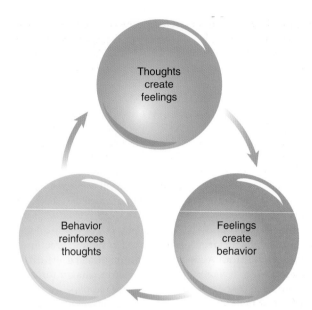

FIGURE 7.2 Cognitive Behavioral Theory. (Redrawn from Stangor, C. [2015]. *Introduction to psychology.* [v. 1.0]. Washington, DC: Flat World Education.)

from an acute event. The following sections describe the role of self-management in nursing care for each of these areas.

Health Enhancement and Wellness

Across the lifespan, nurses help patients and their caregivers engage in positive behaviors that optimize health and promote well-being. A critical component of patient self-management for health enhancement and wellness is that patients must schedule and attend wellness visits and screening appointments that have been determined to be necessary. They must also engage in the lifestyle behaviors that promote good health, including maintaining a normal body mass index (BMI), eating a healthy diet, getting regular exercise, getting sufficient sleep, managing stress, and reducing unintentional injuries through safety measures such as wearing a seat belt or helmet and using age-appropriate car seats for children. Nurses may impart some of this information to patients during one-to-one clinical visits; however, community-based and public health initiatives also serve as a source of information on how individuals can self-manage their daily decisions to maximize health.

Predisease/Disease Prevention

Predisease is a state in which individuals do not meet the full diagnostic criteria for a diagnosis but have one or more clinical markers indicating that they are not completely healthy.[26] Some common predisease states include prediabetes, prehypertension, and precancerous lesions, and these are most often diagnosed as a result of age-, sex-, and risk-based screening. For many predisease states, there are some important self-management tasks for patients to initiate, such as changes in diet or physical activity, quitting smoking, using sunscreen, or even starting a low-dose medication. Nurses play an important role in helping patients to understand both the predisease state and the ultimate disease, including family, lifestyle, and environmental factors that contribute to the disease, their risk of developing the disease based on their current health status and risks, and the potential benefit of making changes to reduce the risk of developing the full disease. A core component of this education is assessing patients' capacity for making changes. That is, nurses need to understand the social and environmental contexts in which patients are trying to self-manage in order to partner with them to help them decide how to approach the necessary changes. For example, if a patient must exercise but lives in an unsafe neighborhood, the nurse and patient will have to work collaboratively to identify a safe means for exercising, such as walking in place at home while watching television.

Disease/New Diagnosis

When patients receive a new disease diagnosis, frequently they must make significant lifestyle changes. Helping patients to self-manage a new disease requires nurses to provide education regarding both the disease and its management. Education about the causes and consequences of the disease helps patients to understand the importance of self-management in general and the specific self-management tasks in which they will need to engage. Much of the information about chronic disease that nurses provide is conveyed individually or in groups in ambulatory clinical areas and community-based settings. However, broader public health initiatives from voluntary healthcare entities, such as the American Heart Association or the American Diabetes Association, also serve as a source of important information for individuals with chronic disease, and nurses can leverage these sources when they are working with patients and their caregivers. As with predisease states, considering patients with chronic disease holistically and understanding their capacity for making changes is critical to successful management over time.

Acute Event Management

An acute event—such as a stroke, myocardial infarction (MI), asthma exacerbation, or hip fracture—is frequently a life-changing occurrence, especially for individuals who were unaware of or did not understand their risk for the event. Self-management after an event is critical to the patient's full recovery, including achieving the best health possible given his or her disease state and preventing a recurrence of the event, the development of comorbidities, or even mortality. As with a new diagnosis, recovery from an acute event requires the patient to self-manage new medications; changes in lifestyle behaviors; and greater healthcare utilization due to increased monitoring, specialty care, and ancillary health services (e.g., dietician and exercise physiologist). If the patient was already managing a chronic disease, these changes may not be as significant as they might be for a patient who was unaware of his or her risk for the event. Thus nursing interventions will involve tailoring self-management education to the patient's pre-event state.

For example, a patient with diagnosed coronary artery disease (CAD) who was already taking lipid-lowering drugs and daily low-dose aspirin and has an MI will need different self-management education than a patient who did not have diagnosed CAD prior to the MI.

INTERRELATED CONCEPTS

A number of concepts within nursing care are interrelated with self-management; these are presented in Fig. 7.3. Adherence to treatment recommendations and self-management tasks is necessary in order to sustain optimal management as evidenced by few or no symptoms and limited interferences with quality of life or activities of daily living. As previously discussed, Patient Education is a central feature of self-management. Healthcare professionals must provide patients with education that helps them to understand the causes and consequences of their disease and the strategies for managing their condition long term. Self-management education does not replace general health education but rather complements it with a specific focus on building capacity for ongoing self-care practices that promote optimal health for the individual. Health Promotion is related to self-management in that it focuses on helping individuals and communities to take control of their health and ultimately improve it.[10] Whereas some health-promotion efforts focus primarily on individuals and how they might manage their behaviors and choices, many approaches move beyond the individual to address a broad range of community, social, and environmental determinants of health that also require management at various levels.[10] Collaboration between patients and providers has also been identified earlier in this chapter as a central feature of self-management. Optimal self-management of chronic conditions depends on patients and providers working together to identify priorities, goals, and specific plans of action to achieve those goals.[5] Care Coordination is also essential for patients with chronic disease to self-manage effectively. Frequently patients need additional information about their disease from specialists and/or must acquire more knowledge and skills regarding diet, physical activity, smoking cessation, medication adherence, and other lifestyle behaviors that affect their condition. Thus, the care of chronic disease becomes a team-based approach wherein multiple providers work together to support patients in their ongoing self-management. These providers can range from specialty physicians and nurse practitioners to registered nurses and other allied health professionals such as nutritionists, exercise physiologists,

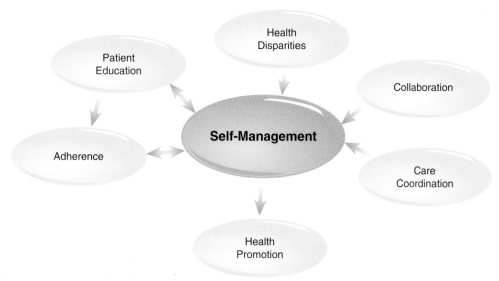

FIGURE 7.3 Self-Management and Related Concepts.

and health behavior specialists. Coordination among these providers regarding services and recommendations is essential for patients to effectively self-manage their conditions without becoming overwhelmed by the amount of information they receive. Finally, Health Disparities populations have been shown to have higher rates of chronic disease and poorer self-management practices, leading to worse health outcomes.[27] Self-management education for these patients must consider how a lack of resources or education may be exacerbating poor self-management; strategies should be tailored to the specific needs of these populations.

CLINICAL EXEMPLARS

Self-management cuts across all areas of health care and populations served—from wellness and health promotion to chronic disease management. For this reason, there are far more exemplars of self-management than could possibly be presented in this text. Box 7.1 presents a list of the most common exemplars by age group and context

that represent the concept. Next, six of these exemplars are featured, with short descriptions.

Featured Exemplars
Prenatal Care

Regular prenatal care helps to inform women about the steps they can take to ensure a healthy pregnancy. These include consuming a healthy diet, taking a prenatal vitamin with minimum daily folic acid requirements, getting regular exercise, avoiding exposure to harmful environmental substances, avoiding alcohol and drugs, and managing preexisting conditions. Ongoing monitoring of the mother's weight, blood pressure, and urine along with results from evidence-based screenings serve as the basis for recommended changes in self-management practices to reduce risk for maternal and infant complications.[28] Women who develop complications of pregnancy—such as gestational diabetes, gestational hypertension, or preeclampsia—will need education about their condition and learn how to manage it through changes in diet, physical activity levels, stress, and medication.

❧ BOX 7.1 EXEMPLARS OF SELF-MANAGEMENT

Health Enhancement/Wellness
- Pediatric well-child visit
- Prenatal care
- Adult/older adult annual wellness visit

Prediisease/Disease Prevention
Pediatric
- Prediabetes
- Overweight
- Prehypertension

Prenatal
- Prehypertension
- Preeclampsia
- Excess gestational weight gain early in pregnancy

Adults
- Prehypertension
- Prediabetes
- Overweight
- Precancerous lesions
- Osteopenia
- Vision impairment
- HIV infection

Disease/New Diagnosis
Pediatric
- Asthma
- Overweight/obesity
- Diabetes
- Malnutrition
- Developmental disabilities
- Behavioral/mental health

Prenatal/Maternal
- Pregnancy-induced hypertension
- Eclampsia
- Gestational diabetes
- Depression

Adult/Older Adult
- Coronary artery disease
- Type 2 diabetes
- Obesity
- Coronary obstructive pulmonary disease
- Osteoporosis
- Arthritis
- Glaucoma
- Dementia
- Depression
- AIDS

Acute Medical Events
Pediatric
- Orthopedic (sprains, ligament tears, broken bones)
- Accidental ingestion (e.g., poison substance, medication)
- Trauma
- Burns
- Sports-related head injuries (concussions)

Prenatal Care
- Premature labor
- Premature rupture of the membranes
- Trauma

Adult/Older Adult
- Congestive heart failure
- Myocardial infarction
- Stroke
- Falls (hip fracture)
- Pneumonia
- Acute renal failure
- Infection/sepsis
- Trauma
- Suicide attempt

 ACCESS EXEMPLAR LINKS IN YOUR GIDDENS EBOOK

Pediatric Asthma

Asthma is one of the most common and costly chronic disorders in children, affecting nearly 10% of all youth younger than age 18 years and accounting for nearly $56 billion annually in healthcare expenditures.[29,30] It is also one of the leading causes of school absenteeism. If not managed properly, asthma can be life-threatening. Proper self-management includes helping patients and their parents/caregivers to adhere to daily medications, understand triggers, know how to self-monitor and assess symptoms for rescue treatment, and make changes to the environment (reduce/eliminate secondhand smoke exposure, place dust mite covers on bedding, etc.).

Type 2 Diabetes

Type 2 diabetes is one of the most prevalent preventable chronic diseases among adults in the United States and worldwide. In addition, the number of children being diagnosed with type 2 diabetes is increasing with the growing prevalence of pediatric overweight and obesity.[31] Self-management of weight through regular physical activity and a healthy diet is the most cost-effective means of preventing or delaying the onset of type 2 diabetes. Once diagnosed, self-management becomes equally critical to the prevention of complications, morbidities, and mortality. Self-management tasks include regular visits to a provider, medication adherence, and health-promoting lifestyle behaviors (e.g., physical activity and a balanced diet).

HIV/AIDS

More than 1.1 million people ages 13 years or older in the United States are infected with HIV, and approximately 14% of them do not know that they are infected.[32] Every year, nearly 40,000 people are newly diagnosed with HIV, and another 18,000 are diagnosed with AIDS.[32] Risk for HIV/AIDS is highest among men who have sex with men, injection drug users, blacks/African Americans, and Latinos. Regular healthcare visits to monitor viral load, opportunistic infections, cardiovascular health, medication adherence, and safe sex practices are among the critical self-management practices individuals with HIV/AIDS must undertake to minimize their risk for morbidity and mortality.[33]

Heart Failure

Heart failure is one of the most common complications of CAD. Approximately 5 million U.S. adults live with heart failure; it is the most common diagnosis for hospital patients 65 years of age or older.[34] Sudden death is common among heart failure patients; more than half of these individuals die within 5 years of diagnosis, and it contributes to nearly 275,000 deaths annually. As with most chronic conditions, patients with heart failure benefit from education about their disease and self-managing diet, physical activity, weight, and medication adherence.

Depression

Depression is a common mental health disorder affecting approximately 8.1% of U.S. adults. Individuals most affected by depression are midlife adults between the ages of 45 and 64 years, women, minorities, individuals without a high school education, and those without health insurance. Treatment for depression includes the use of medication and psychotherapy. In addition, patients must learn to manage their moods, including suicidal thoughts; to recognize triggers and relapses; and to set goals for the management of their disease.[35]

CASE STUDY

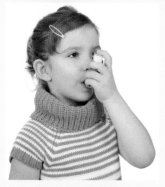

Case Presentation

Margaret is a 5-year-old with a past medical history of an acute asthma attack at age 3 years requiring 5 days of hospitalization, 2 of which were in the pediatric intensive care unit. Her parents made an appointment with the nurse practitioner (NP) to get advice on how to better manage Margaret's asthma. In the previous year, they had taken Margaret to the emergency department three times and to urgent care twice. She has been on oral steroids (prednisolone) four times in the previous 12 months, and she uses her rescue inhaler (albuterol) at least twice weekly when she is well. In the first 4 months of the school year, Margaret missed 12 days of kindergarten due to asthma.

The NP evaluates Margaret. Her vital signs and BMI are within the normal rage. Her parents report that Margaret receives her maintenance medications most days, missing on average 1 or 2 days per week. The NP asks about the family's living situation and learns that Margaret lives with her biological parents and a 7-year-old Labrador retriever, which is an indoor dog. Her paternal grandmother, a smoker, also lives with the family during the winter months. The family's house is 76 years old with carpeted living and sleeping areas and a basement. The parents do not have Margaret's bedding encased with dust mite protectors. The parents deny any mold, mice, or cockroaches in the home. The parents report that Margaret occasionally wheezes during activity, but she does not pretreat with her rescue inhaler.

The NP discusses with Margaret's parents the importance of daily medication adherence as the first line of defense. When she investigates further, she learns that the nebulizer administration sometimes gets in the way of her parents adhering to their daily schedule. The NP discusses with them increasing the daily dose and changing the administration route to the metered dose inhaler with spacer, which they already use for the rescue medications. The parents agree this would make daily adherence easier. The NP also educates the family on asthma triggers and the role of smoking. She asks the parents to discuss with the grandmother smoking outdoors when she is visiting. The parents agree that they will discuss with each other how to approach the conversation. The NP educates the parents about bedding encasements for mattresses and pillows and provides a flyer listing online stores that sell them. The parents agree to purchase these encasements. Due to the parents' report of coughing with physical activity, the NP recommends pretreating Margaret with two puffs of the rescue inhaler before exercise, and the parents agree. Finally, the NP discusses the importance of keeping track of medication administration and symptoms using an application on a phone or paper-based recording tool in order to determine triggers and patterns in symptoms. The mother downloads a tool in the office to begin tracking. Based on the conversation, the parents and NP together update the asthma action plan and agree on a follow-up plan. The NP asks the family to follow up in 3 months or sooner if Margaret needs to go to the emergency department or urgent care.

Case Analysis Questions

1. What information exists suggesting that Margaret's condition is not being managed optimally?
2. What specific measures are described that would improve the management of Margaret's asthma?

From goce risteski/iStock/Thinkstock

🍃 **ACCESS EXEMPLAR LINKS IN YOUR GIDDENS EBOOK**

REFERENCES

1. Buttorff, C., Ruder, T., & Bauman, M. (2017). *Multiple chronic conditions in the United States*. Santa Monica, CA: RAND Corporation.
2. Holman, H., & Lorig, K. (2004). Patient self-management: A key to effectiveness and efficiency in care of chronic disease. *Public Health Reports, 119*(3), 239–243.
3. Lawn, S., & Schoo, A. (2010). Supporting self-management of chronic health conditions: Common approaches. *Patient Education and Counseling, 80*(2), 205–211.
4. Barlow, J., Wright, C., Sheasby, J., et al. (2002). Self-management approaches for people with chronic conditions: A review. *Patient Education and Counseling, 48*(2), 177–187.
5. Battersby, M., Von Korff, M., Schaefer, J., et al. (2010). Twelve evidence-based principles for implementing self-management support in primary care. *Joint Commission Journal on Quality and Patient Safety, 36*(12), 561–570.
6. Clark, N. M., Becker, M. H., Janz, N. K., et al. (1991). Self-management of chronic disease by older adults: A review and questions for research. *Journal of Aging and Health, 3*(1), 3–27.
7. Modi, A. C., Pai, A. L., Hommel, K. A., et al. (2012). Pediatric self-management: A framework for research, practice, and policy. *Pediatrics, 129*(2), e473–e485.
8. Leventhal, H., Phillips, L. A., & Burns, E. (2016). The Common-Sense Model of Self-Regulation (CSM): A dynamic framework for understanding illness self-management. *Journal of Behavioral Medicine, 39*(6), 935–946.
9. Newman, S., Steed, L., & Mulligan, K. (2004). Self-management interventions for chronic illness. *Lancet, 364*(9444), 23–29.
10. World Health Organization. (2002). *Innovative care for chronic conditions: Building blocks for actions: Global report*. Geneva: Author.
11. Lawn, S., McMillan, J., & Pulvirenti, M. (2011). Chronic condition self-management: Expectations of responsibility. *Patient Education and Counseling, 84*(2), e5–e8.
12. Chiauzzi, E., Rodarte, C., & DasMahapatra, P. (2015). Patient-centered activity monitoring in the self-management of chronic health conditions. *BMC Medicine, 13*(1), 77.
13. Warsi, A., Wang, P. S., LaValley, M. P., et al. (2004). Self-management education programs in chronic disease: A systematic review and methodological critique of the literature. *Archives of Internal Medicine, 164*(15), 1641–1649.
14. Wilson, D. (2017). An overview of the application of wearable technology to nursing practice. *Nursing Forum, 52*(2), 124–132.
15. Lindsay, S., Kingsnorth, S., & Hamdani, Y. (2011). Barriers and facilitators of chronic illness self-management among adolescents: A review and future directions. *Journal of Nursing and Healthcare of Chronic Illness, 3*(3), 186–208.
16. Bodenheimer, T., Lorig, K., Holman, H., et al. (2002). Patient self-management of chronic disease in primary care. *JAMA: The Journal of the American Medical Association, 288*(19), 2469.
17. Hibbard, J. H., Stockard, J., Mahoney, E. R., et al. (2004). Development of the patient activation measure (PAM): Conceptualizing and measuring activation in patients and consumers. *Health Services Research, 39*(4 Pt. 1), 1005–1026.
18. Hibbard, J. H., Mahoney, E. R., Stock, R., et al. (2007). Do increases in patient activation result in improved self-management behaviors? *Health Services Research, 42*(4), 1443–1463.
19. World Health Organization: *Health education*. (2018). Retrieved from: http://www.who.int/topics/health_education/en.
20. Lorig, K. R., & Holman, H. R. (2003). Self-management education: History, definition, outcomes, and mechanisms. *Annals of Behavioral Medicine: A Publication of the Society of Behavioral Medicine, 26*(1), 1–7.
21. Care Continuum Alliance: *Definition of disease management*. (2018). Retrieved from: http://www.carecontinuum.org/dm_definition.asp.
22. Bandura, A. (1977). Self-efficacy: Toward a unifying theory of behavioral change. *Psychological Review, 84*(2), 191–215.
23. Bandura, A. (1986). The explanatory and predictive scope of self-efficacy theory. *Journal of Social and Clinical Psychology, 4*(3), 359–373.
24. Hupp, S. D., Reitman, D., & Jewell, J. D. (2008). Cognitive–behavioral theory. *Handbook of Clinical Psychology, 2*, 263–288.
25. Schwarzer, R. (2001). Social–cognitive factors in changing health-related behaviors. *Current Directions in Psychological Science, 10*(2), 47–51.
26. Viera, A. J. (2011). Predisease: When does it make sense? *Epidemiologic Reviews, 33*(1), 122–134.
27. National Center for Health Statistics. (2017). *Health, United States, 2016, With chartbook on long-term trends in the health*. Hyattsville, MD: Author.
28. NICHD/NIH: *What is prenatal care and why is it important? Pregnancy: Condition information*. (2018). Retrieved from: https://www.nichd.nih.gov/health/topics/pregnancy/conditioninfo/prenatal-care.
29. American Lung Association: *Asthma & children fact sheet*. (2018). Retrieved from: http://www.lung.org/lung-disease/asthma/resources/facts-and-figures/asthma-children-fact-sheet.html.
30. Barnett, S. B. L., & Nurmagambetov, T. A. (2011). Costs of asthma in the United States: 2002–2007. *The Journal of Allergy and Clinical Immunology, 127*(1), 145–152.
31. Centers for Disease Control and Prevention. (2014). *National diabetes statistics report: Estimates of diabetes and its burden in the United States*. Atlanta, GA: Author.
32. U.S. Department of Health and Human Services: U.S. Statistics – HIV. (2018). Retrieved from: https://www.hiv.gov/hiv-basics/overview/data-and-trends/statistics.
33. Centers for Disease Control and Prevention. (2016). Estimated HIV incidence and prevalence in the United States, 2010-2015. *HIV Surveillance Report, 23*(1).
34. Emory Healthcare: *Heart failure statistics*. (2018). Retrieved from: http://www.emoryhealthcare.org/heart-failure/learn-about-heart-failure/statistics.html.
35. Centers for Disease Control and Prevention: *Prevalence of depression among adults aged 20 and over: United States, 2013-2016*. (2018). Retrieved from: https://www.cdc.gov/nchs/products/databriefs/db303.htm.

Health and Illness Concepts

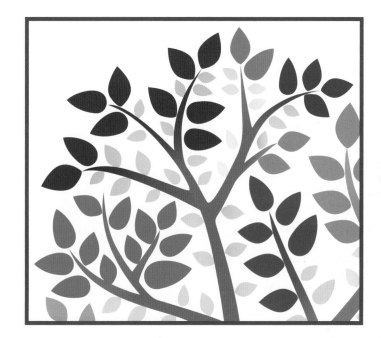

The provision of health care is geared toward three general goals: to promote health, to prevent disease, and to treat illness when it arises. These do not represent three separate and competing goals; rather, these goals characterize the health and illness continuum and apply to all people across the life span. The concepts presented in Unit II are related to these goals within the context of the patients who receive our care.

Health and illness concepts are complex and represent a multitude of health-related conditions. These concepts are presented similarly and include concept definition, scope of concept, physiologic processes, variations and context, consequences, risk factors, assessment, clinical management inter-related concepts, clinical exemplars, and a case study. Presented from a life span and health-continuum perspective, these concepts focus on the commonalities of conditions represented as opposed to specific disease conditions. For each concept, nurses should understand the concept and notice situations that place an individual at risk for less than optimal function; furthermore, nurses should know how to recognize alterations when they occur, and they should have a general understanding of interventions both to promote optimal health and to restore health if an alteration occurs.

The following six themes are used to organize 29 concepts in this unit:
- Homeostasis and Regulation
- Sexuality and Reproduction
- Protection and Movement
- Resilience
- Mood and Cognition
- Maladaptive Behavior

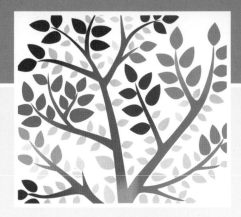

CONCEPT
8

Fluid and Electrolytes

Linda Felver

Fluid in the body circulates in the blood and lymph vessels, surrounds the cells, and provides the environment inside cells in which cellular chemistry occurs. The amount, concentration, and composition of the fluid in the body influence function at all levels from the cell to the whole person. The body continuously adjusts the characteristics and location of its fluid through specific physiological processes that nurses must understand in order to help individuals maintain or restore their fluid and electrolyte balance and function optimally. This chapter presents a conceptual analysis of fluid and electrolytes including the process of maintaining balance and the recognition and management of imbalances when they occur.

DEFINITION

The concept Fluid and Electrolytes refers to the *process of regulating the extracellular fluid volume, body fluid osmolality, and plasma concentrations of electrolytes*. Fluid is water plus the substances dissolved and suspended in it. Important characteristics of fluid are its volume (amount) and its degree of concentration (osmolality), which are discussed in this chapter. Another important characteristic of body fluid is its pH, which is discussed in Concept 9, Acid–Base Balance. Electrolytes are substances that are charged particles (ions) when they are placed in water. Examples of electrolytes are sodium ions (Na^+), potassium ions (K^+), calcium ions (Ca^{2+}), and magnesium ions (Mg^{2+}). In healthcare settings, people often omit the word "ion" when they discuss electrolytes, referring to K^+ as "potassium," for example. All body fluids contain electrolytes; body fluids in different locations normally contain different concentrations of electrolytes that are necessary for optimal function.

The maintenance of physiological balance of body fluid and electrolytes is a dynamic interplay between three processes: intake and absorption, distribution, and output. *Intake and absorption* refers to the addition of fluid and electrolytes to the body (intake) and their movement into the blood (absorption). *Distribution* is the process of moving fluid and electrolytes between the various body fluid compartments. These fluid compartments include those inside the cells (holding *intracellular* fluid) and those outside the cells (holding *extracellular* fluid). The extracellular fluid (ECF) compartment holds fluid between the cells (*interstitial* fluid) and fluid inside blood vessels (*vascular* fluid).[1] *Output* is the removal of fluid and electrolytes from the body through normal or abnormal routes.

Fluid and electrolyte balance is a dynamic interplay because fluid and electrolyte output occurs continuously. Intake of fluid and electrolytes influences output to some degree, but intake can easily become less than or more than output. Fluid and electrolyte distribution can shift rapidly when conditions change. Optimal fluid and electrolyte balance keeps the volume, osmolality, and electrolyte concentrations of fluid in the various body fluid compartments within their normal physiological ranges.

SCOPE

From the most abstract perspective, the concept of Fluid and Electrolytes is quite simple: One has either an optimal balance or an imbalance. Fluid and electrolyte imbalances can be too little, too much, or misplaced. Conceptually, *fluid balance* has two aspects: extracellular volume and osmolality. *Electrolyte balance* requires separate consideration. Extracellular fluid volume (ECV), body fluid osmolality, and plasma electrolyte concentrations can each be visualized as a continuum with three categories: optimal balance and two types of imbalances (Fig. 8.1).

NORMAL PHYSIOLOGICAL PROCESS

An understanding of the physiological processes of fluid and electrolyte balance provides the foundation for understanding the consequences of imbalances or disruptions. The three physiological processes whose interplay creates fluid and electrolyte balance were defined previously: intake and absorption, distribution, and output. This discussion describes these processes in more detail. Optimal balance occurs when both of the following characteristics are present:

- Intake and absorption of fluid and electrolytes matches the output of fluid and electrolytes.
- Volume, osmolality, and electrolyte concentrations of fluid in the various body fluid compartments are within their normal ranges.

To maintain optimal fluid and electrolyte balance, output must be matched by appropriate intake, and the intake must be absorbed (Fig. 8.2).

Intake and Absorption

The most common route of fluid and electrolyte intake is oral. Other routes include intravenous (IV) administration and less common avenues such as insertion into the rectum, introduction through nasogastric or other tubes into the gastrointestinal (GI) tract, instillation into body cavities, and infusion into subcutaneous tissues (hypodermoclysis)[2] or bone marrow (intraosseous).[3] The amount and type of intake can be manipulated deliberately to maintain fluid and electrolyte balance. Habit,

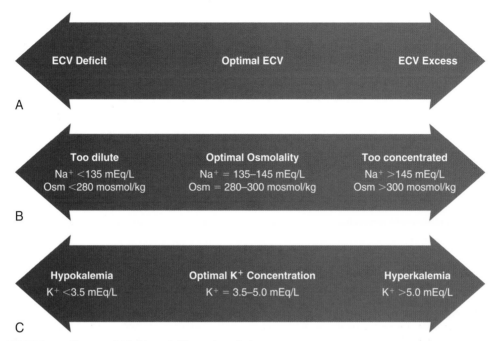

FIGURE 8.1 Scope of Fluid and Electrolyte Balance. (A) Scope of extracellular fluid volume *(ECV)* balance. (B) Scope of body fluid osmolality balance. (C) Scope of electrolyte balance. Potassium (K⁺) is used as an example.

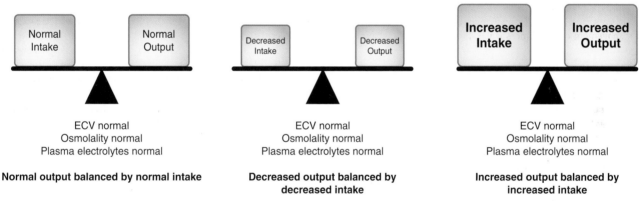

FIGURE 8.2 Optimal Balance of Fluid and Electrolytes With Fluid and Electrolyte Output Balanced by Intake. *ECV,* extracellular fluid volume.

anticipation of need for fluid, and thirst are strong influences on oral fluid intake. The most important stimulus to thirst is increased osmolality of body fluids, although dry oral mucous membranes, angiotensin II, angiotensin III, and arterial baroreceptor stimulation during severe hypovolemia also trigger thirst.[4]

Fluid and electrolytes that enter the body by all routes except IV must be absorbed into the bloodstream. IV fluid and electrolytes do not need absorption because they enter the bloodstream directly. Absorption is especially important to consider for oral intake of the electrolytes Ca^{2+} and Mg^{2+}, which have specialized absorption mechanisms in the intestines. Ca^{2+} absorption in the duodenum, its most important absorptive site, is dependent on adequate availability of vitamin D.[1] A healthy intestinal epithelium in the terminal section of the ileum is necessary for Mg^{2+} absorption. If fluid and electrolytes are not absorbed, they remain in the GI tract and leave the body in the feces.

Distribution

After fluid and electrolytes enter the blood, they are distributed to various body compartments. Normal fluid and electrolyte distribution is necessary for optimal function. The process of filtration distributes the ECF between the two major extracellular compartments: vascular and interstitial. The process of osmosis distributes water between the ECF and cells because of osmotic forces. Numerous factors distribute electrolytes between the ECF and electrolyte pools.[5]

Fluid Distribution Between Vascular and Interstitial Compartments

Fluid distribution between the vascular and interstitial compartments occurs by *filtration*, the net result of simultaneous opposing forces at the capillary level. Two forces tend to move fluid out of capillaries and two other forces tend to move fluid into capillaries.[1] The forces that are stronger at any particular time determine which way the fluid moves. *Hydrostatic pressure* pushes fluid out of its compartment. Capillary blood hydrostatic pressure (a relatively strong force) pushes fluid out of the capillaries; interstitial fluid hydrostatic pressure (a relatively weak force) pushes fluid out of the interstitial compartment back into capillaries. *Colloid osmotic pressure*, caused by large protein particles in the fluid, pulls fluid into its compartment. Thus capillary blood colloid osmotic pressure (normally a relatively strong force) pulls fluid into the capillaries; interstitial fluid colloid osmotic pressure (normally a very weak force) pulls fluid out of the capillaries and into the interstitial compartment. With normal fluid distribution, the net result of these opposing forces filters some of the ECF from capillaries into the interstitial compartment at the arterial end of capillaries, bringing oxygen and nutrients to cells. At the venous end of capillaries, some interstitial fluid filters back into the capillaries, carrying waste products to be excreted.

Water Distribution Between Extracellular and Intracellular Fluid

The structure of cell membranes allows water to cross the membrane readily, but Na^+ enters with difficulty. This is the reason why cell membranes are called *semipermeable*. The process of *osmosis* is the movement of water across a semipermeable membrane that separates compartments with different concentrations of particles. As noted previously, the osmolality of a fluid is its degree of concentration. Technically it is the number of particles per kilogram of water.[1] Osmosis occurs almost instantaneously when the osmolality changes on one side of the semipermeable cell membrane. This rapid equilibration keeps the ECF and intracellular fluid at the same osmolality.

Electrolyte Distribution

With the exception of Na^+, which has a high ECF concentration that reflects osmolality, electrolytes have low concentrations in the ECF compared with their concentrations in electrolyte pools.[5] The K^+ pool is inside cells; it contains almost 98% of total body potassium.[5,6] Bone is an important Ca^{2+} pool. Mg^{2+} pools are inside cells and in bones.[7] Physiologically inactive forms of Ca^{2+} and Mg^{2+} bound to albumin or organic anions such as citrate can also be considered electrolyte pools.[8]

Numerous opposing factors influence the distribution of electrolytes between the ECF and the electrolyte pools. For example, two hormones influence Ca^{2+} distribution: parathyroid hormone (PTH) from the parathyroid glands and calcitonin from the thyroid. Calcitonin moves Ca^{2+} into bone; PTH shifts Ca^{2+} from bone into the ECF.[1,9] Unusual amounts of factors that shift electrolytes can alter their distribution and cause plasma electrolyte deficits or excesses, which are discussed later in this chapter.

Output

The normal excretory routes of fluid and electrolytes are renal (urine), gastrointestinal (feces), through the skin (insensible perspiration and sweat), and the lungs (water vapor). Some of these routes (urine, sweat, and, to some degree, feces) are regulated physiologically to maintain optimal balance, but the regulatory mechanisms can be overwhelmed. Other excretory routes, including insensible water exiting through skin and lungs, are mandatory, regardless of fluid balance.[1] Insensible water excretion increases when a person has a fever. Abnormal routes of fluid and electrolyte output include emesis, hemorrhage, drainage through tubes or fistulas, and other routes of fluid and electrolyte loss often seen in clinical situations.[5] These abnormal output routes do not have physiological regulatory mechanisms.

Renal excretion provides the largest output of fluid and electrolytes in normal circumstances. The hormone aldosterone (along with natriuretic peptides not discussed in this concept presentation) regulates renal excretion of Na^+ and water (isotonic fluid), whereas antidiuretic hormone (ADH) regulates the excretion of water.[1] Aldosterone increases the renal excretion of K^+ directly and probably Mg^{2+} indirectly.[10]

Aldosterone

The adrenal cortex secretes aldosterone in response to angiotensin II, one of the components of the renin-angiotensin system. When the ECV is low, the resulting decreased blood flow through the renal arteries increases the release of renin, formation of angiotensin I, and then formation of angiotensin II, thus increasing aldosterone secretion. Aldosterone acts on the kidneys to remove Na^+ and water from the renal tubules and return them to the blood, which restores or even expands the ECV.[1] The liver cells normally metabolize aldosterone, which stops its action. Decreased renin release or damage to the adrenal cortex will decrease aldosterone secretion, thus increasing renal Na^+ and water excretion. Aldosterone is the major hormonal regulator of ECV.[1] Conditions involving excessive or insufficient secretion of aldosterone cause ECV imbalances.

Aldosterone also facilitates renal excretion of K^+. Increased concentration of plasma K^+ stimulates aldosterone secretion, which causes the kidneys to excrete more K^+ and helps return the plasma K^+ concentration to normal. If plasma K^+ concentration decreases, aldosterone secretion is suppressed and the kidneys excrete less potassium. Another influence on renal excretion of K^+ is the amount of flow in the distal nephrons, where K^+ is secreted into renal tubular fluid. More flow in the distal nephrons increases K^+ output in urine.[6] This situation is clinically important with osmotic diuresis and with the use of potassium-wasting diuretics, both of which cause excessive K^+ output. Cortisol and other glucocorticoids have some aldosterone-like action on the kidneys.

Antidiuretic Hormone

ADH regulates renal excretion of water but not Na^+. Its name describes its action on the kidneys; the antidiuretic effect removes water from the renal distal tubules and collecting ducts and returns it to the blood, which dilutes the ECV and other body fluids. The posterior pituitary normally releases ADH at a level that maintains osmolality (degree of concentration) within normal limits. When body fluids become too concentrated (osmolality too high), osmosensitive cells in the hypothalamus trigger more release of ADH from the posterior pituitary. Increased renal action of ADH retains more water and dilutes body fluids back to their normal osmolality.[1] On the other hand, when body fluids become too dilute (osmolality too low), the osmosensitive cells in the hypothalamus suppress release of ADH from the posterior pituitary. Less ADH action on the kidneys allows more water excretion in the urine and concentrates body fluids back to their normal osmolality. The serum Na^+ concentration usually reflects the osmolality of body fluids. Conditions that cause excessive or deficient ADH release cause plasma Na^+ concentration imbalances.

Age-Related Differences
Infants and Children

Neonates and infants are not able to communicate thirst except by crying, which can affect their fluid intake if their caregivers are not vigilant. They also have a high percentage of body weight as water and more ECF than intracellular fluid. As infants grow, creating more cells, the percentage of body weight as water decreases and the amount of intracellular fluid exceeds the amount of ECF. Those conditions persist throughout the rest of the lifespan. Because both neonates and infants have large body and lung surface areas compared with body mass, they have higher fluid exchange ratios than any other age group. In addition, neonates and infants have immature kidneys that have little reserve capacity, reaching maturation only during childhood.[11]

Older Adults

The thirst sensation is blunted in older adults. Thus they may have a decreased fluid intake because the osmolality of their body fluids can rise higher before they become thirsty.[12] Older adults also have a decreased lean body mass, which decreases the percentage of their body weight that is water compared with that of young and middle-aged adults. Although older adults who do not have renal disease have functioning kidneys, they have decreased renal reserve due to the decrease in the number of nephrons that occurs with normal aging.

VARIATIONS AND CONTEXT

As mentioned previously, the primary problems are imbalance of fluids and imbalance of electrolytes (see Fig. 8.1). The term *imbalance* is often used to indicate disrupted fluid or electrolyte balance. Fluid imbalances can reflect imbalance of fluid volume or imbalance of fluid concentration. Any electrolyte can be out of balance, but for the purposes of this concept presentation, the two most important electrolytes are sodium and potassium. This section explains the categories of imbalances and the common causes that lead to imbalances.

Categories of Fluid and Electrolyte Imbalances
Extracellular Fluid Volume Imbalances

As the name indicates, ECV imbalances are abnormal amounts of fluid in the extracellular compartment (vascular plus interstitial). Fluid that has the same effective concentration as normal body fluid is called isotonic fluid.[1] Normal ECF is isotonic Na^+-containing fluid. The Na^+ is necessary to hold the water in the extracellular compartment.

There are two types of ECV imbalances. ECV deficit is too little Na^+-containing isotonic fluid in the extracellular compartment; ECV excess is too much Na^+-containing isotonic ECF. With ECV imbalances, the amount of isotonic fluid changes but its concentration remains the same unless an osmolality imbalance is present at the same time.

Osmolality Imbalances

Osmolality imbalances are changes in the degree of concentration of body fluid. If osmolality changes, it equilibrates rapidly between ECF and intracellular fluid as a result of osmotic shifts of water across cell membranes. Although osmolality can be measured directly, in many clinical settings it is tracked using the serum Na^+ concentration, which usually rises or falls in parallel with osmolality.[13] Na^+ stays in the ECF when water moves into or out of cells, which is why the serum Na^+ concentration changes when the osmolality changes.

There are two types of osmolality imbalances: hypernatremia and hyponatremia. Hypernatremia (increased serum Na^+ concentration) indicates that body fluids are too concentrated (osmolality is too high). Hyponatremia (decreased serum Na^+ concentration) indicates that body fluids are too dilute (osmolality is too low).[13] Osmolality imbalances can occur alone or with ECV imbalances. The combination of ECV deficit and hypernatremia is known as clinical dehydration.[5]

Electrolyte Imbalances

Electrolyte imbalances are abnormal plasma concentrations of electrolytes such as K^+, Ca^{2+}, and Mg^{2+}. Although Na^+ is also an electrolyte, its concentration reflects the osmolality, as discussed previously. Electrolyte concentrations are measured from blood samples and do not necessarily correlate with the concentrations inside cells.

There are two types of electrolyte imbalances: deficits and excesses in plasma concentration. Names of electrolyte imbalances are constructed from a prefix that indicates whether the concentration is too low (*hypo-*) or too high (*hyper-*), a combining form that indicates the specific electrolyte involved (e.g., *-kal-* for K^+, *-calc-* for Ca^{2+}, and *-magnes-* for Mg^{2+}), and the suffix *-emia* that signifies "in the blood." Electrolyte imbalances can occur alone or with ECV and/or osmolality imbalances.

Causes of Fluid and Electrolyte Disturbances

Practically speaking, there are only three overarching causes leading to fluid and electrolyte imbalances. All of these imbalances involve at least one of the following conditions:

- Fluid and electrolyte output is *greater than* intake and absorption.
- Fluid and electrolyte output is *less than* intake and absorption.
- Fluid and electrolyte distribution is altered.

Output Greater Than Intake and Absorption

When fluid and electrolyte output is greater than intake and absorption, ECV deficit, increased osmolality (hypernatremia), and various plasma electrolyte deficits can occur (Fig. 8.3). Two situations cause output to exceed intake and absorption (see Fig. 8.3A):

- Normal output but deficient intake or absorption
- Increased output not balanced by increased intake

Normal output but deficient intake or absorption. Body fluid output through the combination of urine, feces, skin, and respirations is dilute Na^+-containing fluid. Therefore daily intake of some Na^+ and considerable water is necessary to maintain optimal fluid balance. Although the kidneys are able to reduce their fluid output to some degree in response to decreased fluid intake, some renal output is obligatory, as is water output through the skin and from the lungs (respiration).[1,13] When intake is less than normal output, the fluid imbalance a person develops depends on the type of fluid that is deficient. For example, people who do not drink enough water to match their water output can make their body fluids too concentrated (osmolality too high; hypernatremia). See hypernatremia in Box 8.1 for examples.

Deficient electrolyte intake and absorption with normal output can cause plasma electrolyte deficits such as hypokalemia or hypomagnesemia. Box 8.2 lists specific causes of electrolyte deficits due to normal output but decreased intake or absorption.

Increased output not balanced by increased intake. Another situation in which fluid and electrolyte output becomes greater than intake arises when output increases but intake does not increase enough to balance it. For example, diarrhea increases output of Na^+, water, and K^+. During diarrhea, an intake of Na^+, water, and K^+ that does not balance the increased output creates a high risk for ECV deficit, increased osmolality (hypernatremia), and hypokalemia.[13] Boxes 8.1 and 8.2 show other examples of imbalances due to increased output not balanced by increased intake. To prevent these imbalances, fluid and electrolyte intake must increase to balance increased output.

Output Less Than Intake and Absorption

When fluid and electrolyte output is less than intake and absorption, ECV excess, decreased osmolality (hyponatremia), and plasma electrolyte excesses can occur. Two situations cause intake to be greater than output (Fig. 8.3B):

- Output less than excessive or too rapid intake
- Decreased output not balanced by decreased intake

Output less than excessive or too rapid intake. Individuals with normal renal function may overwhelm their output capacity by excessive or very rapid intake of fluid and electrolytes. This situation most commonly occurs with IV infusions. Any person receiving IV fluid is at risk for developing fluid and electrolyte imbalances from excessive or too rapid infusion of the solution, even if the infusion is intended to replace a fluid or electrolyte deficit. The specific imbalance that

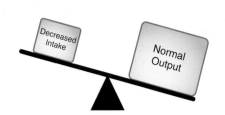

ECV deficit
Osmolality too high
Plasma electrolyte deficits

A **Normal output but deficient intake or absorption**

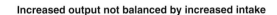
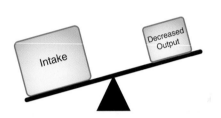

ECV deficit
Osmolality too high
Plasma electrolyte deficits

Increased output not balanced by increased intake

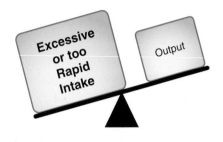

ECV excess
Osmolality too low
Plasma electrolyte excesses

B **Output less than excessive or too rapid intake**

ECV excess
Osmolality too low
Plasma electrolyte excesses

Decreased output not balanced by decreased intake

FIGURE 8.3 Disrupted Balance of Fluid and Electrolytes. (A) Imbalance from fluid and electrolyte output greater than intake and absorption. (B) Imbalance from fluid and electrolyte output less than intake and absorption. *ECV,* extracellular fluid volume.

develops depends on the type of IV solution being administered.[14] Nurses must be especially alert when infusing IV solutions that contain K^+ because hyperkalemia caused by too rapid infusion can cause dangerous cardiac dysrhythmias.[10,13]

Excessive oral intake that overwhelms normal output mechanisms is also possible. The most common example is the mild ECV excess that occurs when people eat salty foods and drink water. They may notice that their rings or shoes feel tight and that they have gained weight overnight. These changes resolve in a day or two as the kidneys excrete the excess Na^+ and water. People who have conditions that cause chronic ECV excess, such as severe cirrhosis, often are prescribed Na^+-restricted diets to avoid exacerbating their ECV excess.[15]

When people drink a lot of water without salt, they normally produce less antidiuretic hormone and their kidneys excrete the extra water. However, massive rapid oral intake of water can overwhelm renal water excretion capacity and make body fluids too dilute (osmolality too low; hyponatremia).[16,17] See hyponatremia in Box 8.1 for examples. Oral intake of electrolyte-rich foods by people who have normal renal function is usually not a problem because the kidneys excrete any excess.

Decreased output not balanced by decreased intake. People who have oliguria from any cause have decreased output of fluid and electrolytes; they must decrease their intake to prevent imbalances. For example, people who have oliguric renal disease develop ECV excess, hyperkalemia, and hypermagnesemia unless their intake is decreased appropriately.[13] See other examples in Boxes 8.1 and 8.2.

Combining excessive or too rapid intake of fluid and electrolytes with decreased output creates a potentially dangerous situation in which imbalances can develop rapidly. An IV solution that infuses excess amounts or too rapidly into an individual who is oliguric can cause life-threatening ECV excess (Na^+-containing fluid) or hyperkalemia (K^+-containing fluid).[5,13,15]

Altered Fluid and Electrolyte Distribution

Alterations of distribution, the process of moving fluid and electrolytes between their various compartments, can create fluid or electrolyte imbalances (Fig. 8.4):

- Shift of vascular fluid into the interstitial space causes edema.
- Rapid shift of ECF into a "third space" can create ECV deficit.
- Electrolyte shift from ECF into an electrolyte pool causes plasma electrolyte deficits.
- Electrolyte shift from an electrolyte pool into ECF causes plasma electrolyte excesses.

Shift of vascular fluid into interstitial space. As explained previously, fluid distribution between the vascular and interstitial compartments occurs by filtration, the net result of simultaneous opposing forces at the capillary level. Altered filtration can allow too much fluid to accumulate in the interstitial compartment, which is called edema. For example, ECV excess causes edema by increasing the capillary blood hydrostatic pressure. Inflammation causes edema because it involves local vasodilation (increases capillary blood hydrostatic pressure) and increased microvascular permeability (protein leakage increases the interstitial fluid colloid osmotic pressure). The edema of hypoalbuminemia is caused by decreased blood colloid osmotic pressure.

Rapid extracellular fluid shift into "third space." The term *third space* refers to a location where ECF accumulates abnormally (becomes misplaced)—a location that is neither the vascular nor the interstitial

BOX 8.1 Causes of Disrupted Fluid Balance

ECV Deficit (Too Little Extracellular Volume)
Normal Output but Deficient Intake of Na⁺ and Water

- Lack of access to Na⁺ and water

Increased Output Not Balanced by Increased Intake of Na⁺ and Water

- Vomiting
- Acute or chronic diarrhea from any cause, including laxative abuse
- Draining GI fistula, gastric suction, or intestinal decompression
- Hemorrhage or burns
- Overuse of diuretics
- Lack of aldosterone (adrenal insufficiency, Addison disease)

Rapid Fluid Shift From ECV Into a Third Space

- Acute intestinal obstruction
- Ascites that develops rapidly

ECV Excess (Too Much Extracellular Volume)
Output Less Than Excessive or Too Rapid Intake of Na⁺ and Water

- Excessive IV infusion of Na⁺-containing isotonic solution (0.9% NaCl, Ringer)
- High oral intake of salty foods and water with renal retention of Na⁺ and water

Decreased Output Not Balanced by Decreased Intake of Na⁺ and Water

- Oliguria (e.g., acute kidney injury, acute glomerulonephritis, end-stage renal disease)

- Aldosterone excess (e.g., cirrhosis, chronic heart failure, primary hyperaldosteronism)
- High levels of glucocorticoids (e.g., corticosteroid therapy, Cushing disease)

Hypernatremia (Body Fluids Too Concentrated; Osmolality Too High)
Normal Output but Deficient Intake of Water

- No access to water or inability to respond to or communicate thirst (e.g., aphasia, coma, infancy)
- Tube feeding without additional water intake

Increased Output Not Balanced by Increased Intake of Water

- Vomiting or diarrhea with replacement of Na⁺ but not enough water
- Diabetes insipidus (lack of antidiuretic hormone)

Hyponatremia (Body Fluids Too Dilute; Osmolality Too Low)
Output Less Than Excessive or Too Rapid Intake of Water

- IV 5% dextrose in water (D₅W) infusion with excess rate or amount
- Rapid oral ingestion of massive amounts of water (e.g., child abuse, club initiation, psychiatric disorder)
- Overuse of tap water enemas or hypotonic irrigating solutions
- Massive replacement of water without Na⁺ during vomiting or diarrhea

Decreased Output Not Balanced by Decreased Intake of Water

- Excessive antidiuretic hormone

ECV, Extracellular fluid volume; GI, gastrointestinal.

BOX 8.2 Causes of Disrupted Electrolyte Balance

Hypokalemia (Plasma K⁺ Deficit)
Normal Output but Deficient K⁺ Intake

- Prolonged anorexia or diet lacking K⁺-rich foods
- No oral intake plus IV solutions not containing K⁺

Increased Output Not Balanced by Increased K⁺ Intake

- Vomiting
- Acute or chronic diarrhea from any cause, including laxative abuse
- Use of K⁺-wasting diuretics or other drugs that increase renal K⁺ excretion
- Excessive aldosterone effect (e.g., large amounts of black licorice, cirrhosis, chronic heart failure, primary hyperaldosteronism)
- High levels of glucocorticoids (e.g., corticosteroid therapy, Cushing disease)

Rapid K⁺ Shift From ECF Into Cells

- Alkalosis, excessive β-adrenergic stimulation, or excessive insulin

Hyperkalemia (Plasma K⁺ Excess)
Output Less Than Excessive or Too Rapid K⁺ Intake

- IV K⁺ infusion with excess rate or amount
- Massive transfusion (>8 U for adults) of stored blood

Decreased Output Not Balanced by Decreased K⁺ Intake

- Oliguria (e.g., severe hypovolemia, circulatory shock, acute kidney injury, end-stage renal disease)
- Use of K⁺-sparing diuretics, angiotensin-converting enzyme (ACE) inhibitors, or other drugs that decrease renal K⁺ excretion
- Lack of aldosterone (e.g., adrenal insufficiency, Addison disease)

Rapid K⁺ Shift From Cells Into ECF

- Lack of insulin or acidosis due to mineral acids
- Massive sudden cell death (e.g., crushing injuries, tumor lysis syndrome)

Hypocalcemia (Plasma Ca²⁺ Deficit)
Normal Output but Deficient Ca²⁺ Intake or Absorption

- Diet lacking Ca²⁺-rich foods
- Poor Ca²⁺ absorption (e.g., chronic diarrhea, lack of vitamin D)

Increased Output Not Balanced by Increased Ca²⁺ Intake and Absorption

- Steatorrhea (binds Ca²⁺ in GI secretions as well as dietary Ca²⁺)

Ca²⁺ Shift From ECF Into Bone or Physiologically Unavailable Form

- Hypoparathyroidism
- Large load of citrate from massive blood transfusion (binds Ca²⁺)
- Alkalosis (more Ca²⁺ binds albumin) or elevated plasma phosphate level
- Acute pancreatitis (Ca²⁺ binds necrotic fat in abdomen)

Hypercalcemia (Plasma Ca²⁺ Excess)
Output Less Than Excessive Ca²⁺ Intake and Absorption

- Vitamin D or Ca²⁺ overdose (includes shark cartilage supplements)

Decreased Output Not Balanced by Decreased Ca²⁺ Intake

- Use of thiazide diuretics

Continued

BOX 8.2 Causes of Disrupted Electrolyte Balance—cont'd

Ca²⁺ Shift From Bone Into ECF
- Hyperparathyroidism
- Cancers that secrete bone-resorbing factors

Hypomagnesemia (Plasma Mg²⁺ Deficit)
Normal Output but Deficient Mg²⁺ Intake or Absorption
- Diet lacking Mg²⁺-rich foods
- Poor Mg²⁺ absorption (e.g., chronic diarrhea, ileal resection, chronic alcoholism)

Increased Output Not Balanced by Increased Mg²⁺ Intake and Absorption
- Prolonged vomiting, gastric suction, or draining GI fistula
- Steatorrhea (binds Mg²⁺ in GI secretions as well as dietary Mg²⁺)
- Use of diuretics or other drugs that increase urinary Mg²⁺

Mg²⁺ Shift Into Physiologically Unavailable Form
- Large load of citrate from massive blood transfusion (binds Mg²⁺)
- Alkalosis (more Mg²⁺ binds albumin)

Hypermagnesemia (Plasma Mg²⁺ Excess)
Output Less Than Excessive Mg²⁺ Intake and Absorption
- Overuse of Mg²⁺-containing laxatives or antacids

Decreased Output Not Balanced by Decreased Mg²⁺ Intake
- Chronic oliguric renal disease

Ca²⁺, calcium ions; *ECF*, extracellular fluid; *GI*, gastrointestinal; *IV*, intravenous; *K⁺*, potassium ions; *Mg²⁺*, magnesium ions.

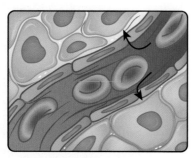

Shift of vascular fluid into the interstitial space

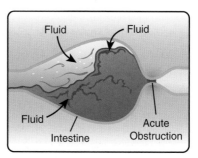

Rapid ECF shift into "third space"

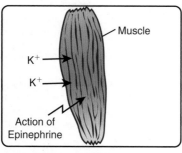

Electrolyte shift from ECF into its electrolyte pool

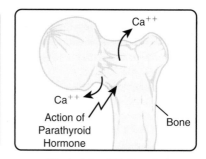

Electrolyte shift from its electrolyte pool into ECF

FIGURE 8.4 Imbalance From Altered Fluid and Electrolyte Distribution. *ECF*, extracellular fluid.

compartment. The peritoneal cavity and the intestinal lumen are examples of third spaces. ECF accumulating in the peritoneal cavity creates ascites. An acute intestinal obstruction may cause ECF to shift rapidly into the intestinal lumen (see Fig. 8.4). Rapid shift of ECF into a third space can cause ECV deficit. If the shift occurs gradually, there is time for the ECV to be replenished without causing symptomatic ECV deficit.

Electrolyte shift from **extracellular fluid into an electrolyte pool.** The electrolytes K⁺, Ca²⁺, and Mg²⁺ have low concentrations in the ECF and high concentrations in other locations, such as inside cells or in bone, that are called *electrolyte pools.* Many factors influence the distribution of these electrolytes between the ECF and their electrolyte pools, with some factors moving electrolytes from the ECF into their pools and others moving them in the opposite direction. Abnormal concentrations of the factors that shift electrolytes into their pools can cause plasma electrolyte deficits (see Fig. 8.4).[5] Although these distribution shifts may not change whole-body electrolyte concentration, they cause signs

and symptoms by changing the ratio of electrolytes inside and outside cells or the amount of physiologically active electrolyte. See hypokalemia, hypocalcemia, and hypomagnesemia in Box 8.2 for examples.

Electrolyte shift from an electrolyte pool into extracellular fluid. The factors that distribute electrolytes between the ECF and electrolyte pools can be altered in a way that shifts electrolytes from their pools into the ECF, causing plasma electrolyte excesses (see Fig. 8.4).[5] These distribution shifts may not change whole-body electrolyte concentration but cause signs and symptoms by changing the ratio of electrolytes inside and outside cells. See hyperkalemia and hypercalcemia in Box 8.2 for examples.

CONSEQUENCES

Disruptions of fluid and electrolyte balance have different physiological consequences, depending on the type of imbalance. ECV, K⁺, Mg²⁺, and

Ca^{2+} imbalances can interfere with perfusion and oxygenation. Osmolality imbalances impair cerebral function.[17,18] K^+, Mg^{2+}, and Ca^{2+} imbalances impair neuromuscular function.[5,9,19]

Impaired Perfusion and Oxygenation

A normal volume of ECF is necessary to provide tissue perfusion and oxygenate cells. Moderate or severe ECV deficit reduces tissue perfusion by decreasing arterial blood pressure (BP). Very severe ECV deficit leads to hypovolemic shock, a condition that severely impairs perfusion and oxygenation.[20] ECV excess can also impair oxygenation. Edema fluid from ECV excess pushes cells farther from capillaries, creating a larger distance for oxygen to diffuse before it reaches cells. This subtle change is part of the reason for the delayed healing of injuries to edematous tissue. A more dramatic example of impaired oxygenation from ECV excess is pulmonary edema that arises from sudden or very severe ECV excess. Fluid in the alveoli interferes with gas exchange and thus oxygenation.

K^+, Mg^{2+}, and Ca^{2+} imbalances can cause cardiac dysrhythmias, some of which can impair perfusion by reducing cardiac output.[9,10,13,19] Severe hyperkalemia causes cardiac arrest.[9]

Impaired Cerebral Function

Osmolality imbalances cause shriveling (hypernatremia) or swelling (hyponatremia) of cells, including brain cells. Impaired cerebral function occurs with either condition.[13] The most common cerebral impairment with osmolality imbalances is a decreased level of consciousness (LOC), which occurs on a continuum from drowsiness to coma. Seizures may occur if the osmolality changes very rapidly, rises very high, or falls very low.[13,15] Brain cell dysfunction caused by osmolality imbalances is reversible with a well-managed return of osmolality to normal, avoiding rapid changes that can injure fragile brain structures.[15,16]

Impaired Neuromuscular Function

Plasma concentration imbalances of K^+, Ca^{2+}, and Mg^{2+} impair neuromuscular function, although they do so in different ways. The ratio of K^+ inside to outside cells is a major determinant of resting membrane potential of muscle cells.[10] Plasma K^+ deficit and excess change the resting membrane potential of skeletal muscle by altering that ratio. Although the state of the resting potential is different in hypokalemia and hyperkalemia, the effect on skeletal muscles is similar: flaccid muscle weakness.[10,13]

Extracellular Ca^{2+} concentration is a major determinant of the speed of ion movement through the membranes of nerve and muscle cells. Mg^{2+} suppresses release of the neurotransmitter acetylcholine at neuromuscular junctions. Plasma concentration imbalances of Ca^{2+} and Mg^{2+} impair neuromuscular function by altering these processes. Plasma deficits of Ca^{2+} and Mg^{2+} increase neuromuscular excitability, which is why hypocalcemia and hypomagnesemia have similar signs and symptoms: muscle twitching and cramping, hyperactive reflexes, and seizures if very severe. In contrast, plasma excesses of Ca^{2+} and Mg^{2+} decrease neuromuscular excitability, causing similar manifestations of muscle weakness, depressed reflexes, and lethargy.[9,13,19]

RISK FACTORS

Populations at Risk

Optimal fluid and electrolyte balance is necessary for the physiological function for all individuals, regardless of race, culture, age, or socioeconomic status. Populations at greatest risk for imbalance are the very young and the very old. Preterm infants are at great risk for fluid and electrolyte disturbances due to their very immature kidneys and large surface area of skin and lungs; the degree of risk is related to the infant's weight and gestational age at the time of birth. Term infants and young

BOX 8.3   Common Risk Factors for Fluid and Electrolyte Disturbances

Conditions
- Vomiting
- Diarrhea
- Malabsorption
- Fever
- Inadequate or excessive intake of fluid or electrolytes
- Inadequate or excessive water intake

Adverse Effects From Medications
- Diuretics
- Laxatives
- Antacids
- Corticosteroids
- Infusion of IV fluids
- Blood transfusions

Acute Medical Conditions, Injury, and Trauma
- Hemorrhage
- Burns
- Crush injuries
- Head injuries
- Acute pancreatitis
- Acute kidney injury

Chronic Medical Conditions
- Heart failure
- Diabetes mellitus
- Cancer
- Chronic oliguric renal disease
- Chronic liver disease
- Chronic alcoholism
- Eating disorders (anorexia nervosa, bulimia)

children also have higher risk than adults due to immature kidneys, high metabolic rate, and large fluid exchange ratio.[11] Older adults have a blunted thirst sensation and decreased renal reserve due to a normal gradual loss of nephrons, which make them more susceptible to fluid and electrolyte disturbances.[12]

Individual Risk Factors

The greatest individual risk factors are associated with serious injury or significant health conditions. Because so many different disease processes and behaviors can disrupt fluid and electrolyte balance, it is more useful to think about risk factors in terms of what the disease or behavior is causing rather than focus on the disease itself. Nurses can deduce logically the individual risk factors for fluid and electrolyte imbalances by considering the dynamic interplay of the processes involved in fluid and electrolyte balance. Box 8.3 lists common situations and conditions that place an individual at risk for fluid and electrolyte imbalances.

ASSESSMENT

Assessments for fluid and electrolyte imbalances often occur in the context of other conditions that cause such imbalances. Nurses can use the risk factors for these imbalances to guide their assessment.

History

Because many of the presenting signs and symptoms of fluid and electrolyte imbalances have other causes, taking a careful history is

TABLE 8.1   Clinical Manifestations of Disrupted Fluid Balance

EXTRACELLULAR VOLUME IMBALANCES		OSMOLALITY IMBALANCES	
Too Little Volume (ECV Deficit)	Too Much Volume (ECV Excess)	Too Dilute (Hyponatremia)	Too Concentrated (Hypernatremia)
Sudden weight loss, skin tenting, dry mucous membranes, vascular underload: rapid thready pulse, postural BP drop with concurrent HR increase, lightheadedness, flat neck veins when supine, oliguria, syncope, circulatory shock if severe	Sudden weight gain, dependent edema, vascular overload: bounding pulse, distended neck veins when upright, dyspnea, pulmonary edema if severe	Impaired cerebral function: decreased LOC, nausea, seizures if severe; serum Na^+ <130 mEq/L	Impaired cerebral function: decreased LOC, thirst (less with older adults), seizures if severe; serum Na^+ >145 mEq/L

BP, blood pressure; *ECV*, extracellular fluid volume; *HR*, heart rate; *LOC*, level of consciousness.

TABLE 8.2   Clinical Manifestations of Disrupted Electrolyte Balance

PLASMA K^+ IMBALANCES		PLASMA Ca^{2+} IMBALANCES		PLASMA Mg^{2+} IMBALANCES	
Hypokalemia	Hyperkalemia	Hypocalcemia	Hypercalcemia	Hypomagnesemia	Hypermagnesemia
Bilateral ascending flaccid muscle weakness, abdominal distention, constipation, postural hypotension, polyuria, cardiac dysrhythmias; serum K^+ <3.5 mEq/L	Bilateral ascending flaccid muscle weakness, cardiac dysrhythmias, cardiac arrest if severe; serum K^+ >5.0 mEq/L	Increased neuromuscular excitability: positive Chvostek and Trousseau signs, muscle cramps, twitching, hyperactive reflexes, carpal and pedal spasms, tetany, seizures, laryngospasm, cardiac dysrhythmias; serum total Ca^{2+} <9 mg/dL (4.5 mEq/L)	Decreased neuromuscular excitability: anorexia, nausea, constipation, muscle weakness, diminished reflexes, decreased LOC, cardiac dysrhythmias; serum total Ca^{2+} >11 mg/dL (5.5 mEq/L)	Increased neuromuscular excitability: positive Chvostek and Trousseau signs, insomnia, hyperactive reflexes, muscle cramps and twitching, nystagmus, tetany, seizures, cardiac dysrhythmias; serum Mg^{2+} <1.5 mEq/L	Decreased neuromuscular excitability: flushing, diaphoresis, diminished reflexes, hypotension, decreased LOC, muscle weakness, respiratory depression, bradycardia, cardiac dysrhythmias; serum Mg^{2+} >2.5 mEq/L

LOC, level of consciousness.

important. The standard questions for history taking are not repeated here, but they are expected. In addition to focusing on renal, endocrine, or other conditions that may cause the fluid or electrolyte imbalance, the history must include questions regarding fluid and electrolyte intake and output. Recent vomiting or diarrhea should be explored as to frequency and quantity, as well as the type and quantity of water, Na^+, and K^+ replacement. Medication history, including dietary supplements, is an important focus because numerous medications influence fluid and electrolyte balance.[5,13,15]

Examination Findings

Clinical manifestations of fluid and electrolyte imbalances are often part of a larger clinical picture of the underlying disease process that caused the imbalance. For example, the ankle edema, bounding pulse, and distended neck veins caused by ECV excess in individuals who have heart failure will be noted as part of the wider cardiac, respiratory, and functional examination.[15] However, unless they are assessed specifically, the quadriceps muscle weakness and constipation of hypokalemia may escape detection until these manifestations become severe.

A specific assessment to detect or monitor ECV excess or deficit is weighing the person daily, because 1 L of body fluid weighs 1 kg (2.2 lb). A gain or loss of 1 or more kg in 24 hours for adults is a gain or loss of body fluid. A similar gain or loss in a longer period may be a change in body fat or muscle rather than fluid, so daily weights are necessary for assessing ECV changes.[21]

Astute clinicians incorporate assessment for the individual's most likely fluid and electrolyte imbalances into every physical assessment rather than waiting until the signs and symptoms become severe. For example, a person who has chronic diarrhea needs assessment for ECV

deficit, hypernatremia, hypokalemia, hypocalcemia, and hypomagnesemia in addition to assessments related to the cause of the diarrhea and its consequences on skin integrity.[5,13]

Table 8.1 and 8.2 present signs and symptoms of fluid and electrolyte imbalances. These manifestations arise from the physiological consequences described previously in this chapter. Interpretation of assessment findings may be complicated by the presence of acid–base imbalances (see Concept 9, Acid–Base Balance).

Diagnostic Tests

Diagnosis of ECV deficit and excess usually is made on the basis of history and clinical examination. Laboratory tests performed on blood samples provide the definitive diagnosis for osmolality and electrolyte imbalances. Normal ranges are provided in Tables 8.1 and 8.2.

CLINICAL MANAGEMENT

Primary and secondary prevention strategies as well as interventions for people who have fluid and electrolyte imbalances are useful in all clinical settings.

Primary Prevention

Primary prevention of fluid and electrolyte imbalances is based on the principle that intake must balance output to maintain optimal fluid and electrolyte balance. For example, teaching people to replace body fluid output from vomiting or diarrhea with Na^+-containing fluid can prevent ECV deficit. Teaching physically active individuals optimal fluid replacement during and after exercise can prevent both ECV deficit and hyponatremia.[22] Similarly, teaching individuals who take potassium-wasting diuretics how to increase their dietary K^+ intake and the importance of taking prescribed K^+ supplements helps prevent hypokalemia. Teaching for people who have oliguric renal disease focuses on decreasing their intake of Na^+, K^+, and Mg^{2+} because their output is decreased.[13]

In addition to teaching people how to maintain optimal fluid and electrolyte balance, nurses engage in primary prevention in clinical settings when they see risk factors for various imbalances and intervene to modify intake or output appropriately. For example, nurses provide accessible and palatable fluids at a patient's preferred temperature as an independent nursing intervention; they request an order for an antiemetic or antidiarrheal medication as a collaborative intervention.[23]

Secondary Prevention (Screening)

Screening to detect disrupted fluid and electrolyte balance is not performed in the general population except as part of a routine physical exam that would include assessment for physical signs of ECV excess or deficit and standard laboratory tests including measurement of serum Na^+, K^+, and Ca^{2+} levels.

Collaborative Interventions

Because fluid and electrolyte intake is easier to modify than output, interventions to restore optimal fluid and electrolyte balance often focus on intake, although diuretics or dialysis may be used to increase output in specific situations.[24]

Fluid and Electrolyte Support

ECV deficit, hypernatremia, and plasma electrolyte deficits are treated by fluid or electrolyte replacement and by treatment of any underlying cause. ECV deficit requires isotonic Na^+-containing fluid; hypernatremia requires water; and electrolyte deficit usually requires replacement of the deficient electrolyte.[13,25] A person who has clinical dehydration will need both isotonic Na^+-containing fluid and extra water. These fluids and electrolytes can be administered orally, by IV infusion, or through other routes, depending on patient status and the resources of the setting.[26] Nursing responsibilities during fluid and electrolyte replacement include safely administering the replacement, measuring fluid intake and output, monitoring for complications of therapy, and teaching patients and families about the therapy.[27,28]

Treatments for ECV excess, hyponatremia, and plasma electrolyte excesses usually involve some type of restriction: Na^+ restriction for ECV excess; water restriction for hyponatremia; and decreased intake of the electrolyte that is excessive.[13,15] Nurses must be sure that people know the reason for the restriction and receive culturally appropriate teaching regarding how to change their diet or fluid intake.[29] In addition to the appropriate restrictions, medications may be used to treat ECV excess, hyponatremia, and plasma electrolyte excesses.

Medication Management

In addition to the fluid and electrolyte replacements mentioned previously, people who have disrupted fluid and electrolyte balance may receive other medications. Depending on the situation, these medications are directed toward various goals: to treat the underlying cause (e.g., antiemetic for imbalances due to vomiting or vasopressin for ADH deficiency); to increase the output of fluid or electrolytes (e.g., diuretics for ECV excess or hyperkalemia); to shift electrolytes into their pools to decrease plasma concentration (e.g., insulin and glucose for acute hyperkalemia or calcitonin for acute hypercalcemia)[6,30]; or to counteract life-threatening effects of the imbalance (e.g., calcium salts to counteract the effect of hyperkalemia on cardiac function).[6] In addition, medications that can contribute to the individual's fluid and electrolyte imbalances must be discontinued or their dosage modified.

BOX 8.4   Nursing Interventions for People With Disrupted Fluid and Electrolyte Balance

- Provide safety and comfort.
- Facilitate oral intake if appropriate.
- Administer collaborative interventions:
  - Adjustment of fluid intake or output
  - Treatment of the underlying cause
- Monitor for complications of therapy.
- Teach how to prevent imbalances or when to seek help (if chronic imbalance).

Independent Nursing Interventions

Independent nursing interventions to provide safety and comfort are foundational for people who have fluid and electrolyte imbalances. For example, safety is high priority for patients with a decreased LOC due to osmolality imbalances or substantial muscle weakness from severe hypokalemia. Comfort measures are especially important for people who must restrict fluid or Na^+. People who have fluid restrictions frequently are uncomfortable from thirst. Interventions such as performing frequent oral hygiene, lubricating the lips, keeping fluids out of sight, providing the allowed liquids in insulated containers, and instructing people to swish fluids in their mouths before swallowing promote comfort during fluid restriction. Individuals who need to restrict Na^+ intake because of chronic ECV excess can be comforted with the knowledge that salt taste often changes after a few weeks of salt restriction, so that the food that seems tasteless at first probably will have a more enjoyable flavor in a few weeks.[15] Learning about herbs and spices can also be helpful to individuals restricting sodium.

Nurses use many different interventions to facilitate the oral intake of fluid. People who have mild ECV deficits need Na^+-containing fluid, but those who have mild hypernatremia need oral water intake. Nurses can make the appropriate fluids available frequently, provide fluids at the individual's preferred temperature, and teach patients to keep their own intake records. Increased fluid intake is also important for individuals with hypercalcemia to prevent renal damage. Teaching people how to prevent fluid and electrolyte imbalances by balancing output with appropriate intake is extremely important. Box 8.4 summarizes nursing interventions for people with disrupted fluid and electrolyte balances.

INTERRELATED CONCEPTS

The concept of fluid and electrolytes has many interrelationships with other concepts discussed in this book. Fluid and electrolytes and Acid–Base Balance are closely related; changes in one can cause changes in the other, and situations such as vomiting and diarrhea can lead to both. Hormonal Regulation has a powerful influence on fluid and electrolytes because of the significant role hormones play in maintaining balance. Nutrition greatly influences fluid and electrolyte intake. Elimination creates fluid and electrolyte output; changes in elimination, such as oliguria and diarrhea, can disrupt fluid and electrolyte balance. Fluid and electrolyte imbalances can influence Perfusion and Gas Exchange (ECV imbalances), Cognition (osmolality imbalances), and Mobility (electrolyte imbalances that cause muscle weakness). These interrelationships are illustrated in Fig. 8.5.

CLINICAL EXEMPLARS

An exemplar of optimal fluid and electrolyte balance is a person of any age whose fluid and electrolyte output is balanced by an appropriate type and amount of intake and whose fluid and electrolyte distributions

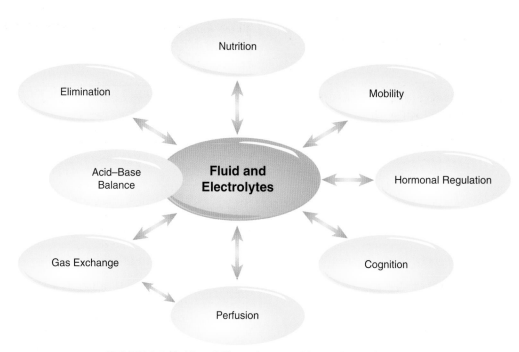

FIGURE 8.5 Fluid and Electrolytes and Interrelated Concepts.

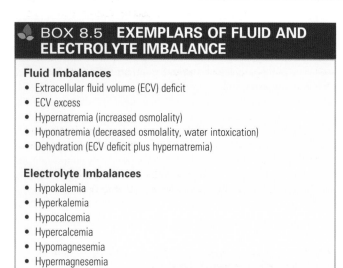

BOX 8.5 EXEMPLARS OF FLUID AND ELECTROLYTE IMBALANCE

Fluid Imbalances
- Extracellular fluid volume (ECV) deficit
- ECV excess
- Hypernatremia (increased osmolality)
- Hyponatremia (decreased osmolality, water intoxication)
- Dehydration (ECV deficit plus hypernatremia)

Electrolyte Imbalances
- Hypokalemia
- Hyperkalemia
- Hypocalcemia
- Hypercalcemia
- Hypomagnesemia
- Hypermagnesemia

ACCESS EXEMPLAR LINKS IN YOUR GIDDENS EBOOK

are normal. This person has ECV, osmolality, and plasma electrolyte values within the normal range.

Box 8.5 lists exemplars of disrupted fluid and electrolyte balance. Using the general individual risk factors presented previously in this concept presentation, nurses can understand the risk factors for each exemplar. For example, hypokalemia can occur from normal output at the same time as deficient K^+ intake, increased output not balanced by increased K^+ intake, or rapid K^+ shift from ECF into cells. Specific causes of each exemplar are organized in Boxes 8.1 and 8.2 under these general individual risk factors.

Featured Exemplars

Extracellular Volume Excess

ECV excess is too much fluid volume in the vascular and interstitial compartments. Signs and symptoms of ECV excess include weight gain of 1 kg or more in 24 hours for an adult, distended neck veins when upright (vascular fluid overload), and dependent edema (interstitial

fluid overload). People at high risk for ECV excess often have decreased excretion of Na^+ and water because they have oliguria or excessive amounts of aldosterone. For example, chronic heart failure decreases cardiac output, which stimulates excessive renin release, which then increases aldosterone secretion, causing ECV excess.[15] People who receive IV isotonic Na^+-containing solutions also develop ECV excess if the infusion is excessive.

Dehydration

Dehydration is the clinical combination of ECV deficit and hypernatremia, although the term is sometimes used loosely in clinical settings to indicate ECV deficit alone. ECV deficit is not enough fluid volume in the vascular and interstitial compartments; hypernatremia is abnormally increased serum Na^+ concentration, denoting increased body fluid osmolality (too concentrated). Clinical dehydration causes signs and symptoms of both conditions: weight loss of 1 kg or more in 24 hours for an adult, rapid thready pulse, postural hypotension, and flat neck veins when supine (vascular fluid underload); skin tenting (interstitial fluid underload); and decreased level of consciousness caused by osmotic shift of water out of brain cells. Although dehydration may occur in people of any age, those with highest risk for clinical dehydration are infants, children, and older adults who have gastroenteritis (vomiting and diarrhea) and whose fluid and Na^+ output is not replaced sufficiently.[26]

Hyponatremia

Hyponatremia is abnormally decreased serum Na^+ concentration; body fluids have decreased osmolality (are too dilute). Water moves into cells by osmosis, causing them to swell. Swollen brain cells impair cerebral function, the basis of the signs and symptoms of hyponatremia.[7] People with a high risk of hyponatremia usually have had a rapid intake of large amounts of water that overwhelms their ability to excrete it renally. For example, they may receive too much intravenous 5% dextrose in water (D_5W) or drink massive amounts of water in a few hours.[13,16,17] People who secrete excessive ADH also develop hyponatremia because ADH causes renal retention of water that dilutes the blood.[18,31]

Hypokalemia

Hypokalemia is abnormally decreased plasma K^+ concentration. Intracellular K^+ may be low, normal, or even high. Skeletal muscle weakness, constipation, and cardiac dysrhythmias occur from the abnormal K^+ distribution. People at high risk for hypokalemia usually have increased K^+ output that they have not balanced with increased K^+ intake. For example, diarrhea increases fecal K^+ output; aldosterone excess, K^+-wasting diuretics, and cortisol excess all increase renal K^+ output.[6,10,15] Other people at high risk for hypokalemia have chronically low K^+ intake or rapid shifts of K^+ from the ECF into cells.[32]

Hypercalcemia

Hypercalcemia is abnormally increased plasma Ca^{2+} concentration. Signs and symptoms include constipation and decreased LOC. People at high risk for hypercalcemia usually have a shift of Ca^{2+} from their bones into the ECF. The two most common examples are hyperparathyroidism and cancer that secretes circulating substances that act like PTH and remove Ca^{2+} from bones.[29,33]

Hypomagnesemia

Hypomagnesemia is an abnormally decreased plasma Mg^{2+} concentration. It increases neuromuscular excitability, causing muscle cramps, hyperactive reflexes, cardiac dysrhythmias, and even seizures, depending on its severity.[34] The people most at risk for hypomagnesemia have low Mg^{2+} intake or absorption or have increased Mg^{2+} output that is not balanced by increased Mg^{2+} intake. For example, people who abuse alcohol on a chronic basis are at very high risk for hypomagnesemia from a combination of decreased Mg^{2+} intake, Mg^{2+} malabsorption, and increased Mg^{2+} output through vomiting and increased renal excretion.[34] People who receive massive citrated blood transfusions are also at high risk for hypomagnesemia because the citrate binds Mg^{2+}, making it physiologically unavailable.[8]

CASE STUDY

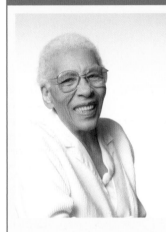

Case Presentation

Mrs. Malone, age 83 years, lives in an apartment with her cat. She has hypertension, hyperlipidemia, and chronic heart failure, which are managed with the diuretic furosemide, KCl, several other medications, and dietary Na^+ restriction. Mrs. Malone volunteers at a nearby elementary school, where earlier in the week several students were sent home sick after vomiting. Mrs. Malone developed vomiting and diarrhea. Although the vomiting stopped, the diarrhea persisted. She drank more water than usual, ate rice and dry toast, and stopped taking her KCl to avoid upsetting her stomach. After 2 days of diarrhea, Mrs. Malone became lightheaded when she got out of bed and had difficulty standing up after using the toilet because her legs were so weak. She telephoned her nurse practitioner (NP), who advised her to drink some broth with salt in it as well as some orange juice. Mrs. Malone needed considerable teaching regarding the importance of Na^+ intake to replace her increased Na^+ output in diarrhea, but eventually she did agree to try the rehydration schedule her NP advised. After checking back by telephone later in the day and learning that Mrs. Malone was no longer lightheaded but still had "weak legs," the NP advised Mrs. Malone to restart her KCl, continue drinking orange juice, and make an appointment to have her plasma K^+ concentration checked.

Case Analysis Questions

1. Review Fig. 8.1. Based on the information presented in the case, where do you suspect Mrs. Malone falls on the ECV and potassium continuums?
2. What risk factors for fluid and electrolyte balance does Mrs. Malone have?
3. Describe the mechanisms that led to her fluid and electrolyte imbalances.

From Barbara Penoyar/Photodisc/Thinkstock.

🔷 ACCESS EXEMPLAR LINKS IN YOUR GIDDENS EBOOK

REFERENCES

1. Hall, J. E. (2016). *Guyton and Hall textbook of medical physiology* (13th ed.). Philadelphia: Saunders.
2. Santillanes, G., & Rose, E. (2018). Evaluation and management of dehydration in children. *Emergency Medicine Clinics of North America, 36*(14), 259.
3. Whitney, R., & Langhan, M. (2017). Vascular access in pediatric patients in the emergency department: Types of access, indications, and complications. *Pediatric Emergency Medicine Practice, 14*(6), 1.
4. Gizowski, C., & Bourgue, C. W. (2018). The neural basis of homeostatic and anticipatory thirst. *Nature Reviews. Nephrology, 14*, 11.
5. Felver, L. (2019). Fluid and electrolyte homeostasis and imbalances. In J. L. Banasik & L. C. Copstead (Eds.), *Pathophysiology* (6th ed.). St Louis: Saunders.
6. Kovesdy, C. P., Appel, L. J., Grams, M. E., et al. (2017). Potassium homeostasis in health and disease: A scientific workshop cosponsored by the national kidney foundation and the American society of hypertension. *American Journal of Kidney Diseases, 70*, 844.
7. Costello, R. B., & Nielsen, F. (2017). Interpreting magnesium status to enhance clinical care: Key indicators. *Current Opinion in Clinical Nutrition and Metabolic Care, 20*, 504.
8. Lim, F., Chen, L. L., & Borski, D. (2017). Managing hypocalcemia in massive blood transfusion. *Nursing, 47*(5), 26.
9. Turner, J. J. P. (2017). Hypercalcemia - presentation and management. *Clinical Medicine (London, England), 17*, 270.
10. Rodan, A. L. (2017). Potassium: Friend or foe? *Pediatric Nephrology (Berlin, Germany), 32*, 1109.
11. Blackburn, S. (2018). *Maternal, fetal, and neonatal physiology* (5th ed.). Philadelphia: Elsevier.
12. Begg, D. P. (2017). Disturbances of thirst and fluid balance associated with aging. *Physiology & Behavior, 176*, 28.
13. Kamel, K., & Halperin, M. (2017). *Fluid, electrolyte, and acid–base physiology* (5th ed.). St. Louis: Elsevier.
14. Okada, M., Egi, M., Yokota, Y., et al. (2017). Comparison of the incidence of hyponatremia in adult postoperative critically ill patients receiving intravenous maintenance fluid with 140 mmol/L or 35 mmol/L of sodium: Retrospective before/after observational study. *Journal of Anesthesia, 31*, 657.
15. Jameson, J. L., Fauci, A., Kasper, D. K., et al. (2019). *Harrison's principles of internal medicine* (20th ed.). New York: McGraw-Hill.
16. Boehm, E., Kumar, S., Nankervis, A., & Colman, P. (2017). Managing hyponatremia secondary to primary polydipsia: Beware too rapid correction of hyponatremia. *Internal Medicine Journal, 47*, 956.
17. Pai, R., Das, L., Dutta, P., & Bhansali, A. (2017). Secondary parkinsonism in a patient of psychogenic polydipsia. *BMJ Case Reports, 2017.*

18. Filippatos, T. D., Makri, A., Elisaf, M. S., et al. (2017). Hyponatremia in the elderly: Challenges and solutions. *Clinical Interventions in Aging, 12,* 1957.

19. Kala, J., & Abudayyeh, A. (2017). Magnesium: An overlooked electrolyte. *The Journal of Emergency Medicine, 52,* 741.

20. Gidwani, H., & Gomez, H. (2017). The crashing patient: Hemodynamic collapse. *Current Opinion in Critical Care, 23*(533), 1.

21. Park, L. G., Dracup, K., Whooley, M. A., et al. (2017). Symptom diary use and improved survival for patients with heart failure. *Circulation. Heart Failure, 10,* e003874.

22. McDermott, B. P., Anderson, S. A., Armstrong, L. E., et al. (2017). National athletic trainers' association position statement: Fluid replacement for the physically active. *Journal of Athletic Training, 52,* 877.

23. Beales, A. (2017). An innovative approach to hydration for a patient with dementia. *Nursing Older People, 29*(4), 26.

24. Johnston, C. T., Maish, G. O., 3rd, Mindard, G., et al. (2017). Evaluation of an intravenous potassium dosing algorithm for hypokalemic critically ill patients. *JPEN. Journal of Parenteral and Enteral Nutrition, 41,* 796.

25. Heckle, M., Agarwal, M., & Alsafwah, S. (2018). ST elevations in the setting of hyperkalemia. *JAMA Internal Medicine, 178,* 133.

26. Carson, R. A., Mudd, S. S., & Madati, P. J. (2017). Evaluation of a nurse-initiated acute gastroenteritis pathway in the pediatric emergency department. *Journal of Emergency Nursing, 43,* 406.

27. Gorski, L. A., Hadaway, L., Hagle, M., et al. (2016). Infusion therapy standards of practice. *Journal of Infusion Nursing, 39*(1 Suppl.), S1–S2016.

28. Geurts, D., Steyerberg, E. W., Moll, H., & Oostenbrink, R. (2017). How to predict oral rehydration failure in children with gastroenteritis. *Journal of Pediatric Gastroenterology and Nutrition, 65,* 503.

29. Rong, X., Peng, Y., Yu, H. P., & Li, D. (2017). Cultural factors influencing dietary and fluid restriction behaviour: Perceptions of older Chinese patients with heart failure. *Journal of Clinical Nursing, 26,* 717.

30. Wagner, J., & Arora, S. (2017). Oncologic metabolic emergencies. *Emergency Medicine Clinics of North America, 31,* 941.

31. Shepshelovich, D., Schnecter, A., Calvarysky, B., et al. (1801). Medication-induced SIADH: Distribution and characterization according to medication class. *British Journal of Clinical Pharmacology, 83,* 2017.

32. Curran, K. A., & Middleman, A. B. (2017). An unusual etiology of hypokalemia in a patient with an eating disorder. *The Journal of Adolescent Health, 60,* 124.

33. Akirov, A., Gorshtein, A., Shraga-Slutzky, I., et al. (2017). Calcium levels on admission and before discharge are associated with mortality in hospitalized patients. *Endocrine, 57,* 344.

34. Palmer, B. F., Deborah, J., & Clegg, D. J. (2017). Electrolyte disturbances in patients with chronic alcohol-use disorder. *The New England Journal of Medicine, 377,* 1368.

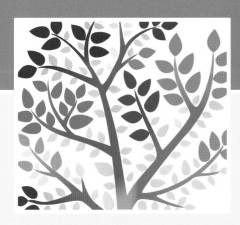

Acid–Base Balance

Linda Felver

The human body requires precise control of multiple physiological processes for optimal function. The concentration of hydrogen ions in body fluids influences cellular function and thus organ, system, and whole person function. An abnormal hydrogen ion concentration impairs cellular and organ function and can be fatal. The body maintains the hydrogen ion concentration within the normal range by continuously making adjustments through specific processes. Nurses providing care to acutely and chronically ill patients must understand these processes in order to optimize their function. This concept presents an analysis of acid–base balance, including the recognition and management of acid–base imbalances when they occur.

DEFINITION

For the purposes of this concept presentation, acid–base balance is defined as *the process of regulating the pH, bicarbonate concentration, and partial pressure of carbon dioxide of body fluids*. The definitions of acid and base are the foundation for the concept of acid–base balance. An *acid* is a substance that releases hydrogen ions (H^+), and a *base* is a substance that takes up H^+. The most important base in the body is bicarbonate (HCO_3^-). The pH of a solution, technically defined later in this concept presentation, is a measure of its degree of acidity. A low pH means the solution is acidic; a high pH means it is basic (alkaline).

Acid–base balance is a dynamic interplay between three processes: acid production or intake, acid buffering, and acid excretion. *Acid production* is the generation of acid through cellular metabolism. Our cells continuously generate two kinds of acid during metabolism: carbonic acid (H_2CO_3) and metabolic acids. Although the chemical structures of metabolic acids vary, both normal and abnormal types of cellular metabolism generate metabolic acids. Occasionally, *acid intake* occurs, which involves entry into the body of acids or substances that the body converts to acids (acid precursors). *Acid buffering* is a process by which body fluids resist large changes in pH when acids or bases are added or removed. Body fluids normally have buffers, which are pairs of chemicals that take up H^+ or release it to keep pH in the normal range. *Acid excretion* is the removal of acid from the body. These concepts are described in greater detail later in this concept presentation.

Acid–base balance is described as a dynamic interplay because acid production is occurring constantly, the body fluids constantly have cellular acids added to them that must be buffered to preserve function, and the acid excretion mechanisms must function continuously to keep acids from accumulating in the body. Optimal acid–base balance keeps the pH of the blood and body fluids within the normal physiological range (7.35 to 7.45).[1]

SCOPE

Considered conceptually, the scope of acid–base balance is on a continuum from acidotic (lower than normal pH) on one end to optimal balance (normal pH and other parameters) in the middle and alkalotic (higher than normal pH) on the other end (Fig. 9.1). These link to three categories associated with this concept: optimal acid–base balance and two types of disrupted acid–base balance—acidosis (too much acid) and alkalosis (too little acid). The term acid–base imbalance often is used to indicate disrupted acid–base balance.

NORMAL PHYSIOLOGICAL PROCESS

The processes whose dynamic interplay is involved in acid–base balance are acid production, acid buffering, and acid excretion. When optimal acid–base balance is occurring, the buffers are not overwhelmed by the amount of acid that is generated and acid excretion keeps pace with acid production. The blood pH and other measures of acid–base status are in the normal range (7.35 to 7.45 for adults; a wider range for infants). This section explains these functions in detail. The process is illustrated in Fig. 9.2.

Acid Production

Cellular metabolism continuously generates carbonic acid and metabolic acids. Increased cellular metabolism produces more of these acids.

Carbonic Acid Production

Cellular metabolism generates carbonic acid (H_2CO_3) in the form of carbon dioxide (CO_2) and water (H_2O). The enzyme carbonic anhydrase in erythrocytes and other cells facilitates the conversion in either direction, depending on the location in the body. In the tissues, in which CO_2 is abundant because it is being produced, the excess CO_2 in the

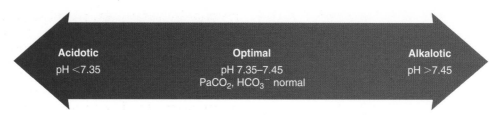

FIGURE 9.1 Scope of Concept of Acid–base Balance Ranges from Optimal Balance to Acidotic and Alkalotic Imbalances.

blood drives the equilibrium toward making H_2CO_3. H_2CO_3 is a weak acid, which means that it dissociates (separates into H^+ and HCO_3^-) only partially in solution:

$$CO_2 + H_2O \leftrightarrows H_2CO_3 \leftrightarrows HCO_3^- + H^+$$
carbon dioxide +   carbonic acid   bicarbonate + hydrogen ion
water

Bicarbonate in the blood is transported to the lung capillaries, where the CO_2 level is low because CO_2 diffuses into the alveoli and is exhaled. Carbonic anhydrase in the lungs converts H_2CO_3 back to CO_2 and H_2O, the form in which it is excreted through exhalation.

Metabolic Acid Production

Metabolic acid, the other type of acid produced by cellular metabolism, is a general term that includes all acids except carbonic acid. Examples of metabolic acid are citric acid, pyruvic acid, and lactic acid. Cells can produce abnormal metabolic acids, such as the ketoacid β-hydroxybutyric acid, when cellular metabolism is disrupted or incomplete. The symbol that represents all metabolic acids is HA. The A indicates anion, which means negatively charged particle. Because these are weak acids, some, but not all, of these molecules dissociate into H^+ and A^-. Metabolic acids move from the cells that produce them into the body fluids, where they are buffered before they reach the kidneys, where they are excreted.

Acid Buffering

Buffers help keep the pH of the blood and other body fluids in the normal range despite the metabolic acid continuously produced by the cells. A buffer is a pair of chemicals (a weak acid and its base) that are in equilibrium in a solution. These two parts of a buffer system must be present in a specific ratio to keep the pH normal. The most important buffer in the extracellular fluid is the bicarbonate buffer system, which consists of carbonic acid (the weak acid) and bicarbonate (its base).[1] When the bicarbonate-to-carbonic acid ratio is 20:1, the blood pH is in the normal range. If the ratio changes significantly, the blood pH becomes abnormal.

The bicarbonate buffer system buffers metabolic acid that is produced by cells or ingested. The bicarbonate portion of the buffer combines with the H^+ from the metabolic acid to make carbonic acid:

$$H^+ + HCO_3^- \leftrightarrows H_2CO_3$$

This process could decrease the available bicarbonate and increase the concentration of carbonic acid, but normally the 20:1 ratio of bicarbonate to carbonic acid is restored immediately because the lungs excrete the carbonic acid as CO_2 and water. Most of the function of bicarbonate buffers in normal physiology is buffering metabolic acid. Bicarbonate buffers cannot buffer carbonic acid because carbonic acid is part of the buffer. If too much metabolic acid is present, the plasma bicarbonate concentration decreases below its normal range because so much bicarbonate was used in buffering.

In abnormal circumstances in which too little metabolic acid is present, the carbonic acid portion of the bicarbonate buffer system will release H^+. This process simultaneously raises the bicarbonate concentration and may restore the pH. However, if entirely too little metabolic acid is present, the plasma bicarbonate concentration increases above its normal range. Thus, the plasma bicarbonate concentration is an indicator of the metabolic acid status in the blood.

Acid Excretion

The two types of acid produced by cellular metabolism differ in that carbonic acid is converted to gases and metabolic acid is not. The lungs excrete the gaseous form of carbonic acid, and the kidneys excrete metabolic acid.

Carbonic Acid Excretion

The lungs serve as the excretory organ for carbonic acid. The lungs are not able to excrete metabolic acid because it cannot be converted into a gaseous form. Changes in rate and depth alter the amount of carbonic acid that is excreted. Hyperventilation (increased rate and depth of respiration) excretes more carbonic acid; hypoventilation (decreased rate and depth of respiration) excretes less carbonic acid. The chemoreceptors influence respiratory rate and depth in response to blood levels of CO_2 and H^+ and, in some situations, oxygen. When the amount of CO_2 increases in the blood, the chemoreceptors increase the respiratory rate and depth,[2] which excretes more CO_2 and H_2O (carbonic acid) and helps restore the CO_2 level to its normal range. If the blood has too little CO_2, the chemoreceptors decrease the respiratory rate and depth, which enables the CO_2 level to rise to its normal range because the cells constantly are producing it. These are examples of *correction:* fixing the problem and returning the blood values to their normal range.

Because chemoreceptors respond to H^+ concentration as well as to blood levels of CO_2, they modify respiratory rate and depth in response to the level of metabolic acid as well as carbonic acid. If too much metabolic acid accumulates, the chemoreceptors trigger hyperventilation (increased respiratory rate and depth).[3] This does not correct the problem because the lungs cannot excrete metabolic acid, but hyperventilation removes more carbonic acid from the body, thus making the blood less acidic. The result is too little carbonic acid, which helps balance the too much metabolic acid. The technical term for this process is *compensation:* moving the pH toward its normal range while making other blood values abnormal. If too little metabolic acid is present, the chemoreceptors cause hypoventilation.[2] This compensatory process moves the pH down toward its normal range by allowing too much carbonic acid to help balance the too little metabolic acid.

Metabolic Acid Excretion

The kidneys excrete metabolic acid but are unable to excrete carbonic acid. They have several mechanisms for excreting metabolic acid. Glomerular filtrate that enters the renal tubules contains HCO_3^- from blood. Cells that line the renal proximal tubules perform chemical processes that essentially take H^+ from the blood and secrete it into renal tubular fluid while moving HCO_3^- in the opposite direction, from the renal

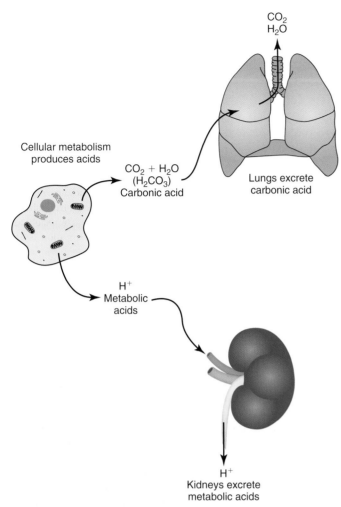

FIGURE 9.2 Acid Production and Excretion. (From Potter, P. A., Perry, A. G., Stockert, P., & Hall, A. [2013]. *Fundamentals of nursing.* 8th ed. St Louis: Mosby.)

tubules into blood. The A⁻ portion of metabolic acids enters renal tubular fluid in the proximal tubules as well. Infants and older adults have reduced ability to excrete large amounts of metabolic acids.[4,5]

The secretion of metabolic acid into the renal tubules adds free H^+ to the fluid, which potentially could damage renal cells. However, many of these H^+ combine with other molecules in the renal tubular fluid, and they no longer influence the pH. For example, renal tubular fluid contains buffers, especially phosphate buffers that were filtered at the glomerulus. Many of the secreted H^+ are buffered; buffered H^+ in urine are called *titratable acid.*[6] Additional H^+ bind to ammonia (NH_3) that distal renal tubular cells produce when additional metabolic acid needs to be excreted. The H^+ that become part of ammonium ions (NH_4^+) do not contribute to the pH. NH_4^+ ions do not return to the cells but remain in the renal tubular fluid and are excreted in the urine:

$$H^+ + NH_3 \leftrightarrows NH_4^+$$

By adjusting their H^+ secretion rate and the amount of NH_3 they make, the kidneys are able to excrete more or less metabolic acid, which assists in maintaining optimal acid–base balance. If too much metabolic acid is present in the blood, the kidneys increase their secretion of H^+ and make more NH_3. These mechanisms correct the problem by removing more H^+ and A⁻ from the blood and simultaneously increasing blood HCO_3^- concentration (moves the opposite direction from the

H^+). Similarly, if too little metabolic acid is present, the kidneys decrease their secretion of H^+ and make less NH_3 so that more metabolic acid remains in the blood and more HCO_3^- is excreted in the urine. These corrective mechanisms normalize the pH by fixing the problem.

If too much carbonic acid accumulates, the kidneys cannot excrete it, but they can excrete more metabolic acid than usual.[2] This renal response to decreased pH compensates for the problem by causing too little metabolic acid in the blood, which somewhat balances the too much carbonic acid. Similarly, if the pH increases because there is too little carbonic acid, the renal compensatory response is less secretion of H^+ and less generation of NH_3. The resulting increase of metabolic acid is an attempt to balance the lack of carbonic acid, normalizing the pH by making other blood values abnormal.

Age-Related Differences
Infants and Children

Infants have several pertinent physiological differences. An infant has a much greater percentage of total body weight attributed to fluid (75%) compared to an adult (60%), more extracellular fluid than intracellular fluid, and an immature renal system that is inefficient in excreting a sudden acid load.[5] In addition, an infant's metabolic rate is higher and the fluid exchange ratio is far greater than those of an adult. These differences place infants at higher risk for metabolic acidosis, as well as fluid and electrolyte imbalances, compared to older children and adults.

Older Adults

A normal physiological change associated with aging is reduced size and function of the kidneys, which play a critical role in maintaining acid–base balance. Despite this age-related gradual loss of nephrons, the kidneys of the older adult typically are able to manage their role in fluid, electrolyte, and acid–base balance under normal circumstances. However, older adults have reduced renal reserve. They are less able to excrete a large acid load renally, and their ability to compensate may be less effective.[4] This makes older adults more susceptible to acid–base disturbances, as well as to fluid and electrolyte imbalances.

VARIATIONS AND CONTEXT

Conceptually, variations in acid–base balance are referred to as acid–base imbalance, of which there are two major categories: acidosis and alkalosis. Each of these categories has two underlying subtypes: respiratory and metabolic (Fig. 9.3). When these conditions are developing, the body attempts to manage the changing acid–base balance through the corrective and compensatory responses described previously. Table 9.1 summarizes the corrective and compensatory responses to disrupted acid–base balance.

Acidosis (Too Much Acid)

In a situation of too much acid, the buffers have been overwhelmed and body fluids have too much acid. Acid excretion is not able to keep up with acid production or intake. Conditions of too much acid are called *acidosis* and are given an additional descriptor that explains whether there is too much carbonic acid or too much metabolic acid. Because the lungs excrete carbonic acid, the condition of too much carbonic acid is called *respiratory acidosis.*[2] Similarly, because the kidneys excrete metabolic acid, the condition of too much metabolic acid is called *metabolic acidosis.* In some cases of metabolic acidosis, the base bicarbonate has been lost from the body, which causes relatively too much metabolic acid. In situations of too much acid, the pH is below the normal range (or in the low part of the normal range), and some other measures of acid–base status are abnormal. These laboratory values are explained in the Assessment section.

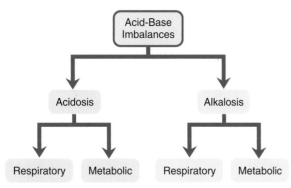

FIGURE 9.3 Categories of Acid–Base Imbalances.

TABLE 9.1 Respiratory and Renal Responses to Disrupted Acid–Base Balance

Stimulus	Respiratory Response	Renal Response
Too much carbonic acid (respiratory acidosis)	Cause of Problem Hypoventilation Correction Hyperventilation	Compensation Increased secretion of H^+ More NH_3 production
Too little carbonic acid (respiratory alkalosis)	Cause of Problem Hyperventilation Correction Hypoventilation	Compensation Decreased secretion of H^+ Less NH_3 production
Too much metabolic acid (metabolic acidosis)	Compensation Hyperventilation	Cause of Problem More metabolic acid than kidneys can excrete Correction Increased secretion of H^+ More NH_3 production
Too little metabolic acid (metabolic alkalosis)	Compensation Hypoventilation	Cause of Problem More bicarbonate than kidneys can excrete (too little metabolic acid) Correction Decreased secretion of H^+ Less NH_3 production

Alkalosis (Too Little Acid)

In situations of too little acid, the buffers also are not able to keep the pH in the normal range and body fluids do not have enough acid. Too much of the base HCO_3^- has been added to the buffer system or acid excretion is greater than acid production. Conditions of too little acid are called *alkalosis*—either *respiratory alkalosis* when there is too little carbonic acid or *metabolic alkalosis* when there is too little metabolic acid. In these situations of too little acid, the pH is above the normal range (or in the high part of the normal range) and some other measures of acid–base status are abnormal. The Assessment section explains these measures.

CONSEQUENCES

A firm grasp of the physiological processes that comprise acid–base balance makes it possible to understand the consequences when these processes are disrupted. Acid–base imbalances trigger compensatory mechanisms, as described previously. The time course of those mechanisms has important clinical implications. In addition to triggering compensatory mechanisms, pH changes impair cellular and organ function.

Time Course of Compensatory Mechanisms

Disruptions of acid–base balance cause the blood pH to move outside its normal range. In these situations, the buffers have been overwhelmed and the acid excretion mechanisms must work to keep the pH from reaching the fatal limits. If the pH falls abnormally low from too much acid, both the lungs and the kidneys will excrete more acid, even though only one of these organs will be excreting the type of acid that is excessive. The other organ is compensating. Depending on the time course and the severity of the problem, the disruption may be uncompensated, partially compensated, or fully compensated.[1]

As explained in the previous section, if a problem with the respiratory system disrupts acid–base balance and the lungs are unable to correct it, renal compensatory mechanisms adjust the pH toward normal. It takes several days for renal compensatory mechanisms to become clinically significant[1,2]; therefore a short-lived respiratory acidosis or alkalosis will not become compensated. Rapid treatment of an acute respiratory acidosis will correct the problem before renal compensation can occur. On the other hand, people who have chronic respiratory acidosis or an acute episode that lasts several days do develop some degree of renal compensation, either partial or full. Episodes of respiratory alkalosis occur from hyperventilation and it is uncommon, but possible, for them to last long enough for renal compensation to occur.[6]

Analogously, if a problem with the kidneys disrupts acid–base balance and the kidneys are unable to correct it, respiratory compensatory mechanisms adjust the pH toward normal.[7] Respiratory compensation begins a few minutes after the pH becomes abnormal, so it is common to have some degree of compensation for a disruption of acid–base balance that involves too much or too little metabolic acid. When the disruption is severe, it will be only partially compensated.[1,2] In cases of metabolic alkalosis (too little metabolic acid), compensatory hypoventilation is limited by the respiratory drive for oxygen so that full compensation usually does not occur.[2] It is important to realize that even if compensatory mechanisms do not return the pH to the normal range, they do prevent pH from becoming more abnormal.

Impaired Cellular and Organ Function

Disruptions of acid–base balance alter cell function, especially in the brain. The disorders involving carbonic acid (respiratory acidosis and alkalosis) generally cause more neurologic signs and symptoms than those involving metabolic acid (metabolic acidosis and alkalosis).[1] This difference occurs because CO_2 from carbonic acid crosses the blood–brain barrier easily and changes the pH of cerebrospinal fluid rapidly. Metabolic acid and HCO_3^- cross the blood–brain barrier with difficulty and produce fewer neurologic manifestations or cause them more slowly.

The enzymes inside cells work most effectively when pH is normal. Abnormal extracellular pH can cause intracellular pH to change, especially with respiratory acidosis and alkalosis. The resulting change in enzyme activity contributes to cell dysfunction. Acidosis decreases the level of consciousness (LOC). With alkalosis, initial excitation may occur, followed by decreased LOC if the pH increase becomes more severe.[6] In addition to brain cell dysfunction that causes altered LOC and other neurologic manifestations, cardiac cell dysfunction from acid–base imbalances can cause dysrhythmias.[1,2] Concurrent potassium imbalances caused by acid–base imbalances also cause cardiac dysrhythmias.

RISK FACTORS

Populations at Risk

All individuals, regardless of race, culture, age, or socioeconomic status, need optimal acid–base balance for physiological function. From a population perspective, those at greatest risk for acid–base disturbances are the very young and the very old. Preterm infants are at great risk for acid–base disturbances due to immature lungs, kidneys, thermoregulation, and metabolic processes; the degree of risk is largely related to the weight and gestational age at the time of birth. Term infants also have greater risk than adults due to immature kidneys, elevated metabolic rate, and large fluid exchange ratio.[5]

Older adults have decreased renal reserve due to a normal gradual loss of nephrons, making their ability to correct and to compensate for imbalances less effective.[4] Thus, they are more susceptible to acid–base disturbances than younger adults.

Individual Risk Factors

Acid–base imbalances usually occur as a consequence of another underlying condition. The most common underlying conditions associated with acid–base disturbances are presented in Box 9.1. These are organized under general causes that provide a framework for remembering the conditions. For example, respiratory acidosis (too much carbonic acid) can arise from alveolar hypoventilation, ineffective neuromuscular action of the chest respiratory pump, or suppression of the neural drive from the brain stem that triggers respirations. Nurses can use these categories to understand specifically how the exemplars cause respiratory acidosis and to generalize their knowledge to other conditions that cause respiratory acidosis by similar mechanisms. Nurses can also deduce logically the risk factors for acid–base imbalance by considering the processes whose dynamic interplay creates acid–base balance. Those at greatest risk for acid–base imbalances are individuals who have at least one of the following risk factors[8]:

- Excessive production or intake of metabolic acid
- Altered acid buffering due to loss or gain of bicarbonate
- Altered acid excretion
- Abnormal shift of H^+ into cells

Excessive Production or Intake of Metabolic Acid

The cells are capable of making excessive amounts of metabolic acid that overwhelm the acid buffering and excretory capacities. A common clinical example of too much metabolic acid due to acid production is diabetic ketoacidosis (DKA), in which abnormal cellular metabolism caused by lack of insulin produces ketoacids faster than the kidneys are able to excrete them.[1,2] DKA is a type of metabolic acidosis; it most commonly occurs with type 1 diabetes, but may occur with type 2 diabetes also. Other high-risk populations for ketoacidosis are people who do not have enough carbohydrate intake and people who abuse alcohol.[9] In addition to the production of excessive metabolic acid within the body, excessive intake of acid or acid precursors also causes metabolic acidosis. Although metabolic acidosis from intake of acid or acid precursors is less common, it is significant clinically in people who accidentally ingest boric acid (intended for ant poisoning) or who drink methanol or antifreeze (acid precursor).[10,11]

In summary, risk factors for excessive production or intake of metabolic acid include the risk factors for ketoacidosis or poisoning with acids or substances the body converts to acid. All of these situations place people at risk for metabolic acidosis. The cells cannot stop producing metabolic acid, so decreased acid production is not a risk factor.

BOX 9.1 COMMON UNDERLYING CONDITIONS LEADING TO ACID–BASE IMBALANCE

Respiratory Acidosis (Too Much Carbonic Acid)
Alveolar Hypoventilation
- Type B COPD (chronic bronchitis)
- End-stage type A COPD (emphysema)
- Severe asthma episode
- Bacterial pneumonia
- Pulmonary edema

Ineffective Respiratory Pump
- Guillain–Barré syndrome

Central Suppression of Respiration
- Opioid overdose

Metabolic Acidosis (Too Much Metabolic Acid)
Excessive Production or Intake of Metabolic Acid
- Diabetic ketoacidosis
- Starvation ketoacidosis
- Alcoholic ketoacidosis
- Lactic acidosis (from tissue anoxia)
- Thyroid storm

Decreased Excretion of Metabolic Acid
- Oliguria from any cause

Loss of Bicarbonate
- Prolonged diarrhea
- Draining intestinal or pancreatic fistula

Respiratory Alkalosis (Too Little Carbonic Acid)
Hyperventilation
- Acute hypoxia
- Acute pain
- Acute anxiety or emotional distress
- Central stimulation of respirations by inflammation from head injury or meningitis

Metabolic Alkalosis (Too Little Metabolic Acid)
Gain of Base (Bicarbonate)
- Excessive ingestion or infusion of $NaHCO_3$
- Massive blood transfusion (citrate metabolized to HCO_3^-)
- Diuretic therapy (contraction alkalosis)

Excessive Excretion of Metabolic Acid
- Repeated vomiting
- Mineralocorticoid excess

COPD, Chronic obstructive pulmonary disease.

Altered Acid Buffering Due to Loss or Gain of Bicarbonate

The base bicarbonate is a component of the major buffer system that buffers metabolic acids. It is possible to lose or gain bicarbonate and thus alter the buffering capacity. People who lose a significant amount of bicarbonate, such as through prolonged diarrhea, lose buffering capacity and have relatively too much metabolic acid. Thus, bicarbonate loss causes metabolic acidosis.[1,12] Conversely, gaining a significant amount of bicarbonate, such as by ingesting baking soda (sodium bicarbonate) as an antacid or by receiving excessive intravenous (IV) sodium bicarbonate, makes too much bicarbonate buffer available and thus creates too little metabolic acid. Thus, bicarbonate gain causes metabolic alkalosis.[1,2] In summary, risk factors for altered acid buffering include prolonged diarrhea and excessive sodium bicarbonate intake in people of any age.[8] These conditions place them at risk for metabolic acidosis or metabolic alkalosis.

Altered Acid Excretion

Cellular metabolism generates two types of acid that are excreted by two different organ systems. For this reason, altered acid excretion occurs in many disease processes that affect lung and kidney function. Carbonic acid excretion occurs by gas exchange in the lung alveoli followed by exhalation; thus, it is possible to decrease or increase carbonic acid excretion. People at high risk for decreased carbonic acid excretion have acute or chronic respiratory diseases or other conditions that interfere with alveolar ventilation.[8] The cells continue producing carbonic acid, but the respiratory system is unable to excrete enough of it. The result is respiratory acidosis—too much carbonic acid. For example, people who have type B chronic obstructive pulmonary disease (COPD) (chronic bronchitis) have decreased carbonic acid excretion due to structural changes in their lungs and excessive mucus production that obstructs airflow.[1] They develop chronic respiratory acidosis, as do people of any age who have severe acute respiratory conditions such as asthma or bacterial pneumonia. Infants and small children have increased risk of respiratory acidosis with acute conditions because their airways have such small diameters.

Although decreased carbonic acid secretion is the most common problem with carbonic acid secretion, it is possible to excrete excessive carbonic acid through hyperventilation.[1,2] This situation causes too little carbonic acid, creating respiratory alkalosis. High-risk populations for too little carbonic acid due to hyperventilation include people who are hypoxic, are experiencing acute pain, or are upset and anxious. These conditions that cause respiratory alkalosis tend to be more short-term than many causes of respiratory acidosis.

Excretion of metabolic acid also may be altered, either decreased or increased. People who have prolonged oliguria for any reason cannot excrete enough of the metabolic acids that their cells continue to produce. Thus, they develop metabolic acidosis. These high-risk populations include people of any age with acute or chronic oliguric renal disease and those with circulatory shock.[13–16] Infants have immature kidneys that are not yet fully effective in excreting metabolic acid; older adults often have reduced ability to excrete a metabolic acid load.[4,5] These difficulties in excreting metabolic acid make them vulnerable to metabolic acidosis, especially in conjunction with increased acid production or intake.

Increased excretion of metabolic acid through the kidneys can occur in people with excessive aldosterone; however, the most common condition involving excessive removal of metabolic acid from the body is vomiting,[17] which removes hydrochloric acid. Vomiting also triggers bicarbonate retention by the kidneys, which alters the buffering capacity and contributes to the resulting metabolic alkalosis.

In summary, risk factors for altered acid excretion include respiratory or other conditions that interfere with the ability to excrete enough carbonic acid, conditions causing hyperventilation that excretes too much carbonic acid, kidneys that are unable to excrete enough metabolic acid, and situations in which the kidneys or repeated episodes of vomiting remove too much metabolic acid from the body.[8]

Abnormal Shift of H⁺ into Cells

Factors that shift substantial numbers of H^+ into cells can cause too little acid to be in the blood. The most common example in this category of risk factors is hypokalemia (abnormally low plasma potassium concentration).[12] When hypokalemia is present, some potassium ions (K^+)

leave cells and H^+ enter cells to maintain a balance of electrical charge. The result is too little metabolic acid in the blood, known as metabolic alkalosis. The primary risk factor for abnormal shift of H^+ into cells is hypokalemia. Risk factors for hypokalemia are discussed in Concept 8, Fluid and Electrolytes.

ASSESSMENT

Disruptions of acid–base balance almost always result from other conditions. For this reason, assessments of acid–base status usually are performed in the context of other conditions.

History

Clinical manifestations associated with disrupted acid–base balance often are caused by an underlying condition and associated fluid and electrolyte imbalances. Acid–base imbalances cause nonspecific signs such as decreased LOC that have many possible causes. It is critical that nurses consider presenting symptoms in the context of other current health conditions. The history focuses on the respiratory, renal, or other conditions that could cause the acid–base problem. The standard questions for any history apply and are not repeated here. Other areas to explore in the history include the following: a recent history of vomiting or diarrhea (repeated vomiting causes metabolic alkalosis; prolonged diarrhea causes metabolic acidosis); use of heartburn or indigestion medications (a few days of baking soda/sodium bicarbonate ingestion can cause metabolic alkalosis); recent attempts to lose weight and methods employed (high-fat, low-carbohydrate diet or fasting predispose to starvation ketoacidosis); and use of medications, dietary supplements, illicit drugs, and alcohol.[18,19]

Examination Findings

Unless the acid–base imbalance is severe, specific signs and symptoms of disrupted acid–base balance often are overshadowed by the clinical manifestations of the underlying cause. For example, in a person who has type B COPD (chronic bronchitis), the dyspnea and excessive mucus production usually are more obvious than the mild drowsiness from partially compensated respiratory acidosis. With severe acute asthma, the chest tightness, coughing, wheezing, use of accessory respiratory muscles, and poor oxygenation typically overshadow the manifestations of acute respiratory acidosis.[1] People who have end-stage renal disease experience many clinical manifestations from this chronic oliguric condition that predominate over lethargy from the metabolic acidosis that may occur between dialysis sessions, unless it becomes severe.[1]

With substantial rapid changes of pH, such as with ketoacidosis, dramatic changes in LOC can overshadow the signs and symptoms of the underlying condition. For example, a person who develops DKA typically will have been experiencing the polyuria, polydipsia, polyphagia, and weight loss of hyperglycemia before the onset of ketoacidosis. These manifestations often are realized only in retrospect, after abdominal pain and decreased LOC from the ketoacidosis have become the focus of attention and the metabolic acidosis is resolved.

Table 9.2 presents signs and symptoms of the various disruptions of acid–base balance. These manifestations arise from the impaired cellular and organ function described previously in this concept analysis. Decreased LOC occurs on a continuum from decreased attention span and drowsiness on one end to stupor and coma on the other. Interpretation of assessment findings may be complicated by the presence of fluid and electrolyte imbalances (see Concept 8, Fluid and Electrolytes).

Diagnostic Tests

Arterial blood gas measurement is the definitive diagnostic test for acid–base balance.[5,20,21] In some settings, venous blood gas values are

TABLE 9.2   Clinical Manifestations of Disrupted Acid–Base Balance

Type of Problem	TOO MUCH ACID		TOO LITTLE ACID	
	Too Much Carbonic Acid (Respiratory Acidosis)	Too Much Metabolic Acid (Metabolic Acidosis)	Too Little Carbonic Acid (Respiratory Alkalosis)	Too Little Metabolic Acid (Metabolic Alkalosis)
Common clinical findings	Headache Decreased LOC Hypoventilation (cause of problem) Cardiac dysrhythmias If severe: hypotension	Decreased LOC Hyperventilation (compensatory mechanism) Abdominal pain Nausea and vomiting Cardiac dysrhythmias	Excitation and belligerence, lightheadedness, unusual behaviors; followed by decreased LOC if severe Perioral and digital paresthesias, carpopedal spasm, tetany Diaphoresis Hyperventilation (cause of problem) Cardiac dysrhythmias	Excitation followed by decreased LOC if severe Perioral and digital paresthesias, carpopedal spasm Hypoventilation (compensatory mechanism) Signs of volume depletion and hypokalemia if present
Blood gas findings	Blood gases: pH decreased (or low normal if fully compensated); $PaCO_2$ increased; HCO_3^- increased from compensation	Blood gases: pH decreased (or low normal if fully compensated); $PaCO_2$ decreased from compensation; HCO_3^- decreased	Blood gases: pH increased; $PaCO_2$ decreased; HCO_3^- decreased if compensation	Blood gases: pH increased; $PaCO_2$ increased from compensation; HCO_3^- increased

LOC, Level of consciousness.

used instead of arterial.[20] This section provides the conceptual basis for interpreting arterial blood gas results related to acid-base status. The commonly used values are pH, $PaCO_2$, HCO_3^- concentration, and base excess. The partial pressure of oxygen in arterial blood (PaO_2) and the saturation of oxygen in arterial blood (SaO_2), which are measures of oxygenation, are not discussed here.

pH

The pH is defined technically as the negative logarithm of the H^+ concentration. H^+ ions arise from dissociation of acids, both carbonic acid and metabolic acid. The H^+ concentration is very small and awkward to write[22]; for that reason, the pH is calculated. The pH scale ranges from 1 to 14, with a pH of 7 being neutral. Because pH is a negative logarithm, a low pH indicates a solution that is acidic (has a high H^+ concentration). A high pH indicates a solution that is alkaline (has a low H^+ concentration). The pH of the blood has a normal range of 7.35 to 7.45 in adults, which is slightly alkaline. The normal range is lower in neonates and infants. In clinical settings, the term *acidemia* is used when the pH declines below the lower limit of normal (becomes *acidotic*). Even though the blood still may be slightly alkaline (>7.0), it is more acidic than the normal range. The term *alkalemia* denotes a blood pH that is above the normal range (becomes *alkalotic*).

$PaCO_2$

$PaCO_2$ is the partial pressure of CO_2 in the arterial blood. It indicates how well the lungs are excreting carbonic acid (CO_2 and H_2O).[8] The normal range of $PaCO_2$ is 35 to 45 mm Hg (4.7 to 6.0 kilopascals [kPa]) for adults (lower in infants). Increased $PaCO_2$ level indicates CO_2 accumulation in the blood (too much carbonic acid) caused by primary or compensatory hypoventilation; decreased $PaCO_2$ level indicates excessive CO_2 excretion (too little carbonic acid) caused by primary or compensatory hyperventilation.

HCO_3^- Concentration

The serum HCO_3^- concentration indicates how well the kidneys are excreting metabolic acid.[8] The normal adult range is 22 to 26 mEq/L (22 to 26 mmol/L); the range is lower in infants. Increased

HCO_3^- concentration indicates that the blood has too little metabolic acid; decreased HCO_3^- concentration indicates that the blood has too much metabolic acid.

Base Excess

Base excess, which normally ranges from −2 to +2 mmol/L, is an indicator of how well the buffers are managing metabolic acid.[21] Values less than −2 mmol/L (negative base excess) indicate too much metabolic acid; values greater than +2 mmol/L indicate too little metabolic acid. When people develop metabolic acidosis, clinicians may calculate other values, such as the anion gap and the Stewart strong ion difference, to assist in diagnosing the specific cause.[23,24]

CLINICAL MANAGEMENT

Clinical management of acid–base balance encompasses all clinical settings with primary and secondary prevention as well as interventions for people with acid–base imbalances.

Primary Prevention

The primary prevention for a disrupted acid–base balance focuses on prevention of the major risk factors previously discussed rather than on prevention of the disrupted acid–base balance itself. For example, prevention of respiratory diseases helps to prevent risk factors for accumulating too much carbonic acid. Thus, efforts to convince people not to begin smoking or to assist them to stop smoking, although targeted directly at the prevention of respiratory disease, also indirectly prevent respiratory acidosis. Similarly, careful diabetes teaching and management help prevent ketoacidosis as well as other potential complications of diabetes. Teaching people how to lose weight safely without totally eliminating carbohydrates can help to prevent starvation ketoacidosis as well as to achieve weight management goals. Poison prevention efforts can help prevent excessive ingestion of acids or acid precursors. Instruction regarding hand hygiene and safe food storage helps prevent diarrhea and vomiting—two common risk factors for disrupted acid–base balance. In summary, many of the primary prevention strategies aimed at specific disease processes and behaviors detrimental to health in general also help to prevent disrupted acid–base balance that can arise from these risk factors.

Secondary Prevention (Screening)

Screening measures to detect disrupted acid–base balance are not performed in the general population.

Collaborative Interventions

Patients experiencing acid–base imbalance require aggressive collaborative management aimed at treating the underlying condition. If left untreated, or not treated effectively, acid–base imbalances can be fatal.[25]

Most medical and nursing management is directed at the disease process that disrupts the acid–base balance. In general, collaborative interventions to manage acid–base imbalances caused by an underlying respiratory condition include respiratory support. Likewise, collaborative interventions to manage acid–base imbalances caused by an underlying metabolic condition usually include fluid and electrolyte support.

Respiratory Support

People who have too much or too little carbonic acid usually receive some type of respiratory support, such as airway management and oxygen therapy. For example, with primary respiratory acidosis (too much carbonic acid), the focus of collaborative interventions is treatment of the disease process that is impairing alveolar ventilation. By treating the underlying cause of the disruption, acid–base balance may return to normal, or at least to a more stable state. People who are hyperventilating develop respiratory alkalosis (too little carbonic acid). Collaborative interventions for these people focus on treating the underlying factor (e.g., hypoxia, acute pain, or acute anxiety) that drives the hyperventilation. Hyperventilation that is a compensatory response to metabolic acidosis (too many metabolic acids) should be allowed to continue while the metabolic acidosis is treated.

Fluid and Electrolyte Support

People whose acid–base balance is disrupted by too much or too little metabolic acid usually receive fluid and electrolyte support as part of collaborative interventions to treat the underlying problem. For example, providing insulin and fluids to treat DKA removes the original problem and normalizes acid–base balance. Dialysis for a person who accumulates too much metabolic acid from oliguric renal disease treats multiple aspects of the condition, including the disrupted acid–base balance.[26]

Very low pH can be fatal; therefore in situations of very severe metabolic acidosis in which pH is dangerously low, the collaborative focus occasionally expands to adjusting the pH itself. The most common agent used for pH adjustment is IV sodium bicarbonate, but its use is controversial.[27] The administration of IV sodium bicarbonate may cause extracellular fluid volume (ECV) excess or hypernatremia, may delay renal excretion of ketoacids, or may even lead to metabolic alkalosis from excessive administration. Monitoring for signs and symptoms of these complications, in addition to monitoring the patient's acid–base balance, is crucial.

Independent Nursing Interventions

Independent nursing interventions provide safety and comfort for people who have disrupted acid–base balance. Safety is high priority for patients with decreased LOC. In addition, interventions can promote compensatory mechanisms. For example, patients who are hyperventilating in compensation for metabolic acidosis need careful positioning to facilitate

---

BOX 9.2   NURSING INTERVENTIONS FOR PEOPLE WITH DISRUPTED ACID–BASE BALANCE

- Ongoing assessment
- Implement safety measures
- Implement comfort measures
- Support compensatory mechanisms
- Implement collaborative interventions focused on
  - Treatment of the underlying cause
  - Adjustment of the pH (controversial)
- Monitor for complications of therapy
- Patient teaching
  - Management of chronic underlying conditions
  - Recognition of early problems; when to seek help

---

chest expansion and frequent oral care to prevent drying and cracking of their lips and the drying of oral mucous membranes. Another important type of intervention is teaching culturally appropriate ways to prevent disruptions of acid–base balance or when to seek help if they have chronic problems. Box 9.2 summarizes nursing interventions for people with disrupted acid–base balance.

INTERRELATED CONCEPTS

Numerous concepts discussed in this book have interrelationships with acid–base balance. For example, Fluid and Electrolytes and acid–base balance are closely related because changes in one of them can cause changes in the other. Gas Exchange, Perfusion, and Nutrition facilitate optimal acid–base balance by allowing normal acid production, whereas alterations such as ischemia, hypoxia, starvation, and high-fat, low-carbohydrate diets can disrupt that process. Similarly, Elimination facilitates optimal acid–base balance through acid excretion; changes such as oliguria and diarrhea can disrupt acid–base balance. An individual who has a disrupted acid–base balance can experience altered Cognition. These interrelationships are illustrated in Fig. 9.4.

CLINICAL EXEMPLARS

An exemplar of optimal acid–base balance is a healthy person of any age. This person's acid production is balanced by acid excretion with adequate buffering. Optimal acid–base balance also can occur in a person with acute or chronic illness (e.g., osteoporosis) that does not seriously impair respiratory, gastrointestinal, endocrine, or renal function. The four exemplars representing acid–base disturbances are presented in Box 9.3 and are summarized briefly in the following Featured Exemplars section.

Featured Exemplars
Respiratory Acidosis

Respiratory acidosis is excess carbonic acid (measured as elevated $PaCO_2$) in the blood. Cellular metabolism continually produces carbonic acid, which must be excreted by the lungs or it accumulates in the blood. People with high risk of primary respiratory acidosis have acute or chronic respiratory diseases or other conditions that interfere with alveolar ventilation. These conditions arise from problems in the alveoli or airways (e.g., type B COPD and severe acute asthma), problems

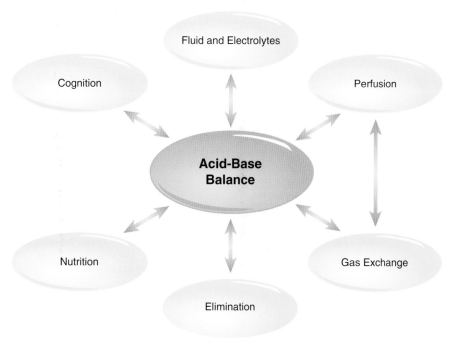

FIGURE 9.4 Acid–Base Balance and Interrelated Concepts.

 BOX 9.3   EXEMPLARS OF ACID–BASE IMBALANCE

- Respiratory acidosis
  - Bacterial pneumonia
  - Acute asthma
  - Type B chronic obstructive pulmonary disease
- Metabolic acidosis
  - Diabetic ketoacidosis
  - Severe hypovolemia
  - Circulatory shock
  - Oliguric renal disease
- Respiratory alkalosis
  - Hyperventilation from acute pain
  - Hyperventilation from acute anxiety
- Metabolic alkalosis
  - Prolonged vomiting
  - Mild hypovolemia
  - Hypokalemia

ACCESS EXEMPLAR LINKS IN YOUR GIDDENS EBOOK

with respiratory muscle function (e.g., Guillain–Barré syndrome), or problems with the brain stem control of respirations (e.g., overdose of opioids or other central nervous system depressants). People develop mild compensatory respiratory acidosis if they have primary metabolic alkalosis.[2]

Respiratory Alkalosis

Respiratory alkalosis is too little carbonic acid (measured as decreased $PaCO_2$) in the blood. People at high risk for primary respiratory alkalosis are hyperventilating, which excretes carbonic acid faster than it is produced by cellular metabolism. Common causes of hyperventilation are acute hypoxia, acute pain, and emotional distress.[8] People develop compensatory respiratory alkalosis if they have primary metabolic acidosis.

Metabolic Acidosis

Metabolic acidosis is excess metabolic acid (measured as decreased HCO_3^-) in the blood. Cellular metabolism continually produces metabolic acid, which must be buffered in the blood by the HCO_3^- buffer system and excreted by the kidneys or the acid accumulates in the blood. People with high risk of primary metabolic acidosis have excessive production or intake of metabolic acid (e.g., ketoacidosis or boric acid ingestion), decreased renal excretion (e.g., acute or chronic oliguria), or lose HCO_3^- buffers from the body (e.g., prolonged diarrhea).[13] These high-risk people include those with undiagnosed or inadequately treated type 1 diabetes, chronic alcohol abuse with malnutrition, untreated hyperthyroidism, circulatory shock, acute kidney injury, and oliguric chronic kidney disease.[9–13,28] In addition, people who have large rapid infusion of IV isotonic saline may develop metabolic acidosis, partly because their bicarbonate levels are decreased by dilution.[29–32] People develop compensatory metabolic acidosis if they have a primary respiratory alkalosis that lasts for at least several days.

Metabolic Alkalosis

Metabolic acidosis is too little metabolic acid (measured as increased HCO_3^-) in the blood. People at high risk of primary metabolic alkalosis most frequently have excessive intake of HCO_3^- through the use of baking soda as antacid, receiving IV $NaHCO_3$, or from metabolizing the citrate in massive blood transfusions.[1] Mild metabolic alkalosis is common with diuretic therapy.[2] People who have prolonged vomiting excrete metabolic acid more rapidly than it is produced while also retaining HCO_3^- renally.[2] People develop compensatory metabolic alkalosis if they have a primary respiratory acidosis that lasts for at least several days.

CASE STUDY

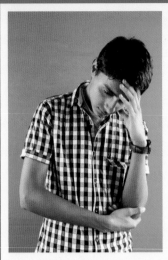

Case Presentation

Kevin Harney, age 14 years, did not appear for breakfast when his mother called him. "That is unusual," she thought, "He has been so hungry lately, and he is so skinny, he really needs the food!" She found Kevin lying on his bed, breathing rapidly and deeply. He responded slowly with one or two words at a time to her increasingly frantic questions. Some of his answers did not make sense. Kevin's parents took him to the nearest emergency department, where his laboratory tests showed arterial blood pH 7.20, $PaCO_2$ 21 mm Hg (2.8 kPa), serum HCO_3^- concentration 8 mEq/L (8 mmol/L), and glucose concentration 450 mg/dL (25 mmol/L). Kevin was diagnosed with DKA arising from previously undiagnosed type 1 diabetes. During Kevin's hospitalization, interventions focused initially on intensive collaborative management of his disrupted acid–base balance with insulin and IV fluid to treat

the diabetes. As a safety intervention, Kevin was positioned on his side to prevent aspiration if he vomited. During this phase of management, attention also was given to supporting his parents, explaining that Kevin's unusual breathing pattern actually was beneficial to him, and coaching his mother to assume the task of protecting Kevin's lips by keeping them lubricated. Careful monitoring of blood values and physical assessment parameters was used to follow his progress and to modify therapy when his condition changed. As Kevin began to be more responsive and stable, the focus of nursing interventions expanded to teaching Kevin and his parents about type 1 diabetes: how to manage it, and how to recognize the signs of hyperglycemia. Although not directed specifically at the acid–base balance, this teaching helped to prevent future episodes of DKA through disease management.

Case Analysis Questions

1. Review Fig. 9.1. Based on the information presented in the case, where does Kevin fall on the continuum?
2. Review Box 9.1, examining the three categories that can cause metabolic acidosis. In which category does Kevin's situation definitely fall? Explain the mechanisms by which this occurs in undiagnosed type 1 diabetes. Is there an additional category that also may have played a part?
3. Explain the mechanisms that caused Kevin's decreased $PaCO_2$ and decreased HCO_3^- concentration.

From samer chand/iStock/Thinkstock.

 ACCESS EXEMPLAR LINKS IN YOUR GIDDENS EBOOK

REFERENCES

1. Jameson, J. L., Fauci, A., Kasper, D. K., et al. (2019). *Harrison's principles of internal medicine* (20th ed.). New York: McGraw-Hill.
2. Kamel, K., & Halperin, M. (2017). *Fluid, electrolyte, and acid–base physiology* (5th ed.). St. Louis: Elsevier.
3. Lands, L. C. (2017). Dyspnea in children: What is driving it and how to approach it. *Pediatr Resp Rev, 24*, 29.
4. Hietavala, E. M., Stout, J. R., Frassetto, L. A., et al. (2017). Dietary acid load and renal function have varying effects on blood acid-base status and exercise performance across age and sex. *Applied Physiology, Nutrition, and Metabolism, 42*, 1330.
5. Morgan, J. L., Nelson, D. B., Casey, B. M., et al. (2017). Impact of metabolic acidemia at birth on neonatal outcomes in infants born before 34 weeks gestation. *J Mat Fetal Neonat Med, 30*, 1902.
6. Batile, D., Chin-Theodorou, J., & Tucker, B. M. (2017). Metabolic acidosis or respiratory alkalosis? Evaluation of a low plasma bicarbonate using the urine anion gap. *Am J Kid Dis, 70*, 440.
7. Nagami, G. T., & Hamm, L. L. (2017). Regulation of acid-base balance in chronic kidney disease. *Adv Chr Kid Dis, 24*, 274.
8. Felver, L. (2019). Acid–base homeostasis and imbalances. In J. L. Banasik & L. C. Copstead (Eds.), *Pathophysiology* (6th ed.). St. Louis: Saunders.
9. Palmer, B. F., & Clegg, D. J. (2017). Electrolyte disturbances in patients with chronic alcohol-use disorder. *The New England Journal of Medicine, 377*, 1368.
10. Collister, D., Duff, G., Palatnick, W., et al. (2017). A methanol intoxication outbreak from recreational ingestion of fracking fluid. *Am J Kid Dis, 69*, 696.
11. Hodgman, M., Marraffa, J. M., Wojcik, S., et al. (2017). Serum calcium concentration in ethylene glycol poisoning. *J Med Toxicol, 13*(2), 153.
12. Ferrari, M. C., Miele, L., Guidi, L., et al. (2017). Watery stools and metabolic acidosis. *Intern Emer Med, 12*, 487.
13. Chen, W., & Abramowitz, M. K. (2017). Epidemiology of acid-base derangements in CKD. *Adv Chr Kidney Dis, 24*(5), 280.
14. Goraya, N., & Wesson, D. E. (2017). Management of the metabolic acidosis of chronic kidney disease. *Adv Chr Kid Dis, 24*, 298.
15. Kraut, J. A., & Madias, N. E. (2017). Adverse effects of the metabolic acidosis of chronic kidney disease. *Adv Chr Kid Dis, 24*, 289.
16. Norton, J. M., Newman, E. P., Romancito, G., et al. (2017). Improving outcomes for patients with chronic kidney disease: Part 2. *The American Journal of Nursing, 117*(3), 26.
17. Nissen, M., Cernalanu, G., Thranhardt, R., et al. (2017). Does metabolic alkalosis influence cerebral oxygenation in infantile hypertrophic pyloric stenosis? *The Journal of Surgical Research, 212*, 229.
18. Gupta, S., Gao, J. J., Emmett, M., et al. (2017). Topiramate and metabolic acidosis: An evolving story. *Hospital Practice, 45*(5), 192.
19. Olson, K. R., Anderson, I. B., Benowitz, N. L., et al. (2018). *Poisoning & drug overdose*. New York: McGraw-Hill.
20. Martin, C. M., & Priestap, F. (2017). Agreement between venous and arterial blood gas analysis of acid-base status in critical care and ward patients: A retrospective cohort study. *Canadian Journal of Anaesthesia, 64*, 1138.
21. Berend, K. (2018). Diagnostic use of base excess in acid-base disorders. *The New England Journal of Medicine, 378*, 1419.
22. Hall, J. E. (2016). *Guyton and Hall textbook of medical physiology* (13th ed.). Philadelphia: Saunders.
23. Glasmacher, S. A., & Stones, W. (2017). A systematic review and diagnostic test accuracy meta-analysis of the validity of anion gap as a screening tool for hyperlactatemia. *BMC Res Notes, 10*, 556.
24. Bell, S. G. (2017). Minding the gap: Utility of the anion gap in the differential diagnosis of metabolic acidosis. *J Neonatal Nurs, 36*, 229.
25. Ross, S. W., Thomas, B. W., Christmas, A. B., et al. (2017). Returning from the acidotic abyss: Mortality in trauma patients with a pH <7.0. *American Journal of Surgery, 214*, 1067.

26. Liu, L., Zhang, L., Liu, G. J., et al. (2017). Peritoneal dialysis for acute kidney injury. *Cochrane Database Sys Rev*, (12), CD011457.

27. Collins, A., & Sahni, R. (2017). Uses and misuses of sodium bicarbonate in the neonatal intensive care unit. *Sem Fetal Neonat Med*, 22(5), 336.

28. Harambat, J., Kunzmann, K., Azukaitis, K., et al. (2017). Metabolic acidosis is common and associates with disease progression in children with chronic kidney disease. *Kid Int*, 92, 1507.

29. Hoorn, E. J. (2017). Intravenous fluids: Balancing solutions. *Journal of Nephrology*, 30, 485.

30. Self, W. H., Semler, M. W., Wanderer, J. P., et al. (2018). Balanced crystalloids versus saline in noncritically ill adults. *The New England Journal of Medicine*, 378, 819.

31. Semler, M. W., Self, W. H., Wanderer, J. P., et al. (2018). Balanced crystalloids versus saline in critically ill adults. *The New England Journal of Medicine*, 378, 829.

32. Sen, A., Keener, C. M., Sileanu, F. E., et al. (2017). Chloride content of fluids used for large-volume resuscitation is associated with reduced survival. *Critical Care Medicine*, 45(2), e146.

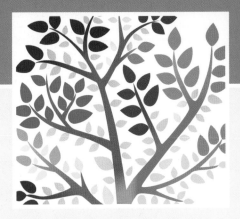

Thermoregulation

L. Jane Rosati and Amy Szoka

The human body has the capability of regulating body temperature at a near constant value, a process known as thermoregulation. Temperature regulation is critical for optimal physiological function. Thermoregulation is a foundational nursing concept; thus, it is essential that nurses apply this concept in nursing practice.

DEFINITION

Optimal physiological function of the human body occurs when a near-constant core temperature is maintained. Normal body temperature ranges from 36.2°C to 37.6°C (97.0°F to 100°F), or an average of 37°C (98.6°F).[1] Fluctuation outside this range is an indication of a disease process, strenuous or unusual activity, or extreme environmental exposure. Thermoregulation is defined as *the process of maintaining core body temperature at a near constant value.*[1] The term *normothermia* refers to the state in which body temperature is within the "normal" range. The term *hypothermia* refers to a body temperature below normal range (<36.2°C), and *hyperthermia* refers to a body temperature above normal range (>37.6°C). An extremely high body temperature is referred to as *hyperpyrexia*.

SCOPE

Thermoregulation is an aspect of homeostasis that balances heat gain and heat loss. The known circadian variation of body temperature usually has an amplitude of 0.8°C to 1.0°C. It is regulated by a circadian variation in the hypothalamic "set point." Body temperature in the middle of a person's usual sleeping time will normally be lower, then begins to rise with their normal waking time, and peaks again late in their usual activity period, decreasing again around the person's usual bedtime. Body temperatures can range from above normal to below normal; thus, the scope of this concept is considered in this way (Fig. 10.1). Physiological adjustments to body temperature are controlled by the hypothalamus—often considered the thermostat center of the body. The nurse uses the average target temperature of 37°C (98.6°F) to assess this state.

NORMAL PHYSIOLOGICAL PROCESS

Thermoregulation occurs through a dynamic and complex physiological process controlled by the hypothalamus that balances heat loss and gain. The hypothalamus establishes a "set point"—meaning the temperature range for optimal physiological functioning. The average hypothalamic set point for core body temperature is 37°C (98.6°F). Compensatory and regulatory actions maintain a steady core temperature. When a person sits or stands, walks or runs, digests food, or even changes his or her respiratory rate, regulation of body functions takes place as the body compensates. A basic review of heat production, heat conservation, and heat loss is foundational to an understanding of thermoregulation. Body temperature is controlled by the dynamic balance of heat production, conservation, and heat loss.

Heat Production and Conservation

Body heat is continually produced through metabolic activity by chemical reactions occurring in the cells. The greatest amount of heat is produced by muscles and through metabolic activity in the liver. Metabolic activity involves the ingestion and metabolism of food and the basal metabolic rate—or the energy required to maintain the body at rest. Basal metabolic rate tends to be higher among younger individuals and decreases as the body ages. Food consumption, physical activity, and hormone levels affect the amount of heat produced. The contraction of muscles produces heat through muscle tone and shivering. Chemical thermogenesis occurs as a result of epinephrine release, which increases metabolic rate. In addition to heat production, the body conserves heat through peripheral vasoconstriction. This process shunts warm blood away from the superficial body tissues and skin surfaces, and increases muscle activity to minimize heat loss.

Heat Loss

Not only does the body continually produce heat through metabolic activity but also it continuously loses heat. Heat loss occurs as a result of multiple mechanisms, including radiation, conduction, convection, vasodilation, evaporation, reduced muscle activity, and increased respiration.

Heat loss to *radiation* occurs through a process of electromagnetic waves that emit heat from skin surfaces to the air. The degree of heat loss through radiation is directly related to the difference between ambient air temperature, skin temperature, and exposure. *Conduction* is a transfer of heat through direct contact of one surface to another; warmer surfaces lose heat to cooler surfaces. A loss of heat by air currents (caused by wind or a fan) moving across the body surface is referred to as *convection*.[2] Warmer air at the body surface is replaced by the cooler air, resulting in cooling of the skin surface. Wet skin or clothing accelerates this process.

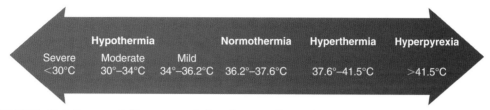

FIGURE 10.1 Scope of Thermoregulation Ranges From Hypothermia to Normothermia to Hyperthermia.

Heat loss can be increased through peripheral *vasodilation*, which brings a greater volume of blood to the body surface. Increased heat loss occurs by conduction (explained previously). However, this process is not effective if ambient air temperature is greater than body temperature. A reduction in muscle tone and muscle activity occurs as another mechanism to minimize heat production. This process explains the fatigue or "washed out" feeling experienced in hot weather or after sitting in a hot tub for a period of time.[3] Perspiration is yet another mechanism involved with heat loss; this process is explained by evaporation of moisture from the skin surface. This provides a significant source of heat reduction and normally accounts for 600 mL of water loss per day. In extreme heat, an individual can lose as much as 4 L of fluids in an hour; for this reason, replacement of fluids and electrolytes is essential to prevent dehydration. Heat is also lost during the process of respiration. Cool ambient air is inhaled and warmed in the respiratory tract and by the microcirculation within the alveoli. The warmed air is then exhaled. For this reason, elevated respiratory rates are seen among individuals with elevated temperature, and lower respiratory rates are seen in individuals with hypothermia.

Temperature Control

Temperature control is mediated by the hypothalamus through neural and hormonal control. The hypothalamus is located below the thalamus in an area of the brain called the diencephalon. This is a small but important area of the brain located between the midbrain and the cerebrum (Fig. 10.2).

Thermoregulation involves a negative feedback system, which reverses or opposes a change in a controlled condition.[3] Multiple thermoreceptors are located throughout the body. Peripheral thermoreceptors (located in the skin) and central thermoreceptors (located in the spinal cord, abdominal organs, and hypothalamus) provide skin and core temperature information to the hypothalamus. The hypothalamus activates a series of responses to lower or raise body temperature based on information received by the thermoreceptors.

When the thermoreceptors signal a lowering of body temperature, the hypothalamus initiates a series of heat-producing and heat-conserving mechanisms through endocrine and sympathetic nervous system connections. Thyrotropin (or thyroxine)-stimulating hormone–releasing hormone (TSH-RH) is secreted by the hypothalamus, which in turn stimulates the anterior pituitary to release thyroid-stimulating hormone (TSH). TSH acts on the thyroid gland to release thyroxine (T_4), which activates the adrenal medulla to cause the release of epinephrine into the blood. Epinephrine increases heat production by increasing the metabolic rate, stimulating glycolysis, and causing vasoconstriction (see Fig. 10.2). The hypothalamus also stimulates the sympathetic nervous system, which triggers the adrenal cortex to increase muscle tone and initiate a shivering and vasoconstriction response.

When the thermoreceptors signal an increase in body temperature, the same mechanisms are reversed (the classic feature of a negative feedback system). The release of TSH-RH is discontinued (thus stopping the T_4 and epinephrine responses), and the sympathetic nervous system is signaled to induce vasodilation, decrease muscle tone, and initiate sweat production (see Fig. 10.2). Sweat glands rapidly produce and release increased levels of perspiration; heat dissipates from the body as sweat evaporates from its surface.

Age-Related Differences

Ineffective thermoregulation occurs at both ends of the age spectrum. Infants and older adults have less efficient physiological mechanisms for heat production and conservation.

Infants

Several important physiological differences among infants exist related to thermoregulation. Newborns do not have heat-conserving capacity; thus, thermoregulation is linked closely with metabolism and oxygen consumption. The newborn infant has a unique source of heat from brown adipose tissue (or brown fat). This tissue is associated with intensified metabolic activity, thus creating greater heat production capacity compared to normal adipose tissue. Brown fat provides an important mechanism for heat production. Because newborn infants generally do not shiver, a process referred to as *non-shivering thermogenesis* (involving increased metabolism and oxygen consumption) helps to offset heat loss.[4] Although newborn infants produce sufficient body heat, they have a propensity for heat loss due to a greater body surface area to weight ratio. The flexed posture of newborns moderates heat loss somewhat by reducing surface area exposure. Another physiological difference leading to newborn heat loss is limited insulation due to a thin layer of subcutaneous fat. Blood vessels are closer to the skin, further contributing to heat loss tendencies.

Thermoregulation becomes more efficient as the infant becomes older. Advanced physiological responses to temperature variations emerge that include the ability of muscles to contract, shivering response, vasoconstriction and vasodilation, and increased adipose tissue.

Older Adults

Several physiological changes associated with aging affect thermoregulation among older adults. Slower circulation, including decreased vasoconstrictor responses, reduced function of thermoregulatory capacity of the skin (including decreased or absent sweating), and reduced heat production (associated with slower metabolic and physical activity), decreased shivering response, and reduced perception of environmental temperature, are seen among older adults.[3]

VARIATIONS AND CONTEXT

Variations in body temperature are represented by higher or lower body temperature from normal and are classified into three major categories: fever, hyperthermia, and hypothermia.

Fever

Fever represents a complex pathophysiological reaction involving the immune system in response to *pyrogens* (fever-producing agents) that

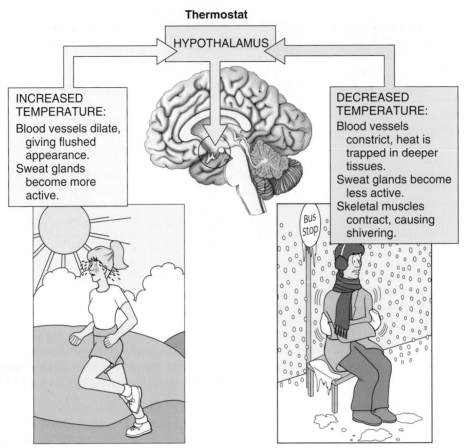

FIGURE 10.2 Temperature Regulation. The hypothalamus controls body temperature and signals for mechanisms to increase heat production or facilitate heat loss. (From Herlihy, B. [2014]. *The human body in health and illness* [5th ed.]. St Louis: Elsevier.)

trigger the hypothalamus in the brain to adjust heat production, heat conservation, and heat loss mechanisms to maintain a higher core temperature, representing an increased hypothalamic set point. (Recall that *set point* is the established value determined by the hypothalamus for optimal physiological function.) There are two kinds of pyrogens. *Exogenous pyrogens* (those of external origin) include bacterial endotoxins, viruses, antigen–antibody complexes, etc. *Endogenous pyrogens* are produced by phagocytic white blood cells as part of the immune response and include interleukin-1, interleukin-6, tumor necrosis factor, and interferon. When exogenous pyrogens invade the body, endogenous pyrogens are released that trigger the production of prostaglandin E_2, which in turn elevates the thermal set point and increases core body temperature.[2]

Hyperthermia

Although elevated body temperature occurs in both hyperthermia and fever, the underlying processes are quite different. Hyperthermia occurs when the body temperature rises above 37.6°C with an unchanged hypothalamic set point. The three physiological mechanisms that coordinate body temperature are also the three mechanisms that can lead to hyperthermia: excessive heat production, inadequate ability to cool, or hypothalamic regulator dysfunction. When heat-related conditions occur, the body's natural ability to dissipate heat is interrupted, resulting in an increase in body temperature that exceeds heat loss. This can occur as a result of several factors, including environment (temperature, humidity, and lack of air movement), excessive physical exertion (particularly in hot, humid environments without sufficient water replacement), genetic

abnormality, metabolic diseases, injury to the hypothalamus, and as a result of pharmacologic agents.

Hypothermia

Hypothermia occurs when the core body temperature declines below 36.2°C and is further classified as mild (34°C to 36°C or 93.2°F to 96.8°F), moderate (30°C to 34°C or 86°F to 93°F), or severe (<30°C or <86°F). Three physiological factors can lead to hypothermia: excessive heat loss, insufficient production of heat, or dysfunction of hypothalamic regulatory mechanisms. Hypothermia may be either accidental or therapeutic. Accidental hypothermia results from environmental exposure (including staying out in the cold too long, wearing insufficient clothing for weather conditions, wet clothing, and cold-water submersion) or as a complication from serious systemic disorders. Therapeutic hypothermia, also called targeted temperature management, is intentionally induced to reduce metabolism and thereby preserve tissue by preventing tissue ischemia such as after a cardiac arrest. Therapeutic hypothermia counteracts the overstimulation of the neuro cells thereby stabilizing calcium and glutamate release reducing cell death.

CONSEQUENCES

Although the body tolerates some variation in body temperature, physiological consequences can occur as a result of elevated or lowered temperature. The two variables that affect the extent of consequences for hypothermia and hypothermia are (1) the extent of temperature change, and (2) the duration of temperature variation.

Consequences of Elevated Body Temperature

A significant increase in body temperature leads to many physiological changes that can be fatal as a result of cardiovascular collapse and damage to the nervous system. Mentioned previously, one compensatory response to elevation in body temperature is sweating—a measure that helps to cool the body. Excessive and prolonged sweating coupled with a sustained high body temperature can result in sodium loss and dehydration if fluid replacement does not occur. Over time, excessive body temperature can lead to hypotension, tachycardia, and decreased cardiac output, progressing to reduced perfusion and coagulation within the microcirculation and cardiovascular collapse. Sustained high core body temperature coupled with reduced perfusion leads to cerebral edema, central nervous system degeneration, and renal necrosis.

Consequences of Hypothermia

The physiological consequences of hypothermia are dependent on the severity and duration of exposure. As core body temperature decreases, compensatory mechanisms including shivering (muscle contraction to simulate warmth) and vasoconstriction (to reduce heat loss) occur. However, because prolonged vasoconstriction would lead to peripheral tissue ischemia, intermittent reperfusion of peripheral tissues occurs. Prolonged hypothermia eventually leads to reduced perfusion in the microcirculation attributable to increased viscosity of the blood and reduced blood flow and coagulation. Also, the vasoconstrictive efforts controlled by the hypothalamus eventually fail, causing vasodilation and thus accelerating the loss of body heat. Individuals experiencing significant hypothermia have been known to remove clothing because of reduced cognition and because the vasodilation can create a false warming sensation.

RISK FACTORS

Risk factors can be described in terms of both populations at risk and individual risk factors. Recognition of risk factors is essential so that appropriate preventive measures can be initiated. Risk factors that affect thermoregulation include age, environment, and physiological condition of the individual.

Populations at Risk

Although all humans are at risk for alterations in thermoregulation, certain population groups have significantly greater risk—particularly the very young and the very old.

Infants and Young Children

Infants (particularly premature infants) have undeveloped temperature regulation capacity. Infants usually produce sufficient body heat, but they lack the ability to conserve heat produced; a large surface area relative to body mass makes them susceptible to excessive temperature loss.[4] Infants and young children are also at risk because they are unable to independently take measures to correct changes in temperature. They are completely dependent on the appropriate actions of caregivers for maintenance of a normothermic temperature range. One of the most visible examples is when infants and young children are trapped inside vehicles, resulting in heat-related deaths.[5]

Older Adults

The elderly experience fluctuations in temperature because of a diminished ability to regulate body temperature due to a less effective thermoregulatory response (described previously).[2] The elderly also have a reduced perception of heat and cold; thus, they may not recognize when to take appropriate action in a timely manner. Elderly who lack resources to stay warm or cool in temperature extremes are also at risk

for thermoregulation. According to the Centers for Disease Control and Prevention (CDC), heat- and cold-related deaths drastically rise among adults older than age 75 years.[6]

Other Population Groups

The risk for heat- and cold-related deaths is twice as high for non-Hispanic black males. Black males have higher rates of heat-related and cold-related deaths than any other race and ethnic group. The CDC reported that non-Hispanic Blacks had a heat-related mortality rate 2.5 times that of non-Hispanic Whites; likewise, non-Hispanic Blacks had a cold-related mortality rate 2.0 times that of non-Hispanic Whites.[6] People of low socioeconomic status may lack resources for adequate clothing, heating, and cooling. The homeless population (because of their frequent exposure to the elements and lack of adequate shelter) is particularly at high risk for hyperthermia or hypothermia. Populations living in certain geographic areas in the United States that have hot or cold climates are also at increased risk. Most heat-related deaths occur in the southern and western states; western states also have the highest cold-related death rates.[6]

Individual Risk Factors

Impaired Cognition

Individuals with impairments in cognition (either acute or chronic) are at risk for imbalanced temperature because of the potential inability to recognize dangerous environmental exposures or the inability to react appropriately. Persons under the influence of drugs or alcohol are at risk because sensory alterations affect judgment or there may be a loss of consciousness, thus increasing the risk for environmental exposure. Because alcohol acts as a vasodilator (dilation of surface blood vessels leads to loss of body heat), it is a common underlying factor in hypothermic deaths.[6]

Underlying Health Conditions

A number of heath conditions are associated with altered thermoregulation (Box 10.1). Individuals with preexisting medical conditions (e.g., congestive heart failure, diabetes, or gait disturbance) are at increased risk for hypothermia because their bodies have a reduced ability to generate heat. Individuals who undergo surgical procedures are also at risk for hypothermia, particularly if the procedure is long as patients

---

BOX 10.1 HEALTH CONDITIONS AS RISK FACTORS FOR ALTERED THERMOREGULATION

- Autoimmune conditions
- Burns
- Chronic conditions
- Hypothalamic injury
  - Traumatic brain injury
  - Stroke
  - Brain neoplasm
- Infection
- Inflammation
- Long surgical procedures
- Metabolic conditions
  - Hyperthyroidism
  - Hypothyroidism
- Prematurity/preterm birth
- Protein calorie malnutrition
- Traumatic injury

may not have adequate covering to conserve heat loss.[7,8] Individuals who have experienced traumatic brain injury are at risk for problems with thermoregulation, particularly if the area of the brain damaged leads to hypothalamic dysfunction.[1]

Several health conditions (infections, autoimmune disorders, trauma, and thyroid disturbances) place individuals at risk for elevated body temperature. Dehydration also may be associated with elevated body temperature because of the need for fluids to cool the body. Some medications, both prescribed and over-the-counter, may impact thermoregulation. Therefore, a complete medication list is needed to further assess risk.

Genetics

A less common risk factor for impaired thermoregulation is genetic predisposition. The classic example of this is malignant hyperthermia (MH), a condition associated with an inherited autosomal dominant pattern. MH is often considered a surgical complication because it is actually a biochemical chain reaction triggered by commonly used general anesthetics and succinylcholine.

Recreational or Occupational Exposures

Individuals may suffer impairments in thermoregulation as a consequence of participating in recreational activities or working in conditions associated with temperature extremes. Strenuous activity in high ambient temperatures, particularly with high humidity, can lead to hyperthermia. Winter recreational activities, such as hiking, snowmobiling, and skiing, can lead to hypothermia if an individual has inadequate clothing for the activity or if the individual becomes lost or injured. Cold water exposure also quickly leads to hypothermia, particularly if the air temperature is also cold.[9]

ASSESSMENT

Body temperature is included in nearly all assessments because this provides baseline information about homeostasis and general health. When problems associated with thermoregulation present, a history and examination are warranted. Assessment begins with the outward appearance of patient, noting sweating and/or shivering, color of skin, and touching the skin for temperature of skin.

History

Typically, a history does not include specific questions related to normal body temperature or thermoregulation. However, in the event of thermoregulation imbalance, a history provides valuable information needed to understand the problem. The age, health history, family history (for MH), and social history provide necessary information to establish risk factors. Additional questions include the presence of recent injury, illnesses, or environmental exposure. If there has been recent environmental exposure, the type, severity, and length of exposure should be determined.

Symptoms associated with hyperthermia vary depending on the degree of elevated temperature and underlying conditions. Reported symptoms may include "feeling feverish" or "feeling hot," chills, general malaise, lethargy, weakness, dizziness, loss of appetite, or muscle cramps. The primary symptom most commonly associated with hypothermia is feeling cold.

Examination Findings
Vital Signs

Nursing assessment begins with measuring vital signs. Body temperature can impact on all vital signs. Therefore, the assessment findings must be considered as a whole and attention given to the accuracy of the measurement method. Body temperature is measured using a thermometer.

The most common routes to measure temperature include oral, rectal, auxiliary, temporal artery, and tympanic.[10] However, when an individual has hyperthermia or hypothermia, the most reliable means available for assessing core temperature is a rectal temperature. A lubricated probe is inserted into the rectal canal at a depth of 1 to 1.5 in. in the adult and 0.5 to 1 in. in the child. Some core temperature sites include the esophagus and urinary bladder.[11] Temperature measurement among infants and children can be accomplished with a tympanic thermometer, an oral thermometer (a pacifier thermometer), an axillary or temporal artery, although the temporal artery method may not be as reliable in children younger than 2 years.

Elevated Body Temperature

Although the general appearance of an individual experiencing hyperthermia varies (depending on the underlying cause and the degree of temperature elevation), several common clinical findings are observed. Vasodilation occurs, causing the skin to appear flushed and warm or hot to touch. If the sweat mechanism has been activated, the individual will be diaphoretic, although this finding may be absent. Patients will often present with dry skin and mucous membranes, decreased urinary output, and other signs of dehydration and electrolyte imbalance. Because of the effects of high body temperature on the brain and central nervous system, seizures may occur, and the patient's cognitive status may range from slightly confused or delirious to coma.

Hypothermia

The clinical presentation of hypothermic patients also varies, depending on the severity of the condition. Peripheral vasoconstriction causes the skin to feel cool and have slow capillary refill; skin color is pale and becomes cyanotic. Muscle rigidity and shivering is typically present in an effort to generate heat. The shivering response diminishes or ceases when the core temperature decreases to 30°C. Cognition is affected because of a gradual reduction in cerebral blood flow.[12] A person may experience poor coordination and sluggish thought processes at 34°C; this progresses to confusion and eventually stupor and coma by the time the temperature decreases to 30°C. Dysrhythmias (e.g., atrial and ventricular fibrillation) may occur due to myocardial irritability. As hypothermia progresses, the metabolic rate declines and perfusion of blood is significantly reduced, leading to diminished urinary function, coma, and cardiovascular collapse.

CLINICAL MANAGEMENT
Primary Prevention

Most cases of hyperthermia and hypothermia are preventable by reducing risk. Primary prevention measures include environmental control and shelter, appropriate clothing for different conditions, and level of physical activity. The nurse's role in primary prevention is through patient education.

Environmental Control and Shelter

Maintaining optimal ambient temperature in the home or having adequate shelter during temperature extremes is essential. If a home does not have air conditioning in the summer months, opening windows and using fans are encouraged. If home heating is inadequate during cold weather, patients should be advised to wear adequate and/or additional clothing and use blankets for additional warmth. Wind drafts should be blocked, and curtains hung at windows to improve insulation.

Community resources, including homeless shelters, can be used to assist those who are unable to stay cool during warm months and warm during the cold months. Individuals also can be encouraged to go to public buildings, such as indoor shopping malls or libraries, where ambient temperatures are usually adequately regulated. For those exposed to the elements, seeking adequate shelter can be life-saving. Shelter includes finding shade and ideally a breeze when temperatures are high, and avoiding the wind and precipitation when temperatures are low.

Appropriate Clothing

The selection of appropriate clothing is another primary prevention strategy. Although this applies to both types of temperature extremes, adequate clothing is essential to prevent hypothermia with cold temperatures. Evaporative heat loss is five times greater when clothing is wet; thus, dry clothing is essential. A newborn is susceptible to rapid heat loss directly after birth, and hypothermia may result. Immediately after delivery, the infant should be dried quickly, wrapped in blankets, and moved to a heated environment. Care should be taken to limit the time the infant's skin is wet (e.g., bathing and wet diapers or clothing).

The infant should be dressed in layers and the head covered for warmth. New parents should be instructed about heat loss in newborns and young children; dressing the infant and child appropriately for the weather and adequate regulation of temperature in the home are essential. When the environmental temperature is low, infants should be provided with a hat to guard against heat loss, just as the elderly patient may need a sweater or clothing with long sleeves for comfort. The elderly (or their caregivers) may need to be reminded to dress in clothing appropriate for the weather.

Physical Activity

Physical activity increases body temperature. Increasing physical activity helps to warm the body when exposed to low temperatures and can prevent hypothermia. Physical exertion in hot conditions increases the risk for hyperthermia because the heat gains may exceed heat loss. Resting, maintaining adequate hydration, wearing appropriate clothing, and seeking shelter will help to reduce risk under such conditions.

Secondary Prevention (Screening)

The goal of secondary prevention refers to the detection of a disease or condition. The only screening mechanism that applies to the concept of thermoregulation is screening for MH. Because susceptibility to MH is inherited (autosomal dominant disorder), genetic screening is available and recommended for individuals who have relatives with genetic mutations.

Collaborative Interventions

Management of the patient with altered thermoregulation is dependent on the core body temperature and the overall physical condition of the individual. Generally, infants and young children, the elderly, and individuals in poor health not only have greater risk factors but also have less physical capacity for physiological compensation when changes in core body temperature occur.

Elevated Body Temperature

The underlying cause of the elevated body temperature should be identified (e.g., a fever associated with an inflammatory process or hyperthermia associated with exposure). Regardless of the cause, the goal is to minimize cardiovascular and neurologic complications associated with excessive body temperature. Care of the individual whose temperature has exceeded 37°C should include removal of excess blanketing and clothing while observing for continued signs of hyperthermia (increased respiration, increased or decreased perspiration, high fever, and seizures). Signs and symptoms that persist beyond 1 hour require further intervention. Hydration, nutritional support, and other palliative measures to reduce core temperature should be implemented. Cool packs may be placed in the axillary and groin areas; a cooling blanket or lukewarm bath may also facilitate temperature reduction. Care should be taken not to induce shivering. More aggressive cooling efforts include gastric or colonic lavage with cool fluids.

The presence of fever is considered an expected finding with a systemic inflammatory response. Mild to moderate fever generally does little harm and may actually have beneficial effects to counteract the inflammation. However, complications such as dehydration and increased metabolic demand can occur.[13] Symptomatic relief of persistent or intermittent fevers can be treated with antipyretics such as nonsteroidal anti-inflammatory drugs (e.g., naproxen or ibuprofen and aspirin) and acetaminophen. Aspirin is also useful for reducing fever but should be used with caution; aspirin is not recommended for children because of the risk of Reye syndrome. The use of a drug called dantrolene sodium can reverse the effects of MH. Intracellular calcium levels are elevated in MH; dantrolene counteracts this abnormality by reducing muscle tone and metabolism. Administration of dantrolene intravenously has dramatically reduced the mortality rate of MH.[14]

Hypothermia

The goal of managing hypothermic patients is to increase the body temperature to the normal range. An initial step is to remove the individual from the cold. If hypothermia is mild, passive and active external rewarming measures are indicated. Passive measures include dry and warm clothing, warm drinks, and exercise, and these may be enough. However, active rewarming measures may be necessary and include providing warm blankets or heating pads, drawing a warm water bath, and placing the patient in a heated environment. The use of heated intravenous fluid helps with hypothermia if the patient is receiving more than 500 mL.

CLINICAL NURSING SKILLS FOR THERMOREGULATION

- Assessment
- Monitoring vital signs
  - Temperature measurement
  - Heart rate
  - Respiratory rate
  - Blood pressure
- External warming devices
  - Warm blankets
  - Administer warm oral fluids
- Active core warming
  - Warm intravenous fluids
  - Heated humidified oxygen
  - Warm fluid lavage
- Cooling measures
  - Cool water bath
  - Cool intravenous fluids
  - Cool fluid lavage
  - Cooling blankets

When core body temperature falls below 35°C, active core rewarming measures are indicated—meaning there is an application of heat directly to the core. Core rewarming should be done slowly and carefully to minimize the risk of triggering dysrhythmias; thus, continuous cardiac monitoring and core body temperature observation are necessary. Active core rewarming strategies include infusion of warm intravenous solutions, gastric lavage with warm fluid, peritoneal lavage with warm fluid, and inhalation of warmed oxygen. In cases of accidental hypothermia with cardiac deterioration, extracorporeal membrane oxygen may be indicated.[15–16]

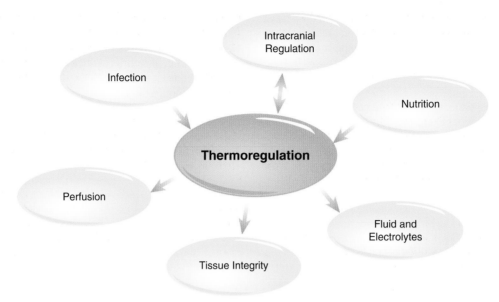

FIGURE 10.3 Thermoregulation and Interrelated Concepts.

INTERRELATED CONCEPTS

A large number of concepts are clearly interrelated to thermoregulation. Those that have greatest importance are presented in Fig. 10.3.

Infection is defined as the invasion and multiplication of microorganisms in body tissues, which may be clinically unapparent or may result in local cellular injury due to competitive metabolism, toxins, intracellular replication, or antigen–antibody response. When infection is present, physical symptoms often include fever and chills. Because the hypothalamus regulates body temperature, Intracranial Regulation is closely associated with thermoregulation. Traumatic brain injury, with its associated cerebral edema, ischemia, energy failure, oxidative stress, and neuronal death, may directly affect the temperature control center.[17] Often, when injury occurs to the brain or spinal cord, there is interruption of the sympathetic nervous system that prevents peripheral temperature sensations from reaching the hypothalamus. Perfusion is impacted by body temperature. Measures to minimize or maximize heat loss include vasodilation and vasoconstriction within the blood vessels; severe extremes in body temperature can result in cardiovascular collapse. The skin plays an important role in body temperature regulation. The skin acts as a protective layer to reduce heat loss. In addition, thermoreceptors in the skin alert all individuals to extremes in temperatures, thus preventing injury. These mechanisms require intact skin and Tissue Integrity. Metabolism of nutrients provides the body with fuel needed for the generation of heat and body activities. Malnutrition increases the risk for hypothermia because of an inability to generate adequate heat. For this reason, Nutrition is interrelated with thermoregulation. Fluid and Electrolytes are affected by thermoregulation. Efficient perspiration requires adequate fluid balances. Fluid and electrolyte imbalances can occur when excessive body temperature exhausts available fluids for perspiration.

CLINICAL EXEMPLARS

Although there are many situations and conditions that can cause altered thermoregulation, the distinct exemplars are fairly straightforward (Box 10.2). It is beyond the scope of this book to describe all possible causative factors and exemplars in detail, although brief descriptions of featured exemplars are presented next. Refer to medical surgical,

BOX 10.2 EXEMPLARS OF ALTERED THERMOREGULATION

- Fever
- Hyperthermia
- Heat cramps
- Heat exhaustion
- Heatstroke
- Malignant hyperthermia
- Hypothermia
- Frostbite
- Therapeutic hypothermia

ACCESS EXEMPLAR LINKS IN YOUR GIDDENS EBOOK

pediatric, geriatric, critical care, and other textbooks for detailed information about exemplars.

Featured Exemplars
Fever

The most common exemplar of thermoregulation is fever. Fever is a temporary elevation in body temperature caused by the immune system's release of endogenous pyrogens (a protein produced by leukocytes) in response to an invasion of bacteria, viruses, fungi, toxins, or drugs.[18] Specifically, pyrogens trigger the hypothalamus to increase the thermostatic set point. The elevated body temperature is thought to increase the production of white blood cells, thus enhancing the immune system response. Fever can also occur due to an exaggerated immune response such as autoimmune disorders or allergic reaction.

Malignant Hyperthermia

MH is a hypermetabolic disorder of skeletal muscle triggered by the induction of anesthetic agents and leads to severe hyperthermia. Susceptibility to MH is inherited as an autosomal dominant disorder; several forms of genetic mutations increase susceptibility. Many of these gene mutations are linked to inherited muscle diseases such as central core disease and multi-minicore disease. Epidemiologic studies reveal that

MH complicates 1 in approximately 100,000 surgeries in adults and 1 in approximately 30,000 surgical procedures in children.[14]

Heatstroke

Heatstroke occurs as a result of exposure to excessively high temperatures in the environment. The condition often occurs when performing physical exertion in a hot environment without proper ventilation. Hyperthermia results because the body cannot adequately cool itself and keep the temperature at the correct level. The central nervous system may not be functioning properly due to disease or injury. The condition is characterized by alterations in mental status, an increase in body temperature, with hot dry skin; severe conditions can be fatal.

Preterm and Newborn Hypothermia

Preterm and newborn hypothermia occurs with heat loss by radiation, evaporation, and conduction. Mechanisms of heat loss cause the newborn to be dependent on environmental temperature to keep warm. It is recommended that a newborn's axillary temperature be regulated at 36.5°C or 97.8°F. A subnormal temperature requires a radiant warmer for additional heat. Preterm infants are often kept under a radiant warmer or in an incubator with protection from draft air. Swaddling, a cap for the head, and/or skin-to-skin contact are additional ways to keep the infant warm.

Environmental Exposure Hypothermia

Environmental exposure hypothermia occurs from exposure to cold temperatures or immersion in cold water; it is exacerbated by weather elements such as precipitation, humidity, and wind. Without proper clothing or shelter, environmental exposure presents a challenge to the thermoregulatory systems of the body. The body compensates by initiating thermoregulatory mechanisms, such as shivering and vasoconstriction, but eventually a hypothermic state occurs if the exposure is extensive in time and/or severity. Hypothermia due to environmental exposure can occur at any age, although very young and older adults are at greatest risk.[6]

CASE STUDY

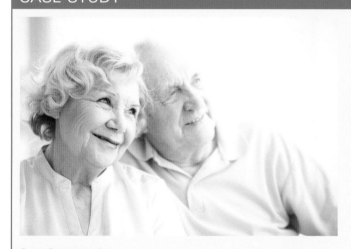

Case Presentation

Tom Anderson is an 86-year-old white male who lives with his 82-year-old wife in their home in upstate New York. During the past few years, Mrs. Anderson has noticed a decline in her husband's mental status. Early on a January morning, Mrs. Anderson was awakened at 4 a.m. by the doorbell. When she opened the door, a neighbor was standing with her husband, who was wearing nothing but his pajamas. The neighbor explained that he saw Mr. Anderson wandering outside on the snowy street. Tom was shivering uncontrollably and confused; the outdoor temperature was only 19°F. Mrs. Anderson immediately called 911 and had her husband transported to the hospital.

From Shironosov/iStock/Thinkstock.

Upon arrival to the emergency department, the nurse noted the following assessment findings:

- Mental status: Confused; not oriented to person, place, or time
- Vital signs: Temperature, 33.1°C rectally; pulse, 62 beats/min; respirations, 12 breaths/min; blood pressure, 100/62 mm Hg
- Skin: Pale, cyanosis around lips and extremities
- Uncontrollable shivering

The nurse immediately placed Mr. Anderson in a dry gown, covered him with warming blankets, and placed him in a warm room. The findings were immediately reported to the physician, and the following measures were implemented:

- Stat electrocardiogram followed by continuous cardiac monitoring
- Continuous vital sign and pulse oximeter monitoring
- Cover patient with warming blanket set at 98.6°F
- Apply warm oxygen at 3 L/min via nasal cannula
- Blood draw for hemoglobin and hematocrit, electrolytes, blood gases, blood urea nitrogen and creatinine, blood glucose, and toxicology screen

After several hours in the emergency department, Mr. Anderson's core body temperature slowly increased to 35.4°C; he stabilized but remained confused. He was admitted to the medical unit for further evaluation.

Case Analysis Questions

1. What risk factors for impaired thermoregulation are represented by this case?
2. Review the treatment measures described in the clinical management section of this chapter and compare these to this case. How are the interventions similar?

 ACCESS EXEMPLAR LINKS IN YOUR GIDDENS EBOOK

REFERENCES

1. Sund-Levander, M., & Grodzinsky, E. (2013). Assessment of body temperature. *British Journal of Nursing, 22*(16), 942–950.
2. McCance, K., & Huether, S. (2015). *Pathophysiology* (ed. 7). St Louis: Mosby.
3. Thibodeau, G., & Patton, K. (2016). *Structure and function of the body* (ed. 15). St Louis: Elsevier.
4. Hockenberry, M., & Wilson, D. (2015). *Wong's nursing care of infants and children* (ed. 10). St Louis: Mosby.
5. Vanos, J. K., Middel, A., Poletti, M. N., & Selover, N. J. (2018). Evaluating the impact of solar radiation on pediatric heat balances within enclosed hot vehicles. *Journal of Temperature, 5*(3), 276–292.
6. Centers for Disease Control and Prevention: Deaths attributed to heat, cold, and other weather events in the United States, 2006–2010, *National*

Health Statistics Reports, 76, July 2014, http://www.cdc.gov/nchs/data/nhsr/nhsr076.pdf.

7. Uzoigwe, C. E., Khan, A., Smith, R. P., et al. (2014). Hypothermia and low body temperature are common and associated with high mortality in hip fracture patients. *Hip International*, *24*(3), 237–242.

8. Thomas, J. (2015). Preventing postoperative hypothermia. *Pennsylvania Nurse*, *70*(2), 14–20.

9. Watson, J. (2018). Inadvertent postoperative hypothermia prevention: Passive versus active warming methods. *ACORN*, *31*(1), 43–46.

10. Ball, J. W., Dains, J. E., Flynn, J. A., et al. (2015). *Seidel's guide to physical examination* (ed. 8). St Louis: Elsevier.

11. Niven, D., Gaudet, J., Laupland, K., et al. (2015). Accuracy of peripheral thermometers for estimating temperature: A systematic review and meta-analysis. *Annals of Internal Medicine*, *163*(10), 768–777.

12. Open Anesthesia. *Cerebral blood flow: Temperature effect*, 2018. https://www.openanesthesia.org/cerebral_blood_flow_temperature_effect/.

13. Mayo Clinic. *Fever*, 2018. Retrieved from https://www.mayoclinic.org/diseases-conditions/fever/symptoms-causes/syc-20352759.

14. Malignant Hyperthermia Association of the United States (MHAUS): *Managing a crisis*, 2018. Retrieved from https://www.mhaus.org/healthcare-professionals/managing-a-crisis/.

15. Niehaus, M. T., Pechulis, R. M., Wu, J., et al. (2016). Extracorporeal membrane oxygenation (ECHMO) for hypothermic cardiac deterioration: A case series. *Prehospital Disaster Medicine*, *31*(5), 570–571.

16. Mazur, P., Kosinski, S., Podsiadlo, P., et al. (2019). Extracorporeal membrane oxygenation for accidental deep hypothermia—current challenges and future perspectives. *Annals of Cardiothoracic Surgery*, 8(1), 137–142.

17. Tran, L. V. (2014). Understanding the pathophysiology of traumatic brain injury and the mechanisms of action of neuro-protective interventions. *Journal of Trauma Nursing*, *21*(1), 30–35.

18. Blomqvist, A., & Engblom, D. (2018). Neural mechanisms of inflammation-induced fever. *The Neuroscientist*, *24*(4), 381–399.

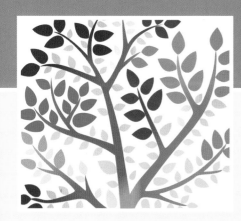

Sleep

Beth Rodgers

Sleep is an essential component of life. The adequacy of sleep affects physiological, psychological, and social functioning. Sufficient quality sleep is crucial to metabolic regulation, cognitive functioning, quality of life, mood, and nearly every other aspect of existence. Sufficient quality of sleep is required to decrease risks for devastating chronic conditions that affect the respiratory, cardiovascular, metabolic, and endocrine systems. Despite the critical nature of sleep, a large percentage of people report that their sleep is inadequate either in quantity or in quality.[1] This widespread problem with sleep deprivation constitutes a significant public health concern because people are at greater risk for chronic illness, decreased quality of life, and accidents and injuries due to what often are very treatable problems with sleep.[2–9] Nurses in all settings have an important role in identifying sleep problems, instituting effective strategies to improve sleep, and promoting healthy sleep as part of an overall program of wellness and disease management.

DEFINITION

People tend to think they have a good understanding of sleep, especially because everyone does it and, in fact, every living mammal engages in sleep. It does not seem very complicated to close your eyes and drift into a state detached from the busy day of wakefulness. However, sleep really is quite complex—even more so because the activities and events associated with sleep take place completely outside of the individual awareness. The very nature of sleep means that the person who is sleeping is not aware of the process. Historically, sleep was considered to be merely a period of inactivity. However, with the development of the ability to monitor brain activity it became apparent that sleep really is a period of considerable action. In more recent years, researchers have discovered that a large number of physiological processes take place during sleep, including neurologic, metabolic, and endocrine activity.

Sleep is a relatively new field of study, and specialization and dictionary definitions often do not match the prevailing state of science. The *Oxford Dictionary of English*, for example, presents a definition of sleep as "a condition of body and mind such as that which typically recurs for several hours every night, in which the nervous system is relatively inactive, the eyes closed, the postural muscles relaxed, and consciousness practically suspended."[10] This definition is partially accurate, but it fails to acknowledge the essential processes that take place during sleep. Merriam–Webster presents a similar approach, with the definition of sleep as "the natural periodic suspension of consciousness

during which the powers of the body are restored."[11] All definitions have in common a change in consciousness that includes loss of awareness of the surrounding environment. More detailed definitions can be very specific about what is happening in the brain or in differentiating specific stages of sleep. For general purposes, the most important idea is that sleep is *natural, necessary, involves a shift in physiologic and neurologic activity, and is intended to be restorative.*

SCOPE

Sleep occurs in a cyclic pattern following intermittent periods of wakefulness for the majority of humans. The time spent in sleep varies across individuals, as does the time of day during which sleep occurs. Despite such natural variation, there is a recurring need in all humans for a period of physical inactivity and a change in level of consciousness that allows for restoration and for specific physiological mechanisms to take place. Ideally, after a quality period of sleep, the individual returns to an alert state feeling refreshed and restored.

For a variety of reasons, some people may not feel restored and refreshed after a period of sleep. This may be due to lifestyle or behavior patterns that prevent the individual from receiving the needed volume and quality of sleep. Lack of restorative sleep also may be indicative of a "sleep disorder," which is a diagnosis of a specific pattern of sleep that is not compatible with the health needs of the individual.

Thus, from a broad perspective, the scope of sleep ranges from restorative sleep that results in an individual feeling rested to impaired sleep leaving the individual not feeling rested or refreshed. Impaired sleep can be intermittent or chronic, with chronic sleep being associated with physical, cognitive, and social challenges (Fig. 11.1).

NORMAL PHYSIOLOGICAL PROCESS

Following a period of wakefulness, humans need to enter a period of rest and sleep that enables them to experience physiological restoration. Sleep occurs in stages and, under normal circumstances, in a fairly consistent pattern of movement through the stages. In general, the stages of sleep can be divided into two major categories: non-rapid eye movement (NREM) and rapid eye movement (REM). In normal sleep, the individual proceeds through four stages of NREM sleep and then to the REM stage (Fig. 11.2). Movement must be through all four stages before reaching REM. Each stage lasts generally from 5 to 15 minutes, and the entire cycle through all four stages plus REM typically takes

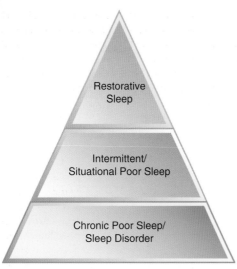

FIGURE 11.1 Scope of Sleep.

90 to 110 minutes. The duration of REM sleep gets progressively longer during the night, producing more deep sleep consistent with this state.

Non-Rapid Eye Movement Sleep

In stage 1 (N1 or NREM stage 1), referred to as light sleep, the individual can be awakened easily. In this stage, brain waves slow and, on electroencephalogram (EEG), the slower wave pattern known as alpha (α) waves appears. The individual at this point is likely to drift in and out of sleep and can be awakened easily. Sensations known as hypnagogic hallucinations can occur during this stage. A common sensation of this type is the feeling of falling. Uncontrolled muscle jerks sometimes occur at this stage along with sudden movements that can startle the individual and restore wakefulness.

In stage 2 (N2), eye movement ceases; brain waves become even slower, with the exception of an occasional burst or more rapid brain waves. Pulse rate and respirations slow, and body temperature decreases as the individual moves toward deeper stages of sleep. Stage 3 (N3) and stage 4 (N4) are the periods of deep sleep. N3 is characterized by very slow brain waves called delta waves interspersed with smaller, faster waves. In N4, the EEG shows almost exclusively delta waves. In this type of sleep, it is difficult to awaken the individual and muscle activity is very limited or may be completely absent. A person awakened from stage 3 or 4 of sleep could be disoriented for a brief period of time before regaining awareness.

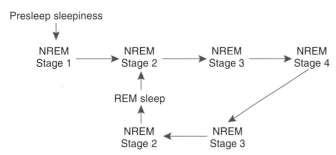

FIGURE 11.2 **Stages of Adult Sleep Cycle.** *NREM,* Nonrapid eye movement; *REM,* rapid eye movement. (From Potter, P. A., & Perry, A. G. [2013]. *Fundamentals of nursing* [8th ed]. St Louis: Mosby.)

Rapid Eye Movement Sleep

REM sleep commonly begins approximately 90 minutes after the onset of sleep. The first REM period may be rather short, sometimes lasting only 10 minutes. Periods of REM become progressively longer as the individual completes successive sleep cycles, and the final period of REM may last as long as 1 hour. EEGs of REM sleep show patterns of brain activity that are very similar to those produced when an individual is awake. In individuals who have normal sleep patterns (i.e., no sleep disorder), cardiac and respiratory rates increase and become uneven, and the REM for which this stage is named takes place. This also is the stage of active dreaming related to the increase in brain activity. Although the brain is more active, there is a form of muscular paralysis that prevents the individual, in normal circumstances, from engaging in movement or other action that could be very dangerous given the activity of the brain during this time.

Restorative Processes of Sleep

Deep sleep is essential for the body to accomplish important restorative processes. Not only does such restoration contribute to wakefulness and alertness during nonsleeping hours but also the body undertakes a number of important physical processes, including tissue regeneration, muscle and bone development, and immune enhancement. Regulation of body metabolism and fat deposition also are affected by the depth and duration of deep sleep. Other hormones associated with sleep and that are essential for health include cortisol, human growth hormone, and leptin and ghrelin—the hormones that regulate appetite and body fat deposition. Sex and reproductive hormones also are affected by sleep and include secretion of testosterone and hormones associated with fertility—follicle-stimulating hormone and luteinizing hormone. An increase in the hormone melatonin at the onset of sleep helps to promote and maintain sleep, and a decrease in levels leads to eventual awakening. The immune system is enhanced as well during sleep as proteins associated with fighting illness are produced. The circadian rhythm, or the typical 24-hour (more or less) cycle through which the body passes, including both awake and sleep cycles, is responsible for regulating all of the physiological processes in the body. Therefore an adequate amount and quality of sleep is essential to all of the regulatory mechanisms that take place in the body.

Age-Related Differences

Sleep is quite consistent throughout the lifespan with regard to physiological processes and the need for restoration and renewal. There also is general consistency in the circadian rhythm. Normal variations that occur with aging pertain primarily to the amount of total sleep needed and the amount of time spent in the various stages of sleep. Individual variation does occur and, in many cases, can be considered within normal limits. Such variation is discussed later. The most noticeable changes associated with age include the amount of sleep and the sleep architecture (the constitution of the sleep pattern). The amount of sleep typically needed by people in each age group is as follows[12–15]:

- *Infants:* 14 to 16 hours each day
- *Toddlers:* 9 or 10 hours at night in addition to 2 or 3 hours of daytime naps
- *School-age children:* 9 to 11 hours
- *Teenagers:* 9 hours
- *Adults:* 7 to 9 hours

It is important to remember that these are general recommendations and some variation will occur. Infants tend to sleep in shorter periods but with multiple episodes of sleep throughout the day. Sleep time gradually decreases during the first several months of life so that by approximately age 6 months, the infant can sleep throughout the night with at least one nap during the day. Infants spend as much as 50% of their sleep time in REM compared to approximately 20% in adults. EEG differences have been documented to show changes in brain activity that occur in sleep at different stages of life.[15]

Older adults may have more difficulty falling asleep, an occurrence referred to as increased sleep latency. They also may experience more awakenings during the night, which leads to a fragmented sleep pattern. Older adults often will awaken more quickly when aroused from sleep. The amount of time spent in deep sleep may decrease, with a corresponding increase in the time spent in N2. These are not necessarily age-related changes; it is likely that medical conditions, such as pain, discomfort, and medication side effects, interfere with the quality of sleep in older adults. Nonetheless, this pattern of changes in latency and time spent in various stages of sleep is very common as adults age.[16]

VARIATIONS AND CONTEXT

The National Sleep Foundation[1] conducts periodic studies of sleep habits and outcomes in the United States. Results of the 2015 poll revealed that approximately one-half of the population does not receive the amount or quality of sleep necessary for good health. The 2018 poll was focused primarily on the relationship between pain and other health conditions and sleep, but still revealed that while the majority of the respondents acknowledged that sleep is important, 41% indicated they did not make sleep a priority when they made plans for each day. In its 2008 study, 49% of people reported not feeling well rested at least several nights per week in the prior month, 65% reported experiencing some type of sleep problem several nights or more per week in the prior month, and 28% reported sleepiness interfering with their daily functioning at least a couple of days per week. This survey has shown consistently that sufficient quality and quantity of sleep are ongoing problems for adults in the United States.

Poor Sleep Patterns

Although the amount of sleep needed by each individual varies, research has shown that those who claim they function well on minimal sleep actually respond to tests in a manner consistent with someone who is sleep-deprived. In addition, they are at greater risk of physical problems consistent with inadequate sleep regardless of their subjective assessment of functioning and sleep quality.[1]

Many variations in sleep are the result of controllable phenomena: personal choices about bedtime; dietary habits, ingestion of alcohol or stimulants, frequent napping, and so on. The environment in which someone sleeps can lead to poor sleep quality as well; for example, noise or disruptive light, a television left on, a bed partner who moves frequently or snores, or a lack of safety in the home environment. Caregiving responsibilities, such as ill or elderly housemates or infants and children with interrupted sleep patterns, can affect the sleep of others in the vicinity. Work and job responsibilities may result in poor sleep due to fragmentation as a result of working more than one job or problems associated with shift work. Any of these can result in a substantial disturbance in sleep. Situational challenges such as worry or stress also can contribute to periodic episodes of ineffective sleep. In such situations, it is common for an individual to have difficulty falling asleep or remaining asleep. Waking several times during the night to deal with worries or stress easily can lead to ineffective sleep. Most people experience ineffective sleep at some, or multiple, points in their lives. When the problem is recurrent or ongoing, the individual may be said to have a sleep disorder.

Research also is showing that exposure to blue light or light-emitting diodes (LEDs) close to bed time interferes with restorative sleep as it alters the body's normal regulatory mechanisms.[17] This relationship is so significant that manufacturers of common handheld computer equipment, such as tablets and smartphones, have added capability for the user to set specific times for the device to filter blue light. Research also has shown that some of the age-related disturbances in sleep may be due to the yellowing of the lens of the eye, which affects the transmission of blue light to the retina.[18] This provides additional support for the impact of light and other environmental factors on sleep quality.

Sleep Disorders

Many individuals have a sleep disorder defined in accordance with existing diagnostic standards such as those set by the American Academy of Sleep Medicine. Variations in sleep can occur along several different dimensions. There may be insufficient time spent sleeping, poor quality of sleep despite adequate time, problems falling or staying asleep, intermittent or situational disturbances in sleep, and any number of situations that result in a lack of feeling rested and refreshed on awakening. Problems with sleep become a "sleep disorder" when the difficulty is recurring or chronic. Sleep disorders are fairly common and similar regardless of age. Disorders in children are similar to those of adults, although enuresis (bed-wetting) is more a factor in children, as are sleep-onset anxiety, night terrors, and behavioral problems around bedtime. Obstructive sleep apnea (OSA) occurs in an estimated 1% to 3% of children, although the causative factors may differ, with tonsillar enlargement being a significant component in children.[19]

Primary Sleep Disorders

Primary sleep disorders are those that exist as an independent condition. The most common categories of primary disorders include insomnia, sleep-related breathing disorders, sleep-related movement disorders, parasomnias, circadian rhythm sleep disorders, and hypersomnia:

- Insomnia exists when there is difficulty falling asleep or staying asleep.
- Sleep-related breathing disorders involve either a problem with the airway, as seen in OSA, or a problem with the neurologic drive to breathe during sleep (central sleep apnea).
- Sleep-related movement disorders include restless leg syndrome and periodic limb movement disorder.
- Parasomnias include a variety of behaviors, such as sleepwalking, sleep terror, and REM behavior disorder.
- Circadian rhythm sleep disorders occur when the drive to sleep does not occur according to what would be considered a normal sleep–wake pattern, such as someone who stays awake until early morning and does not have the drive to fall asleep as nighttime progresses.
- Hypersomnia is characterized by excessive sleepiness or falling asleep at inappropriate times. Narcolepsy is an example of hypersomnia as a primary sleep disorder.

Secondary Sleep Disorders

Secondary sleep disorders occur as the result of some other situation, and correcting that situation should resolve the problem with sleep. Secondary disorders are often caused by medical conditions, mental health conditions, and side effects of medical treatments. Box 11.1 presents medical conditions that are commonly known to interfere with sleep. A secondary sleep disorder also may be associated with the use of any medication that has either a sedative or a stimulating effect because either of these actions can interfere with restorative sleep (Box 11.2). Prematurity in infants also may lead to problems with sleep secondary to the state of neurologic or cardiovascular development.

> ## BOX 11.1 COMMON CONDITIONS THAT AFFECT SLEEP
>
> - Alzheimer disease
> - Anxiety
> - Arthritis
> - Asthma
> - Cancer
> - Chronic obstructive pulmonary disease
> - Chronic kidney disease
> - Depression
> - Diabetes
> - Epilepsy
> - Febrile conditions
> - Fibromyalgia
> - Gastroesophageal reflux disease
> - Heart failure
> - Hyperthyroidism
> - Menopause
> - Pain
> - Parkinson disease
> - Stroke

> ## BOX 11.2 COMMON PHARMACEUTICAL CATEGORIES THAT IMPAIR SLEEP
>
> - Antiarrhythmics
> - Antihistamines
> - β-blockers
> - Corticosteroids
> - Diuretics
> - Nicotine products
> - Selective serotonin reuptake inhibitors
> - Theophylline
> - Thyroid hormone

CONSEQUENCES

Excessive daytime sleepiness is a very distressing side effect of insufficient or poor quality sleep. In addition to the psychological and emotional challenges of sleepiness, the physiological consequences of poor sleep are widespread and can be serious. When sleep is inadequate, a large number of basic regulatory mechanisms of the body do not function effectively. Commonly occurring physiological consequences of poor sleep include hypertension, heart disease, heart failure, stroke, obesity, and developmental disorders that may be related to physiological factors such as alternations in growth hormone. Reproductive disorders can occur due to disruption in hormonal regulation. Mortality is increased significantly for people who report less than 6 or 7 hours of sleep per night, and studies have shown that sleep is a greater risk factor for mortality than smoking, high blood pressure, and heart disease.[2–6] Sleep apnea particularly increases the risk for metabolic syndrome, diabetes, hypertension, and heart disease, and it has been identified as a potential causative factor for these conditions. Research has revealed that the common stereotype of individuals having sleep apnea because of obesity is not accurate and that the obesity may actually be the outcome. Sleep, therefore, is essential to effective weight management, and anything that diminishes the amount or quality of sleep can have significant consequences. Immune function also is diminished in cases of inadequate sleep. Sleep is essential for all of the body's physiological

mechanisms, so results of poor sleep are widespread and significant. It is quite common clinically to see individuals with multiple health problems, including diabetes, heart disease, and hypertension, who have a concomitant sleep disorder as a potential causative or aggravating factor in the physical problems. In children, poor sleep quality or insufficient sleep may be manifested primarily by developmental and behavioral abnormalities that may have physiological components as well.[2–6]

RISK FACTORS

Every human being is at risk for sleep problems. Wherever sleep exists as a part of the life pattern, there is the potential for challenges with sleep or diagnosable sleep disorders. Although the risk for sleep problems is widespread, several known factors place individuals or groups at greater risk; also, risk factors are not easily generalizable because some risk factors are unique for specific sleep problems. Assessment of sleep can be made easier by recognizing common risk factors associated with various conditions.

Populations at Risk

As a population, middle-aged and older individuals are at greater risk for nearly all adult sleep disorders. Hormonal changes, changes in routine and lifestyle with advancing age, and the development of medical conditions (and subsequent symptoms and treatments) are all common among people as they age.[14–16,19] Women tend to be at greater risk for some sleep disorders, including insomnia and restless leg syndrome. Pregnant and perimenopausal women often experience sleep disturbances as a result of hormone fluctuations that can disrupt sleep through night sweats or lead to symptoms of insomnia. Pregnant women have the additional challenge of changes in body shape that create discomfort and difficulty breathing when lying down, along with pressure on the bladder that can lead to frequent awakenings. Men are at higher risk for OSA than women until menopause, at which point the risk for women increases to near that of men. African Americans, Hispanics, and Pacific Islanders are at greater risk for OSA than Caucasian populations. Children also have a greater risk for OSA than the general population, primarily as a result of tonsillar enlargement. Obesity can increase the risk for OSA in children as well.[19–24]

Individual Risk Factors

The most notable individual risk factors are related to family history, individual behaviors, and underlying conditions.

Family History

Family history is a significant factor in the occurrence of most sleep disorders, including OSA, narcolepsy, and insomnia. However, the nurse is not likely to have this information unless a thorough history is obtained. The completion of a thorough history is complicated by the fact that it is quite common for people not to know that a family member did, in fact, have a sleep disorder.

Individual Behavior

Individuals who work variable shifts, particularly involving night shifts (e.g., emergency medical technicians and firefighters), are at risk for ineffective sleep and sleep disorders, especially if they try to maintain a typical daytime period of wakefulness on days they are not working. Also at risk for sleep disorders are those who work very long hours and have monotonous routines such as truck drivers.

Individuals who have undergone a recent life change or are experiencing increased stress are at high risk for sleep problems, particularly insomnia. Those who have irregular daily routines often experience problems with inadequate sleep or poor sleep quality, and the idea that it is possible to "catch up" is believed by many; however, research shows that such attempts to catch up are not effective and do not compensate for poor sleep at other times. Drug and alcohol use along with dietary behaviors, such as consumption of stimulants, also interfere greatly with sleep. Other dietary habits, television watching in bed, disturbance from light, or a bed partner who is restless or has different sleep times all can interfere with the quality of sleep an individual receives. Child care and other responsibilities can disrupt sleep as well. Many people live in environments in which they do not feel safe either for domestic reasons or because of the environment surrounding their residence. An overwhelming number of people who report poor "sleep hygiene" experience insufficient and poor quality sleep.[1,22]

Underlying Medical Conditions

A significant risk factor for ineffective sleep is having one or more underlying medical conditions, pharmaceutical agents used to treat medical conditions that interfere with sleep, or the treatments for those conditions interfere with sleep (see Boxes 11.1 and 11.2). Symptoms that commonly interfere with sleep include pain, problems breathing, and anxiety.

Persons with retrognathia (receding jaw) and micrognathia (small jaw structure) or with craniofacial abnormalities are at greater risk for OSA, as are children with tonsillar enlargement. Obesity commonly is reported as a risk factor for OSA as well, although it is important to note that the obesity may occur as a consequence of OSA and not necessarily as a cause. The association of OSA and obesity means that OSA should be considered as a possibility in anyone who is obese, particularly as the obesity advances to more severe levels. Sleep disorders also are commonly associated with heart disease and respiratory conditions as both an outcome and a risk factor. Therefore individuals with heart and respiratory problems should be evaluated for sleep quality. In women, polycystic ovarian syndrome has been found to be highly associated with sleep disorders, including OSA.[17–25]

ASSESSMENT

Although assessment of sleep is a component of health assessment, this is not addressed consistently by healthcare personnel. Practitioners do not always ask patients about sleep, and when concerns are discussed, clinicians may have difficulty differentiating fatigue or tiredness from sleepiness. In view of the importance of sleep to overall health, nurses should incorporate sleep assessment with all patients with whom they interact to determine if individuals are getting sufficient restorative sleep.

Assessment of sleep is complicated by the fact that individuals cannot subjectively determine the quality of their sleep. Individuals with OSA, for example, might say they "sleep" 10 hours each night and do not understand why they are so "tired." However, during that 10 hours, they have no way of knowing what is happening to their bodies. People also quite commonly report feeling "tired," but "tired" may be the result of many different conditions or factors. Tired, fatigued, and sleepy are very different in origin. Someone who has difficulty falling asleep or awakens frequently might complain of "insomnia," but awareness of what actually happens during sleep is usually limited. In terms of assessment, then, it is important to recognize that time spent in bed is not a good indicator of amount or quality of sleep. Problems with sleep result in "sleepiness," which can be differentiated from tiredness or fatigue. There are instruments that, with a few questions, can determine someone's sleepiness or likelihood of falling asleep under certain circumstances. These are not typically applied outside of specialty centers, but they are a good example of how attention to "sleepiness" can help to identify sleep problems.[26–31] More recently, a variety of apps have been developed to work on Smartphones as a convenient way for people to monitor their own sleep behaviors and sleep quality. Many of these have been adapted for clinician use as well or can generate reports to be evaluated by a health professional.[26–31]

History

Start by asking the individual how he or she feels upon awakening. Ideally, the person awakens feeling rested and refreshed. Any response to the contrary indicates less than ideal sleep. The individual may not feel rested and refreshed on awakening, may lack energy to do the things he or she enjoys, or may feel less productive at work. Statements indicating weakness, malaise, lack of appetite, and so on may accompany reports of fatigue.

A description of what happened while trying to sleep should come next. If the individual reports difficulty falling asleep, assessment should include a discussion of what happens when the individual tries to sleep. Are thoughts racing? Is there discomfort that prevents sleep? Does the individual feel safe while sleeping? Does the individual awaken during the night or awaken early in the morning? What awakens him or her? What happens around any awakening? Inquire about the sleeping environment, including the bedroom and comfort factors such as light and temperature. Specific inquiry regarding physical symptoms, including discomfort or need to urinate that might lead to awakening, can be helpful, along with any other symptoms such as headache, dry mouth, or nasal stuffiness. Inquire about the thoughts, worries, or concerns the individual might be aware of when awakening. Can the person return to sleep quickly after being awakened? What position is the individual in when awakening? Is the bed in disarray, indicating the person has been very active while sleeping? If there is a bed partner, any observations made about the person's behavior while asleep can be very informative.

A detailed history of behavior prior to sleep is key to determining whether or not a sleep problem exists and what the nature of that problem might be. Fatigue is an extremely common symptom of impaired sleep, and, in many cases, the cause is behavioral in origin. The individual stays up late during the week, perhaps to watch television or have some quiet time after tasks are completed, and then arises early the next morning. The use of medications, recreational drugs, stimulants, alcohol, sedentary or active lifestyle, and dietary habits can be associated with sleep problems. Daytime napping may contribute to poor sleep at night, as may other possible factors, such as stress, dietary habits, lack of exercise, and exposure to LEDs near bedtime.[17,18]

A thorough review of systems is important to identify problems that might indicate an underlying sleep disorder, such as pins and needles feelings in the legs or pain or nocturnal urination that disrupt the pattern of sleep. Headache, respiratory problems, dry mouth or sore throat, heartburn or reflux, a feeling of the heart beating either very fast or irregularly, a pins and needles feelings, or pain in any part of the body are all possible findings on the history and review that may be indicative of a sleep disorder. Also, family history is significant because there is a strong familial predisposition for most of the sleep disorders.

Examination Findings

Relatively few physical exam findings directly indicate a sleep disorder. However, sleep disorders are more common in people with upper airway or craniofacial construction that can lead to a more easily obstructed upper airway. Micrognathia, retrognathia, enlarged tonsils, somewhat thicker tongue, and a generally smaller upper airway are common in people with OSA. A measurement known as the Mallampati score is a determination of the difficulty of inserting an oral airway and reflects the openness of the upper airway. This measurement is used in assessment of sleep disorders. A Mallampati score of 3 or 4 is common in individuals with OSA. Neck circumference of 16 or greater in women and 17 or greater in men also is associated with OSA. Although obesity may be a result of sleep problems and not a cause, there is a higher incidence of OSA in people with higher body mass index (BMI). Therefore, a BMI of 30 or greater may indicate a possibility of OSA. OSA also can occur in people with normal or lower BMI, so it should not be relied on as an exclusive screening tool for OSA. People who are obese often have OSA, but not everyone with OSA is obese.[32,33]

Physical examination of respiratory and cardiac function is helpful because such conditions often are associated with sleep disorders either as sequelae or by raising problems with circulation and oxygenation that then interfere with sleep. Cardiac function and general skin and mucous membrane color can indicate oxygenation status and thus can alert the nurse to possible sleep problems. Neurologic changes also tend to have an impact on sleep quality; therefore abnormalities detected on examination of this system might point to the existence of challenges to sleep.

Diagnostic Tests

A variety of tests can be conducted that might identify conditions that have occurred as a result of sleep problems. The only definitive tests for sleep problems are those that measure activity and events related to sleep and wakefulness. These are most often done after referral to a sleep medicine specialist who can determine the most likely cause of the sleep problem and order appropriate tests. There are tests that are focused on determining ability to stay awake, time needed to fall asleep, actigraphy that monitors time spent in awake and sleeping states, and an array of other related tests. An actigraph is a device that is worn on the wrist to record general movement. Analysis of the recording using special software can provide an estimate of sleep patterns and may be a helpful adjunct to subjective reports and sleep diaries. Actigraphy has been found to be a valid measure in a variety of populations, although it is not a definitive diagnostic tool.[34]

Polysomnogram

One of the most important tests to identify sleep disorders is the polysomnogram (PSG). A PSG is conducted while an individual sleeps, and includes the monitoring of an array of physical parameters. PSGs can be used to evaluate a variety of sleep disorders, including difficulty falling asleep, difficulty staying awake, and sleep-related breathing disorders. PSGs are conducted using an array of electrodes and monitoring devices that can vary depending on the specific reason for conducting the study. Generally, however, a PSG will involve EEG-type electrodes to monitor sleep patterns and stages, stretching belts to measure respiratory effort, leads to monitor muscle activity (typically on the limbs but also for chin/jaw and eye movement), nasal and oral airflow, and pulse oximetry. Monitors to document body position also may be indicated, and the entire experience often is recorded on videotape. Registered PSG technicians conduct these studies in clinical facilities designed specifically for overnight sleep studies; this also includes video monitoring and, if indicated, the capability for initiating and titrating positive airway pressure therapy for people found to have OSA during the PSG. Individuals who work at night and sleep during the day should have their studies done during the daytime to match their usual routine. A limited version of an overnight sleep study can be done outside of a sleep lab, typically in the home setting. Although home studies typically lack some of the monitoring capability of lab studies, they are effective in documenting sleep-related breathing problems and are used in some settings as an alternative to more costly studies or in cases of long waits for an overnight study.

Sleep Journals

Other means of data collection to help in the diagnosis of sleep problems are subjective in nature, particularly the maintenance of a sleep journal.

Individuals may be asked to record a summary of their daily activities, dietary intake, bedtime, discussion of what happened during the night, and time of awakening. Subjective assessment on awakening, such as whether or not the individual feels refreshed and restored on awakening, can be an important adjunct to other means of measuring and assessing sleep. As noted previously, subjective assessment of sleep is fraught with difficulties because an individual who is sleeping is not aware of what is happening during sleep.

CLINICAL MANAGEMENT

Clinical management of sleep problems varies with the nature and type of problem or disorder. Regardless of more specific interventions that might be indicated, improvement in sleep begins with understanding and implementing behaviors that are conducive to quality sleep, an approach that is referred to generally as sleep hygiene. The major components of sleep hygiene are the sleeping environment and personal behavior. Proper sleep hygiene often is enough to remedy problems with sleep and is the foundation for quality sleep. It is also something that nurses can work with independently and make a significant difference in the lives of people with whom they work (and in their own).

Primary Prevention

Sleep hygiene is a critical link in healthy sleep and either avoiding or managing sleep problems. Sleep hygiene includes attention to the environment for sleep and to personal behavior. The sleeping environment should be comfortable, well ventilated, quiet, and as dark as possible. The optimal temperature for sleep usually is a bit cool; either cold or too warm a temperature can interfere with sleep quality. The bed should be used only for sleep and sexual activity. Bedding and blankets should be evaluated along with other factors of the environment to determine if something in the bed or environment overall is detracting from the quality of sleep.

Personal behaviors and habits are widespread causes of sleep problems. A lack of time spent in sleep often contributes to daytime sleepiness. A large number of sleep complaints and problems stem from not allocating enough time to sleep or not making sleep a priority. Too often sleep is done only when everything else in the person's busy life has been completed. The healthiest pattern is to have a consistent bedtime and awakening time and to adhere to that pattern at all times. Sleep also needs to be a priority; the motivation to sleep, and placing a priority on sleep, usually are associated with good sleep habits and sleep quality. Napping generally is discouraged except in cases in which the naptime is short (30 minutes or so) and the individual has no problem falling asleep at bedtime. Dietary habits, particularly alcohol and stimulants, should be avoided as bedtime approaches, generally 4 to 6 hours before bed. Alcohol, stimulants, eating a heavy meal, spicy foods, or sugary foods should be avoided 4 to 6 hours before bedtime. Regular exercise is very conducive to healthy sleep, although many people find that it is not beneficial to exercise close to bedtime.[35–38]

Use of over-the-counter sleep products can interfere significantly with quality sleep patterns, and it is easy for an individual to feel dependent on the product for sleep. Older adults, particularly, may consume products that contain antihistamines and other sedating drugs without being aware that these actually can contribute to persistent sleep problems. Many products marketed for nighttime pain relief contain other drugs that may interfere with quality sleep. Even those advertised to help with sleep can, with regular use, negatively affect healthy sleep patterns. Therefore primary prevention focuses on good sleep hygiene and the elimination, when possible, of factors that may interfere with or limit the quality of sleep.[35–38]

Secondary Prevention (Screening)

A number of instruments can be used for more focused screening of sleep problems. The American Academy of Sleep Medicine has a screening tool that addresses a variety of sleep problems. Selected aspects of this tool can be adapted and used for screening as appropriate to the population and as screening reveals aspects of sleep that warrant a more specific focus.[39]

Other professional organizations that are focused on sleep, along with a number of clinical agencies, have developed their own screening tools for use in assessing sleep quality and the presence of sleep problems specific to the populations with which they work. Nurses will not have difficulty finding age and developmentally appropriate screening tools. Because of the subjective nature of sleep quality, considerable screening can be accomplished with some fairly simple questions that determine whether the individual awakens rested and refreshed and whether some lifestyle or behavioral factors might be responsible for any problems in this area.

Collaborative Interventions
Sleep Hygiene

Sleep hygiene, as noted previously, is the foundation of any approach to improving sleep and thus is applicable as a prevention strategy and an intervention for sleep disturbances. Without a good foundation of appropriate lifestyle and behavioral approaches to sleep, other interventions will fall short of the desired outcome of quality and restorative sleep. Despite the importance of a solid foundation of sleep hygiene, that alone is not always sufficient to resolve existing sleep problems. Collaboration with individuals capable of prescribing other interventions, then, becomes necessary. In most cases, referral should be made to a sleep specialty center for more thorough assessment and diagnosis.

Pharmacologic Agents

Pharmaceutical preparations also may be needed in some situations related to poor sleep quality. In general, sleep aids and other medications designed to address sleep problems should be used only after a thorough assessment, and after measures related to improved "sleep hygiene" have been implemented. Common pharmacologic agents used to treat sleep disorders are presented in Box 11.3. These should be used with caution, and the patient should be monitored for effectiveness. For some conditions, such as restless leg syndrome, specific agents targeting the nervous system are used. These would require referral to a neurologist or sleep specialist for assessment and determination of an appropriate treatment regimen. Melatonin can be used in cases of circadian rhythm problems and difficulties associated with maintaining a functional sleep–wake pattern. Pharmaceutical-grade (standardized) melatonin should be used to ensure quality and consistency in strength and only the lowest dose possible for a short period of time should be consumed.[40–50]

Invasive Procedures

For individuals with upper respiratory system obstructions such as upper airway resistance syndrome or OSA, dentists and oral surgeons with additional and specialized education in sleep disorders can perform surgical procedures to provide more openness to the airway or construct oral appliances that aid in keeping the airway open during sleep.[51,52]

INTERRELATED CONCEPTS

A number of concepts are related to sleep through their essential role in healthy sleep patterns. The number of concepts that are related to

---

BOX 11.3 COMMON PHARMACOLOGIC AGENTS USED TO TREAT SLEEP DISORDERS

Anticonvulsants
- Gabapentin (Neurontin)

Antidepressants
- Amitriptyline (Elavil)
- Bupropion (Wellbutrin)
- Doxepin (Sinequan)
- Fluoxetine (Prozac)

Antihistamines
- Diphenhydramine (Benadryl)

Benzodiazepines
- Diazepam (Valium)
- Flurazepam (Dalmane)
- Lorazepam (Ativan)
- Triazolam (Halcion)

Benzodiazepine Receptor-Like Agents
- Zolpidem (Ambien)
- Zaleplon (Sonata)
- Eszopiclone (Lunesta)

Melatonin-Receptor Agonists
- Ramelteon (Rozerem)

---

sleep is quite extensive. The concepts of greatest concern in discussing sleep directly are presented in Fig. 11.3.

Perfusion and Gas Exchange are shown with bidirectional arrows in Fig. 11.3 because poor perfusion can cause problems sleeping and poor sleep exacerbates many cardiac and respiratory conditions, such as coronary artery disease, chronic obstructive pulmonary disease, and asthma. Cognition is also shown with a bidirectional arrow because many individuals with impaired cognition experience sleep disturbances and impaired sleep can affect cognitive function. Individuals experiencing Pain often have problems sleeping—unless the pain can be adequately managed. Changes in Hormonal Regulation, such as increased thyroid secretion, can alter stages of sleep, and altered sleep can affect hormone regulation. Problems with Elimination are known to be disruptive to sleep, particularly in adults; enuresis (bed-wetting) is an example of a childhood sleep dysfunction. Fatigue is a common outcome associated with impaired sleep. Stress and Coping can be affected significantly by quality of sleep as well, with lack of sleep creating difficulties with daily functioning and resilience.

CLINICAL EXEMPLARS

There are many types of sleep disorders that serve as exemplars of this concept. Exemplars are presented in Box 11.4, organized by the disorder category as appropriate. Although a detailed discussion of each of these exemplars is beyond the scope of this text, several are briefly described next. Refer to pediatric, medical, surgical, and geriatric references for additional information.

Featured Exemplars
Insomnia

The term insomnia refers to the inability to fall asleep or stay asleep and can last a few days (transient) or can occur over time. Insomnia

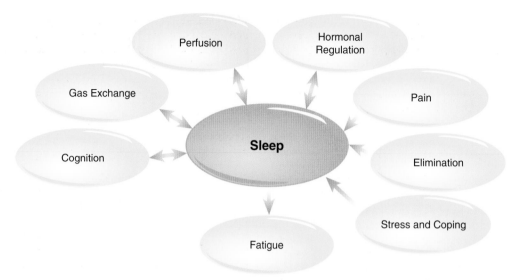

FIGURE 11.3 Sleep and Interrelated Concepts.

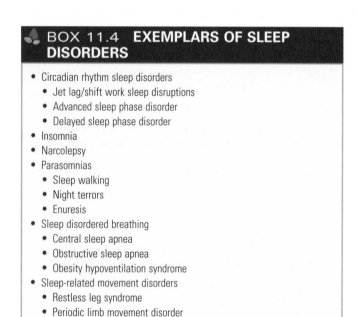

ACCESS EXEMPLAR LINKS IN YOUR GIDDENS EBOOK

can be associated with any number of conditions, including acute stress, pain, depression, and underlying medical conditions, and it can occur as a result of drug or alcohol use. A common scenario involves an individual who is stressed by work or life events, lies in bed with thoughts racing, cannot stop thinking about the events of the day or concerns, and consequently cannot fall asleep or cannot maintain sleep, waking up in the middle of the night only to have the disturbing thoughts gathering attention again.

Jet Lag/Shift Work Sleeping Disorders

The most common circadian rhythm sleep disorder occurs among individuals who work variable shifts (particularly night shifts) and those who do extensive travel. This condition is characterized by disruptions in the sleep–wake cycle, thus affecting the individual's ability to sleep. For those who travel across time zones, the term "jet lag" is often used because the individual's body time is not synchronized with the environmental time, thus affecting the sleep–wake cycle. There is a direct

correlation between the severity of symptoms and the number of time zones crossed.

Narcolepsy

Narcolepsy is a poorly understood chronic neurologic disorder caused by a deficiency of a neuropeptide (hypocretin) that results in the inability of the brain to properly regulate sleep–wake cycles. This condition is most common among adults and is characterized by overwhelming daytime sleepiness; individuals with this condition often find it difficult to stay awake for long periods of time, and they may experience brief periods of falling asleep throughout the day. This condition can lead to poor school and work performance, creating significant challenges, including reduction in functional ability.

Obstructive Sleep Apnea

Obstructive sleep apnea is a condition characterized by interruption of sleep due to temporary airway obstruction by the soft palate, base of the tongue, or both. These structures collapse against the pharyngeal walls due to reduced muscle tome during sleep. The episodes, lasting up to 30 seconds, result in decreased oxygen saturation and fragmented sleep. A person with OSA typically will describe being extremely tired despite having spent sufficient time in bed. Other symptoms include heavy snoring, chronic daytime sleepiness, and fatigue; a sore throat or headache on awakening may also be reported.

Obesity Hypoventilation Syndrome

Obesity hypoventilation syndrome (OHS), one of the most severe forms of sleep-disordered breathing, is characterized by poor gas exchange (resulting in reduced oxygen and increased carbon dioxide levels in the blood) during sleep. Although the exact cause is unknown, OHS is thought to be caused by impaired respiratory mechanics (due to excessive weight against the chest wall) and depressed respiratory control during sleep. Most individuals with OHS are overweight or obese and often have a short, thick neck. Common symptoms include reports of poor sleep quality, daytime sleepiness, fatigue, and headaches.

Somnambulism

The common term for somnambulism is sleep walking. This condition occurs most frequently among children (especially school-aged children) but can occur among adults as well. Somnambulism is characterized by getting out of bed and doing an activity in a partial-wakefulness state during NREM sleep. The activity is often goal-directed and can range from sitting up in bed to walking around the house, moving objects, and even driving a car with no recall of the event on awakening.

Sleep Terrors

Sleep terrors (also known as night terrors) are a parasomnia characterized by sudden episodes of intense fear, screaming, panic, and confusion while still asleep. The episode can last from just a few seconds to several minutes. There is usually increased respiratory rate, heart rate, dilated pupils, and diaphoresis. Night terrors are not associated with dreams during REM sleep, and there is usually no recall of the awakening. Night terrors occur most often during early to middle childhood, although they can occur among adults, particularly those under significant stress or those associated with substance use.

CASE STUDY

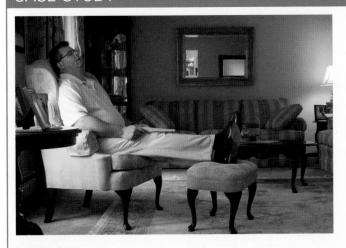

Case Presentation

Jim Wyatt is a 42-year-old Caucasian male, 5 ft. 11 in. and 200 pounds, with a BMI of 27.9 (considered overweight according to BMI tables). He reports being tired "all the time." Other health problems include hypertension that is poorly controlled with three prescription medications and an HgbA1C level that has been rising, with the most recent measure at 6.2. On a typical day, he awakens at 6:30 a.m., often with a significant headache and feeling like he has not gotten a good night's sleep. He adds that on most mornings, he has a dry mouth as well. He is worried that his work performance is suffering, and he has trouble staying awake at meetings. He had one minor traffic accident recently when his car went off the road after he fell asleep at the wheel. He often will nap when he gets home from work, and he falls asleep watching television after dinner. He attempts to go to bed at approximately 9:30 or 10:00 p.m. each night with the hope of getting enough sleep so he will not be so tired the next day. He has stopped going to social events in the evening due to the difficulty he has staying awake. On a recent camping trip, his companions teased him about his loud snoring. He explains that his father "was the same way." On physical exam, the nurse notes that he is having difficulty staying awake while he is talking and he has a neck circumference of 17 ½ in. On examination of his oropharynx, the nurse cannot visualize the uvula or tonsils.

Case Analysis Questions

1. Consider Fig. 11.1. Where on the scope of sleep does Mr. Wyatt fall?
2. What risk factors does Mr. Wyatt have that are associated with impaired sleep?
3. How would you describe the impact of Mr. Wyatt's sleep issues on his quality of life?

From Michael Greenberg/Digital Vision/Thinkstock.

 ACCESS EXEMPLAR LINKS IN YOUR GIDDENS EBOOK

REFERENCES

1. National Sleep Foundation. *Sleep in America Poll (2002–2018)*. Retrieved from https://sleepfoundation.org/sleep-polls.
2. Agaronov, A., Ash, T., Sepulveda, M., et al. (2018). Inclusion of sleep promotion in family-based interventions to prevent childhood obesity. *Childhood Obesity*, doi:10.1089/chi.2017.0235. [Epub ahead of print].
3. Ogilvie, R. P., & Patel, S. R. (2018). The epidemiology of sleep and diabetes. *Current Diabetes Reports*, 18, 82.
4. Twig, G., Shina, A., Afek, A., et al. (2016). Sleep quality and risk of diabetes and coronary artery disease among young men. *Acta Diabetologica*, 53(2), 261–270.
5. May, A. M., & Mehra, R. (2014). Obstructive sleep apnea: Role of intermittent hypoxia and inflammation. *Seminars in Respiratory and Critical Care Medicine*, 35(5), 531–544.
6. Colten, H. R., & Altevogt, B. M. (Eds.), (2006). *Sleep disorders and sleep deprivation: An unmet public health problem*. Washington, DC: Committee on Sleep Medicine and Research, Board on Health Sciences Policy, National Academies Press.
7. Bin, Y. S., Marshall, N. S., & Glozier, N. (2012). Secular trends in adult sleep duration: A systematic review. *Sleep Medicine Reviews*, 16, 223–230.
8. Chattu, V. K., Sakhamuri, S. M., Kumar, R., et al. (2018). Insufficient sleep syndrome: Is it time to classify it as a major noncommunicable disease? *Sleep Science*, 11(2), 55–64.
9. Hublin, C., Partinen, M., Koskenvuo, M., et al. (2007). Sleep and mortality: A population-based 22-year follow-up study. *Sleep*, 30(10), 1245–1253.
10. Oxford University Press. (2005). Sleep. In *Oxford Dictionary of English*. Oxford: Oxford University Press.
11. Merriam–Webster (n.d.). *Sleep*. Retrieved from http://www.merriam-webster.com/dictionary/sleep.
12. Novelli, L., Ferri, R., & Bruni, O. (2013). Sleep cyclic alternating pattern and cognition in children: A review. *International Journal of Psychophysiology: Official Journal of the International Organization of Psychophysiology*, 89(2), 246–251.
13. Moraes, W., Piovezan, R., Poyares, D., et al. (2014). Effects of aging on sleep structure throughout adulthood: A population-based study. *Sleep Medicine*, 15(4), 401–419.
14. Iglowstein, I., Jenni, O. G., Molinari, L., et al. (2003). Sleep duration from infancy to adolescence: Reference values and generational trends. *Pediatrics*, 111(2), 302–307.
15. Redeker, N. S. (2011). Developmental aspects of normal sleep. In N. S. Redeker & G. P. McEnany (Eds.), *Sleep disorders and sleep promotion in nursing practice* (pp. 19–32). New York: Springer.
16. Gulia, K. K., & Kumar, V. M. (2018). Sleep disorders in the elderly: A growing challenge. *Psychogeriatrics: the Official Journal of the Japanese Psychogeriatric Society*, 18(3), 155–165.
17. Shechter, A., Kim, E. W., St-Onge, M. P., et al. (2018). Blocking nocturnal blue light for insomnia: A randomized controlled trial. *Journal of Psychiatric Research*, 96, 196–202.
18. Kessel, L., Siganos, G., Jorgensen, T., et al. (2011). Sleep disturbances are related to decreased transmission of blue light to the retina caused by lens yellowing. *Sleep*, 34, 1215–1219.

19. Baweja, R., Calhoun, S., Baweja, R., et al. (2013). Sleep problems in children. *Minerva Pediatrica*, *65*(5), 457–472.

20. Hiestand, D. M., Britz, P., Goldman, M., et al. (2006). Prevalence of symptoms and risk of sleep apnea in the US population: Results from the National Sleep Foundation Sleep in America 2005 Poll. *Chest*, *130*(3), 780–786.

21. Chen, X., Wang, R., Zee, P., et al. (2015). Racial/ethnic differences in sleep disturbances: The Multi-Ethnic Study of Atherosclerosis (MESA). *Sleep*, *38*(6), 877–888.

22. Ralls, F. M., & Grigg-Damberger, M. (2012). Roles of gender, age, race/ ethnicity, and residential socioeconomics in obstructive sleep apnea syndromes. *Current Opinion in Pulmonary Medicine*, *18*(6), 568–573.

23. Koo, B. B. (2015). Restless leg syndrome across the globe: Epidemiology of the restless legs syndrome/Willis-Ekbom disease. *Sleep Medicine Clinics*, *10*(3), 189–205.

24. Moran, L. J., March, W. A., Whitrow, M. J., et al. (2015). Sleep disturbances in a community-based sample of women with polycystic ovary syndrome. *Human Reproduction*, *30*(2), 466–472.

25. Won, C., & Guilleminault, C. (2015). Gender differences in sleep disordered breathing: Implications for therapy. *Expert Review of Respiratory Medicine*, *9*(2), 221–231.

26. Gulia, K. K., & Kumar, V. M. (2018). Sleep disorders in the elderly: A growing challenge. *Psychogeriatrics: the Official Journal of the Japanese Psychogeriatric Society*, *18*(3), 155–165.

27. Fino, E., & Mazzetti, M. (2018). Monitoring healthy and disturbed sleep through smartphone applications: A review of experimental evidence. *Sleep and Breathing*. Retrieved from https://doi.org/10.1007/ s11325-018-1661-3.

28. Damiani, M. F., Quaranta, V. N., Falcone, V. A., et al. (2013). The Epworth Sleepiness Scale: Conventional self vs physician administration. *Chest*, *143*(6), 1569–1575.

29. Ulasli, S. S., Gunay, E., Koyuncu, T., et al. (2014). Predictive value of Berlin Questionnaire and Epworth Sleepiness Scale for obstructive sleep apnea in a sleep clinic population. *The Clinical Respiratory Journal*, *8*(3), 292–296.

30. Billings, M. E., Rosen, C. L., Auckley, D., et al. (2014). Psychometric performance and responsiveness of the Functional Outcomes of Sleep Questionnaire and Sleep Apnea Quality of Life Index in a randomized trial: The HomePAP study. *Sleep*, *37*(12), 2017–2024.

31. Borsini, E., Ernst, G., Salvado, A., et al. (2015). Utility of the STOP-BANG components to identify sleep apnea using home respiratory polygraphy. *Sleep and Breathing*, *19*(4), 1327–1333.

32. Leitzen, K. P., Brietzke, S. E., & Lindsay, R. W. (2014). Correlation between nasal anatomy and objective obstructive sleep apnea severity. *Otolaryngology–Head and Neck Surgery: Official Journal of American Academy of Otolaryngology-Head and Neck Surgery*, *150*(2), 325–331.

33. Laratta, C. R., Ayas, N. T., Povitz, M., et al. (2017). Diagnosis and treatment of obstructive sleep apnea in adults. *CMAJ: Canadian Medical Association Journal = Journal de l'Association Medicale Canadienne*, *189*(48), E1481–E1488.

34. Kawada, T. (2013). Sleep parameters from actigraphy and sleep diary: Is the agreement important for sleep study? *Sleep Medicine*, *14*(3), 298–299.

35. Irish, L. A., Kline, C. E., Gunn, H. E., et al. (2015). The role of sleep hygiene in promoting public health: A review of empirical evidence. *Sleep Medicine Reviews*, *22*, 23–36.

36. Kline, C. E., Irish, L. A., Buysse, D. J., et al. (2014). Sleep hygiene behaviors among midlife women with insomnia or sleep-disordered breathing: The SWAN Sleep Study. *Journal of Women's Health*, *23*(11), 894–903.

37. Hood, H. K., Rogojanski, J., & Moss, T. G. (2014). Cognitive–behavioral therapy for chronic insomnia. *Current Treatment Options in Neurology*, *16*(12), 321.

38. Kloss, J. D., Nash, C. O., Walsh, C. M., et al. (2016). A "Sleep 101" program for college students improves sleep hygiene knowledge and reduces maladaptive beliefs about sleep. *Behavioral Medicine (Washington, D.C.)*, *42*(1), 48–56.

39. American Academy of Sleep Medicine (n.d.). *Screening questions–Sleep history & physical.* Retrieved from https://aasm.org/resources/medsleep/ (harding)questions.pdf.

40. Earley, C. J. (2014). Latest guidelines and advances for treatment of restless legs syndrome. *The Journal of Clinical Psychiatry*, *75*(4), e08.

41. Philip, P., Chaufton, C., Taillard, J., et al. (2014). Modafinil improves real driving performance in patients with hypersomnia: A randomized double-blind placebo-controlled crossover clinical trial. *Sleep*, *37*(3), 483–487.

42. Pergolizzi, J. V., Jr., Taylor, R., Jr., Raffa, R. B., et al. (2014). Fast-acting sublingual zolpidem for middle-of-the-night wakefulness. *Sleep Disorders*, doi:10.1155/2014/527109.

43. Idzikowski, C. (2014). The pharmacology of human sleep, a work in progress? *Current Opinion in Pharmacology*, *14*, 90–96.

44. Victorri-Vigneau, C., Gérardin, M., Rousselet, M., et al. (2014). An update on zolpidem abuse and dependence. *Journal of Addictive Diseases*, *33*(1), 15–23.

45. Schwartz, T. L., & Goradia, V. (2013). Managing insomnia: An overview of insomnia and pharmacologic treatment strategies in use and on the horizon. *Drugs in Context*, *2013*, 212257.

46. Vellante, F., Cornelio, M., Acciavatti, T., et al. (2013). Treatment of resistant insomnia and major depression. *La Clinica Terapeutica*, *164*(5), 429–435.

47. Shah, C., Sharma, T. R., & Kablinger, A. (2014). Controversies in the use of second-generation antipsychotics as sleep agent. *Pharmacological Research*, *79*, 1–8.

48. Schroeder, A. M., & Colwell, C. S. (2013). How to fix a broken clock. *Trends in Pharmacological Sciences*, *34*(11), 605–619.

49. Tamrat, R., Huynh-Le, M. P., & Goyal, M. (2014). Non-pharmacologic interventions to improve the sleep of hospitalized patients: A systematic review. *Journal of General Internal Medicine*, *29*(5), 788–795.

50. FDA-approved drugs to treat sleep disorders. (2013). *Journal of Psychosocial Nursing and Mental Health Services*, *51*(10), 9–10.

51. Mintz, S. S., & Kovacs, R. (2018). The use of oral appliances in obstructive sleep apnea: A retrospective cohort study spanning 14 years of private practice experience. *Sleep and Breathing*, *22*(2), 541–546.

52. Basyuni, S., Barabas, M., & Quinnell, T. (2018). An update on mandibular advancement devices for the treatment of obstructive sleep apnoea hopopnoea syndrome. *Journal of Thoracic Disease*, *10*(Suppl.), S48–S56.

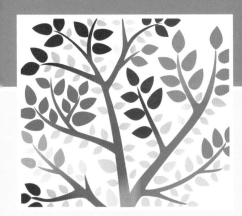

Cellular Regulation

Kevin Brigle

The cell is always speaking—the secret is to learn its language.

Andrew S. Bajer, Cell Biologist

Cells are the smallest form of life; they are the functional and structural units of all living things. The regulation of cellular activity is an intricate and tightly regulated process not only through the lifespan of an *individual* cell but also between cells. To maintain health, cells are constantly working, changing, sending and responding to chemical cues, and correcting mistakes whenever possible. When this is not possible, specific cellular pathways are activated to remove individual cells that are no longer functioning as they have been programmed to do. Although the complex interconnected circuits of cellular regulation have tremendous fidelity, irreparable errors can occur at many steps along these pathways, leading to permanent abnormal changes that can significantly impact biophysical and psychosocial health and functional status. Nurses should be familiar with the scope and process of cellular regulation, the consequences of altered cellular regulation, and the healthcare priorities to implement when conditions of altered cellular regulation develop.

DEFINITION

The term cellular regulation refers to all functions carried out within a cell to maintain homeostasis, including its responses to extracellular signals (e.g., hormones, cytokines, and neurotransmitters) and the way it produces an intracellular response.[1] Included within these functions is cellular replication and growth. Common terms used to describe detailed aspects of cellular reproduction and growth include proliferation and differentiation. Proliferation refers to the production of new cells through cell growth and cell division. Differentiation refers to the acquisition of a specific cell function, a normal process by which a less specialized cell becomes a more specialized cell type. These terms are further described later. Another important term associated with this concept is neoplasia, an abnormal and progressive multiplication of cells, leading to the formation of a neoplasm (also known as a tumor). A neoplasm refers to new but abnormal tissue growth that is uncontrolled and progressive. Neoplasms are categorized as either benign or malignant (cancerous).

SCOPE

The concept of cellular regulation is very broad and represents all aspects of cellular function. Some of the basic functions that cells have in common include creating fuel for the body, manufacturing a complex array of proteins, transporting materials, and disposing of wastes. Included in cellular regulation is cellular division and reproduction—processes that are strictly controlled for normal cells. The scope of this concept analysis focuses on the *cellular growth and reproduction* aspect of cellular regulation and the development of malignant neoplasms described previously. In this context, normal cellular growth is at one end of the spectrum, whereas malignant neoplasia is at the opposite end. Within this continuum is dysplasia, which describes morphologically abnormal cells having high risk of becoming malignant (Fig. 12.1).

NORMAL PHYSIOLOGICAL PROCESS

Normal Cellular Reproduction and Growth

Cellular replication is an extraordinarily efficient process with millions of cells generated daily over the course of one's life. New cells are formed through a process of cell division referred to as proliferation. The rate of proliferation varies according to the needs of the tissue involved. For example, rapid proliferation occurs within epithelial cells, bone marrow, and the gastrointestinal tract, whereas slower proliferation occurs in muscles, cartilage, and bone.

There are two kinds of normal cell division: mitosis and meiosis. Mitosis is essentially a duplication process: Two genetically identical "daughter" cells are produced from a single "parent" cell. Mitosis may take place in cells in all parts of the body, keeping tissues and organs in optimal working order. Normal cells capable of mitosis divide for only one of two reasons: to develop normal tissues or to replace lost or damaged normal tissues. Meiosis generates "daughter" cells that are purposely distinct from one another and from the original "parent" cell. Essentially all cells are capable of mitosis, but only a few special cells are capable of meiosis—those that will become eggs in females and sperm in males. Basically, mitosis is necessary for growth and maintenance of normal tissues, whereas meiosis is utilized for sexual reproduction.

Replication

Cellular replication is activated in the presence of cellular degeneration and death or based on physiological need. That is, when replication is functioning normally, new cells are created at the same rate as older cells die. The determination and timing of cellular division are strictly

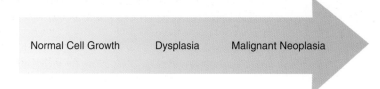

FIGURE 12.1 Scope of Cellular Regulation.

controlled by molecular "stop" and "go" signals. For example, when a wound occurs, injured cells send "go" signals to the surrounding cells, which respond to the extracellular signals by activating intracellular proliferation pathways. This results in controlled cellular growth and division that, in time, seals the wound. Conversely, "stop" signals are sent by the newly formed tissue when the wound healing process nears completion and cell replacement is no longer required. However, in a pathologic process, these signals can function abnormally whereby a "go" signal can be produced when it should not be or a "stop" signal may be ignored by surrounding cells. Such errors could result in uncontrolled growth and the development of neoplasms. However, due to the redundancy of error-correcting mechanisms in cellular regulation, it takes more than one incorrect "stop" or "go" signal for neoplasia to develop. The human body is quite efficient at protecting its essential systems, and it generally requires multiple errors compounded over time for healthy cells to become malignant.[2]

With normal reproduction, cells proceed through a cycle (known as the cell cycle) whereby the entire cellular contents of the parent cell are duplicated, after which it undergoes mitosis (cell division) and splits into two identical daughter cells. This pathway follows an orderly progression whereby certain steps need to precede others for the process to continue. Initially, the cell must leave the resting state, G_0 (gap 0), in order to enter the cell cycle. This initial entry into the cell cycle is an irreversible act, and it commits the cell to either mitosis or death. Cells cannot reverse the process and go backward to G_0; thus, the most fundamental aspect of cell cycle control is this regulation of entry and exit. The cell cycle is divided into four distinct phases: G_1 (gap 1), S (synthesis), G_2 (gap 2), and M (mitosis). Phases G_1 through G_2 are known as interphase, during which chromosomes (the genetic material) are copied and the cell typically doubles in size. During the M phase, mitosis occurs, leading to the formation of two identical cells. Surveillance checkpoints exist at the junction of each phase to ensure that damaged or incomplete DNA is not passed on to daughter cells. Abnormal cells may be removed through error-correcting or cell death pathways. In neoplastic tumors, the duration of the cell cycle is equal to or longer than that of normal cells. However, the proportion of cells that have committed to the cell cycle and are in active cell division is much higher than that in normal tissue. This results in a net increase in cell number and the formation of a tumor.

Differentiation

Most mature normal cells are functionally and morphologically differentiated into a specialized cell type. *Differentiation* means that a cell acquires functions that are *different* from those of the original cell from which it derived. Differentiation is a normal process by which a less specialized cell develops to possess a distinct form and specialized function. Differentiation dramatically changes a cell's size, shape (morphology), and its responsiveness to extracellular signals. These specialized changes are largely due to highly controlled modifications in gene expression specific to each differentiated cell type. Thus, different cells can have very different physical characteristics despite having the exact same complement of human genes. *Morphology* refers to the science

of structure and form without regard to function. Each cell type has a specific morphology and at least one specific function.

Surveillance of Cellular Replication and Growth

Normal cellular replication and growth requires precise, error-free interpretation of both extra- and intracellular cell signals. Cell signaling is a complex communication system, requiring accurate communication pathways within the cell (intracellular signaling) and among cells (extracellular signaling). Intracellular signaling is a multistep pathway often initiated by an extracellular signal provided by a nearby or even distant cell. Many factors can cause dysregulated cellular signaling, including genetic mutations and aberrant protein expression or function. When a signaling mistake occurs in the cell cycle, a host of surveillance mechanisms are present to recognize and repair the error. If it cannot be repaired, the cell can be destroyed through a process known as *apoptosis* or programmed cell death. These error-recognition processes help ensure accurate replication of daughter cells.

VARIATIONS AND CONTEXT

Despite the exquisite fidelity of cellular reproduction and growth, mistakes may occur at almost any point in the cell cycle. Surveillance mechanisms usually recognize and correct these errors or, if unable to do so, destroy the cells to avoid passing the errors to subsequent daughter cells. However, when a mistake goes undetected, a repair is ineffective, or an aberrant cell is not destroyed, mutations become fixed, leading to neoplasia and the formation of tumors. These tumors can be benign or malignant, and comparisons between these two categories of neoplasms are presented in Table 12.1.

Benign Neoplasm

Benign neoplastic cells tend to retain most of the morphologic and functional characteristics of the normal cells from which they were derived but represent groups of abnormal cells with excessive growth. Benign neoplastic cells are capable of replication and mitosis, but they are not capable of metastasis (the spread to locations outside their site of origin). Examples of common benign neoplastic tissues include endometriosis, nevi, and hypertrophic scars.

While benign tumors do not invade adjacent tissue or metastasize to distant organs, they can result in significant health consequences. A benign tumor can obstruct or mechanically press on body structures, resulting in pain, physiological dysfunction, or even death. For example, a benign brain tumor may compress brain structures, leading to neurologic symptoms and dysfunction. Other benign tumors, such as lipomas, may have more of a psychosocial impact because they may be outwardly visible and thus affect physical appearance of an individual.

Malignant Neoplasm

A malignant neoplasm (cancer) is characterized by cells having abnormal growth patterns, multiple abnormal functions, and the ability to disseminate to distant sites. These abnormal characteristics give the malignant cell advantages that allow it and its offspring to thrive and survive,

TABLE 12.1   Comparison of Benign and Malignant Neoplasms

Characteristic	Benign	Malignant
Encapsulated	Usually	Rarely
Differentiated	Normally	Poorly
Metastasis	Absent	Capable
Recurrence	Rare	Possible
Vascularity	Slight	Moderate to marked
Mode of growth	Expansive	Infiltrative and expansive
Cell characteristics	Fairly normal; similar to parent cells	Cells abnormal, become more unlike parent cells

From Lewis, S. L., Bucher, L., Heitkemper, M. M., Harding, M. M., Kwong, J., & Roberts, D. (2017). *Medical–surgical nursing: Assessment and management of clinical problems* (10th ed.). St Louis: Mosby.

TABLE 12.2   Targeting the Hallmarks of Cancer and the Enabling Characteristics

Cancer Cell Phenotype[a]	Targeting Agent
Sustaining proliferative growth signaling	Cyclin-dependent kinase inhibitors[b]
Evading growth suppressors	Epidermal growth factor inhibitors[b]
Resisting cell death	Programmed death receptor blocking antibodies[b]
Avoiding immune destruction	Immune activators of cytotoxic T cells[b]
Enabling replicative immortality	Telomerase inhibitors[b]
Inducing angiogenesis	Inhibitors of vascular endothelial growth factor (VEGF) signaling[b]
Activating invasion and metastases	Inhibitors of hepatocyte growth factor (HGF)/c-Met[b]
Deregulating cellular energetics	Aerobic glycolysis inhibitors[b]
Genome instability and mutation	Poly-ADP-ribose polymerase inhibitors[b]
Tumor-promoting inflammation	Selective anti-inflammatory drugs[b]

[a]The first eight phenotypes represent acquired functional capabilities of cancer cells that are necessary for tumor growth and progression. The last two phenotypes represent the enabling characteristics that help the cancer cell acquire these functional capabilities.
[b]A class of antineoplastic agents in which there is a drug with Food and Drug Administration approval.
Data from Hanahan, D., & Weinberg, R. A. (2011). Hallmarks of cancer: the next generation. *Cell, 144*(5):646–674.

even in unfavorable conditions. Malignant neoplastic cells arise from previously normal cells due to unrepaired errors in multiple cancer-causing genes. The identity of these genes varies from one cancer type to another, and in fact, they vary even within a given type of cancer. All cancers, however, evolve to acquire a similar set of functional capabilities, referred to as the "eight hallmarks of cancer" aided by two "enabling characteristics" (Table 12.2).[3] Acquisition of these eight individual capabilities depends on a multistep succession of mutations, eventually resulting in a progressive expansion of subclones, one or more of which will evolve into a tumor of increasing growth dominance. Tumors are much more than insulated masses of identical proliferating tumor cells. Rather, they are very complex tissues composed of many distinct cell types (including nonmalignant "normal cells") that interact with one another and with the cancer cells. In this complex tumor microenvironment, cancer cells are able to recruit the associated "normal" cells to serve as contributors to support their proliferation, invasion, and metastases. In fact, an important part of modern cancer therapy has been the development of antineoplastic agents that target these normal "helper cells" rather than the cancer cells themselves.[4] Because cancer cells are often resistant to single-agent treatment modalities, new agents have been developed for use in combination to target each of these eight common capabilities of cancer cells and the associated enabling characteristics (see Table 12.2).

CONSEQUENCES

Malignant tumors acquire characteristics that allow them to spread, invade, and destroy normal tissue. Like any other tissue, cancer tumors require oxygen and nutrition to sustain their rapid growth. For this to happen, the tumor releases factors that encourage tumor neovascularization. This process, known as tumor angiogenesis, facilitates further growth and invasion capability. When neovascularization is not possible or is halted, cancer cells are able to reprogram their energy metabolism, allowing for sustained and rapid growth under anaerobic conditions as well.[5] Regardless of the energy source, as the tumor increases in size and metastasizes, it acts like a parasite, robbing normal body tissues of nutrients and oxygen and destroying invaded tissues. Unless treatment is successful, the result is fatigue, weight loss, pain, organ failure, and eventual death.

Even though many cancers are curable, people often associate the disease with inevitable pain and death. The most common psychosocial consequences associated with a cancer diagnosis are fear, stress, and anxiety. When a malignant tumor is first discovered, patients and their family members often experience tremendous stress for days to weeks during the diagnostic and staging process. Often, the fear of the unknown can be as anxiety provoking as the diagnosis itself. Some individuals cope with the stress through a mechanism of denial, whereas others become very proactive and are interested in every aspect of the diagnostic and treatment process. In instances in which a child is diagnosed with cancer, the entire family is impacted. Parents often exhibit depression, stress, and anxiety, whereas children commonly experience fear, anger, guilt, and grief, often expressed through behavioral changes.[6]

In addition to fear and anxiety, changes in family dynamics are common. Financial challenges often occur as a result of medical expenses and reduced income associated with lost time at work, both for the patient and the caregivers. Changes in self-image and self-identity may result if patients experience a significant change in their physical appearance or their family role due to the disease process. This, in turn, can lead to alterations in interpersonal relationships and the development of mood disorders. The psychosocial effects of cancer are particularly pronounced for cancer survivors and their families when cancer recurs.[7]

RISK FACTORS

As of January 2016, there were an estimated 15.5 million Americans living with a history of cancer. In 2018, an estimated 1,735,350 new cancer cases (excluding basal and squamous cell skin cancers) will be diagnosed, and an estimated 609,640 patients will die from their disease.[8] While cancer deaths have declined by 1.5% per year since the 1990s it remains the second most common cause of death in the United States, exceeded only by heart disease. Among men, the three most common new cancer diagnoses are prostate, lung/bronchus, and colon/rectum. For women, the three most common sites are breast, lung/bronchus, and colon/rectum. Lung cancer is the most common cause of cancer deaths among both men and women, followed by breast cancer and colorectal cancer for women and prostate cancer and colorectal cancer for men. In contrast to the high number of cancer diagnoses in adults, only 10,590 children (ages 0 to 14 years) are expected to be diagnosed with cancer in 2018 (fewer than 1% of all cancer diagnoses). Leukemia and cancers affecting the brain or central nervous system are the most common childhood cancers, accounting for 29% and 26% of all childhood cancers, respectively. Although it is relatively uncommon, cancer remains the second leading cause of death in this age group, exceeded only by accidents. An estimated 1180 cancer deaths are expected to occur among children in 2018.

Populations at Risk

When cancer death rates were evaluated across populations, certain racial and ethnic minorities appeared to be at higher risk, and for years this was attributed to biologic differences. In recent years, it has been shown that these disparities in cancer burden largely reflect obstacles to receiving healthcare services related to cancer prevention, early detection, and high-quality treatment, with poverty as the overriding factor. In addition, racial and ethnic minorities tend to receive lower-quality health care than whites even when insurance status, age, severity of disease, and health status are comparable. In minority groups, communication barriers and provider assumptions can affect interactions between patients and physicians, which further contributes to miscommunication and the delivery of substandard care.

Individual Risk Factors

Age

Although it is not a modifiable risk factor, the risk for developing an invasive cancer increases significantly as a person ages. It is estimated that 87% of new cancer diagnoses occur among those ages 50 years or older. Between the ages 50 and 59 years, the probability of developing cancer (among those who were previously cancer free) is 6% for both men and women, and the probability increases to 32% for men and 26% for women age 70 years or older. Lifetime risk of developing cancer is slightly higher for men (39.7%) than for women (37.6%).[8]

Smoking/Tobacco

Another known risk factor for cancer is smoking. At least 30% of all cancer-related deaths and 80% of all lung cancer deaths can be attributed to smoking. In addition, smoking is a known risk factor for 18 different types of cancers. Nonsmokers exposed to environmental tobacco smoke are also at increased risk of lung cancer, and secondhand smoke is estimated to cause 21,400 lung cancer deaths worldwide each year. Nontraditional tobacco products such as snuff, lozenges, and chewing tobacco are promoted as alternatives in smoke-free environments, but these products are associated with increased risk of oral cavity, esophageal, and pancreatic cancers.[9]

Infectious Agents

Bacteria and viruses are known to cause cancer and examples include the *Helicobacter pylori* bacteria (gastric cancer), hepatitis B and hepatitis C viruses (liver cancer), and human papillomavirus (cervical, oropharyngeal, and anal cancer). Vaccines are available to prevent infection by hepatitis B and the human papillomavirus and thus provide immediate opportunities for preventing cancers, especially in at-risk populations.[10]

Genetic Risk

Only approximately 5% of all cancers result from an inherited genetic alteration that is associated with an increased risk of developing certain types of cancer. In some cases, a specific gene mutation results in an extraordinarily high risk of cancer, such as women with a *BRCA1* gene mutation that confers a 70% lifetime risk of developing either breast or ovarian cancer. Fortunately, these types of mutations are rare in the population. Although approximately 20 other "cancer syndromes" are known (e.g., Lynch syndrome), more common are the generally unexplained genetic susceptibilities and familial tendencies that increase cancer risk in certain families. Likely, many familial cancers arise not exclusively from genetic makeup, but from the interplay between common gene variations and lifestyle and environmental risk factors. The development of breast cancer among first-degree relatives is an example.[11]

Radiation

There are two main types of radiation (ultraviolet and ionizing) exposure that are linked to an increased risk of developing certain types of cancer. Ionizing radiation includes medical radiation from tests used to both diagnose (x-rays and computed tomography scans) and treat (radiation therapy) disease, and it is responsible for an increased risk of developing leukemia, breast, and thyroid cancer. An equally important source of ionizing radiation is from radon gas, which is a natural decay product of uranium in the earth. Exposure to radon gas dramatically increases risk for lung cancer. Ultraviolet radiation from the sun is the main cause of melanoma and the ubiquitous nonmelanoma skin cancers (basal and squamous). Although the latter of these is highly curable, the obvious intervention to decrease risk is to avoid sun exposure and to use protective measures.[12]

Carcinogens

Environmental carcinogens have been associated with the development of many types of cancer. Exposure to these carcinogens is often due to lifestyle choices (e.g., smoking), but other carcinogens are present as environmental pollutants in the air, water, soil, or food. Although the risk level per person is thought to be quite low (accounting for only 6% of cancer deaths), the large number of people involuntarily exposed to these pollutants leads to a large population effect. Probably more significant are high levels of exposure to agents (e.g., asbestos, dioxins, tetrachloroethylene, and arsenic) that disproportionately increase risk in specific low-income occupations and in some poor and disenfranchised communities.[12]

Nutrition and Physical Activity

Diet, body weight, and activity levels are interrelated and act in complex ways to either promote or reduce the risk of cancer. Combined, more than 20% of all cancer cases are attributed to poor nutrition, a sedentary lifestyle, and excessive weight. It is difficult to absolutely define the effects of diet on cancer because an individual's diet typically includes foods that may protect against cancer as well as foods that may increase the risk of cancer. However, a number of epidemiologic studies suggest that high intake of fresh fruits and vegetables are associated with lower cancer rates. Obesity is associated with increased risk for both developing new cancers and cancer recurrence. Weight loss has been shown to reduce cancer risk, although the exact mechanism is not well understood. In addition to their risk for developing cancer, these factors are also responsible for significant disability and death from other causes, such as heart disease, hypertension, stroke, diabetes, and arthritis.[13]

ASSESSMENT

Assessment involves the collection of data from the health history, a physical examination, and diagnostic studies. It is not the intention of this text to describe the process of assessment or to describe the specific findings of all problems associated with cellular reproduction and growth because these are highly variable based on the involved tissue, organ, or body system. However, on initial diagnosis, several presenting symptoms and clinical findings often serve as "red flags" that are unusual and worthy of further investigation. The nurse should have an awareness of the significance of these symptoms and findings.

History

Individuals are usually asymptomatic when neoplasms are early in their development. As the tumor grows, an individual may become aware of its physical presence or may notice symptoms caused by the tumor. The most common presenting complaints include discovery of a lump, mass, or lesion; the onset of new symptoms (e.g., unusual or unexplained bleeding, pain, cough, or fatigue); changes in appearance of a body part; or signs associated with alterations in major body functions (e.g., appetite, weight, mental status, swallowing, or elimination). Often, the presenting symptoms are vague, and the nurse should conduct a symptom analysis to collect as much information as possible. This includes questions regarding the duration of the symptom, its location, characteristics, aggravating and relieving factors, and treatments undertaken, if any. In addition to documenting the symptoms, these questions also provide early information about the patient's coping skills or potential denial of the problem. A medical history, family history, and psychosocial history will provide additional information that may later prove valuable (e.g., history of smoking or a family history of cancer).

Examination Findings

When a patient presents with a specific symptom that raises concern, the examination should be focused to learn more about the presenting problem. However, patients do not always experience symptoms and, thus, the nurse needs be aware of possible indicators of neoplastic growth when conducting the physical exam. Abnormal findings that may suggest the presence of a neoplasm include visible lesions, physical asymmetry, palpable masses, abnormal sounds, or the presence of blood such as on pelvic exam or in a guaiac test for occult blood.

Diagnostic Tests

A diagnostic workup is indicated when a symptom, examination finding, or screening test suggests the presence of a tumor. The tests discussed here are those most commonly used in the detection and diagnosis of tumors.

Radiographic Tests

Radiographic tests provide an image of tumors so that size, location(s), and activity can be assessed. The most common radiographic tests used for the diagnostic process related to cellular regulation include radiographs (x-rays), magnetic resonance imaging, computed tomography, radioisotope scans, ultrasound, and diagnostic mammography.

Direct Visualization

Some tumors can be evaluated by insertion of a lighted scope into a lumen or body cavity (e.g., colonoscopy, endoscopy, or cystoscopy). These tests not only provide visualization of the tumor but also allow for biopsy to provide tissue samples for pathologic analysis.

Laboratory Tests

Several laboratory tests are useful in the diagnostic process. Perhaps the two most useful tests are the complete blood count and the chemistry panel. Although these tests are not diagnostic in themselves (except in the case of some hematologic malignancies), they may provide information about the overall health status of the patient or provide clues as to the presence of neoplasm. For example, an undiagnosed malignancy might first be detected in a patient having unexplained anemia or changes in his or her white blood cells. A limited number of tumor markers (e.g., carcioembryonic antigen and prostate-specific antigen) or cancer-specific genetic changes (e.g., Philadelphia chromosome) can be detected in blood samples that may help provide a diagnosis. If a certain type of cancer is suspected, specific studies may be ordered that would be helpful in determining risk, such as genetic tests for the *BRCA1* and *BRCA2* genes that are linked to breast cancer.

Pathology

Pathology is the study of the origin and course of disease and is moreover the branch of medicine that deals with the laboratory examination of cells and tissues for diagnostic purposes. Pathologic evaluation of a tissue sample is the only definitive way to determine if a tumor is malignant or benign. It may also provide information such as the tissue type (histology), the degree of differentiation (grade), the presence or absence of certain markers on the cell surface, and increasingly (in the era of precision medicine) the presence or absence of genetic or molecular markers.

Cytology is the microscopic study of cells obtained either by aspiration (a fine-needle biopsy) or from a smear, washing, or scraping. A surgical biopsy involves removal of larger amounts of tissue for pathologic review. An incisional biopsy removes just part of the tumor or affected tissue, whereas excisional biopsy removes the entire tumor or tissue for evaluation. The type of biopsy done is based on the type of tissue to be removed, its location, and the amount of tissue required to make a diagnosis. Different biopsy approaches include going through the skin (percutaneous), through a scope (endoscopic), or directly during surgery. Percutaneous and endoscopic biopsy procedures are often facilitated with stereotactic approaches that allow for exact positioning of the biopsy instruments directly at the site of the tumor.

Classification: Grading and Staging

When a malignancy is identified, clinical staging is done as part of the diagnostic workup to define the extent or spread of the disease and to aid as a guide to treatment. Staging includes determining the size of the tumor, its location(s), and the presence or absence of metastasis. Grading of the tumor includes determining both the tissue origin of the malignancy and its histologic grade (i.e., the degree of differentiation).

Grading Cellular Differentiation

Grading is the measure of the degree of differentiation of a neoplasm. Some pathology grading systems apply only to malignant neoplasms, whereas others apply to benign neoplasms as well. The neoplastic grading system is a measure of a cell's *anaplasia* or how different it appears from its tissue of origin. A cancer cell that is well differentiated looks more like the normal cell from which it derived, whereas a poorly differentiated cell has little resemblance to the original normal cell and typically represents a more advanced and aggressive cancer. For solid tumors, different grading systems are used to classify the appearance of malignant cells, although the most common is that recommended by the American Joint Committee on Cancer (Box 12.1).[14]

BOX 12.1   Grading System of the American Joint Committee on Cancer

- GX—Grade cannot be assessed
- G1—Well differentiated (low grade)
- G2—Moderately differentiated (intermediate grade)
- G3—Poorly differentiated (high grade)
- G4—Undifferentiated (high grade)

From Amin, M. B., Edge, S. B., Greene, F., Compton, M. D., Gershenwald, J. E., Brookland, R. K., et al. (2017). *AJCC cancer staging manual* (8th ed.). New York: Springer.

Cancer-specific grading scales are also used for certain types of solid tumor malignancies, such as the Gleason score[15] (prostate cancer) and the Bloom-Richardson grading system[16] (breast cancer). For the myriad of complex hematologic malignancies, the World Health Organization has developed detailed classification systems for these neoplasms and leukemias.[17]

Clinical Staging

For all solid tumors, the TNM classification system is used to determine the stage of the disease.[14] This system assesses the growth and spread of the tumor based on three factors: *Tumor* size and invasiveness, the presence or absence of spread to regional lymph *Nodes*, and the presence or absence of *Metastasis* to distant organs (Table 12.3). Once the T, N, and M categories are determined, a stage (I to IV) is assigned, with stage I representing early stage disease and stage IV representing the most advanced disease. The actual assignment into these stages is specific to the cancer type. Hematologic cancers (i.e., liquid tumors) cannot be staged using the TNM classification system, and each of these malignancies has its own unique staging system often incorporating factors to assign risk. In recent years, unique genetic changes and molecular markers have been identified in many solid and liquid tumor types and this new information has been incorporated into the staging and prognostic systems specific to those cancers.

TABLE 12.3 TNM Classification System

Primary Tumor (T)[a]

TX	Tumor cannot be measured.
T0	No evidence of primary tumor (tumor cannot be found).
Tis	Tumor *in situ*, meaning malignant cells only within superficial layer of tissue; no extension into deeper tissue.
T1	Description of primary tumor based on size and/or invasion
T2	into nearby structures; the higher the T number, the larger
T3	the tumor and/or the more it has grown into nearby
T4	tissues.

Regional Lymph Nodes (N)[b]

NX	Nearby lymph nodes cannot be evaluated.
N0	No evidence of cancer cells in regional lymph nodes.
N1	Description of size, location, and/or number of lymph nodes
N2	involved; the higher the N number, the more extensive the
N3	lymph node involvement.

Metastases (M)[c]

MX	Metastases cannot be evaluated.
M0	No evidence of metastases can be found.
M1	Description of extent of metastasis; the higher the M number,
M2	the more extensive the metastasis.
M3	
M4	

[a]Describes the primary (original) tumor based on size (measured in centimeters).
[b]Describes whether or not the cancer has spread into regional (nearby) lymph nodes.
[c]Describes whether or not the cancer has metastasized (spread) to other parts of the body.
Adapted from American Cancer Society: http://www.cancer.org.

CLINICAL MANAGEMENT

Primary Prevention

Preventing cancer from occurring is the most definitive way to lessen the burden of cancer. Risk factors can be eliminated or reduced through behavior modification, modification of the environment, vaccination, or treatment of infections. Major risk reduction is possible through smoking cessation, avoiding excessive sun exposure, participating in regular physical activity, and eating a balanced diet.[12] Combined, these four risk factors account for nearly 60% of all cancers. Although it is not a common approach, another primary prevention strategy is prophylactic surgery for individuals at risk. For example, a woman with the *BRCA1* genetic marker has a 70% lifetime risk of developing breast or ovarian cancer, and thus, she might elect to have a bilateral mastectomy and oophorectomy to prevent development of these two cancers.

Secondary Prevention (Screening)

The goal of secondary prevention is early disease detection so that prompt treatment can be initiated. Screening refers to the application of a test to a population that has no overt signs or symptoms of the disease in question in order to detect disease at a stage when treatment is more effective. Screening tests identify individuals who require further investigation to determine the presence or absence of disease, but they are not primarily diagnostic tests. Whereas some screening tests may positively identify a malignancy (e.g., colonoscopy), others often only identify suspected problems (e.g., mammography). Individuals who a have positive screening test of any type need to be referred for a full diagnostic workup.

There are multiple types of cancer screening, and a discussion of each is beyond the scope of this text. Examples of common screening tests for cancer include mammography for breast cancer, prostate-specific antigen testing for prostate cancer, and colonoscopy and guaiac testing for occult blood in the stool for colon cancer. The U.S. Preventive Services Task Force establishes evidence-based screening recommendations for the general population.[18] Because the recommendations are based on the latest scientific evidence, screening recommendations will periodically change, as noted most recently with prostate and colon cancer screening.

Collaborative Interventions

Interventions for neoplasia are addressed in terms of treatment goals, which include cure, control, and palliation. The interventions discussed here may be used in various sequences or combinations.

Surgery

Surgery is the oldest intervention for cancer treatment. In addition to primary treatment, surgical intervention is also used for diagnosis, staging, and cytoreduction (debulking). Surgery may also be used to prevent cancer, to relieve the symptoms of cancer, or to enhance functional and cosmetic outcomes. Primary surgical resection is rarely curative, and it is frequently combined with other treatment modalities to improve cure rates and increase disease-free intervals. Additional therapies that are done following surgery are called *adjuvant* therapy and may include any of the following therapies outlined below. If these therapies occur prior to the surgical procedure, they are considered *neoadjuvant* therapy.

Nursing care associated with the patient undergoing surgical procedures for any aspect of cancer (prevention, cure, palliation, and reconstruction) includes patient education, pre- and post-operative care, infection prevention, pain management, and psychosocial care.[19]

Radiation Therapy

Radiation therapy is a local treatment for cancer and may be used anytime in the disease trajectory. It can take the form of either palliative or potentially curative treatment. Radiation is essentially a small packet of energy in the form of photons (e.g., x-rays and ultraviolet light) or particles (e.g., protons, neutrons, α-particles, and electrons) that is delivered directly to the site of the neoplasm. When these packets of energy penetrate the tissue, ionization induces direct biologic damage to the cells. Because these packets often pass through healthy tissue on their way to the neoplasm, damage to unaffected cells is an unintended consequence.[20] Radiation therapy may be delivered in several ways, the most common of which is external beam therapy using a linear accelerator. Another delivery technique, known as brachytherapy, delivers a high dose of radiation to a limited volume of tissue. Using this technique, short-range radiation sources are enclosed in a protective capsule and placed directly at the site of the tumor. Thus, the radiation affects only a very localized area and limits exposure of radiation to healthy tissues. The nursing management of patients receiving either type of radiation therapy largely involves patient education and the management of symptoms associated with the therapies.[21]

Chemotherapy

The word *chemotherapy* means treatment with chemicals, but the term has evolved over time to mean the systemic treatment of cancer (although there are a few instances when chemotherapy can be applied locally to treat cancers). The general goal of chemotherapy is to prevent cancer cells from multiplying, invading, and metastasizing to distant sites. Unlike surgery or radiation, which are local and regional treatments, systemic chemotherapy agents act at the site of the tumor as well as at distant sites where tumor cells may have already metastasized. The principle of chemotherapy is based on the phases of the cell cycle, and most chemotherapeutic drugs are classified according to the specific phase of the cell cycle in which they exert their cytotoxic effects.[22] The role of the nurse in cancer chemotherapy is vast, pivotal, and rewarding. Nurses are responsible for assessment and education of the patient, handling and administration of chemotherapeutic agents, management of side effects, and management of psychosocial issues. Before they can administer chemotherapy in the clinic, nurses must undergo specialized training and certification through the Oncology Nursing Society.[23]

Hormonal Therapy

Another effective form of cancer treatment involves the use of antihormonal agents to treat malignancies that are responsive to hormones, such as breast, prostate, and endometrial cancers. Current approaches use agents that are hormonal agonists or antagonists, depending on type of cancer and the nature of the disease process. Hormonal therapies were developed based on their ability to target and block specific receptors and their various associated feedback loops. Thus, these agents are considered the first form of targeted cancer therapy.[24]

Targeted Therapy

Targeted therapy is the most rapidly evolving and expanding class of anticancer agents due to their specificity at targeting cancer cells and their generally reduced side effect profile. These agents act on both intra- and extra-cellular targets and are designed to interfere with molecules that are necessary for tumor growth, progression, and metastasis. This is in contrast to chemotherapy agents that act against all actively dividing cells. These agents take several forms but generally fall into the categories of antibodies, antibody-drug conjugates, or small molecule inhibitors, of which there are many different classes. Targeted therapies have been developed that prevent growth signaling, interfere with tumor blood vessel formation, stimulate the immune system to destroy cancer cells, or even deliver toxic drugs directly to cancer cells. In all, more than 85 of these agents have been approved by the U.S. Food and Drug Administration for use in the treatment of a wide variety of cancers and there are many more in development. They are the cornerstone of the treatment arm of precision medicine, a medical model that seeks to use high resolution genetic information about a person's disease to prevent, diagnose, and precisely tailor treatment.[25]

Biologic Therapy

Biotherapy (also known as immunotherapy) refers to modulation of the immune response for a therapeutic goal. Biotherapy is a global term used to describe the use of biologic agents to activate the immune system (biologic response modifiers) and more recently includes approaches that manipulate cells within immune system to recognize cancer cells. Within the scope of the biologic response modifiers is the broad class of drugs that are extracted or produced from biologic material. Such agents include colony-stimulating factors, monoclonal and bispecific monoclonal antibodies, checkpoint inhibitors, angiogenesis inhibitors, vaccines, and chimeric antigen receptor T-cell therapies (CAR-T). Note that many of these agents also fall into the category of targeted therapy because they have very specific targets within the immune system.[26] These agents often have unique side effects that are quite different from those of traditional chemotherapy agents. As with chemotherapy, nurses wishing to administer and manage the side effects of these novel agents must receive specialized training and certification through the Oncology Nursing Society.[23] Due to the unique nature of biotherapy, nurses play a significant role in patient education and psychosocial support. As with many of the targeted therapies, these agents can be quite expensive, and there are frequently economic issues for the patient receiving biotherapy.[27]

Bone Marrow and Hematopoietic Stem Cell Transplantation

Hematopoietic (blood-forming) pluripotent stem cells are found in the bone marrow and when given the proper signals, these cells mature and give rise to fully formed erythrocytes, leukocytes, and platelets. Stem cells can be collected from the blood through a process called apheresis, or they may be harvested directly from multiple bone marrow biopsy samples. When these stem cells are infused into a patient, the procedure is called a "stem cell" or "bone marrow" transplant, with the nomenclature essentially reflecting the source of the stem cells. Regardless of the source, the principle of the procedure is to replace diseased hematopoietic cells with these highly specialized stem cells that will then give rise to the full spectrum of healthy hematopoietic cells. The transplant can be autologous (by harvesting and using one's own stem cells) or allogeneic (whereby the stem cells come from a matched family donor or matched unrelated donor).[28] Stem cell transplantation is usually done for the purpose of cure or quality-of-life years gained. Patients undergoing transplantation can have many complex medical issues, and nurses working with these patients require very specialized training.

Symptom Management Resulting from Cancer and Cancer Treatment

Patients who undergo cancer treatment or who have an advanced cancer diagnosis experience multiple complications related to both the disease and its treatment. For these patients, nursing interventions are geared toward managing both the physical and the psychosocial aspects of these complications. Nurses can support the patient and family members by identifying coping mechanisms and resources. Although identifying all the specific complications and adverse effects associated with the

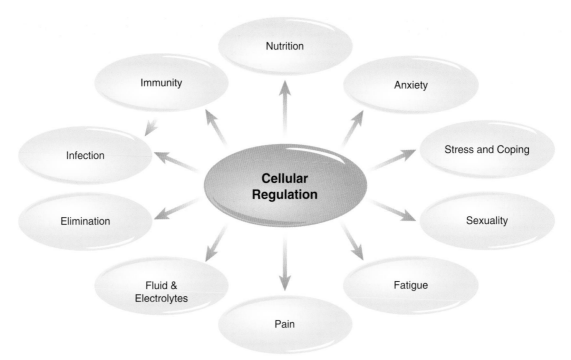

FIGURE 12.2 Cellular Regulation and Interrelated Concepts.

previously discussed treatment modalities is beyond the scope of this text, the most common and important complications and side effects are briefly presented in the following section.

INTERRELATED CONCEPTS

Cellular regulation is closely related to many of the concepts presented in this textbook. The interrelated concepts may be associated with the disease process, as consequence of treating the disease, or a combination of both. The most important interrelated concepts are presented in Fig. 12.2, and they are briefly described here. Nutrition is an important interrelated concept because many patients with cancer experience calorie and especially protein malnutrition. Cancer cells divert nutrients from normal cells to sustain their cellular growth and expansion. In addition, many patients undergoing cancer treatment lose weight due to reduced or lost appetite (anorexia), nausea, vomiting, stomatitis, diarrhea, or physical inability to eat as part of the disease process.[29] Compromised Immunity is a concern especially among patients with a hematologic malignancy and is a common side effect of the myelo-suppressive effects of chemotherapy or radiation. Although this is typically transient, patients are vulnerable to many opportunistic infections. Disease- or treatment-related immunodeficiency puts cancer patients at significant risk for Infection. Moreover, due to their immuno-compromised status, they may not present with the typical signs and symptoms of infection that are present in healthy patients. This can be fatal if it results in a delay in recognizing and treating an infection. In fact, infection is a common cause of death for cancer patients undergoing treatment.[30] Pain is a common symptom associated with cancer and is among the most feared. It may result directly from cancer-caused tissue destruction, or it may be treatment related. It is a complex symptom to manage because of the wide variability in pain perception among patients. Unfortunately, pain is often underassessed and undertreated in cancer patients.[31] Fatigue is a common symptom associated with cancer and its treatment. Fatigue in patients with cancer, known as

cancer-related fatigue (CRF), is distinct and more debilitating than general fatigue. The unique and more debilitating symptoms associated with CRF are thought to be related to high levels of circulating inflammatory cytokines present in patients with cancer. A multitude of additional contributing factors may include side effects from medications, anemia, anorexia, weight loss, depression, and general organ dysfunction often associated with later-stage cancer.[32] Many cancer patients experience an altered pattern of Elimination—the most common of which is diarrhea. Conversely, some chemotherapy agents and most pain medications (opioids) cause significant issues with constipation. Bowel obstructions may occur as a result of the disease process, such as in the case of colorectal cancer, or urinary flow may be impaired by the presence of an enlarged malignant prostate.

Fluid and Electrolyte imbalances can occur as a result of cancer or its treatment. Early in treatment when the disease burden is high, patients are at risk for tumor lysis syndrome manifested by elevated levels of uric acid, phosphate, and potassium. Other imbalances such as dehydration, hypercalcemia, and third spacing of fluids are common in patients with more advanced disease. Anxiety, Stress and Coping, and Sexuality have important and interrelated impacts on patients with cancer due to the significant psychosocial issues associated with their diagnosis and treatment.[33]

CLINICAL EXEMPLARS

There are many examples of abnormal cellular reproduction and growth and, in fact, there are more than 200 different types of cancer. Although it is beyond the scope of this text to describe all types of abnormalities related to cellular regulation, some of the most common are presented in Box 12.2 and are featured here. Specific and detailed information related to each of these exemplars is readily available in nursing and medical textbooks, as well as on reputable websites, such as those of the American Cancer Society (http://www.cancer.org) and the National Cancer Institute (http://www.cancer.gov).

BOX 12.2   EXEMPLARS OF ALTERED CELLULAR REGULATION

Benign Tumors
- Adenoma
- Benign prostate hypertrophy
- Benign brain tumor
- Fibroma
- Lipoma
- Meningioma
- Papilloma
- Rhabdomyoma

Malignant Tumors
Carcinoma and Adenocarcinoma (Originate from Skin, Glands, and Mucous Membrane Lining of Respiratory, Gastrointestinal, and Genitourinary Tracts)
- Breast cancer
- Prostate cancer
- Lung cancer
- Colon cancer

Sarcoma (Originates from Muscle/Bone/Connective Tissues)
- Chondrosarcoma
- Ewing sarcoma
- Fibrosarcoma
- Kaposi sarcoma
- Rhabdomyosarcoma
- Osteosarcoma

Lymphomas (Originates from Lymph System)
- Hodgkin lymphoma
- Non-Hodgkin lymphoma

Leukemia (Originates from Hematopoietic System)
- Chronic lymphocytic leukemia (CLL)
- Chronic myeloid leukemia (CML)
- Acute lymphocytic leukemia (ALL)[a]
- Acute myeloid leukemia (AML)[a]

[a]Common among children.

 ACCESS EXEMPLAR LINKS IN YOUR GIDDENS EBOOK

Featured Exemplars

Breast Cancer

Breast cancer originates in the tissues of the breast and the most common subtype is ductal carcinoma, which begins in the lining of the milk ducts. Invasive breast cancer describes disease that has spread from where it began in the breast ducts into surrounding normal breast tissue. Lymphatic vessels in the breast drain to the axillary lymph nodes; thus, lymph nodes are often sampled to detect the presence of cancer cells. Risk factors include gender, age, family history, menstrual and pregnancy history, obesity, and hormone replacement therapy. Treatment for breast cancer is dependent on stage and includes surgery, radiation, hormonal, and targeted therapies.[34]

Lung Cancer

Lung cancer is characterized by uncontrolled cell growth of tissues of the lung. The main types of lung cancer are small-cell lung carcinoma (SCLC) and non-small-cell lung carcinoma (NSCLC), the latter of which comprises 85% of lung cancers. Subtypes of NSCLC include adenocarcinoma, squamous cell carcinoma, and large cell carcinoma. Prognosis is generally quite poor because it is usually detected at later stages of the disease. Common symptoms include coughing (including coughing up blood), weight loss, shortness of breath, and chest pain. The vast majority (80%) of lung cancers are due to long-term exposure to tobacco smoke.[35]

Prostate Cancer

Prostate cancer, a malignancy that originates in the prostate, usually grows slowly and initially remains confined to the prostate gland, where it rarely causes serious harm. In later stages, however, the cancer cells often spread to the bones and nearby lymph nodes. Because it grows slowly it may require minimal or no treatment. However, some subtypes can be quite aggressive and will spread quickly if left unattended. Prostate cancer is the most common type of cancer in men; risk factors include older age, family history of the disease, and race. Approximately 99% of all cases of prostate cancer occur in men older than age 50 years.[36]

Acute Lymphocytic Leukemia

Acute lymphocytic leukemia (ALL) is a malignancy of the white blood cells characterized by the overproduction and accumulation of malignant immature white blood cells known as blasts. As blasts accumulate in the bone marrow, they inhibit the production of normal cells such as red and white blood cells and platelets, resulting in symptoms such as fever, infection, shortness of breath, tachycardia, bleeding, and bruising. Blasts can leave the blood and bone marrow and infiltrate other organs. ALL is the most common type of cancer in children, and treatment generally results in a cure. When it occurs in adults, treatment is not nearly as successful. ALL was one of the first cancers for which an effective chemotherapeutic treatment was developed.[37]

Fibroma

A fibroma is a benign tumor mostly composed of fibrous or connective tissue that can form anywhere in the body and most commonly occur in adults. Common types of fibroma include angiofibromas, dermatofibromas, ovarian fibromas, and plantar fibromas. Most are harmless, and treatment is not required unless there are disturbing symptoms or cosmetic concerns. Depending on the site and size of the fibroma, removal may be accomplished by a simple surgical procedure or by cryotherapy. Neurofibromas, associated with an autosomal dominant mutation in the *NF1* gene, are associated with extensive lesion formation and can result in symptoms ranging from physical disfiguration to cognitive disability.[38]

Lipoma

A lipoma is a benign tumor composed of adipose or body fat and is the most common benign soft tissue tumor. It occurs in approximately 1 in every 1000 people and usually in adults. Lipomas are generally slow growing, often arising over a period of months or years. Most are small, soft to the touch, movable, and painless. They can occur almost anywhere in the body, including muscles and internal organs. In most cases, lipomas do not need to be treated, although they may be surgically removed if there is concern about location, they are causing pain, or they are impacting physical appearance.[39]

CASE STUDY

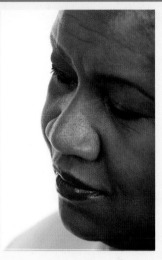

Case Presentation

Katrina Wells, a 54-year-old African American female, works a sedentary job in telecommunications. She has been overweight most of her life and has never engaged in physical activity on a regular basis. Because of limited finances and limited healthcare coverage, Katrina seeks health care only when she is ill.

Through a community outreach program, Katrina met Lydia Robinson, a nurse who helped her gain access to basic preventive healthcare services. Acting on the advice of Lydia, Katrina agreed to have a screening mammogram. The radiologist who reviewed the mammography films discovered a small mass in the upper outer quadrant of Katrina's left breast. She was contacted by the radiologist and told she had an abnormal mammography result and that she needed to return to the imaging center for further workup. Katrina, not knowing what this meant, asked if she had cancer. She was told that cancer was a possibility but that further testing was needed to determine if this was the case.

Katrina was upset by this information, and she was not sure she wanted any additional tests. Her mother had breast cancer, and Katrina watched her lose her breast and hair, in addition to becoming very sick from the medications. Lydia helped Katrina understand the need for the additional workup. During the next 4 weeks, Katrina underwent several tests as part of her diagnostic workup. Lydia helped Katrina by explaining the process and providing emotional support. The diagnostic mammogram and ultrasound examination of the breast revealed a 7.4 mm lesion, and a needle biopsy confirmed the diagnosis of breast cancer. The pathology showed it to have low-risk features and that it would be responsive to hormonal therapy. Katrina was referred to a surgical and medical oncologist at the local cancer center for treatment.

An oncology clinical nurse specialist at the cancer center met with Katrina at her first oncology appointment to begin guiding her through the treatment process. Due to the small size of the lesion and the low-risk features, she was told she would not need chemotherapy. Her treatment would involve only surgery and radiation, followed by 5 to 10 years of hormonal therapy to decrease the risk of recurrence. She underwent a lumpectomy followed by 5 weeks of radiation to the left breast and axillary region. Following completion of radiation, she was started on an oral aromatase inhibitor, which she was to take daily for at least the next 5 years. She was to continue visiting the medical oncologist at the cancer center every 3 to 6 months during that time. At those visits, she would get a clinical breast exam and reinforcement about how to do a breast self-exam between visits. The staff at the cancer center also arranged for her to get yearly mammograms to screen for a new or recurrent breast cancer.

Case Analysis Questions

1. What were a Katrina's risk factors for developing breast cancer?
2. How did Katrina's nurses help navigate her journey from diagnosis through treatment and follow up?

From Jeremy Woodhouse/Blend Images/Thinkstock.

 ACCESS EXEMPLAR LINKS IN YOUR GIDDENS EBOOK

REFERENCES

1. Gomes, A. P., & Blenis, J. (2015). A nexus for cellular homeostasis: The interplay between metabolic and signal transduction pathways. *Current Opinion in Biotechnology, 34,* 110–117.
2. Hanahan, D., & Weinberg, R. A. (2000). The hallmarks of cancer. *Cell, 100*(1), 57–70.
3. Hanahan, D., & Weinberg, R. A. (2011). Hallmarks of cancer: The next generation. *Cell, 144*(5), 646–674.
4. Hanahan, D., & Coussens, L. M. (2012). Accessories to the crime: Functions of cells recruited to the tumor microenvironment. *Cancer Cell, 21*(3), 309–322.
5. Pavlova, N. N., & Thompson, C. B. (2016). The emerging hallmarks of Cancer Metabolism. *Cell Metabolism, 23,* 27–47.
6. Peek, G., & Melnyk, B. M. (2010). Coping interventions for parents of children newly diagnosed with cancer: An evidence review with implications for clinical practice and future research. *Pediatric Nursing, 36*(6), 306–313.
7. Vivar, C. G., Canga, N., Canga, A. D., et al. (2009). The psychosocial impact of recurrence on cancer survivors and family members: A narrative review. *Journal of Advanced Nursing, 65*(4), 724–736.
8. Siegel, R. L., Miller, K. D., & Jemal, A. (2018). Cancer statistics, 2018. *CA: A Cancer Journal for Clinicians, 68*(1), 7–30.
9. Balogh, E. P., Dresler, C., Fleury, M. E., et al. (2014). Reducing tobacco-related incidence and mortality: Summary of an Institute of Medicine Workshop. *The Oncologist, 19,* 21–31.
10. Plummer, M., de Martel, C., Bignat, J., et al. (2016). Global burden of cancers attributable to infections in 2012: A synthetic analysis. *The Lancet. Global Health, 4,* e609–e616.
11. Garber, J. E., & Offit, K. (2005). Hereditary cancer predisposition syndromes. *Journal of Clinical Oncology: Official Journal of the American Society of Clinical Oncology, 23*(2), 276–292.
12. Anand, P., Kunnumakkara, A. B., Sundaram, C., et al. (2008). Cancer is a preventable disease that requires major lifestyle changes. *Pharmaceutical Research, 25*(9), 2097–2116.
13. Kohler, L. N., Garcia, D. O., Harris, R. B., et al. (2016). Adherence to diet and physical activity cancer prevention guidelines and cancer outcomes: A systematic review. *Cancer Epidemiology, Biomarkers and Prevention: A Publication of the American Association for Cancer Research, Cosponsored by the American Society of Preventive Oncology, 25*(7), 1–11.
14. Amin, M. B., Edge, S. B., Greene, F., et al. (2017). *AJCC cancer staging manual* (8th ed.). New York: Springer.
15. Egevad, L., Granfors, T., Karlberg, L., et al. (2002). Prognostic value of the Gleason score in prostate cancer. *BJU International, 89*(6), 538–542.
16. Genestie, C., Zafrani, B., Asselain, B., et al. (1998). Comparison of the prognostic value of Scarff–Bloom–Richardson and Nottingham histological grades in a series of 825 cases of breast cancer: Major importance of the mitotic count as a component of both grading systems. *Anticancer Research, 18*(1B), 571–576.
17. Arber, D. A., Orazi, A., Hasserjian, R., et al. (2016). The 2016 revision to the World Health Organization classification of myeloid neoplasms and acute leukemia. *Blood, 127*(20), 2391–2405.
18. U.S. Preventive Services Task Force. (2018). *Recommendations.* Retrieved from http://www.uspreventiveservicestaskforce.org/Page/Name/recommendations.
19. Lewis, S. L., Bucher, L., Heitkemper, M. M., et al. (2017). *Medical–surgical nursing: Assessment and management of clinical problems* (ed. 10). St Louis: Mosby.
20. Baskar, R., Lee, K. A., Yeo, R., et al. (2012). Cancer and radiation therapy: Current advances and future directions. *International Journal of Medical Sciences, 9*(3), 193–199.

21. Iwamoto, R. R., Haas, M., & Gosselin, T. K. (2012). *Manual for radiation oncology nursing practice and education*. Pittsburgh, PA: Oncology Nursing Society.

22. Fernando, J., & Jones, R. (2015). The principles of cancer treatment by chemotherapy. *Surgery, 33*(3), 131–135.

23. Neuss, M. N., Gilmore, T. R., Belderson, K. M., et al. (2016). 2016 updated American Society of Clinical Oncology/Oncology Nursing Society chemotherapy administration safety standards, including standards for pediatric oncology. *Journal of Oncology Practice, 12*(12), 1262–1277.

24. Abraham, J., & Staffurth, J. (2011). Hormonal therapy for cancer. *Medicine, 39*(12), 723–727.

25. Wujcik, D. (2014). Science and mechanism of action of targeted therapies in cancer treatment. *Seminars in Oncology Nursing, 30*(3), 139–146.

26. Smith, E. L., Zamarin, D., & Lesokhin, A. (2014). Harnessing the immune system for cancer therapy. *Current Opinion in Oncology, 26*(6), 600–607.

27. Wujcik, D. (2016). Scientific advances shaping the future roles of oncology nurses. *Seminars in Oncology Nursing, 32*(2), 87–98.

28. Singh, N., & Loren, A. W. (2017). Overview of hematopoietic cell transplantation for the treatment of hematologic malignancies. *Clinics in Chest Medicine, 38*, 575–593.

29. Holder, H. (2003). Nursing management of nutrition in cancer and palliative care. *British Journal of Nursing (Mark Allen Publishing), 12*(11), 667–674.

30. Lyman, G. H., & Rolston, K. V. I. (2010). How we treat febrile neutropenia in patients receiving cancer chemotherapy. *Journal of Oncology Practice, 6*(3), 149–152.

31. Canivet, D., Delvaux, N., Gibon, A. S., et al. (2014). Improving communication in cancer pain management nursing: A randomized controlled study assessing the efficacy of a communication skills training program. *Supportive Care in Cancer, 22*(12), 3311–3320.

32. Bower, J. E. (2014). Cancer-related fatigue: Mechanisms, risk factors and treatments. *Nature Reviews. Clinical Oncology, 11*, 597–609.

33. Pedersen, B., Koktved, D. P., & Nielsen, L. L. (2013). Living with side effects from cancer treatment? A challenge to target information. *Scandinavian Journal of Caring Sciences, 27*(3), 715–723.

34. National Cancer Institute. (n.d.). *Breast cancer*. Retrieved from http://www.cancer.gov/cancertopics/types/breast.

35. National Cancer Institute. (n.d.). *Lung cancer*. Retrieved from http://www.cancer.gov/types/lung.

36. National Cancer Institute. (n.d.). *Prostate cancer*. Retrieved from http://www.cancer.gov/cancertopics/types/prostate.

37. National Cancer Institute. (n.d.). *Acute lymphocytic leukemia*. Retrieved from http://www.cancer.gov/cancertopics/types/leukemia.

38. Romano, R. C., & Fritchie, K. J. (2017). Fibrohistiocytic tumors. *Clinics in Laboratory Medicine, 37*, 603–631.

39. Balach, T., Stacy, G. S., & Haydon, R. C. (2011). The clinical evaluation of soft tissue tumors. *Radiologic Clinics of North America, 49*, 1185–1196.

CONCEPT

13

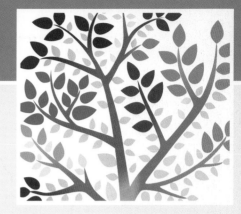

Intracranial Regulation

Debra J. Smith

The brain is a highly complex organ that processes internal and external stimuli and controls body functions. As the largest component of the central nervous system (CNS), the brain lies within the cranium and is protected by the skull. The intracranial regulation (ICR) concept includes normal and abnormal processes of intracranial function. Nurses care for individuals experiencing a wide variety of ICR issues in both community and inpatient settings.

DEFINITION

The term *cranium* refers to the collective bone structure that encloses the brain—also known as the skull.[1] The prefix *intra-* refers to within. Thus, the term intracranial refers to those components that lie within the skull, which include the brain, circulatory system, and dura mater. *Regulation* is a term that refers to compliance and maintenance of balance. In the case of ICR, it is referring to maintaining a balance to promote an environment that is conducive to optimal brain functioning. The concept of ICR includes anything that affects the contents of the cranium and affects the regulation of maintaining an optimally functioning brain. For the purpose of this concept presentation, ICR is defined as *mechanisms or conditions that impact intracranial processing and function.* Although the brain receives input from outside the cranium, specifically through the peripheral nervous system and the spinal cord component of the CNS, this concept does not include problems with the peripheral nervous system or spinal cord. ICR focuses on those conditions that specifically affect the contents of the cranium. As will be discussed further, many variables can upset this balance with potentially devastating results.

SCOPE

The scope of this concept ranges from normal to impaired function (Fig. 13.1). When functioning optimally, ICR allows individuals to function normally. Impairment is caused by a number of factors including reduced blood flow to the brain, compromised neurotransmission, and damage to brain tissue. The resulting neurologic dysfunction can range from minimal to severe.

NORMAL PHYSIOLOGICAL PROCESS

The brain is the primary structure associated with ICR and is part of the CNS, serving as the primary control center for the body. Anatomically, the brain is divided into the following areas: the cerebrum, the diencephalon, the cerebellum, and the brain stem (Fig. 13.2). Normal ICR involves interaction among these structures through a complex communication system. Table 13.1 presents general functions of these structures. Neurons are cells within the nervous system designed for the transmission of information within the brain and throughout the body. Neurons direct signals from cell to cell through dendrites and axons. Optimal ICR is dependent on the transmission of nerve impulses across neuronal synapses by neurotransmitters.

Brain function depends on a consistent supply of blood delivering oxygen and nutrients. A sufficient volume of blood and cardiac function is required for adequate perfusion. The level of oxygen in the blood is dependent on gas exchange in the lungs and hemoglobin capacity. Likewise, because carbohydrates are the main source of fuel for the brain, optimal ICR is dependent on blood glucose levels. Several other unique physiological processes are in place to protect and preserve critical brain functions, which are described next.

Cranial Vault/Skull

The skull is composed of multiple bones that act as a rigid, noncompliant protective covering of the brain. Within the skull are three components: brain tissue (80%), blood (10%), and cerebrospinal fluid (CSF) (10%).

Intracranial pressure (ICP) is the sum of the pressure exerted by these three volumes in the skull. In adults, ICP is normally ≤15 mm Hg; a sustained ICP of ≥20 mm Hg is considered intracranial hypertension. Because the total volume inside the skull cannot change, a change in one compartment necessitates a change in another. This interrelationship of volume and compliance of the three cranial components is known as the Monro-Kellie doctrine.[2]

Blood-Brain Barrier

Between the arterial and venous network of the brain is a unique capillary system called the blood-brain barrier (BBB), which consists of a tight layer of endothelial cells. This restrictive barrier makes it difficult for neurotoxic substances to pass into the brain.[3] This barrier may become compromised secondary to decreased perfusion.

Meninges

There are three layers of a tough protective membrane that surrounds the brain and spinal cord: dura mater, arachnoid layer, and pia mater. The area between the arachnoid layer and the pia mater is referred to as the subarachnoid space, which contains CSF (Fig. 13.3).

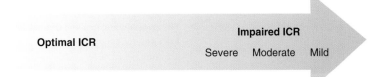

FIGURE 13.1 Scope of Intracranial Regulation *(ICR)*.

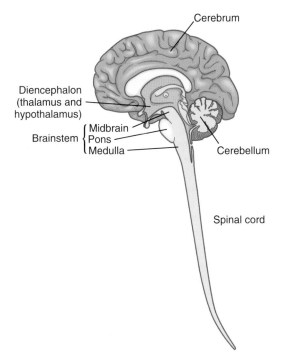

FIGURE 13.2 **Structures of the Brain.** (Modified from Lewis, S. L., Bucher, L., Heitkemper, M. M., Harding, M. M., Kwong, J., & Roberts, D. [Eds.]. [2017]. *Medical–surgical nursing: Assessment and management of clinical problems* [10th ed.]. St Louis: Elsevier.)

TABLE 13.1 Structures of the Brain and General Functions		
Brain Structure	Description	Functions
Cerebrum	Largest brain structure located at the top; divided into two hemispheres (right and left) and four lobes (frontal, parietal, temporal, occipital)	Thinking, consciousness, sensory perception, movement, emotions, memory
Cerebellum	Located under occipital lobe of the cerebrum	Balance, muscle coordination, posture
Diencephalon	Located between the cerebrum and the midbrain; consists of two structures—the thalamus and hypothalamus	Sensory relay, emotions, alerting mechanism (thalamus); regulation of body temperature, fluid balance, sleep, appetite (hypothalamus)
Brain stem	Located at the base of the brain; consists of the medulla oblongata, pons, and midbrain	Conduction pathway between brain and spinal cord for movement, cardiac, respiratory, and vasomotor control; conduction pathway for visual and auditory impulses

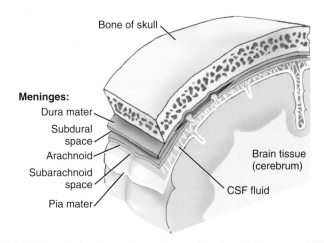

FIGURE 13.3 **Meninges: Dura Mater, Arachnoid Layer, and Pia Mater.** *CSF,* Cerebrospinal fluid. (From Shiland, B. J. [2019]. *Mastering healthcare terminology* [6th ed.]. St. Louis: Elsevier.)

ICR problems are frequently referred to in relation to the meningeal layer location—for example, subarachnoid hemorrhage, subdural hematoma, or epidural hematoma. Meningitis is an inflammatory condition of the meninges.

Autoregulation

Cerebral blood flow (CBF) is normally maintained at a relatively constant rate by intrinsic cerebral mechanisms referred to as autoregulation. Autoregulation adjusts regional CBF in response to the brain's metabolic demands by changing the diameter of cerebral blood vessels. Cerebral arterial walls are thinner than those in the systemic circulation because of a lack of smooth muscle and a decreased thickness of the tunica media. They also do not have the ability to develop collateral circulation in response to ischemia. Autoregulation allows the cerebral circulation to deliver a constant supply of blood despite wide fluctuations in systemic blood pressure.

Cerebral Spinal Fluid

CSF is produced at a rate of approximately 20 mL/hour, circulates within the subarachnoid space, and then is absorbed into the venous system.

It acts to cushion and support the brain and other structures of the CNS and provides nutrients. CSF analysis provides useful diagnostic information related to certain nervous system conditions (see "Diagnostic Tests" under "Assessment").

Hyperventilation

Another protective mechanism in response to increasing cerebral volume is spontaneous hyperventilation. Carbon dioxide is a potent vasodilator. Hyperventilation is a compensatory mechanism that causes vasoconstriction, which reduces cerebral blood volume and ICP.

Age-Related Differences

The brain undergoes significant development during infancy and childhood. At birth, brain function is primarily limited to primitive reflexes and is sufficiently developed to sustain life. Extensive development occurs thereafter during the first few years, not only in size but also in function. Throughout childhood, a child's growth and development are influenced by evolving cognitive, emotional, and motor functions within the brain. Cranial sutures are ossified by age 12 years, with no expansion of the skull after age 5 years.[4] Before the sutures are entirely closed, there is some room for expansion in the case of cerebral edema and increasing ICP.

Aging is associated with a reduction in brain size, weight, and number of neurons. Atrophy of neuronal dendrites causes a slowing of neurotransmission and neural processes. These changes, however, are not directly associated with mental function, and cognitive abilities remain intact in the absence of disease, although cognitive function is enhanced with continued stimulation.

VARIATIONS AND CONTEXT

There are several categories that describe impairment or dysfunction associated with ICR. These include problems associated with perfusion, neurotransmission, glucose regulation, and pathologic processes. These categories are briefly described next, and the pathologic consequences of these impairments are detailed in the sections that follow. All these impairments can occur across the lifespan, although some are more prevalent in particular age groups.

Impaired Perfusion

For the brain to function, there must be a consistent supply of blood delivering oxygen and nutrients. Impairment in blood flow, reduced oxygenation of the blood, or reduced blood glucose can lead to significant dysfunction. Intracerebral perfusion can be disrupted in a number of different conditions, such as internal blockage of a vessel, severe hypotension, or loss of vessel integrity attributable to damage or excessive external pressure on a vessel that exceeds perfusion pressure. For example, an ischemic stroke is the result of inadequate perfusion past the thrombus or embolus. Perfusion can also be disrupted as the result of an intracranial hemorrhage, such as a subdural hematoma or subarachnoid hemorrhage caused by a traumatic brain injury (TBI). A disruption of cerebral perfusion leads to a wide variety of ICR problems depending on the area of the brain that is affected and the length of time before perfusion is restored.

Compromised Neurotransmission

Optimal functioning of the brain is dependent on the transmission of nerve impulses across neuronal synapses by neurotransmitters. Normal transmission requires fully functioning neurons, nerves, and neurotransmitters. Presynaptic neurons release neurotransmitters that travel to postsynaptic neurons. Neurotransmitters can be either excitatory or inhibitory. Many components of this process can be disrupted. Degenerative diseases (see "Pathology") disrupt brain functioning by the loss of neurons, which also disrupts neurotransmission. The concentration of the neurotransmitter acetylcholine is reduced in Alzheimer disease (AD) secondary to the destruction of acetylcholine-secreting neurons. Neurotransmitters can be affected by drugs and toxins, which can modify their function or block their attachment to receptor sites on the postsynaptic membrane. For example, heroin binds to presynaptic endorphin receptors and reduces pain by blocking the release of the neurotransmitter that causes pain.[3] Seizures are aberrant neuronal activity that can manifest clinically as disrupted motor control, sensory perception, behavior, and/or autonomic function.

Glucose Regulation

Because the brain cannot store glucose, a constant supply is needed to maintain optimal functioning. Areas of the brain that are particularly sensitive to hypoglycemia are the cerebral cortex, hippocampus, and cerebellum. Prolonged hypoglycemia may cause widespread neuronal injury. Children, who have smaller glycogen stores, are particularly susceptible to hypoglycemia, which can adversely affect brain tissue.

Hyperglycemia (glucose level >126 mg/dL) can also cause problems by augmenting brain injury in acute stroke. Some of the deleterious effects of hyperglycemia are increased tissue acidosis from anaerobic metabolism, free radical generation, and increased blood-brain barrier permeability. The American Heart Association/American Stroke Association guidelines for acute ischemic stroke recommend treatment for hyperglycemia to achieve serum glucose concentrations in the range of 140 to 180 mg/dL.[5]

Pathology

There are many pathologic states that disrupt intracranial functioning and regulation. Pathology of the brain can take many forms, such as brain tumors, degenerative diseases, and inflammatory conditions.

Many degenerative diseases of the brain are clinical exemplars of the ICR concept. Alzheimer's disease is a degenerative process that results in the loss of neurons primarily in the gray matter of the brain. Parkinson's disease is a result of damage to the basal ganglia, and Huntington's disease is a degeneration of striatal neurons. Although the degenerative process varies with each of these diseases, the result is the same—disruption of brain regulation and function.

The most common inflammatory conditions of the brain are abscesses, meningitis, and encephalitis. Although the etiology varies with each condition, the result is an inflammatory response that can result in disrupted cerebral function and regulation.

CONSEQUENCES

Regardless of the specific condition or cause, when there is impaired blood flow, compromised neurotransmission, and damage to brain tissue from trauma or other pathologic conditions, significant pathophysiologic consequences can occur.

Cerebral Edema

Cerebral or brain parenchymal edema occurs for many reasons. Box 13.1 shows common causes of cerebral edema. It is a symptom that is common to many ICR conditions. Cerebral edema may be classified as vasogenic, cytotoxic, or interstitial. Regardless of the classification or origin of cerebral edema, the result is an increase in brain size that will negatively affect perfusion and oxygenation to the brain. As discussed next, signs and symptoms will become evident to varying degrees based on the location and amount of cerebral edema.

BOX 13.1   CAUSES OF CEREBRAL EDEMA

Mass Lesions
- Brain abscess
- Brain tumor (primary or metastatic)
- Hematoma (intracerebral, subdural, epidural)
- Hemorrhage (intracerebral, cerebellar, brain stem)

Head Injuries and Brain Surgery
- Contusion
- Hemorrhage
- Post-traumatic brain swelling

Cerebral Infection
- Meningitis
- Encephalitis

Vascular Insult
- Anoxic and ischemic episodes
- Cerebral infarction (thrombotic or embolic)
- Venous sinus thrombosis

Toxic or Metabolic Encephalopathic Conditions
- Lead or arsenic intoxication
- Hepatic encephalopathy
- Uremia

From Lewis, S. L., Bucher, L., Heitkemper, M. M., Harding, M. M., Kwong, J., & Roberts, D. (Eds.). (2017). *Medical–surgical nursing: Assessment and management of clinical problems* (10th ed.). St Louis: Elsevier.

Increased Intracranial Pressure

Elevated ICP is a potentially devastating complication of neurologic injury caused by many different conditions. Pathologic intracranial hypertension (ICH) is evident at sustained pressures ≥20 mm Hg. Several conditions may cause increased ICP, such as TBI, ruptured aneurysm, CNS infections, hydrocephalus, and brain tumors. Symptoms of increased ICP include headache, decreased level of consciousness, and vomiting. Signs may include cranial nerve VI palsies, papilledema, and periorbital bruising; a late sign is Cushing triad (see increased intracranial pressure later in this concept presentation).[2] The untoward consequence of increased ICP is impaired perfusion (see "Measurement of Cerebral Perfusion Pressure").

Brain Tumors

A tumor can occur in any part of the brain and spinal cord. Brain tumors are most commonly a result of metastasis from another primary site outside the brain. Clinical manifestations will depend on the size and location of the tumor.

RISK FACTORS

Populations at Risk

All populations are potentially at risk for problems with ICR because there are such a wide variety of conditions included in this concept. Depending on the condition, some populations are at a higher risk. ICR problems related to degenerative pathology have a higher incidence in the elderly population. Injury-related ICR problems are more commonly seen in the adolescent and young adult age groups. The leading cause of TBI is falls which disproportionately affect the youngest and oldest age groups. Being struck by or against an object is the second leading cause of TBI. Among all age groups, motor vehicle crashes were the third overall leading cause of TBI.[6]

Individual Risk Factors

Individual risk factors are dependent on the cause of injury or pathology. For example, the risk factors for stroke include age, hypertension, diabetes, smoking, obesity, and cardiovascular disease. Some of the degenerative pathologic conditions have a strong genetic component and put certain individuals at higher risk.

ASSESSMENT

History

A thorough history should be solicited from the patient or a family member if the patient is unable to provide information. Patient presentation will help direct the practitioner to the most relevant areas of inquiry. Information in a history that provides data about intracranial function can relate to multiple systems. Asking pertinent questions will provide clues to the examiner of ICR problems and will help to focus the physical examination. Potential ICR areas on which to focus include the following:
- Numbness, paralysis, tingling, neuralgia
- Loss of consciousness, dizziness, fainting, confusion
- Changes in recent or remote memory
- Changes in vision, hearing, balance, gait
- Speech problems (expressive and/or receptive)
- Chewing/swallowing problems
- Muscle weakness or loss of bowel or urinary control
- Onset of unexplained tremors or other motion disturbances
- Unexplained, severe headache
- Vomiting
- Symptom onset
- History of head injury

Examination Findings

Objective examination findings that convey neurologic status are found throughout a physical examination. Specific signs of dysfunction vary depending on the ICR problem. Many age-related degenerative changes occur in the CNS. When assessing an older adult, it is important to distinguish between the expected changes and changes potentially related to an ICR problem that could improve with appropriate treatment. Findings common to most conditions are a change in mental status and motor function. Some of the more common examination techniques and tools are discussed next, but these are not all-inclusive.

Mental Status

A complete mental status examination includes assessment of the individual's emotional responses, mood, cognitive functioning, and personality. Depending on the patient's presenting condition, the nurse will decide which components of the exam are relevant.[7] If it is not practical or necessary to do a complete mental status exam, the Mini-Mental Status Examination is an option, which is a simplified scored form of the cognitive portion of the mental status examination. It consists of 11 questions and takes only 5 to 10 minutes to administer.[8]

Cognitive functioning should be intact in the healthy elderly client, although some changes may occur as individuals grow older.[7] When assessing an elderly patient, it is essential to determine the patient's baseline neurologic functioning in order to establish if there are significant changes.

Glasgow Coma Scale

The Glasgow Coma Scale (GCS) is used to give a standardized numeric score of the neurologic patient assessment. This is a widely used measurement tool that consists of three components: eye opening, verbal response, and motor response. Although this is an objective measurement tool, there is room for subjective interpretation of assessment findings. To minimize subjectivity and facilitate consistency, when transferring care of a patient, nurses should complete the GCS together and agree on the values. Changes in the GCS will help to determine treatment methods and priorities. Table 13.2 describes the components of the GCS.

TABLE 13.2	Glasgow Coma Scale	
Appropriate Stimulus	**Response**	**Score**
Eyes Open	Spontaneous response	4
• Approach to bedside	Opening of eyes to name or	3
• Verbal command	command	
• Pain	Lack of opening of eyes to previous stimuli but opening to pain	2
	Lack of opening of eyes to any stimulus	1
	Untestable[a]	U
Best Verbal Response	Appropriate orientation, conversant; correct identification of self, place, year, and month	5
• Verbal questioning with maximum arousal	Confusion; conversant, but disorientation in one or more spheres	4
	Inappropriate or disorganized use of words (e.g., cursing), lack of sustained conversation	3
	Incomprehensible words, sounds (e.g., moaning)	2
	Lack of sound, even with painful stimuli	1
	Untestable[a]	U
Best Motor Response	Obedience of command	6
• Verbal command (e.g., "raise your arm, hold up two fingers")	Localization of pain, lack of obedience but presence of attempts to remove offending stimulus	5
• Pain (pressure on proximal nail bed)	Flexion withdrawal,[a] flexion of arm in response to pain without abnormal flexion posture	4
	Abnormal flexion, flexing of arm at elbow and pronation, making a fist	3
	Abnormal extension, extension of arm at elbow usually with abduction and internal rotation of arm at shoulder	2
	Lack of response	1
	Untestable[a]	U

[a]Added to the original scale by some centers.
Modified from Lewis, S. L., Bucher, L., Heitkemper, M. M., Harding, M. M., Kwong, J., & Roberts, D. (Eds.). (2017). *Medical–surgical nursing: Assessment and management of clinical problems* (10th ed.). St Louis: Elsevier.

Cranial Nerves

As the name implies, the cranial nerves originate in the cranium; therefore, assessment of the cranial nerves should be included in a thorough neurologic assessment. Abnormal findings will help to locate the affected area of the brain. Assessment techniques can be found in nursing assessment textbooks.

Intracranial Pressure

The earliest sign of increased ICP is a change in level of consciousness. Another early sign is headache. Headache characteristics associated with increased ICP include nocturnal awakening, pain worsened by cough/defecation, recurrent and localized, and progressive increase in frequency or severity. Vomiting, usually not preceded by nausea, is often a nonspecific sign of increased ICP.[9]

For children, the clinical manifestations of elevated ICP varies by the age of the child and whether the rise in pressure is gradual or acute.[10] Nausea and vomiting are common presenting symptoms at any age.[10]

ICP is measured using a catheter placed in one of the following locations in the cranium: intraventricular, intraparenchymal, subarachnoid, or epidural (Fig. 13.4). The most common placement is in the lateral ventricle. Patients must be in an intensive care environment for this type of monitoring. Most commonly, ICP monitoring is done in trauma patients with a closed head injury. Some other indications include stroke, intracerebral hemorrhage, hydrocephalus, and subarachnoid hemorrhage. Guidelines for management of severe head injury recommend that ICP monitoring is indicated in comatose head injury patients with a GCS score of 3 to 8 and with an abnormal computerized tomography (CT) scan. Treating ICP above 22 mm Hg is recommended because values above this level are associated with increased mortality.[9] Catheters are available that monitor ICP, drain CSF, and measure brain oxygenation. When the patient has increased ICP, the catheter may be used for therapeutic drainage of CSF in order to reduce ICP.

If hydrocephalus is present, a ventriculostomy may be used to remove CSF. In some instances, a permanent catheter is placed to drain CSF, which is known as a ventriculoperitoneal (VP) shunt.

Cushing triad is useful in explaining the late signs of increased ICP. It is an ominous late sign of increased ICP and an indication of impending herniation. The triad consists of hypertension (with widened pulse pressure), bradycardia, and changes in respiratory pattern in the presence of increased ICP. Pupil and vision changes may become apparent as edema impinges on cranial nerves II, III, IV, and/or VI.[7]

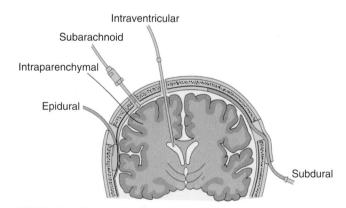

FIGURE 13.4 Coronal Section of Brain Showing Potential Sites for Placement of Intracranial Pressure Monitoring Devices. (Modified from Lewis, S. L., Bucher, L., Heitkemper, M. M., Harding, M. M., Kwong, J., & Roberts, D. [Eds.]. [2017]. *Medical–surgical nursing: Assessment and management of clinical problems* [10th ed.]. St Louis: Elsevier.)

Measurement of Cerebral Perfusion Pressure

Cerebral blood flow increases with hypercapnia and hypoxia. Ischemia results from inadequate cerebral perfusion or increased cerebral oxygen consumption. To maintain adequate perfusion, it is necessary to optimize cerebral perfusion pressure (CPP), which is calculated by subtracting the ICP from the mean arterial pressure. When CPP is less than 60 mm Hg, cerebral blood flow is compromised and autoregulation is impaired.[2] CPP should be kept between 60 and 70 mm Hg in patients with elevated ICP to avoid ischemic injury. CPP greater than 70 mm Hg should be avoided because of an increased risk for adult respiratory failure.[9]

Normal CPP range for children is not well established, but it is likely lower than that of adults because systolic blood pressure is lower in children. Appropriate CPP values are probably 40 to 60 mm Hg.[10]

The National Institutes of Health Stroke Scale

The National Institutes of Health Stroke Scale (NIHSS) is an example of one type of specific tool for nurses to use when assessing a patient following stroke. This scale, composed of 11 items, has been widely used and validated. The NIHSS score on admission has been correlated to stroke outcome and is recommended for all patients with suspected stroke.[11]

Diagnostic Tests

When an ICR problem is suspected, time is of the essence. Diagnostic tests that can quickly give the most pertinent information are recommended initially.

Neuroimaging Studies

Imaging studies are essential to obtain in patients presenting with sudden neurologic deterioration, and they may also be utilized with nonemergent conditions such as suspected brain tumor. A non-contrast CT or magnetic resonance imaging (MRI) scan should be performed as soon as possible to determine the origin of a neurologic injury. Current guidelines recommend a head CT for all TBI patients with a GCS of 14 or lower, which can detect skull fractures, intracranial bleeding, and cerebral edema.[9] Advanced CT and MRI technologies, such as magnetic resonance angiography and positron emission tomography, are available that can distinguish between brain tissue that is irreversibly infarcted and that which is potentially salvageable, which will help when deciding appropriate treatment.

Skull Radiograph

Depending on the mechanism of action and patient presentation, a skull x-ray may be ordered to detect fractures, bone erosion, calcification, and/or abnormal vasculature.

Electroencephalogram

An electroencephalogram (EEG) measures and records the brain's electrical activity through multiple electrodes placed on the scalp. Video EEG monitoring refers to continuous EEG monitoring over a prolonged period while simultaneously recording the patient's movements and activity. This monitoring combination is useful in diagnosing and localizing the area of seizure origin. The EEG is also helpful in identifying psychogenic nonepileptic seizures. The origin of these seizures may be associated with psychological conditions or other physical problems, but they are not caused by electrical activity in the brain.[12]

Brain Biopsy

To determine the type and stage of a brain tumor, a biopsy is performed, usually during a surgical procedure. Preliminary histologic type can usually be determined quickly in the operating room; then the tumor is sent to pathology for complete analysis and final determination.

Lumbar Puncture

The lumbar puncture (spinal tap) may be indicated when infection is suspected. A lumbar puncture should be deferred until after the head CT scan if intracranial hypertension is suspected because brain herniation may be precipitated by increasing the pressure gradient between the cranial vault and the spinal cord.

CLINICAL MANAGEMENT

Primary Prevention

Primary prevention strategies are intended to maintain optimal health and prevent injury or disease. This applies to intracranial regulation in many ways. Leading a healthy lifestyle, which includes smoking cessation, maintaining a healthy weight, controlling blood pressure, and exercising, can decrease the risk of vascular disease affecting the cerebral arteries. This is linked to stroke risk reduction. Injury prevention measures such as proper use of seat belts and/or helmets, knowledge of firearm safety, and participation in violence prevention programs reduce the risk of TBI. *Healthy People 2030*[13] has one specific objective to reduce fatal traumatic brain injuries.

Secondary Prevention (Screening)

There are no true screening tests available related to ICR. In the event of injury or the presence of clinical findings suggesting intracranial dysfunction, specific diagnostics tests are initiated to determine a cause.

Collaborative Interventions

There are many interventions related to caring for patients with ICR issues. A few of the most common examples are discussed. The overarching goal of caring for patients is to prevent secondary injury (damage to the vulnerable adjacent tissues) by improving cerebral perfusion. This is primarily achieved by decreasing cerebral edema and ICP, which will improve oxygenation to prevent cell death.

Pharmacotherapy

Because impairments in intracranial regulation represent a large number of conditions, there are many classes of pharmacologic agents associated with this concept. Table 13.3 presents these agents, and they are described further here.

Osmotic diuretics. Osmotic diuretics create an osmolar gradient that draws water across the blood-brain barrier, leading to a decrease in interstitial volume and a subsequent decrease in ICP. Mannitol is the agent used most commonly to achieve ICP control in a variety of conditions, and it has been shown to improve cerebral blood flow. Hypertonic saline is increasingly being used, but research has not clearly determined the volume, tonicity, or most effective method of administration.[14]

Sedatives. Sedatives can decrease ICP by reducing metabolic demand. Propofol (Diprivan) is frequently used in the intensive care unit setting because it has a short half-life and is easily titrated, permitting frequent neurologic assessment. Barbiturate coma is sometimes used as a final effort to control increased ICP, but there is little clinical evidence to support its use.[14] Benzodiazepines, such as lorazepam (Ativan), are another sedative option.

Analgesics. Pain increases oxygen demand; therefore, in addition to controlling pain for patient comfort, it is controlled to avoid

TABLE 13.3 Pharmacologic Agents Commonly Used to Treat Problems with Intracranial Regulation

Classification	Indications Specific for Intracranial Regulation	Most Common Agents Used
Osmotic diuretics	Reduction of ICP by reducing fluid	Mannitol
Sedatives	Reduction of metabolic demand to reduce ICP	Propofol, lorazepam
Analgesics	Pain control to reduce oxygen demand	Fentanyl, morphine
Antiepileptics	Seizure control	Phenytoin, valproic acid
Glucocorticoids	Cerebral edema associated with pathologies	Dexamethasone
Antipyretics	Fever control to reduce metabolic demand	Acetaminophen
Antihypertensives	Reduce blood pressure in hemorrhagic stroke	Labetalol, transdermal nitroglycerin paste, nicardipine
Antiparkinsonian agents	Restore balance of dopamine in brain	Levodopa, pramipexole, ropinirole, bromocriptine, selegiline
Cholinesterase inhibitors	Mild to moderate dementia	Donepezil, rivastigmine, galantamine
	Moderate to severe dementia	Memantine

ICP, Intracranial pressure.

compromising sufficient oxygen delivery to ischemic neuronal cells. The use and choice of sedative agents should be individualized according to specific clinical circumstances and provider expertise. Short-acting narcotics, such as fentanyl or morphine, are generally preferable to allow for periodic neurologic assessments.

Antiepileptics. Seizures can exacerbate or cause increased ICP and increase oxygen demand. Antiepileptics may be used as a prophylactic or treatment measure. These medications act by stabilizing nerve cell membranes and preventing the distribution of the epileptic discharge. Initial seizure management of TBI patients includes phenytoin (Dilantin) or valproic acid (Depakote). Patient education is important because there are many serious side effects associated with antiepileptic medications.

Glucocorticoids. Glucocorticoids may be indicated for use in some ICR problems and are contraindicated in others. Dexamethasone (Decadron) may be effective in reducing cerebral edema related to tumors, abscesses, and CNS infections. Steroids are not recommended for improving outcome or reducing ICP. In patients with severe TBI, high-dose methylprednisolone is associated with increased mortality.[9]

Antipyretics. Fever may worsen the outcome after stroke and severe head injury by aggravating secondary brain injury caused by increased metabolic demand. Normothermia should be maintained through the use of antipyretic medications, such as acetaminophen, or by implementation of other treatment modalities such as mechanical cooling.

Antihypertensive medications. Depending on the ICR condition, antihypertensive medications may be detrimental or beneficial. Mean arterial pressure must be adequate to maintain sufficient CPP to limit secondary injury. Because of this, higher systemic blood pressures are tolerated in patients with ICR conditions that impair CPP. In these patients, antihypertensive medications are not recommended, and medications may be initiated in order to sufficiently raise the systemic pressure, particularly if the ICP is elevated. Several studies have shown

that lowering the systemic blood pressure in patients with acute ischemic stroke has been associated with clinical deterioration. Conversely, reducing blood pressure in patients with a hemorrhagic stroke may be beneficial by minimizing further bleeding and continued vascular damage.[4]

Antiparkinsonian medications. Antiparkinsonian medications attempt to restore the balance of dopamine through one of several mechanisms, depending on drug type. The most effective drugs, called dopaminergic drugs, replace dopamine, or mimic its action in the brain. Another group of drugs delays the breakdown of dopamine, thus increasing the level in the brain.

Levodopa (Sinemet) is the most commonly used antiparkinsonian medication; it is converted to dopamine in the CNS, where it serves as a neurotransmitter. To minimize the side effects of dopamine in the periphery, another medication is administered with levodopa. In the United States, this drug is carbidopa, which prevents the conversion of levodopa to dopamine until it reaches the brain.

Dopamine agonists mimic the effect of dopamine by stimulating the same cells as dopamine. Monoamine oxidase B (MAO-B) is an enzyme that breaks down levodopa in the brain. MAO-B inhibitors prolong the effectiveness of dopamine and levodopa.

Cholinesterase inhibitors. Cholinesterase inhibitors are prescribed to patients with mild to moderate dementia to make acetylcholine more available, improving cortical function. In moderate to severe dementia, an *N*-methyl-D-aspartate (NMDA) receptor antagonist may have a neuroprotective function as well as decrease dementia symptoms. However, it does not slow progression of the disease.[15]

Surgical Interventions

Many types of cranial surgery are available to address ICR problems. Some examples are craniotomy, craniectomy, and shunt and stereotactic procedures.

A *decompressive craniectomy* removes the rigid confines of the skull, allowing for expansion of the cranial contents and lowering the ICP. Potential complications of this surgery include herniation through the skull defect, spinal fluid leakage, wound infection, and epidural and subdural hematoma.

A *craniotomy* may be performed to remove a lesion or tumor; repair a damaged area; or relieve pressure and/or drain blood secondary to epidural, subdural, or intracerebral hematomas.

Frequently, the origin of seizures is either the hippocampus or the amygdala, which is located in the temporal lobe of the brain (see "Diagnostic Tests, Electroencephalogram"). If seizures are found to arise from these areas, a temporal lobectomy surgery is performed to resect the identified area. This surgery is becoming more common and has been successful in obtaining seizure control.

Stereotactic procedures allow precise localization of a specific area of the brain and may be utilized for dissection or to obtain a biopsy.

Shunt procedures place an artificial pathway for excessive CSF to be drained from an area of the brain to an extracranial location using a tube or implanted device. Accumulation of CSF may be due to overproduction, obstruction, or problems with normal reabsorption. Placement of a ventriculoperitoneal (VP) shunt is a common example of this type of procedure.

Ongoing Assessment

With prevention of secondary injury being the goal of patient care, it is of upmost importance to recognize changes in the patient's condition early. For this reason, thorough and frequent neurologic assessment is critical in the care of a patient with ICR problems. A complete neurologic assessment includes determination of level of consciousness and measurement of GCS score along with cognitive, motor, sensory, and reflex testing.

Vital signs should be monitored consistently on all patients with an ICR problem. The frequency will be dictated by the condition and acuity of the patient. Assessment should be frequent enough to detect significant changes early so that the appropriate interventions can be implemented to prevent patient deterioration (see the discussion of Cushing triad in the "Intracranial Pressure" section).

Intracranial Pressure/Cerebral Perfusion Pressure Monitoring

As discussed previously, it is imperative that the brain receive a constant, adequate blood supply to optimize brain functioning. Severely head-injured patients should receive continuous ICP and CPP monitoring. If these values are not optimal, several possible collaborative and nursing interventions are available. Most guidelines recommend that treatment for elevated ICP should be initiated when ICP is greater than 22 mm Hg.

Interventions to Lower Intracranial Pressure

Positioning. The intracranial venous system consists of canals and sinuses, and unlike the peripheral venous system, it lacks valves. Interventions promoting venous outflow from the head decrease cerebral volume and help to lower ICP. Such interventions include head-of-bed elevation and proper alignment of the head and neck with the body. Head-of-bed elevation of 30 degrees is usually recommended to decrease ICP. It is also important to keep the head and neck midline (to prevent compression of jugular veins) and to limit hip flexion. Head-of-bed elevation potentially could decrease cerebral perfusion by increasing venous return. Therefore, head-of-bed elevation is recommended as long as the CPP remains at an appropriate level.

Activity management. Balance between being efficient and not increasing oxygen demand when providing nursing care is crucial. Clustering of many nursing tasks at once will increase oxygen demand and may compromise cerebral perfusion. Distribution of care procedures over a longer period is preferable.

Airway management. Endotracheal suctioning stimulates coughing, which increases ICP. Patients with increased ICP should undergo endotracheal suctioning only when suctioning is indicated. In addition, these patients may need to be sedated before the procedure. Careful assessment is necessary to maintain an adequate airway and minimize complications of increased ICP.

Hyperventilation. Prophylactic hyperventilation ($PaCO_2$ ≤25 mm Hg) in TBI is not recommended because it decreases perfusion, which will negatively affect oxygen delivery. Hyperventilation is recommended only as a temporary measure to reduce elevated ICP.[9] A 1 mm Hg change in $PaCO_2$ is associated with a 3% change in cerebral blood flow.[2] Hyperventilation can also increase extracellular lactate and glutamate levels, which may contribute to secondary brain injury.[14]

Bowel management. Constipation increases intra-abdominal pressure and causes straining when defecating, thereby raising ICP. Stool softeners or laxatives may be necessary to minimize these untoward effects on ICP.

Nutrition Management

Nutrition management is a high priority when caring for patients with ICR conditions. The nurse should advocate for an early dietary consultation in order to ensure prompt and adequate nutrition to facilitate healing. Depending on the ICR impairment and patient condition, enteral or parenteral feeding may be appropriate. Swallowing function should be assessed before initiation of enteral feeding for certain patients, particularly following a stroke.

Patient Education

Patient education is always a primary nursing function, which is no exception when caring for patients with ICR conditions. Education should be focused on all levels of health promotion. Problems involving the brain can have devastating and long-lasting effects. Nurses are uniquely qualified and available to assist patients and their families throughout the course of their care.

Rehabilitation

Particularly after a stroke or head injury, rehabilitation is an important part of patient care. The focus is on returning the patient to optimal functioning. The composition of the rehabilitation team will depend on the patient's needs, which may include speech therapy, physical therapy, and occupational therapy along with medical and nursing care as needed. As soon as the patient is stabilized in the acute care setting, rehabilitation should begin. Because recovery is dependent on the formation of new neural networks, it may take months to years to determine how much function will be regained.

INTERRELATED CONCEPTS

Many concepts are closely related to ICR. Those considered most important are shown in Fig. 13.5.

Cognition is dependent on an optimally functioning brain. If ICR is disrupted, depending on the area of the brain affected, cognitive function may be impaired either temporarily or permanently. The degree of cognitive function impairment is dependent on the number of neuronal cells affected.

The brain controls movement, coordination, and balance. Thus, optimal Mobility is dependent on an intact neurologic system and effective intracranial regulation. Individuals who have intracranial

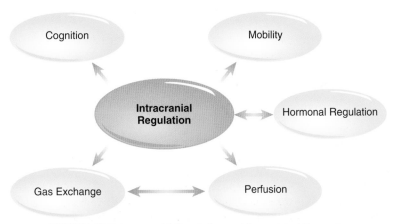

FIGURE 13.5 Intracranial Regulation and Interrelated Concepts.

regulation problems may become immobile because of unsteadiness; imbalance; or the inability to initiate or execute purposeful movement to the arms, legs, or trunk.

Perfusion and Gas Exchange are intimately involved with intracranial regulation and have been discussed thoroughly in the Normal Physiological Process and Physiological Consequences sections. Without adequate perfusion of oxygen- and nutrient-rich blood, the neurons are unable to function. Hormonal Regulation is dependent on normal intracranial regulation because of the location of the hypothalamus and pituitary glands within the brain. Damage to these structures or surrounding brain tissue (from trauma or disease) can have disastrous effects on hormonal regulation.

CLINICAL EXEMPLARS

There are many clinical exemplars of intracranial regulation. Common exemplars are presented in Box 13.2. Although exemplars are listed under a specific category, there are instances in which an exemplar could fit under more than one category. For example, brain tumors can be considered *pathology* and can also cause problems with *neurotransmission*. Similarly, if a brain tumor is large enough and exerts enough pressure, it can also disrupt *perfusion*. The categories are not meant to be all-inclusive or exclusive but, rather, a suggested organization framework for ICR conditions. A brief discussion of common clinical exemplars follows. For detailed explanations and the nursing care for all the exemplars, see medical-surgical, pediatric, and gerontology textbooks.

Featured Exemplars
Stroke
A stroke occurs when there is a loss of blood flow to an area of the brain, causing the neurons to die. Two major classifications of stroke are ischemic stroke and hemorrhagic stroke. Ischemic stroke is the most common. Stroke is the third leading cause of death and serious long-term disability. Nearly three-fourths of all strokes occur in people older than age 65 years. The risk of having a stroke more than doubles each decade after age 55 years. In the United States, stroke death rates are higher for African Americans than for Caucasians, even at younger ages (see "Case Study").[16]

Traumatic Brain Injury
Traumatic brain injury occurs when a blow to the head causes injury to the brain. The most common causes are motor vehicle accidents, falls, and violence. Brain injury can range from mild to severe. With significant injury, the brain tissue swells, leading to cerebral edema and increased ICP; intracranial bleeding may also occur, further contributing to increased ICP. Traumatic brain injury is a major cause of death and disability in the United States.[9]

Epilepsy
Epilepsy, also known as seizure disorder, is a brain disorder characterized by recurrent unprovoked seizures. A seizure happens when abnormal electrical activity in the brain causes an involuntary change in body movement, sensation, awareness, or behavior. Risk factors are more common in children younger than age 2 years and adults older than age 65 years.[17]

Alzheimer's Disease
Alzheimer's disease (AD) is one of many degenerative conditions that affect ICR. It is the most common form of dementia, affects more than 5 million Americans, and is the sixth leading cause of death in the United States. Almost two-thirds of those with AD are women. The most common form occurs in individuals older than age 65 years.[18] The exact cause of AD is unknown, but it is thought to be associated with abnormal plaque formation in the brain tissue and neuron tangles.

Meningitis
Meningitis is a pathologic condition affecting ICR that is caused by inflammation of the protective membranes covering the brain and spinal cord. The types are viral, bacterial, fungal, parasitic, amebic, and noninfectious.[19] Viral meningitis is the most common type and less severe; bacterial meningitis is less common but is usually severe and associated with higher mortality. The populations at risk, transmission, and treatment vary widely, depending on the cause.

BOX 13.2 EXEMPLARS OF INTRACRANIAL REGULATION

Perfusion
Ischemic Stroke
- Embolic stroke
- Thrombotic stroke

Hemorrhagic Stroke
- Intracerebral hemorrhage
- Intraventricular hemorrhage
- Ruptured aneurysm
- Subarachnoid hemorrhage

Head Injury
- Epidural hematoma
- Skull fractures
- Subdural hematoma
- Traumatic brain injury

Neurologic Transmission
- Epilepsy
- Seizure

Pathology
Brain Neoplasm
- Benign brain tumor
- Malignant brain tumor

Degenerative Conditions
- Alzheimer disease
- Dementia
- Huntington disease
- Multiple sclerosis
- Parkinson disease

Inflammatory Conditions
- Bacterial meningitis
- Brain abscess
- Encephalitis
- Viral meningitis

 ACCESS EXEMPLAR LINKS IN YOUR GIDDENS EBOOK

CASE STUDY

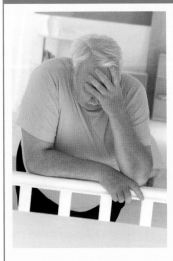

Case Presentation

Mr. James Hobson is a 69-year-old male with a history of hypertension that is fairly well controlled on medication. He has been smoking one or two packs of cigarettes a day for the past 52 years and has a body mass index of 37.3. He awoke yesterday morning complaining of blurry vision and some weakness on the left side of his body. He thought he had just slept wrong, so he was not concerned. Later in the morning, he was having trouble walking and his wife convinced him to call his physician. The physician's office called 911, and Mr. Hobson was transported to the nearest hospital.

Upon arrival to the emergency department, the physical exam findings were as follows: heart rate, 112 beats/min; blood pressure, 172/90 mm Hg; respiratory rate, 24 breaths/min; O_2 saturation, 90%; arm and leg weakness (3/5); and somewhat decreased sensation. He was awake and responding to questions appropriately, although slowly. The following diagnostics tests were ordered: noncontrast CT (NCCT) of the head; electrocardiogram; complete blood count with platelets, cardiac enzymes, and troponin; electrolytes; blood urea nitrogen; creatinine; glucose; prothrombin time/international normalized ratio; and partial thromboplastin time. An NCCT can exclude or confirm the presence of hemorrhage. The sensitivity of an NCCT to show ischemia increases after 24 hours. This patient's CT scan did not show any signs of hemorrhage. Because it was unclear exactly when the symptoms began, the decision was made not to administer a thrombolytic.

Case Analysis Questions

1. What is the core feature of the onset of hemorrhagic and ischemic strokes?
2. What are other conditions that mimic a stroke presentation?
3. What diagnostic test is performed to determine if a suspected stroke is hemorrhagic or ischemic?

From JPC-PROD/iStock/Thinkstock.

🔹 ACCESS EXEMPLAR LINKS IN YOUR GIDDENS EBOOK

REFERENCES

1. Merriam–Webster. (n.d.). *Cranium*. Retrieved from http://www.merriam-webster.com/dictionary/cranium.
2. Smith, E. R., & Amin-Hanjani, S. (2017). *Evaluation and management of elevated intracranial pressure in adults*. Retrieved from http://www.uptodate.com/contents/evaluation-and-management-of-elevated-intracranial-pressure-in-adults?source=search_result&search=elevated+icp&selectedTitle=1~150.
3. Lewis, S. L., Bucher, L., Heitkemper, M. M., et al. (2017). *Medical–surgical nursing: Assessment and management of clinical problems* (10th ed.). St Louis: Mosby.
4. Perry, S., Hockenberry, M., Lowdermilk, D., et al. (Eds.) (2014). *Maternal child nursing care* (5th ed.). New York: Mosby.
5. Oliveira-Filho, J., & Mullen, M. T. (2018). *Initial assessment and management of acute stroke*. Retrieved from http://www.uptodate.com/contents/initial-assessment-and-management-of-acute-stroke?source=search_result&search=acute+stroke&selectedTitle=1~120.
6. Centers for Disease Control and Prevention. (2017). *Traumatic brain injury in the United States: Fact sheet*. Retrieved from http://www.cdc.gov/TraumaticBrainInjury/get_the_facts.html.
7. Ball, J., Dains, J., Flynn, J., et al. (2017). *Seidel's guide to physical examination – E book: An Interprofessional Approach* (9th ed.). St. Louis: Elsevier.
8. Alzheimer's Society. (2018). *Mini-Mental Status Examination (MMSE)*. Retrieved from http://www.alzheimers.org.uk/site/scripts/documents_info.php?documentID=121.
9. Brain Trauma Foundation. (2016). *Guidelines for the management of severe traumatic brain injury*, 4th ed. Retrieved from https://braintrauma.org/guidelines/guidelines-for-the-management-of-severe-tbi-4th-ed#/.
10. Tasker, R. C. (2018). *Elevated intracranial pressure (ICP) in children*. Retrieved from http://www.uptodate.com/contents/elevated-intracranial-pressure-icp-in-children?source=search_result&search=elevated+ICP+children&selectedTitle=1~150.
11. National Institute of Health National Institute of Neurological Disorders and Stroke. (2003). *NIH stroke scale*. Retrieved from https://stroke.nih.gov/resources/scale.htm.
12. Epilepsy Foundation. (2018). *Types of seizures*. Retrieved from https://www.epilepsy.com/learn/types-seizures.
13. Healthy People 2030. *Proposed Objectives for Inclusion In Healthy People 2030*. Retrieved from https://www.healthypeople.gov/sites/default/files/ObjectivesPublicComment508.pdf.
14. Hemphill, J. C. (2017). *Management of acute severe traumatic brain injury*. Retrieved from http://www.uptodate.com/contents/management-of-acute-severe-traumatic-brain-injury?source=search_result&search=management+of+acute+severe+traumatic+brain+injury&selectedTitle=1~150.
15. Press, D., & Alexander, M. (2018). *Treatment of dementia*. Retrieved from http://www.uptodate.com/contents/treatment-of-dementia?source=search_result&search=treatment+of+dementia&selectedTitle=1~150.
16. Internet Stroke Center. (2018). *U.S. stroke statistics*. Retrieved from http://www.strokecenter.org/patients/about-stroke/stroke-statistics.
17. Centers for Disease Control and Prevention. (2017). *Epilepsy: One of the nation's most common neurological conditions at a glance*. Retrieved from https://www.cdc.gov/chronicdisease/resources/publications/aag/epilepsy.htm.
18. Alzheimer's Association. (2018). *Alzheimer's disease facts and figures*. Retrieved from http://alz.org/alzheimers_disease_facts_and_figures.asp#prevalence.
19. Centers for Disease Control and Prevention. (2018). *Meningitis*. Retrieved from http://www.cdc.gov/meningitis/index.html.

CONCEPT
14

Hormonal Regulation

Jean Giddens

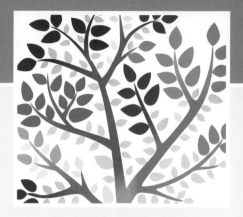

Hormonal regulation is a complex physiological process with integrated responses involving various glands, hormones (produced and secreted by the glands), and the action of hormones on the target tissues. Although each gland and hormone has a specific function, collectively hormonal regulation has five overarching functions: fetal differentiation of the reproductive and central nervous system, sequential growth and development during childhood and adolescence, reproduction, metabolic activity, and adaptive responses.[1] Imbalances of hormonal regulation can lead to significant health and social consequences. This concept presentation focuses on the normal process of hormonal regulation, hormonal imbalance, assessment, and interventions to optimize hormone balance.

DEFINITION

The term *hormonal regulation* is often used in the context of describing a specific group of hormones or metabolism. The focus of this concept presentation is broad, encompassing the general regulatory process including hormone production, secretion, and action. Clearly, the function and physiological action of each hormone are unique, and a presentation of details for each gland, each hormone, and conditions associated with imbalances is not intended; rather, a global perspective is proposed. Given this perspective, what is meant by hormonal regulation? For the purposes of this concept presentation, hormonal regulation is defined as *physiological mechanisms that regulate the secretion and action of hormones associated with the endocrine system.*

Several additional terms are important to fully understand this concept. An *endocrine gland* refers to a specialized cluster of cells, tissue, or an organ that produces and secretes hormones directly into the bloodstream. This distinction is important because there are also other types of glands (known as exocrine glands) that excrete other nonhormonal substances or fluids through ducts to body organs, cavities, or the skin. Examples include sweat glands, salivary glands, mammary glands, and Bartholin glands. Exocrine glands are excluded from this concept presentation because they do not secrete hormones. A *hormone* is a chemical substance that stimulates cellular action in target tissues. *Target tissue* refers to the specific tissue that hormones can influence. A final term worth mentioning is *receptor site*, which refers to a location on the surface of a cell where hormones attach and gain access to the cell, allowing for physiological influence.

SCOPE

The scope of hormonal regulation ranges from the normal range of circulating hormone (based on physiological need) to abnormal secretion, in either excess or deficient amounts. This range, shown in Fig. 14.1, is presented as a continuum because the secretion of hormones is variable, and it changes in response to physiological feedback. Typically the prefix "hypo" before reference to the gland or hormone involved is used to describe deficient states, and the prefix "hyper" is used to describe states of excess. The scope of hormonal regulation can also be thought about from the perspective of the hormones and glands represented. Hormonal regulation represents the hormones produced and secreted from the hypothalamus, anterior pituitary, posterior pituitary, thyroid, parathyroid, adrenal cortex, ovary, testes, and pancreas.

NORMAL PHYSIOLOGICAL PROCESS

Hormones are produced by glands. The structural categories of hormones include protein and peptide hormones, steroid hormones, and monoamine hormones, with the majority being protein or peptides.[2] Fig. 14.2 presents the locations of various adrenal glands, and Box 14.1 summarizes these glands, the hormones they produce, the target tissue, and the physiological effect.

Hormone Production, Secretion, and Transport

Many physiological functions are directed by hormones, which serve as chemical messengers that influence or control functions of other organs or body tissues. Hormones are produced and secreted by endocrine glands. The secretion of a hormone by the gland is in response to a certain level of a substance (e.g., sodium or glucose level) or in response to an alteration within the cellular environment. Once secreted from the gland, hormones are transported to their target tissue. In some cases, the target tissue is adjacent to the endocrine gland that produces the hormone, but more often the hormone is transported to one or more target tissues throughout the body by the circulatory system.[3] Water-soluble hormones circulate in the blood in free form, whereas most lipid-soluble hormones bind to a carrier (e.g., a protein) for transportation.

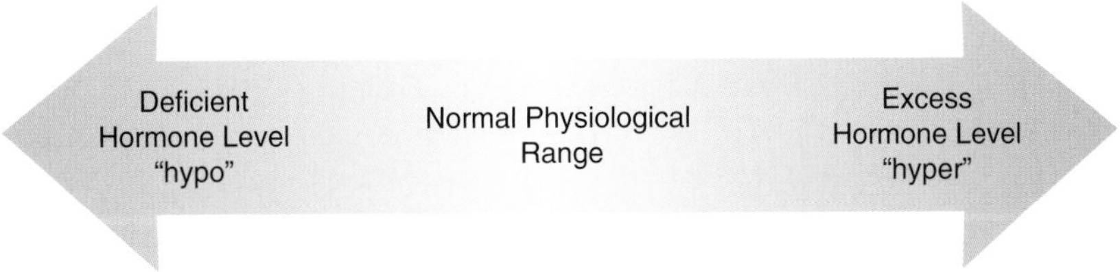

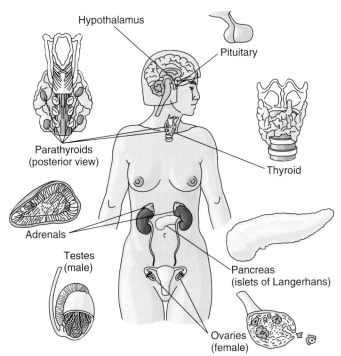

FIGURE 14.1 Scope of Hormonal Regulation.

FIGURE 14.2 Location of Various Endocrine Glands. (From Ignatavicius, D. D., & Workman, M. L. [2013]. *Medical-surgical nursing: Patient-centered collaborative care* [7th ed]. St Louis: Elsevier.)

Hormone Action on Target Tissue

Hormones have very specific cellular effects but only on designated cells within the target tissue. Hormones depend on receptor sites to gain access and exert their specific physiological action within the cell.[4] Target cells have unique receptor sites for the designated hormone, much like a specific key is needed for a lock. For this reason, hormones are unable to influence cells unless the cell has the appropriate receptor site allowing a hormone to act on the cell. The more receptors on the cell, the higher affinity or sensitivity the cell has for that particular hormone. The cell has the ability to adjust the number of receptors (or sensitivity) based on the concentration of circulating hormone. When the circulating concentration of a hormone increases, fewer receptor sites are needed; when the concentration decreases, more receptor sites become available.

Control of Hormone Secretion

Maintaining hormone levels in normal physiological range is accomplished through feedback systems, although the specific mechanism varies depending on the gland or hormone involved. Hormonal regulation occurs through four types of feedback control: negative feedback, positive feedback, biological rhythms, and central nervous system control.

Negative Feedback

The most common type of feedback system for hormonal regulation is the negative feedback system, whereby information regarding a hormone level or the effect of a hormone is communicated back to the gland that secrets the hormone which directs the need for hormone secretion or suppression.[1] One of the simplest examples is the secretion of insulin based on serum glucose levels. When serum glucose rises, the pancreas secretes insulin. Insulin has an effect on transporting glucose into the cell. As serum glucose levels drop, the pancreas inhibits insulin secretion. In this example, serum glucose levels trigger or inhibit the release of insulin.

Negative feedback is more complex when multiple glands and hormones are involved, but the same general process applies. For example, the secretion of thyroid hormones involves three glands (hypothalamus, anterior pituitary gland, and the thyroid gland). The hypothalamus secretes thyroid-releasing hormone, which triggers the release of thyrotropin, which in turn stimulates the secretion of triiodothyronine (T_3) and thyroxine (T_4) from the thyroid gland. As plasma levels of T_3 and T_4 rise, this information is communicated back to the hypothalamus and anterior pituitary gland to inhibit thyroid-releasing hormone and thyroid-stimulating hormone (TSH) secretion.

Positive Feedback

Positive feedback occurs when an increasing level of hormone triggers further elevation of hormone stimulation. The classic example of positive feedback is seen with the menstrual cycle, in which luteinizing hormone (LH) is secreted by the pituitary gland, which triggers the ovaries to secrete estradiol, which in turn stimulates the pituitary gland to secrete more LH.[2]

Biological Rhythms

The secretion of some hormones is controlled by biological rhythms. One example of this is the influence of the circadian rhythm on cortisol secretion. Cortisol secretion is highest in the morning and lowest in the late evening. Disruptions in biological rhythms and sleep deprivation can affect the normal secretion patterns of some hormones.[5]

Central Nervous System Stimulation

Another type of control mechanism for the secretion of hormones is through central nervous system stimulation.[1] For example, when an individual experiences a stressful situation, the sympathetic division of the autonomic nervous system is activated, triggering the release of epinephrine from the adrenal medulla (the fight-or-flight response). When the perceived stress is resolved, the adrenal medulla reduces the release of epinephrine.

Age-Related Differences

Glands and the action of hormones are influenced by the aging process, particularly during adolescence and among older adults.

BOX 14.1   Endocrine Glands, Hormones Secreted, and Physiological Effects

Hypothalamus

- Corticotropin-releasing hormone (CRH)/*anterior pituitary*/release of corticotropin hormone
- Thyrotropin-releasing hormone (TRH)/*anterior pituitary*/release of thyrotropin
- Gonadotropin-releasing hormone (GNHRH)/*anterior pituitary*/release of LH and FSH
- Growth hormone-releasing hormone (GHRH)/*anterior pituitary*/release of GH
- Growth hormone-inhibiting hormone (GHIH)/*anterior pituitary*/inhibition of GH
- Prolactin-inhibiting hormone (PIH)/*anterior pituitary*/inhibition of PRL
- Melanocyte-inhibiting hormone (MIH)/*anterior pituitary*/inhibition of MSH

Anterior Pituitary

- Thyrotropin/*thyroid*/stimulates synthesis and release of thyroid hormone
- Corticotropin/*adrenal cortex*/stimulates synthesis and release of cortisol
- Luteinizing hormone (LH)/*ovary and testis*/stimulates ovulation and progesterone secretion in females; testosterone secretion in males
- Follicle-stimulating hormone (FSH)/*ovary and testis*/stimulates estrogen secretion and follicle maturation in females; spermatogenesis in males
- Prolactin (PRL)/*mammary glands*/stimulates breast milk projection
- Growth hormone (GH) (also known as somatotropin)/*bone, muscle, and soft tissue*/promotion of growth and metabolism
- Melanocyte-stimulating hormone (MSH)/*skin*/pigmentation

Posterior Pituitary

- Antidiuretic hormone (AHD)/*kidney and blood vessels*/promotes water reabsorption
- Oxytocin/*uterus and mammary glands*/stimulates uterine contractions

Thyroid

- Triiodothyronine (T_3) and thyroxine (T_4)/*body-wide*/increased metabolism
- Calcitonin/*bones and kidneys*/lowers serum calcium and phosphate

Parathyroid

- Parathyroid hormone (PTH)/*bone, kidney, and gastrointestinal tract*/increases serum calcium and phosphate

Adrenal Cortex

- Glucocorticoids (cortisol)/*body-wide*/stress response, glucose regulation, immunity
- Mineralocorticoids (aldosterone)/*kidney*/retains water and Na^+, exertion of K^+

Adrenal Medulla

- Catecholamines (epinephrine and norepinephrine)/*heart, blood vessels, lung, kidney, liver, pancreas, and skin*/stress response: fight-or-flight reaction

Gonads

- Estrogen/*uterus, ovary, and breast*/reproduction
- Progesterone/*uterus, ovary, breast, and skin*/development of ova, female sex characteristics
- Testosterone/*sex organs, muscle, and skin*/development of sperm, male sex characteristics

Pancreas

- Insulin/*liver, muscles, and fat tissue*/regulates metabolism, lowers blood glucose
- Glucagon/*liver, muscles, and fat tissue*/elevates blood glucose

Adolescence

Reproductive glands and hormones lie mostly dormant during childhood and become active at the onset of adolescence.[6] During puberty, the anterior pituitary increases secretion of gonadotropins (LH and follicle-stimulating hormone). In the male, this stimulates the maturation of the testes, production of testosterone, and development of external genitalia. In the female, this stimulates estrogen production, the maturation of ovaries leading to ovulation, and development of external genitalia.

Older Adults

In response to advancing age, most glands become smaller with reduced hormone production.[1] This does not necessarily lead to hormonal regulation impairments, but the physiological activity of the hormone is reduced, which is linked to some common physiological changes associated with aging. For example, frailty has been shown to be associated with a pattern of hormonal changes in elderly men.[7] Also, menopause in women occurs as a normal response to aging and is associated with a reduction of estrogen produced by the ovaries. Reduced metabolism results in cold intolerance and reduced appetite. A reduction in the production of antidiuretic hormone (ADH) also occurs, leading to a more dilute urine and thus leaving the older adult more at risk for dehydration.

VARIATIONS AND CONTEXT

Many problems can lead to hormone imbalance. Two general categories of hormonal imbalance can occur for each hormone secreted by endocrine glands: hormonal deficiency or excess. Problems with hormone deficiency or excess are usually associated with an issue in production/secretion or in the regulatory mechanisms directing the glands. Glands can be affected in a number of ways, including by trauma; congenital, genetic, and inflammatory conditions (including autoimmune conditions); and tumors. Damage to a gland can result in a reduction or loss of the ability of that gland to produce and secrete a hormone.

For example, damage to the thyroid gland can result in the inability to produce thyroid hormones. A number of other conditions can result in excessive production and secretion of a hormone. Signaling errors, caused by improper levels of other hormones or ineffective negative feedback mechanisms, can lead to excessive production or inhibition of hormone secretion. Other physiological triggers can result in undesired elevations or deficiencies in hormones. For example, excessive and sustained stress can result in chronic elevated circulating cortisol; interruption of the circadian cycle (e.g., from sleep deprivation) can result in reduced secretion of melanin.

Although hormonal deficiency or excess is often caused by a production/secretion problem, other variations can occur if the hormone loses its effect on the tissue or is unable to gain access to the cells due to a problem with receptor sites—often referred to as insensitivity.[8] A classic example of this is seen in type 2 diabetes, in which insulin insensitivity develops at the receptor sites.

CONSEQUENCES

Understanding the physiological consequences of hormone imbalance requires an understanding of the physiological effects of the hormones, presented in Box 14.1. Thus an excess or deficiency of any hormone can create significant physiological challenges. The severity of such effects can vary widely—from the devastation a partnered couple experiences with infertility to life-threating states such as seen in thyroid storm, diabetes insipidus, or diabetic ketoacidosis. Common consequences

BOX 14.2 Common Risk Factors for Hormonal Imbalance

- Age
- Autoimmune conditions
- Cancer treatment
- Chromosomal deficiencies
- Chronic medical conditions
- Family history
- Genetics
- Hormonal supplement therapy
- Obesity
- Sedentary lifestyle
- Stress
- Trauma

from impaired hormonal regulation can include alterations in growth and development, alterations in cognition, alterations in metabolism, alterations in reproduction, changes in growth, and altered adaptive responses. The disruption of any hormone production may result in potential complications associated with the underlying condition and the potential for lifetime hormonal replacement therapy.

RISK FACTORS

All individuals of all population groups have the potential for problems with hormonal regulation. Risk factors for hormonal imbalance are usually considered in the context of the specific gland and hormone involved. For example, risk factors involving the anterior pituitary gland and the secretion of growth hormone (GH) differ significantly from risk factors associated with the hormonal imbalance involving the pancreas and secretion of insulin. Although risk factors are typically described at the level of each gland and hormone dysfunction, there are several risk factors that are shared by many hormonal imbalances (Box 14.2). One of the most obvious is hormone supplement therapy. Exogenous supplementation of any hormone places an individual at risk for excess or deficient hormone levels due to the variability in dosing needs and medication adherence. In response to advanced age, most glands become smaller with reduced hormone production, which increases the risk for certain hormonal deficiencies and reduced metabolism. Obesity and sedentary lifestyle are associated with many hormonal imbalances, such as diabetes and polycystic ovarian syndrome.[8] Genetics, chromosomal abnormalities, and family history, particularly a history of autoimmune responses, increase risk for several hormone deficiencies.

ASSESSMENT

Because hormonal regulation affects all body systems, and because each hormone has a specific role, there are not standard questions and examination procedures for all glands and hormones. Instead, hormonal function is considered adequate unless the patient, a parent, or other family members report a symptom or a clinical finding presents itself that suggests an abnormality. Such a situation triggers an in-depth history, examination, and diagnostic tests based on the presenting sign and/or symptom. For this reason, this section provides a very broad discussion regarding endocrine assessment.

History

The history provides the foundation for assessment. Baseline history always includes gender, age, marital status, past medical history (including age at menarche, last menstrual period, and reproductive history for females), current conditions, current medications, psychosocial history, and family history.[9] Often, these baseline data provide important clues if a hormonal imbalance is suspected. For example, some hormonal imbalances are more common in men than in women; some are more common among older adults than in children.

From a functional perspective, the symptoms or problems most likely reported by a parent of a child, an adolescent, or an adult patient are often associated with basic physiological functions. These include abnormal growth patterns, physical development, activity, energy level, sleep, nutrition, elimination, sexual response or reproductive problems, and unexplained changes in weight. Any of these types of symptoms warrants a symptom analysis of the presenting problem.

Examination Findings

Because of the anatomic location of the glands, most glands, with the exception of the thyroid gland and testes, are inaccessible to direct examination. Thus most of the examination focuses on evidence of physiological or clinical effects of hormonal function.

Vital Signs, Height, and Weight

Physical examination begins with an assessment of vital signs, height, and weight. For children, the height and weight should be analyzed based on standardized growth charts. Many hormones can affect changes in weight and vital signs, especially those secreted by the thyroid, pancreatic, and adrenal glands. Abnormal growth patterns may be associated with growth hormone (or growth hormone-inhibiting or -releasing hormone).

Inspection

Many clues about hormonal balance (or imbalance) may be noted during a general inspection, particularly by a healthcare professional with a critical eye.[9] Note the overall skin color and texture, hair texture, body posture, facial characteristics, and affect. Findings associated with one or more hormonal imbalances include unusual dryness, pigmentation, wounds, or other lesions; malformation of the fingernails; unusual hair texture; and excessive hair growth in unexpected areas (e.g., on the face of women) or excessive hair loss. Note anxious or fidgety behavior, a flat affect or an overly animated affect, puffiness around the face, and protrusion of the eyes (exophthalmos). Notice the neck and determine if there is a thickening or enlargement that might be caused by an enlarged thyroid gland. Abnormal findings of the external genitalia (e.g., size, shape, color, and pubic hair distribution) for the patient's age/developmental level may also reveal important clues associated with hormonal imbalance.

Palpation and Auscultation

The thyroid gland and testes are anatomically positioned to allow for direct palpation; ovaries can be palpated through bimanual palpation. The thyroid gland, located on the anterior neck just below the cricoid cartilage, is not particularly easy to palpate unless it is abnormally large or has nodules. An enlargement of the thyroid (goiter) or the presence of nodules are abnormal findings. If the thyroid is enlarged, the area should be auscultated for bruits, which would indicate increased vascular flow. The testes are palpated through the scrotal sac. They should be firm, small, and smooth.[9] An irregular shape or texture are abnormal findings. Ovaries can be indirectly palpated through a bimanual examination as part of a pelvic examination. This examination is usually done by an advanced practice nurse (e.g., a nurse practitioner) or a physician.

Diagnostic Tests
Laboratory Tests

A number of laboratory tests are used to determine hormonal function.

Hormone level. One of the most common ways to assess hormonal function is a direct measure of the hormone level in the blood (or other body fluids such as urine). If a hormone is secreted at a consistent rate (e.g., thyroid hormone), then a single sample can be drawn at any time. However, some glands secrete hormones on a cyclic pattern; thus the specific time the sample is drawn is critical for test analysis. For example, a cortisol level tests adrenal function. Secretion of cortisol is highest in the morning and lowest in the evening; thus blood sample should be drawn at 8 a.m. and 4 p.m.[10] When the test involves the collection of urine, this is often done as a 24-hour urine sample. This often requires specific handling of the sample during the collection period.

An indirect assessment of the hormone function involves evaluating the blood or urine for components affected by the hormone function. For example, blood glucose provides an indirect measure of the pancreatic cells that produce insulin or insulin usage.

Stimulation and suppression testing. These tests are done to evaluate the process for hormone secretion and inhibition. Stimulation testing involves giving the patient a stimulus substance or hormone to stimulate the targeted gland to trigger hormone release. A measure of the hormone level follows, with an elevation in hormone level as the normal (expected) finding. A suppression test involves giving the patient a suppression substance or hormone to suppress the targeted gland from producing hormone. A measure of the hormone level follows, with a decrease in hormone level as the normal (expected) finding.[10]

Imaging

In some cases, imaging of the gland is necessary for diagnostic purposes. Ultrasound imaging can be used for imaging the thyroid, parathyroid, ovaries, and testes. Magnetic resonance imaging or computed tomography scans are very effective to evaluate pituitary, adrenal glands, pancreas, and ovaries. These scans may involve the injection of a radioactive isotope that allows imaging of the substance in the target tissue.[11]

Biopsy

In some cases, pathology analysis of the gland tissue is needed. A biopsy may be performed to collect tissue sample of the gland involved. Because of the relative ease of accessibility, the thyroid gland is the most common gland for this analysis.

CLINICAL MANAGEMENT

Primary Prevention

Primary prevention refers to strategies aimed to optimize health and prevent disease. Primary prevention strategies typically include education, diet, exercise, weight control, injury avoidance, and avoidance of environmental hazards.[12] These basic primary prevention strategies affect hormonal regulation as well. Maintaining a healthy lifestyle optimizes overall health and thus provides an optimal physiological environment for hormonal regulation to occur. For example, diet, exercise, and weight control affect the production and function of some hormones, such as insulin, glucagon, and thyroid hormones.[13] Measures to manage stress can prevent excess secretion of cortisol. Maintaining routine sleep–wake patterns optimizes the secretion of hormones dependent on a circadian cycle. Preventing head injury through the use of helmets reduces risk of injury to the hypothalamus and pituitary glands.

Secondary Prevention (Screening)

Secondary prevention refers to the early identification of a disease so that prompt treatment can be initiated. The two primary endocrine-related screening recommendations are for hyroid and diabetic conditions and include recommendations for infants and adults.

Infants

A routine congenital thyroid screening in infants is recommended as part of the uniform screening panel. This recommendation includes the screening of every newborn for 31 core conditions, including two endocrine disorders—congenital adrenal hyperplasia and congenital hypothyroidism.[14]

Adults

The two pertinent areas for screening include thyroid and diabetes. According to the U.S. Preventative Services Task Force (USPSTF), there is insufficient evidence to recommend routine screening for thyroid problems among asymptomatic adults.[15] Regarding gestational diabetes screening, the USPSTF found insufficient evidence to recommend routine screening before 24 weeks of gestation, but it does recommend routine screening in all asymptomatic women after 24 weeks of gestation.[16] The USPSTF also recommended screening for abnormal blood glucose among adults aged 40 to 70 who are overweight or obese (grade B recommendation).[17]

Collaborative Interventions

The management of individuals with endocrine disturbances is complex, and a detailed discussion for each is beyond the scope of this concept presentation. However, common underlying care principles include a combination of diet, fluid management, pharmacotherapy, surgical options, radiation, and psychosocial support. This section presents the common interventional categories associated with hormonal disturbances and is not intended to be comprehensive for any specific endocrine disorder.

Pharmacotherapy

Pharmacologic treatment for individuals with hormone imbalance typically involves hormone replacement (for deficiencies) or drugs that block production or use of hormones in states of excess hormone production. For this reason, the pharmacologic agents are presented with the underlying problem.

Hypopituitarism. Synthetic human growth hormone (GH) is used for GH deficiencies caused by pituitary insufficiency, as well as other conditions such as Turner syndrome, chronic kidney disease, and children small for gestation age. Testosterone is used as supplement for men with gonadotropin deficiency. Estrogen and progesterone supplements, also referred to as *hormone replacement therapy*, are indicated for women with gonadotropin deficiency and for the relief of postmenopausal symptoms.[18] Estrogen is also known to regulate secretion and action of GH in men and women.[19]

Hyperpituitarism. Dopamine agonists (bromocriptine mesylate, cabergoline, and pergolide) inhibit release of GH; octreotide (somatostatin) and pegvisomant (Somavert) block GH receptors.

Posterior pituitary antidiuretic hormone deficiency. Desmopressin (DDAVP) and vasopressin (Pitressin) represent replacement therapy for ADH. Chlorpropamide (Diabinese) has antidiuretic action and increases ADH production in the hypothalamus.

Posterior pituitary antidiuretic hormone excess. Tolvaptan (Samsca) and conivaptan (Vaprisol) are vasopressin antagonists that promote water excretion without loss of sodium.

Adrenal insufficiency (Addison disease). Cortisone, hydrocortisone (Cortef), prednisone, and fludrocortisone (Florinef) are used for the treatment of adrenocorticoid deficiency.

Hypercortisolism (Cushing disease). Aminoglutethimide (Elipten and Cytadren), metyrapone (Metopirone), and cyproheptadine (Periactin) interfere with adrenocorticotropic hormone (ACTH) production.

Hypothyroidism. Levothyroxine sodium (Synthroid) is a synthetic hormone preparation that represents the most common form of thyroid replacement therapy.

Hyperthyroidism. Propylthiouracil (PTU) and methimazole (Tapazole) block thyroid hormone production.

Hypoparathyroidism. Because parathyroid regulates calcium, therapy involves calcium, vitamin D, and magnesium sulfate supplements.

Diabetes. A variety of insulin preparations are used for individuals with type 1 diabetes and represent hormone replacement. In type 2 diabetes, several agents are used to increase insulin secretion and/or improve insulin receptor sensitivity. These include sulfonylurea agents glipizide (Glucotrol) and glimepiride (Amaryl); meglitinide analogs repaglinide (Prandin) and nateglinide (Starlix); and insulin sensitizers, which include biguanides (metformin [Glucophage]) and thiazolidinediones (rosiglitazone [Avandia] and pioglitazone [Actos]).[3]

Nutrition Therapy

Nutrition management is the cornerstone of many endocrine disorders, with diabetes being the most obvious (and which is discussed in detail in Concept 15, Glucose Regulation).

Fluid and Electrolyte Management

Some hormone imbalances or associated treatments can lead to an actual or potential for fluid and electrolyte imbalances. This is particularly true with antidiuretic hormone imbalances, hypercortisolism, aldosterone imbalances, parathyroid hormone disturbances, and as a result of insulin deficiency (diabetic ketoacidosis).[8] Thus monitoring fluid intake and output and monitoring serum electrolytes is a central component of care for many of these conditions.

Surgery

Hypophysectomy. A hypophysectomy is the surgical removal of the pituitary gland and often an associated tumor. The most common cause of hyperpituitarism is a benign tumor within the anterior pituitary gland (pituitary adenoma).[3] This procedure may also be done when there is hypersecretion of ACTH from the pituitary gland, leading to adrenocortical hypersecretion.

Adrenalectomy. Removal of one or both adrenal glands is a treatment option for three different types of hormonal regulation problems. Adrenocortical hypersecretion and hyperaldosteronism are often caused by a benign adrenal tumor affecting the adrenal cortex, although some cases are bilateral.[20] A pheochromocytoma is a catecholamine-producing tumor of the adrenal medulla and leads to excessive release of epinephrine and norepinephrine. Patients require lifelong glucocorticoid and mineralocorticoid replacement if both adrenal glands are removed. If only one gland is removed, replacement therapy is needed temporarily until the remaining adrenal gland can sufficiently increase hormone production.

Thyroidectomy. A complete removal or partial removal of the thyroid gland is indicated for individuals with an excessively large goiter (causing compression on the esophagus or trachea) or who do not have adequate response to pharmacotherapy with antithyroid agents or with radioactive iodine therapy (RAI). The variations in procedures include partial thyroid lobectomy (removal of one part of a lobe), thyroid lobectomy (removal of an entire lobe), thyroid lobectomy with isthmusectomy (removal of one entire lobe and the isthmus), bilateral subtotal thyroidectomy (removal of all of one lobe, the isthmus, and a portion of another lobe), and total thyroidectomy (removal of the entire gland).[21] The patient must be monitored for serious complications (hemorrhage, respiratory distress, hypocalcemia, tetany, thyroid storm, and laryngeal nerve damage) in the postoperative period.[22] Patients who undergo a total thyroidectomy require lifelong thyroid replacement therapy.

Parathyroidectomy. Hyperparathyroidism is often caused by a benign tumor in the parathyroid glands. Removal of one or more of the four parathyroid glands may be indicated for hyperparathyroidism. The minimally invasive radio-guided technique shows promise as a surgical option.[23] Because the parathyroids are located on the thyroid gland, similar concerns for postoperative monitoring apply. In addition, calcium levels are monitored to avoid hypocalcemic crisis.

Radiation

Radioactive iodine therapy (RAI) is indicated for the treatment of hyperthyroidism. It is given as an oral preparation, usually as a single dose. Radioactive iodine therapy makes its way to the thyroid gland, where it destroys some of the cells that produce thyroid hormone. Radioactive iodine therapy is completely eliminated from the body after approximately 4 weeks. The extent of thyroid cell destruction is variable; thus the patient has ongoing monitoring of thyroid function. If thyroid production remains too high, a second dose may be needed.[3]

Psychosocial Support

A hormonal imbalance often represents a change in an individual's lifestyle and can affect an individual's physical appearance, libido, sexual functioning, and mood. Combined, these changes can affect interpersonal relationships, self-confidence, and often require an adjustment (particularly if it is a chronic condition). Patients may benefit from individual counseling and support groups as a means for effective coping.

Patient Education

The complexity of many hormonal imbalances requires significant patient education regarding diet, activity, and medications to achieve optimal disease management. Patients who undergo hormone replacement therapy must understand the need to take medications regularly, consistently, and within the dosing parameters established for their condition. Patients must also know the signs and symptoms of excessive or insufficient hormone supplements. Patients with conditions requiring specific dietary and/or fluid management must be taught how to incorporate dietary patterns into their culture and lifestyle.

INTERRELATED CONCEPTS

All body systems are affected by hormones; for this reason, all health and illness concepts are interrelated in some way. However, concepts with the closest interrelationships are presented in Fig. 14.3. Intracranial Regulation has a significant role in hormonal regulation because of its influence on the function of the hypothalamus and pituitary glands. Many hormonal imbalances occur as a result of brain injury or damage to these glands located in the brain. Likewise, optimal intracranial regulation and cognitive function depend on normal regulation of hormones. Maintaining balance of Fluid and Electrolytes is highly dependent on the secretion and regulation of aldosterone and ADH. Glucose Regulation and Nutrition are highly dependent on the regulation of insulin and glucagon. Because of the role that glucocorticoids and catecholamines play in the stress response, the Stress and Coping concept is closely aligned. The processes of Development and Reproduction are dependent on hormones such as GH, estrogen, progesterone, testosterone, LH, follicle-stimulating hormone, prolactin, and oxytocin.

CLINICAL EXEMPLARS

There are clearly many exemplars of hormonal regulation. The classic exemplars are presented in Box 14.3, organized by the glands producing

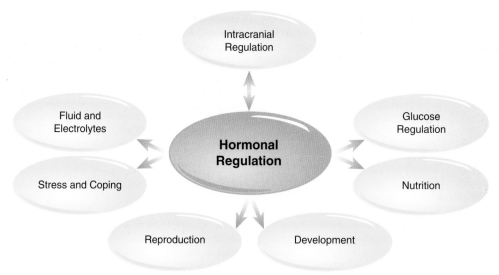

FIGURE 14.3 Hormonal Regulation and Interrelated Concepts.

 BOX 14.3   EXEMPLARS OF IMPAIRED HORMONAL REGULATION

Thyroid and Parathyroid
- Thyrotoxicosis (hyperthyroidism)
- Primary hypothyroidism
- Congenital hypothyroidism
- Hyperparathyroidism
- Hypoparathyroidism

Pancreas
- Type 1 diabetes mellitus
- Type 2 diabetes mellitus
- Gestational diabetes mellitus

Pituitary Gland
- Pituitary adenoma (hypopituitarism)
- Gigantism
- Acromegaly
- Hypopituitarism
- Pituitary dwarfism
- Diabetes insipidus
- Syndrome of inappropriate antidiuretic hormone

Adrenal Gland
- Hypercortisolism (Cushing syndrome)
- Hyperaldosteronism
- Adrenal insufficiency (Addison disease)
- Pheochromocytoma

ACCESS EXEMPLAR LINKS IN YOUR GIDDENS EBOOK

hormones. It is beyond the scope of this text to discuss each endocrine condition, and this information is easily found in pathophysiology, adult health, and pediatric textbooks. A brief description of some of the most important or common exemplars is featured next.

Featured Exemplars
Hypothyroidism
Hypothyroidism refers to insufficient secretion of thyroid hormones. Typically this is caused by reduced production of thyroid hormone by the thyroid gland, but it can also be a result of dietary intake of substances (e.g., iodide and tyrosine) enabling thyroid hormone production. Because thyroid hormones influence metabolic rate, thyroid insufficiency has a significant effect on systemic cellular metabolism, creating body-wide symptoms including fatigue, weight gain, depression, reduced cardiac and respiratory rates, as well as myxedema. This condition occurs most often among women between ages 30 and 60 years, with increased incidence with age.[24]

Type 1 Diabetes Mellitus
Type 1 diabetes mellitus is a metabolic condition resulting from the destruction of pancreatic beta cells, leading to a loss of insulin production. Insulin is a hormone that is necessary to facilitate movement of glucose into the cell for metabolic activity. Insulin deficiency is clinically associated with hyperglycemia, with significant systemic effects over time. The cause of type 1 diabetes is unknown, but it may be associated with an autoimmune response with genetic predisposition. Native Americans, non-Hispanic blacks, and Hispanics have significantly higher rates of diabetes compared to non-Hispanic whites and Asian Americans.[25]

Hypercortisolism (Cushing Syndrome)
Cushing syndrome affects an estimated 1 to 15 per 1 million people each year[26] and is characterized by chronic excess glucocorticoid (cortisol) secretion from the adrenal cortex. This is caused by the hypothalamus, the anterior pituitary gland, or the adrenal cortex. Cushing syndrome can also be caused by taking corticosteroids in the form of medication (e.g., prednisone) over time—referred to as *exogenous Cushing syndrome*. Regardless of the cause, excess secretion of cortisol has a systemic effect, affecting immunity, metabolism, and fat distribution (truncal obesity), and causing reduced muscle mass, loss of bone density, hypertension, fragility to microvasculature, as well as thinning of the skin.

Syndrome of Inappropriate Antidiuretic Hormone
Antidiuretic hormone is responsible for fluid balance and is normally secreted by the posterior pituitary gland in response to elevated plasma osmolarity. As the name suggests, the syndrome of inappropriate antidiuretic hormone (SIADH) is a condition in which ADH is secreted despite normal or low plasma osmolarity, resulting in water retention and dilutional hyponatremia. In response to increased plasma volume, aldosterone secretion increases and further contributes to sodium loss.[3]

A large number of clinical conditions can cause SIADH, including malignancies, pulmonary disorders, injury to the brain, and certain pharmacologic agents.

Adrenal Insufficiency (Addison Disease)

Adrenal insufficiency, also known as Addison disease, occurs with an insufficient secretion of adrenocortical steroids (cortisol and aldosterone). Adrenal insufficiency can occur from dysfunction of the pituitary gland and insufficient secretion of ACTH, which signals adrenocortical steroid release from the adrenal glands, or from damage to the adrenal cortex, in which adrenocortical steroids are produced.[8] Adrenal insufficiency results in fluid and electrolyte imbalances—particularly hyponatremia, hyperkalemia, and hypovolemia. This condition can be life-threatening if the physiological requirement for cortisol and aldosterone exceeds supply—often association with severe physiological stress such as surgery, trauma, or sepsis.

CASE STUDY

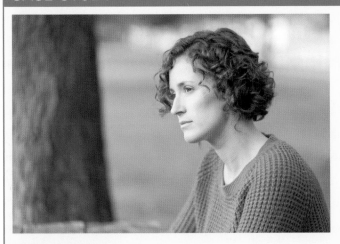

Case Presentation

Marci Myers, a 38-year-old female, presented to a community-based clinic with generalized complaint of feeling "odd" for the past few months. Michael, a nurse practitioner, evaluated her. Marci denied any previous medical conditions and takes no medications other than vitamin supplements. When Marci was asked to explain her symptoms further, she described a variety of sensations, including palpitations in her chest, shortness of breath, generalized weakness and fatigue, heat intolerance, and insomnia. She described often feeling restless and was told by her coworkers that she is irritable, but in her opinion she is not—she just does not feel herself. When asked about recent weight loss, Marci was unsure, but admitted that her clothes might be a bit looser than they used to be and she had not been dieting. During the interview, Marci appeared somewhat restless, and a slight trembling to her hands was noted. Her vital signs were as follows: heart rate, 106 beats/min; respiratory rate, 24 breaths/min; blood pressure, 132/80 mm Hg; and temperature, 36.9°C. Marci's skin was very warm and slightly damp. The thyroid gland felt somewhat enlarged when palpated, and the rest of the examination was unremarkable. Laboratory tests for T_3, T_4, and free T_4 index were ordered to assess thyroid hormone regulation. All three of these tests were elevated. Because the nurse practitioner suspected Marci had hyperthyroidism, he referred her to an endocrinologist.

Further diagnostic testing done by the endocrinologist included thyrotropin-stimulating test (which was low), thyroid-releasing hormone stimulation test (showed no response), thyroid antibodies titer (was elevated), thyrotropin receptor antibodies (TSH-RAb) test (showed high titers), and a thyroid scan (showed an enlarged thyroid gland and increased radioactive iodine uptake). These tests confirmed a diagnosis of hyperthyroidism caused by Graves disease.

Case Analysis

1. In what way does the case exemplify hormonal regulation?
2. What clinical findings exhibited by Marci are indicative of altered hormonal regulation?
3. How are the diagnostic tests described in the case consistent with what was described for assessment of hormonal regulation?

From NADOFOTOS/iStock/Thinkstock.

 ACCESS EXEMPLAR LINKS IN YOUR GIDDENS EBOOK

REFERENCES

1. McCance, K., & Huther, S. (2014). *Pathophysoiology: The biologic basis for disease in adults and children* (7th ed.). St Louis: Elsevier.
2. Wu, J., & McAndrews, J. (2012). Introduction to the endocrine system. Part 1: Basic concepts and anatomy. *American medical writers association journal, 27*(4), 153–156.
3. Ignatavicius, D., Workman, M., & Rebar, C. (2019). *Medical–surgical nursing: Concepts for interprofessional collaborative care* (9th ed.). St Louis: Elsevier.
4. McAndrews, J., & Wu, J. (2013). Introduction to the endocrine system. Part 2: Physiology. *Am Medical Writers Association Journal, 28*(2), 51–56.
5. Konishi, M., Takahaski, M., Naoya, E., et al. (2013). Effects of sleep deprivation on autonomic and endocrine functions throughout the day and on exercise tolerance in the evening. *Journal of Sports Sciences, 31*(3), 248–255.
6. Hockenberry, M., Wilson, D., & Rodgers, C. (2017). *Wong's essentials of pediatric nursing* (10th ed.). St Louis: Elsevier.
7. Tajar, A., O'Connell, M., Mitnitski, A. B., et al. (2011). Frailty in relation to variations in hormonal levels of the hypothalamic–pituitary–testicular axis in older men: Results from the European Male Aging Study. *Journal of the American Geriatrics Society, 59*(5), 814–821.
8. Lewis, S., Bucher, L., Heitkemper, M., et al. (2017). *Medical–surgical nursing: Assessment and management of clinical problems* (10th ed.). St Louis: Elsevier.
9. Wilson, S., & Giddens, J. (2017). *Health assessment for nursing practice* (6th ed.). St Louis: Elsevier.
10. Fischbach, F., & Dunning, M. B. (2014). *A manual of laboratory and diagnostic tests* (9th ed.). Philadelphia: Lippincott Williams & Wilkins.
11. Pagana, K., Pagana, T., & Pagana, T. (2015). *Mosby's diagnostic laboratory test reference* (12th ed.). St Louis: Mosby.
12. Pender, N., Murdaugh, C., & Parson, M. A. (2015). *Health promotion in nursing practice* (7th ed.). Upper Saddle River, NJ: Pearson.
13. Schubert, M., & Sabapathy, S. (2014). Acute exercise and hormones related to appetite regulation: A meta-analysis. *Sports Medicine (Auckland, N.Z.), 44*(3), 387–403.
14. Advisory Committee on Heritable Disorders in Newborns and Children. (2016). *Recommended uniform screening panel*. Retrieved from http://www.hrsa.gov/advisorycommittees/mchbadvisory/heritabledisorders/recommendedpanel/index.html.
15. U.S. Preventative Services Task Force. (2015). *Thyroid dysfunction: Screening*. Retrieved from http://www.uspreventiveservicestaskforce.org/Page/Topic/recommendation-summary/thyroid-dysfunction-screening.

16. U.S. Preventative Services Task Force. (2014). *Gestational diabetes mellitus, Screening*. Retrieved from http://www.uspreventiveservicestaskforce.org/Page/Topic/recommendation-summary/gestational-diabetes-mellitus-screening?ds=1&s=gestational%20diabetes.

17. U.S. Preventative Services Task Force. (2015). *Final Recommendation Statement, Abnormal glucose and type 2 diabetes mellitus: Screening*. Retrieved from https://www.uspreventiveservicestaskforce.org/Page/Document/RecommendationStatementFinal/screening-for-abnormal-blood-glucose-and-type-2-diabetes.

18. Archer, D., Sturdee, D., Baber, R., et al. (2011). Menopausal hot flashes and night sweats: Where are we now? *Climacteric: The Journal of the International Menopause Society, 14*(5), 515–528.

19. Birzniece, V., Sutanto, S., & Ho, K. (2012). Gender difference in neuroendocrine regulation of growth hormone axis by selective estrogen receptor modulators. *The Journal of Clinical Endocrinology and Metabolism, 97*(4), E521–E527.

20. Lacroix, A. (2013). Heredity and cortisol regulation in bilateral macronodular adrenal hyperplasia. *The New England Journal of Medicine, 369*(22), 2147–2149.

21. Kaplan, E., Angelos, P., Applewhite, M., et al. (2015). Surgery of the thyroid. In *Endotext*. Retrieved from https://www.ncbi.nlm.nih.gov/books/NBK285564/.

22. Massick, D., & Garrett, M. (2014). Hypocalcemia after minimally invasive thyroidectomy. *ENT. Ear, Nose, and Throat Journal, 93*(9), 414–417.

23. Rubello, G. (2013). Minimally invasive parathyroidectomy. *Journal of Postgraduate Medicine, 59*(1), 1–3.

24. National Institute of Diabetes and Digestive and Kidney Diseases. (2013). *Hypothyroidism*. Retrieved from http://www.niddk.nih.gov/health-information/health-topics/endocrine/hypothyroidism/Pages/fact-sheet.aspx.

25. Centers for Disease Control and Prevention. (2017). *National diabetes statistics report*. Retrieved from https://www.cdc.gov/diabetes/pdfs/data/statistics/national-diabetes-statistics-report.pdf.

26. Guaraldi, F., & Salvatori, R. (2012). Cushing syndrome: Maybe not so uncommon of an endocrine disease. *Journal of the American Board of Family Medicine: JABFM, 25*(2), 199–208.

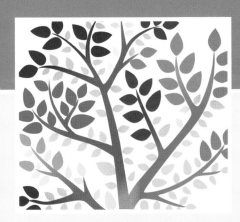

Glucose Regulation

Katherine Pereira

Glucose is fundamental to the process of human life. Glucose is the preferred energy source for most cells in the body, and the neurologic system is dependent on glucose for energy needs. When glucose metabolism becomes impaired, serious health consequences occur. Because this concept represents a foundational basis of health, the nurse must possess a solid understanding of energy and glucose regulation, including the ability to recognize and respond to situations in which this process is impaired.

DEFINITION

Glucose regulation is achieved through a delicate balance between nutrient intake, hormonal signaling, and glucose uptake by the cell. Once glucose enters the cell, it is oxidized through cellular respiration into adenosine triphosphate (ATP). The efficiency of glucose metabolism is reflected in circulating blood glucose (BG) levels. For the purposes of this concept presentation, glucose regulation is defined as *the process of maintaining optimal blood glucose levels.*

A few other key terms are important to mention. *Glycogen* is the major form of stored glucose, primarily in the liver and muscle cells. *Glycogenolysis* refers to the breakdown of glycogen to glucose. *Gluconeogenesis* refers to the process of producing glucose from noncarbohydrate sources (e.g., proteins and fats).

SCOPE

The scope of glucose regulation can conceptually be represented by the categories of normal/optimal regulation and impaired regulation throughout the lifespan. Normal BG levels range between 70 and 99 mg/dL in the fasting state and 100 and 140 mg/dL in the 2-hour postprandial state, otherwise referred to as *euglycemia*. Impaired regulation can be further categorized by the etiology and is reflected in abnormally high or low BG levels. *Hyperglycemia* refers to a state of elevated BG levels, generally defined as greater than 100 mg/dL in the fasting state as or greater than 140 mg/dL 2 hours postprandial. *Hypoglycemia* refers to a state of insufficient or low BG levels, defined as less than 70 mg/dL. Fig. 15.1 shows the spectrum of glucose metabolism and regulation: hypoglycemia, euglycemia, and hyperglycemia.

NORMAL PHYSIOLOGICAL PROCESS

In the healthy individual, glucose regulation occurs with little awareness given to the process. To help maintain glucose homeostasis, a variety of hormones are required. Insulin is the only hormone produced that lowers elevated BG levels after carbohydrate intake. Several counterregulatory hormones (hormones that oppose the action of other hormones) are required to raise BG if levels begin to decrease or in anticipation of increased needs. When this system works efficiently, glucose levels remain normal, even in the setting of extreme stress.

After the consumption of food, insulin is released in response to rising glucose levels. Insulin facilitates glucose metabolism by binding to insulin receptors on the cell wall, *signaling* glucose transporter molecules that facilitate glucose entry into the cell. Insulin suppresses glucagon secretion and facilitates glycogen storage.

Glucagon is one of several counterregulatory hormones released in response to cellular deficiency of glucose. Glucagon suppresses insulin and stimulates hepatic glucose production (from glycogen), resulting in elevated glucose levels. Gluconeogenesis is required if blood glucose and glycogen stores are insufficient and can also occur with stress conditions, or from use of steroid medications, with resulting increased risk of loss of muscle mass. Other counterregulatory hormones released include cortisol, growth hormone, norepinephrine, and epinephrine. Counterregulatory hormones all lead to utilization of glycogen stores, and these hormones are also increased with stress-related conditions, both physical (e.g., pain, illness, and injury) and emotional, and are therefore often referred to as stress hormones.

VARIATIONS AND CONTEXT

Problems with glucose regulation arise when glucose-regulating hormones are either deficient or excessive, or when the timing of production is not balanced with blood glucose needs. An imbalance of glucose regulation results in either too much or insufficient glucose.

Hyperglycemia

Hyperglycemia occurs as a result of insufficient insulin production or secretion, excessive counterregulatory hormones secretion, or from deficient hormone signaling. The word *diabetes* means "sweet urine," and the term *diabetes mellitus* describes a group of disorders characterized by chronic hyperglycemia and disturbances in carbohydrate, protein, and fat metabolism.

Insufficient Insulin Production/Secretion

Insulin is produced, stored, and released by pancreatic β cells (located in pancreatic islets). Damage or destruction of the β cells results in insufficient or cessation of insulin secretion. Insufficient insulin secretion

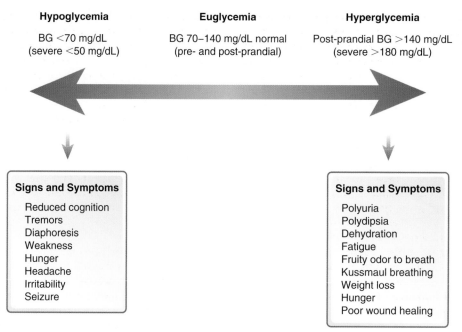

Hypoglycemia	**Euglycemia**	**Hyperglycemia**
BG <70 mg/dL (severe <50 mg/dL)	BG 70–140 mg/dL normal (pre- and post-prandial)	Post-prandial BG >140 mg/dL (severe >180 mg/dL)

Signs and Symptoms

Reduced cognition
Tremors
Diaphoresis
Weakness
Hunger
Headache
Irritability
Seizure

Signs and Symptoms

Polyuria
Polydipsia
Dehydration
Fatigue
Fruity odor to breath
Kussmaul breathing
Weight loss
Hunger
Poor wound healing

FIGURE 15.1 Scope of Glucose Regulation.

results in a hyperglycemic state because glucose is unable to enter the cells for cellular metabolism. Damage to the β cells is usually caused by an autoimmune response with genetic disposition, or can occur secondarily from other diseases such as pancreatitis or pancreatic cancer.

Deficient Hormone Signaling

The term *insulin resistance* refers to a state in which the body cells respond abnormally to the signaling action of insulin; in other words, there is not a problem with insulin supply but, rather, with how the cell responds to insulin signaling due to a reduction of insulin receptors or glucose transporter molecules,[1] resulting in sluggish glucose uptake by the cell. The pancreas overproduces insulin to compensate for reduced cellular glucose update, resulting in hyperinsulinemia. When insulin resistance persists for long periods of time, the insulin producing capacity of the pancreas is exhausted and hyperglycemia ensues.[2]

Excessive Counterregulatory Hormone Secretion

Excessive secretion of any of the counterregulatory hormones can result in hyperglycemia. These include glucagon (previously described) and cortisol, a hormone that raises blood glucose through gluconeogenesis. Causes of increased cortisol secretion include chronic stress, pain, sleep deprivation, and acute injury or illness. It can also occur as an adverse effect of medications (particularly with high doses of corticosteroids) or due to Cushing disease. Elevated cortisol levels also exacerbate insulin resistance (described previously).

Hypoglycemia

Hypoglycemia is a state of low glucose levels and typically occurs as a result of insufficient nutritional intake, adverse reaction to medications, excessive exercise, and/or as a consequence of disease states. Often, hypoglycemia occurs due to a combination of these factors.

Insufficient Nutritional Intake

Malnutrition leads to depletion of glucose stores in the liver and adipose tissue and thus prevents hepatic mechanisms for maintenance of normal glucose levels. Free fatty acids are mobilized as substrates for glucose production and resulting production of ketone bodies. Prolonged starvation and malnutrition can eventually lead to life-threatening hypoglycemia.

Adverse Reaction to Medication

Hypoglycemia is generally attributed to inappropriate dosing of exogenous insulin or the sulfonylurea form of oral hypoglycemic agents, which increases endogenous insulin production. Once an individual requires insulin therapy to maintain glucose control, creating a physiological insulin replacement regimen while avoiding hypoglycemia can be difficult, and this is one of the great challenges of caring for patients with diabetes.

Excessive Exercise

The work of muscle contraction requires energy, and initially this energy is derived from glucose stored in muscle cells as glycogen. As an exercise interval lengthens, glucose stores are quickly depleted, and then glucose from the circulation and hepatic glucose stores is utilized for energy, lowering blood glucose levels. During post exercise recovery, muscle cells then replenish glycogen stores with additional glucose from the circulation also lowering glucose levels, and this is sometimes referred to as "lag effect."

CONSEQUENCES

A number of significant physiological consequences are associated with poor glucose regulation. Hyperglycemia and insulin resistance are known to be toxic and proinflammatory states, causing cellular changes, cell death, and contributing to the various long-term health problems. Likewise, hypoglycemia can result in impaired function of the neurological system and thus grave danger to the patient. The consequences of hyperglycemia and hypoglycemia are discussed separately.

Physiological Consequences of Hyperglycemia

Insulin resistance is understood to be a proinflammatory state, thus contributing to atherogenesis and plaque formation,[3] and is also thought to be associated with increased cancer risk, with hyperinsulinemia appearing to act as a cellular growth factor. Hypertension is present in 50% of insulin-resistant individuals and 80% of those with type 2 diabetes, both sharing a common mechanism of high oxidative stress and inflammation.[4] Hyperinsulinemia causes hypertension through its role in reducing elasticity of blood vessels.[5] Insulin resistance may alter glucose uptake in the cerebrum, thus increasing the chance of impaired memory in older adults.[6] Other conditions associated with insulin resistance and proinflammatory states are nonalcoholic steatohepatitis and sleep apnea.[7]

Angiopathy

Individuals with long-standing or chronic hyperglycemia are at risk for developing several significant physiological complications attributable to angiopathy (damage to blood vessels). Chronic elevations of blood glucose damage the basement membrane of small blood vessels and impair adequate oxygenation to the tissues. These are known microvascular effects and directly lead to end-organ disease, including damage to the eye (retinopathy and vision loss) and the kidney (chronic kidney disease that can lead to end-stage renal disease).

Chronic hyperglycemia further damages medium and larger blood vessels, leading to hypertension and cardiovascular and peripheral vascular disease. The risk for myocardial infarction and stroke is two to four times higher for those with type 2 diabetes compared with those without diabetes.[8] The vascular damage to small blood vessels in the lower extremities leads to impaired blood supply to the lower extremities and peripheral vascular disease, increasing the risk of foot ulcers and chronic wound infection (sometimes leading to amputation).

Peripheral Neuropathy

Hyperglycemia is toxic to nerves, resulting in nerve damage and leading to peripheral neuropathy causing symptoms such as burning and numbness in the lower extremities. Once protective sensation is lost in the feet, the risk for foot ulcers and foot lesions greatly increases. Peripheral neuropathy is seen with prediabetes and may be the presenting symptom of impaired glucose utilization.[9]

Fluid, Electrolyte, and Acid–Base Imbalances

A potential consequence of severe hyperglycemia is dehydration because of a water deficit resulting from osmotic diuresis. Hyperosmolar hyperglycemic state (HHS) usually presents as severe hyperglycemia (>600 mg/dL), dehydration, and accompanied impaired mental status, and is more common in elders with type 2 diabetes.[10] There is also an increasing incidence of HHS in children with type 2 diabetes, in direct correlation with increasing type 2 diabetes rates in children.[11] An acid–base disturbance, diabetic ketoacidosis (DKA), is a hyperglycemic state (associated type 1 diabetes), whereby an absolute insulin deficiency is accompanied by the use of fatty acids and subsequent excess of ketone bodies and metabolic acidosis.

Physiological Consequences of Hypoglycemia

To a large degree, the impact of the body's processes to contend with and overcome adverse effects of inadequate glucose availability is largely unknown. Because the brain depends on glucose as its only source of fuel, hypoglycemia can progress from mild symptoms of nervousness, irritability, diaphoresis, anxiety, and palpitations to neurological changes, seizures, loss of consciousness, and death. Recurrent hypoglycemia can lower the glucose level that typically stimulates counterregulatory hormones; thus symptoms of hypoglycemia do not occur until glucose levels are dangerously low, and also carries a higher risk of chronic cognitive impairment and accelerated cognitive decline. The risk of fatal hypoglycemia is estimated to be 4% to 10% in those with type 1 and type 2 diabetes.[12]

Chronic hypoglycemia leads to the condition of hypoglycemia unawareness in which the counterregulatory hormonal response is blunted, describing a state of autonomic failure. This includes diabetes neuropathy and other symptoms of gastroparesis with associated symptoms of early satiety, poor food absorption, constipation, fecal incontinence, and diarrhea. The spectrum of autonomic neuropathy includes impaired pupil response to light, erectile dysfunction, loss of vaginal lubrication, painless cardiac ischemia, impaired exercise tolerance, orthostatic hypotension, resting tachycardia, dry skin, and impaired temperature regulation.[13] Hypoglycemia occurs two or three times more frequently in those with type 1 diabetes, and remains a challenge for those of all ages.[14]

RISK FACTORS

Impaired glucose regulation can potentially occur in any individual regardless of age, race, cultural identity, or gender. However, there are well-known risk factors for impaired glucose regulation.

Populations at Risk
Pregnant Women

Pregnancy and the associated hormonal changes (specifically hormones produced by the placenta) produce a state of insulin resistance and associated risk for hyperglycemia, especially postprandial hyperglycemia. All pregnant women are screened for gestational diabetes during the 24- to 28-week gestational mark, and women with known prediabetes or multiple risk factors for type 2 diabetes are screened at the first prenatal visit.[15]

Infants

The large for gestational age infant is at high risk for hypoglycemia after birth. The prevalence of neonatal hypoglycemia is also higher among infants whose mothers had diabetes during pregnancy.[16] Hypoglycemia is generally attributed to neonatal hyperinsulinemia that occurs in response to elevated glucose levels in utero. Small for gestational age and premature infants are at risk of hypoglycemic states because of increased energy needs and insufficient glycogen stores.

Older Adults

Older adults as a group are at greater risk for impaired glucose metabolism and hyperglycemia because of an increase in visceral fat and associated reduction in lean muscle mass, where most glucose is metabolized. This is often accompanied by age-related reduced insulin production and resulting reduced capacity to regulate and metabolize glucose concentration.[17]

Racial/Ethnic Groups

Certain racial and ethnic populations have greater genetic predisposition to insulin resistance, leading to a higher risk for type 2 diabetes, especially American Indians/Alaska Natives (age-adjusted percentile of 15.1%), African Americans (12.7%), Hispanic/Latino (12.1%, with Puerto Ricans and Mexican Americans having the highest rate), and Asian Americans (8.5%) compared with 7.4% among whites.[18] There is a growing trend of increased diabetes prevalence seen in societies that are less burdened with infectious disease prevalence and the resulting increase in noncommunicable diseases. In addition, the urbanization of countries results in a more sedentary population, as seen in China.[19] Other ethnic groups, particularly those of northern European descent, have a genetic tendency for the autoimmune form of diabetes.[20] Other autoimmune disorders are found in increased frequency among persons with type 1 diabetes, including celiac disease, adrenal insufficiency, pernicious anemia, vitiligo, and autoimmune thyroid disorders.[21]

Individual Risk Factors
Genetic Risk Factors

Research is rapidly expanding our understanding of the genetics of diabetes. Currently there are at least 120 known genetic markers, including *HLA* genes, associated with the risk of type 2 diabetes.[22] Insulin resistance is the common feature associated with metabolic syndrome and type 2 diabetes. Persons with a family history of type 2 diabetes, obesity, or factors associated with metabolic syndrome are at increased risk of insulin resistance and type 2 diabetes.[23]

Lifestyle Risk Factors

While there are clear genetic links for diabetes, a number of lifestyle choices promote and worsen insulin resistance. One of these is a poor diet with a high intake of saturated and trans-fatty acids (with the excess caloric intake leading to obesity) and a low fiber intake. An inappropriately high intake of calories, particularly carbohydrates, will also adversely affect glucose metabolism, regardless of the presence of insulin resistance or type 2 diabetes. Obesity and a lack of physical activity also contribute to insulin resistance.

Medications

Many medications used for treatment of health conditions are known to affect glucose regulation, which can place an individual at risk for hyperglycemia or hypoglycemia. Although there are too many to list, some of the most common include insulin, oral hypoglycemic agents, corticosteroids, estrogen, ACE inhibitors, β-blockers, potassium-depleting diuretics, bronchodilators, antipsychotics, and many antibiotics.

ASSESSMENT

History

The relevant history pertaining to glucose homeostasis includes personal medical history (including a list of current medications), social history, family history, and a review of systems. In each area of the assessment, the nurse considers data consistent with actual or potential problems with glucose regulation. Central obesity and diabetes are two clear conditions to note in a personal or family history. As previously mentioned, certain medications may place an individual at greater risk for impaired glucose regulation.

The nurse should recognize common clinical manifestations of impaired glucose regulation (Table 15.1). Individuals may or may not have symptoms of hyperglycemia. Individuals in ketoacidosis may display *polyphagia* (excess hunger), which may occur due to cells not receiving adequate glucose, and *polydipsia* (excess thirst) and consequent *polyuria* (excess urination) due to an osmotic diuresis (when the renal glucose threshold of 180 mg/dL is exceeded, water is pulled along with it).

Other symptoms to ask about in a history include complications associated with long-standing hyperglycemia. Those with retinopathy might describe reduced vision. Those with peripheral neuropathy may report reduced sensation or pins-and-needles sensation in the lower extremities. Wounds that do not heal or generalized lower extremity pain may be suggestive of poor peripheral perfusion. Insulin-resistant individuals and those with type 2 diabetes may experience sleep apnea, which can result in worsening glucose control, worsening hypertension and chronic fatigue.[24] It is also well established that individuals with diabetes are at higher risk for developing depression.[25] "Diabetes Distress" is a term coined to described the chronic grieving process and worries related to the complexity of caring for diabetes.[26] Individuals with diabetes should be screened for depressive symptoms (lack of interest, feelings of sadness or worthlessness, difficulty with sleep, appetite or weight changes, suicidal thoughts, and difficulty concentrating).

Examination Findings

The examination should always include vital signs and anthropometric measurements such as height and weight to determine body mass index and waist/hip measurements (to determine waist-to-hip ratio). These

TABLE 15.1 Comparison of Clinical Presentation of Hypoglycemia and Hyperglycemia		
	Hypoglycemia	**Hyperglycemia**
Symptoms	Symptoms related to degree of hypoglycemia and can include weakness, dizziness, headache, hunger, blurred vision, difficulty concentrating, feeling shaky, palpitations	No specific symptoms for elevated blood glucose, but symptoms may be associated with dehydration or acidosis and may include nausea, vomiting, abdominal cramps, fatigue, excessive hunger (polyphagia), excessive thirst (polydipsia)
Mental status	Anxious, irritability, confusion, seizures, unconsciousness, coma	Can range from alert to confused and coma, particularly if in untreated ketoacidosis
Skin	Diaphoresis, cool, clammy	Warm, moist
Respiratory/cardiovascular	Tachycardia; no change in respirations	Deep, rapid respirations; acetone odor to breath; tachycardia if dehydrated
Other	Muscle tremors, normal hydration, no ketones	Dehydration, polyuria, ketones

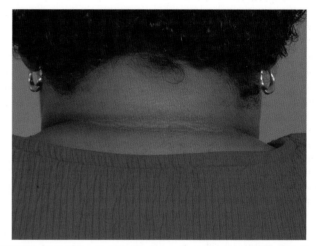

FIGURE 15.2 Acanthosis Nigricans is a Physical Exam Finding Frequently Seen in Individuals Who are Insulin Resistant. (Courtesy of Dr. Ann Brown, Duke University School of Medicine.)

measurements assess for hypertension and determine overweight or obesity as well as central obesity. Obesity and central obesity are both associated with insulin-resistant states.

Several physical findings are common among individuals with long-standing states of impaired glucose metabolism. Acanthosis nigricans, a velvety darkening of the skin, sometimes seen on the posterior neck, axillae, and skin folds of the groin, is a cutaneous marker of insulin resistance and a "red flag" for diabetes risk (Fig. 15.2). Skin tags are often seen with insulin resistance, commonly seen on the neck and axillae.

The lower extremities should be examined for evidence of peripheral vascular disease (poor perfusion and chronic wounds).

A foot exam includes inspection of skin for blisters, ulcers, skin lesions, nail abnormalities, and excessive callusing. Sensation and motor strength of the extremities should be assessed to evaluate for neuropathy. Assessing visual acuity and inspection of intraocular structures may provide important information associated with retinopathy, although a dilated eye exam provides a more detailed retinal exam.

Diagnostic Tests

Diagnostic testing is an essential component associated with assessment for impairments in glucose regulation and metabolism. Laboratory tests can help reveal the etiology of impaired glucose metabolism, measure and assess blood glucose management, and evaluate consequences of impaired glucose metabolism on other disease conditions.

Blood Glucose Testing

Measurement of blood glucose (BG) is used widely for screening and monitoring glucose metabolism. A fasting glucose level greater than 100 and less than 126 mg/dL is indicative of prediabetes or impaired fasting glucose, a level of 126 mg/dL or greater on two separate occasions is indicative of diabetes, and a random BG measurement greater than 200 mg/dL with signs and symptoms of diabetes is conclusive. The glucose tolerance test (GTT) is the most sensitive measure of glucose metabolism and can often detect early diabetes.

Glycosylated hemoglobin (also known as the A1C) is a laboratory measurement reflecting the average BG reading and estimates glucose control for the prior 3 months. The A1C is used for diagnostic screening and monitoring disease management. A reading of 6.5% or greater is indicative of diabetes and can be measured even if the patient has not been fasting. The A1C is not as sensitive as GTT for diagnosing diabetes. In addition, A1C has been associated with significant variability related to ethnicity and conditions that alter the turnover of red blood cells, such as end stage renal disease, severe thalassemia, hereditary spherocytosis, splenomegaly, autoimmune hemolytic anemia, and some hemoglobin variants.[27] An A1C of ≤7.0% has been associated with reduced risk for complications from diabetes and is the recommended goal for glucose control.[28]

Antibody Testing

The assessment of antibodies is used to confirm type 1 diabetes. The most common test is the glutamic acid decarboxylase (GAD) antibody test. A C-peptide test (an indirect measure of insulin levels) and fasting insulin level may also be measured to help determine the quantity of residual insulin production.

Lipid Analysis

The most common lipid assessments include measurements of total cholesterol, high-density lipoprotein (HDL) cholesterol, and triglycerides. From these results, the low-density lipoprotein (LDL) cholesterol level is calculated, which is referred to as calculated LDL. Triglyceride levels are generally a reflection of glycemic control, meaning that when glucose levels are high, triglycerides will also be high. HDL levels indicate severity of insulin resistance, and low HDL cholesterol is seen frequently in insulin-resistant individuals.

Renal Function Tests

An early indication of renal disease associated with diabetes is microscopic protein loss in the urine, measured by the amount of albumin (microalbuminuria). Significant loss of albumin into the urine (>300 mcg/dL) is associated with renal damage and the risk for development of end-stage renal disease. Two other standard laboratory tests to assess renal function are blood urea nitrogen and creatinine.

C-Reactive Protein

C-reactive protein (CRP) is made by the body during times of stress or infection. It is often elevated in those with diabetes, and it is associated with the inflammatory process of insulin resistance and cardiovascular disease risk. CRP can also be elevated in those with inflammatory processes such as rheumatoid arthritis or infection.

CLINICAL MANAGEMENT

Primary Prevention

Primary prevention measures for optimal glucose regulation emphasize healthy lifestyle behaviors. The general measures include maintaining optimal body weight, regular physical activity, and eating a balanced diet. The Diabetes Prevention Program found that those with prediabetes could reduce the progression to type 2 diabetes by 58% through the combination of exercise for 30 minutes, 5 days a week, and a modest weight loss of 7% body weight. Metformin can also reduce progression to diabetes by 31%, and it is a recommended diabetes prevention strategy for those younger than age 60 years with prediabetes and a BMI ≥35 kg/m^2, and women with a history of gestational diabetes.[29]

Maintaining Optimal Body Weight

Obesity is directly linked to insulin resistance and the development of diabetes. In 2016, 18.4% of children ages 6 to 11 years were classified as obese, as were 20.6% of those ages 12 to 19 years, and in addition 93.9 million adults (39.8% of the population) in the United States were classified as obese.[30] The increase in diabetes prevalence in recent years correlates directly with the increase in overweight and obesity, and the decline in regular physical activity during the past two decades.

Exercise

Exercise dramatically improves insulin resistance and cellular metabolism by increasing the number of GLUC4 transporter molecules within muscle cells,[31] thus facilitating glucose diffusion into the cell and lowering glucose levels. The American Diabetes Association recommends moderate-intensity aerobic exercise for at least 150 minutes per week and additional moderate resistive training 2 or 3 days per week for those with diabetes and for diabetes prevention.[32] Resistive training works large muscle groups that often are not used during aerobic activities such as walking, but contraction of these muscles dramatically improves insulin resistance and insulin-mediated glucose uptake.

Diet

Primary prevention further includes avoiding excess caloric intake, avoiding sweet drinks, and striving for a healthy weight. ChooseMyPlate.gov and the *2015–2020 Dietary Guidelines* should be promoted; these emphasize consuming a diet high in whole grains, fruits, and vegetables that are deep orange in color, leafy green vegetables, and legumes/beans, along with low-fat milk and a variety of lean protein sources.[33] These foods contribute to optimal cellular metabolism through provision of vitamin, minerals, fiber, and appropriate amounts of macronutrients and kilocalories needed for health. In addition, lower sodium guidelines can help lower blood pressure and reduce the risk of cardiovascular disease.

Secondary Prevention (Screening)

Secondary prevention refers to the early detection of disease through screening. Population-based screening recommendations vary across organizations, although blood glucose screening among adults with risk factors for diabetes and among all pregnant women after 24 weeks of gestation is widely recommended. There are no specific recommendations for population-based screening for hypoglycemia.

For individuals with diabetes, there are several regular screening measures for early detection of complications. The American Diabetes Association recommends A1C measurements at least twice per year (or every 3 months if not meeting glycemic targets); annual renal function and lipid tests; and annual dental, foot, and dilated eye examinations.[34] Individuals with type 1 diabetes are at higher risk for other autoimmune processes, and therefore thyroid function is monitored annually.

Collaborative Interventions

Management of conditions within the diabetes syndrome requires an interdisciplinary approach, with glycemic control as the goal to which all interventions are geared. The Diabetes Control and Complications Trial (DCCT) was the first randomized controlled trial to prove that improved glycemic control could lead to a significant reduction in diabetes-related complications in patients with type 1 diabetes.[35] The United Kingdom Prospective Diabetes Study (UKPDS) noted similar results in reducing complications for type 2 diabetes with good glycemic control.[36] These two landmark trials are the basis of diabetes treatment goals, with the end aim to prevent complications and improve the quality of life for those with diabetes. Specific collaborative interventions include patient education for self-management, glucose monitoring, nutrition therapy, and pharmacologic agents.

Patient Education for Self-Management

Diabetes self-management education (DSME) is aimed at promoting self-care behaviors for those with diabetes. Healthcare professionals can provide insight into management decisions, but the diabetic patient is involved in daily decision making for disease management. Self-care behaviors as a component of diabetes management includes diet, exercise, weight control, medication management, getting adequate rest, and maintaining awareness of complications.

Monitoring and Managing Blood Glucose

Monitoring and managing BG involves regular monitoring of BG level and using these data to determine medication or dietary action (if needed) to correct an imbalance. Two approaches to BG monitoring are incorporated in diabetes management: self-monitoring of blood glucose (SMBG) and A1C.

Self-monitoring of blood glucose. Self-monitoring of blood glucose is done with a standard BG meter or a continuous glucose monitor that can measure BG concentration changes that occur every 5 minutes. Blood glucose meters measure finger-stick capillary glucose levels and are calibrated to read equivalent to plasma glucose with a variance of approximately 10% from the laboratory setting. Because BG concentration fluctuates throughout the day, SMBG assists with decisions related to carbohydrate intake and medications. Patient or caregiver teaching is essential for accurate SMBG and is most helpful if the patient records readings regularly, along with other details related to diet, activity, and stress. Most glucose monitors allow data to be downloaded at a clinic or office for viewing during a patient encounter, or to upload to a website for sharing with a provider. Glucose logs are helpful in identifying glucose trends that allow for provider medication adjustment.

Monitoring glycosylated hemoglobin (A1C). A person with prediabetes or diabetes can benefit from regular monitoring of A1C levels to determine progression to overt diabetes. The goal A1C for most patients is 7.0% or less, although higher glucose (~8.0%) may be appropriate for certain individuals to minimize the risk for episodes of hypoglycemia. Specifically, young children, elderly patients with impaired renal function, and patients taking β-blockers should have less stringent glycemic goals.[37]

Correcting hypoglycemia. One of the ongoing risks associated with glucose-lowering agents is hypoglycemia. The *15/15 rule* is recommended for correcting hypoglycemia: 15 g of quick-acting carbohydrate can

---

BOX 15.1   Optimal 15 Gram Carbohydrates for Treatment of Hypoglycemia

- ½ cup regular soda or juice
- 1 cup milk
- ½ ampule of dextrose 50% (D50)
- 1 mg of glucagon
- 3–4 glucose tablets
- 1 tablespoon honey
- 4–6 pieces hard candy
- 15 jelly beans

---

raise blood glucose levels by approximately 50 mg/dL. Some examples of quick-acting, 15-g portions of carbohydrate are shown in Box 15.1. The blood glucose level should be checked after 15 minutes to determine effectiveness. If hypoglycemia is not corrected, the process is repeated until euglycemia is achieved (15 g of quick-acting carbohydrate followed by a repeat BG check after 15 minutes). Exceptions to the 15/15 rule include severe hypoglycemia, whereby 30 g of quick-acting carbohydrate is provided (for the conscious individual). If the patient is unconscious, either intravenous dextrose or glucagon is given. Patients receiving glucagon should be rolled onto their side or face down to reduce the risk of aspiration (nausea and vomiting are side effects of high-dosage glucagon).

It is not uncommon for patients to experience a "rebound" of blood sugar to very high levels after an episode of hypoglycemia (sometimes referred to as the *Somogyi effect*). During the stress of a hypoglycemic event, counterregulatory hormones (including growth hormone, cortisol, epinephrine, and norepinephrine) are released, all of which promote glycogenolysis and gluconeogenesis, resulting in elevated glucose levels after a hypoglycemic episode. For example, a patient can have a drop in glucose to 40 to 70 mg/dL and then experience a rebound high up to 300 to 400 mg/dL, creating a "roller coaster" of glucose levels.

Nutrition Therapy

Nutrition therapy is a cornerstone of diabetic management. Individualized dietary strategies should be developed in conjunction with the patient in accordance with his or her needs, preferences, readiness, and ability to alter lifestyle. For patients with type 2 diabetes, education often includes strategies to facilitate weight loss. Most individuals with insulin resistance, reactive hypoglycemia, or type 2 diabetes tolerate a range of up to 50 to 60 g of carbohydrate (three or four servings) per meal very well, especially if the meal is low in glycemic index. Nutrition education for those with type 1 diabetes is focused on knowledge of various nutrient components of each meal (carbohydrates, protein, and fats) to optimize nutrition in concert with insulin therapy.

Pharmacologic Agents

The American Diabetes Association and the American Association of Clinical Endocrinologists emphasize an individualized approach to medication therapy for those with diabetes. Factors such as life expectancy, support system, comorbidities, patient engagement and understanding of the disease process, risk for hypoglycemia, disease duration, and vascular complications are considered when creating a medication management plan.[38]

Oral hypoglycemic agents. Oral hypoglycemic agents are used in the treatment of type 2 diabetes, and help manage glycemic control by reducing insulin resistance and enhancing insulin secretion. These agents are as follows:

- *Insulin sensitizers:* The first-line oral agent for type 2 diabetes is the insulin sensitizer metformin in the biguanide class. Pioglitazone is in the thiazolidinedione class. Both metformin and pioglitazone help correct the defect of insulin resistance seen in type 2 diabetes.
- *Insulin secretagogues:* Sulfonylureas and the shorter acting non-sulfonylurea secretagogues enhance insulin secretion from the pancreas, but they are effective only for those who have effective insulin-secreting capacity in the pancreas. As the duration of diabetes diagnosis lengthens, these agents typically become increasingly less useful.
- *Incretin agents:* The incretin drugs (both the GLP-1 agonists and DPP-4 inhibitors) reduce postprandial glucose levels, and they are weight neutral or facilitate weight loss.
- *SGLT-2 inhibitors:* These agents increase the amount of glucose excreted by the kidneys and are associated with weight loss. They can also cause an osmotic diuresis and increase risk for dehydration and orthostatic hypotension.

Insulin. Patients who require insulin replacement need both basal (or long-acting) insulin and mealtime (or short-/fast-acting) insulin to achieve euglycemia. Normal insulin secretion patterns consist of a steady secretion of very small amounts of insulin throughout the day and night, with pulsations of insulin secretion at mealtimes. Insulin replacement therapy attempts to mimic this normal pattern by using basal and mealtime insulin. The following types of insulin replacement therapy are used:

- *Basal insulin therapy:* Basal insulin therapy can be provided with either neutral protamine hagedorn (NPH) insulin, glargine, detemir, degludac insulin.
- *Mealtime insulin therapy:* Mealtime insulin therapy can be provided with regular insulin or rapid-acting analogs such as lispro, aspart, and glulisine insulin.
- *Mixed preparations:* Mixed insulin preparations combine long-acting basal insulin with mealtime insulin. Examples of mixed insulin include 70/30 NPH/lispro, 70/30 NPH/regular, and 75/25 NPH/aspart.

The onset of action, peak of action, and length of action of various insulin preparations are shown in Table 15.2.

Statin agents. Statin medications are used for the primary prevention of cardiovascular disease (CVD) in all individuals with diabetes ages 40 to 75 years and an LDL cholesterol of 70 to 189 mg/dL without any evidence of CVD. Evidence strongly suggests statin agents reduce the rate of myocardial infarction, stroke, and death in those with diabetes.[39] It is thought that statin medications possess anti-inflammatory properties that confer additional CVD risk reduction beyond their LDL-lowering properties.[40]

Glucose Control

Glucose control in the hospitalized patient has taken on new importance due to landmark clinical trials that note significant reduction in mortality, wound infections, and length of stay when glucose levels are kept near glycemic goals of 140 to 180 mg/dL.[41]

In the outpatient setting, pattern management based on carbohydrate counting can be effective in stabilizing BG level with reduced frequency of hypo- and hyperglycemia, and it is now the recommended approach. In this approach, assessments of home glucose readings, grams of carbohydrate consumed, and the number of insulin units used help to verify the needed ratio of insulin to carbohydrate intake. Typically most adults with type 1 diabetes require 1 unit per every 15 g of carbohydrate, or 1 carb serving. A very active adult or a young child may need as little as 1 unit for every 30 g of carbohydrate, whereas an obese, insulin-resistant individual with type 2 diabetes may need as much as 1 unit for every 2 or 3 g of carbohydrate intake. If there is a consistent pattern of hyper- or

TABLE 15.2   Characteristics of Various Insulin Preparations

Insulin	Onset of Action	Peak of Action	Duration of Action
NPH	1.5–4 h	4–12 h	Up to 24 h
Glargine (Lantus)	45 min to 4 h	Minimal	Up to 24 h
Detemir (Levimir)	45 min to 4 h	Minimal	Up to 24 h
Regular Humulin R Novolin R	30–60 min	2–5 h	Up to 12 h
Aspart (Novolog)	10–30 min	0.5–3 h	3–5 h
Lispro (Humalog)	10–30 min	0.5–3 h	3–5 h
Glulisine (Epidra)	10–30 min	0.5–3 h	3–5 h
Degludec (Tresiba)	1 h	12 h	42 h

Premixed Preparations
Humulin 50/50 50% NPH/50% regular
Humulin 70/30 70% NPH/30% regular
Novolin 70/30 70% NPH/30% regular
Humalog mix 50/50 50% NPH/50% lispro
Novolog mix 50/50 50% NPH/50% aspart
Novolog mix 75/25 75% NPH/50% aspart

NPH, Neutral protamine hagedorn.
From Beaser, R. S. (2013). *Joslin's diabetes deskbook: A guide for primary care providers* (3rd ed.). Boston: Joslin Diabetes Center.

hypoglycemia by this time period, or by the next meal, the amount of insulin or carbohydrate can be adjusted up or down as needed. Once a ratio is determined, this will generally apply to other meals, although exceptions do occur. For example, the "dawn phenomenon" causes the early morning BG level to rise through increased production of cortisol and growth hormone, which are both counterregulatory hormones. Consequently, early morning glucose levels can be elevated without clear reason, and there is often a decreased tolerance to carbohydrate intake with increased need for insulin endogenous or exogenous.

An insulin correction factor can be used to correct hyperglycemia in addition to using the mealtime insulin-to-carbohydrate ratio. The *1800 rule* predicts the drop in BG level for each 1 unit of extra regular insulin beyond the bolus insulin needed to cover meal carbohydrate intake. The insulin correction factor is determined by dividing the total daily dose (TDD) of insulin units into the number 1800. For example, if a person is taking a usual TDD of 100 units, the predicted insulin correction factor is 18 (1800/100 = 18). In other words, each additional unit of insulin taken will decrease the BG level by 18 points. The higher the TDD, the lower the insulin correction factor, and thus the patient will require higher doses of correction insulin. Likewise, the lower the TDD, the less correction insulin required by the patient. Another person may be taking only 10 units of TDD insulin, which predicts that 1 extra unit of rapid-acting insulin would drop the BG 180 points (1800/10 = 180). The insulin correction factor is also referred to as the insulin sensitivity factor. The calculation factor for regular insulin in 1800/TDD, and for aspart/glulisine/lispro it is 1500/TDD.

INTERRELATED CONCEPTS

Glucose regulation affects and is affected by most, if not all, physiological processes. As the primary energy substrate, all life processes are dependent on normal glucose metabolism and regulation. Fig. 15.3 shows some of the most important interrelated concepts.

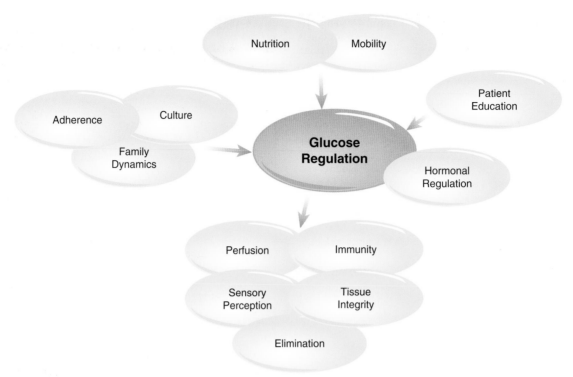

FIGURE 15.3 Glucose Regulation and Interrelated Concepts.

Hormonal Regulation is shown as a close interrelated concept because of the significant influence that hormones have on the regulation of glucose. Proper **Nutrition** and regular physical activity (**Mobility**) are needed for optimal regulation of glucose concentration and management of conditions in which regulatory mechanisms are impaired. Long-term consequences of hyperglycemia lead to micro- and macrovascular changes (**Perfusion**), poor wound healing (**Tissue Integrity**), impaired immune function (**Immunity**), reduced renal function (**Elimination**), and changes in vision and peripheral sensation (**Sensory Perception**).

The concepts **Family Dynamics**, **Adherence**, and **Culture** influence the behavioral changes needed for optimal health promotion or disease management. Family relationships can suffer when attempts to regulate the diet of one individual have an adverse impact on mealtime that affects other family members. This can result in mealtime-associated stress if optimal family dynamics are not present. **Patient Education** is a cornerstone of treatment and has a tremendous impact on outcomes for those with impaired glucose regulation.

CLINICAL EXEMPLARS

Although much of the attention in this concept presentation has focused on diabetes, glucose regulation represents a number of other clinical exemplars characterized by hyperglycemic and hypoglycemic states and are presented in Box 15.2. Several of these exemplars are briefly featured here.

Featured Exemplars
Type 2 Diabetes Mellitus

Type 2 diabetes mellitus is characterized by the features of insulin resistance paired with β cell failure resulting in hyperglycemia. Chronic hyperglycemia leads to damage of blood vessels and nerves, leading to the complications of retinopathy, nephropathy, neuropathy, and cardiovascular disease. Previously common in adults only, type 2 diabetes is now more common in children and adolescents due to increasing rates of obesity and overweight in this population. Ninety-five percent of individuals with diabetes have type 2 diabetes.

Type 1 Diabetes Mellitus

Type 1 diabetes mellitus is an autoimmune disorder in which the body's immune system destroys the β cells in the pancreas, resulting in absolute insulin deficiency. These patients require lifelong insulin replacement therapy to maintain normal metabolism and nutrition. Most individuals with type 1 diabetes are thin or normal weight, and although it is more common in children and adolescents, approximately 13% of all newly diagnosed type 1 diabetes occurs in people ages 30 to 50 years.

Polycystic Ovary Syndrome

Polycystic ovary syndrome (PCOS) is the most common endocrine disorder in women of reproductive age. PCOS is characterized by infrequent menses (longer than 35 days apart) and signs of higher than normal androgen levels (hirsutism, acne, and male pattern hair loss). Infertility is common due to lack of regular menses caused by anovulation. Women with PCOS are very insulin resistant, and approximately 40% of women with PCOS who are obese or overweight will have diabetes or prediabetes before the age of 40 years; therefore, diabetes prevention efforts in these women are crucial.[42]

Diabetic Ketoacidosis

Diabetic Ketoacidosis (DKA) is an acute event that results from insulin deficiency and is sometimes the presenting symptom of type 1 diabetes. The combination of hyperglycemia, ketosis, and acidosis leads to dehydration, and fluid resuscitation and insulin therapy are required to correct this state. Other symptoms include abdominal pain, vomiting, poor skin turgor, tachycardia, and hypotension. Stress or illness is a frequent trigger for DKA.

BOX 15.2   EXEMPLARS OF IMPAIRED GLUCOSE REGULATION

Hyperglycemia

- Conditions of excess counterregulatory hormones: Cushing syndrome
- Cystic fibrosis
- Diabetic ketoacidosis
- Hyperosmolar hyperglycemic nonketotic syndrome
- Type 1 diabetes
- Type 2 diabetes
- Overcorrection of hypoglycemia
- Rebound hyperglycemia ("Somogyi effect")
- Corticosteroid therapy
- Gestational diabetes
- Insulin resistance
- Polycystic ovary syndrome
- Hemochromatosis
- Pheochromocytoma
- Pancreatitis
- Stress response

Hypoglycemia

- Addison disease
- Insulin treatment
- Gastroparesis
- Glycogen storage diseases
- Prematurity
- Starvation
- Large for gestational age infant
- Liver failure
- Nesidioblastoma
- Insulinoma

ACCESS EXEMPLAR LINKS IN YOUR GIDDENS EBOOK

Hyperosmolar Hyperglycemic Nonketotic Syndrome

Hyperosmolar hyperglycemic nonketotic syndrome (HHNS) is a state characterized by hyperglycemia, hyperosmolarity, and dehydration without acidosis. HHNS is more common in elderly patients and can present with glucose levels greater than 600 mg/dL. This condition accounts for less than 1% of hospital admissions, and treatment emphasizes correction of dehydration and lowering of blood glucose with insulin. HHNS typically has a trigger of stress or illness, and treatment of the underlying cause is a priority of care.

Gestational Diabetes Mellitus

Gestational diabetes mellitus (GDM) is a hyperglycemic condition associated with pregnancy seen in 5.7% to 8.7% of pregnancies in the United States in 2014.[43] Placental hormones increase insulin resistance, especially as the pregnancy progresses, and postprandial hyperglycemia is the common presentation. Risk factors include obesity, past history of GDM, age older than 25 years, and family history of type 2 diabetes. Approximately 5% to 10% of women who develop gestational diabetes will have persistent hyperglycemia after pregnancy and be subsequently diagnosed with type 2 diabetes.[44]

Cushing Syndrome

Cushing syndrome is a rare disorder resulting in excessive corticosteroid secretion leading to hyperglycemia. This condition can be primary (caused by corticosteroid-secreting tumor of the adrenal cortex), secondary (caused by adrenocorticotroic hormone (ACTH)-secreting pituitary tumor or ectopic ACTH secretion), or iatrogenic (when symptoms are related to administration of supraphysiological doses of corticosteroids). Symptoms include hyperglycemia, elevated blood pressure, hypokalemia, central fat distribution, dark purple striae, ruddy facial complexion, hirsutism, weight gain, easy bruising, and muscle weakness. Only 10 to 15 of every 1 million people are diagnosed with primary or secondary Cushing syndrome annually.

CASE STUDY

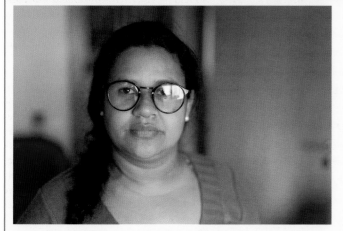

Case Presentation

Marla is a 34-year-old woman with who presents to a healthcare provider to establish primary care and management of her diabetes. She was diagnosed with type 2 diabetes 3 years ago, and has a history of polycystic ovary syndrome and hypertension. She works as a pharmacy technician at a local pharmacy chain, and has been married for 1 year. She lives with her husband and recently moved to the area from across the country for better job opportunities. Her A1C 1 year ago was at the recommended goal of 7.0%. Her current medications include metformin ER 2000 mg daily, enalapril 10 mg daily, and a prenatal vitamin daily. She has no allergies, and does not smoke or drink alcohol. She has been checking his glucose levels at home once daily, and readings vary from 110 to 165 mg/dL. She walks for 30 minutes 2 days a week (her days off), as she feels she is on her feet enough when she is at work. She would also like a referral to obstetrics/gynecology, as she and her husband want to start a family in the coming year and are not using any contraception.

Vital signs are as follows: weight, 72.5 kg; height, 63 in.; body mass index, 29.5; temperature, 98.4°F; pulse, 84 beats/min; respiratory rate, 20 breaths/min; and blood pressure, 140/82 mm Hg.

Lab results are as follows: A1C, 7.6%; glucose, 155 mg/dL; sodium, 135; blood urea nitrogen, 19; creatinine, 0.8; total cholesterol, 186 mg/dL; triglycerides, 186 mg/dL; HDL, 44; and LDL, 104.

Case Analysis Questions

1. What is your overall assessment of Marla's current diabetes management status?
2. What considerations should be made regarding Marla's desire to get pregnant?
3. How should Marla focus her self-management activities prior to becoming pregnant?

🌿 **ACCESS EXEMPLAR LINKS IN YOUR GIDDENS EBOOK**

REFERENCES

1. DeFronzo, R. A., et al. (2015). Type 2 diabetes mellitus. *Nature Reviews. Disease Primers, 1*(15019).
2. Chen, C., Cohrs, C. M., Stertmann, J., et al. (2017). Human beta cell mass and function in diabetes: Recent advances in knowledge and technologies to understand disease pathogenesis. *Molecular Metabolism, 6*(9), 943–957.
3. Laakso, M., & Kuusisto, J. (2015). Insulin resistance and hyperglycemia in cardiovascular disease development. *Nature Reviews. Endocrinology, 10*(5), 293.
4. Kobayashi, J. (2015). Nitric oxide and insulin resistance. *Immunoendocrinology, 2*(1), 657–666.
5. Soleimani, M. (2015). Insulin resistance and hypertension: New insights. *Kidney International, 87*(3), 497–499.
6. Arnold, S. E., Arvanitakis, Z., Macauley-Rambach, S. L., et al. (2018). Brain insulin resistance in type 2 diabetes and Alzheimer disease: Concepts and conundrums. *Nature Reviews. Neurology, 14*(3), 168.
7. Lam, D. C., Lam, K. S., & May, S. M. (2015). Obstructive sleep apnea, insulin resistance and adipocytokines. *Clinical Endocrinology, 82*(2), 165–177.
8. Centers for Disease Control and Prevention. (2017). *National diabetes statistics report, 2017*. Atlanta, GA: US Department of Health and Human Services.
9. Ziegler, D., Papanas, N., Vinik, A. I., & Shaw, J. E. (2014). Epidemiology of polyneuropathy in diabetes and prediabetes. *Handbook of Clinical Neurology, 26*, 3–22.
10. Stoner, G. D. (2017). Hyperosmolar hyperglycemic state. *American Family Physician, 96*(11).
11. Bagdure, D., Rewers, A., Campagna, E., & Sills, M. R. (2013). Epidemiology of hyperglycemic hyperosmolar syndrome in children hospitalized in USA. *Pediatric Diabetes, 14*(1), 18–24.
12. Seaquist, E. R., Anderson, J., Childs, B., et al. (2013). Hypoglycemia and diabetes: A report of a workgroup of the American Diabetes Association and the Endocrine Society. *Diabetes Care, 22*, DC_122480.
13. Freeman, R. (2014). Diabetic autonomic neuropathy. *Handbook of Clinical Neurology, 126*, 63–79.
14. Gubitosi-Klug, R. A., Braffett, B. H., White, N. H., et al. DCCT Epidemiology of Diabetes Interventions and Complications (EDIC) Research Group. (2017). The risk of severe hypoglycemia in type 1 diabetes over 30 years of follow-up in the DCCT/EDIC Study. *Diabetes Care, 24*, dc162723.
15. Gupta, Y., Kalra, B., Baruah, M. P., et al. (2015). Updated guidelines on screening for gestational diabetes. *International Journal of Women's Health, 7*, 539.
16. Mitanchez, D., Yzydorczyk, C., Siddeek, B., et al. (2015). The offspring of the diabetic mother–short-and long-term implications. *Best Practice & Research. Clinical Obstetrics & Gynaecology, 29*(2), 256–269.
17. Gong, Z., & Muzumdar, R. H. (2012). Pancreatic function, type 2 diabetes and metabolism in aging. *International Journal of Endocrinology, 2012*, 320482.
18. Centers for Disease Control and Prevention. (2017). *National diabetes statistics report, 2017*. Atlanta, GA: US Department of Health and Human Services.
19. Guariguata, L., Whiting, D. R., Hambleton, I., et al. (2014). Global estimates of diabetes prevalence for 2013 and projections for 2035. *Diabetes Research and Clinical Practice, 103*(2), 137–149.
20. Pociot, F., & Lernmark, Å. (2016). Genetic risk factors for type 1 diabetes. *Lancet, 387*(10035), 2331–2339.
21. Kahaly, G. J., & Hansen, M. P. (2016). Type 1 diabetes associated autoimmunity. *Autoimmunity Reviews, 15*(7), 644–648.
22. Prasad, R. B., & Groop, L. (2016). Genetics of type 2 diabetes—pitfalls and possibilities. *Genes, 6*(1), 87–123.
23. American Diabetes Association. (2018). Classification and diagnosis of diabetes: Standards of medical care in diabetes—2018. *Diabetes Care, 41*(Suppl. 1), S13–S27.

24. Lee, S. W., Ng, K. Y., & Chin, W. K. (2017). The impact of sleep amount and sleep quality on glycemic control in type 2 diabetes: A systematic review and meta-analysis. *Sleep Medicine Reviews, 31*, 91–101.
25. Holt, R. I., De Groot, M., & Golden, S. H. (2014). Diabetes and depression. *Current Diabetes Reports, 14*(6), 491.
26. Stuart, J., McCarthy, K., Dennick, K., et al. (2015). What characterizes diabetes distress and its resolution? A documentary analysis. *International Diabetes Nursing, 12*(2), 56–62.
27. Sacks, D. B. (2016). Hemoglobin A1c and race: Should therapeutic targets and diagnostic cutoffs differ among racial groups? *Clinical Chemistry, 62*(9), 1199–1201.
28. American Diabetes Association. (2018). Glycemic targets: Standards of medical care in diabetes—2018. *Diabetes Care, 41*(Suppl. 1), S55–S64.
29. American Diabetes Association. (2018). Prevention or Delay of Type 2 Diabetes: Standards of medical care in diabetes—2018. *Diabetes Care, 41*, S51–S54.
30. Hales, C. M., Carroll, M. D., Fryar, C. D., et al. (2017). *Prevalence of obesity among adults and youth: United States, 2015–2016* NCHS data brief, no 288. Hyattsville, MD: National Center for Health Statistics.
31. Stanford, K. I., & Goodyear, L. J. (2014). Exercise and type 2 diabetes: Molecular mechanisms regulating glucose uptake in skeletal muscle. *Advances in Physiology Education, 38*(4), 308–314.
32. American Diabetes Association. (2018). Lifestyle management: Standards of medical care in diabetes—2018. *Diabetes Care, 41*(Suppl. 1), S38–S50.
33. U.S. Department of Health and Human Services and U.S. Department of Agriculture. (2015). *2015–2020 Dietary Guidelines for Americans*, 8th Edition. Retrieved from https://health.gov/dietaryguidelines/2015/guidelines/.
34. American Diabetes Association. (2018). Comprehensive medical evaluation and assessment of comorbidities: Standards of medical care in diabetes—2018. *Diabetes Care, 41*(Suppl. 1), S28–S37.
35. Nathan, D. M., DCCT/Edic Research Group. (2014). The diabetes control and complications trial/epidemiology of diabetes interventions and complications study at 30 years: Overview. *Diabetes Care, 37*(1), 9–16.
36. Hayward, R. A., Reaven, P. D., Wiitala, W. L., et al. (2015). Follow-up of glycemic control and cardiovascular outcomes in type 2 diabetes. *The New England Journal of Medicine, 372*(23), 2197–2206.
37. American Diabetes Association. (2018). Pharmacologic approaches to glycemic treatment: Standards of medical care in diabetes—2018. *Diabetes Care, 41*, S73–S85.
38. Inzucchi, S. E., Bergenstal, R. M., Buse, J. B., et al. (2015). Management of hyperglycemia in type 2 diabetes, 2015: A patient-centered approach: update to a position statement of the American Diabetes Association and the European Association for the Study of Diabetes. *Diabetes Care, 38*(1), 140–149.
39. Lloyd-Jones, D. M., Morris, P. B., Ballantyne, C. M., et al. (2016). 2016 ACC expert consensus decision pathway on the role of non-statin therapies for LDL-cholesterol lowering in the management of atherosclerotic cardiovascular disease risk: A report of the American College of Cardiology Task Force on Clinical Expert Consensus Documents. *Journal of the American College of Cardiology, 68*(1), 92–125.
40. Oesterle, A., Laufs, U., & Liao, J. K. (2017). Pleiotropic effects of statins on the cardiovascular system. *Circulation Research, 120*(1), 229–243.
41. American Diabetes Association. (2018). Diabetes care in the hospital: Standards of medical care in diabetes—2018. *Diabetes Care, 41*(s1), S144–S151.
42. Goodman, N. F., Cobin, R. H., Futterweit, W., et al. (2015). American Association of Clinical Endocrinologists, American College of Endocrinology, and Androgen Excess and PCOS Society disease state clinical review: Guide to the best practices in the evaluation and treatment of polycystic ovary syndrome-part 2. *Endocrine Practice, 21*(12), 1415–1426.
43. Bardenheier, B. H., Elixhauser, A., Imperatore, G., et al. (2013). Variation in prevalence of gestational diabetes mellitus among hospital discharges for obstetric delivery across 23 states in the United States. *Diabetes Care, 36*, 1209–1214.
44. American Diabetes Association. (2018). Management of diabetes in pregnancy: Standards of Medical Care in Diabetes—2018. *Diabetes Care, 41*(Suppl. 1), S137–S143.

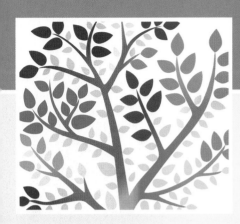

Nutrition

Sylvia Escott-Stump

Nutrition encompasses the process by which food and nutrients affect growth and development, cellular function and repair, health promotion, and disease prevention. As a science, nutrition delineates the requirements as well as the functions of macro- and micronutrients for optimal physiological functioning. Most nutrients are needed daily to achieve short-term and long-term health goals. Nutritional status impacts a variety of health conditions and disorders. In turn, many diseases adversely affect nutritional status by altering the ability to ingest, digest, absorb, and metabolize nutrients in their intact form or at the cellular level. Because nutrition and health are directly linked, this represents a fundamental concept for nursing practice.

DEFINITION

The concept of nutrition is complex, involving several physiological processes. For this concept presentation, nutrition is defined as *the science of optimal cellular metabolism and its impact on health and disease.* Several other terms are essential to an understanding of this concept that merit definition. *Macronutrients* are the *kilocalorie (kcal)* energy-containing nutrients known as carbohydrates, proteins, and fats. Alcohol also provides kilocalories, but it is not considered a macronutrient because it cannot support or maintain bodily functions. Vitamins and minerals are *micronutrients* because they are required in minute amounts. Some minerals are needed in such small amounts that they are called "ultra" trace mineral requirements. Water is the final product considered to be an essential nutrient. *Phytochemical* refers to a plant compound that has antimicrobial, antioxidant, anti-inflammatory, and immune-boosting properties. Examples of phytochemicals include lutein (associated with the green color of vegetables) and lycopene (found in high amounts in tomato products). Another popular phytochemical is resveratrol in red grapes and peanuts.

SCOPE

Nutritional status can be viewed as either *optimal* or *suboptimal*. An optimal nutritional status is one in which all nutrients are available in balanced amounts for cellular metabolism and physiological function for the individual. A suboptimal state (or malnourished state) reflects either insufficient or excessive quantity or quality of macronutrients or micronutrients. The scope of this concept is represented as a continuum with malnutrition on both ends (insufficient nutrition and excess nutrition) and optimal nutrition in the middle (Fig. 16.1). The

continuum representation is important because nutritional status has the potential to change in either direction due to several factors and can be corrected with successful measures. Nutritional health status is also an issue of balance or imbalance. Poor nutritional status negatively impacts health, and poor health can negatively impact nutritional status (Fig. 16.2).

NORMAL PHYSIOLOGICAL PROCESS

Oral Intake

Normal intake requires appropriate ingestion of necessary foods to meet macronutrient, micronutrient, and fluid needs. Required macronutrients and micronutrients are presented in Table 16.1. The amount of nutrient intake needed for optimal function changes throughout the lifespan. National guidelines for recommended intake, referred to as Dietary Reference Intakes (DRIs), are available on the U.S. Department of Agriculture website (http://fnic.nal.usda.gov).

Adequate oral intake of nutrients (and water) involves access to food sources, informed food choices, and efficient chewing (mastication) and swallowing abilities. In general, the philosophy is "If the gut works, use it." Evidence shows that much immunity begins in the intestine, so it is important to provide nutrients using the gastrointestinal (GI) tract whenever possible.

Digestion

Digestion is the process of mechanical and chemical breakdown of food matter and complex macronutrients. Mechanical breakdown includes chewing in the mouth, as well as the mixing motions and muscular (peristaltic) action of propelling food through the stomach and intestines. Digestive enzymes are responsible for the chemical breakdown of food matter; this process is most efficient when food is thoroughly chewed, thus increasing the surface of food particles for enzyme action.

Chemical breakdown begins in the oral cavity. Saliva is a mucous-like fluid that contains the digestive enzyme amylase, which assists with the process of food breakdown and aids in the chewing and swallowing process. In the stomach, gastric enzymes begin to break down proteins into amino acids and carbohydrates into simple sugars. Pancreatic enzymes finalize digestion in the small bowel, with fats being broken down into fatty acids. Bile, produced in the liver and stored in the gallbladder, is involved in fat digestion by modifying dietary fats into emulsions for better absorption.

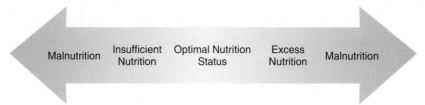

FIGURE 16.1 Scope of Nutrition Concept.

TABLE 16.1	**Required Nutrients**		
Macronutrients and Primary Role	**Fat-Soluble Vitamins**	**Water-Soluble Vitamins**	**Major Minerals**
Carbohydrates	Vitamin A	Vitamin C	Calcium
Primary source of fuel and energy	Vitamin D	B Vitamins	Phosphorus
	Vitamin E	Thiamin	Magnesium
Protein	Vitamin K	Riboflavin	Sodium
Facilitates growth and repair of tissues; energy source		Niacin	Potassium
		Pyridoxine	Chloride
		Pantothenic	
Fat		Biotin	
Source of fatty acid, necessary for growth and development; energy		Folate	
		Cobalamin	

Absorption

Once food matter has been digested, the microscopic hair-like projections (villi) that line the intestinal tract absorb nutrients into capillaries, which are then transported by the vascular system. The upper portion of the small intestinal tract (duodenum) is the primary site for absorbing trace minerals. The middle section (jejunum) is the primary site for absorbing water-soluble vitamins and proteins. The lower section (ileum) is the site of fat and fat-soluble vitamin absorption. Water is primarily absorbed in the colon.

Elimination

Large food particles and undigested fibers are not absorbed—they are eliminated from the colon. A healthy GI tract with efficient peristaltic action is required for optimal elimination. Bulky stools, from adequate fiber intake, stimulate peristalsis. Elimination is enhanced with adequate fluid, fiber intake, and physical activity.

Cellular Metabolism

Cellular metabolism includes the hormonal and enzymatic processes that occur within cell structures that allow proteins, carbohydrates, or fats to be used for energy or made into new products or tissues. Adequate intake of both macro- and micronutrients is required for optimal cellular metabolism. Proteins (in the form of essential amino acids) must be available for cells to manufacture other proteins, such as carrier proteins, and to enable tissue growth and repair. Adequate carbohydrate intake provides the energy for protein to do its many jobs. Carbohydrates are also required to provide glucose for the unique fuel needs of the brain, the neurologic system, and the red blood cells. Essential fatty acids maintain the integrity of the phospholipid-based cell membranes, found around every cell. Many metabolic enzymes assist in cellular metabolism. Zinc and magnesium are each part of more than 200 different metabolic enzymes. Both zinc and folic acid are critical in the production of proteins and cellular structures; without these micronutrients, growth and tissue repair are severely impaired.

Age-Related Differences

Although the general physiological process of nutrition is consistent throughout life, there are specific age-related considerations worth noting.

Infants and Children

Significant changes in growth and development occur in the first year of life. Birth weight triples, and length increases by an average of 50%. Infants have very different nutrient needs (compared with adults) to support this rapid growth. Due to the lack of teeth, chewing capability, and immature GI tract, the nutritional intake of infants should be limited to breast milk (or formula) and water for the first 4 to 6 months of life. Newborn infants depend on a strong suck–swallow reflex for adequate nutritional intake. As the child's GI tract develops, solid foods that do not require chewing can be gradually introduced (ideally starting at 6 months of age). As teeth emerge, the older infant and young child can be offered foods with various textures. The small oropharynx places young children at risk of choking; thus the need to provide foods in small bites is particularly important. Specific nutrient requirements for infants and children can be found by referring to DRIs.

Pregnancy and Lactation

Significant changes in nutrition needs occur during pregnancy and lactation to account for the body composition changes during pregnancy (hormonal, metabolic, and anatomic), growing fetus (before birth), and the production of breast milk after delivery. Increases in carbohydrates, proteins, fats, and most micronutrients are recommended. Expected weight gain during pregnancy ranges from 15 to 40 pounds, depending on prepregnancy weight and stature. Specific nutrient requirements for pregnant women and during lactation can be found by referring to DRIs.

Older Adults

Physiologically, the effects of aging can be associated with a reduced ability to ingest, absorb, and metabolize nutrients. In the mouth, reduced chewing ability, less saliva production, and altered sense of taste are common concerns. The esophagus may be elongated (due to kyphosis), and atrophic changes occur, particularly in the lower esophagus. Atrophic changes and intestinal microflora occur in aging, resulting in reduced efficiency in absorption. In the absence of disease, the liver, gallbladder, and pancreas continue to function, although there is a decrease in metabolic efficiency.

VARIATIONS AND CONTEXT

Malnutrition is a comprehensive term that refers to two major categories of nutritional conditions: insufficient nutrition and excess nutrition. Within each of these two categories, nutritional problems are represented by the specific nutrient or nutrients involved. The causes of problems vary widely and include problems with access, intake, absorption, and metabolism.

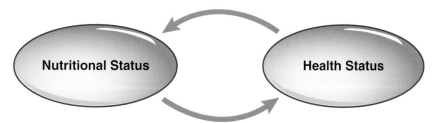

FIGURE 16.2 Interrelationship Between Nutritional Status and Health Status.

Insufficient Nutrition

Insufficient nutrition occurs when there is inadequate intake, impaired nutrient absorption, or ineffective nutrient utilization, leading to a state of malnutrition. The malnutrition can be associated with insufficient calorie intake leading to unintended weight loss and/or insufficient intake of one or more nutrients, yielding a number of nutritional deficiencies. The state of being underweight is described as a body mass index (BMI) less than 18.5. *Starvation-related malnutrition* describes conditions such as anorexia nervosa, whereas *acute disease-related malnutrition* occurs after burn injury or trauma. The third type of adult malnutrition (*chronic disease-related malnutrition*) is exemplified by sarcopenic obesity or pancreatic cancer.

Excess Nutrition

At the opposite end of the spectrum is the situation in which excessive nutritional intake progresses to weight gain or nutritional toxicities. The most common form of excess nutrition is associated with excessive calorie intake leading to weight gain. Standardized categories, based on BMI, are used to describe overweight and obesity. For adults, overweight is described as a BMI between 25.0 and 29.9. Three classes of obesity are class I (BMI of 30 to 34.9), class II (BMI of 35 to 39.9), and class III (BMI >40). Child obesity is described in terms of BMI compared with percentiles on standardized growth charts. A child whose BMI is between the 85th and 95th percentile for children of the same age and sex is classified as overweight; obesity is defined as a BMI greater than the 95th percentile.

Excess micronutrient intake most often occurs with the use of high-dose fat-soluble vitamin and mineral supplements or when consuming foods that have 100% of the DRI levels of a nutrient, plus an oral supplement, and a liquid enhanced beverage all in the same day. The outcomes of excessive food or supplement intake on physiological processes can be detrimental, especially if prolonged over time.

CONSEQUENCES

Several physiological consequences are associated with a poor nutritional state on both ends of the spectrum: nutritional deficiencies and nutritional excess. These are best understood by considering the specific nutrients involved. Malnutrition is highly devastating for infants and children because it limits their growth, brain development, ability to learn, and, later, their ability to participate effectively in society.

Nutritional Deficiencies

Macronutrient Deficiencies

Protein is a component of every cell of the body. Thus protein deficiency has diverse consequences, and the effects can be subtle or dramatic, depending on the severity, amount of inflammation, and length of time. In children, an inadequate intake of protein and kilocalories (*marasmus*) impairs growth and development, stunting height and brain development most evidently. The condition in which the insufficiency is protein

alone, with adequate energy (*kwashiorkor*), is seen in developing countries after an infant is weaned to a diet that contains mostly grains.

At any age, inadequate protein intake will adversely impact the body's ability to repair or replace body tissues or produce other constituents such as immune factors. In older adults, the loss of muscle mass (in sarcopenia) is difficult to replace. A spiraling decline in health may occur if not corrected through rapid and effective interventions. Insufficient circulating protein in the blood (hypoalbuminemia) can also lead to anasarca (severe generalized edema).

Inadequate carbohydrate intake can alter cellular metabolism and results in the use of dietary protein as a fuel substrate, diminishing cell growth and repair. Ultimately, if inadequate carbohydrate intake continues, there is a shift to use body fat and protein for energy resulting in weight loss and accumulation of ketones, especially if insulin is unavailable.

Essential fatty acid deficiency affects all cellular membranes and is particularly a problem with premature infants. Docosahexaenoic acid (DHA) and eicosapentaenoic acid (EPA) are long-chain omega-3 fatty acids that support retinal development, neurotransmitter production, and brain function.

Vitamin and Mineral Deficiencies

Deficiency of vitamin C was one of the first recognized nutrient deficiency diseases, with the severe form (scurvy) being a cause of death among early sea voyagers. British sailors were called "limeys" because their intake of limes while onboard sea vessels prevented this condition. In the early twentieth century, processed grains were becoming popular. Soon, a mysterious syndrome appeared as the "4 Ds": dermatitis on sun-exposed areas, diarrhea, dementia, and death. This condition (pellagra) was determined to be from a B vitamin deficiency. The government mandated that processed white flour products had to be enriched with the nutrients that were removed during processing—vitamins B_1, B_2, and B_3 (thiamin, riboflavin, and niacin, respectively).

The role of folic acid in the development of the central nervous system had been known for decades, but not until the 1990s did it become clear that most neural tube defects (NTDs) could be prevented by fortifying grains. Folic acid is now added to flour processed in the United States and in many countries; an important reduction in NTDs has been shown in these countries.

Lutein and zeaxanthin are carotenoids found in yellow and orange foods (cantaloupe, corn, carrots, salmon, and egg yolks) that help prevent macular degeneration. The intact form of vitamin A is also essential for vision; deficiency begins with loss of night vision and progresses to total blindness.

Vitamin D insufficiency is known to lead to osteoporosis, hip fracture, and hyperparathyroidism. Studies also suggest links with cardiovascular disease, cancer, multiple sclerosis, tuberculosis, and muscular and immune system disorders. Table 16.2 summarizes key nutrient deficiency and toxicity concerns.

TABLE 16.2 Common Vitamin and Mineral Deficiencies and Toxicities

Nutrient	Consequences of Deficiencies	Consequences of Toxicities
Vitamin A	Night blindness	Loss of appetite, bone pain, hypercalcemia
Vitamin B₁ (thiamine)	Wernicke encephalopathy with neurodegeneration	Toxicity rare
Vitamin B₃	Pellagra with 4 Ds: dermatitis, diarrhea, dementia, death	Abnormal glucose metabolism, flushing, nausea and vomiting
Vitamin B₁₂	Pernicious anemia, psychiatric disorders	Toxicity unknown
Biotin	Hair loss	Toxicity unknown
Vitamin C	Bleeding tendency, scurvy	Inhibits zinc absorption, urinary stones
Vitamin D	Rickets, bone disease, muscle pain, falls	Hypercalcemia, renal stones, calcification of soft tissues
Copper	Anemia, skin lesions, neurologic disease, bone fragility	Found in Wilson disease; neuron and liver cell damage
Iron	Anemia, fatigue, poor growth	Hemochromatosis (genetic) with liver, pancreatic, and cardiac damage
Magnesium	Hypertension, dysrhythmia, preeclampsia	Increased calcium excretion
Zinc	Dermatitis, impaired taste, impaired growth, low level of alkaline phosphatase enzyme	Copper deficiency, renal damage, nausea and vomiting, diarrhea

Nutritional Excess

Malnutrition also occurs from excess macronutrient (energy) intake that leads to weight gain. Often, obese individuals have micronutrient insufficiency while consuming excess calories from the macronutrients.

The consequences of excessive weight have been well documented and can include type 2 diabetes, coronary heart disease, hypertension, stroke, fatty liver disease, gallbladder disorders, sleep apnea, asthma and other respiratory problems, musculoskeletal disorders, as well as some cancers (breast, prostate). With more obesity in children and teens, these medical conditions are now seen at younger ages, with similar health challenges and high risks for early mortality.

RISK FACTORS

All individuals have a potential risk for malnutrition. Some risk factors are more common in population groups or during certain life stages, but individual choices and circumstances also play a role.

Populations at Risk
Age or Life Stage

At the beginning of life and again at the later stages, nutritional deficits are a significant concern. Pregnancy is a very important stage because of the long-term effects on the health of both infant and mother. The very young are at risk because of immature organ development and total dependence on others for feeding. Particularly at risk are premature infants because of their impaired oral intake. With parenteral or tube feeding, the use of breast milk may be impossible, eliminating the

benefits of cost savings, immunological protection, ideal nutrient content, and microbial support.[1,2]

Senior citizens are also at high risk for nutritional inadequacies. Factors such as reduced organ function, limited income, interactions between nutrients and medications, isolation, decreased interest in meal preparation, changes in appetite, fatigue, and altered taste sensations are common. Those elderly who are institutionalized are at even greater risk. Severe dietary restrictions, rigid mealtimes, generally poor health status, and feeding dependency can lead to inadequate oral intake. Physiological risk factors include frailty, low BMI (BMI <21 is associated with a high risk of mortality despite nutritional intervention), and neurologic deficits from a stroke or Alzheimer disease.[3–5]

Ethnicity/Race

Nutritional deficits and genetic predispositions have triggered many chronic diseases of the modern world.[6] Vitamin D deficiency is more frequently found among Hispanics and Americans of African heritage than those of European heritage.[7,8] Type 2 diabetes also seems to affect Hispanic, Native American, and African Americans in higher percentages than Europeans. Diseases more common in European heritage include type 1 diabetes, celiac disease, and neurodegenerative disorders such as Huntington disease and multiple sclerosis.[9]

The Poor and Underserved

As a population group, those of low socioeconomic status are at risk for malnutrition because of food insecurity and food availability. Lack of access to healthy foods because of insufficient funds, distance to supermarkets, limited options for food preparation, high prices of quality foods, cheap prices of fast food, and limited transportation are some of the reasons why individuals with low incomes may eat poorly and become obese.[10] Where access to healthy, affordable food is limited, the community is designated as a "food desert." Creative approaches are often needed to help families learn to budget their food dollars wisely and nutritiously. The homeless who experience food insecurity over a prolonged period of time are particularly at risk.

Individual Risk Factors
Genetics

Many conditions that impact nutrition are linked to genetics. Inherited metabolic defects include phenylketonuria (PKU), a deficiency in the enzyme responsible for the metabolism of the amino acid phenylalanine. PKU allows phenylalanine to accumulate in the brain, blood, and tissues, leading to cognitive dysfunction unless the affected individual follows a low-phenylalanine diet for life. Other rare inherited metabolic defects include galactosemia and maple syrup urine disease. In cystic fibrosis (CF), thick secretions block pancreatic ducts, eventually leading to impaired digestion and absorption of fats and fat-soluble vitamins.

Lifestyle and Patterns of Eating

How one chooses foods, shops, plans, and prepares meals ultimately affects his or her nutritional status. Factors that influence these decisions include interpersonal relationships, learned stress-coping mechanisms, and alterations in mood. Weight gain can occur when food habits change to match those of the partner, such as during dating and marriage.

Family food offerings can positively or negatively influence nutritional intake. Mothers who avoid high-fat, high-sugar foods but emphasize a variety of vegetables, fruits, whole grains, lean meats, and low-fat milk can send the right message to their families. Family influences that may negatively impact nutritional status include lack of home-prepared meals, eating meals on the go, restricting multiple food groups because of allergies or dislikes, or limited choices because of financial challenges.

The influence of peers is common among adolescents. Skipping meals, following fad diets, choosing salty and sugary snacks over healthy foods, eating super-sized portions, and drinking alcohol are examples. Here, mood swings are common. Coping mechanisms often include eating large amounts of sweets or comfort foods, or reducing intake altogether during periods of depression. Peer influences are especially strong among young people with lower self-esteem.[11]

Personal Food Choices

Personal choice is the major internal influence over food intake. Women tend to experience cravings around their menstrual periods and during pregnancy.[12] If they give in to these cravings regularly, obesity may result.

Occasionally, individuals may experience nutritional disorders because of erroneous understandings or perceptions about foods. Some fad diets require the omission or limitation of whole food groups; others allow only certain foods (e.g., the grapefruit diet, the cabbage soup diet). The person who follows such restrictions may unknowingly miss out on important nutrients.

If a vegan diet is undertaken without adequate knowledge, the intake may be insufficient for essential amino acids, calcium, zinc, and vitamins D and B_{12}. Inadequate vitamin B_{12} has been associated with anemia and with neurologic damage, especially dangerous in children.[13] Calcium and vitamin D levels tend to be low unless fortified foods or supplements are used. Without adequate planning of foods containing the various amino acids, protein deficiency can occur. Fortunately, a carefully planned vegan diet offers protection against obesity, hypertension, type 2 diabetes, and cardiovascular disease, especially in men.[14]

Underlying Medical Conditions

A wide range of medical conditions place individuals at risk for various nutritional problems. Some of these are shown in Table 16.3.

Impaired oral intake. Adequacy of oral intake is associated with the ability to chew and swallow. Thus the inability to chew or swallow properly can easily lead to malnutrition. Pain from dental caries, poorly fitting dentures, and loss of teeth can impair the ability to chew and limit diet quality. Cleft palate impacts an infant's sucking ability, thereby limiting successful breast-feeding. Difficulty swallowing (dysphagia) is common in neurologic conditions, especially after a stroke. Not all patients require altered food consistency, but patients should be seated as upright as possible to prevent aspiration. In conditions such as Parkinson or Alzheimer disease, the sense of smell diminishes, leading to decreased food intake. Unbalanced food intake also occurs in mental health conditions such as anorexia nervosa, mood disorders, anxiety, and depression.

Impaired digestion and absorption. Many conditions interfere with digestion or absorption and place the affected individual at risk for malnutrition. Examples of such conditions include lactose intolerance, gastroparesis, gastric surgery, intestinal resection, and inadequate gastric acidity. Some genetic conditions lead to defects in metabolism of nutrients, such as PKU (as described previously) or CF. Impaired digestion and absorption can also occur as an adverse effect from some medications.

Increased metabolic demand. A variety of conditions increase metabolic rate and energy needs, thus increasing the risk for protein–calorie malnutrition (PCM). Examples include cancer, chronic obstructive pulmonary disease, Parkinson disease, trauma, burns, stroke, and HIV/AIDS. Depending on the severity of the disease state, it may be difficult to meet the increased nutrient needs without enteral or parenteral nutrition support.

Altered organ function. The failure of organs involved in digestion and metabolism are associated with nutritional deficiencies. Hepatic disease adversely impacts the ability to reassemble amino acids into the various proteins needed for physiological function. A damaged liver

TABLE 16.3 Impact of Medical Conditions on Risk for Malnutrition

Medical Conditions or States	Impact on Nutritional Status
Oral/GI problems with limited protein–calorie intake (e.g., sensory issues, allergies, dental problems, dysphagia)	Hypoalbuminemia/ impaired protein nutrition
Impaired intestinal absorption of proteins (diarrhea/malabsorption: e.g., celiac disease, Crohn disease, short-bowel syndrome, bariatric surgery)	
Hepatic disease with impaired protein synthesis	
Chronic kidney disease with proteinuria	
Nephrotic syndrome	
Cancer with increased metabolic needs	
Burns with loss of protein in body fluids	Hypocalcemia
Hypoalbuminemia (lack of carrier proteins)	
Hyperphosphatemia (in chronic kidney disease, end stage)	
Malabsorption/diarrhea	
Hypoparathyroidism	
Hypomagnesemia	
Vitamin D deficiency	
Hyperparathyroidism	Hypercalcemia
Hyperthyroidism	
Adrenal insufficiency	
Cancer	
Hypervitaminosis A and D	
Wound healing protocol with excess supplementation of zinc	Copper deficiency anemia
GI bleed	Iron deficiency anemia/ microcytic anemia
Hemochromatosis	Iron overload
Hepatic disease	
Gastrectomy	Vitamin B_{12} deficiency
Pernicious anemia/lack of intrinsic factor	
Primary hypothyroidism	
Achlorhydria	
Epilepsy with use of antiseizure medications	Folic acid deficiency/ megaloblastic anemia
Chronic kidney disease (end stage) and dialysis treatments	
Edema/hypertension with K^+-depleting diuretics	Hypomagnesemia
Malabsorption/diarrhea	
Hepatic disease	
Pancreatitis	
Chronic kidney disease with limited ability to convert to active form	Vitamin D deficiency
Malabsorption	
Hypoalbuminemia	Zinc deficiency
Chronic kidney disease (end stage) and dialysis treatments	
Alcoholic cirrhosis/hepatic disease	
Inflammatory bowel disease	
Sickle cell anemia	

GI, Gastrointestinal.

TABLE 16.4   Interpreting Body Mass Index in Children and Adults

Age Group and Approach	BMI	Interpretation
Children (Percentile)	<5th	Underweight; may be acceptable if bone growth is adequate and child "follows the curve"; promote increased kilocalorie intake as needed if weight curve is declining.
BMI percentile for children: Apply calculated BMI (weight in pounds/ height in inches/height in inches × 703) to percentile growth chart (see http://www.cdc.gov/growthcharts)	5th to 85th	Optimal weight; still important to "follow the curve" and meet goals for bone growth.
	85th to 95th	Overweight; goal to prevent obesity without causing risk to bone growth or emotional development.
	≥95th	Childhood obesity; goal for young children is not to exceed percentile growth curve; promote physical activity and healthy eating to help "grow into weight."
Adults (Calculated BMI)	<19	Underweight; severe level <15 indicative of anorexia.
BMI calculated by weight in pounds/ height in inches/height in inches × 703	19–24.9	Optimal body weight composition; elderly persons should strive for BMI >21.
	25–29.9	Overweight; may be appropriate given health status.
	30–34.9	Class I obesity; slow weight loss advised to promote permanent weight loss; not appropriate for older populations to lose weight.[19-21]
	35–39.9	Class II obesity; slow weight loss advised; may be a candidate for bariatric surgery if comorbidities present and not able to achieve long-term weight loss through diet and exercise.
	≥40	Class III or "extreme" obesity (formerly known as morbid obesity); may be a candidate for bariatric surgery based on health status, age, and level of obesity and history of not being able to achieve long-term weight loss through diet and exercise.

BMI, Body mass index.

will also be unable to metabolize and excrete drugs properly, thus altering nutrient absorption and utilization even further. In chronic kidney disease (CKD), nutritional status is adversely impacted through a variety of mechanisms. Protein is lost through the urine and can lead to impaired skin integrity, slow wound healing, suppressed immunity, sarcopenia, and altered osmotic pressure. As CKD progresses, phosphorous levels can increase and lead to hypocalcemia. Renal disease further reduces nutrient levels, especially vitamin D because the kidney metabolizes vitamin D_2 into the bioactive D_3 form. With lowered vitamin D status, bone health is impacted because vitamin D is required to absorb calcium.

The kidneys are involved in producing red blood cells; therefore, in patients with CKD, an anemia can develop that is unresponsive to iron intake due to an insufficient level of erythropoietin, a protein-based hormone. Even nutrition therapy can have adverse nutritional consequences; limited fluid or food intake and phosphorus/protein/potassium restrictions can be challenging. This is especially true when CKD is compounded by an acute illness. Thus organ damage and illnesses can seriously impact nutritional status, as shown in Table 16.3.

ASSESSMENT

All nurses should know how to perform a basic assessment of nutritional status. Maintaining an awareness of the risk factors helps to focus the interview and examination.

History

In the interview of the patient or family members, it should be remembered that food has a strong emotional component. Actual food or eating practices may not be revealed unless there is trust and rapport. This is especially true when interviewing parents of a child whose growth and development are not within expected ranges. In general, adults respond more openly to health providers if they are aware of the rationale for the questions. Mentioning some potential nutritional complications of a condition, or asking about the individual's personal health concerns, allows for focused interviewing.

The basic elements of this form of history include nutritional intake, diet restrictions, changes in appetite and intake, changes in weight, medical history, current medical conditions, current medications and treatments, allergies, family history, and social history. In addition, it

is important to consider the chief complaint/presenting symptoms because they might relate to nutrition and may warrant closer analysis. The most important screening problems or presenting symptoms include the following: unplanned changes in weight, changes in appetite or intake, nausea and/or vomiting, difficulty chewing or swallowing, abdominal pain or discomfort, changes in bowel habits, and recent history of prolonged constipation or diarrhea.

Examination Findings

Several techniques are used to assess nutritional status, including general observation, anthropometric measurements, and other various clinical findings from systems' assessment. Measuring actual height and weight and determining BMI are the initial steps in assessing nutritional status. General goals and interpretation guidelines for BMI are presented in Table 16.4. If BMI is within normal limits and weight has been stable, it is still important to have at least a brief assessment of oral intake to verify that macronutrients and micronutrients are being consumed in appropriate amounts. If there is any suspicion of poor nutritional status, lab work should be ordered by the attending provider to help assess status more completely.

General physical appearance, level of orientation, and demeanor will give insight into health and nutritional status. Assess skin integrity and turgor. The skin should be smooth and elastic without cracks or bruising. The hair should be shiny and not brittle. Nail beds should be smooth, pink, and firm. The teeth should be free of cavities, and oral tissues should be moist, pink, and firm. Mucous membranes around the eyes should be pink, moist, and free of lesions; the sclera should be white. The cornea should be clear and shiny.

Diagnostic Tests

Nurses need to understand common nutrition-related tests, and they need to know when to alert the physician or dietitian if malnutrition is suspected.

Laboratory Tests

Serum albumin, prealbumin, and C-reactive protein. Serum albumin measures circulating protein in the blood. Low albumin can reflect protein-calorie malnutrition. However, other conditions (such as chronic or acute inflammation, blood loss, altered fluid status) can also cause low serum albumin levels. Elevated high-sensitive C-reactive protein (hsCRP) is useful for identifying inflammation in conjunction with low serum albumin.

Very low albumin levels indicate severity of illness and are also predictors of mortality in adults older than age 60 years.[15] Prealbumin reflects recent dietary protein intake. Thus low prealbumin is more closely related to nutritional status than albumin is.

Blood glucose and hemoglobin A_{1c}. Blood glucose reflects metabolism of carbohydrates, and this test is generally used to screen or monitor impaired glucose metabolism. Hypoglycemia may suggest inadequate caloric intake and hyperglycemia may be an indication of diabetes mellitus or an acute illness. Hemoglobin A_{1c} is a test that shows average blood glucose levels over time and is used in the management of diabetic patients. It indicates how well glucose levels are controlled. Note that for anemia of renal disease, false readings of the A_{1c} level may occur; finger-stick glucose tests may be more reliable in these situations.

Lipid profile. A lipid profile includes several tests that assess lipid metabolism. Tests included are low-density lipoprotein (LDL), high-density lipoprotein (HDL), cholesterol, and triglycerides. High triglyceride levels generally reflect hyperinsulinemia, although an individual with newly diagnosed type 1 diabetes may have temporary elevations.

Electrolytes. Electrolytes provide information about general health status and specific information about sodium, potassium, calcium, magnesium, and phosphorus. These are usually ordered as part of a chemistry profile blood test. Electrolytes can become imbalanced with inadequate dietary intake or many other conditions, such as renal disease, liver disease, and diabetes. See the Fluid and Electrolytes concept for further information.

Hemoglobin and hematocrit. Hemoglobin (Hgb) and hematocrit (Hct) is a blood test that examines red blood cells (including the number, size, shape, and color) to diagnose anemia caused by dietary deficiency, such as iron, folate, and vitamin B_{12}. Hgb and Hct also provide information about the hydration status of the patient.

CLINICAL MANAGEMENT

Primary Prevention

Primary prevention measures are aimed at preventing the onset of disease through risk reduction and behavior modification. The foundation of primary prevention efforts, as it relates to this concept, includes healthy eating and physical activity.

Healthy Eating

A person who follows the current *Dietary Guidelines for Americans* and MyPlate (see ChooseMyPlate.gov) can achieve a healthy diet. The inclusion of the minimum number of servings in MyPlate will meet the DRI micronutrient and macronutrient needs for general health needs. The *Dietary Guidelines* are aimed more at preventing chronic health diseases associated with excess intake of macronutrients, especially solid fats (saturated/trans fats), sugar, and salt. Food labels with DRI values reinforce the Dietary Guidelines. Food labels include four marker nutrients: calcium, iron, vitamin A, and vitamin C. In general, if these micronutrients are included in adequate amounts from foods naturally high in them, the other key micronutrients will also be obtained.

Exclusive breast-feeding is recommended for optimal nutrition of infants for the first 4 to 6 months of life. Breast milk contains all the essential nutrients and has immunologic benefits that protect the infant from acute and chronic disease.

Physical Activity

Physical activity helps to prevent obesity. The general goals include 30 minutes of physical activity on most days of the week or 150 or more minutes weekly. Weight loss may require at least twice this amount of exercise. However, guidelines for exercise need to be individualized. A sedentary person or one who has sarcopenia or cardiovascular disease needs limited intervals of exercise more frequently.

Secondary Prevention (Screening)

Secondary prevention involves screening tests to detect disease. Screening for nutritional status in the general population is limited primarily to lipid screening, blood glucose screening, and BMI. Blood glucose screening is advised for persons with evidence of insulin resistance, such as central obesity found with metabolic syndrome. Lipid screening is recommended for those with specific risk factors. Although not an essential nutrient, it often becomes necessary to supplement coenzyme Q10 with long-term statin use.

For infants, routine screening that occurs at birth includes the following: glucose levels; at least 40 different genetically linked metabolic disorders, including PKU and maple syrup urine disease; carbohydrate disorders, including galactosemia; other congenital disorders that can affect nutritional status, including cystic fibrosis; and HIV. The number of screenings will vary from state to state.

Collaborative Interventions

There are several interventions for nurses to manage individuals who have nutrition-related health conditions. Interventions are classified into the following groups: dietary interventions, pharmacologic agents, and surgical interventions. Coordination of care often involves working with the registered dietitian-nutritionist (RDN), with home care services, or with a community agency (e.g., referral to Meals-On-Wheels for home-delivered meal services). Discharge planning is an essential team effort on behalf of the patient.

CLINICAL NURSING SKILLS RELATED TO NUTRITION

Assessment
- Physical signs of malnutrition
- Weight and height records—accuracy, frequency; scale calibrations

Education: Basic nutrition and modified diet guidance

Feeding-dependent patient assistance
- Dysphagia management
- Hydration, intake–output records
- Nursing assistant training

Nutrition support
- Enteral nutrition: Tube feedings
  - Nasogastric tube
  - Gastrostomy tube
  - Jejunostomy tube
- Parenteral nutrition

Nourishment administration
- Documentation

Red flags: Referral to the registered dietitian–nutritionist
- Pressure ulcers, weight loss
- Inadequate oral intake or changes in appetite
- NPO, nausea or vomiting >3 days

Dietary Interventions

As part of the healthcare team, nurses often work with other health professionals for optimal nutritional outcomes. *Registered dietitian-nutritionists* are health professionals who have a background in biochemistry and metabolism, with knowledge about the macronutrient and micronutrient contents of foods and how the body uses them. Another health professional, the *dietetic technician*, assists the RDN with menu planning, nutrition education, and management of food services. Nutrition therapy is a term used to describe the typical services of the RDN or registered dietetic technician, whereas "medical nutrition therapy (MNT)" is a legal term for reimbursable services provided by the RDN.

The nutrition care process includes documentation with standardized language and codes established for the dietetics professional. Complex assessments, nutrition diagnosing, and diet therapy interventions are the role of the RDN. A qualified RDN may have diet order-writing privileges as determined by competency assessment, licensure laws, and facility protocols. Thus the RDN can adjust a patient's meal plan so that it is appropriate for health goals, realistic, economical, and feasible for the family. Nurses should understand basic modified diets to reinforce messages provided by the RDN and encourage referrals as needed.

The concept of *personalized nutrition* is replacing the old paradigm that "one diet fits all" through the science of nutrigenomics—in other words, how genetics will influence nutritional interventions. Individuals differ in how nutrients are assimilated, metabolized, stored, and excreted; these differences are often significant. Further, individualized dietary plans are needed to address unique dietary needs of patients based on their age, calorie needs, and underlying health condition. For example, not all hypertensive individuals respond to sodium (salt) restriction, not all individuals with high serum cholesterol levels respond to a low saturated fat diet, and sugar alone is not the culprit in diabetes management.

Another aspect of dietary interventions is ensuring that the food provided matches the patient's ability to eat. A patient who has his or her original teeth (none missing) and good oral hygiene, or well-fitting dentures plus adequate saliva, represents the ideal patient who can chew all kinds of foods. Unfortunately, many hospitalized or aging patients require assistance because they have missing teeth or ill-fitting dentures. Nurses can make note of these concerns early in treatment so that diets may be altered or oral health services can be provided.

Enteral Nutrition

Nurses administer nutrition support via tube feedings. Tube feedings are indicated for an individual who is unable to eat or swallow but has an intact/functional GI tract. Feeding tubes are inserted directly into the stomach (gastrostomy) or small intestine (jejunostomy) for the delivery of enteral feedings. A specific formula is selected by the physician and RDN based on patient needs. In some hospitals, the RDN may be qualified to write the diet orders or even to insert the tube. The tube feeding is administered either by gravity or through a feeding pump.

A common procedure is a percutaneous endoscopic gastrostomy (PEG) feeding. A PEG tube requires a small incision into the stomach. Fortunately, the procedure is relatively safe, simple, and reversible. Although unused formula must be discarded after 24 hours, the tubes can be maintained longer with strict infection control procedures according to facility protocols.

Parenteral Nutrition

Parenteral nutrition is used to provide either total or supplemental nutrition intravenously. These intravenous feedings are generally used for patients who have intestinal failure and cannot be fed orally or by enteral feeding. Here, nutrition consists of a glucose-based intravenous solution (various dextrose concentrations) with electrolytes, minerals, and amino acids. Fat emulsions (lipids) may also be included or administered as a separate solution.

Because parenteral nutrition is indicated for individuals who are unable to process nutrients via the GI tract for more than 4 or 5 days, therapy can be short term or long term. For short term, it may be administered peripherally, whereas for long term, it can be administered centrally. Sepsis and electrolyte and metabolic imbalances can occur; thus meticulous nursing care of the vascular access is required.

Excessive infusion of enteral or parenteral nutrition solutions can be dangerous. The critically ill patient is vulnerable because metabolic shifts occur throughout each day from sepsis and various procedures. Ideally, indirect calorimetry is used to determine energy needs so overfeeding can be avoided. Extra caution should be used in pediatric and neonatal units.

Surgical Interventions

The most common surgical intervention affecting nutrition is bariatric surgery. It is increasingly being used to control obesity and diabetes. In general, bariatric surgery has demonstrated good success for weight loss, improved glucose level, and normalized blood pressure. However, complications include macro- and micronutrient deficiencies that are not easily managed, either because of lack of adherence to dietary and supplement guidelines or because of limited knowledge of actual needs.[16] In addition, weight gain can occur if the patient is noncompliant with calorie control. The most malabsorptive bariatric surgical procedure is the Roux-en-Y gastric bypass. In this procedure, most of the stomach and the proximal small intestine are bypassed, with food entering a Y-shaped reconnection between the upper stomach and the distal portion of the duodenum or jejunum. Lap-band procedures are much less invasive, although nutritional deficits are still possible.

Pharmacologic Agents

Many supplements are available to enhance the nutritional status of individuals, and most are available over the counter. Supplement examples include vitamin supplements (e.g., multivitamins, niacin, B vitamins, and vitamin C), mineral supplements (e.g., iron and calcium folic acid), and protein and nutrient supplements (Ensure, nutrition bars, enhanced puddings, even coffees).

For the use of pharmacologic agents in obesity management, research continues. There have been complications with previous forms of weight loss medications, and currently these medications have limitations on duration of use. Statins (e.g., atorvastatin, fluvastatin, lovastatin, pravastatin, and rosuvastatin) are the drugs of choice for treatment of lipid and cholesterol reduction because of their ability to inhibit the synthesis of cholesterol, leading to reductions in LDL and HDL. There are a variety of pharmacologic agents that address other nutrient-based problems, including dietary supplements, statins to control lipid levels, and agents to control glucose levels (see Concept 15, Glucose Regulation).

INTERRELATED CONCEPTS

Nutrition is interrelated with nearly all the health and illness concepts as a preventive or disease management intervention. In addition, nutrition has an interrelated role with many body functions, as presented in Fig. 16.3. **Glucose Regulation** (closely linked to **Hormonal Regulation**) is dependent on caloric intake and is critical to adequate metabolism of nutrients; glucose regulation is much like a subconcept of nutrition. Nutrition influences other metabolic processes, such as **Immunity**, **Tissue Integrity**, and **Thermoregulation**; these all depend on adequate nutrients for optimal functioning. **Development**, **Culture**, and **Spirituality** are also interrelated based on the influence of these concepts on dietary patterns, religious observances, rituals, and preferences.

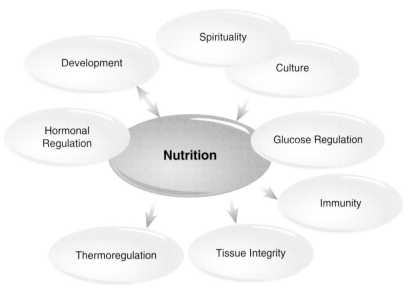

FIGURE 16.3 Nutrition and Interrelated Concepts.

BOX 16.1 EXEMPLARS OF IMPAIRED NUTRITION

Conditions Associated with Insufficient Nutrition
- Anorexia nervosa
- Bulimia
- Fat malabsorption syndrome
- Iron deficiency anemia
- Protein–calorie malnutrition
- Vitamin deficiencies (A, B-complex, C, D, K)
- Zinc deficiency

Conditions Associated with Excessive Nutrition
- Obesity
- Hyperlipidemia
- Obesity-related conditions
  - Metabolic syndrome
  - Type 2 diabetes mellitus
  - Heart diseases
  - Stroke
  - Hypertension
  - Colon and hormonal cancers (prostate, breast)

Conditions Associated with Altered Digestion/ Metabolism
- Lactose intolerance
- Celiac disease
- Gastroesophageal reflux
- Phenylketonuria

 ACCESS EXEMPLAR LINKS IN YOUR GIDDENS EBOOK

CLINICAL EXEMPLARS

Clinical exemplars of nutrition represent conditions associated with insufficient nutrition and excessive nutrition. Although it is beyond the scope of this concept to list all possible conditions that have a link to nutrition, Box 16.1 presents common exemplars seen in clinical practice. A brief discussion of a few common clinical exemplars follows. For detailed explanations and the nursing care for exemplars, see nutrition, medical–surgical, pediatric, and gerontology textbooks.

Featured Exemplars
Protein–Calorie Malnutrition
Protein–calorie malnutrition refers to an extended state of insufficient protein and calorie intake. Protein–calorie malnutrition is one of the most common nutritional deficiency conditions associated with insufficient intake, wasting disease, or a combination of both, and it has multisystem effects. This can affect individuals of all ages, but it especially affects patients with extended hospitalization with acute illness or injury or the institutionalized elderly. Among children, protein–calorie deficiencies are serious concerns because of the potential for delays in cognitive and physical development. Protein–calorie malnutrition is characterized by muscle wasting, loss of subcutaneous fat, and protein deficiency.

Anorexia Nervosa
Anorexia nervosa is one of a group of psychiatric conditions associated with a fear of weight gain and distortion of body image. It is character-ized by an avoidance of food consumption often combined with excessive exercise with the intent to lose weight. Untreated, patients with anorexia nervosa experience extreme weight loss and muscle wasting, represent-ing a condition of insufficient nutrition. This condition is most common among adolescent females, but it is seen in both genders and can occur in childhood and adulthood.

Celiac Disease
Celiac disease is an autoimmune disorder, whereby an inflammatory reaction occurs in the intestine when the mucosa is exposed to gluten, a protein found in wheat, rye, and barley. Among the most commonly reported symptoms are abdominal discomfort, bloating, diarrhea, and nausea. A long-term consequence of untreated celiac disease involves dietary deficiencies due to malabsorption of nutrients. It is diagnosed based on the presence of flattened villi, as well as specific antibodies in the blood.

Less severe forms of gluten sensitivity have fewer symptoms, but there is still an autoimmune response to the grain proteins that requires a strict gluten-free diet. One consequence of not following the diet includes non-Hodgkin lymphoma, later in life. Because true celiac disease has a serious prognosis, it is important that a medical diagnosis distinguishes between the disease and the sensitivity so that a lifelong strict diet can prevent comorbidities.[17] The use of a gluten-free diet for weight loss in healthy individuals is not advisable, as it leads to malnutrition.

Obesity

The most common form of excessive nutrition, obesity occurs when there is a chronically high intake of calories. Obesity is multifactorial and can include overeating, inactivity, and genetics. Obesity is associated with systemic, chronic low-grade inflammation and conditions related to the metabolic syndrome.[18] Consequences such as type 2 diabetes, heart disease, and stroke affect individuals of all ages and can lead to medical complications or a shortened lifespan. It is estimated that more than 66% of the U.S. population (including adults and children) is classified as overweight or obese. Overweight is defined as having a BMI greater than 25; obesity is associated with a BMI greater than 30, or being more than 20% over ideal body weight.

Hyperlipidemia

Another example of excess nutrition is hyperlipidemia, characterized by an elevation of serum lipids (cholesterol, triglycerides, and/or phospholipids). Individuals are thought to have a genetic predisposition to hyperlipidemia. Hyperlipidemia primarily affects adults but can occur associated with chronic inflammation and even with childhood obesity.

CASE STUDY

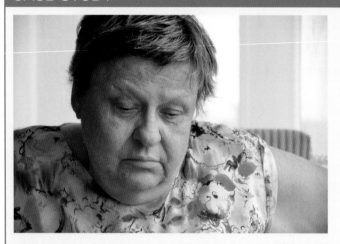

Case Presentation

Mary Williams is a 62-year-old female who is 5'4" and weight 223 lbs. Mary has stage 4 CKD, poorly controlled type 2 diabetes, and class II obesity. She was "chunky" as a child and adolescent, with a lifetime habit of having consumed a relatively high-fat, high-calorie diet. As she recalls, her entire family was overweight, and she believed she had little control over the obesity.

After marriage, she gained excess weight with each of her three pregnancies and was never able to lose all the weight. Throughout her career, she worked as a legal assistant. She spent most of her free time watching her children do various activities or watching television, and she freely admits she has not really exercised since high school.

Following the death of her husband 5 months ago, Mary moved into a one-bedroom apartment within a long-term senior healthcare center. Soon after moving to her new residence, she experienced acute heart failure, which was subsequently resolved. She was also told by her physician that her kidneys were "on the verge of failing." The episode of acute heart failure and the realization that she could have renal failure frightened Mary, so she has become very engaged in her care, making an effort to follow medical recommendations.

She has met with a registered dietitian nutritionist who has devised a specific nutrition therapy plan for Mary. As part of the plan Mary has been advised to follow a controlled carbohydrate diet with a protein limit of 1 g of protein/kg and moderate intake of sodium, potassium, and phosphorus. She was also switched to a basal/bolus insulin regimen. She takes insulin at mealtimes based on the percentage of meal intake corresponding to the insulin-to-carbohydrate ratio. For 3 months, she has successfully adhered to the treatment strategies, maintaining optimal blood glucose levels, meeting dietary goals, and maintaining a stable weight.

Case Analysis Questions

1. Consider the scope of the concept nutrition. Where does this case fit within the scope of Nutrition?
2. In her history profile, it is mentioned that Mary has class II obesity. What does this mean, and how was it determined that she has class II obesity?
3. Based on this case, what physiological consequences is Mary experiencing as a result of her nutritional state?
4. How does the clinical management strategies outlined in Mary's case compare to those presented in the concept? Are there other strategies that might be helpful to Mary?

From berna namoglu/iStock/Thinkstock.

 ACCESS EXEMPLAR LINKS IN YOUR GIDDENS EBOOK

REFERENCES

1. Herrman, K., & Carroll, K. (2014). An exclusively human milk diet reduces necrotizing enterocolitis. *Breastfeeding Medicine: The Official Journal of the Academy of Breastfeeding Medicine, 9*(4), 184–190.
2. Su, B. H. (2014). Optimizing nutrition in preterm infants. *Pediatrics and Neonatology, 55*(1), 5–13.
3. Martone, A. M., Onder, G., Vetrano, G. L., et al. (2013). Anorexia of aging: A modifiable risk factor for frailty. *Nutrients, 5*(10), 4126–4133.
4. Wang, Y. F., Tang, Z., Tao, L. X., et al. (2017). BMI and BMI Changes to all-cause mortality among the elderly in Beijing: A 20-year cohort study. *Biomedical and Environmental Sciences, 30*(2), 79–87.
5. Wirth, R., Smoliner, C., & Jager, M. (2013). Guideline clinical nutrition in patients with stroke. *Experimental & Translational Stroke Medicine, 5*(1), 14.
6. Collins, J., Bertrand, B., Hayes, V., et al. (2013). The application of genetics and nutritional genomics in practice: An international survey of knowledge, involvement and confidence among dietitians in the US, Australia, and the UK. *Genes & Nutrition, 8*(6), 523–533.
7. Batai, K., Murphy, A. B., Shah, E., et al. (2014). Common vitamin D pathway gene variants reveal contrasting effects on serum vitamin D levels in African Americans and European Americans. *Human Genetics, 133*(11), 1395–1405.
8. Taksler, G. B., Cutler, D. M., Giovanucci, E. L., et al. (2015). Vitamin D deficiency in minority populations. *Public Health Nutrition, 18*(3), 379–391.
9. Hollingworth, S., Walker, K., Page, A., et al. (2013). Pharmacoepidemiology and the Australian regional prevalence of multiple sclerosis. *Multiple Sclerosis (Houndmills, Basingstoke, England), 19*(13), 1712–1716.
10. Ghosh-Dastidar, B., Cohen, D., Hunter, G., et al. (2014). Distance to store, food prices, and obesity in urban food deserts. *American Journal of Preventive Medicine, 47*(5), 587–595.

11. Bevelander, K. E., Anshutz, D. J., Creemers, D. H., et al. (2013). The role of explicit and implicit self-esteem in peer modeling of palatable food intake: A study on social media interaction among youngsters. *PLoS ONE, 8*(8), 72481.

12. Orloff, N. C., & Hormes, J. M. (2014). Pickles and ice cream! Food cravings in pregnancy: Hypotheses, preliminary evidence, and directions for future research. *Frontiers in Psychology, 23*(5), 1076.

13. Demir, N., Koc, A., Ustoyl, L., et al. (2013). Clinical and neurological findings of severe vitamin B_{12} deficiency in infancy and importance of early diagnosis and treatment. *Journal of Paediatrics and Child Health, 49*(10), 820–824.

14. Le, L. T., & Sabate, J. (2014). Beyond meatless, the health effects of vegan diets: Findings from the Adventist cohorts. *Nutrients, 6*(6), 2131–2147.

15. Hannan, J. L., Radwany, S. M., & Albanese, T. (2012). In-hospital mortality in patients older than 60 years with very low albumin levels. *Journal of Pain and Symptom Management, 43*(3), 631–637.

16. Freeland-Graves, J. H., Lee, J. J., Mousa, T. Y., et al. (2014). Patients at risk for trace element deficiencies: Bariatric surgery. *Journal of Trace Elements in Medicine and Biology: Organ of the Society for Minerals and Trace Elements (GMS), 28*(4), 495–503.

17. Leonard, M. M., Sapone, A., Catassi, C., & Fasano, A. (2017). Celiac disease and nonceliac gluten sensitivity: A review. *JAMA: The Journal of the American Medical Association, 318*(7), 647–656.

18. Everard, A., & Cani, P. D. (2013). Diabetes, obesity and gut microbiota. *Best Practice & Research. Clinical Gastroenterology, 27*(1), 73–83.

19. Parto, P., & Lavie, C. J. (2017). Obesity and cardiovascular diseases. *Current Problems in Cardiology, 42*(11), 376–394.

20. Zanni, G. R., & Wick, J. Y. (2011). Treating obesity in older adults: Different risks, different goals, different strategies. *The Consultant Pharmacist: The Journal of the American Society of Consultant Pharmacists, 26*(3), 142–148, 153–154.

21. Chapman, I. M. (2011). Weight loss in older persons. *The Medical Clinics of North America, 95*(3), 579–593.

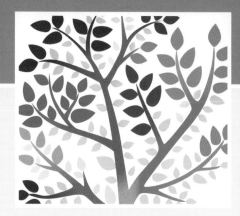

Elimination

Jean Giddens

Elimination is a concept that has various applications across multiple disciplines, including mathematics, economics, chemistry, and biology. From a biological perspective, elimination is a concept applicable to all living organisms—from the smallest of microbes to plants, animals, and humans. This concept presentation focuses on elimination as a physiological concept, as it applies to humans and includes normal or expected elimination patterns and problems associated with elimination.

DEFINITION

Broadly speaking, the term *elimination* refers to the removal, clearance, or separation of matter. From a human physiological perspective, the term elimination is defined as *the excretion of waste products.*[1] The human body eliminates various forms of waste through the skin, kidneys, lungs, and intestines. This concept presentation focuses on elimination of waste from the urinary system and the gastrointestinal system. For the purposes of this concept presentation, bowel elimination is defined as *the process of expelling stool* (also referred to as feces). Terms used to describe the process of bowel elimination include defecation, defecate, or bowel movement. Urinary elimination is defined as *the process of expelling urine.* Terms used to describe this process include *micturition* or *urination.* The term *continence* refers to the purposeful control of urinary or fecal elimination.

   Impaired elimination refers to one or more problems associated with the elimination process. There are many terms associated with impaired urinary elimination including *anuria* (absence of urine), *dysuria* (painful urination), *polyuria* (multiple episodes of urination, as with diabetes), urinary *frequency* (multiple episodes of urination with little urine produced in a short period of time), and urinary *hesitancy* (the urge to urinate exists, but the person has difficulty starting the urine stream).

SCOPE

The scope of this concept includes the normal or expected physiological process of waste formation and excretion by the gastrointestinal and renal systems as well as problems associated with this process (Fig. 17.1). Each of these body systems are complex and differ significantly from an anatomical and physiological perspective. The kidneys are responsible for the removal of metabolic waste and other elements from the blood in the form of urine, and gastrointestinal tract is responsible for the removal of digestive waste in the form of stool.

Despite these differences, similarities are clear when considering this from a conceptual lens. In both systems, the process involves the formation and excretion of waste. The scope of this concept also includes impairment of urinary and bowel elimination, representing a wide range of problems and conditions.

NORMAL PHYSIOLOGICAL PROCESS

Because of the significant differences between urinary and bowel elimination, an overview of the normal physiological process for each is presented separately.

Normal Urinary Elimination

Urinary elimination involves the process of waste formation (production of urine) and the excretion of urine involving several specific structures. The kidneys, ureters, bladder, and urethra must all function adequately for normal urination to occur.

Formation of Urine

The removal of metabolic waste from the blood by the urinary system represents an essential process needed to maintain physiologic homeostasis and regulation. The main functional unit of the kidneys is the nephron; each kidney has more than 1 million nephrons. Each nephron is composed of two parts—blood vessels and renal tubules. Optimal physiological effect depends on continuous perfusion of a large volume of blood (an average of 1 L/min) to the kidneys and functioning nephrons.

   The formation of urine is complex and involves three main processes: glomerular filtration, tubular reabsorption, and tubular secretion. Blood enters the kidney through the renal artery, which then branches into progressively smaller arteries, arterioles, and finally to a cluster of capillaries known as the glomerulus (Fig. 17.2). The glomerulus is a semipermeable membrane that serves to filter blood into a C-shaped structure of the renal tubule known as the Bowman capsule. This process *(glomerular filtration)* represents the beginning of urine formation.

   The filtrate contains water, electrolytes, and waste that have been removed from the blood. As the filtrate passes through a sequence of renal tubules (from the Bowman capsule to the proximal convoluted tubule, the loop of Henle, and the distal convoluted tubule; see Fig. 17.2), a network of capillaries surrounding the renal tubules reabsorb most of the water, electrolytes, and other necessary elements back into

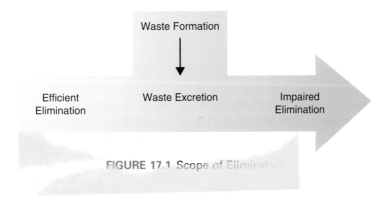

FIGURE 17.1 Scope of Elimination.

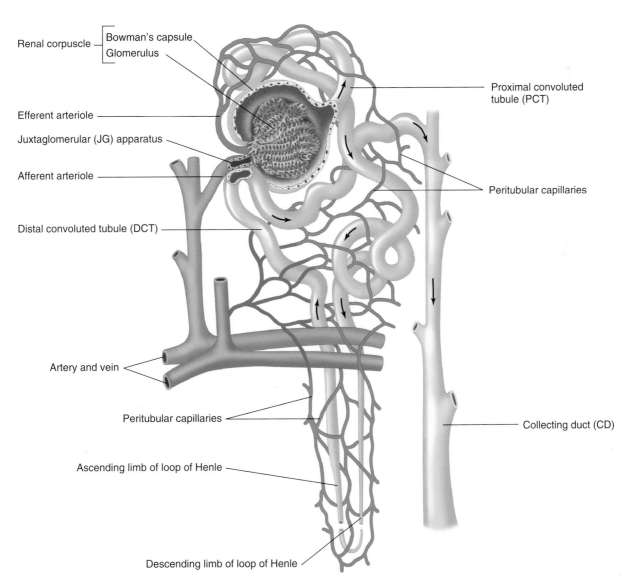

FIGURE 17.2 The Nephron. (Modified from Patton, K. T., & Thibodeau, G. A. [2014]. *The human body in health and disease* [6th ed.]. St Louis: Mosby.)

the blood. This process is referred to as *tubular reabsorption*. The third process, *tubular secretion*, involves a secondary process for small amounts of select substances (e.g., potassium, hydrogen, ammonia, and drugs) to be moved from the blood in the capillaries surrounding the tubules into the tubules. The amount of water and electrolytes reabsorbed into the blood or excreted in the renal tubules is controlled by several hormones, particularly aldosterone, antidiuretic hormone, parathyroid hormone, renin, and atrial natriuretic factor.

Excretion of Urine

Urine formed in the renal tubules moves into the collecting duct and then into the renal pelvis, the ureter, and the bladder, where it is stored until urination occurs (Fig. 17.3). The bladder holds approximately 300 to 500 mL in adults (much less volume in children) before the pressure stimulates stretch receptors in the bladder wall. The stretch receptors send nerve impulse through the spinal cord to signal the need for urination. An internal sphincter, composed of smooth muscle, contracts involuntarily to prevent urine from leaking out of the bladder. The external sphincter, located just below the internal sphincter and surrounding the upper part of the urethra, is composed of skeletal muscle and is voluntarily controlled. Thus the process of urination involves a series of nerve signals between the bladder and spinal cord to trigger the micturition reflex; this causes the internal sphincter muscles to relax and bladder wall contraction. With the voluntary relaxation of the external urinary sphincter, urine passes out of the body through the urethra. The external urinary sphincter must be under the individual's control in order for urinary control (continence) to be successful.

Normal Bowel Elimination
Digestion and the Formation of Stool

The gastrointestinal system has two overarching functions: the breakdown and absorption of nutrients from foods ingested and the elimination

of waste from this process. The gastrointestinal system extends from the esophagus to the anus. The first part of the gastrointestinal tract (esophagus, stomach, and small intestines) is involved in the digestion and absorption of nutrients, a process that also involves other digestive organs, including the liver, gallbladder, and pancreas (Fig. 17.4). The digestive process is described further in Concept 16, Nutrition.

The process of waste formation occurs in the colon. The waste product, known as stool or feces, are comprised of water, bile, undigested food matter, unabsorbed mineral, bacteria, mucous, and epithelial cells

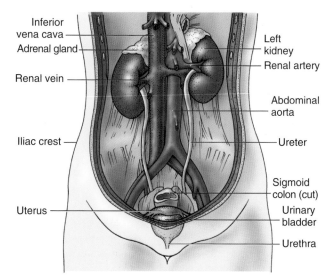

FIGURE 17.3 Urinary Elimination. (From Ignatavicius, D. D., & Workman, M. L. [2013]. *Medical surgical nursing: Patient-centered collaborative care* [7 ed.]. St. Louis: Elsevier.)

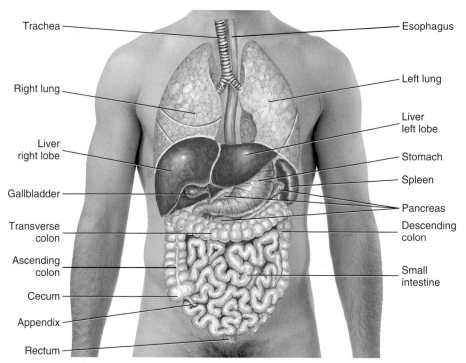

FIGURE 17.4 The Gastrointestinal Tract. (From Wilson, S., & Giddens, J. [2017]. *Health assessment for nursing practice* [6th ed.]. St Louis: Elsevier.)

from the lining of the intestines. Smooth muscles within the intestinal tract stimulate peristalsis, which helps move the fecal matter through the gastrointestinal tract. The large intestine, which is 5 or 6 feet long and approximately 2 inches in diameter, has four parts: the cecum (and appendix), the colon, the rectum, and the anus (see Fig. 17.4). The function of the large intestine is to absorb water and electrolytes as fecal matter moves through its walls. Mucus in the intestine helps lubricate the walls and aids in the expulsion of the stool. If there is excessive peristalsis and the stool moves through the large intestine quickly, less water is absorbed, resulting in a loose stool. If the peristalsis is reduced, feces pass through the large intestine slowly, resulting in greater absorption of water and a harder stool.[2]

Elimination of Stool

The process of expelling stool is referred to as defecation, which is a reflexive action involving both voluntary and involuntary control. When the stool reaches the rectum, pressure stimulates parasympathetic nerve fibers in the sacral aspect of the spinal cord, which then produces contraction of the rectum with a relaxation of the internal anal sphincter. These actions result in an urge to defecate. The urge to defecate can be suppressed until the person is in an appropriate environment. At that time, the individual voluntarily relaxes the external anal sphincter to allow passage of the stool.

Age-Related Differences
Infants, Toddlers, and Children
Patterns of elimination change in the first few years of life. Infants and toddlers initially lack control over the sphincters and muscles that control urination and bowel elimination, but control is attained during early childhood as a normal developmental milestone. Children are typically 18 to 24 months of age before they are able to identify the urge to urinate and defecate.[3] Toilet training by the parent or caregiver helps the child obtain conscious control of his or her bowel and bladder functions. Most children are ready for "potty training" between ages two and three.[2]

Pregnant Women
Pregnancy can affect elimination patterns because the fetus in the abdominal cavity affects both bowel and bladder function. As the fetus grows, increased pressure is placed on the bladder, and frequent urination is required. The woman will have larger volumes of urine because she has a larger blood volume during the gestation. The growing fetus can also interfere with intestinal peristalsis and can cause constipation. The use of prenatal vitamins with iron can also contribute to constipation in the pregnant female.[4]

Older Adults
A number of physiological changes associated with aging affect elimination. By age 80 years, renal blood flow reduces to an estimated 600 mL/min, and the kidneys lose up to 50% of functioning nephrons for a variety of reasons, including changes in size of the kidney and sclerosis. In the absence of disease, this does not change the older adult's ability to produce urine sufficiently to maintain normal composition of body fluids, although it represents reduced renal reserve, making the older adult more susceptible to fluid and electrolyte imbalances and kidney damage due to medications. Although the bladder retains tone with age, the volume of urine that can be held reduces, leading to urinary frequency. In many older adults, muscles around the urethra become weak, thus increasing the risk of incontinence.

Age-related changes affecting bowel elimination include atrophy of smooth muscle layers in the colon and reduced mucous secretions. Reduced tone of the internal and external sphincter as well as reduced neural impulses (reducing the sensation of bowel evacuation) can make the older adult more susceptible to constipation or incontinence.

VARIATIONS AND CONTEXT

Alterations in elimination can occur with urinary or gastrointestinal function and represent a wide spectrum of problems. Most problems and conditions can be grouped by common themes and include incontinence, retention, discomfort, infections and inflammation, neoplasms, and organ failure.

Control
The ability to control the elimination of urine and stool is an important physiologic function. The term *incontinence* refers to the loss of control of either urine or bowel elimination. Control issues arise as a result of undeveloped elimination mechanisms, malfunctions in the mechanism of elimination, alterations in cognition, or with significant urge and the inability to access a bathroom. Nearly all individuals experience either fecal or urinary incontinence during their lifetime. Individuals who are incontinent are at risk for skin breakdown (particularly if bedridden) and can potentially experience changes in daily activities, functional activities, and social relationships.

Urinary incontinence is a disruption in the storage or emptying of the bladder with involuntary release of urine usually associated with dysfunction of the external and/or internal urinary sphincters.[5] It can range from light urine leakage when coughing or laughing (stress incontinence) to full loss of continence. Factors affecting urinary incontinence may be psychological or physical, such as depression, anxiety, cognitive impairments, or acute injury or surgical procedures.[6,7] Types of urinary incontinence are listed in Table 17.1.

Fecal incontinence is the involuntary passage of stool and ranges from an occasional leakage of stool while passing gas (flatus) to a complete loss of bowel control. Fecal incontinence most commonly occurs with diarrhea, particularly when it is associated with forceful intestinal peristalsis (cramping). Complete fecal incontinence occurs with the loss of sphincter control—usually as a result of traumatic injury, pathologic changes to the rectum, or neurologic injury. Fecal incontinence also can occur as a result of cognitive changes.[8,9]

TABLE 17.1	Types of Urinary Incontinence
Type of Incontinence	**Description**
Stress	Leakage of small amounts of urine during physical movement (coughing, sneezing, exercising)
Urge	Leakage of large amounts of urine at unexpected times, including during sleep
Overactive bladder	Urinary frequency and urgency, with or without urge incontinence
Functional	Untimely urination because of physical disability, external obstacles, or cognitive problems that prevent person from reaching toilet
Overflow	Unexpected leakage of small amounts of urine because of full bladder
Mixed	Usually occurrence of stress and urge incontinence together
Transient	Leakage that occurs temporarily because of a situation that will pass (infection, taking a new medication, colds with coughing)

Retention

Retention refers to the unintentional retention of urine or stool. Retention problems can occur at any age. The primary mechanisms causing retention are usually associated with obstructions, inflammation, or ineffective neuromuscular activation within the bladder or the gastrointestinal tract.

Urinary retention occurs as either incomplete emptying of the bladder after urination or a complete inability to urinate and is caused by a number of factors. Incomplete emptying can occur due to malfunction in nervous system innervation to the bladder or mechanical change in the shape of the bladder that causes retention.[10] For example, women may experience urinary retention if there is hard stool that presses against the bladder or rectoceles or cystoceles that cause prolapse of the bladder and trapping of urine. Retention can also occur when an obstruction blocks the passage of urine (e.g., an enlarged prostate) or when the external sphincter of the bladder does not relax, allowing the urine to be expelled from the bladder. Medications that may cause urinary retention include antidepressants, anticholinergics, and antihistamines.[11] Postoperative patients may have problems with urinary elimination as a result of the effects of anesthetics or the use of catheters during the surgical procedure. Psychosocial factors (e.g., fear or anxiety) may also affect the ability to successfully void.

Retention of stool occurs when the person is unable to pass stool successfully from the rectum. This condition is not normal for the young, but it may occur if the "urge to defecate" is ignored and stool becomes difficult to eliminate. Stool retention may occur as a side effect to many medications, including narcotic pain medications or can occur secondarily to reduced peristalsis or intestinal blockage. Stool retention usually results in constipation, defined as the difficult passage of hard, dry stool. Ongoing retention of stool causes loss of appetite, discomfort, and potentially fecal impaction.[12]

Discomfort

The process of elimination should normally be free of pain or discomfort; in the case of significant urgency, the process of elimination can actually relieve discomfort. The most common causes for urinary discomfort are associated with inflammation (often associated with infection) of the urinary tract or bladder distention associated with urinary retention. Pain associated with urinary tract infection is often described as a burning pain. Pain also can be associated with irritation when urine comes in contact with lesions on the genitalia.

Common causes of discomfort associated with bowel elimination include constipation, excessive flatus, abdominal cramping, and diarrhea. Other causes of discomfort include inflammation or injury to the anus, the presence of hemorrhoids (both internal and external), anal fissure, and gastrointestinal infection or inflammation. Chronic conditions such as colitis or irritable bowel syndrome are also commonly associated with discomfort. In children, there can be telescoping of the bowel back into itself (intussusception) that can result in abdominal pain from obstruction and retention of stool.[2]

Infections and Inflammation

Elimination problems also can be caused by inflammatory or infectious conditions. Infection in the urinary system is often referred to as urinary tract infection, but specific structures in the urinary system can become inflamed or infected, including the kidney (nephritis), the renal pelvis (pyelonephritis), and the bladder (cystitis).

Acute intestinal inflammation and infection are most commonly associated with viral infections or food poisoning. Chronic inflammatory conditions of the intestinal tract include colitis and diverticulitis or autoimmune disorders. Inflammation and infections are usually associated with abdominal pain and discomfort (sometimes severe) and can potentially lead to nutritional deficits or intestinal perforation.

Neoplasms

Neoplasms are tumors and can have an effect on urinary and bowel elimination. Benign and malignant neoplasms of the prostate often lead to blockage of urinary flow in men. Tumors can also occur in the kidney or bladder, but these are less common. Neoplasms in the intestinal tract are also common and include benign growths (e.g., polyps) and cancerous lesions in the intestine, colon, or rectum.[13]

Organ Failure

One additional category of problems related to elimination is organ failure. The most obvious organ that comes to mind is the kidney. Renal failure can occur suddenly, usually associated with an injury to the kidney (referred to as acute kidney injury), or it can occur as a slow, chronic process (referred to as chronic kidney disease), whereby the kidneys lose functional capacity over months to years. The inability to remove metabolic waste and fluid creates significant physiological challenges. The failure of other key organs, such as the heart, the liver, and the pancreas, also hampers elimination efforts. For example, heart failure and shock reduce blood flow to the kidneys and gastrointestinal system, thereby reducing the efficiency of urine production and removal as well as formation of stool. Removal of the small or large intestines because of injury or disease also results in significant changes in elimination.

CONSEQUENCES

A number of consequences occur associated with impaired elimination processes and are linked to the underlying problem.

- Consequences associated with incontinence range from the potential for skin breakdown and falls (if associated with urgency) to social, lifestyle, and relationship consequences and depression and withdrawal.
- The consequences of urinary retention include pain, chronic bladder infection, and bladder distention. Bladder distention can lead to urinary reflux (a backflow of urine from the bladder into the ureters), causing dilation of the ureters and renal pelvis, and can lead to pyelonephritis and renal atrophy.
- The complete loss of renal function represents significant physiological consequences. The inability to remove toxins and metabolic waste results in fluid and electrolyte and acid–base disturbances and leads to death if untreated.
- The consequence of excessive fecal retention includes pain, loss of appetite, nausea, and vomiting.
- An ileus refers to a loss of peristaltic activity in the gastrointestinal tract. This can occur subsequent to abdominal trauma or surgery and is associated with nausea, vomiting, and distention. Although rare, rupture of the colon can occur, representing a life-threatening situation.

RISK FACTORS

Elimination represents normal physiological function; thus problems with the elimination of urine and stool and can affect any person regardless of age, gender, or race. It is a challenge to adequately summarize all risk factors for problems affecting elimination because each condition has its own unique risk factors. However, there are a few universal risk factors for the majority of problems affecting normal elimination. The single greatest risk factor for altered elimination is advanced age because of physiologic changes associated with aging process. Other general risk

TABLE 17.2 Common Risk Factors for Incontinence and Retention

	Persistent Incontinence	Retention
Urinary	Advanced age	Advanced age
	Female	Male
	Menopause	Prostate enlargement, inflammation, or infection
	Multiparity	
	Obesity	Pelvic organ prolapse
	Smoking	Pelvic mass
	Impaired mobility	Pelvic trauma/surgery
	Trauma or surgery pelvic region	Medications (anticholinergics, sympathomimetics)
	Impaired cognitive, debilitated state	
	Neurologic disorders (such as stroke, spinal injury, brain tumor)	
Fecal	Advanced age	Advanced age
	Diarrhea	Female
	Impaired mobility	Pregnancy
	Impaired cognitive, debilitated state	Lower income
		Poorly educated
	Injury, chronic condition affecting rectal neuropathway	Sedentary lifestyle
		Dehydration
		Chronic conditions (inflammatory bowel syndrome, depression)
		Medications (opioids, diuretics, antidepressants, aluminum-based antacids)

factors common to most elimination problems include individuals with altered cognition, impaired mobility, the debilitated, injuries or pathology affecting the neurologic system, spine, or pelvic organs. There is also a high correlation between some elimination problems—urinary and fecal incontinence, as one example.[14] Also, many medications are known to cause changes in elimination—general anesthesia[15] and opioids as common examples. Table 17.2 presents specific risk factors for retention and incontinence.

ASSESSMENT

Assessment of elimination includes taking a history, conducting a physical examination, and performing diagnostic testing when problems are identified.

History

Conducting a history is the first step to understanding problems associated with elimination. Ask about patterns of urinary and bowel elimination, including frequency, appearance of stool and urine, and associated symptoms. Common symptoms directly related to elimination include alterations in elimination patterns; changes in the appearance, frequency, or quality of stool or urine; or discomfort and difficulty associated with elimination. A symptom analysis approach is helpful to fully understand the symptom. Determine if there have been changes in diet, recent changes in health status (e.g., cognition, mobility, functional ability, or other medical conditions), and if there are new medications or changes in medications. Voluntary or involuntary (incontinence) emptying of the bowel or bladder also must be assessed to determine the impact of the condition on the individual. Adults of all ages should be asked about urinary continence because it is an underreported phenomenon.

Examination Findings

Physical assessment incorporates four examination techniques: inspection, auscultation, palpation, and percussion.

Inspection

The abdomen is inspected for contour; abdominal or bladder distention is an abnormal finding. The genitalia are also inspected to examine the urinary meatus for evidence of redness, lesions, or discharge. Discharge from the urinary meatus is an abnormal finding and may suggest infection, especially if the patient reports pain with voiding. Observe the perianal area. The area should be free from redness or lesions; the presence of hemorrhoids or an anal fistula may be observed if the patient complains of pain with defecation.

Inspection also includes looking at a stool or urine sample if available. Urine should be clear and yellow with mild odor. Very dark urine may be indicative of dehydration, may be a side effect of medication, or may indicate the presence of blood. Stool should be brown and formed. Stools that are black and tarry in appearance often signal gastrointestinal bleeding. Loose stools or diarrhea may be associated with diet, inflammation, or infection.

Auscultation

Auscultation is limited to the abdomen to listen to bowel sounds. Bowel sounds should be heard in all four quadrants. An absence of bowel sounds may be associated with paralytic ileus; hyperactive bowel sounds may be noted with gastrointestinal inflammation or with an intestinal obstruction.[16] Auscultation is not indicated in urinary assessment.

Palpation

Abdominal palpation is a physical examination technique for both urinary and bowel elimination. The abdomen should be soft and non-tender with palpation over the entire abdomen and over the urinary bladder. Abdominal or urinary distention is considered an abnormal finding and may be associated with reduced peristalsis or retention of stool or urine.

Rectal palpation is done to assess the rectal sphincter and to examine for the presence of masses, lesions, or impacted stool. Digital palpation is also part of the prostate examination.[16] Although this is not directly an examination associated with elimination, prostate enlargement can result from a tumor (benign or malignant) or inflammation; both can contribute to urinary retention.

Diagnostic Tests

There are a number of diagnostic tests associated with elimination. In general, the diagnostic tests are classified into one of three categories: laboratory, radiographic, and direct observation.

Laboratory Tests

Urinalysis. A urinalysis is one of the most common of all laboratory tests. It is useful for screening a number of conditions not associated with a problem in elimination and is obtained with either a sterile urine specimen or a clean-catch specimen. Bacteria indicate infection, whereas blood may indicate damage from infection or trauma to the urinary system. Urinary analysis that indicates the presence of bacteria or blood components in the urine may require further assessment of the urinary tract by a physician specialist in the field of urology.

Renal function tests. Laboratory tests assessing renal function include blood urea nitrogen, blood creatinine, and creatinine clearance tests.

Creatinine and blood urea nitrogen are excreted entirely by the kidneys and therefore provide a measure of renal function.

Culture. Urine and stool cultures are relatively common laboratory tests. When a urinary tract infection is suspected, a urine culture determines the presence and type of organism causing the urinary infection. Stool cultures are indicated when a parasitic infection is suspected.

Occult blood. When blood is suspected in stool, an occult blood test is indicated. It also represents a basic screening that should be performed as part of a rectal examination. The presence of blood in the stool could be related to a gastrointestinal bleed (inflammation and infection), hemorrhoids, or tumors.

Pathology

A biopsy is a sample of tissue or cells that undergoes pathologic evaluation. A biopsy can be taken from the rectum, colon, bladder, or kidney. Biopsies provide information associated with tumors or with general organ function.

Radiographic Tests and Scans

Numerous radiographic tests are used to assess elimination. Common radiographic tests include x-rays, computerized tomography, magnetic resonance imaging, and ultrasound. These are used to detect a variety of problems, including the presence of an intestinal tumor, a congenital renal abnormality, or kidney stones. Angiography is used to assess renal blood flow and can detect renal artery stenosis.

Direct Observation Tests

The ability to directly observe internal organs can be accomplished with scopes. With regard to the concept of elimination, scopes can be used to visualize the colon (*colonoscopy*), the sigmoid colon (*sigmoidoscopy*), the bladder (*cystoscopy*), or the urethra or ureters (*uroscopy*).

Direct visualization of the colon is done for screening or diagnostic purposes for polyps, cancer, and inflammatory conditions such as Crohn disease. Direct visualization of the bladder or ureters is done with a special scope as part of diagnostic or surgical procedures.

Other Diagnostic Tests

Several special tests are available to evaluate urinary elimination, including bladder stress testing, uroflowmetry and other urine flow studies, and postvoid residual measurement through the use of bladder scans or postvoid catheterization.

CLINICAL MANAGEMENT

Primary Prevention

Primary prevention measures are aimed at maintaining optimal health and preventing the onset of disease through the reduction of risks. The foundation of primary prevention efforts, as it relates to this concept, includes awareness of environmental factors, maintaining a healthy diet, hydration, physical activity, and following optimal toileting practices.

Environmental Factors

Avoidance of contaminated water and foods can assist in maintaining consistent bowel habits. Bacteria in water or food can cause diarrhea and colitis. Parasites can be present in water or food that is not properly prepared. Parasites not only can cause elimination problems but also can affect overall health. Laboratory testing can determine if parasites are present in the gastrointestinal system that may be causing problems with bowel elimination.

Maintaining Hydration

Water is a key element for prevention of bowel and urinary elimination problems. Water is absorbed by the stool to soften it and promote intestinal motility, which assists in the elimination of stool. Water serves the urinary system in that it increases volume, reduces bladder irritation, and helps eliminate toxins from the body.

Dietary Fiber

Fiber intake has been shown to prevent stool retention, especially when combined with adequate water intake and exercise. Fiber creates enough friction along the bowel surface that it can assist in the production of a bowel movement. Adequate fluid intake with the fiber is imperative. Fiber should be slowly added to the diet to prevent abdominal discomfort and excessive gas formation in the intestine. The U.S. Food and Drug Administration recommends 25 g of fiber/day, based on a 1000 kcal diet.[17]

Physical Activity

Physical activity is known to increase intestinal peristalsis which reduces the time for food matter to move through intestines. By decreasing the time it takes feces to move through the large intestine, less water is reabsorbed. For this reason, exercise helps prevent constipation.[12]

Maintenance of Regular Toileting Practices

Maintaining a consistent time of defecation is important in the regulation of bowel movements. The use of familiar toileting facilities may also encourage defecation. Avoidance of foods that cause discomfort during digestion and absorption or are known to cause constipation can also help maintain regular patterns of bowel elimination. To prevent urinary incontinence or retention, there should be timely and complete emptying of the bladder. Holding urine should be discouraged because this encourages bacterial growth in the bladder and consequent urinary tract infection.

Secondary Prevention (Screening)

Two common screening tests associated with elimination are screening for occult blood and colonoscopy—both are considered effective for the detection of colon cancer. The U.S. Preventive Services Task Force (USPSTF) recommends screening for colorectal cancer beginning at age 50 years until 75 years of age (recommendation grade A).[18] The two categories of screening are stool-based testes and direct visualization tests. Stool-based tests (guaiac-based fecal occult blood test, fecal immunochemical test, or multitargeted stool DNA test) are recommended annually; the guaiac-based test is routinely done as part of a rectal exam. Direct visualization tests include colonoscopy or sigmoidoscopy. These are recommended every 10 years (or more often with certain risk factors). Such tests allow direct visualization of the colon and removal of precancerous lesions, averting the development of colon cancer.

Screening for prostate cancer is the only screening associated with urinary elimination. The recently revised recommendation is for periodic prostate-specific antigen (PSA)–based screening of men ages 55 to 69 to be an individualized decision, after weighing risks and benefits associated with screening with their healthcare provider (recommendation grade C). The USPSTF recommends against screening for prostate cancer in men over the age of 70.[19] The USPSTF reports insufficient evidence to support routine screening for bladder cancer.[20]

Collaborative Interventions

Problems with elimination represent a wide range of conditions involving two major body systems—the gastrointestinal system and the urinary system. For the purposes of this concept, common interventions are only briefly described; detailed information is available in various nursing textbooks.

Pharmacologic Agents

Antibiotics. Infections of the kidney and urinary tract are treated with antibiotics. Antibiotics are selected based on the results of culture and sensitivity testing and the provider's best judgment. Although a variety of agents are used, trimethoprim, trimethoprim with sulfamethoxazole, or nitrofurantoin are commonly prescribed for urinary tract infections; parenteral antibiotics are indicated for more severe infections such as pyelonephritis. Antibiotics may also be used prophylactically with urinary retention or recurrent urinary tract infection.

Diuretics. Diuretics increase the volume of urine produced along with excreting sodium and potassium from the body by affecting the water resorption in the renal tubules. Loop diuretics prevent reabsorption of sodium in the loop of Henle. Thiazide diuretics prevent sodium from being reabsorbed at the beginning of the distal convoluted tubules. Potassium-sparing diuretics stop the extensive loss of potassium at the distal convoluted tubules. Excessive use to treat certain conditions requires careful monitoring and frequent lab testing of the electrolytes.

Antispasmodics. Anticholinergics are often used to relieve smooth muscle spasms in the bowel or bladder. Bladder spasms can occur as a consequence of neurologic injury. Anticholinergics can reduce bladder spasms and can provide relief from urinary incontinence. Bowel spasms commonly occur with irritable bowel syndrome. Some antispasmodic medications, such as Imodium (loperamide), are effective for the treatment of diarrhea because they cause a reduction in peristalsis and slow the passage of stool.

Agents to manage constipation. Pharmacologic management to treat stool retention includes both prescribed and over-the-counter versions of laxatives, bulk-forming agents, bowel stimulants, lubricants, stool softeners, saline laxatives, and enemas. The drawback in using these medications is that the bowel can become dependent on laxatives and stimulants for the impulse to defecate. Medications for stool retention should be a last resort and discontinued as soon as the bowel elimination is achieved.

Analgesics. Analgesics are indicated for relief of mild discomfort to severe pain for select urinary or bowel elimination conditions. Examples of conditions causing pain with elimination include kidney stones, cystitis, urinary tract infections, bladder spams, hemorrhoids, and rectal fissures.

Incontinence Management

Multidisciplinary management of the person with alterations in elimination must occur in order to successfully control the condition. The need for retraining the bowel and bladder is of paramount importance. Providing a regular toileting schedule, managing fluid intake, modifying the environment, avoiding indwelling catheters, providing high-quality skin care and assessment, and avoiding medications that contribute to incontinence are nursing actions that will promote urinary continence. Personal absorbent pads or bed-protecting pads may be used to catch episodes of incontinence in both mobile and immobile individuals. Biofeedback may be used to assist the person in gaining improved control over the muscles of elimination. Biofeedback involves placement of sensors onto the affected area of bowel so that the person can receive feedback regarding which muscles are being used to control bowel function. Among those with dementia, toilet assistance (including timed voiding and prompted voiding) along with protective pads and skin care are standard interventions.[21]

Invasive Procedures and Surgical Interventions Involving Urinary Elimination

A variety of procedures are performed as treatment for urinary elimination problems. The benefits must outweigh the risks for utilization of these interventions because they can be invasive and sometimes lifestyle-altering procedures.

Dialysis. Dialysis is indicated for acute or chronic renal failure. It involves filtration of the blood to remove toxins through an external process. Two types of dialysis are hemodialysis and peritoneal dialysis. A dialysis machine is used in hemodialysis to filter a patient's blood to remove excess toxins and water. The blood is circulated from the patient to the dialysis machine and then back to the patient over several hours. In peritoneal dialysis, a dialysate solution is introduced into the peritoneal cavity that absorbs the toxins over several hours; the solution and waste are then removed.

Procedures relieving urinary retention. The most common procedure to relieve urinary retention is urinary catheterization.[22] This can be intermittently performed with a straight catheter, or an indwelling catheter can be inserted. Measures must be taken to prevent complications (e.g., infection) when urinary drainage systems are used for long periods of time.[23]

Surgical intervention may be needed to treat other forms of obstructions, including surgery on the bladder, prostate, or ureters. Many procedures are conducted through a cystoscope. Stents, which are rigid tubes that provide an opening that is not normally present, may be used internally in the urethra and externally as part of anastomosis procedures performed for bladder cancer. Stents maintain the patency of pathways for urinary elimination.

Removing renal calculi. Renal calculi (also known as kidney stones) often require surgical intervention if the stones are unable to pass through the urinary tract. A variety of surgical procedures are available to treat renal calculi, including *lithotripsy* (fragmentation of the stones through sound wave technology); *endourologic procedures* (insertion of a ureteroscope and crushing the stones with a surgical instrument called a lithotrite); or open procedures (*nephrolithotomy, pyelolithotomy, ureterolithotomy,* or *cystotomy*), in which an incision is made and the stone is surgically removed.

Nephrectomy. Occasionally, surgical removal of the kidney is required, as with renal cancer. Other conditions, such as polycystic kidney disease, may also require surgical intervention.

Prostate surgery. An enlarged prostate can cause significant urinary obstruction. A transurethral resection of the prostate is a surgical procedure done for benign prostate hypertrophy when other noninvasive treatment measures have failed. *Prostatectomy* refers to the removal of the prostate and is usually performed among younger men diagnosed with prostate cancer, particularly if diagnosed in early disease stage.

Bladder surgeries. Surgical interventions of the bladder include a wide variety of procedures to treat many types of conditions, such as prolapsed bladder or bladder cancer. Surgical treatment options include laser surgery, transurethral resection, and partial or total cystectomy. If the bladder is removed, urinary diversion is required.

Urinary diversion. Urinary diversion procedures involve diverting the ureters to a urinary stoma on the skin (usually on the abdomen).

There are multiple types of diversion procedures that are described in greater detail in many nursing textbooks. Urinary diversion is required with a cystectomy and is also used in the treatment of other conditions, such as bladder cancer, neurogenic bladder, or trauma to the bladder. Maintenance of skin integrity at the stoma site is of great importance. External urinary pouches are used in many cases to collect urine in these types of situations.

Invasive Procedures and Surgical Interventions Involving Bowel Elimination

Surgical procedures for bowel elimination problems are primarily associated with the colon, rectum, and anus, and they treat pathologic conditions or traumatic injury.

Colectomy. A colectomy (also referred to as a *colon resection*) involves removing a portion of the bowel. This may be done because of disease to a portion of the bowel (e.g., a cancerous tumor) or as treatment for traumatic injury. The two ends of the remaining colon are reattached (anastomosed).

Colostomy/ileostomy. Diversion of the intestines (colon or small intestine) through a stoma on the skin is occasionally needed temporarily or permanently as a result of injured or diseased intestine, colon, or rectum. The use of external devices (e.g., a colostomy pouch) is required for the collection of stool. Maintenance of skin integrity around the stoma is of utmost importance.[21]

Rectal prolapse repair. Rectal prolapse is a condition that occurs when the rectum falls into or through the anal opening. This is most common among young children and the elderly. Prolapse can occur from weak pelvic floor muscles or from excessive straining during bowel movements, as with chronic constipation. Surgical repair is indicated if prolapse occurs regularly or is associated with significant discomfort.

Hemorrhoidectomy. This procedure involves the excision of internal or external hemorrhoids. Hemorrhoids may require surgical intervention if topical treatments and changes in diet do not eliminate their associated discomfort. Thus this procedure is usually only performed for patients with severe pain and multiple thrombosed hemorrhoids or when there is significant prolapse.

Fecal collection systems. A fecal collection system uses a flexible tube inserted into the rectum that is used to collect liquid stool in patients with incontinence who are not candidates for bowel retraining or have *Clostridium difficile* and its resulting diarrhea. These are fecal management systems for liquid stool only and help prevent skin breakdown in cases of severe diarrhea.

INTERRELATED CONCEPTS

A number of interrelated concepts presented in this text are associated with elimination (Fig. 17.5). **Nutrition** has a close interrelationship with bowel and urinary elimination. The types of foods and fluids ingested impact stool formation and urinary elimination. The kidneys play a vital role in maintaining homeostasis of **Fluid and Electrolytes** and **Acid–Base Balance**. Under the direction of hormones, the kidneys retain or eliminate water and electrolytes, which are critical for these balances to be maintained. Also, changes in electrolyte balance can influence neuromuscular transmission of smooth muscles, thus reducing or increasing intestinal peristalsis.

A lack of **Mobility** can result in both urinary and bowel elimination problems. Mobility helps with stimulation of peristalsis. Immobility, particularly when an individual is in a supine position, can lead to ineffective bladder emptying. Finally, changes in **Cognition** increase the potential for complications in both elimination mechanisms and can result from the inability to obtain and maintain adequate food and fluid intake. They can also lead to an inability to recognize cues for elimination—thus leading to incontinence.

CLINICAL EXEMPLARS

Exemplars of alterations in urinary elimination include conditions across the lifespan—ranging from bed-wetting, which may occur as a child is learning to control urinary elimination, to incontinence, which may occur as a person ages and the muscles supporting the bladder become less efficient. Bowel function also spans the life cycle; a variety of issues may affect function as an infant, such as structural problems in the bowel (e.g., strictures and fissures), whereas functional issues such as constipation may occur as a person advances in age. Box 17.1 presents common exemplars of conditions associated with the concept of elimination. Some of the most common exemplars of impaired elimination, urinary, and fecal incontinence have previously been described in the variations and context section of this concept presentation.

Featured Exemplars
Urolithiasis

Urolithiasis refers to the presence of stones called calculi within the urinary tract. Although it is not entirely clear how stones are formed, most contain calcium. Stones can form in the kidney (nephrolithiasis)

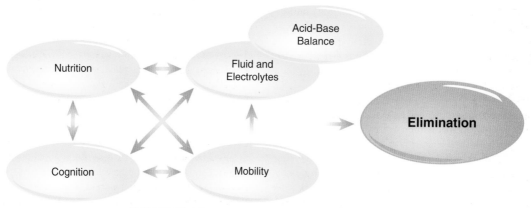

FIGURE 17.5 Elimination and Interrelated Concepts.

BOX 17.1 EXEMPLARS OF IMPAIRED ELIMINATION

Incontinence
- Bed-wetting
- Stress incontinence
- Urge incontinence
- Fecal incontinence

Retention
- Benign prostatic hyperplasia
- Bladder cancer
- Bowel obstruction
- Colorectal cancer
- Constipation
- Fecal impaction
- Prostatitis
- Prostate cancer
- Spinal cord injury
- Urethral stricture

Discomfort
- Anal fissure
- Anorectal abscess
- Hemorrhoids
- Interstitial cystitis
- Pilonidal cyst
- Urolithiasis

Infections and Inflammation
- Crohn's disease
- Diarrhea
- Gastritis
- Gastroenteritis
- Glomerulonephritis
- Pyelonephritis
- Ulcerative colitis
- Urinary tract infection

Renal Failure
- Acute kidney injury
- Chronic kidney disease

Neoplasms
- Benign prostate hyperplasia
- Bladder cancer
- Colorectal cancer
- Prostate cancer
- Renal cancer

ACCESS EXEMPLAR LINKS IN YOUR GIDDENS EBOOK

or within the ureters (ureterolithiasis). The stones are associated with severe pain when they move down the ureter, into the bladder, and through the urethra (referred to as "passing the stone").[21] Hematuria is a common finding. If the stone becomes lodged in the ureter, a blockage can occur, leading to hydronephrosis and impaired kidney function.

Benign Prostatic Hyperplasia

Benign prostatic hyperplasia is an enlargement of the prostate gland commonly seen among older men. It is estimated that 30% of men age 60 years have moderate symptoms and 50% of men age 80 years or older have symptoms.[24] If untreated, the enlarging prostate, which surrounds the urethra at the base of the bladder, can obstruct urine flow, creating urinary retention. Common symptoms include frequency of urination, increased frequency of urinating at night, difficulty starting urinary flow, and a weak urinary stream. Chronic retention of urine can lead to urinary tract infection.

Urinary Tract Infection

Urinary tract infection (UTI) is caused by an infection in the urinary tract, representing the second most common bacterial infection in individuals. The symptoms associated with UTI include nausea and vomiting, chills, suprapubic or low back pain, bladder spasms, dysuria, burning with urination, frequency, urgency, hesitancy, or nocturia. UTIs are seen more frequently in pregnant women, females, and older men and women. These infections may cause sepsis and can result in death if not treated, especially in the elderly.[21]

Renal Failure

Renal failure occurs when there is a partially or complete cessation of kidney function. Renal failure can be acute or chronic. Acute kidney injury (AKI) is associated with a loss of renal function over a few days and can typically be reversed. Chronic kidney disease (CKD) involves a process of renal failure that occurs over a long period of time. It is characterized by a gradual decrease in renal functioning and a gradual increase in metabolic waste. Regardless of the cause, untreated renal failure results in fluid overload, electrolyte imbalances, and metabolic acidosis, and ultimately leads to death.

Constipation

Constipation refers to difficulty passing stool and is usually associated with the passage of hard, dry stool; it can occur among individuals of any age. Constipation may be painful due to the bloating and flatus that may occur and also with trying to pass the stool itself. Chronic constipation may be caused by a lack of dietary fiber, certain medications (narcotic pain medications), chronic decreased intestinal peristalsis, or decreased fluid intake.[21]

Diarrhea

Diarrhea is the frequent passing of watery, liquid, or loose stools and occurs among individuals across the lifespan. It can be acute or chronic. Acute diarrhea is usually associated with inflammation within the gastrointestinal tract due to a virus or bacteria and usually resolves in a few days. Chronic diarrhea persists for a longer period of time, such as several weeks. Because diarrhea is associated with the loss of water and electrolytes, dehydration and electrolyte imbalance may occur quickly, particularly among infants, children, and older adults.[21]

Colorectal Cancer

Colorectal cancer is the third leading cause of cancer in men and women in the United States, estimated to caused 51,651 deaths in 2014.[25] Colorectal incidence and mortality rates are highest among African American men and women. Colorectal screening can prevent the development of cancer by removing precancerous colon polyps and has been credited with reducing the incidence and mortality during the past decade.

CASE STUDY

Case Presentation

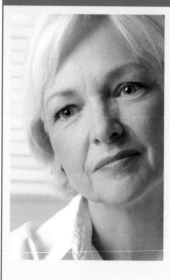

Ms. Amanda Doyle is a 67-year-old white female with a history of type 1 diabetes and osteoarthritis in her left hip. Her diabetes is well controlled with diet and insulin. Although she takes ibuprofen to treat the arthritic pain, her mobility has declined and now uses a walker. Because of a past bad experience with anesthesia, she has been resistant to having hip replacement surgery and instead opted to increase the dosage of ibuprofen to 600 mg four times a day and just learn to live with the pain.

For the past 3 months, Ms. Doyle has experienced intermittent abdominal pain, cramping, and bloating with diarrhea. She also has had a reduced appetite and has frequently felt tired.

On several occasions she has experienced fecal incontinence because she was unable to get to the bathroom in time and was unable to "hold it." On two occasions, she experienced fecal incontinence in a public setting and was completely embarrassed by the situation. She is now afraid to leave the house because she fears it will happen again.

Ms. Doyle's daughter took her to her primary care provider who ordered several diagnostic tests. An occult blood test showed blood in her stool. A stool culture was done to rule out parasitic infections; this was negative. Because it had been 9 years since her last colonoscopy, a colonoscopy was ordered to rule out pathology within the colon such as ulcerations, inflammation, or tumors. The colonoscopy revealed inflammation to the lining her colon. Her physician made the diagnosis of inflammatory bowel disease.

Case Analysis

1. In what way does the case exemplify the concept of elimination?
2. What risk factors for altered elimination (fecal incontinence) and inflammatory bowel disease does Ms. Bowel have?
3. How are the diagnostic tests described in the case consistent with what was described for assessment of elimination?

Hemera Technologies/AbleStock.com/Thinkstock.

 ACCESS EXEMPLAR LINKS IN YOUR GIDDENS EBOOK

REFERENCES

1. Venes, D. (Ed.), (2013). *Taber's cyclopedic medical dictionary* (21st ed.). Philadelphia: Davis.
2. Kimball, V. (2016). The perils and pitfalls of potty training. *Pediatric Annuals, 45*(6), e199–e201.
3. Hockenberry, M. J., & Wilson, D. (2012). *Wong's pediatric nursing* (9th ed.). St Louis: Mosby.
4. Trottier, M., Erebara, A., & Bozzo, P. (2012). Treating constipation during pregnancy. *Canadian Family Physician, 58*(8), 836–838.
5. Demir, O., Sen, V., Irer, B., et al. (2017). Prevalence and possible risk factors for urinary incontinence. *Urologia Internationalis, 99*(1), 84–90.
6. Seshan, V., Alkhasawneh, E., & Hashmi, I. (2016). Risk factors of urinary incontinence in women: A literature review. *International Journal of Urologic Nursing, 10*(3), 118–126.
7. Mayo Clinic. (2017). Urinary incontinence. Retrieved from https://www.mayoclinic.org/diseases-conditions/urinary-incontinence/symptoms-causes/syc-20352808.
8. Whitehead, W., Borrud, L., Goode, P., et al. (2009). Fecal incontinence in U.S. adults: Epidemiology and risk factors. *Gastroenterology, 137*(2), 512–517.
9. National Institute of Diabetes and Digestive and Kidney Diseases. (2017). *Bowel Control Problems:* Fecal incontinence. Retrieved from https://www.niddk.nih.gov/health-information/digestive-diseases/bowel-control-problems-fecal-incontinence/definition-facts.
10. National Institute of Diabetes and Digestive and Kidney Diseases. (2014). *Urinary retention.* Retrieved from http://kidney.niddk.nih.gov/kudiseases/pubs/UrinaryRetention.
11. Selius, B., & Subedi, R. (2008). Urinary retention in adults, diagnosis and initial management. *American Family Physician, 77*(5), 643–650.
12. Uduak, A., Camille, V., Burgio, K., et al. (2016). Shared risk factors for constipation, fecal incontinence, and combined symptoms in older U.S. adults. *Journal of the American Geriatrics Society, 64*(11), e183–e188.
13. Centers for Disease Control and Prevention. (2018). *Colorectal (colon) cancer.* Retrieved from http://www.cdc.gov/cancer/colorectal/index.htm.
14. Wu, J., Matthews, C., Vaughan, C., & Markland, A. (2015). Urinary, fecal, and dual incontinence in older U.S. adults. *Journal of the American Geriatrics Society, 63*(5), 947–953.
15. Simsek, Y., & Sureyya, K. (2016). Postoperative urinary retention and nursing approaches. *International Journal of Caring Sciences, 9*(2), 1154–1161.
16. Wilson, S., & Giddens, J. (2017). *Health assessment for nursing practice* (6th ed.). St Louis: Elsevier.
17. U.S. Food and Drug Administration. (n.d). *Dietary Fiber.* Retrieved from https://www.accessdata.fda.gov/scripts/interactivenutritionfactslabel/factsheets/Dietary_Fiber.pdf.
18. U.S. Preventive Services Task Force. (2017). *Colorectal cancer: Screening.* Retrieved from https://www.uspreventiveservicestaskforce.org/Page/Document/RecommendationStatementFinal/colorectal-cancer-screening2.
19. U.S. Preventive Services Task Force. (2017). *Prostate Cancer Screening.* Retrieved from https://www.uspreventiveservicestaskforce.org/Page/Document/RecommendationStatementFinal/prostate-cancer-screening1.
20. U.S. Preventive Services Task Force. (2011). *Bladder Cancer Screening.* Retrieved from https://www.uspreventiveservicestaskforce.org/Page/Document/UpdateSummaryFinal/bladder-cancer-in-adults-screening.
21. Lewis, S., Bucher, L., Heitkemper, M., et al. (2017). *Medical–surgical nursing* (10th ed.). St Louis: Elsevier.
22. National Kidney and Urologic Disease Clearinghouse. (2014). *Urinary retention.* Retrieved from http://kidney.niddk.nih.gov/kudiseases/pubs/urinaryretention/index.aspx.
23. Newman, D. K. (2007). The indwelling catheter: Principles for best practice. *Journal of Wound, Ostomy, and Continence Nursing, 34*(6), 655–663.
24. Mayo Clinic. (2017). *Benign prostatic hyperplasia (BPH).* Retrieved from http://www.mayoclinic.org/diseases-conditions/benign-prostatic-hyperplasia/basics/definition/CON-20030812.
25. Center for Disease Control. (2018). *Colorectal Cancer Statistics.* Retrieved from https://www.cdc.gov/cancer/colorectal/statistics/index.htm.

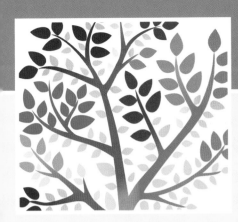

Perfusion

Susan F. Wilson

Cells need a consistent blood supply to obtain oxygen and nutrients and to discard waste products. When the blood supply or perfusion is impaired, ischemia develops and can progress to necrosis, if prolonged. The purpose of this concept presentation is to help the nurse acquire an understanding about perfusion across the lifespan. Nurses should be able to promote an individual's healthy behaviors that optimize perfusion, identify individuals at risk of impaired perfusion, recognize when individuals are experiencing an impairment of perfusion, and respond with appropriate interventions.

DEFINITION

For the purpose of this concept presentation, perfusion refers to *the flow of blood through arteries and capillaries delivering nutrients and oxygen to cells.* Perfusion is a normal physiological process that requires the heart to generate sufficient cardiac output to transport blood through patent blood vessels for distribution in the tissues throughout the body. Thus maintaining cardiovascular health is essential to optimal perfusion.

SCOPE

The concept of perfusion and problems associated with impaired perfusion represents a wide range of physiological processes and conditions. The scope of perfusion ranges from optimal perfusion to no perfusion (Fig. 18.1). Variations in perfusion are seen among individuals across the lifespan with multiple causative factors and a wide range of impact and duration. Changes in perfusion can be temporary, long term, or permanent. Disorders that lead to changes in perfusion include acute conditions (such as myocardial infarction, stroke, or shock) and chronic disorders (such as hypertension, heart failure, sickle cell, or hemophilia). Conditions that specifically involve perfusion include neurologic (interfering with blood flow within the brain), pulmonary (impairing blood flow to and from the lungs), and cardiovascular (interfering with blood flow in heart, arteries and veins). Causes of these disorders include congenital defects, genetic disorders, injury, inflammation, and infections.

NORMAL PHYSIOLOGICAL PROCESS

From a conceptual lens, the process of perfusion can be thought of in two general categories: central perfusion and tissue perfusion. The normal physiological process of perfusion is presented from this perspective.

Central Perfusion

Central perfusion is generated by cardiac output—the amount of blood pumped by the heart each minute. Cardiac output is an outcome of coordinated effects of electrical and mechanical factors that move blood through the heart into the peripheral vessels. This central perfusion propels blood to all organs and their tissues from patent arteries through capillaries and returns the blood to the heart through patent veins.

Central perfusion begins when the heart is stimulated by an electrical impulse that originates in the sinoatrial (SA) node and travels to the atrioventricular (AV) node. From the AV node, the impulse moves through a series of branches (bundle of His) and Purkinje fibers in the myocardium, which causes the ventricles to contract. The phase of the cardiac cycle during which the ventricles contract is called *systole.* As the ventricles contract, they create pressure that closes the mitral and tricuspid valves, preventing the backflow of blood into the atria. This ventricular pressure forces the aortic and pulmonic valves to open, resulting in ejection of blood into the aorta (from the left ventricle) and the pulmonary arteries (from the right ventricle). As blood is ejected, the ventricular pressure decreases, causing the aortic and pulmonic valves to close. The ventricles relax to fill with blood. The movement of blood from the atria to the ventricles is accomplished when the pressure of the blood in the atria becomes higher than the pressure in the ventricles. The higher atrial pressures passively open the mitral and tricuspid valves, allowing blood to fill the ventricles. The phase of the cardiac cycle when ventricles fill with blood is called *diastole.* Normal cardiac output ranges from 4 to 6 L/min in the adult. Two variables that influence cardiac output are stroke volume and heart rate. *Stroke volume* is the amount of blood ejected from each ventricle during contraction. It is affected by three factors: preload, contractility, and afterload. *Preload* is the amount of blood in the ventricles at the end of diastole, called the end diastolic pressure. *Contractility* refers to the strength of myocardial contraction. The greater the volume of blood in the ventricles (preload), the greater the stretch of the myocardium, and the stronger the myocardial contraction. *Afterload* is the force the ventricles must exert to open the semilunar valves (aortic and pulmonic). It is influenced by resistance to the ejected blood created by the diameter of blood vessels receiving the blood, also called *systemic vascular resistance (SVR).* The smaller or more constricted the blood vessels, the greater the pressure required to open the semilunar valves to eject the blood. This increased pressure increases the workload of the heart. Hypertension, for example, increases the afterload and therefore the workload of the heart. Alternatively, the larger or more dilated the blood vessels, the

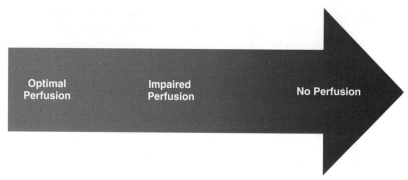

FIGURE 18.1 The Scope of Perfusion Ranges from Optimal to Impaired and a Total Lack of Perfusion.

less pressure required to eject blood; thereby reducing the workload on the heart. For example, during anaphylactic shock an allergic reaction causes a massive vasodilation, reducing the afterload. Heart rate is influenced by the autonomic nervous system. The sympathetic nervous system increases the heart rate while the parasympathetic nervous system decreases it. Fig. 18.2 shows the flow of blood through the right and left sides of the heart.

Tissue Perfusion

Tissue perfusion refers to blood that flows through arteries and capillaries to target tissues. Arterial blood pressure is determined by the cardiac output and SVR. Ventricular contraction creates a pressure, which pushes blood through arteries, into capillaries, and into the interstitial spaces allowing delivery of oxygen, fluid, and nutrients to cells. The tough and tensile arteries and their smaller branches, the arterioles, are subjected to remarkable pressure from the cardiac output. They maintain blood pressure by constricting or dilating in response to stimuli. Blood is returned to the heart through veins and their smaller branches, the venules. These vessels are less sturdy but more expansible, enabling them to act as a reservoir for extra blood, if needed to decrease the workload of the heart. Pressure within the veins is low compared to that of arteries. The valves in each vein keep blood flowing in a forward direction toward the heart.

When vascular injury occurs, a complex coagulation process involving platelets, and clotting factors work together to stop bleeding. Vasoconstriction reduces blood flow and allows the clotting process to start. Platelets are activated and stick to the injured blood vessel to form a platelet plug. Next, clotting factors are activated and proceed in a coagulation cascade to the common final pathway where thrombin stimulates fibrinogen to form insoluble fibrin that stabilizes the clot.

Age-Related Differences
Infants and Adolescents

In infancy, the size of the heart in relation to the total body size is larger. The systolic blood pressure after birth is low due to the weaker left ventricle of the neonate. The left side of the heart develops strength and the systolic pressure rises rather sharply during the first 6 weeks. Soon after puberty, the systolic pressure rises to adult levels. An increase in heart size occurs during the adolescent growth spurt with increase in blood pressure and decrease in heart rate. Arteries and veins lengthen to keep pace with growth.[1]

Older Adults

The most relevant age-related changes are stiffening and thickening of the myocardial tissue and decreased elasticity of arterial walls. Heart valves tend to calcify and become fibrose. Collectively these changes lead to reduced cardiac efficiency (decreased stroke volume and cardiac output) during exercise and with other factors contributing to increased oxygen demand. Arterial stiffening contributes to an increase in blood pressure. A decrease in blood pressure upon standing (orthostatic hypotension) may contribute to falls. The valves in the veins become less efficient contributing to lower extremity edema.[2]

VARIATIONS AND CONTEXT

The two broad categories used to describe the normal physiological process of perfusion are also used to describe problems associated with perfusion: impaired central perfusion (mechanisms for blood delivery) and impaired tissue perfusion (amount of blood available to target tissues). Both of these categories are described in the following sections.

Impaired Central Perfusion

Many conditions associated with impaired perfusion result in decreased cardiac output. Cardiac output can be reduced by altered myocardial contraction, changes in myocardial conduction, ineffective heart valves, and congenital defects. Central perfusion impairment can also result from increased SVR, attributed to vasoconstriction of the arteries, or increased viscosity of the blood. An increased SVR requires the heart to compensate by increasing the contractile force and/or increasing heart rate to maintain adequate cardiac output. Likewise, cardiac output is affected by a reduction in SVR, attributed to vasodilation of the arteries or blood loss. Specific examples of conditions that lead to impaired central perfusion are presented later.

Impaired Local/Tissue Perfusion

Interference with tissue perfusion reduces blood flow through capillaries reducing delivery of oxygen, fluid, and nutrients to cells. Different organs and tissues require different volumes of blood to maintain adequate function. Some organs, such as the brain and intestines, require larger volumes of blood compared to skeletal tissue, for example. Inadequate tissue perfusion can result from poor central perfusion or from a mechanism within the vessel or organ itself, such as a blocked or narrowed blood vessel leading to or from the tissue or from excessive edema within the tissue interfering with the cellular oxygen exchange. Specific examples of conditions that lead to impaired local/tissue perfusion are presented later.

PHYSIOLOGIC CONSEQUENCES

Physiologic Consequences of Impaired Central Perfusion

Impairment of central perfusion occurs in conditions that decrease cardiac output or cause shock. Any occlusion or constriction of coronary

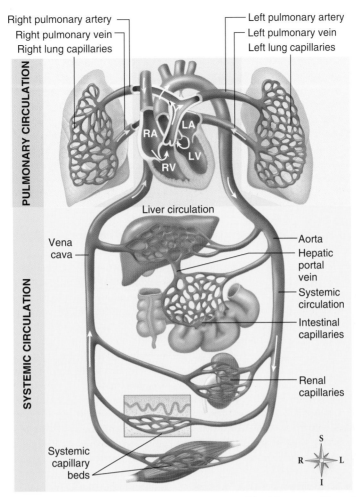

FIGURE 18.2 Circulatory Routes. The pulmonary circulation routes blood flow to and from the gas exchange tissues of the lungs. The systemic circulation, on the other hand, routes blood flow to and from the oxygen-consuming tissues of the body. (From Patton, K. T., & Thibodeau, G. A. [2016]. *Anatomy & physiology* [9th ed.]. St. Louis: Mosby.)

arteries that reduces blood flow to the myocardium can result in a myocardial infarction that decreases cardiac output. This impairment prevents the myocardium from performing the mechanical function of pumping blood to the body. Also, altered impulse conduction through the heart (from the SA node through the AV node to the right and left bundle branches and Purkinje fibers) interrupts the electrical function necessary for the myocardium to contract and causes ineffective contractions. Malfunction of heart valves, either stenosis or insufficiency, impairs flow of blood through the heart. Congenital defects also interrupt the blood flow through the heart. Shock, the inadequate blood flow to peripheral tissues, occurs as a consequence of impaired central perfusion when the heart is unable to act as a pump (cardiogenic shock), as well as a consequence of impaired local perfusion when fluid is lost (hypovolemic shock) or systemic vasodilation occurs (anaphylactic, neurogenic, or septic shock).

Physiologic Consequences of Impaired Tissue Perfusion

Impairment of tissue perfusion is associated with occlusion, constriction, or dilation of arteries or veins as well as blood loss. Atherosclerosis or thrombi can occlude arteries (which reduce the blood flow to tissues) and thrombi can occlude veins (which interrupt the return of blood to the heart). Vasoconstriction can result in hypertension, which increases

the risk for stroke or myocardial infarction. Examples of dilation are aneurysms in arteries and varicose veins. Blood loss occurs with bleeding or hemorrhage. Impaired tissue perfusion interferes with blood flow, resulting in ischemia to localized tissue and, if uncorrected, infarction and cellular death.

Ischemia is a *reversible* cellular injury that occurs when the demand for oxygen exceeds the supply because of a reduction or cessation of blood flow. When ischemia is prolonged, it may result in a lack of oxygen to tissues followed by necrosis and irreversible cellular injury. Examples are myocardial ischemia causing angina or chest pain from reduced blood flow and myocardial infarction causing cardiac arrest and cardiogenic shock with permanent damage to affected areas of the myocardium. Hypoxia and anoxia are examples of the interrelationship between the cardiovascular and respiratory systems because cells are deprived of oxygen from the lack of blood flow, from the lack of oxygen, or both.

RISK FACTORS

Adequate perfusion is required for life therefore, all individuals, regardless of age, sex, race, or socioeconomic status, are potentially at risk for impaired perfusion. Some risk factors are modifiable through lifestyle behaviors, whereas others are not. Nurses need to recognize populations and individuals at risk so that changes can be made to reduce that risk.

Populations at Risk
Older Adults

Older adults have many risk factors for impared perfusion. Coronary artery blood flow, stroke volume, and cardiac output decrease, increasing the risk for heart failure. Also the stiffening and thickening of the heart tissues decreases the ability to respond to the need for increased circulation and prolongs the time needed for the heart to return to a resting state after stress. Decreased elasticity of arteries limits the consistent forward movement of blood to organs. The valves in veins become less efficient, contributing to peripheral edema, and the sluggishness of blood flow contributes to deep vein thrombosis.[2]

Social and Environmental Factors

Low family income and low educational level are contributing factors to adverse cardiovascular disease outcomes. Social and psychological factors such as access to health care, medical compliance, eating habits, depression, and stress are thought to play a role in this relationship.[3]

Individual Risk Factors

A number of individual risk factors are associated with perfusion. Table 18.1 presents some of the most common modifiable and unmodifiable risk factors; many of these are described in more detail as follows.

Genetics

Although the focus on risk reduction for cardiovascular disease has traditionally centered around management of lifestyle factors, genetic risk factors appear to predispose individuals to cardiovascular disease as well. The risk for illness is even greater when unhealthy lifestyle habits are combined in individuals with genetic risk factors. A few examples are presented here.

Genetics is thought to play some role in hypertension.[4] African Americans tend to develop hypertension more often than people of any other racial background in the United States. It often is more severe in this group and some medications are less effective.[5]

Familial hypercholesterolemia, a defect that does not allow the body to remove low density lipoproteins (LDLs), contributes to atherosclerosis characterized by plaques of cholesterol and other lipids lining the inner layers of arteries to obstruct blood flow.[6] Other conditions are thought to have inherited risk include coronary artery disease, heart failure, diabetes, as well as certain arrhythmias. Hemoglobinopathies are inherited blood disorders resulting in abnormal hemoglobin, such as sickle cell disease. In this disorder, the abnormal hemoglobin clumps together and occludes blood vessels when the person experiences hypoxia, dehydration, or acidosis.[7]

Genetic disorders causing bleeding include hemophilia A and B and von Willebrand disease. People with these disorders bleed longer than others. Bleeding can be internal into joints and muscles, or externally from minor cuts, dental procedures, and trauma. Hemophilia A and B are recessive sex-linked genetic defects affecting males. Each type has a deficiency of a specific clotting factor. Von Willebrand disease is a genetic disorder caused by a missing or defective clotting protein; while it affects men and women, women experience more symptoms during menses and childbirth.[8]

Lifestyle

A number of risk factors are associated with lifestyle choices—and these may exacerbate disease among those who have genetic predisposition to cardiovascular disease. Among the most important risk factors include smoking, inactivity, an unhealthy diet, and obesity. These lifestyle factors are known to increase their risks for hypertension, obesity, and type 2 diabetes mellitus, which impair perfusion.[9]

Immobility

Individuals who are immobile are at risk for impaired tissue perfusion. This includes those who are paralyzed, are unconscious or have an impaired cognitive state, or are on bed rest to recover from an illness, injury, or surgery. Sitting in one position for a prolonged time can interrupt blood flow of the legs. Perfusion impaired by immobility can cause two problems: pressure ulcers and venous thrombi. When individuals remain in one position for a prolonged time, their perfusion is impaired by the external pressure on the dependent areas. If the prolonged pressure exceeds the capillary pressure, then ischemia occurs resulting in anoxia and necrosis causing skin breakdown.[10] Being immobile also contributes to blood clot formation by slowing the return of venous blood to the heart. Slow blood flow results in stasis, a risk factor for thrombi formation. Individuals who are confined to a sitting position for long periods (e.g., long airplane flights) are susceptible to formation of venous clots.

ASSESSMENT

Assessment of perfusion includes obtaining a history, conducting a physical examination, and analyzing results of diagnostic tests.

History
Baseline History

When collecting subjective data, nurses ask patients about their present health status, past health history, family history, and personal and psychosocial history. Present health status includes questions about chronic diseases, such as diabetes mellitus, renal failure, hypertension, or hemophilia. Nurses ask patients for a list of medications they take, both prescription and over-the-counter, including the reason for each medication and its effectiveness. Patients are asked about their use of recreational or street drugs such as cocaine, because it is associated with myocardial infarction and stroke. Past health history includes questions about heart disease, heart defects, rheumatic fever, or sickle cell disease. Data are collected about family members with cardiovascular and clotting disorders. Personal and psychosocial history includes diet, exercise, smoking, and alcohol consumption. A diet high in fat and carbohydrates together with minimal or infrequent exercise contributes to atherosclerosis and obesity. The patient is asked about the kind of exercise and how often it is performed and for what length of time, because exercise

TABLE 18.1 **Individual Risk Factors for Impaired Perfusion**	
Modifiable Risk Factors	**Unmodifiable Risk Factors**
• Smoking: Nicotine vasoconstricts	• Age: Increases with age
• Elevated serum lipids: Contribute to atherosclerosis	• Gender: Men > women
• Sedentary lifestyle: Contributes to obesity	• Genetics: Family history
• Obesity: Increases risk for type 2 diabetes mellitus and atherosclerosis	
• Diabetes mellitus: Increases risk of atherosclerosis	
• Hypertension: Increases work of myocardium	

Adapted from Wilson, S., & Giddens, J. (2017). *Health assessment for nursing practice* (5th ed.). St. Louis: Elsevier.

increases blood flow. Information about smoking habits is important, because nicotine causes vasoconstriction and is a toxin that damages the endothelium, contributing to atherosclerosis. Excessive alcohol intake is associated with dysrhythmias.[11]

A health history of an infant should include data about feeding problems and weight gain. Feeding difficulties accompanied by fatigue, rapid breathing, sweating with feeding, and poor weight gain are common symptoms in infants with heart disease.[1] Respiratory infections and breathing problems should be noted as well as onset and frequency of skin tone changes, especially cyanosis.

For older children and adolescents, a history should include questions about exercise tolerance, edema and respiratory problems, chest pain, palpitations, fainting, and headaches.[1]

Problem-Based History

When providing their history, patients may describe pain, fainting (syncope), dizziness, shortness of breath (dyspnea), swelling (edema), bleeding, or fatigue. When these symptoms are reported, the nurse follows up with a symptom analysis to obtain additional data, including the onset of the symptom; the location, duration, and severity of the symptom; a description of the symptom; factors that alleviate or aggravate the symptom; other associated symptoms; and actions taken by the patient to relieve the symptom.[11]

Pain. A common symptom reported by patients with impaired tissue perfusion is pain. When there is inadequate perfusion to carry oxygen needed to meet tissue needs, patients experience ischemic pain. This type of pain occurs by the same process, whether it is occurring in coronary arteries affecting central perfusion or in femoral arteries affecting tissue perfusion.

Chest pain may be due to impaired blood flow to the myocardium or pulmonary emboli. Patients experience myocardial ischemia, also called stable angina, when there is an increased demand for oxygen on the heart. They often report a precipitating event, such as physical exertion, exposure to cold temperatures, or emotional stress. Patients with angina pectoris often describe their chest pain as a constricting or squeezing sensation that is relieved with rest and/or by taking one or more nitroglycerin tablets (a vasodilator). By contrast, patients with acute coronary syndrome (unstable angina advancing to myocardial infarction) report severe chest pain that is not relieved by rest or nitroglycerin, shortness of breath, and radiating pain to the jaw or arms. Related symptoms may be nausea, vomiting, dizziness, and diaphoresis. Although men and women may experience similar symptoms, some women have had acute myocardial infarction with no chest pain; instead they may report shortness of breath, dizziness, and neck, jaw, shoulder, upper back, or abdominal discomfort.[12]

Pulmonary embolism causes chest pain by blocking the pulmonary arteries with emboli that travelled from the legs. The chest pain is often worse when breathing deeply (pleurisy), coughing, bending, or stooping. The pain becomes worse with exertion and is not relieved by rest. Related symptoms may include cyanosis, fever, irregular heart rate, and dizziness.[13]

Pain in the legs attributable to impaired tissue perfusion may be caused by peripheral arterial disease (PAD) or deep vein thrombus. PAD develops from atherosclerosis that causes vessel occlusion. Signs and symptoms vary depending on the number and location of arteries affected, degree of impairment, presence of collateral circulation, and the patient's activity level. Patients may report pain when walking that is relieved with rest, called intermittent claudication. This pain indicates an inadequate blood supply to transport oxygen needed to meet the demands of the leg muscles. Thus, the pain stops when the increased demand of oxygen from walking stops. As the arterial occlusion increases, patients may report "rest pain," which is leg pain while walking that is

not relieved with rest.[14] By contrast, deep vein thrombosis occurs when a blood clot (thrombus) forms in one or more deep veins, usually in the legs, that occludes the vein thereby impairing the blood return to the heart. The pain is described as soreness or cramping.[15]

Patients experiencing a sickle cell crisis report mild to severe localized or generalized pain due to ischemia that may last minutes to days. Joints and bones are commonly involved. Associated symptoms are low-grade fever and edema of soft tissues over hands and feet.[16]

Syncope. Syncope is the transient loss of consciousness due to inadequate cerebral perfusion. Nurses ask about symptoms experienced before the syncope to help determine the cause. For example, reports of headache, numbness, and confusion may indicate a stroke caused by cerebral emboli. Slowing of the pulse may suggest a cardiac rhythm disorder. Reports of ringing in the ears may indicate an inner ear problem.[11]

Dizziness. Patients may report feeling dizzy. Using a symptom analysis, nurses collect data to learn when this lightheadedness occurs as well as aggravating and alleviating factors. If the dizziness occurs when the patient sits up suddenly, it is called *orthostatic hypotension*, which is defined as a 20- to 30-mm Hg drop in systolic blood pressure when a patient moves from a lying to a sitting or standing position. Nurses inquire about the duration of the dizziness. For many patients, the dizziness subsides if they sit for a few seconds before standing. In contrast, dizziness unrelated to position changes may be caused by inadequate blood flow to the brain. The carotid arteries may be obstructed from atherosclerosis, preventing adequate blood flow to the brain.[11]

Dyspnea. Inadequate circulation of blood interferes with oxygen transport to tissues, making patients dyspneic or short of breath during activity. This symptom may be reported by patients with primary perfusion problems, such as heart failure, or by those with primary gas exchange problems, such as chronic obstructive pulmonary disease. Patients may report having to sleep sitting up or using several pillows to prop up during the night. Lightheadedness may be reported, attributable to inadequate oxygen transport to the brain. Nurses inquire about the duration of patients' shortness of breath, as well as if the dyspnea occurs on inhalation or exhalation, or both. Related symptoms include chest pain or swelling of the feet and ankles.[11] When an infant is being evaluated for heart disease, the mother or caretaker may report the infant needing to stop sucking "to catch his or her breath" or the infant exhibiting a bluish color around the lips when sucking.[17]

Edema. Patients may report their socks leaving an indentation around their legs or edema in their feet that is worse at the end of the day. This edema reflects excessive fluid in the interstitial spaces, which indicates a fluid overload or an accumulation of fluids; a related symptom is weight gain. When present in both legs, edema may be caused by fluid overload from diseases (e.g., heart failure, renal failure, or liver disease). The excessive fluid may occur from renal disease when blood cannot be filtered by the kidneys. Right-sided heart failure is another cause of peripheral edema that develops if the right ventricle is unable to eject its usual volume of blood. Reflux of blood occurs from the right ventricle into the right atrium and then into the inferior and superior venae cavae. Because of the buildup of blood, the veins are unable to transport blood back to the heart, resulting in an accumulation of blood in the venous system that pushes fluid into the interstitial spaces, causing edema.[11] Unilateral edema of an extremity may be lymphedema caused by occlusion of lymph channels (e.g., elephantiasis or trauma) or surgical removal of lymph channels (e.g., after mastectomy). Localized edema of one leg may be caused by venous insufficiency from varicosities or deep vein thrombosis.

Bleeding and bruising. Nurses ask about unusual bleeding and bruising (ecchymosis). Patients may describe bleeding that takes longer than usual to stop. They may report bleeding from various areas of the body, including bleeding gums after brushing teeth; nosebleeds; black, tarry stools; blood from rectum (hematochezia); blood in the urine (hematuria); blood in emesis (hematemesis); coughing up blood (hemoptysis); bleeding from the mouth; or new bruising, a discoloration of the skin caused by blood in the dermal tissues.[18] Indications of intracranial bleeding may include a headache, changes in vision, sudden difficulty talking, or weakness of one arm or leg. Patients may report fatigue or dyspnea from anemia caused by blood loss. When applicable, women are asked about the amount of blood lost during menses and whether the length of menses has increased.

Parents of children with hemophilia may report that the children bleed after minor trauma such as from a circumcision, during loss of deciduous teeth, or after a slight fall. Bleeding into a joint (hemarthrosis) may produce complaints of stiffness, tingling, or ache of knees, elbows, and ankles. Hematuria may also be reported.[18]

Fatigue. Fatigue is another common symptom associated with impaired perfusion. Patients may report feeling more tired than usual or having a lack of energy. Nurses ask whether the onset was gradual or sudden, at what time of day onset occurred, and about the duration. Fatigue experienced during daily activities such as shopping or climbing stairs occurs because the heart cannot pump enough blood to meet the body tissue needs. Both right-sided and left-sided heart failure cause a gradual onset, while acute blood loss produces fatigue more rapidly. Anemia causing fatigue may occur in patients with heart failure due to impaired nutritional intake caused by dyspnea during meals, renal disease resulting from reduced blood flow to kidneys, or medication adverse effects such as from taking angiotensin-converting enzyme inhibitors (e.g., enalapril). Fatigue from anemia lasts all day.[11]

Examination Findings

Physical assessment is performed by measuring vital signs, including oxygen saturation, and by using the examination techniques of inspection, palpation, and auscultation.

Vital Signs

When measuring blood pressure and peripheral pulses, nurses may notice changes such as hypotension or hypertension, bradycardia, or tachycardia. For example, severe bleeding may result in hypotension and tachycardia. The pulse rhythm may be irregular when conduction problems are present. When assessing for orthostatic hypotension, blood pressure is measured with the patient in three positions: lying, sitting, and standing. Nurses compare these three blood pressure readings to confirm position changes as a contributing factor to the dizziness or fainting.

Peripheral pulse rates should be equal bilaterally. In adults the respiratory rate may be increased and breathing labored with a low oxygen saturation when perfusion is inadequate to provide oxygenated blood to cells. A child's pulse rate may normally increase on inspiration and decrease on expiration. Congenital heart disease in infants produces elevations in heart and respiratory rates when feeding.[11]

Inspection

Inspect the overall skin tone and for evidence of skin discoloration. Petechiae, ecchymosis, and purpura from bleeding into the subcutaneous tissue may be observed. Subcutaneous and intramuscular hemorrhages are common among patients with hemophilia.[11] Pale skin may indicate anemia.

Inspect the anterior chest and neck. A marked retraction on the chest near the apical space may indicate pericardial disease or right ventricular hypertrophy. Jugular vein pulsations are an expected finding;

however, fluttering or prominent pulsations may indicate right-sided heart failure.

Inspect the upper and lower extremities for symmetry, skin integrity, and color. Arms and legs should be symmetric with skin intact and color uniform and appropriate for race. If one arm or leg appears larger than the other, measure the circumference of each arm or leg and compare. Lymphedema may cause one arm to be larger. Venous thrombi may cause redness and an increased circumference of the extremity from edema. Skin ulcerations may indicate arterial or venous perfusion abnormalities. Patients with arterial occlusion may have pallor and lack of hair on the legs.

Palpation

Palpate the apical pulse or point of maximal impulse (PMI) at the fifth intercostal space, midclavicular line. The apical pulse should be felt at that location and have a regular rhythm. When patients have ventricular hypertrophy, their enlarged myocardium may move the PMI laterally. An apical pulse rate that is faster than the radial pulse rate indicates a pulse deficit, which is calculated by subtracting the radial rate from the apical rate. This deficit should be 0 (zero), meaning the rates are equal. Pulse deficits occur when patients have dysrhythmias, commonly atrial fibrillation. When irregular pulses are palpated, notice whether the irregularity has a rhythm. A regular irregularity is felt when patients have premature atrial contractions (PACs)—for example, an extra beat after every third beat. An irregular irregularity is felt in patients who have atrial fibrillation when no pattern is noted in the irregularity.

When palpating the chest, the nurse may feel a slight thrust during systole called a *lift*. A more prominent thrust during systole is called a *heave*. Lifts and heaves may occur from left or right ventricular hypertrophy due an increased workload. A thrill is a palpable vibration over the precordium associated with a loud murmur.

Palpate upper and lower extremities for skin turgor, temperature (using the back of the hands), capillary refill, and peripheral pulses. Skin turgor should be elastic; temperature should be warm with capillary refill of fingers and toes <2 seconds and pulses (brachial, radial, posterior tibial and dorsalis pedis) 2+ strength and regular rhythm. If the skin does not immediately fall back into place after palpation, it is termed *tenting* and indicates reduced fluid in the interstitial space from a fluid volume deficit. By contrast, when the indentation of the nurse's thumb or finger remains in the skin, it is termed *pitting edema* indicating increased fluid in the interstitial spaces. Skin temperature may feel cool, called *poikilothermia*, due to impaired arterial perfusion. Capillary refill greater than 2 seconds indicates poor perfusion. The strength of the pulse, also called the *amplitude*, is an indication of perfusion. Absence of a pulse is indicated as 0; a diminished or barely palpable pulse is 1+, indicating poor perfusion or fluid/blood loss; a full or strong pulse is 3+, indicating fluid excess; and a bounding pulse is 4+, indicating fluid overload.[11] Lower extremity pain and paresthesia, as well as weak or absent dorsalis pedis and posterior tibial pulses, are indications of arterial occlusion. When this is suspected, the nurse calculates an ankle-brachial index (ABI) by dividing the ankle systolic blood pressure by the brachial systolic blood pressure. Those with peripheral arterial disease have an ABI less than the normal value of 1.0 or above. By contrast, venous occlusion is indicated when leg pain is accompanied by redness and edema.[11]

Auscultation

Auscultation of the patient's heart may reveal S_1 and S_2 heart sounds, as expected, as well as abnormal heart sounds such as S_3, S_4, and murmurs. The S_3 sound is heard in early diastole and may be due to left ventricular failure, volume overload, or regurgitation of the mitral, aortic, or tricuspid valves. The S₄ sound is heard in late diastole and may be due to resistance to ventricular filling from hypertension, ventricular hypertrophy, aortic stenosis, or coronary artery disease. Murmurs create a blowing sound indicating turbulent blood flow through the heart. When a patient has a history of atherosclerosis or reports dizziness, the nurse auscultates the carotid artery for bruits.[12]

When auscultating the heart of an infant and child, the nurse uses a pediatric stethoscope. A venous hum heard over the jugular vein caused by turbulent blood flow is considered a normal variation in children. Characteristic heart murmurs are heard in infants with congenital heart disorders such as atrial septal defect, ventricular septal defect, and patent ductus arteriosus. Infants with coarctation of the aorta have high blood pressure and bounding pulses in the arms but lower blood pressure, weak to absent pulses, and cool lower extremities.[1]

Diagnostic Tests
Laboratory Tests
Cardiac enzymes/markers. Enzymes released from damaged cells circulate in the blood and can be measured to confirm a number of cardiovascular conditions.

- Creatine kinase (CK) is an enzyme present in myocardium (CK-MB), in muscle (CK-MM), and in brain (CK-BB) tissues. When enzymes are isolated, the level of CK-MB is elevated 3 to 6 hours after a myocardial infarction.[19]
- Cardiac troponins are myocardial muscle proteins released after myocardial injury. This test is used to evaluate patients with suspected acute coronary syndromes and predict the likelihood of future cardiac events. Cardiac troponins become elevated sooner and remain elevated longer than CK-MB.[19]
- Myoglobin is an oxygen-binding protein found in cardiac and skeletal muscles. Increased myoglobin levels indicating cardiac injury or death occur about 3 hours after infarction.[19]
- Homocysteine (Hcy) is an amino acid. Evidence suggests that elevated levels of homocysteine may act as an independent risk factor for ischemic heart disease, cerebrovascular disease, peripheral arterial disease, and venous thrombosis.[19]
- C-reactive protein (CRP) is produced by the liver during acute inflammation. The level of CRP correlates with peak levels of the CK-MB, but CRP peaks occur 1 to 3 days earlier. Failure of CRP to normalize may indicate ongoing damage to the heart.[19]

Serum lipids. Serum lipids are measured to detect hyperlipidemia and include cholesterol lipoproteins (low-density lipoproteins [LDLs], high-density lipoproteins [HDLs], very low-density lipoproteins [VLDs]), and triglycerides. Lipoproteins are an accurate predictor of heart disease. High levels of LDL adhere to the endothelium obstructing blood flow. The function of HDL is to remove lipids from the endothelium to provide a protective effect against heart disease.[19]

Complete blood count. Elements of the complete blood count provide information regarding the oxygen-carrying capacity of the blood and the risk for clotting. Specifically, the number of red blood cells (RBCs), the hemoglobin, and hematocrit are used to diagnose polycythemia and anemia, as well as determine hydration. Patients with polycythemia have elevated levels of erythrocytes or RBCs, which increases the risk of clotting. Patients may develop anemia due to blood loss, which is indicated by RBC, hemoglobin, and hematocrit values below normal.[19]

Blood coagulability.
- Platelet count is the number of platelets (thrombocytes) per cubic millimeter of blood. Platelet activity is essential for blood clotting. When the platelet count is decreased (thrombocytopenia), the person is at risk for bleeding.[19]
- Fibrinogen (or clotting factor I) is essential to the blood-clotting mechanism. It is used primarily to aid in the diagnosis of suspected bleeding disorders. Produced by the liver, fibrinogen rises sharply during tissue inflammation or necrosis and has been associated with an increased risk or coronary heart disease, stroke, myocardial infarction, and peripheral arterial disease.[19]
- Prothrombin time (PT) measures the adequacy of the extrinsic system and common pathways in the clotting mechanism, which include clotting factors I (fibrinogen), II (prothrombin), V, VII, and X. When these clotting factors are found in decreased amounts, the PT is prolonged, meaning more time is needed for blood to clot. PT results are reported in seconds along with a control value. The patient's value should be approximately equal to the control. A normal finding is 11 to 12.5 seconds.[19]
- The international normalized ratio (INR) was established by the World Health Organization to standardize the INR results regardless of the reagents or methods used to analyze the blood. The INR is used to monitor the effectiveness of anticoagulant therapy such as warfarin (Coumadin) that is given to inhibit the formation of blood clots.[19]
- Partial thromboplastin time (PTT) measures the intrinsic system and common pathway of clot formation, which includes factors I (fibrinogen), II (prothrombin), V, VIII, IX, X, XI, and XII. Factors II, VII, IX, and X are vitamin K–dependent factors. When there are reduced amounts of these clotting factors, the PTT is prolonged, meaning more time is needed for blood to clot. Like the PT values, the PTT results are reported in seconds along with a control value. Activators were added to PTT reagents to shorten normal clotting time and provide a narrow normal range. This shortened time is called *activated PTT*, or *APTT*. The PTT is used to monitor the therapeutic ranges of patients taking anticoagulants such as heparin.[19]
- The D-dimer test assesses the activity of both thrombin, used to form blood clots, and plasmin, used to break down blood clots. While plasmin breaks down fibrin clots, fibrin degradation products and D-dimer are produced. The D-dimer assay provides a highly specific measurement of the amount of fibrin degradation that occurs as the clot is dissolved. Plasma normally does not have detectable amounts of fragment D-dimer. This test is used to confirm a diagnosis of disseminated intravascular coagulation (DIC).[19]

Bone marrow biopsy. A bone marrow biopsy allows examination of bone marrow, which is used to evaluate patients with hematologic diseases. Indications include evaluating anemias, leukopenias, and thrombocytopenias; diagnosing leukemia; and documenting abnormal iron stores.[19]

Electrocardiogram

An electrocardiogram (ECG) is performed by placing 12 leads on the patient's chest and extremities to record the electrical impulses through the heart. The waveforms generated detect cardiac dysrhythmias by documenting on a screen or paper the electrical impulses generated by the heart during contraction and relaxation of atria and ventricles. A 12-lead ECG is obtained to detect myocardial ischemia or infarction when patients complain of chest pain. An ECG also is used to continuously monitor the heart rhythm using one or more leads.[19]

Cardiac Stress Test

A cardiac stress test is used to detect issues with cardiac perfusion in the presence of a stressor. It is usually indicated for individuals with symptoms (chest pain with activity or unexplained shortness of breath) or significant risk factors. Two types of stress tests include an exercise stress test and a pharmacologic stress test.

Exercise cardiac stress test. The exercise cardiac stress test is one of the most common cardiac stress tests because it is relatively simple and noninvasive. The patient exercises on a treadmill with a progressive increase in speed and elevation or pedals a stationary bike to increase heart rate and workload. During the test, an ECG is recorded along with regular monitoring of heart rate and rhythm, blood pressure, and respiratory rate.[20] If coronary artery disease is present, changes in electrical conduction or other symptoms such as chest pain may occur.

Pharmacologic stress test. Another common cardiac stress test involves the administration of certain pharmacologic agents that stimulate the physiological effects of exercise such as dilating the coronary arteries. This is often done when patients are unable to perform the exercise stress test due to underlying conditions or when a treadmill or stationary bike is not available. Agents often administered include dobutamine and adenosine. ECG monitoring (or radionuclide imaging) is performed, while the pharmacologic agents are given to detect problems with conduction, heart rate, or strength of contractions.[7]

Radiographic Studies

Chest x-ray. Chest x-rays provide visualization of the lungs, ribs, clavicles, vertebrae, heart, and major thoracic vessels. For patients with impaired perfusion, x-rays are taken to visualize the size of the heart and lung fields.[19]

Ultrasound. An ultrasound of the heart is called *echocardiography*; a noninvasive ultrasound procedure is used to evaluate the structure and function of the heart. It is used in the diagnosis ventricular hypertrophy, endocarditis, septal defects, and valvular disorders such as valvular stenosis, valvular regurgitation, and mitral valve prolapse. Vascular ultrasound uses a Doppler to identify occlusion or thrombosis of veins and arteries of an extremity. Doppler ultrasound uses a probe that directs high-frequency sound waves to indicate blood flow in the artery.[19]

Arteriogram. This diagnostic procedure allows visualization of arteries by injecting radiopaque contrast into them so that the location and extent of occlusion can be identified. A cardiac catheterization is one type of arteriogram that allows visualization of coronary arteries and heart chambers. A catheter is passed into the heart through a peripheral vein or artery, depending on whether catheterization of the left or right side of the heart is being performed. Pressures are recorded through the catheter, and radiographic contrast is injected to visualize the patency of coronary arteries.[19]

Venogram. This diagnostic test allows visualization of lower extremity veins to assess blood flow and to determine the size and condition of the veins. The test shows if there is a blockage of blood flow (from a narrowing of the vessel or a thrombi as examples). Radiopaque contrast is injected into veins and then an x-ray is taken to visualize the veins under examination. If thrombi are present, the location and extent of thrombi can be identified.[19]

CLINICAL MANAGEMENT

Clinical management associated with the perfusion concept involves the prevention of illness, early detection, and appropriate collaborative management of cardiovascular problems.

Primary Prevention

Primary prevention includes measures to promote health and prevent disease. For the concept of perfusion, these measures include promoting heart and peripheral vascular health, as well as preventing abnormal clotting and bleeding. Promoting heart and peripheral vascular health involves controlling modifiable risk factors by eating a healthy diet exercising most days of the week and not smoking.[21] Common primary prevention strategies are presented in Box 18.1.

> **BOX 18.1   Health Promotion Recommendations: Perfusion**
>
> 1. Eat a healthy diet.
>   - Choose foods low in sodium, saturated fat, and trans fats.
>   - Eat plenty of fruits, vegetables, fiber-rich whole grains, legumes, nuts.
>   - Choose fish and skinless poultry; avoid red meat; if you choose to eat meat, choose lean cuts of meat.
>   - Select lower fat dairy products: fat-free or low-fat dairy products.
>   - Limit sugar-sweetened beverages.
> 2. Participate in physical activity.
>   - Adults >20 years of age should engage in 150 min of moderate-intensity activity/week or 75 min of vigorous intensity activity every week.
>   - Children 12–19 years of age should engage in at least 60 min of moderate intensity activity every day.
> 3. Refrain from smoking and have no exposure to environmental tobacco smoke.
> 4. Maintain blood pressure in recommended range.
>   - Adults >20 years of age: <120/<80 mm Hg
>   - Children 1–13 years of age: <90th percentile
>   - Children aged ≥13 years of age: <120/<80 mm Hg
> 5. Achieve and maintain desirable weight.
>   - Adults >20 years of age: 18.5–24.9 BMI
>   - Children 12–19 years of age: <85th percentile

Data from American Heart Association (2019). Understanding your risks to prevent a heart attack. Retrieved from https://www.heart.org/en/health-topics/heart-attack/understand-your-risks-to-prevent-a-heart-attack?s=q%3Drisk%2520factors%2520for%2520coronary%2520artery%2520disease%26sort%3Drelevancy.

Strategies for prevention of blood clotting include minimizing the risks for blood stasis, increased blood viscosity, and vessel injury. Patients at risk for venous stasis or those with clotting disorders are encouraged to enhance blood flow by performing leg exercises, engaging in regular walking, or wearing compression stockings. High-risk patients (e.g., those following knee or hip replacement surgery) take anticoagulant therapy as a prophylactic measure. Women with an increased risk for clots may be advised to avoid taking birth control pills because of their adverse effect on clotting. Maintaining adequate hydration reduces the potential for increased blood viscosity. For problems associated with excessive bleeding, the only true primary prevention measure is genetic counseling, which is advised for couples who have a family history of bleeding disorders and want to start a family. Genetic counseling assists couples to understand risks and options and make an informed decision.[22]

Secondary Prevention (Screening)

Secondary prevention includes screening and early diagnosis and prompt treatment of existing health problems. Its purpose is to shorten the duration and severity of consequences. Routine screening involves monitoring blood pressure and serum lipids.

Blood Pressure Screening

Blood pressure screening is a simple and cost-effective screening recommended across the lifespan. Beginning in infancy, blood pressure screening is recommended at every well-child visit and at least annually.[23] The U.S. Preventative Services Task Force (USPSTF) recommends screening for high blood pressure in adults aged 18 to 39 every 3 to 5 years, and annually for adults 40 years or older and for those who are at increased risk for high blood pressure.[24] Persons at increased risk

TABLE 18.2 Blood Pressure Guidelines for Adults

Normal range	SBP <120
	and
	DBP <80
Elevated blood pressure	SBP 120–129
	and
	DBP <80
Stage 1 hypertension	SBP 130–139
	or
	DBP 80–89
Stage 2 hypertension	SBP ≥140
	or
	DBP ≥90
Hypertensive crisis	SBP >180
	and/or
	DBP >120

DBP, Diastolic blood pressure; *SBP*, systolic blood pressure.
From Whelton, P. K., Carey, R. M., Aronow, W. S., Casey, D. E., Jr., Collins, K. J., Dennison Himmelfarb, C., et al. (2018). 2017 ACC/AHA/ABC/ACPM/AGS/APhA/ASH/ASPC/NMA/PCNA Guideline for the prevention, detection, evaluation, and management of high blood pressure in adults: Executive summary: A report of the American College/American Heart Association task force on clinical practice guidelines. *Hypertension, 71*(6), 1269–1324.

include those who have elevated blood pressure (Table 18.2), those who are overweight or obese, and African Americans.

Collaborative Interventions

The management of individuals with impaired perfusion is highly dependent on the specific condition. The following sections describe common interventions implemented in the treatment of conditions resulting in impaired perfusion. Some of these conditions are also listed as primary prevention measures. They are listed again here because these same measures are useful to improve health for those with impaired perfusion.

Nutrition Therapy

Nutrition therapy should meet the recommendations described under Primary Prevention, but the goal of the heart-healthy diet is tertiary prevention—to lower serum lipid levels, lose weight, and maintain an optimal weight. For this reason, nutrition therapy is considered an intervention in both primary prevention and disease management.

Smoking Cessation

Smoking cessation is also considered both primary prevention and collaborative intervention for disease management. For interventions directed at smoking cessation, refer to Concept 19, Gas Exchange.

Activity and Exercise

Activity and exercise are a regular part of any treatment regimen. Specifically, they are included in the following applications:
- For the purpose of weight loss and weight maintenance
- Cardiac rehabilitation after acute coronary syndrome
- Progressive activity for patients with peripheral arterial disease

Pharmacotherapy

Pharmacotherapy represents one of the most common collaborative interventions for individuals with conditions associated with cardiovascular disease. The following are the general classifications of drugs; there are many types of drugs within each of these categories:

- *Vasodilators* increase the diameter of blood vessels in a variety of ways that block normal mechanisms. They are used to treat hypertension as well as angina. Common examples include angiotensin-converting enzyme inhibitors (captopril, lisinopril, and losartan), nitrates (amyl nitrite, nitroglycerine, and nitroprusside), potassium channel activators (diazoxide and minoxidil), and smooth muscle relaxants (hydralazine).[25]
- *Vasopressors* decrease or vasoconstrict the diameter of blood vessels. They are used to treat hypotension resulting from hemorrhage, myocardial infarction, septicemia, or drug reactions. Examples include epinephrine, norepinephrine, and dobutamine.[25]
- *Diuretics* promote the formation and excretion of urine by preventing the reabsorption of sodium in the kidneys. They are used to reduce blood volume to treat hypertension. Common examples include loop (furosemide), thiazide (hydrochlorothiazide), potassium-sparing (spironolactone), and osmotic (mannitol).[25]
- *Antidysrhythmics* correct erratic electrical impulses to create regular cardiac rhythms. They are used to treat premature ventricular contractions (PVC), tachycardia, hypertension, and atrial fibrillation. These agents act by blocking electrolytes that affect electrical conduction in the heart, such as potassium (amiodarone) and calcium (diltiazem), or by blocking β-adrenergic receptors (atenolol).[26]
- *Cardioglycosides* have a positive inotropic effect with a lowering of heart rate to increase cardiac output and are used for the treatment of heart failure, atrial fibrillation, and cardiogenic shock. The classic example is digoxin.[25]
- *Anticoagulants* prevent blood clotting at several locations in the clotting cascade. They are most effective in preventing venous thrombosis. Common examples include heparin, warfarin sodium, enoxaparin, dabigatran, and rivaroxaban.[25]
- *Antiplatelet* agents prevent platelets from aggregating to form clots. They are most effective in preventing arterial thrombosis. Classes of antiplatelet agents are glycoprotein inhibitors (tirofiban), platelet adhesion inhibitor (dipyridamole), thrombin inhibitor (bivalirudin), and platelet aggregation inhibitors (aspirin and clopidogrel).[25]
- *Thrombolytics* disrupt blood clots that are impairing perfusion by lysing fibrin. Common examples include tissue plasminogen activator, alteplase, and urokinase.
- *Antilipidemics* decrease the levels of lipids that contribute to atherosclerosis and result in blood vessel occlusion by reducing the synthesis of cholesterol. The primary group of drugs used are the statins (e.g., atorvastatin, fluvastatin, lovastatin, and pravastatin).[25]

Procedures and Surgical Interventions

A variety of procedures and surgical interventions are used to improve central perfusion as well as tissue perfusion. Myocardial contractions can be improved by performing defibrillation or inserting a pacemaker. Blood flow through the heart can be improved by replacing heart valves.

Blood flow through coronary and peripheral arteries is improved in several ways: by surgically bypassing the obstruction, compressing the obstruction (e.g., angioplasty and inserting stents to maintain patency) or removing the obstruction (e.g., endarterectomy or thrombectomy).

Defibrillation. Defibrillation is used to change abnormal cardiac rhythms by the passage of an electric shock through the heart that is sufficient to depolarize myocardial cells so that the SA node will resume the role as pacemaker. Defibrillation is used for emergency treatment during cardiac arrest when ventricular fibrillation or ventricular tachycardia is present. Synchronized cardioversion is a therapeutic procedure using defibrillation on a nonemergent basis to convert an abnormal rhythm, such as ventricular tachycardia with a pulse or atrial fibrillation, to a normal sinus rhythm.[26]

Pacemaker. This electronic device used to increase the heart rate in severe bradycardia by electronically stimulating the myocardium. The basic pacing circuit consists of a battery-operated pulse generator and one or more conducting leads that pace the atrium and one or both ventricles. Pacemakers can be external (temporary) or surgically implanted (permanent).[26]

Heart valve replacement. Heart valve replacement is indicated for patients with valves that have stenosis (do not open completely) or insufficiency (do not close completely). Heart valves are repaired or replaced with a prosthetic valve. Valves may be mechanical or biological. Mechanical valves are constructed of metal alloys, pyrolytic carbon, and Dacron, whereas biological valves are constructed from bovine, porcine, or human (cadaver) cardiac tissue, and usually contain some man-made materials.[27]

Arterial bypass graft. The two most common areas for arterial bypass include coronary bypass and peripheral artery bypass. Coronary revascularization is accomplished with a coronary artery bypass graft (CABG). This procedure surgically implants patent blood vessels to transport blood between the aorta and the myocardium distal to the obstructed coronary artery or arteries. The internal mammary artery, radial artery, and saphenous vein from the patient are used frequently as bypass grafts. CABG requires a sternotomy to gain access to the heart and cardiopulmonary bypass (CPB) to divert the patient's blood from the heart to the CPB machine. The CPB machine oxygenates the patient's blood and returns it to the patient, allowing the surgeon to operate on a nonbeating, bloodless heart while perfusion to organs is maintained.[28]

Peripheral artery revascularization is a surgical procedure using an autogenous vein or synthetic graft to bypass the lesion in the artery that is impairing perfusion. Femoropopliteal bypass is an example of this procedure, in which a graft is attached to the femoral artery to divert blood around the occlusion and attached to the popliteal artery.[29] The femoral artery is clamped proximal to the insertion of the graft, allowing the surgeon to attach the graft to a bloodless artery.

Angioplasty with stent placement. Cardiac catheterization and coronary angiography provide images of coronary circulation to identify lesions blocking coronary arteries. If appropriate, revascularization can be performed using balloon angioplasty. During this procedure, a catheter equipped with an inflatable balloon tip is inserted into the affected coronary artery. When the blockage is located, the catheter is passed through it, the balloon is inflated, and the blockage (atherosclerotic plaque) is compressed, which dilates the artery. Intracoronary stents are often inserted into the artery during an angioplasty to hold the artery open. A stent is an expandable meshlike structure designed to expand the artery to maintain patency.[28]

Endarterectomy. This surgical procedure removes obstructing plaque or blockage from the lining of an artery to improve perfusion. The carotid artery is a common site for this procedure, resulting in improved perfusion to the brain and thereby preventing an ischemia stroke.[29]

Thrombectomy. This procedure removes a thrombus from a vessel through a catheter placed percutaneously or as an open surgical procedure (e.g., direct arteriotomy or venous thrombectomy).[29]

Cardiac transplant. This procedure involves the replacement of a diseased heart with a healthy donor heart (from a person after death). A cardiac transplant is indicated in a variety of terminal or end-stage heart conditions.[30] It has become a relatively common procedure with 3244 individuals undergoing this procedure in 2017.[31]

CLINICAL NURSING SKILLS FOR PERFUSION

- Assessment
  - Measure vital signs
  - General inspection for color, respiratory effort, distress
  - Inspect the thorax
  - Auscultate heart and vascular sounds
  - Inspect extremities for skin color
  - Palpate extremities for edema
  - Palpate peripheral pulses
  - Assess capillary refill
  - When indicated, calculate the ankle-brachial index, measure leg circumferences, calculate pulse deficit
- Cardiac monitoring
- Hemodynamic monitoring
  - Continuous arterial blood pressure monitoring
  - Pulmonary artery pressure monitoring
- Medication administration
  - Oral medications
  - Intravenous fluids and medications
- Sequential compression devices and elastic stockings
- Ambulation
- Positioning
- Patient teaching

INTERRELATED CONCEPTS

Because all cells in the body depend on perfusion to carry oxygen and nutrients to cells, this concept is interrelated to nearly all of the health and illness concepts within this textbook. Concepts that most closely interrelate with perfusion are shown in Fig. 18.3 and explained as follows.

Patients complain of **Pain** when perfusion is impaired by clotting or narrowed arteries, whether it be in the coronary arteries, causing chest pain, or in the iliac or femoral arteries, causing leg pain when walking. Impaired tissue perfusion leading to ischemia creates lactic acid that contributes to pain. Because impaired tissue perfusion to the legs causes pain during walking, peripheral arterial disease reduces the **Mobility** of patients due to the pain they experience. Walking is beneficial to exercise the heart and improve central perfusion, an important health promotion behavior. **Nutrition** also is an important health promotion consideration for heart and vessel health—and adequate perfusion in the gastrointestinal system is necessary for the digestion and metabolism of nutrients. **Inflammation** occurs when there is tissue damage, which is linked to ischemia. Also, it is the inflammation that develops after damage to the endothelium of arteries that initiates atherosclerosis. Impaired perfusion results in impaired **Gas Exchange** because the blood carries oxygen from alveoli to cells and carbon dioxide away from cells to alveoli for exhalation. **Elimination** from the kidneys is an indirect indicator of cardiac output because blood flows from the heart through the aorta to the renal arteries and through nephrons that produce urine. While **Stress** creates sympathetic responses that increase heart rate and blood pressure to affect blood flow, implementing adaptive **Coping** behaviors can reduce or eliminate the cardiovascular effects of stress. Because the brain is highly dependent on the steady perfusion of oxygenated blood, **Intracranial Regulation** is an interrelated concept. Interruption of cerebral blood flow either due to cerebral blood clots or due to cerebral hemorrhage can lead to brain tissue injury or death. **Cognition** is also altered when perfusion to the brain is impaired. **Patient Education** is central to the prevention of cardiovascular disease, as well as management of cardiovascular disease.

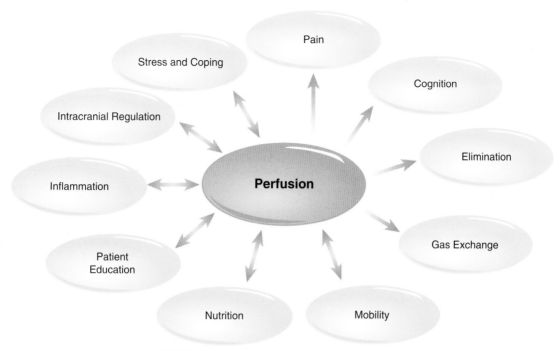

FIGURE 18.3 Perfusion and Interrelated Concepts.

CLINICAL EXEMPLARS

Multiple conditions contribute to impaired perfusion—far more than are described in this text. Box 18.2 lists common conditions associated with impaired perfusion across the lifespan; further details about these conditions can be found in pathophysiology, medical–surgical, and pediatric nursing textbooks.

Featured Exemplars
Atrial Fibrillation

This cardiac dysrhythmia is characterized by disorganized electrical activity due to impulses triggering atrial contraction that are not initiated from the SA node. The result is ineffective atrial contraction, with atrial rates as high as 350 to 600 beats/min. Because the ventricles do not have time to fill, cardiac output is reduced. The pulse rhythm is irregularly irregular. Atrial fibrillation may occur in brief episodes or may be permanent. It is the most common, clinically significant dysrhythmia with respect to morbidity and mortalityrates.[26] Approximately 2% of people younger than age 65 and about 9% of people older than age 65 years have atrial fibrillation. Clots may form in the atria due to blood stasis, which can become emboli that flow to the brain causing strokes. Atrial fibrillation accounts for as many as 15 to 20% of all ischemic strokes.[32]

Acute Myocardial Infarction

When perfusion from the coronary arteries is impaired, sustained ischemia causes irreversible myocardial cell death (necrosis) resulting in acute myocardial infarction (AMI). The AMI is one part of acute coronary syndrome, which also includes unstable angina caused by temporary ischemia to the myocardium as well as specific types of AMI. Most AMIs are caused by a thrombus that impairs blood flow. Risk factors include medical conditions such as hypertension, hyperlipidemia, and diabetes, as well as lifestyle choices such as smoking, excessive alcohol use, physical inactivity, unhealthy diet, and excessive alcohol use. Chest pain; pain or discomfort in one or both arms, jaw, back or stomach; shortness of breath; lightheadedness; and nausea are common symptoms. Coronary artery disease is the most common type of heart disease, with 735,000 Americans diagnosed with an AMI and 370,000 dying annually.[33]

Heart Failure

Heart failure develops when either ventricle fails to pump efficiently. This condition can develop in response to a weak myocardium unable to adequately pump blood or excessive afterload that increases the work of the heart. Heart failure is associated with hypertension, coronary artery disease, diabetes, and obesity. In left-sided failure, the most common type, the impairment, causes blood to back up into the left atrium and pulmonary veins, producing dyspnea; coughing up pink, foamy mucus; and irregular heartbeat (S₃ heart sound). In right-sided failure, the blood backs up into the right atrium and venous circulation, producing edema of legs, feet, and ankles, and weight gain from fluid retention About 5.7 million people in the United States have heart failure.[34]

Hyperlipidemia

Elevated blood levels of cholesterol and triglycerides indicate hyperlipidemia. Diets high in cholesterol and genetic inheritance are common causes of hypercholesterolemia. Triglycerides are a simple fat compound obtained from animal and vegetable fats. High cholesterol has no symptoms, but it thickens arterial walls in coronary or cerebral vessels, leading to myocardial infarction or stroke. An estimated 78 million American adults (35%) have high cholesterol.[35]

Hypertension

Hypertension is associated with excessive pressure or force of blood flowing through arteries. Nearly half of American adults have hypertension, and the risk increases with age. Criteria for normal blood pressure is a systolic pressure less than 120 mm Hg and a diastolic pressure less than 80 mm Hg. Four classifications of hypertension are presented in Table 18.2.[36]

Elevated blood pressure increases the workload of the heart and damages endothelium contributing to atherosclerosis. Because

BOX 18.2   EXEMPLARS OF IMPAIRED PERFUSION

Central Perfusion

Cardiac Dysrhythmias
- Asystole
- Atrial fibrillation
- Third-degree heart block
- Ventricular fibrillation

Valvular Heart Disease
- Aortic stenosis or insufficiency
- Mitral valve stenosis or insufficiency

Congenital Defects
- Atrial septal defect
- Coarctation of the aorta
- Tetralogy of Fallot
- Ventricular septal defect

Shock
- Anaphylactic shock
- Cardiogenic shock
- Hypovolemic shock
- Neurogenic shock
- Septic shock

Other Conditions Associated with Central Perfusion
- Cardiomyopathy
- Cor pulmonale
- Endocarditis
- Heart failure
- Pulmonary hypertension
- Ruptured arterial aneurysm (leading to hemorrhagic shock)

Local/Tissue Perfusion
- Acute myocardial infarction
- Arterial embolism
- Atherosclerosis
- Hyperlipidemia
- Hypertension
- Peripheral artery disease
- Pulmonary embolism
- Raynaud disease
- Sickle cell disease
- Stroke
- Venous thromboembolism

Clotting Disorders
- Disseminated intravascular coagulation
- Hemophilia A and B
- Thrombocytopenia
- Von Willebrand disease

 ACCESS EXEMPLAR LINKS IN YOUR GIDDENS EBOOK

hypertension usually has no symptoms, people should routinely have their blood pressures measured. Nearly half of American adults have hypertension, and the risk increases with age.[36]

Peripheral Artery Disease

The gradual thickening of arterial walls reduces perfusion in upper and lower extremities, resulting in PAD. Risk factors include tobacco use, hyperlipidemia, uncontrolled hypertension, and diabetes mellitus. The risk for PAD increases with age and typically appears in the sixth to eighth decades. Manifestations include decreased to absent peripheral pulses; cool skin temperature; loss of hair and thin, taut, shiny skin on affected extremities; and ischemic pain during exercise (intermittent claudication).[14]

Thromboembolus

A thrombus is a blood clot attached to the interior wall of an artery or vein. The thrombus causes a partial or complete blockage of blood flow to tissue in arteries and away from tissue in veins. Obstruction of an artery is an emergency because of a reduction of oxygenated blood reaching tissues; the outcome is dependent on the degree, length of time, and location of the obstruction. An arterial thrombosis can occur in any artery, but the most common sites are the vessels of the heart (leading to cardiac ischemia or infarction), the brain (leading to ischemic stroke), and the vessels in the legs. Blood clots that form within deep veins are called *deep vein thrombosis* (*DVT*) and produce pain, edema, and warm skin temperature. A venous thrombus can break off and travel to the lungs, causing a pulmonary embolus (PE), which blocks pulmonary circulation and produces rapid onset of dyspnea, chest pain, and hemoptysis. The continuum from DVT to PE is called *venous thromboembolism* (*VTE*). An estimated 60,000 to 100,000 individuals die from VTE each year.[37]

Hemophilia

The word *hemophilia* refers to a group of inherited bleeding disorders caused by a gene mutation leading to the absence of or ineffective production of clotting protein factors. The two most common types of hemophilia are factor VIII deficiency (hemophilia A) and factor IX deficiency (hemophilia B). This genetic recessive disorder of the X chromosome affects only males, although females can be carriers of the hemophilia gene. Approximately 20,000 males in the United States have hemophilia, accounting for approximately 1 in every 5000 male births.[8]

Sickle Cell Disease

The term *sickle cell disease* (SCD) describes a group of inherited blood cell disorders. People with SCD inherit two abnormal hemoglobin genes, one from each parent. In all forms of SCD, at least one of the abnormal genes causes the person's body to make hemoglobin S instead of the normal hemoglobin A. When a person has two hemoglobin S genes (hemoglobin SS), their disease is called *sickle cell anemia*, which is the most common and most severe form of SCD. Normal blood cells live 90 to 120 days, while sickle cells last 10 to 20 days. SCD is present at birth; however, infants don't have symptoms until 5 to 6 months of age. Early symptoms usually begin in childhood and include painful edema of hands and feet and fatigue from anemia. When an affected person experiences dehydration, fever, acidosis, or hypoxia, the hemoglobin S changes its shape to resemble a sickle, causing a sickle cell crisis. The result of the sickle shape is less oxygen-carrying capacity, destruction of the blood cells by the spleen, and clumping of blood cells, impairing perfusion to organs and tissues and causing pain. Sickle cell disease is most common among people whose ancestors come from Africa, Mediterranean countries, the Arabian Peninsula, India, and Spanish-speaking regions in South and Central America. Approximately 100,000 Americans have SCD.[38]

CASE STUDY

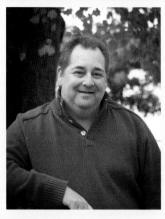

Case Presentation

George Jones is a 59-year-old male who has arrived at the emergency department with chest pain. He had experienced this chest pain for 30 minutes, and it was not relieved after taking four nitroglycerin tablets 5 minutes apart. He reports the pain feels "like an elephant is sitting on my chest." He is diaphoretic and appears anxious. His vital signs are as follows: temperature, 99°F; blood pressure, 100/68 mm Hg; heart rate, 110 beats/min; and respiratory rate, 24 breaths per minute. Mr. Jones is overweight and has type 2 diabetes mellitus, hyperlipidemia, and hypertension. He quit smoking last year after a 40-year history of smoking one pack of cigarettes a day. His troponin level is elevated, and the ECG shows ST segment elevation. The nurse administers oxygen and draws blood for arterial blood gas analysis. Mr. Jones is told he will have a cardiac catheterization to locate the blockage, determine its severity, and evaluate left ventricular function.

The cardiac catheterization revealed a 90% blockage in one coronary artery. The cardiologist performed a balloon angioplasty and placed a stent in Mr. Jones's blocked coronary artery to reestablish perfusion. Mr. Jones was admitted to the cardiovascular surgery unit and was ambulating within 24 h after stent placement. The nurse's goals for Mr. Jones's plan of care are to maintain effective cardiac output, control pain, relieve anxiety, and balance physical activity with energy-conserving activities. The nurse also played a significant role in Mr. Jones's therapy by teaching him and his family about lifestyle changes, including diet and exercise, and the purpose of his prescribed medications, including adverse effects and the importance of following the medication regimen. Mr. Jones is referred for cardiac rehabilitation after discharge.

Case Analysis Questions

1. What risk factors does Mr. Jones have for impaired perfusion?
2. Does this case exemplify an impairment of local perfusion, central perfusion, or both?

joyfnp/iStock/Thinkstock

 ACCESS EXEMPLAR LINKS IN YOUR GIDDENS EBOOK

REFERENCES

1. Schroeder, M., Delaney, A., & Baker, A. (2015). The child with cardiovascular dysfunction. In M. Hockenberry & D. Wilson (Eds.), *Wong's nursing care of infants and children* (10th ed., pp. 1251–1321). St Louis: Elsevier.
2. Jett, K. (2018). Biological theories of aging and age-related physical changes. In T. Touhy & K. Jett (Eds.), *Ebersole and Hess' gerontological nursing & healthy aging* (5th ed., pp. 29–30). St Louis: Elsevier.
3. Erqou, S., Echouffo-Tcheugui, J., Kip, K., et al. (2017). Association of cumulative social risk factor with mortality and adverse cardiovascular disease outcomes. *BMC Cardiovascular Disorders, 17*, 110. Bmccardiovascdisord.biomedcentral.com/articles/10.1186/s12872-017-0539-9.
4. American Heart Association. *Know your risk factors for high blood pressure, 2017.* Retrieved from heart https://www.heart.org/en/health-topics/high-blood-pressure/why-high-blood-pressure-is-a-silent-killer/know-your-risk-factors-for-high-blood-pressure.
5. Go, A. S., Mozaffarian, D., Roger, V. L., et al. The American Heart Association Statistics Committee and stroke Statistics. (2013). *Heart disease and stroke statistics 2013 update: A report from the American Heart Association.* Retrieved from http://circ.ahajournals.org/content/127/1/e6.
6. 2017). *Familial hypercholesterolemia.* Retrieved from https://medlineplus.gov/ency/article/000392.htm.
7. Healthy People 2020. (n.d.). *Blood Disorders and Blood Safety.* Retrieved from https://www.healthypeople.gov/2020/topics-objectives/topic/blood-disorders-and-blood-safety.
8. National Hemophilia Foundation. *Types of bleeding disorders, 2018.* Healthy People 2020. *Blood Disorders and Blood Safety,* n.d. Retrieved from www.hemophilia.org/Bleeding-Disorders/Types-of-Bleeding-Disorders.
9. National Heart, Lung, and Blood Institute. (2017). *Lower heart disease risk.* https://www.nhlbi.nih.gov/health/educational/hearttruth/lower-risk/risk-factors.htm.
10. National Pressure Ulcer Advisory Panel, European Pressure Ulcer Advisory Panel and Pan Pacific Pressure Injury Alliance. (2014). In E. Haesler (Ed.), *Prevention and treatment of pressure ulcers: Quick reference guide.* Osborne Park, Australia: Cambridge Media.
11. Wilson, S., & Giddens, J. (2017). *Health assessment for nursing practice* (6th ed.). St Louis: Mosby.
12. Mayo Clinic. (2018). *Heart disease in women: Understand symptoms and risk factors.* Retrieved from https://www.mayoclinic.org/diseases-conditions/heart-disease/in-depth/heart-disease/art-20046167.
13. Mayo Clinic. (2018). *Pulmonary embolism.* Retrieved from https://www.mayoclinic.org/diseases-conditions/pulmonary-embolism/symptoms-causes/syc-20354647?p=1.
14. Berti-Hearn, L., & Elliot, B. (2018). A closer look at lower extremity peripheral arterial disease. *Nursing, 48*(1), 34–41.
15. Mayo Clinic. (2018). *Deep vein thrombosis (DVT).* Retrieved from https://www.mayoclinic.org/diseases-conditions/deep-vein-thrombosis/symptoms-causes/syc-20352557.
16. Bryant, R. (2015). The child with hematologic or immunologic dysfunction. In M. J. Hockenberry & D. Wilson (Eds.), *Wong's Nursing care of infants and children* (10th ed., pp. 1322–1378). St Louis: Elsevier.
17. Conlon, P., & Wilson, D. (2015). The child with respiratory dysfunction. In M. Hockenberry & D. Wilson (Eds.), *Wong's nursing care of infants and children* (10th ed., pp. 1164–1250). St Louis: Elsevier.
18. Schwartz, A., McCance, K., & Rote, N. (2016). Alterations of Hematologic function. In S. Huether & K. McCance (Eds.), *Understanding pathophysiology* (6th ed., pp. 513–553). St Louis: Elsevier.
19. Pagana, K., et al. (2017). *Mosby's diagnostic and laboratory test reference* (13th ed.). St Louis: Mosby.
20. National Heart, Lung, and Blood Institute. (n.d.). *Stress testing.* Retrieved from www.nhlbi.nih.gov/health-topics/stress-testing.
21. Healthy People 2020. (2018). *Heart disease and stroke.* Retrieved from https://www.healthypeople.gov/2020/topics-objectives/topic/heart-disease-and-stroke.
22. Healthy People 2020. (2018). *Blood disorders and blood safety.* Retrieved from https://www.healthypeople.gov/2020/topics-objectives/topic/blood-disorders-and-blood-safety.
23. Hockenberry, M. J. (2015). Communication, physical, and developmental assessment. In M. J. Hockenberry & D. Wilson (Eds.), *Wong's Nursing care of infants and children* (10th ed., pp. 91–151). St Louis: Elsevier.
24. U.S. Preventive Services Task Force. (April, 2019). *Final Recommendation Statement: Hight Blood Pressure in Adults: Screening.* Retrieved from https://www.uspreventiveservicestaskforce.org/Page/Document/RecommendationStatementFinal/high-blood-pressure-in-adults-screening.

25. Skidmore, L. (2018). *Mosby's 2018 Nursing drug reference* (31st ed.). St. Louis: Elsevier.

26. Bucher, L. (2017). Dysrhythmias. In S. Lewis (Ed.), *Medical-surgical nursing: Assessment and management of clinical problems* (10th ed., pp. 757–779). St. Louis: Mosby.

27. Kupper, N., & Mitchell, D. A. (2017). Inflammatory and structural heart disorders. In S. Lewis (Ed.), *Medical-surgical nursing: Assessment and management of clinical problems* (10th ed., pp. 780–801). St. Louis: Mosby.

28. Shaffer, R., & Bucher, L. (2017). Coronary artery disease and acute coronary syndrome. In S. Lewis (Ed.), *Medical-surgical nursing: Assessment and management of clinical problems* (10th ed., pp. 702–736). St. Louis: Mosby.

29. Wipke-Tevis, D., & Rich, K. (2017). Vascular disorders. In S. Lewis (Ed.), *Medical-surgical nursing: Assessment and management of clinical problems* (10th ed., pp. 802–831). St. Louis: Mosby.

30. Moffa, C. (2017). Heart failure. In S. Lewis (Ed.), *Medical-surgical nursing: Assessment and management of clinical problems* (10th ed., pp. 737–756). St. Louis: Mosby.

31. UNOS. (2019). *Transplants by organ type.* Retrieved from https://unos.org/data/transplant-trends/transplants-by-organ-type/.

32. Center for Disease Control and Prevention. (2017). *Atrial fibrillation fact sheet.* Retrieved from https://www.cdc.gov/dhdsp/data_statistics/fact_sheets/fs_atrial_fibrillation.htm.

33. Center for Disease Control and Prevention. (2017). *Heart disease facts.* Retrieved from https://www.cdc.gov/dhdsp/data_statistics/fact_sheets/fs_atrial_fibrillation.htm.

34. Center for Disease Control and Prevention. (2016). *Heart failure fact sheet.* Retrieved from www.cdc.gov/dhdsp/data_statistics/fact_sheets/fs_heart_failure.htm.

35. Centers for Disease Control and Prevention. (2019). *About cholesterol.* Retrieved from https://www.cdc.gov/cholesterol/about.htm.

36. Whelton, P. K., Carey, R. M., Aronow, W. S., et al. (2018). 2017 ACC/AHA/AAPA/ABC/ACPM/AGS/APhA/ASH/ASPC/NMA/PCNA guideline for the prevention, detection, evaluation, and management of high blood pressure in adults: A report of the American College of Cardiology/American Heart Association Task Force on Clinical Practice Guidelines. *Journal of the American College of Cardiology, 71*(6), e127–e248.

37. American Heart Association. (2017). *What is venous thromboembolism, VTE?* Retrieved from http://www.heart.org/en/health-topics/venous-thromboembolism/what-is-venous-thromboembolism-vte.

38. National Heart, Lung, and Blood Institute. (n.d.). *Sickle Cell Disease.* Retrieved from https://www.nhlbi.nih.gov/health-topics/sickle-cell-disease.

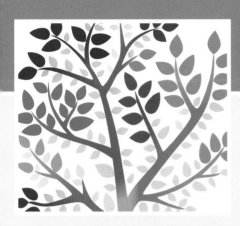

CONCEPT
19

Gas Exchange

Shelly Orr

All cells depend on a consistent supply of oxygen and removal of waste. For this reason, gas exchange is a critical concept for nurses to understand and incorporate into practice. The purpose of this concept presentation is to help nurses acquire an understanding of gas exchange across the lifespan. In practice, nurses promote individuals' healthy behaviors that optimize gas exchange, identify individuals at risk of impaired gas exchange, recognize when individuals are experiencing impairment in gas exchange, and respond with appropriate interventions.

DEFINITION

Gas exchange is defined as *the process by which oxygen is transported to cells and carbon dioxide is transported from cells.* This normal physiological process requires interaction among the neurologic, respiratory, and cardiovascular systems. The lungs deliver oxygen to the pulmonary capillaries, where it is carried by hemoglobin to cells. After cellular metabolism, carbon dioxide is carried in hemoglobin to the lungs, where it is exhaled. Thus, adequate functioning of these systems is essential for optimal gas exchange. Several other terms are important as they relate to this concept. *Ischemia* refers to insufficient flow of oxygenated blood to tissues that may result in hypoxemia and subsequent cell injury or death. *Hypoxia* is insufficient oxygen reaching cells, whereas *anoxia* is the total lack of oxygen in body tissues. *Hypoxemia* is reduced oxygenation of arterial blood.[1,2]

SCOPE

The concept of gas exchange and problems associated with impaired gas exchange represent a variety of physiological processes. Variations in gas exchange are seen among individuals across the lifespan, with multiple causative factors and a wide range of impact and duration. From the broadest perspective, the scope of gas exchange represents a spectrum of optimal gas exchange to impaired gas exchange (Fig. 19.1). The more gas exchange is impaired, the more compromised the body becomes due to insufficient oxygen (hypoxia). Cessation of gas exchange leads to anoxia.

NORMAL PHYSIOLOGICAL PROCESS

The process of gas exchange is presented in Fig. 19.2. Breathing is involuntary because changes in ventilation rate and volume are stimulated and regulated automatically by the nervous system to maintain arterial blood gases (ABGs) within normal ranges. Chemoreceptors in the medulla sense carbon dioxide levels, and when carbon dioxide concentration is elevated, these receptors transmit impulses to the diaphragm and intercostal muscles to contract. As the diaphragm contracts, negative pressure pulls in 21% oxygen from the atmosphere. The nose warms and humidifies the air, which flows to alveoli through patent airways (trachea and bronchi). Alveolar walls are lined with a single layer of epithelial cells, called type I alveolar cells, that provide structure. In between these type I cells are thicker type II alveolar cells that produce surfactant—a lipoprotein that coats the inner surface of alveoli to keep them open. The high pressure of oxygen in alveoli causes it to diffuse into pulmonary capillaries, where it dissolves into the plasma and attaches to hemoglobin in erythrocytes to be transported (perfused) to cells. Oxygen dissolved in plasma is measured clinically by the partial pressure of oxygen in the artery, or PaO_2. Oxygen attached to hemoglobin is measured clinically by the saturation of arterial hemoglobin or oxygen saturation (SaO_2). At the cellular level, oxygen is released from hemoglobin, referred to as hemoglobin desaturation. Oxygen dissolves in plasma and diffuses into the interstitial space, and then diffuses into cells to be used in metabolic processes.[1]

Carbon dioxide, a by-product of cellular metabolism, is transported to the atmosphere in the reverse order of oxygen and lowers the arterial carbon dioxide level. The high pressure of the carbon dioxide in cells causes it to diffuse into plasma, which is measured clinically by the partial pressure of carbon dioxide in the artery, or $PaCO_2$. When $PaCO_2$ decreases, it turns off signals to the medulla to initiate inhalation until the carbon dioxide level rises again to repeat the gas exchange process.

The term gas exchange can be misinterpreted because the word "exchange" can mean "swap, substitute, or trade." However, as described by Dalton's law of partial pressures, the pressure exerted by each gas is independent of the pressure exerted by other gases. Oxygen diffuses from the alveoli to the pulmonary capillaries because the pressure of oxygen in the alveoli is higher than the pressure of oxygen in the capillaries. Gases diffuse from areas of high concentration to areas of low concentration.[1,2] The belief that oxygen diffuses based on the diffusion of carbon dioxide is incorrect. These two gases are independent; they do not exchange with each other.

Age-Related Differences

Babies born after 36 weeks of gestation have sufficient surfactant to prevent alveoli from collapsing after every exhalation. Infants are obligate nose breathers until approximately 3 months. Should their nasal

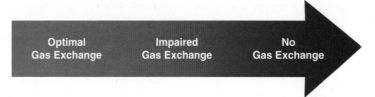

FIGURE 19.1 Scope of Concept: Gas Exchange.

passages become occluded, they may have difficulty breathing. Sneezing occurs commonly as a way to clear the nose. Respiratory patterns for newborns may be irregular, with brief pauses between breaths of no more than 10 to 15 seconds.[3]

For older adults, diminished strength of respiratory muscles reduces the maximal inspiratory and expiratory force. This may result in a weaker cough. The alveoli become less elastic and more fibrous, causing dyspnea more frequently because of a reduction in diffusion across the alveolar-capillary membrane. Older adults experience a reduction in erythrocytes, which increases their risk of anemia.[3]

VARIATIONS AND CONTEXT

Variations in gas exchange may occur in individuals across the lifespan with a wide range of impact. Problems with gas exchange may occur among premature infants born before 36 weeks of gestation (when lungs are not fully developed) and among older adults who experience expected physiologic changes due to aging and the effects of chronic conditions or smoking. Changes in gas exchange can be temporary, long-term, or permanent. Disorders that lead to changes in gas exchange include acute illnesses such as asthma or pneumonia,

and chronic disorders such as chronic obstructive pulmonary disease (COPD), which includes emphysema and chronic bronchitis. Conditions that specifically involve gas exchange include neurologic (including those affecting the brain or spinal cord), cardiovascular (including blood flow in heart, arteries, and veins), and hematologic (including anemia). Conditions in these body systems can be caused from congenital defects, genetic conditions, injury, inflammation, infections, and malignant neoplasms. The three broad categories that represent problems associated with this concept are ventilation, transport, and perfusion.

Ventilation

Ventilation is the process of inhaling oxygen into the lungs and exhaling carbon dioxide from the lungs. Ventilation may be impaired by the unavailability of oxygen, such as at high altitudes, as well as by any disorder affecting the conducting airways, lungs, or respiratory muscles. Impaired ventilation may occur in the following situations:
*   Inadequate bone, muscle, or nerve function to move air into the lungs, such as a rib fracture that reduces inhalation due to pain, muscle weakness that prevents full thoracic expansion, or cervical spinal cord injury that limits movement of the diaphragm

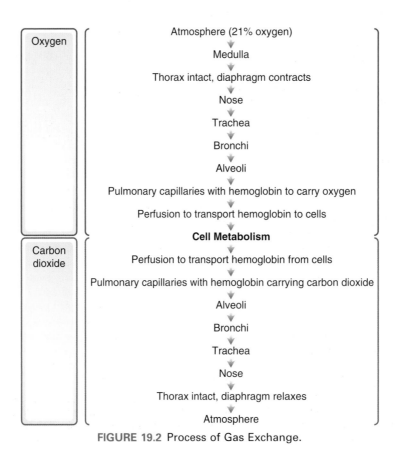

FIGURE 19.2 Process of Gas Exchange.

- Narrowed airways from bronchoconstriction (e.g., in asthma) or from obstruction (e.g., in chronic bronchitis or cystic fibrosis)
- Poor gas diffusion in the alveoli, such as in pulmonary edema, acute respiratory distress syndrome, or pneumonia

Transport

Transport refers to the availability of hemoglobin and its ability to carry oxygen from alveoli to cells for metabolism, and to carry carbon dioxide produced by cellular metabolism from cells to alveoli to be eliminated. *Altered transport of oxygen* occurs when an insufficient number or quality of erythrocytes is available to carry oxygen, or when the amount of hemoglobin in the blood is low. This occurs when patients have anemia for any reason. Blood loss from acute or chronic causes reduces the number of erythrocytes, thus making hemoglobin unavailable to carry oxygen. Finally, destruction of erythrocytes occurs in hemolytic anemias when the spleen destroys these cells prematurely, such as in sickle cell crisis.

Perfusion

Perfusion refers to the ability of blood to transport oxygen-containing hemoglobin to cells and return carbon dioxide-containing hemoglobin to the alveoli. Inadequate or impaired perfusion can be caused by decreased cardiac output, as well as by thrombi, emboli, vessel narrowing, vasoconstriction, or blood loss. (See Concept 18, Perfusion.)

CONSEQUENCES

When gas exchange is compromised for any reason, a reduction or cessation of oxygen occurs that affects the cells, triggering a number of physiological problems depending on the extent of impairment.

With mild impairment, an individual often experiences fatigue. This symptom actually helps the body compensate through rest, thus reducing oxygen demand. Heart rate and respiratory rate also may increase in an attempt to increase oxygen delivery to cells. When impaired gas exchange becomes more pronounced, a reduction of oxygen at the cellular level leads to reduced mitochondrial respiration and oxidative metabolism. Carbon dioxide transport from the cells to the alveoli leads to a buildup of acid. Thus, when the underlying problem is associated with ventilation, respiratory acidosis may result. Metabolic acidosis can occur if the underlying problem is associated with transport or perfusion. If the impairment is prolonged or severe, cellular ischemia and necrosis can occur. A complete cessation of gas exchange occurs when breathing or perfusion stops, and quickly results in death.

RISK FACTORS

Because adequate gas exchange is required for life, all individuals—regardless of age, gender, race, or socioeconomic status—potentially are at risk for gas exchange impairment. Nurses need to recognize, however, that some individuals are at greater risk for impairment. Some of these risk factors are controllable due to lifestyle behaviors, whereas others are not.

Populations at Risk

Populations at greatest risk are infants, young children, and older adults. Infants are at risk because they have fetal hemoglobin. Fetal hemoglobin is present for the first 5 months of life and results in shortened survival of erythrocytes, causing physiological anemia by age 2 or 3 months. Contributing to anemia at approximately 6 months of age is the lower level of hemoglobin caused by gradually diminishing maternal iron stores.[4] Infants and young children are at risk for impaired gas exchange because they have less alveolar surface area for gas exchange, as well as

narrow branching of peripheral airways that are easily obstructed by mucus, edema, or foreign objects.[5]

Older adults are at risk for impaired gas exchange because of anatomic and physiological changes that are expected with advanced age. The chest wall becomes stiffer with loss of elastic recoil. Respiratory muscles become weaker, reducing the effectiveness of coughing which is normally a protective mechanism to prevent aspiration. Additional expected changes are dilation of alveoli, decreased surface area for gas diffusion, and decreased pulmonary capillary network. Finally, the ability to initiate an immune response to infection is decreased in older adults.[1]

Individual Risk Factors

A number of personal risk factors are linked to impairment in gas exchange. Nonmodifiable risk factors include age (as described under Populations at Risk), air pollution, and allergies. *Tobacco use* is the single most preventable cause of death and disease in the United States and is the most significant risk factor for impaired gas exchange. Boxes 19.1 and 19.2 present data about those who use tobacco. The percentages in each of the five categories in Box 19.2 have decreased over the last few years, indicating fewer people smoking. Risk for aspiration is increased during an altered state of consciousness, such as from a chemical alteration (e.g., alcoholism, drug overdose, and anesthesia) or from a neurologic disorder (e.g., head injury, seizure, and stroke). Patients requiring tracheal intubation are at risk because of the bypassing of protective mechanisms for the alveoli. Bed rest and prolonged immobility reduce thoracic expansion, which can increase the risk for atelectasis and pneumonia. Chronic diseases, such as cystic fibrosis, COPD, or heart failure, increase risk because of mucus and fluid accumulation in the airways and alveoli. Immunosuppression alters the body's natural ability to fight infection, whether it is from a systemic disorder (e.g., aplastic anemia), a cancer (e.g., leukemia), or a treatment regimen (e.g., cancer chemotherapy).

BOX 19.1 Use of Tobacco Products by Adolescents in 2018

Percent of Adolescents Using a Tobacco Product
- High school students = 27%
- Middle school students = 7.2%
  Among those who use tobacco products, 73% of high school students and 56% of middle school students use flavored tobacco product

Types of Tobacco Products Used by Adolescents
E-Cigarettes
- High school students = 20%
- Middle school students = 4.9%

Cigarettes
- High school students = 8.1%
- Middle school students = 1.8%

Cigars
- High school students = 7.6%
- Middle school students = 1.6%

Smokeless Tobacco
- High school students = 5.9%
- Middle school students = 1.8%

From Centers for Disease Control and Prevention. (2019). Vital signs: Tobacco product use among middle and high school students—United States, 2011–2018. *Morbidity and Mortality Weekly Report*, 68(06), 157–164.

BOX 19.2 Characteristics of Smokers

By Gender
- 17.5% of men
- 13.8% of women

By Age
- 13.1% of ages 18–24 years
- 17.6% of ages 25–44 years
- 18.0% of ages 45–64 years
- 8.8% of ages 65 years or older

By Race/Ethnicity
- 31.8% of non-Hispanic American Indians/Alaska natives
- 9.0% of non-Hispanic Asians
- 16.5% of non-Hispanic blacks
- 10.7% of Hispanics
- 16.6% of non-Hispanic whites
- 25.2% of non-Hispanic multiple race individuals

By Education
- 24.1% of adults with 12 or fewer years of education (no diploma)
- 40.6% of adults with a General Educational Development (GED) certificate
- 19.7% of adults with a high school diploma
- 18.9% of adults with some college (no degree)
- 16.8% of adults with an associate's college degree
- 7.7% of adults with an undergraduate college degree
- 4.5% of adults with a graduate college degree

By Poverty Status
- 25.3% of adults who live below the poverty level
- 14.3% of adults who live at or above the poverty level

From Centers for Disease Control and Prevention. (2018). Current cigarette smoking among adults in the United States. Retrieved from http://www.cdc.gov/tobacco/data_statistics/fact_sheets/adult_data/cig_smoking/index.htm.

ASSESSMENT

Nurses gather data from the patient's history, physical examination, and diagnostic test results. Assessment of gas exchange involves recognizing indications of adequate and inadequate ventilation, transport, and perfusion. Adequate ventilation is apparent when the following occur:

- Breathing is quiet and effortless at a rate appropriate for age.
- Oxygen saturation (SaO_2) is between 95% and 100%.
- Skin, nail beds, and lips are appropriate colors for the patient's race.
- Thorax is symmetric with equal thoracic expansion bilaterally.
- Spinous processes are in alignment; scapulae are bilaterally symmetric.
- Anteroposterior (AP) diameter of the chest is approximately a 1:2 ratio of AP to lateral diameter.
- Trachea is midline.
- Breath sounds are clear bilaterally.[3]

History
Baseline History

When collecting subjective data from patients, nurses ask about lifestyle behaviors, including diet, exercise, and smoking habits. Nurses ask about patients' work and home environments to identify potential respiratory irritants. Also, patients are asked about any chronic diseases as well as allergies that may affect the respiratory system. Nurses ask patients about medications they take, both prescription and over-the-counter, and the reason each medication is taken as well as its efficacy.[3]

Problem-Based History

The following symptoms are often reported by individuals experiencing gas exchange impairment: cough, shortness of breath, and chest pain with breathing. When a symptom is reported, a symptom analysis is conducted.

Cough. When a cough is reported or observed, the patient should be asked if the cough causes fatigue or interferes with sleep. The patient should also be asked if the cough is productive or nonproductive. Inquire about the color and consistency of productive coughs. Question the patient about factors that aggravate and alleviate the cough as well as any self-treatment measures taken to relieve the cough. Also, the patient should be asked about other symptoms that accompany the cough, such as fever or shortness of breath.[3]

Shortness of breath. Patients may report they have had to stop climbing stairs to "catch their breath." Others may report having to sleep sitting up or using several pillows to prop themselves up during the night. Lightheadedness may be reported as a result of inadequate oxygen transport to the brain. Inquire about what precipitated the shortness of breath and if it occurs during inhalation or exhalation, or both. The patient should be asked what factors aggravate and alleviate the dyspnea and also if there are other symptoms, such as cough, chest pain, or swelling of the feet and ankles.[3]

Chest pain with breathing. The patient should be asked what activity is associated with the chest pain when it occurs and how long the pain lasts. Inquire if the onset of chest pain was gradual or sudden, and ask for a description of the pain, such as sharp or dull, pain radiation, and severity.[3]

Examination Findings
Vital Signs

Inadequate gas exchange causes changes in vital signs such as an increase in respiratory rate, decrease in SaO_2, increase in heart rate, and increase in temperature. An increased respiratory rate may be due to increased work of breathing. The SaO_2 value may drop below 95% when oxygen is not being transported by hemoglobin to cells. Tachycardia may occur either from anxiety caused by not being able to breathe well or from anemia. Temperature may be elevated because of an infection, such as pneumonia or respiratory syncytial virus.

Inspection

If a patient is having difficulty breathing, the nurse may notice the patient assuming a position to ease the work of breathing (e.g., sitting leaning forward). Patients with impaired gas exchange often appear anxious because of the sensation of not getting enough air or a feeling of suffocation. Low SaO_2 may impair mentation as a result of lack of adequate oxygen supply to the brain. Patients may use accessory muscles on inspiration to help get air into the lungs. They may use pursed-lip breathing on exhalation to keep airways open longer. The skin and lips may appear pale because of anemia or hypoxemia. A late sign of hypoxemia is cyanosis. Clubbing of nails develops in patients with chronic hypoxic disorders such as cystic fibrosis or COPD. When patients develop a barrel chest from air trapped in alveoli from emphysema, their AP to lateral diameter ratio changes from a normal of 1:2 to 1:1. The thorax may be asymmetric with unequal thoracic expansion unilaterally attributable to pneumothorax. Scoliosis is a curvature of vertebrae that creates asymmetric expansion of the thorax as well as malalignment of spinous processes and scapulae. The trachea shifts from midline away from the lung that is experiencing a tension pneumothorax.[3]

Additional assessment findings commonly noted in infants and young children with inadequate gas exchange are flaring of the nares, chest wall retractions on inspiration, grunting on inspiration, cyanosis around the lips when sucking, and the need to stop during feeding to breathe.[5]

Auscultation

During auscultation, narrowed bronchi may produce expiratory and/or inspiratory wheezing or stridor. Mucus or secretions in the bronchi may create rhonchi, and fluid in alveoli may generate crackles.[3]

Diagnostic Tests

There are a number of diagnostic tests associated with gas exchange that are used to assess for impairment.

Laboratory Tests

Arterial blood gases. Arterial blood gases (ABGs) reveal measurements of pH, oxygen, carbon dioxide, and bicarbonate concentrations in arterial blood. They are used to detect respiratory acidosis and alkalosis. Respiratory acidosis develops during hypoventilation when carbon dioxide is retained, such as in patients with COPD. Respiratory alkalosis develops during hyperventilation when excessive carbon dioxide is exhaled, such as during anxiety or hysteria. ABGs include the following measures:

- pH is inversely proportional to the actual hydrogen ion concentration. Normal values are between 7.35 and 7.45. A pH value less than 7.35 indicates acidosis, and a value greater than 7.45 indicates alkalosis.[6]
- SaO_2 is an abbreviation for "saturation of arterial oxygen" and represents the percentage of arterial hemoglobin that is saturated with oxygen. This value accounts for approximately 97% of arterial oxygen. The normal value for adults is 95% to 100% and for newborns 40% to 90%.[6]
- PaO_2 is an abbreviation for the "partial pressure of arterial oxygen" and represents the pressure of oxygen dissolved in arterial blood. This value accounts for approximately 3% of oxygen. The normal value for adults is 80 to 100 mm Hg and for newborns 60 to 70 mm Hg.[6]
- $PaCO_2$ is an abbreviation for the "partial pressure of arterial carbon dioxide" and represents the pressure of carbon dioxide dissolved in arterial blood. The normal value for adults is 35 to 45 mm Hg and for children younger than age 2 years is 26 to 41 mm Hg. The CO_2 level and pH are inversely proportional; thus when CO_2 levels increase, the pH decreases, indicating acidosis. When CO_2 levels decrease, the pH increases, indicating alkalosis. $PaCO_2$ is controlled primarily by the lungs; the faster and more deeply one breathes, the more CO_2 is blown off, leading to a reduction in $PaCO_2$ levels.[6]
- HCO_3 is an abbreviation for bicarbonate and represents most of the carbon dioxide in the blood. Normal values are 22 to 26 mEq/L. There is a direct proportional relationship between HCO_3 concentration and pH; thus, when HCO_3 concentration is above normal, the pH increases, indicating alkalosis. When the HCO_3 concentration is below normal, the pH decreases, indicating acidosis. The kidneys compensate for primary respiratory acid-base alterations. For example, in respiratory acidosis, the kidneys compensate by retaining HCO_3 in an attempt to regain acid-base balance. However, in respiratory alkalosis, the kidneys compensate by excreting HCO_3 in an attempt to regain acid-base balance.[6]

Complete blood count. The complete blood count (CBC) reveals measurements of red blood cells (RBCs), hemoglobin (Hb), hematocrit (Hct), and white blood cells (WBCs):

- RBC count determines the oxygen-carrying capacity of the blood. Each RBC carries Hb that transports oxygen to tissues and carbon dioxide from tissues. Patients who have anemia have decreased numbers of RBCs, which reduces the patient's oxygen-carrying ability.
- Hb level reflects the number of RBCs in the blood and determines the oxygen and carbon dioxide transport capability.

- Hct measures the percentage of blood volume that is composed of RBCs. The Hct closely reflects the Hb and RBC values.
- WBC count measures the number of leukocytes in blood. The WBC differential measures the percentage of each leukocyte (e.g., neutrophils, eosinophils, basophils, or monocytes) contained within the total number of WBCs. Elevations in total WBC count occur when there is inflammation, and often the inflammation is due to infection. Decreases in WBC count occur with certain cancers and as an adverse effect of chemical or radiation therapy to treat cancer. Patients with low WBC counts are at risk for newly acquired infection because the immune system is unable to respond optimally.[6] The WBC differential is helpful in suggesting a generalized cause of the abnormal value. For example, elevated neutrophils indicate an acute inflammation, whereas increased monocytes indicate a chronic infection. Eosinophils are elevated during allergies.

Sputum examination. Studying sputum specimens can help in the diagnosis of respiratory disorders. Culture and sensitivity are performed on a single specimen to detect bacteria and determine which antibiotic is most effective. Gram stain of sputum distinguishes gram-positive from gram-negative bacteria. Testing a series of three early morning sputum samples for acid-fast bacillus is diagnostic for tuberculosis. A single sputum specimen for cytologic examination is performed to detect a pulmonary malignancy.[7]

Skin tests. Mantoux skin test is used to detect tuberculosis. A positive reaction to the skin test indicates that patients have developed antibodies to *Mycobacterium tuberculosis*. Allergies detected by skin tests may indicate causes of bronchoconstriction. The sweat chloride test screens for cystic fibrosis, which produces high levels of chloride in the sweat.

Pathologic analysis. Tissue from the lungs or bronchus may be taken for pathologic analysis, particularly if a malignant tumor is suspected.

Radiologic Studies

Chest x-ray. Chest x-ray films are very useful in detecting impaired ventilation because they provide visualization of the lungs, ribs, clavicles, vertebrae, heart, and major thoracic vessels. They are useful in identifying foreign bodies, infiltrations in pneumonia, tubercles in tuberculosis, tumors in cancer, or edema. In patients with COPD, chest x-rays show the flat diaphragm and barrel chest configuration of ribs and vertebrae. Also, chest x-rays can identify pleural effusion, pneumothorax, hemothorax, or empyema.[7]

Computed tomography. Computed tomography (CT) scans of the chest produce three-dimensional images of the lungs and are useful for detecting pulmonary densities, space-occupying tumors, and pulmonary emboli.[7]

Ventilation–perfusion scans. Ventilation–perfusion (V/Q) scans use radioactive particles to diagnose disorders involving both perfusion and ventilation. Radioactive particles are injected into peripheral veins to detect impaired perfusion to the lungs. Also, inhaled radioactive particles are used to detect impaired lung function. This scan is used to diagnose pulmonary emboli.[7]

Positron emission tomography. A positron emission tomography (PET) scan uses an intravenous injection of radioactive chemical compounds to distinguish benign from malignant pulmonary nodules.[7]

Pulmonary Function Studies

Pulmonary function tests assess the presence and severity of diseases in large and small airways. A spirometer measures the volume of air moving in and out of the lungs and then calculates the lung capacities.[7] One example of its use is for patients with asthma. As their bronchoconstriction worsens, they exhale less air. This finding is reported as decreased forced expiratory volume.

Pulmonary function tests are also used to distinguish between obstructive and restrictive pulmonary diseases. Because air trapping increases for patients with obstructive lung disease, such as cystic fibrosis or COPD, more air remains in their lungs, which is reflected as an increase in reserve volume. Obstructive lung diseases impair patients' ability to get air out of the lungs. By contrast, patients may develop restrictive lung diseases from intrapulmonary or extrapulmonary causes. Intrapulmonary causes include pulmonary fibrosis or empyema. Extrapulmonary causes include chest wall trauma or cervical spinal cord injury. Restrictive lung diseases impair the patient's ability to get air into the lungs, as reflected in a decreased tidal volume.

Endoscopy Examination

Bronchoscopy is an endoscopic examination in which a flexible fiberoptic bronchoscope is extended through the bronchi for the purpose of diagnosis, specimen collection, or tissue biopsy.[7]

CLINICAL MANAGEMENT

Clinical management related to gas exchange includes health promotion and the management of emerging or present conditions that compromise gas exchange. The ultimate goal is to optimize gas exchange.

Primary Prevention

Primary prevention includes measures to promote health and prevent development of disease. Several measures prevent conditions known to impair gas exchange.

Infection Control

One of the simplest primary prevention measures is infection control. Proper hand hygiene helps to prevent respiratory tract infections. All individuals should be taught the importance of hand hygiene and proper hand-washing technique; in addition, individuals should be instructed to clean surfaces that are frequently touched, such as doorknobs and countertops. Coughing or sneezing into a tissue or into the elbow or sleeve reduces the particles delivered into the air. Avoiding large groups of people reduces the airborne transmission of microorganisms.

Smoking Cessation

Smoking cessation is important for both primary prevention, discussed here, and an intervention to treat disease. Goals related to tobacco use include reducing both tobacco use and initiation by adolescents and adults; adopting policies and strategies to increase access, affordability, and use of smoking cessation services and treatments; and establishing policies to reduce exposure to secondhand smoke, increase cost of tobacco, restrict tobacco advertising, and reduce illegal sales to minors.[8]

Nicotine in tobacco products is a psychoactive drug that produces dependence and is the most common form of chemical dependence in the United States. The American Lung Association and American Cancer Society have resources to help patients stop smoking.[9,10] Quitting smoking is difficult and may require multiple attempts. Smokers often report lack of success in smoking cessation because of stress, weight gain, and withdrawal symptoms, which include irritability, anxiety, difficulty concentrating, and increased appetite.

People who are successful at smoking cessation greatly reduce their risk for disease and premature death. In addition to nicotine, cigarette smoke contains at least 250 chemicals known to be toxic or carcinogenic.[11] Health benefits of smoking cessation include reducing the risk for lung and other cancers, and reducing the risk for coronary heart disease, stroke, peripheral vascular disease, and COPD. When women

in their reproductive years quit smoking, they reduce the risk for infertility. Smoking cessation in women who are pregnant reduces the risk of delivering a low-birth-weight infant.[11]

Immunizations

Immunizations prevent infection by bacteria or viruses, such as diphtheria, *Haemophilus influenzae* type b (Hib), H1N1 flu, influenza, measles, pneumococcal pneumonia, pertussis, and rubella. Schedules for these immunizations from infancy to adulthood are found on the Centers for Disease Control and Prevention website.[12]

Preventing Postoperative Pulmonary Complications

After a surgical procedure, patients are encouraged to deep breathe and cough at least every 2 hours and/or use an incentive spirometer to prevent pneumonia and atelectasis. This device encourages deep breathing for patients and measures the air inhaled as an outcome indicator that is useful for nursing assessment.

Preventing deep vein thrombosis (DVT) is essential for all patients who are less active than usual so that pulmonary emboli are prevented. This includes patients after a surgical procedure or those whose disease process prevents them from ambulating as much as usual. One intervention is to subcutaneously administer an anticoagulant to reduce clotting of platelets. Another intervention is to apply elastic stockings to the legs or use intermittent compression devices to the lower legs to prevent venous stasis. A third intervention is to encourage ambulation as soon as possible.

Secondary Prevention (Screening)

Secondary prevention includes screening and early diagnosis and prompt treatment of existing health problems. Its purpose is to shorten the duration and severity of consequences. There are few routine screenings for problems associated with gas exchange. A Mantoux skin test may be administered to individuals who have exposure risks to tuberculosis.

Collaborative Interventions
Smoking Cessation

Although smoking cessation is typically considered primary prevention (to prevent respiratory illness), it is also considered an important intervention strategy among individuals who have a disease process because smoking can exacerbate respiratory disease.

Pharmacotherapy

Pharmacotherapy plays a very important role in managing individuals with impaired gas exchange. Agents can be used to open upper and lower airways to improve gas exchange by dilating airways, reducing edema, increasing a cough's effectiveness, and killing or limiting the growth of microorganisms. Depending on the pharmacologic agent, these drugs are administered through a number of routes, including oral, intravenous, and inhalation through inhalers or nebulizers (aerosol). Descriptions of general classifications of agents are presented next; consult a pharmacology textbook for further information about specific agents.

Drugs that affect upper airways. Antihistamines relieve symptoms of sneezing, rhinorrhea, and nasal itching experienced in allergic rhinitis. They are more effective when taken prophylactically. Antihistamines block the histamine$_1$ receptors to cause vasoconstriction and decreased capillary permeability of small arterioles and venules.[13]

Decongestants relieve congestion in passageways and sinuses. Intranasal glucocorticoids exert an antiinflammatory effect to prevent or suppress major symptoms of allergic rhinitis such as congestion, rhinorrhea, sneezing, nasal itching, and erythema. Sympathomimetics act as decongestants by activating the α_1-adrenergic receptors on nasal blood vessels to cause vasoconstriction that shrinks edematous membranes, thereby reducing nasal drainage.[13]

Lower airway bronchodilators. Glucocorticoids reduce bronchial hyperreactivity that occurs in asthma by suppressing inflammation. Specifically, they decrease synthesis and release of inflammatory mediators such as leukotrienes, histamine, and prostaglandins; decrease infiltration of inflammatory cells such as eosinophils and leukocytes; and decrease edema of airway mucosa. They may be given by inhalation, orally, or intravenously.

Sympathomimetic agents are β_2 agonists that act on these receptors to relax the bronchial smooth muscle of the lung to relieve bronchospasm. These agents stimulate the normal sympathetic nervous system to open airways.[13]

Anticholinergics improve lung function by blocking muscarinic receptors in the bronchi, causing bronchodilation. These agents block the normal parasympathetic nervous system so it cannot stimulate constriction of airways.[13]

Agents to help cough up mucus. Two types of agents assist in the removal of mucous. Mucolytics react directly with the mucus to make it more liquid. Expectorants cause the cough to be more productive by stimulating the flow of respiratory tract secretions.

Cough suppressants. Coughing is a protective mechanism and is useful to expectorate sputum. However, when coughing is chronic and nonproductive, it may prevent sleep or tire the patient, making cough suppression therapeutic. Most antitussives act within the central nervous system.

Antimicrobials. Respiratory tract infections are treated with antimicrobials to kill or limit growth of microorganisms.

Agents to aid smoking cessation. Many products available as first-line treatment for smoking cessation are used as nicotine replacement therapy (NRT). They are available in gum, lozenge, patch, inhaler, or nasal spray form. Nicotine replacement therapy allows smokers to substitute a drug source of nicotine for the nicotine in cigarettes and gradually withdraw the replacement nicotine to wean off nicotine completely.[13]

Oxygen Therapy

Delivery of humidified oxygen is a cornerstone of gas exchange intervention. Nurses collaborate with respiratory therapists to supply patients with oxygen and teach them how to use oxygen at home when applicable. Oxygen therapy is provided through a variety of delivery mechanisms when patients require more than 21% oxygen. A standard nasal cannula is used to deliver 24% oxygen (at flow rates of 1 L/min) to 44% oxygen (at flow rates of 6 L/min) through plastic nasal prongs. This is a safe and simple method that can be used for long-term therapy. For greater oxygen needs, high-flow nasal cannulas can deliver up to 40 L/min. The use of a cannula allows patients to eat, talk, and cough while wearing this device. Patients whose pulmonary disease causes retention of carbon dioxide, such as those with COPD, should not use oxygen levels greater than 3 L/min unless necessary.[14] Their bodies have adjusted to chronically high levels of carbon dioxide (hypercapnia) so that carbon dioxide no longer acts as the stimulant to breathe. For these patients, low blood oxygen levels become the stimulant to initiate breathing. Thus, giving these patients oxygen can eliminate their stimulus to breathe, causing hypoventilation and, if prolonged, death.

Oxygen therapy can be provided through a simple face mask that covers the patient's nose and mouth. This mask delivers between 35% and 50% humidified oxygen at flow rates of 6 to 12 L/min and is often used for short-term therapy because of its uncomfortable fit.[14] Partial or non-rebreathing masks are used for short-term therapy when patients need higher levels of humidified oxygen between 60% and 90% at flow rates of 10 to 15 L/min. Oxygen flows into a reservoir bag and mask during inhalation. To attain these high levels of oxygen, the mask must fit snugly over the nose and mouth and may be uncomfortable.[14] Venturi masks can deliver precise, high-flow rates of humidified oxygen. These lightweight, cone-shaped devices are fitted to the face and are able to deliver 24%, 28%, 31%, 35%, 40%, and 50% oxygen. These masks are often used to deliver low-flow, constant oxygen concentrations to patients in need.[14] A tracheostomy collar is available to provide humidified oxygen to patients with tracheostomy tubes.

Airway Management and Breathing Support

Patients with an acute disorder causing impaired gas exchange may need airway support. Before arrival of the emergency team, the nurse may insert a nasopharyngeal or oropharyngeal airway to maintain or open the patient's airway.

Patients may require intubation using an endotracheal or tracheostomy tube. Using these devices, precise quantities of humidified oxygen up to 100% can be delivered to the trachea and bronchi. When breathing support is needed, the patient's respiratory rate and volume can be controlled by a ventilator.

Chest Physiotherapy and Postural Drainage

Chest physiotherapy and postural drainage are performed for the purpose of loosening and moving secretions into large airways where they can be expectorated. Chest physiotherapy includes percussion (cupping and clapping) and vibration to loosen secretions. Postural drainage involves positioning the patient in specific positions (e.g., head down, on left and right sides, and supine and prone) to use the benefit of gravity to remove secretions after they are loosened from specific segments of the lungs. Patients with cystic fibrosis use this procedure frequently to help remove the thick secretions formed by their disorder.

Invasive Procedures

There are a number of invasive therapeutic interventions. The nurse provides care for patients during and after the procedures.

Chest tubes. Chest tubes are placed in the pleura to remove air (pneumothorax) and/or blood (hemothorax) so that the lungs can be reexpanded after thoracic surgery or trauma. Nurses monitor the dressings around these tubes, amount and appearance of drainage from chest tubes, and functioning of drainage collection devices.

Thoracentesis. Thoracentesis is a procedure to relieve a pleural effusion by inserting a needle into the pleural space to remove fluid. Nurses assist physicians with this procedure and monitor the patient's vital signs, lung sounds, and pain level.

Bronchoscopy. Bronchoscopy is a procedure that can be diagnostic or therapeutic. The procedure involves insertion of a bronchoscope through the trachea into bronchi. The diagnostic effect is directly visualizing the airway or taking tissue samples for biopsy. The therapeutic effects can include removing foreign objects and suctioning mucous plugs from airways or airway lavage. Airway patency can also be accomplished using laser therapy, electrocautery, cryotherapy, and stents placed through a bronchoscope.[7]

Nutrition Therapy

Nutrition therapy is needed to provide energy for the increased work of breathing and to support the immune system. High-protein, high-calorie, nutritious foods and drinks meet the needs of these patients. Small meals are advised for patients who become dyspneic while eating. For patients with a productive cough, oral care should be offered before meals to reduce any lingering taste of sputum.[14]

Positioning

Two positions are important interventions for patients with impaired gas exchange. The first position is *sitting up.* Patients with acute or chronic impaired gas exchange breathe more easily in high-Fowler's position, Fowler's position, or semi-Fowler's position. These positions use gravity to move the diaphragm away from the lungs to reduce the work of breathing. Orthopnea refers to an abnormal condition in which a person must sit or stand to breathe comfortably. Patients with chronic pulmonary disease may use a tripod position or prefer sleeping while leaning forward over a table.

The second position is *lying horizontally*, which helps patients who are hypoxemic and have acute lung disease. The distribution of pulmonary capillary blood flow is affected by gravity in different body positions. The greatest volume of pulmonary blood flow occurs in the gravity-dependent areas of the lung. Thus the areas of the lung that are most dependent become the best ventilated and perfused.[1]

Other Interventions

Patients can alternate activity with rest periods. For example, if the patient becomes dyspneic after a bath or shower, allow a rest period before a meal or exercise. Many patients with COPD perceive they can breathe easier when there is an increase in air circulation, which they accomplish by using an electric fan. Patients' coping may be improved by encouraging them to express their feelings about their impaired gas exchange and how it has changed their lives.

CLINICAL NURSING SKILLS FOR GAS EXCHANGE

- Assessment
- Oxygen administration
- Positioning
- Peak expiratory flow rate
- Nebulizers
- Chest physiotherapy
- Airway suctioning
- Endotracheal tube and tracheostomy care
- Chest tube
- Mechanical ventilation
- Medication administration

INTERRELATED CONCEPTS

Gas exchange is interrelated with nearly all of the health and illness concepts within this textbook because all cells in the body depend on gas exchange. Concepts that most closely interrelate with gas exchange are illustrated in Fig. 19.3 and described below.

Acid–Base Balance is affected by gas exchange in several ways. Diseases that retain carbon dioxide, such as COPD, create increased levels of carbonic acid, which causes respiratory acidosis. Conversely, when excessive carbon dioxide is exhaled such as during an anxiety attack, less carbonic acid is formed, causing a respiratory alkalosis. Hypoxia attributable to inadequate **Perfusion**, such as from a myocardial infarction, causes lactic acid formation that causes metabolic acidosis. When patients experience breathlessness, such as during an asthma attack, they may experience anxiety due to the lack of oxygen. **Anxiety** also links to gas exchange because individuals who are unable to get sufficient oxygen become very anxious.

Mobility may be reduced when patients with impaired gas exchange become dyspneic when walking or climbing stairs. **Fatigue** is related to gas exchange in two different ways. When anemia is a cause of impaired gas exchange, fatigue may be a manifestation of the anemia. However, patients who must use accessory muscles and work hard to breathe, such as those with emphysema, exert significant energy to breathe, which contributes to fatigue.

Nutrition is a concern for patients who expend more than usual energy to breathe, such as those with emphysema or cystic fibrosis. They require high-calorie, high-protein, nutritious foods in small servings so they do not tire while eating. When dyspneic, patients focus on getting air in and are thus unable to eat. Patients with anemia need food high in iron to maintain or increase their Hb levels.

CLINICAL EXEMPLARS

There are multiple conditions that contribute to impaired gas exchange—more than are described in this text. Box 19.3 lists common conditions associated with impaired gas exchange across the lifespan; further details about these conditions can be found in medical-surgical and pediatric nursing textbooks.

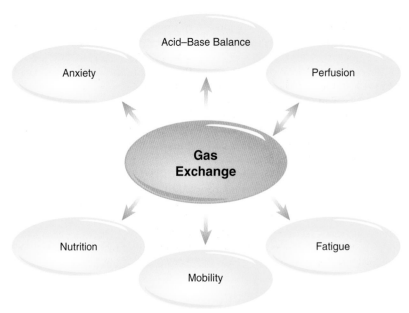

FIGURE 19.3 Gas Exchange and Interrelated Concepts.

BOX 19.3 EXEMPLARS OF IMPAIRED GAS EXCHANGE

Impairment of Ventilation
- Acute respiratory failure
- Acute respiratory distress syndrome
- Asthma
- Atelectasis
- Chronic bronchitis
- Cystic fibrosis
- Emphysema
- Lung cancer
- Pleural effusion
- Pneumonia
- Pneumothorax
- Respiratory syncytial virus
- Trauma and flail chest
- Tuberculosis

Impairment in Perfusion
- Aneurysm
- Heart failure
- Peripheral artery disease
- Pulmonary emboli
- Shock

Impairment in Transportation
- Aplastic anemia
- Folic acid deficiency anemia
- Hemolytic anemia
- Iron deficiency anemia
- Pernicious anemia
- Sickle cell anemia
- Thalassemia

ACCESS EXEMPLAR LINKS IN YOUR GIDDENS EBOOK

Featured Exemplars

Asthma

Asthma is a chronic disorder characterized by periods of reversible airflow obstruction. These *asthma attacks* are caused by hyperreactive airways leading to contraction of the muscles surrounding the airways and inflamed airways. Patients experience wheezing, coughing, dyspnea, and chest tightness. Factors involved in the development of asthma include genetics, inhalation of airborne allergens or pollutants, airway infections, exercise, or emotional stress. Asthma can be controlled with medications and avoidance of triggers for asthma attacks. Prevalence for adults is higher among females, people 18 to 24 years old, and multirace and black persons. Among children, prevalence is higher among males, children 5 to 9 years old, and multirace and black persons.[15]

Chronic Obstructive Pulmonary Disease

Chronic obstructive pulmonary disease is characterized by chronic airflow limitation that is not fully reversible. Chronic obstructive pulmonary disease includes two obstructive airway diseases: chronic bronchitis and emphysema. *Chronic bronchitis* develops when hypersecretion of mucus obstructs the trachea and bronchi, caused by irritants such as cigarette smoke, air pollution, or respiratory infection. Symptoms are productive cough and dyspnea on exertion.[3] *Emphysema* develops when the alveolar walls are destroyed leading to permanent abnormal enlargement. The most common cause is cigarette smoking. Emphysemic patients are often underweight with a barrel chest and become short of breath with minimal exertion.[14] Chronic obstructive pulmonary disease is typically diagnosed in adults approximately 50 years of age after a long history of smoking. It is the third leading cause of death in the United States.[16]

Lung Cancer

Lung cancer is an uncontrolled growth of anaplastic cells in the lung tissue. Common causes include cigarette smoke, pipe and cigar smoke, exposure to radon gas, and occupational and environmental exposures such as secondhand smoke, asbestos, radiation, and air pollution. Cigarette smoking is by far the most important risk factor for lung cancer. The most common initial symptom is persistent cough, but other complaints include chest pain, productive cough, dyspnea, and recurrent lung infections. Lung cancer remains the leading cause of cancer-related deaths in the United States. Incidence and mortality rates have declined in the past decade, attributed to reductions in smoking.[17]

Pneumonia

An inflammation of terminal bronchioles and alveoli results in pneumonia. Microorganisms are the most frequent causes. Viral pneumonia tends to produce a nonproductive cough or clear sputum, whereas bacterial pneumonia causes a productive cough of white, yellow, or green sputum. Other manifestations include fever, chills, dyspnea on exertion, and sharp, stabbing chest pain upon inspiration.[18] Rhonchi or crackles may be heard on auscultation. Children may experience retractions and nasal flaring. Viral pneumonias occur more frequently than bacterial pneumonia in children of all ages.[5] Older adults with pneumonia may experience confusion.[18]

Anemia

Oxygen moves from the alveoli to the cells attached to erythrocytes. When erythrocytes are in short supply, as occurs in anemia, oxygenation is less than optimal. Anemia is caused by disorders that interfere with the formation of erythrocytes (aplastic anemia, folic acid deficiency, iron deficiency, pernicious anemia, and thalassemia), premature destruction of erythrocytes (sickle cell anemia), and loss of erythrocytes (hemolytic anemia). Despite the cause, common manifestations that occur in all anemias include weakness, fatigue, pallor, exertional dyspnea, dizziness, and lethargy.[19] Vitamin B_{12} deficiency may occur in 12% of older people due to inadequate dietary intake or malabsorption due to low stomach acid.[20]

Pulmonary Emboli

A blockage of pulmonary arteries by a thrombus, fat or air embolism, or tumor tissue creates a pulmonary embolism (PE). The embolus travels with blood flow through smaller blood vessels until it obstructs perfusion of alveoli. Manifestations are nonspecific, making diagnosis difficult. The classic triad of dyspnea, chest pain, and hemoptysis occurs in approximately 20% of patients. Hypoxemia with low arterial carbon dioxide is a common finding. Most emboli arise from deep vein thrombosis (DVT) in the legs. Venous thromboembolism is the preferred terminology to describe the spectrum of pathology from DVT to PE. The highest rate of DVT is seen in patients with prolonged bed rest.

CASE STUDY

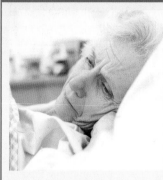

Case Presentation

Martha Moore is an 87-year-old woman with a history of osteoporosis and hypertension. She had an exploratory laparotomy for a small bowel obstruction 2 days ago. Mrs. Moore's hemoglobin level is 9 g and her SaO_2 is 90%. Upon assessment, Martha reports her cough kept her awake last night. Vital signs are as follows: temperature, 101°F; blood pressure, 150/78 mm Hg; heart rate, 100 beats/min; and respiratory rate, 24 breaths/min. On auscultation, the nurse hears crackles in both lungs. The patient reports a sharp pain in her chest when she takes a deep breath. After the deep breath for auscultation, the patient has a productive cough, and the nurse notices the sputum is green with rust-colored tinting. Martha reports she tries not to cough because it causes abdominal pain at her incision site.

The nurse recognizes that Mrs. Moore has symptoms suggesting pneumonia as a postoperative complication. The nurse knows Mrs. Moore needs to deep breathe, increase activity as tolerated, and increase fluid intake. The nurse works with Mrs. Moore to implement the plan of care. The nurse asks Mrs. Moore to use the incentive spirometer and notices she is moving only 800 mL of air. The nurse emphasizes the importance of using the incentive spirometer approximately 10 times every hour while awake to help get air into Mrs. Moore's lungs. Together, they agree on a goal of moving 1500 mL using the spirometer. The nurse also talks with Mrs. Moore about giving her pain medication to relieve the abdominal pain. To further reduce pain when coughing, the nurse recommends that Mrs. Moore hold a pillow over her incision when she coughs to splint the incision site. After receipt of pain medication, Mrs. Moore is assisted to sit on the side of the bed and then walk to a chair for her breakfast (clear liquids). The nurse encourages Mrs. Moore to drink all of the liquids to help liquefy her secretions. When the surgeon makes rounds, the nurse reports the findings from Mrs. Moore's assessment and the plan of care initiated. The surgeon orders a chest x-ray, acetaminophen (Tylenol) as needed for fever, an antibiotic, and iron tablets. After a bath, a nap, pain medication, and use of incentive spirometry with coughing, Mrs. Moore is assisted to walk in the hall. Before discharge, Mrs. Moore is taught about ways to treat her anemia with foods rich in iron and with the daily iron tablet. The outcome of this plan of care is that by discharge, Mrs. Moore will be able to move at least 1500 mL on the spirometer, have clear breath sounds bilaterally, have an SaO_2 greater than 95%, be afebrile, and be able to state the plan to treat her anemia.

Case Analysis Questions

1. What risk factors for impaired gas exchange does Mrs. Moore have?
2. What types of gas exchange impairments are evident in this case?

From Stockbyte/Thinkstock.

 ACCESS EXEMPLAR LINKS IN YOUR GIDDENS EBOOK

REFERENCES

1. Brashers, V. (2017). Structure and function of the pulmonary system. In S. Huether & K. McCance (Eds.), *Understanding pathophysiology* (6th ed., pp. 671–686). St Louis: Elsevier.
2. Brashers, V., & Huether, S. (2017). Alterations of pulmonary function. In S. Huether & K. McCance (Eds.), *Understanding pathophysiology* (6th ed., pp. 687–714). St Louis: Elsevier.
3. Wilson, S., & Giddens, J. (2017). *Health assessment for nursing practice* (6th ed.). St Louis: Elsevier.
4. Wilson, D. (2015). Health promotion of the infant and family. In M. Hockenberry & D. Wilson (Eds.), *Wong's nursing care of infants and children* (10th ed., pp. 413–451). St Louis: Elsevier.
5. Conlon, P., & Wilson, D. (2015). The child with respiratory dysfunction. In M. Hockenberry & D. Wilson (Eds.), *Wong's nursing care of infants and children* (10th ed., pp. 1164–1250). St Louis: Elsevier.
6. Pagana, K., Pagana, T. J., & Pagana, T. N. (2017). *Mosby's diagnostic and laboratory test reference* (13th ed.). St Louis: Mosby.
7. Mondor, E. (2017). Assessment of respiratory system. In S. Lewis, L. Bucher, M. Heitkemper, & M. Harding (Eds.), *Medical-surgical nursing: Assessment and management of clinical problems* (10th ed., pp. 453–474). St Louis: Mosby.
8. Healthy People 2020: *Tobacco use*. Retrieved from http://www. healthypeople.gov/2020/topics-objectives/topic/tobacco-use, 2018.
9. American Lung Association: *Stop smoking*, n.d. Retrieved from http:// www.lungusa.org/stop-smoking.
10. American Cancer Society: *Stay healthy, Stay away from tobacco*, n.d. Retrieved from https://www.cancer.org/healthy/stay-away-from-tobacco. html.
11. Centers for Disease Control and Prevention: *Quitting smoking*, 2017. Retrieved from http://www.cdc.gov/tobacco/data_statistics/fact_sheets/ cessation/quitting.
12. Centers for Disease Control and Prevention: *Immunization schedules*. Retrieved from http://www.cdc.gov/vaccines/schedules/index.html, 2018.
13. Burchum, J., & Rosenthal, L. (2016). *Lehne's pharmacology for nursing care* (9th ed.). St. Louis: Elsevier.
14. Collazo, S. (2017). Obstructive pulmonary diseases. In S. Lewis, L. Bucher, M. Heitkemper, & M. Harding (Eds.), *Medical-surgical nursing: Assessment and management of clinical problems* (10th ed., pp. 538–584). St Louis: Mosby.
15. Centers for Disease Control and Prevention: *Asthma facts: CDC's National Asthma Control Program Grantees*, 2013. Retrieved from http:// www.cdc.gov/asthma/pdfs/asthma_facts_program_grantees.pdf.
16. American Lung Association: *Chronic obstructive pulmonary disease (COPD)*, n.d. Retrieved from http://www.lung.org/lung-health-and-diseases/lung-disease-lookup/copd/.
17. American Cancer Society: *Cancer facts & figures* 2018. Retrieved from https://www.cancer.org/content/dam/cancer-org/research/cancer-facts-and-statistics/annual-cancer-facts-and-figures/2018/cancer-facts-and-figures-2018.pdf.
18. American Lung Association: *Pneumonia symptoms, causes, and risk factors*, 2018. Retrieved from http://www.lung.org/lung-health-and-diseases/lung-disease-lookup/pneumonia/symptoms-causes-and-risk.html.
19. Schwartz, A., McCance, K., & Rote, N. (2017). Alterations of hematologic function. In S. Huether & K. McCance (Eds.), *Understanding pathophysiology* (6th ed., pp. 513–553). St Louis: Elsevier.
20. Rome, S. I. (2017). Hematologic problems. In S. Lewis, L. Bucher, M. Heitkemper, & M. Harding (Eds.), *Medical-surgical nursing: Assessment and management of clinical problems* (10th ed., pp. 606–655). St Louis: Mosby.

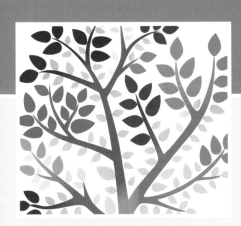

Reproduction

Nancy Jallo and Susan Lindner

The creation of all life occurs as a result of reproduction. As a foundational concept in the biological sciences, reproduction has been studied extensively. Two main types of reproduction described are sexual and asexual reproduction. With asexual reproduction, an organism can create genetic copies of itself. Viruses, bacteria, fungi, and some plants reproduce through such a process. Sexual reproduction is a biological process in which a combination of genetic material from two sources is needed. Mammals, fish, reptiles, and most plants reproduce through this process. The purpose of this concept analysis is to present the concept of reproduction as it applies to humans, and in the context of nursing from the formation of reproductive cells and the creation of a pregnancy through birth.

DEFINITION

There are multiple definitions of human reproduction in the literature. However, the foundational principle of human reproduction is that it is the process by which human beings produce a new individual. Conception of a child occurs when the sperm fertilizes the egg. The sex glands, or gonads (ovaries in the female and testes in the male), produce the germ cells (oocytes and spermatozoa) that unite and grow into a new individual.

During sexual intercourse, the interaction between the male and female reproductive systems may result in fertilization of the woman's ovum by the man's sperm. Fertilization of the ovum may also be achieved outside the uterus without sexual intercourse using a process known as assisted reproductive technology (ART). This includes procedures such as in vitro fertilization and intrauterine insemination. Childbirth follows a typical gestation period of 40 weeks. For the purpose of this concept presentation, reproduction is defined as *the total process by which organisms produce offspring*. In humans, the concept is referred to as human reproduction.[1]

SCOPE

In the broadest sense, the scope of reproduction for a woman falls into one of two states—the non-pregnant state and the pregnant state (Fig. 20.1). However, substantial complexity underlies this simplistic dichotomous perspective.

Non-Pregnant State

The majority of the life of a female is spent in a non-pregnant state. All individuals in a non-pregnant state represent one of two variables: (1) not pregnant by choice, or (2) not pregnant, not by choice. *Not pregnant by choice* is a relatively simple variable, represented by a man, a woman, and/or a sexually engaged couple who are capable of creating a pregnancy and take specific measures to avoid a pregnancy. Pregnancy avoidance behavior is achieved through contraceptive measures or sexual abstinence. By contrast, *not pregnant, not by choice* represents individuals or couples who are unable to create a pregnancy—regardless of whether pregnancy is desired or not. Three categories representing this variable are (1) individuals who have not yet reached sexual maturity, (2) individuals who have reached sexual maturity and are infertile (including women who have reached menopause), and (3) those who have reached sexual maturity but are fertile and partnerless (or lack resources to create a pregnancy by other means).

Pregnant State

The other state is pregnancy and represents individuals or couples who intentionally create a pregnancy and those experiencing an unplanned pregnancy. The pregnant state begins at conception and is sustained until birth or ends with a premature cessation of the pregnant state. Not surprisingly, the range of emotion and acceptance of a pregnancy ranges from significant joy and celebration, to worry and stress (particularly if the pregnancy was unplanned or if complications arise).

NORMAL PHYSIOLOGICAL PROCESS

In order for normal human reproduction to occur, the following complex developmental and physiological events must occur sequentially: the formation of reproductive cells, the menstrual cycle, conception, and pregnancy. Although the majority of this discussion focuses on the female, the male role in reproduction is not to be minimized.

Formation of Reproductive Cells

A physiological discussion of reproduction starts with the formation of reproductive cells known as germ cells. These cells carry the genetic materials needed for conception and the diverse genetic material needed to perpetuate the species.[2] Gametogenesis is a term that refers to the formation and development of germ cells—oocytes and spermatocytes.[1] A specialized form of cell division called meiosis produces cells with a haploid number of 23 chromosomes. Two sequential meiotic cell divisions occur during gametogenesis. Homologous chromosomes pair during prophase and separate during anaphase. The first meiotic division is a reduction division in which each new cell forms a secondary oocyte or spermatocyte retaining the haploid number of

Not Pregnant		Pregnant	
By Choice	Not by Choice	Unplanned	Planned
• Contraceptive measures • Abstinence	• Sexual maturity not reached • Infertility • Partnerless	Conception to birth or pregnancy termination.	

FIGURE 20.1 Scope of Reproduction.

chromosomes. In the second meiotic division, each chromosome divides to form two chromatids that are drawn to a different pole of the cell. The daughter cells that are produced contain a haploid number of chromosomes representative of each pair.[2] The primary spermatocyte contains one X and one Y chromosome; thus during the first reduction division, two secondary spermatocytes are produced—one X and one Y. Therefore spermatocytes have either X or Y chromosomes. Because the primary oocyte contains two X chromosomes, all oocytes have X chromosomes.

Oogenesis

In females, the process of egg formation (ovum) begins during fetal life and is known as oogenesis. The ovaries at birth contain all the cells that may undergo meiosis during a woman's reproductive stage of life. Only 400 to 500 ova out of 2 million oocytes will mature during a woman's reproductive years. Primary oocytes begin their first meiotic division before birth but remain suspended in prophase until puberty. At puberty, at the onset of menarche, monthly cycles begin, and usually one oocyte matures and completes the first meiotic division. The second meiotic division begins at ovulation but progresses only to metaphase when division is arrested. If the zona pellucida (inner layer) is penetrated by a sperm, the second meiotic division is completed.[3]

Spermatogenesis

In males, the formation of a germ cell to a sperm cell is known as spermatogenesis. This process begins at puberty under the influence of testosterone and continues throughout adult life. Spermatogenesis takes place in the seminiferous tubules within the testes. As sperm cells are produced, they travel through efferent tubules to the epididymis, where they mature. Once mature, sperm cells move to the ejaculatory duct through the vas deferens, where they wait until ejaculation.

Menstrual Cycle and Ovulation

The female menstrual cycle represents a physiological preparation for conception. It is regulated by hormonal levels controlled by the hypothalamus, anterior pituitary, and ovaries and occurs in four stages that repeat every 28 days. Stage I (menstrual phase) occurs with the shedding of the endometrium (caused by decreases in estrogen and progesterone), triggering menstrual bleeding. Stage II (follicular phase) is the preovulation phase, whereby the ovary and follicle prepare for the release of an ovum through the influence of follicle-stimulating hormone and estrogen. In stage III (ovulation phase) ovulation occurs, which is the process in which the ovum is expelled from the follicle (triggered by a sharp rise in estrogen and luteinizing hormone) and is drawn into the fallopian tube. During stage IV (luteal phase), cilia in the fallopian tubes are stimulated by high estrogen levels, which propel the ovum toward the uterus. The follicle transforms into the corpus luteum during this phase and releases progesterone, which causes the uterine wall to thicken in anticipation of supporting a fertilized egg. If an ovum is not fertilized by a sperm within 24 hours of ovulation, it is usually reabsorbed by the woman's body.[3] The corpus luteum degenerates and estrogen and progesterone decrease, thus triggering the shedding of the uterine wall and starting the next cycle.

Pregnancy

Pregnancy is considered a normal physiological process that occurs without incident in the large majority of cases. Regardless of whether the pregnancy is planned or unplanned, it is an expected outcome among women of childbearing years who have sexual intercourse in the absence of contraceptive measures, or when contraceptive measures fail. Pregnancy begins with fertilization and, in the absence of complications, involves a 40-week gestation period (measured from the first day of the last menstrual period) and results in a live birth. The trends in pregnancy rates often vary by population subgroups and age and are influenced by factors such as changes in sexual activity and new contraceptive methods; changes in marital/cohabitation trends; and social and economic context of childrearing.[4]

Fertilization

During sexual intercourse, sperm is ejaculated through the penis and into the vagina. Because of their mobility, sperm travel through the cervix into the uterus and into the fallopian tubes in search of an ovum. Fertilization of an ovum by sperm usually occurs in the lower third of the fallopian tube (Fig. 20.2) when a sperm penetrates the ovum membrane. The sperm and ovum are enclosed in a process called the cortical reaction; this prevents other sperm from entering the ovum. The ovum nucleus becomes the female pronucleus, and the second meiotic division is completed. The head of the sperm enlarges to form the male pronucleus and the tail degenerates.

Fertilization results in a new cell called the zygote, which has two sets of chromosomes; half of the zygote genetic material is obtained from the ovum and half is obtained from the sperm.[2] A female develops through the fertilization of the ovum by an X-bearing sperm, producing an XX zygote; a male is produced through the fertilization by a Y-bearing sperm, producing an XY zygote. Therefore at fertilization, chromosomal sex is established.[1]

Within the fallopian tube, a membrane-like sac, known as the zona pellucida, forms around the zygote. Approximately 30 hours after fertilization, division of the zygote (a process known as cleavage) begins. The zygote divides and two blastomeres are produced; soon thereafter, these divide again to form four blastomeres. Rapid cellular division occurs while the blastomeres travel down the reproductive tract. Although there is an increase in the number of cells, there is no increase in mass. Approximately 3 days after fertilization, a cell mass of 12 to 16 blastomeres, known as the morula, enters the woman's uterus.[3]

Implantation

A cavity is formed within the morula 4 days after fertilization. It becomes a blastocyst and floats freely within the uterus for 2 days. Spaces form between the central cells of the morula and fluid passes through the zona pellucida, collecting in these spaces. The cells then separate into

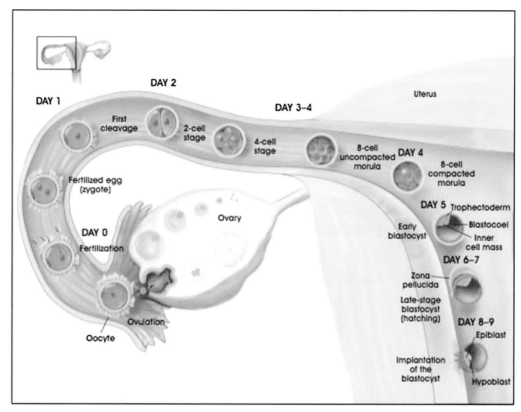

FIGURE 20.2 Fertilization and Implantation. (From National Institutes of Health. [2010]. Blastocyst implantation picture.) https://stemcells.nih.gov/info/2001report/appendixA.htm. © 2001 Terese Winslow.

an outer layer known as a trophoblast and an inner layer known as an embryoblast. The blastocyst receives nourishment from the endometrial glands in the uterus, including carbohydrates, pyrimidines, purines, and amino acids, by active and passive transport. While the blastocyst implants into the endometrium at 6 days following fertilization, the zona pellucida lyses and degenerates (see Fig. 20.2). By 9.5 days following ovulation, the blastocyst is completely embedded into the endometrium, where it is provided nourishment for growth. The idea that the human implantation window is narrow has been challenged. Evidence obtained from in vitro fertilization programs suggests that the window for implantation may be 2 or even 3 days later than expected, but the issue is still being studied.[3]

Embryonic Period

The embryonic period is the stage between weeks 3 and 8 after fertilization. During this time, differentiation of body systems and organs occurs. Teratogenicity is a major concern during this period because all external and internal structures are developing (Fig. 20.3). A pregnant woman should avoid exposure to all potential toxins during pregnancy, especially alcohol, tobacco, radiation, and sources of infection during embryonic development. At the end of this period, the embryo has human features and is referred to as a fetus.[3]

Fetal Period

The fetal period represents the final stage of development beginning on the ninth week after fertilization until birth. This is a period of significant fetal growth; in fact, the normal human fetus grows approximately 1.5% per day. Because differentiation of major organs occurs during the embryonic period, the fetus is less susceptible to congenital malformations. The process of human development presented by stages is shown in Fig. 20.3.

VARIATIONS AND CONTEXT

A number of problems are associated with the concept of reproduction and essentially can be categorized into two major areas: infertility and problems sustaining a pregnancy to term gestation. In addition, for some individuals and couples who were not seeking a pregnant state, unplanned pregnancy could be considered a problem.

Infertility

Infertility is defined as not being able to get pregnant despite having unprotected sex for at least one year. Although difficult to calculate for a number of reasons, it is estimated that infertility affects approximately 15% of reproductive-age couples in the United States.[5]

A number of conditions and factors cause infertility. Contributing factors can originate in both males and females, such as genetic problems (e.g., Turner syndrome or Klinefelter syndrome). Ovarian factors affecting female fertility include developmental anomalies, primary or secondary anovulation, pituitary or hypothalamic hormone disorder, adrenal gland disorder, congenital adrenal hyperplasia, disruption of hypothalamic–pituitary–ovarian axis, amenorrhea after discontinuing oral contraceptive pills (OCPs), premature ovarian failure, and increased prolactin levels. Uterine, tubal, and peritoneal factors affecting female fertility include developmental anomalies, reduced tubal motility, tubal inflammation, tubal adhesions, endometrial and myometrial tumors, uterine adhesions, endometriosis, chronic cervicitis, pelvic inflammatory disease, and inadequate cervical mucus. Other factors affecting female fertility include nutritional deficiencies such as anemia, obesity, thyroid dysfunction, and idiopathic conditions.[5]

Hormonal disorders affecting male fertility include low testosterone levels, hypopituitarism, and endocrine disorders. Structural and anatomical complications affecting male fertility include testicular damage

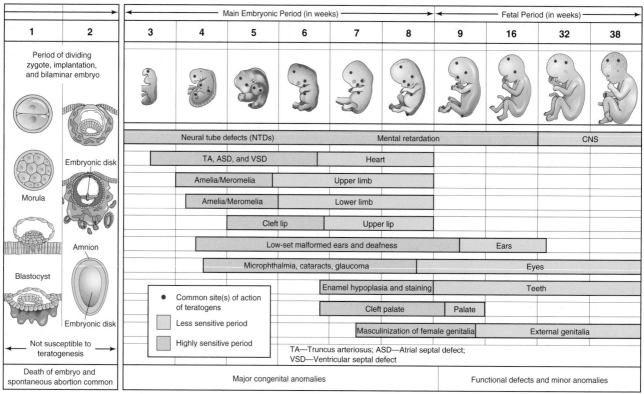

FIGURE 20.3 Critical Periods in Human Development. (From Moore, K., & Persaud, T. [2008]. *Before we are born: Essentials of embryology and birth defects* [7th ed.]. Philadelphia: Saunders.)

caused by mumps, undescended testes, hypospadias, varicocele, obstructive lesions of the vas deferens or epididymis, or retrograde ejaculation. Other factors affecting male fertility include sexually transmitted infections; exposure to environmental hazards such as radiation or toxic substances; exposure of the scrotum to high temperatures; nutritional deficiencies; obesity; the presence of antisperm antibodies; substance abuse; changes in sperm motility; decrease in libido; and impotence caused by alcohol, antihypertensive medications, and idiopathic conditions.[5] With age, male testes become smaller and softer. Sperm shape, quality, quantity, and motility decline. There is also an increased risk of genetic defects in the sperm.[1] Patients with infertility are usually referred to a reproductive endocrinologist or obstetrician who specializes in infertility.

Maintaining a Pregnancy and Optimizing Fetal Growth and Development

Human reproduction may be inefficient with 15% of clinically recognized pregnancies ending in spontaneous losses or miscarriage, with the majority of losses occurring before 12 weeks of gestation.[6] There are a multitude of reproduction problems characterized by failure to maintain a pregnancy. These problems are related to maternal/fetal complications and are categorized by trimester. First-trimester complications may include maternal/fetal infections such as rubella or toxoplasmosis, ectopic pregnancy, trauma, or spontaneous abortion (miscarriage). Spontaneous abortion in the first trimester usually results from chromosomal abnormalities.

Complications of pregnancy that become evident during the second and third trimesters include fetal congenital and chromosomal anomalies, maternal systemic conditions (e.g., gestational diabetes, gestational hypertension, and preeclampsia), and infections. Many other complications can occur later in pregnancy, such as preterm labor, premature

rupture of the membranes, placenta previa, abruptio placentae, trauma, fetal distress, and intrauterine fetal death.

Unplanned Pregnancy

Pregnancy is considered an expected event among persons who engage in intercourse without contraceptive measures. Unplanned pregnancy occurs when contraceptive efforts fail, when consensual or nonconsensual sexual intercourse occurs without contraceptive measures, or when people lack education regarding conception and pregnancy.

CONSEQUENCES

The consequences of reproductive problems are highly variable and can affect the woman, her partner, and the fetus. Consequences of infertility are generally associated with stress, anxiety, and grief, particularly if the treatment options are not successful. Such consequences can be debilitating to individuals and couples.

Complications of pregnancy can lead to several consequences as well, depending on the type of problem and the stage of pregnancy or labor at which the complications occur. Fetal consequences can range from fetal stress to long-term health problems for the infant (e.g., genetic and congenital defects) and fetal demise. Fetal distress may be caused by any number of physiological or mechanical insults; for example, a pregnant woman involved in a motor vehicle collision may sustain abdominal trauma that could then cause fetal distress. Premature infants often have long-term physiological consequences, including developmental and intellectual disabilities or delays, cerebral palsy, or problems with sensory integration. In cases of severe prematurity or fetal distress, fetal death may occur in the intrapartum setting.

Physiological consequences to a mother can range from lacerations sustained to the perineum during childbirth, to postpartum hemorrhage and death. For example, if postpartum bleeding or hemorrhage is severe enough, the mother may require surgical intervention to stop the bleeding, such as a hysterectomy.

RISK FACTORS

Despite the complexity of human reproduction, this process occurs without incident in the majority of individuals. However, as discussed previously, problems do occur and reproduction does not always progress as expected. This section identifies common risk factors for problems associated with reproduction. Risk factors affecting successful human reproduction and fertility transcend all races and nations, with Third World developing countries largely affected because of poverty.

Populations at Risk

The adolescent population worldwide is a reproductive high-risk group. Adolescent pregnancy concerns and complications include impaired nutrition, anemia, infections, depression, social isolation, preeclampsia, protracted labor, cephalopelvic disproportion, premature birth, and cesarean section. The impact on the female is lifelong and includes the risks of higher dropout rates, completing school later or not at all, lower income and dependence on government assistance, and living in poverty. In 2016, there were over 200,000 infants born to adolescent females between the ages of 15 and 19 in the United States.[7] While this represents a decrease in births over the previous few decades, the U.S. teen birth rate remains higher than other developed countries.[7] There are also differences in teen birth rates between ethnicities, with the 2016 birth rates for U.S. blacks at 29.3:1000, Hispanics at 31.9:1000, and whites at 14.3:1000.

Individual Risk Factors

There are numerous risk factors for women and men affecting reproductive health and pregnancy outcomes. These can be categorized into biophysical, psychosocial, sociodemographic, and environmental factors. Some of the risk factors for human reproduction fit into multiple categories.

Biophysical Factors

Genetic concerns encompass altered or mutated genes, inherited disorders, chromosomal anomalies, multiple gestation, large fetal size, and ABO incompatibilities. Nutritional concerns include malnutrition, diets, young age, pre-pregnancy obesity, inadequate or excessive weight gain, and anemia. Medical and obstetric disorders encompass complications of past or current pregnancies, obstetric illnesses, and previous pregnancy losses.[1,8] Although changes in fertility and sexual functioning occur in males as they grow older, there is no maximum age at which a man can father a child.

Psychosocial Factors

Psychosocial factors include smoking, excessive caffeine intake, alcohol consumption, drug abuse, spousal abuse, and addictive lifestyles. In addition, maternal emotional well-being has been found to influence reproductive health.[1,8] Positive affect during pregnancy may be beneficial for outcomes related to the length of gestation.[9] Conversely, negative affective states such as stress, anxiety, and depression during pregnancy are risk factors for shortened gestation and preterm birth.[10]

Sociodemographic Factors

Sociodemographic factors include low income, inadequate prenatal care, age at both ends of the spectrum of reproductive years (younger than age 15 years and older than age 35 years), parity, marital status, geographic location (urban vs. rural), and race/ethnicity.[3,11] It is beyond the scope of this concept presentation to discuss every ethnic group worldwide. However, a disproportionate number of nonwhite women die of pregnancy-related causes annually compared to white women (a 3:1 ratio). African American newborns have the highest rate of prematurity, low birth weight, and infant mortality.[12]

Environmental Factors

Environmental factors affecting reproductive health and pregnancy outcomes include industrial pollution, radiation, chemical exposure, bacterial and viral infections, drugs (over-the-counter, therapeutic, and illicit), and stress.[1,13]

ASSESSMENT

The assessment of human reproduction involves history, examination, and diagnostic testing. Nurses should have a basic understanding of the elements of an assessment; they should also be able to recognize abnormal findings and understand common diagnostic tests related to normal reproduction.

History

Elements of a reproductive and sexual health history include inquiring about sexual history (including number and sex of partners), contraceptive history (including methods previously used and reasons for discontinuation), relevant surgical history (e.g., removal of polyps, fibroids, or neoplasms of the genitourinary system), alterations in pelvic support (including uterine displacement, uterine prolapse, cystocele, or rectocele), Papanicolaou test history (including normal and abnormal results), and menstrual history. Additional pertinent history includes immunization status (including but not limited to hepatitis B, rubella, and tetanus), mental health history, dietary history (including any history of deficiency or disordered eating), alcohol and caffeine intake, drug use (both prescribed and nonprescribed), and known genetic familial disorders. Positive findings that are not expected would alert the nurse that additional testing, screening, or monitoring may be needed.[8]

Subjective assessment of the pregnant woman's data may reveal fatigue, nausea, and vomiting for 4 to 12 weeks of gestation due to increasing levels of human chorionic gonadotropin.[14] Increased levels of estrogen and progesterone can cause breast enlargement, fullness, tenderness, and heightened sensitivity, as well as increased urinary frequency. As the pregnancy progresses, the pregnant woman may feel Braxton Hicks contractions starting at 16 weeks and palpable, "obvious" fetal movements at approximately 20 weeks.[14]

Examination Findings

When conducting a physical examination on a pregnant woman, normal vital signs are expected, including normotension, afebrile state, and normal respiration and pulse. In addition, although many pregnant women experience some degree of varying discomfort during their pregnancy due to musculoskeletal changes, significant pain or discomfort is not expected. Weight gain is expected to be within normal limits depending on the patient's pre-pregnancy body mass index (BMI), pre-pregnancy nutritional status, and current pregnancy. For example, a woman who is underweight or overweight before pregnancy will have specific dietary requirements and should also be under the care of a dietician or nutritionist during the pregnancy. A woman pregnant with twins has a significantly higher daily caloric requirement than a woman carrying a single fetus.[15] Benign physical findings are expected as each body system is examined, including the cardiovascular, respiratory, gastrointestinal, and lymph systems. These findings may be altered based on the woman's past medical history and current state of health.[14]

Typical objective data gathered during an examination of the genitourinary system reflect the following expected and normal changes: softening and compression of the lower uterine segment (Hegar sign), softening of the cervical tip (Goodell sign), and a violet blue vaginal mucosa and cervix at 6 weeks (Chadwick sign).[16] The breasts will also enlarge to prepare for lactogenesis, or the production of breast milk for infant nutrition, and the areola and nipples may darken. The pregnant woman should be reassured that these findings are normal and are her body's way of preparing for birth and subsequent breastfeeding.

Objective assessment data also include visualization of the fetus by real-time ultrasound at 5 weeks, fetal heart activity observed at 6 weeks via transvaginal ultrasound, fetal heart tones auscultated at approximately 8 weeks by external Doppler, and palpable fetal movement by approximately 19 weeks. It is important to reassure women that these times are merely averages. A woman's previous pregnancy history, gestational age, and state of health may alter each of these values.[3,14]

Diagnostic Tests

Several diagnostic tests are performed during pregnancy and for reproductive health. Table 20.1 shows commonly ordered laboratory tests, screening tests, and other diagnostic studies throughout the pregnancy. Not all women need every test listed, and some may choose to defer various tests or screening procedures based on personal belief or need. For example, some women may choose not to have any diagnostic screening that would alert them to the risk of a child with Down syndrome or other trisomy. The type and frequency of testing and screening should be determined with the woman, keeping in mind her values and priorities for her health and pregnancy.[17] Also, based on various risk factors, some women may have additional screening tests done throughout the pregnancy. For example, a woman who is morbidly obese or who has a history of diabetes will require earlier glucose screening.

Various screening tests assess fetal health and development in utero. The maternal serum α-fetoprotein (MSAFP) test analyzes a sample of maternal blood and searches for abnormally high or low hormonal levels that may be indicative of trisomy 21, trisomy 18, or neural tube defects. These values are determined based on the mother's age, ethnicity, and gestational age. Because this test may be done only between 16 and 18 weeks of gestation, it is imperative to have an accurate gestational age when conducting this screening. Amniocentesis is another form of genetic analysis available to pregnant women. A sample of amniotic fluid is collected, and the fetal karyotype is analyzed, providing definitive diagnosis. It is often used as a follow-up to an abnormal screening test, such as the nuchal translucency or MSAFP.[2] If any testing reveals abnormal findings, treatment and further monitoring may be necessary to ensure the health of the woman and her fetus.

Pregnancy Monitoring

During the first and second trimesters, the woman is usually seen once a month. The third trimester (starting at 28 weeks) begins with visits every 2 weeks. At 36 weeks, the visits are weekly until birth. The individual needs of the childbearing family are considered, and the pregnant woman may need fewer or more frequent visits depending on her health status.[17] Prenatal visits are not only important for the health and well-being of the developing child, but are also important to ensure the mother's health and adjustment to the pregnancy and impending birth, as well as the health and well-being of her partner.

CLINICAL MANAGEMENT

The health management related to reproduction includes using interventions to prevent problems and optimize health, screening for problems, and providing collaborative interventions if problems arise. The levels of care related to the concept of human reproductive health are discussed next; for the pregnant female, prenatal care is the cornerstone to nursing care.

Primary Prevention

Primary prevention refers to health-promotion activities that further health and well-being. An example of primary prevention is teaching a group of high school students about reproductive health. Topics to discuss may include abstinence; the importance of safe sex; contraceptive options; tobacco, alcohol, and drug avoidance; avoidance of environmental toxins; folic acid supplementation; and the need for preconception counseling and prenatal care throughout pregnancy.[18]

Nurses should be instrumental in providing anticipatory guidance to women and childbearing families by providing instruction in human sexuality and maternal and newborn care; offering parenting classes; and promoting healthy lifestyles through education about proper nutrition, exercise, and stress management. Education provided during teachable moments—at the right place and time—can change the course of a woman's life and positively affect her reproductive health.

The use of contraceptive agents is also primary prevention, and it is the intentional prevention of pregnancy during sexual intercourse.[19] The effectiveness of contraception varies and depends on both the method and user characteristics. Therefore effectiveness can be measured during "perfect use," when the method is used correctly and consistently as directed, or during "typical use," when the method is used during actual use, including inconsistent and incorrect use. For example, oral contraceptive pills (OCPs) are 99% effective in preventing pregnancy during "perfect use," compared to 91% effective during "typical use."[20] On the other hand, long-acting reversible contraception, such as intrauterine devices (IUDs), have a typical failure rate of 0.05% to 0.8% because they are inserted into the uterus where they can remain for several years, thus reducing the risk of "typical use."[20] Other methods of contraception include abstinence, natural family planning, coitus interruptus, spermicides, male and female condoms, diaphragms,

TABLE 20.1	Routine, Screening, and Diagnostic Tests Performed in Pregnancy	
First Trimester	**Second Trimester**	**Third Trimester**
• Urine or serum pregnancy test • CBC with differential • Blood type and Rh factor • Rubella titer • Hepatitis B titer • Syphilis test (RPR or VDRL) • HIV test • Urinalysis and culture • Pap test • Gonorrhea and chlamydia cultures[a] • Nuchal translucency screening at 10–12 weeks • Amniocentesis as needed • Emotional well-being	• Repeat CBC at approximately 24–26 weeks gestation • 1-h glucose tolerance test • MSAFP screen • Amniocentesis as needed • Emotional well-being	• Group B strep testing at approximately 36+ weeks of gestation • Screening and diagnostic ultrasound • Emotional well-being

[a]Gonorrhea and chlamydia cultures may be repeated at any time exposure is suspected, as well as HIV testing.
CBC, Complete blood count; *MSAFP*, maternal serum α-fetoprotein; *RPR*, rapid plasma reagin; *VDRL*, venereal disease research laboratory.

cervical caps, vaginal sponges, vaginal contraceptive rings, transdermal patches, injectable and implantable progestins, and surgical sterilization of either the male or female.

Secondary Prevention (Screening)

Secondary prevention refers to early detection of disease and disease sequelae. An example of secondary prevention relating to reproductive health is continuing prenatal care in the second trimester of pregnancy. The purpose of prenatal care is to determine the gestational age of the fetus, identify risk for and minimize reproductive complications, define the health status of the fetus and the mother, provide education and counseling, and perform the normal screening done at prenatal clinic visits.[3,14] Screening includes complete blood count (CBC); blood type and Rh; rubella titer; TB skin test; urinalysis; urine culture; Pap smear; glucose tolerance test; and tests for gonorrhea, chlamydia, syphilis, human papilloma virus, and HIV. In addition, each visit provides a valuable opportunity to screen for the mother's emotional health and well-being (e.g., early warning signs of depression), as well as the emotional health of her partner and support people. In addition, each visit should include screening for domestic violence and abuse.

Collaborative Interventions

Collaborative interventions in this specific population include routine pregnancy care. Table 20.2 presents common pharmacologic agents used during pregnancy. Collaborative interventions also include the management and treatment of pregnancy-related conditions or complications. This may include prescribing antibiotics for a sexually transmitted infection, or following up with serial ultrasounds to measure fetal growth in an infant diagnosed with a congenital condition, or referral for mental health services for issues related to maternal distress. More common examples are treatment for gestational diabetes, preeclampsia, and premature cervical dilation. Other collaborative interventions include assistive reproductive technology and abortion.

CLINICAL NURSING SKILLS FOR REPRODUCTION

- Assessment
- Education, support, and anticipatory guidance
- Fetal monitoring
- Breastfeeding education and support
- Contraception education
- Medication administration

Management of High-Risk Pregnancy

Women experiencing a high-risk pregnancy are often managed by an obstetrician/gynecologist or a perinatologist. Factors related to high-risk childbearing are categorized as biophysical, psychosocial, sociodemographic, and environmental. *Biophysical factors* include genetics, nutritional status, and obstetric-related illnesses, including gestational diabetes and preeclampsia. *Psychosocial factors* include effects of nicotine, caffeine, alcohol, and drugs on the developing fetus, and maternal psychological status. *Sociodemographic factors* include low income, lack of prenatal care, pregnant adolescents or older mothers, parity, marital status, place of residence, and race/ethnicity. *Environmental factors* related to high-risk pregnancy may include infections, radiation exposure, chemical exposures such as to lead or mercury, therapeutic and/or illicit drugs, cigarette smoke, industrial pollutants, poor diet, and stress.[21]

Collaborative interventions for the management of high-risk pregnancy include ongoing assessment of maternal and fetal well-being,

TABLE 20.2 Pharmacologic Agents Commonly Used in Pregnancy and the Peripartum

Pharmacologic Agents	Indications for Usage
Analgesics (e.g., acetaminophen)	Pain
Antibiotics (e.g., ampicillin, clindamycin, cefazolin, metronidazole, gentamicin, penicillin, erythromycin)	Infections
Antidepressants (e.g., sertraline, escitalopram)	Mood disorders
Antiemetics (e.g., promethazine, ondansetron)	Nausea/vomiting of pregnancy
Folic acid	Prevention of neural tube defects
Ferrous sulfate (iron)	Important for transfer of iron to fetus and to expand maternal red blood cell mass; used to treat iron deficiency
Flu vaccine	Prevention of influenza
Laxative/stool softeners (e.g., docusate)	Constipation
Magnesium sulfate	Prevention of seizures in preeclamptic patients and fetal neurologic protection in women experiencing preterm labor
Prenatal vitamins	Support maternal nutrition and optimal fetal growth
Progesterone	Support early intrauterine pregnancy; promote uterine relaxation in those at risk for preterm labor
Rho(D) Immune Globulin (e.g., RhoGAM)	Used to prevent hemolytic disease of newborn
Tocolytics (e.g., nifedipine)	Suppress uterine contractions in those with preterm labor

which includes maternal weight, blood pressure, and the presence of protein in the urine. Ongoing fetal assessment may include ultrasound to assess fetal growth and fetal monitoring for heart rate.

Assisted Reproductive Technologies

The inability to conceive a child is a reproductive dilemma that affects more than 15% of all couples worldwide. Couples who are unable to conceive naturally may consult specialists and seek ART procedures such as in vitro fertilization–embryo transfer, gamete intrafallopian transfer, zygote intrafallopian transfer, therapeutic donor insemination, or intracytoplasmic sperm injection.[1] See other resources for discussion of these procedures.

Abortion

Abortion is the elective termination of pregnancy. Indications may include (1) a woman's request, (2) genetic disorders of a fetus, (3) incest or rape, and (4) preserving the health of a woman. The most common planned clinic abortion procedure is vacuum aspiration. It is used up to 16 weeks after a woman's last menstrual period. Other types of abortion procedures include dilation and curettage, in which the cervix is dilated and the products of conception are removed from the uterus, and dilation and extraction, which is typically used in later-aged gestations. This is usually performed later than 16 weeks after a woman's last menstrual period.[19] The woman's health nurse needs to be familiar with state-specific laws regarding abortion for the state(s) in which he or she practices.

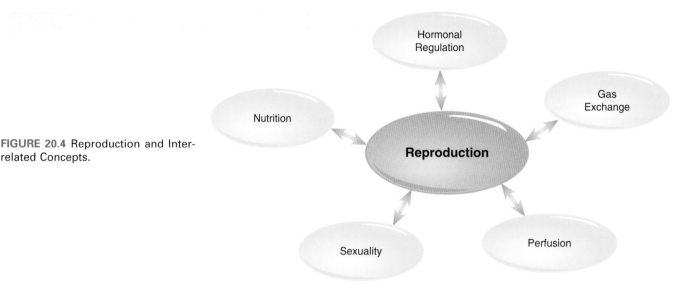

FIGURE 20.4 Reproduction and Inter-related Concepts.

INTERRELATED CONCEPTS

Fig. 20.4 shows the interrelationships of major concepts that influence or are influenced by the process of human reproduction. **Sexuality** is closely related to reproduction. The lesbian, gay, bisexual, transgender and queer or questioning (LGBTQ) population have unique reproductive healthcare needs and may face challenges and barriers related to their reproductive health, putting them at risk for poor health outcomes.[22]

Hormonal Regulation is closely linked to reproduction because the entire reproductive cycle is influenced by hormones, as noted previously. Hormonal imbalance is often an underlying factor in reproductive problems. The discussion of the effects of proper **Nutrition** on human reproduction and pregnancy outcomes is prevalent in the literature. In the 1950s, researchers concluded that prenatal folic acid supplementation prevented pregnancy-induced megaloblastic anemia. In the 1990s, further research studies confirmed that periconceptual folic acid supplementation (400 mcg/day) and folic acid food fortification decreased the incidence of neural tube defects.[23]

Adequate **Perfusion** of maternal blood to the growing fetus is absolutely essential, as is adequate **Gas Exchange**. A female who smokes tobacco may reduce oxygenation to her developing fetus, which can lead to a number of complications. Smoking cessation has been recognized as the most important preventable risk factor for improving reproductive and pregnancy outcomes worldwide.[24]

Understanding the interrelationships of these major concepts helps nurses recognize risk factors and their potential effect on the human reproductive process and pregnancy outcomes. These are important steps in providing anticipatory guidance, clinical judgment, and screening when planning for reproductive health needs of adolescents and childbearing families.

CLINICAL EXEMPLARS

The concept of reproduction represents many clinical situations, from pregnancy prevention to conception and pregnancy. A comprehensive discussion related to all these factors is beyond the scope of this concept, and it is best left to other textbooks devoted to sexual and reproductive health. Box 20.1 presents common exemplars related to reproductive conditions seen in clinical practice.

Featured Exemplars
Gestational Diabetes Mellitus
Gestational diabetes mellitus (GDM) is defined as carbohydrate intolerance of variable severity with onset or first recognition during pregnancy that is often a consequence of the altered maternal metabolism due to changing maternal hormonal levels.[25] Because GDM complicates approximately 7% of all pregnancies, every pregnant woman should be assessed for risk of GDM at the first prenatal visit.[25] Risk factors for GDM include BMI greater than 25, race/ethnicity (Hispanic, black, Asian, Native American), history of cardiovascular disease, prior history of GDM, and over age 40. Women at high risk should be screened for GDM as soon as possible, whereas those of average risk are often tested at the end of the second trimester, typically 24 to 28 weeks.[25]

Preeclampsia

Preeclampsia is a syndrome characterized by an increase in blood pressure after 20 weeks of gestation, accompanied by renal changes such as proteinuria in a previously normotensive woman, possibly due to alternations in vascular remodeling, endothelial dysfunction, an immune response to paternal antigens, and/or an exaggerated systemic inflammatory response.[26] In the United States, preeclampsia complicates approximately 3% to 8% of all pregnancies and can lead to numerous maternal and fetal morbidities, as well as death. Risk factors include nulliparity, age (under the age of 18, or over age 40), African American women, obesity, and pregestational diabetes.[27]

Postpartum Hemorrhage

A postpartum hemorrhage occurs when a mother loses a significant amount of blood after the delivery of the fetus. Postpartum hemorrhage is a life-threatening event and is the cause of 30% of the maternal deaths. Postpartum hemorrhage is defined as a blood loss of 500 mL or more after a vaginal birth and 1000 mL or more after a cesarean section delivery. There are multiple risk factors, including overdistended uterus, anesthesia, high parity, prolonged labor, and chorioamnionitis.[28] Hemorrhage may be managed with a variety of uterotonic drugs.

Shoulder Dystocia

A shoulder dystocia occurs when the fetus's anterior shoulder becomes stuck under the maternal pubic bone preventing vaginal birth. This is most commonly seen in larger infants (e.g., those born to mothers with diabetes). Consequences of prolonged or unresolved shoulder dystocia include increased risk of perineal trauma to the mother, and hypoxia and acidosis in the newborn. Risk factors include macrosomia, diabetes mellitus, and obesity.[29] Dystocia may be managed with a variety of maternal and fetal maneuvers.

BOX 20.1 EXEMPLARS OF REPRODUCTION

Normal Reproductive Health
Contraception
- Intrauterine device
- Hormonal contraception (inplant, injectable, pill, patch, ring)
- Natural family planning
- Cervical cap
- Contraceptive sponge
- Condoms and spermicides
- Sterilization

Pregnancy
- Planned, uncomplicated pregnancies
- Unplanned, uncomplicated pregnancies

Problems Associated with Reproduction
Conception
- Infertility

Gestational Conditions
- Gestational diabetes
- Gestational hypertension
- Iron deficiency anemia
- Preeclampsia

- Eclampsia
- HELLP syndrome
- Hyperemesis gravidarum
- Spontaneous abortion or "miscarriage"
- Premature dilation of the cervix
- Ectopic pregnancy
- Abruptio placentae
- DIC
- Sexually transmitted infections
- Preterm labor
- Dystocia
- Prolapsed umbilical cord
- Uterine rupture
- Postpartum hemorrhage

Fetal Complications/Genetic Congenital Defects
- Neural tube defects (spina bifida)
- Other genetic anomalies
- Intrauterine growth restriction
- Impaired fetal brain development/anencephaly
- Fetal alcohol syndrome
- Premature delivery

DIC, Disseminated intravascular coagulation; *HELLP syndrome*, syndrome of hemolysis, elevated liver enzymes, and low platelet count.

ACCESS EXEMPLAR LINKS IN YOUR GIDDENS EBOOK

CASE STUDY

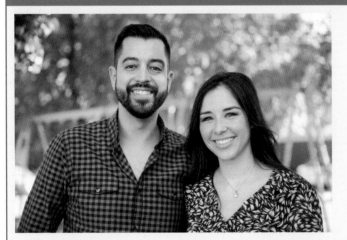

Case Presentation

Katherine Cordova, a 25-year-old female, gravida 4, para 2, with a history of one spontaneous abortion at 8 weeks, presents with her male partner to the community women's clinic for her first prenatal appointment. Last week she took a urine pregnancy test at home, and it was positive. The nurse at the clinic estimates her current gestational age based on Katherine's last menstrual period at approximately 10 weeks and 2 days.

The couple has been together for 4 years; her partner is the father of her other children. Both Katherine and her partner are social drinkers, but they do not smoke cigarettes. They are weight-appropriate for height, although Katherine

does not engage in regular cardiovascular exercise. She estimates that she exercises perhaps twice a week for approximately 20 minutes each time. Both she and her partner work outside the home full-time; she is a teacher's aide in a second-grade elementary school class, and her partner works as a police officer. They both have health insurance, and Katherine denies financial concerns at this time. In addition, Katherine denies domestic violence, and she states that they have support of their extended family and friends. This is a planned pregnancy about which she and her partner are excited.

At this time, she reports slight nausea and vomiting in the mornings, but otherwise she is having no other symptoms of pregnancy. Her medical history is grossly noncontributory, although she has a history of genital herpes simplex virus (HSV), diagnosed at the age of 20 years. She denies recent or current outbreaks, and she is not experiencing prodromal symptoms.

Katherine is prescribed prenatal vitamins that include folic acid 400 mcg daily. She is also educated on proper diet for pregnancy, which includes a diet high in grains and fiber, as well as fruits and vegetables and lean proteins. Katherine is given anticipatory guidance by the nurse practitioner in the clinic that at 36 weeks of gestation, she will need to begin suppressive therapy to help prevent HSV outbreaks during the last 4 or 5 weeks of pregnancy.

Case Analysis Questions

1. Review Fig. 20.1. Where does Katherine fall in the scope of reproduction?
2. Consider the history and clinical findings from the first prenatal visit. Are the findings typical? Is there anything that is abnormal or concerning?
3. Since this is her fourth pregnancy, what differences (if any) occur in screening practices compared to women who are experiencing their first pregnancy?

From Antonio_Diaz/iStock/Thinkstock.

🌿 **ACCESS EXEMPLAR LINKS IN YOUR GIDDENS EBOOK**

REFERENCES

1. Perry, S. E., et al. (2016). Conception and fetal development. In D. L. Lowdermilk, S. E. Perry, & K. Cashion (Eds.), *Maternity & women's health care* (11th ed., pp. 265–282). St Louis: Mosby.
2. Lewis, R. (2010). *Human genetics: Concepts and applications* (9th ed.). Boston: McGraw-Hill.
3. Beckmann, C., Ling, F. W., Herbert, W., et al. (2014). *Obstetrics and gynecology* (7th ed.). Philadelphia: Lippincott Williams & Wilkins.
4. *Pregnancy rate*, n.d. Retrieved from https://www26.state.nj.us/doh-shad/sharedstatic/PregnancyRate.pdf.
5. Gingrich, P. M., et al. (2012). Infertility. In D. L. Lowdermilk, S. E. Perry, & K. Cashion (Eds.), *Maternity & women's health care* (11th ed., pp. 194–210). St Louis: Mosby.
6. Cashion, K., et al. (2016). Hemorrhagic disorders. In D. L. Lowdermilk, S. E. Perry, & K. Cashion (Eds.), *Maternity & women's health care* (11th ed., pp. 669–686). St Louis.
7. U.S. Department of Health and Human Services Office of Adolescent Health. Retrieved from https://www.hhs.gov/ash/oah/facts-and-stats/national-and-state-data-sheets/adolescent-reproductive-health/united-states/index.html.
8. Zdanuk, J. L., et al. (2012). Assessment and health promotion. In D. L. Lowdermilk, S. E. Perry, & K. Cashion (Eds.), *Maternity & women's health care* (11th ed., pp. 307–328). St Louis: Mosby.
9. Voellmin, A., Entringer, S., Moog, M., et al. (2013). Maternal positive affect over the course of pregnancy is associated with the length of gestation and reduced risk of preterm delivery. *Journal of Psychosomatic Research, 75*(4), 336–340.
10. Dunkel Schetter, C., & Tanner, L. (2012). Anxiety, depression and stress in pregnancy: Implications for mothers, children, research, and practice. *Current Opinion in Psychiatry, 25*(2), 141–148.
11. Tucker, J. A., et al. (2016). Assessment of high risk pregnancy. In D. L. Lowdermilk, S. E. Perry, & K. Cashion (Eds.), *Maternity & women's health care* (11th ed., pp. 633–652). St Louis.
12. Farley, C., & Wright, M. (2019). Diversity and inclusiveness in the childbearing year. In R. G. Jordan, C. L. Farley, & K. T. Grace (Eds.), *Prenatal and postnatal care* (2nd ed., pp. 313–321). New Jersey: John Wiley & Sons.
13. Garland, M. (2019). Exercise, sexual, occupational, and environmental health in pregnancy. In R. G. Jordan, C. L. Farley, & K. T. Grace (Eds.), *Prenatal and postnatal care* (2nd ed., pp. 323–340). New Jersey: John Wiley & Sons.
14. Link, D. G., et al. (2016). Nursing care of the family during pregnancy. In D. L. Lowdermilk, S. E. Perry, & K. Cashion (Eds.), *Maternity & women's health care* (11th ed., pp. 301–343). St Louis.
15. Moore, M. C., et al. (2016). Maternal and fetal nutrition. In D. L. Lowdermilk, S. E. Perry, & K. Cashion (Eds.), *Maternity & women's health care* (11th ed., pp. 344–366). St Louis.
16. Alden, K. R., et al. (2016). Anatomy and physiology of pregnancy. In D. L. Lowdermilk, S. E. Perry, & K. Cashion (Eds.), *Maternity & women's health care* (11th ed., pp. 283–300). St Louis.
17. Klima, C. S. (2019). Prenatal care: Goals, structure, and components. In R. G. Jordan, C. L. Farley, & K. T. Grace (Eds.), *Prenatal and postnatal care* (2nd ed., pp. 81–102). New Jersey: John Wiley & Sons.
18. Nypaver, C. (2019). Preconception care. In R. G. Jordan, C. L. Farley, & K. T. Grace (Eds.), *Prenatal and postnatal care* (2nd ed., pp. 59–79). New Jersey: John Wiley & Sons.
19. Ferguson, L. L., Mancuso, P., et al. (2016). Contraception and abortion. In D. L. Lowdermilk, S. E. Perry, & K. Cashion (Eds.), *Maternity & women's health care* (11th ed., pp. 171–196). St Louis.
20. CDC Centers for Disease Control and Prevention. (2017). *Contraception*. Retrieved from https://www.cdc.gov/reproductivehealth/contraception/index.htm#44.
21. Tucker, J. A., et al. (2016). Assessment of high risk pregnancy. In D. L. Lowdermilk, S. E. Perry, & K. Cashion (Eds.), *Maternity & women's health care* (11th ed., pp. 633–652). St Louis.
22. Walker, K., Arbour, M., & Waryold, J. (2016). Educational strategies to help students provide respective sexual and reproductive health care for lesbian, gay, bisexual, and transgender person. *Journal of Midwifery & Women's Health, 61*(6), 737–743.
23. Tsunenobu, T., & Picciano, M. F. (2006). Folate and human reproduction. *The American Journal of Clinical Nutrition, 83*(5), 993–1016.
24. Cnattingius, S. (2010). The epidemiology of smoking during pregnancy: Smoking prevalence, maternal characteristics, and pregnancy outcomes. *Nicotine & tobacco research: Official Journal of the Society for Research on Nicotine and Tobacco, 6*(Suppl. 2), S125–S140.
25. Trout, K. (2019). Gestational diabetes. In R. G. Jordan, C. L. Farley, & K. T. Grace (Eds.), *Prenatal and postnatal care* (2nd ed., pp. 527–539). New Jersey: John Wiley & Sons.
26. Dix, D., et al. (2016). Hypertensive disorders. In D. L. Lowdermilk, S. E. Perry, & K. Cashion (Eds.), *Maternity & women's health care* (11th ed., pp. 653–668). St Louis.
27. Jordan, R., & Gabzdyl, E. (2019). Hypertensive disorders of pregnancy. In R. G. Jordan, C. L. Farley, & K. T. Grace (Eds.), *Prenatal and postnatal care* (2nd ed., pp. 511–526). New Jersey: John Wiley & Sons.
28. Lanning, R. K., et al. (2016). Postpartum complications. In D. L. Lowdermilk, S. E. Perry, & K. Cashion (Eds.), *Maternity & women's health care* (11th ed., pp. 802–815). St Louis.
29. Babini, D. R., et al. (2016). Labor and birth complications. In D. L. Lowdermilk, S. E. Perry, & K. Cashion (Eds.), *Maternity & women's health care* (11th ed., pp. 759–801). St Louis.

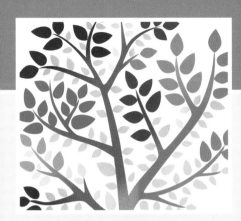

Sexuality

Sue K. Goebel

In general, human sexuality is how people experience and express themselves as sexual beings. It includes our body parts and sex. It is that sense of being "girl" or feminine and "male" or masculine, regardless of the "parts." It includes how we express that sense of gender, whom we are attracted to, and who is attracted to us. It is the nature of relationships with ourselves and others. Sexuality is unique to the individual, is core to who we are, and is dynamic throughout a lifetime. Learning about human sexuality and the sexual well-being of patients is an important part of providing holistic patient-centered nursing care.

DEFINITION

For the purpose of this concept presentation, the World Health Organization (WHO) provides a working definition of sexuality as follows:

> *A central aspect of being human throughout life encompasses sex, gender identities and roles, sexual orientation, eroticism, pleasure, intimacy and reproduction. Sexuality is experienced and expressed in thoughts, fantasies, desires, beliefs, attitudes, values, behaviors, practices, roles and relationships. While sexuality can include all of these dimensions, not all of them are always experienced or expressed. Sexuality is influenced by the interaction of biological, psychological, social, economic, political, cultural, legal, historical, religious and spiritual factors.*[1]

The word "sexuality" has its roots in the word "sex." The word *sexuality*, meaning the action or fact of being sexual, is documented as early as 1789. In 1879, sexuality was further defined to include being capable of sexual feelings, and by 1980 the definition included the idea of sexual identity and sexual orientation.[2] In 2001, the Surgeon General of the United States issued a "Call to Action" to promote sexual health and responsible sexual behavior[3]; sexual health is a function of sexuality and thus needs to be defined. The Centers for Disease Control and Prevention (CDC) offers the following encompassing definition of sexual health based on that of the WHO:

> *A state of physical, emotional, mental and social well-being in relation to sexuality; it is not merely the absence of disease, dysfunction, or infirmity. Sexual health requires a positive and respectful approach to sexuality and sexual relationships, as well as the possibility of having pleasurable and safe sexual experiences, free of coercion, discrimination and violence.*[4]

Other related terms are defined in Table 21.1.

SCOPE

The scope of sexuality as a concept ranges from sexual well-being to sexual ill-being; these can be a measure of sexual function and dysfunction (Fig. 21.1). Well-being is defined as the state of being happy, healthy, or successful (function), and ill-being is defined as a condition of being deficient in health, happiness, or prosperity (dysfunction).[5] Although it is a simplistic definition, sexual well-being can be evidenced by the presence of positive attitudes, the absence of negative emotions, and an "overall satisfaction with life, fulfillment, and positive functioning."[6]

NORMAL PHYSIOLOGICAL PROCESS

Sexuality is more complex than one might initially imagine. To fully understand the physiological process of sexuality, three perspectives are presented: sexual response, age-related considerations, and sexual attitudes and behaviors.

Sexual Response

The human sexual response cycle, first described by Masters and Johnson in 1966, was based on physiological measures of heart rate, blood pressure, changes in genital size, and genital lubrication during stimulation and orgasm.[7] Four consecutive phases were identified to describe human sexual response: excitement, plateau, orgasmic, and resolution phases. Since then, other human sexual response models have been formulated to consider psychological and sociological factors as well, most notably the notions of sexual motivation and desire. The original works of Masters and Johnson continue to inform present-day models of sexual response. Although aspects of each model may vary slightly, the general phases are the same and include motivation, arousal, genital congestion, orgasm, and resolution.[7–10]

Motivation

The desire to engage in sexual activity is also known as libido or sex drive. Libido is biological, psychological, sociological, and spiritual in nature. It can be impacted by medical conditions, medications, personality, temperament, personality, lifestyle, relationships, and environmental stressors.

Arousal

Sexual arousal is the physiological response to the release of neurotransmitters that stimulate specific areas of the brain involved in cognition,

TABLE 21.1 Definitions Related to the Concept of Sexuality

Bisexual	A person who is attracted to two sexes or two genders, but not necessarily simultaneously or equally
Gay	Men attracted to men. Colloquially uses as an umbrella term to include LGBTQ people
Gender identity	The gender that a person sees oneself as
Heterosexuality	Sexual, emotional, and/or romantic attraction to a sex other than your own. Commonly thought of as attraction to the opposite sex.
Homosexuality	Sexual, emotional, and/or romantic attraction to the same sex
Intersex	Clinical term which describes the biological state of having discordance in sexual organs (e.g., having both a penis and ovaries); previously referred to *hermaphrodite*
Lesbian	A woman who is attracted to women
LGBTQ	Lesbian, gay, bisexual, transgender, queer
Pansexual	A person who is fluid in sexual orientation and/or gender or sex identity
Queer	A term to refer to the entire LGBT community
Sex	A biological term; refers to a person based on their anatomy (genitalia, chromosomes, internal reproductive organs). Terms include male, female, transsexual, intersex.
Sex identity	The sex that a person sees themselves as; a person can refuse to label themselves as a sex
Sexual orientation	The deep-seated direction of one's sexual (erotic) attraction. It is on a continuum and not a set of absolute categories, sometimes referred to as *affection orientation* or *sexuality*.
Trans female/woman	A male-to-female transition (MTF)
Transgender	An adjective that applies to people who feel that their assigned sex (biological sex) does not match their true gender identity
Trans male/man	A female-to-male transition (FTM)
Transsexual	A clinical term that has historically been used to describe those transgender people who sought medical intervention for gender affirmation

LGBTQ, Lesbian, gay, bisexual, transgender, and queer.
Data from Deutsch, M. B. (Ed.), (2016). Guidelines for the Primary and Gender Affirming Care of Transgender and Gender Nonbinary People. Retrieved from: http://transhealth.ucsf.edu/protocols; Walker, K., Arbour, M., & Waryold, J. (2016). Education Strategies to Help Students Provide Respectful Sexual and Reproductive Health Care for Lesbian, Gay, Bisexual and Transgender Persons. *Journal of Midwifery and Women's Health, 61*(6), 737–743; Yingling, C. T., Cotler, K., & Hughes, T. L. (2016). Building nurse's capacity to address health inequities: Incorporating lesbian, gay, bisexual and transgender health content in a family nurse practitioner programme. *Journal of Clinical Nursing, 26*(17–18), 2807–2817.

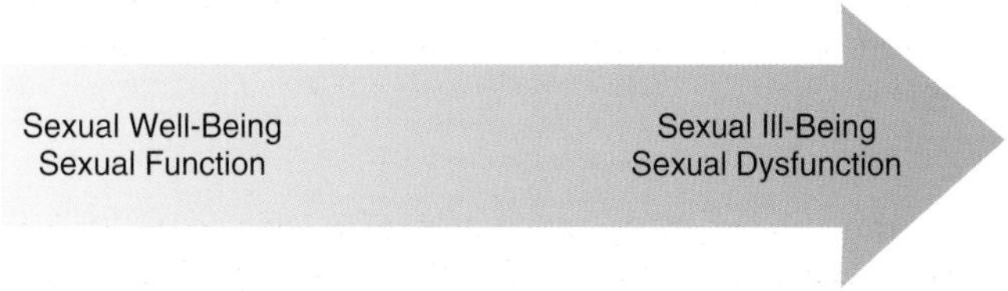

Sexual Well-Being
Sexual Function

Sexual Ill-Being
Sexual Dysfunction

FIGURE 21.1 Scope of Sexuality.

emotion, motivation, and organization of genital congestion. An awareness of being sexually aroused is described as sexual excitement. Human sexuality is a sensual matter; consider the notion that someone can be "turned on" or "turned off" sexually by varying stimuli of sight, smell, sound, taste, and touch. The stimulus–response can be excitatory or inhibitory in action; dopamine, norepinephrine, and melanocortins are excitatory neurotransmitters, whereas serotonin, prolactin, and GABA are inhibitory neurotransmitters.[7–10]

Genital Congestion

Genital congestion is a reflexive autonomic response facilitated by the parasympathetic and inhibited by the sympathetic nervous system responses. This vasocongestion can occur within seconds of a sexual stimulus and results in increased blood flow to the genital area. In a female, clitoral swelling and vulvar engorgement will occur, along with an increase in vaginal lubrication. In a male, this neurovascular response will result in an erection of the penis. Concurrently, flushing of skin throughout the body may occur and can be seen as pinking of the skin in areas of the face, torso, genitals, and even hands and feet.[7–10]

Orgasm

Generally a pleasurable sensation, orgasm produces rapid contractions of the muscles in the genital and anal area and, for some humans, throughout the body; it is the mechanism by which pelvic congestion is relieved slowly. The physical process of orgasm is similar for both sexes. In females, contractions occur in the lower part of the vagina, in the uterus, anus, and pelvic floor. Approximately 10% of women also ejaculate a clear fluid from the urethra at orgasm; the fluid originates from the Skene glands in the wall of the urethra and is much like the prostate fluid found in male ejaculate. In males, the pelvic floor muscle contractions result in a pulsatile ejaculation of seminal fluid. Ejaculation with orgasm is much more common in men than in women. Most of the time, a man will have an orgasm at the same time he ejaculates, but occasionally men have an orgasm without ejaculating or ejaculate without having an orgasm.[7–10]

Resolution

Resolution is described as a sense of well-being, muscular relaxation throughout the body, or fatigue that generally follows orgasm; sexual arousal need not result in orgasm for resolution to occur. Resolution is believed to be directly related to the neurotransmitters prolactin, ADH, and oxytocin that are released during orgasm. In a female, relief of pelvic congestion will occur slowly, and the sense of pelvic and genital fullness will abate. In a male, the penis will decrease in size and return to its flaccid state as pelvic congestion is relieved.[7–10]

Age-Related Differences

Human sexuality can be described as a developmental process, beginning at conception and ending at death. Our early awareness of sexual self as an aspect of self-identity begins in infancy and is influenced by the dynamic combination of *biological*, *societal*, *cultural*, and *familial* factors (Fig. 21.2). The development of human sexuality can be observed through the socially defined stages of childhood, preadolescence, adolescence, and adulthood. Three common attributes of sexual development—gender identity, sexual response, and the capacity for meaningful, intimate relationships—are essential as we move from infancy through adulthood.[11]

Childhood (Birth to 7 Years)

The physiological capacity for sexual response is first observed in infancy: Baby boys get erections and baby girls exhibit increased vaginal lubrication, a result of genital congestion. Infants of both sexes have been

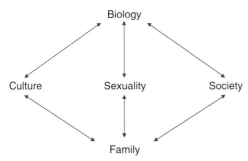

FIGURE 21.2 Factors Influencing the Development of Sexuality. (From Brown, R. T., & Brown, J. D. [2006]. Adolescent sexuality. *Primary Care* 33:373–390.)

observed fondling their own genitals, a natural form of sexual expression and arousal. Attitudes and behaviors conveyed by a child's family during childhood are key in shaping sexuality as each child begins to form a gender identity—the sense of maleness and femaleness. Sexual interest and activity are observed as young children begin to model adult behaviors while they "play house" or "play doctor" as part of their natural curiosity. Facilitated by positive physical contact, the quality of relationships during early childhood is instrumental in shaping sexual and emotional relationships later in life.[11]

Preadolescence (8 to 12 Years)

During this stage, there is often a general social division of boys and girls into separate groups, and thus sexual curiosity and learning occurs between children of the same sex. Research indicates that many children engage in masturbation during this stage, with as many as 40% of females and 38% of males in a sample of college students reporting this activity prior to starting puberty.[12]

Adolescence (13 to 19 Years)

During adolescence, the physical changes associated with puberty become evident. Although these physical changes associated with sexual maturation signal the possibility of adult-like sexual activity, psychosocial factors can facilitate or inhibit such sexual expression. During adolescence, two developmental tasks present: learning to manage physical and emotional aspects of sexuality in order to form intimate relations and resolving the conflict between identity and role confusion.[13] Further development of gender identity, just as sexual identity, emerges as well. Sexual identity, a sense of being attractive and being attracted to others, is described in terms of being heterosexual, lesbian, gay, bisexual, transgender, and queer (LGBTQ). Over the past decade, as a result of increasing visibility and acceptance of those who identify as other than heterosexual, we speak now of sexual fluidity; it is the idea that an individual's sexual orientation and/or gender identification changes over time.[11]

Adulthood (20 Years and Older)

The process of sexual maturation continues throughout a lifetime. Two major developmental tasks for adults are learning to effectively communicate in intimate relationships and making informed decisions about sexual health, such as issues of family planning and prevention of sexually transmitted infections (STIs). Attitudes and behaviors related to sexuality are further defined as adults experience varying lifestyles and social influences. Sexual lifestyle options include celibacy, long-term monogamy, serial monogamy, and polyamory. Although many factors contribute to changes in sexual function, sexual interest and desire may continue well into late adulthood.[11] While there is a prevailing misconception that with increasing age, sexual desire diminishes,

the literature reflects otherwise; sexuality is an ongoing phenomenon throughout the life cycle.[14]

Positive Sexual Attitudes and Behaviors

Practitioners often equate positive sexual functioning with Masters and Johnson's sexual response cycle rather than considering the psychological and emotional components of what truly makes an optimal sexual encounter.[14] Recent research has identified six components of optimal sexuality.

The most predominant component is that of *being present*—in the moment and fully attentive,[14] described as "utter immersion and intensely focused attention" in which they are fully embodied in the experience and able to allow thinking to stop and arousal to take over.[14] Being present is inextricably linked with a second component of *authenticity*, described as "feeling free to be themselves with their partner."[14] A third theme is *intense emotional connection*, described as heightened intimacy during the sexual encounter. Many couples felt that intimacy needed to be present both inside and outside of the bedroom, whereas others noted that "great sex" also occurred in new relationships, with friends or "play partners." Another component of optimal sexuality is *sexual and erotic intimacy*, described as a deep sense of caring for one another regardless of the length of the relationship. Excellent *communication* is also crucial to the success of any sexual encounter, which includes not only verbal communication but also empathy and making one's needs known through touch.[14] The sixth component is *transcendence*, a combination of heightened mental, emotional, physical, relational, and spiritual states of mind.[14] This picture of "great sex" that is painted by these six attributes is certainly different from that touted by mass media. These findings illustrate that optimal sexuality is not necessarily about technique or skill but, rather, about attitude, positive behaviors, and healthy relationships.

VARIATIONS AND CONTEXT

Many individuals experience sexual problems, but it is also important to acknowledge the wide variation, based on individual perceptions and expectations. For example, one individual's desire to have sex daily and another's to have sex every few months does not delineate function versus dysfunction; the difference is not a dysfunction unless it results in a self-identified source of personal or relational distress. As noted by Herdman et al., "The perception of the patient is a critical factor in determining whether the diagnosis is within the domain of nursing and amenable to nursing intervention in the form of teaching and counseling."[15] Recall that the word "normal" in scientific context generally means "average," and there is limited ability to define average when it comes to human sexuality.

Etiology of Sexual Disorders

A number of underlying situations can lead to sexual disorders or sexual dysfunction (SD), including physiological, psychological, maturational, and environmental factors, or some combination thereof. Specifically, categories include sexually transmitted infections, SD, and intimate partner violence. Alterations in sexuality and sexual function can be further categorized as lifelong versus acquired, situational versus generalized, and organic versus psychogenic. These are not necessarily discrete categories; instead, SD is often multifactorial with an overlap between categories.[9,10,16]

Physiological Factors

An alteration in physiological function of a body system(s) (i.e., cardiovascular, respiratory, musculoskeletal, neurological, and endocrine) can result in SD. An acute illness, infection, surgery, trauma, medications, loss of mobility, decreased activity tolerance, hormonal changes, and alcohol or substance abuse are physiological conditions that can contribute to alterations in sexual function.[8] Pregnancy and the process of aging, although not pathological conditions, can also result in SD.

Psychological Factors

Any stressor that impacts the human psyche has the potential to result in SD. Psychological and emotional factors such as fear, anxiety, fatigue, reproductive health concerns, and adverse childhood events can result in SD. Alterations in body image and self-image, role confusion, and personal conflicts (religion, culture, and values) can also contribute to SD. Furthermore, mental health conditions such as psychosis or alterations in cognition related to dementia will impact sexuality.[9,10,16]

Maturational

For some, SD can be a result of a knowledge deficit with regard to sexuality, birth control, safer sex practices, and changes associated with aging. Lack of general social skills can interfere with establishing intimate and social relationships necessary in the growth and development of one's own sexuality.[9,10]

Environmental

There is increasing evidence that environmental pollutants and chemicals can depress sexual function. Situational factors that influence the patient's environment include social isolation and the absence or lack of a partner, disallowing persons to experience the wholeness of their sexuality. Lack of privacy or an appropriate environment in which to be sexual can contribute to SD.[9,10]

Sexually Transmitted Infections

Among the most common sexuality problems are sexually transmitted infections (STIs). These are infections transmitted through sexual contact and can include protozoa, parasites, and viral and bacterial infections. Some STIs are associated with symptoms that cause an individual to seek medical attention, and other STIs can be asymptomatic but lead to longer term problems, such as complications with pregnancies and increased cancer risk. Some STIs (e.g., chlamydia) are curable with treatment, and others (e.g., genital herpes) are chronic.

Female Sexual Disorders

According to the National Institute of Health, as many as 40% of women in America suffer from sexual dysfunction (SD), and it can affect a woman at any age.[17] Although SD may involve many physiological factors (diabetes, neuropathy, paralysis, and hormones), the majority of research and clinical trials on SD in women have focused on psychological causes (stress, anxiety, depression, and anger). In keeping with the stages of the human sexual response cycle of motivation, arousal, genital congestion, orgasm, and resolution, various SDs have been described. The condition of SD includes the medical diagnoses of hyposexual activity disorder, sexual aversion disorder, sexual arousal disorder, orgasmic disorder, sexual pain disorder, and persistent genital arousal disorder; the general nature of the SD can be presumed simply by its name.[9,10,16]

Male Sexual Disorders

Although men can experience sexual dysfunction related to sexual desire (libido), arousal, and pain, the two widely recognized conditions specific to men are erectile dysfunction (ED) and ejaculatory disorders. Erectile dysfunction is an inability to develop or maintain an erection of the penis during sexual activity. Ejaculatory dysfunction is characterized by reduced or absent semen volume, which may be the result of a psychological condition, a medical condition, a medication, or a surgery. Stress, vascular disease, diabetes, antidepressants, antihypertensive medications, alcohol, illicit drugs, and prostate surgery can affect erectile and ejaculatory function. Four categories of ejaculatory disorders are premature ejaculation, delayed ejaculation, retrograde ejaculation, and anejaculation/anorgasmia (no ejaculation/no orgasm).[10]

CONSEQUENCES

A number of consequences can occur as a result of sexual disorders and are based on physiological and psychological concerns. Physiological consequences can include, but are not limited to, unfulfilled sexual desire, unsatisfactory sexual responses, pain, STI infection as a result of a sexual encounter, inability to create a pregnancy, and complications with pregnancies. Psychosocial consequences include problems with relationships (particularly if sexual responses between a couple have changed), low self-esteem, anxiety, and depression. The significance of the consequences is also dependent on the patient's age, interest in sex, and whether the underlying sexual disorder is a temporary or chronic condition.

RISK FACTORS

It is important for nurses to be aware that some groups of patients will be more vulnerable to and at increased risk for alterations in sexual well-being.

Populations at Risk
Adolescents

Addressing adolescent sexuality includes considering critical factors that may influence their behavior: socioeconomic status, family structure, future perspectives for education, and lived experiences. Furthermore, among demographic subgroups of adolescents defined by sex, race/ethnicity, and grade in school, several significant health disparities exist; this is especially so when comparing sexual minority and nonsexual minority groups. Sexual minority youth include those who self-identify as LGBTQ, and those who are unsure about their sexual identity.[18] Many adolescents are at risk for HIV, STIs, unintended pregnancy, and sexual violence. According to the 2017 U.S. Youth Risk Behavior Surveillance System,[18] among U.S. high school students surveyed, 52% had had sexual contact, 10% had four or more sexual partners, and 7% had been physically forced to have unwanted sexual intercourse. Young people (ages 13 to 24) accounted for approximately 21% of all new HIV diagnoses in the United States in 2016, and of these 81% were gay and bisexual males. While teen pregnancy rates have continued to decline since the 1990s, the United States reports a teen pregnancy rate of 57 pregnancies per 1000 females, and a teen birth rate of 41.5 per 1000 females between the ages of 15 to 19 years.[19]

Disabilities: Cognitive, Developmental, and Physical

Sexuality and its expression has long been overlooked as an essential aspect and an inherent right of people with disabilities; there exists an underlying assumption that these individuals are asexual and have no need of sexual fulfillment. All people, including those with disabilities, are entitled to move toward both sexual and social maturity in the same manner.[20] For some with disabilities, ignorance will place them at further risk because sexual behavior is a result of poor decision-making, loneliness, manipulation, or even force instead of being a healthy expression of their sexuality. Special consideration for the geriatric population includes chronic illness (CVD, COPD, cancer), cognitive decline, LGBTQ issues previously not acknowledged, and STIs.[20]

Newly Unpartnered

A unique population at increased risk for negative sequelae are those adults who have recently separated—unpartnered—from their long-term partners because of death or divorce and are now exposed to an entirely new sexual paradigm. These adults may begin dating and suddenly have several new and unknown sexual partners.[21] Depending on their age, HIV, AIDS, and other STIs may not have been of concern when these adults were initially partnered. Although HIV/AIDS infections in the United States are now considered to be chronic conditions, all parties who have intercourse must be cognizant of their risk for exposure to these and other diseases and receive appropriate health education.[21]

Sexual Orientation and Identification: Lesbian, Gay, Bisexual, Transgender, Queer

In comparison to their heterosexual counterparts, LGBTQ gay, lesbian, and bisexual youths have been found to engage in more high-risk sexual practices.[22] Young women who primarily have sex with women also report that they are likely to engage in sexual activity with men who are homosexual, bisexual, or injection drug users.[23] Adolescent boys who participate in sexual activity with bisexual men are at significantly increased risk for possible transmission of HIV and AIDS.[23] New cases of HIV diagnosis are increasing among men who have sex with men (particularly those of racial minorities) perhaps because of the "glamorization" of anal intercourse, misperceptions that partners are at low risk, and the belief that medical advances in the treatment of AIDS have eliminated the need for appropriate protection during sexual activity.[22–24]

Individual Risk Factors

High-Risk Behaviors

Although sexual activity is considered a normative process, some individuals inadvertently place themselves at increased risk for sexual health problems—primarily those who engage in sexual activity with multiple and casual partners and/or refrain from "safe sex" practices.[21] According to the most recent surveys, these individuals are composed of young people (particularly lesbian, gay, bisexual, and transgender youth) and men who have sex with men regardless of race.[23–25]

Of secondary importance is the influence of nonsexual high-risk behavior, such as the use of alcohol, marijuana, or other illicit substances. Prior research has shown that when these substances are ingested close to the time of sexual activity, the rate of sexual risk-taking increases.[22,26] The abuse of alcohol or drugs most often results in impaired judgment and consequently less thoughtfulness related to the sexual act.[21]

Underlying Medical Conditions and Medications

A number of underlying medical conditions, particularly chronic health conditions, and/or medications used to treat underlying conditions can place an individual at risk for sexual disorders. Some of the most common conditions that increase risk include acute or chronic pain, chronic fatigue, anxiety, depression, cardiovascular disease, diabetes, and chronic respiratory conditions. Likewise, many medications can affect sexual health. Common medications that can affect sexual function are presented in Box 21.1.

ASSESSMENT

A majority of nurses believe that sexual assessment is part of their professional responsibility in providing nursing care. In practice, however, most nurses rarely or never address sexuality as a health issue, even though patients have identified it as an expected and appropriate behavior in

---

BOX 21.1 Common Medications that Reduce Sexual Desire or Response

- Antihypertensives (ACE inhibitors, β blockers, β agonists, diuretics)
- Antiulcer medications (cimetidine, omeprazole)
- Antidepressants
- Antipsychotics
- Anticonvulsants
- Diuretics
- Narcotics

ACE, angiotensin-converting-enzyme.

---

the nurse–patient relationship.[27–31] Application of the nursing process in identifying and addressing problems related to sexuality is essential to promoting sexual well-being of individuals, couples, families, and communities.[15,32]

History

A sexual history is elicited as an essential part of a routine health history during an initial visit and annual visits thereafter. Despite the importance of sexual health and patients' expressed desire to be queried about sexual issues, questions related to sexual health are infrequently raised during routine examinations.[33] Barriers identified by nurses include personal discomfort, lack of training, and lack of time; those identified by patients include personal discomfort and beliefs that their concerns would be dismissed and that it is the provider's responsibility to initiate the dialogue.[30–32]

The CDC drafted guidelines for sexual history taking and incorporates five areas that should be broached with patients; these are known as the "the five P's." These stand for *partners*, *practices*, *protection* from infection, *past* history of infection, and *prevention* of pregnancy.[34] *Partners* includes the number and gender of the patient's sexual partners. *Practices* refers to safe sex practices. If the patient reports more than one partner in the past 12 months or if the patient has had sex with a partner who has other sex partners, the nurse should inquire about condom use. *Protection* refers to questions assessing measures that the patient takes to protect himself or herself from STIs. This may include exploring about abstinence, monogamy, and the patient's perception of his or her own risk or his or her partner's risk. These questions are helpful in assessing patient risk for STIs.

Typical health history questions for females include those about menarche, menstruation, pregnancy, contraception, and menopause; for males, questions include those about contraception, penile discharge or lesions, scrotal pain or swelling, and alterations in urine elimination and andropause. Questions about practices for both sexes include those regarding safer sex knowledge and practice, frequency of intercourse, number of partners/lifetime partners, sexual behaviors, preferences, sexual response, and personal safety. Recall it is important to discuss sexual behaviors separately from sexual identity and orientation, as identity and orientation do not define risk.[11]

Examination Findings

The physical examination is guided by the sexual history and the patient's age, gender, and pertinent needs. A physical examination may or may not be a necessary component of nursing care as it relates to sexuality. For example, the report of genital pain will rely on the assessment techniques of history, inspection, and palpation, whereas a report of an alteration in sexual motivation or desire may not warrant physical examination.

Knowledge of the physical changes associated with normal growth and development is essential, and those associated with milestones such as puberty, pregnancy, menopause, and andropause are of particular interest as they relate to sexuality. Described as a sequence of physical changes, sexual maturation can be estimated based on the observed changes of primary and secondary sex characteristics: in females, breast development and pubic hair, and in males, genital development, along with pubic hair. Relying on a scale first suggested in the 1960s as an aide to quantify these physical changes is commonly referred to as "Tanner staging," named after the physician who first proposed it.[35]

Female Physical Examination

The first genital exam should occur at birth with the infant girl in a supine position; it is a relatively easy and noninvasive assessment. A general assessment of the vulva will include inspection of the labia majora, labia minora, clitoris, urethral opening, introitus, hymen, perineum, and anus. The initial assessment should confirm the sex of the infant and the patency of the urethra and anus; this is baseline data. Nurses observe for the passage of urine and meconium to confirm patency of the urethra and anus. Throughout childhood, the sexual history will guide the appropriate physical examination.

The gynecologic examination, generally associated with puberty and beyond, includes inspection and palpation of the external genitalia, internal inspection of the vagina per speculum, collection of specimens as indicated (swabs for cervical smears and STI screening), and bimanual palpation (pelvic exam) if indicated; a rectal exam may be performed if indicated. Physical findings might include the following: healed scars from childbirth or trauma, hymenal tags, bulges (cystoceles or rectoceles), thinning of the vaginal wall, fistulas, masses, lesions, and inflammation. An annual gynecological exam typically includes a clinical breast exam as well.

Male Physical Examination

The first genital exam should occur at birth with the infant male in a supine position. A general assessment will include inspection of the penis, testes, scrotum, perineum, and anus. The initial assessment will confirm the sex of the infant, patency of the anus, and the location of the urinary meatus with any deviation (epispadias and hypospadias) documented; this is baseline data. Throughout childhood, the sexual history will guide the appropriate physical examination.

A general assessment of the male examination includes inspection and palpation of the penis, scrotum, testicles, perineum, and perianal area; a digital rectal examination (DRE) for assessment of the prostate may be indicated. The nurse should begin by examining the penis, scrotum, and testicles. The penis is inspected for discharge and lesions; the scrotum is inspected for lesions and contour. The testicles within the scrotal sac are palpated for size, texture, and tenderness, which may reveal such findings as hydrocele, masses, nodules, tenderness, or inflammation.[36]

Diagnostic Tests

Based on the patient's history and needs, a number of laboratory tests and diagnostic procedures may be indicated. Specimen collection from a variety of sources includes serum, urine, genital discharge/secretions, lesions, and semen. Diagnostic procedures include tissue biopsy, aspiration, ultrasound, x-ray, laparoscopy, colposcopy, and colonoscopy. Diagnostic testing may be performed for screening of genetic issues (ambiguous genitalia noted at birth), cancers (cervical, ovarian, prostate, and anus), infections (chlamydia, gonorrhea, syphilis, HPV, and HIV), and hormonal states (hypogonadism and pregnancy); the type of testing is best determined individually for each patient.

CLINICAL MANAGEMENT

Primary Prevention

Patient education, counseling, and referral are essential components of health promotion and disease prevention for optimal sexual well-being. Focused areas of discussion include abstinence, contraception, safer sex practices, STIs, healthy relationships, and community resources. Although a great diversity of opinion exists regarding how to address sexuality issues in the United States, two common themes have been identified that support a communication framework for sexual health. The first theme is about protecting health through making good choices with regard to sexual behavior. The second theme supports broadening sexual health programs to go beyond disease control prevention to include wellness-related approaches to promote sexual health.[37]

Human papilloma virus (HPV) can be prevented by HPV vaccination. There are currently three vaccines available, of which one is a U.S. Food and Drug Administration–approved HPV vaccine; it can be given in a two or three-dose series. Vaccination is routinely given at 11 or 12 years of age to both girls and boys. HPV vaccination is considered to be safe and effective, and it offers protection from genital warts and cancers caused by HPV, including that of the cervix, vagina, vulva (women), penis (men), anus, and oropharynx (both women and men).[38]

Secondary Prevention (Screening)

In contrast to primary prevention strategies, secondary prevention attempts to diagnose an existing disease in its earliest stages. This is referred to as screening with a goal of reducing morbidity and mortality and preserving quality of life.

Screening for Sexually Transmitted Infection

There is limited consistency in the literature regarding screening recommendations. The U.S. Preventive Services Task Force (USPSTF) recommends screening based on level of risk.[39] Level of risk is based on sexual behavior and includes unprotected intercourse, having sex with multiple partners, adolescent-onset intercourse, sharing of intravenous needles, and history of STIs. Individuals in a mutually monogamous relationship are considered low risk. For individuals who are at increased risk, periodic screening for chlamydia, gonorrhea, syphilis, and HIV is recommended; specific screening intervals vary, but it is common for screenings to occur as part of an annual pelvic examination.

Screening for Intimate Partner Violence

The USPSTF recommends that all women of childbearing age (14 to 46 years) be screened for IPV, whereas others advocate for universal screening of patients across the lifespan.[40] Available screening instruments, including the Hurt, Insult, Threaten, Scream (HITS) screening tool, have been determined to be valid and reliable in the detection of current, past, and risk for abuse in clinical settings. Adequate evidence supports that effective interventions can reduce violence, abuse, and physical or mental harms for women of reproductive age.

Collaborative Interventions

A number of interventions are indicated for individuals experiencing a wide range of sexual problems and disorders.

Pharmacotherapy

Antibiotics. Infections of the reproductive tract are usually caused by STIs. A wide range of antibacterial, antiviral, and antiprotozoal agents are used in the treatment of STIs depending on the microorganism involved.

Hormone replacement therapy. Hormone replacement therapy (HRT) is often used to treat the symptoms of menopause—most notably hot flashes and vaginal dryness. HRT may be given as low-dose estrogen (for women who have had a hysterectomy) or combination therapy (estrogen and progesterone) for women who still have their uterus.

Phosphodiesterase-5 inhibitors. Two phosphodiesterase-5 (PDE-5) drugs (sildenafil and vardenafil) represent the first-line treatment for ED. These drugs act by relaxing smooth muscles in the corpora cavernosa of the penis to increase blood flow and compressing the veins in the corpora to reduce outward blood flow. These combined actions result in penile erection with sexual stimulation.

Surgical Procedures

There are indications for surgical procedures for men and women who are experiencing certain sexual problems.

Hysterectomy. A hysterectomy is the surgical removal of the uterus and may be indicated for a variety of uterine conditions, including menorrhagia, pelvic pain from endometriosis, prolapse of the female reproductive organs (uterus, cystocele, and rectocele), uterine fibroids, myomas, and cancer.

Penile implant surgery. Penile implant surgery involves the insertion of an inflatable device in the penis with a reservoir placed in the scrotum. The device is inflated by squeezing the reservoir. This procedure has become much less common since the introduction of pharmacotherapy for ED. Typically this procedure is done in cases where less invasive treatments are not successful.

Minor procedures. Other surgical procedures include removal of genital lesions (e.g., warts or polyps) or incision and drainage for cysts or abscess.

Cognitive–Behavioral Therapy

For some individuals, cognitive–behavioral therapy (CBT) and sexual counseling have proven effective in the treatment of sexual problems with psychological origins, including some cases of ED. Many psychological and emotional factors, such as fear, anxiety, fatigue, and reproductive health concerns, can impair sexual performance. Individuals with sex addictions may also benefit from CBT.

Other Interventions

An alternative to PDE-5 in the treatment of ED is the vacuum construction device. This is an external cylinder-like device that fits over the penis and uses a vacuum effect to draw blood into the penis to gain an erection. A tension band is placed at the base of the penis to maintain the erection once the cylinder is removed, allowing the individual to have sex. The ring is removed within 1 hour.

INTERRELATED CONCEPTS

The concept of sexual health represents the "integration of somatic, emotional, intellectual and social aspects of sexual being in ways that are enriching and enhance personality, communication and love."[1] Sexuality and interrelated concepts are presented in Fig. 21.3. This model illustrates some concepts that may be impacted by normative sexual functioning and/or have an impact on sexuality.

Reproduction (and reproductive health) are highly interrelated to sexuality. By definition, they include topics of puberty, contraception, STIs, safer sex practices, fertility, infertility, and sexuality. Additional considerations for females are breast and cervical cancer screening, menstruation, preconceptual counsel and screening, pregnancy, and menopause.

One barrier to healthy sexual expression and function is Pain. Regardless of the source or type of pain the patient experiences, it can contribute to sexual dysfunction; pain can be chronic or acute, physical, psychological, or spiritual. For those in pain, sometimes the pain itself makes having sex not possible. It is noteworthy that both positive touch and sexual intimacy are known to stimulate the release of endorphins, the body's natural painkillers.

Medical conditions that lead to alterations in Gas Exchange (e.g., chronic obstructive pulmonary disease, cystic fibrosis, interstitial lung disease, and asthma) can lead to shortness of breath, fatigue, depression, and feelings of anxiousness and thus can inhibit the human sexual response and can result in sexual dysfunction.[41] Individuals who rely on supplemental oxygen may experience impaired body image.

"Being present" is identified as a positive attribute of sexuality; Anxiety can preoccupy the mind, body, and spirit. Patients with anxiety often present with concerns related to sexual dysfunction; those who seek care for SD often report feelings of anxiety. Anxiety is often linked to stress. If a patient is undergoing extreme stress from other life issues, this may have a negative impact on sexual function, particularly among those with insufficient coping strategies (Stress and Coping). Anxiety stimulates the sympathetic nervous system—the stress response is that of fight–flight–freeze—and negatively impacts the sexual response cycle.[42]

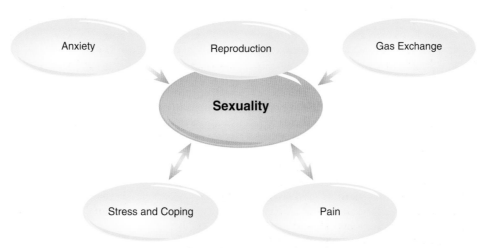

FIGURE 21.3 Sexuality and Interrelated Concepts.

BOX 21.2   EXEMPLARS OF IMPAIRED SEXUALITY

Disorders Affecting Sexual Response
- Anorgasmia
- Coital incontinence
- Dysfunctional uterine bleeding
- Ejaculatory disorders
- Endometriosis
- Erectile dysfunction
- Hyposexual activity disorder
- Menopause
- Orgasmic disorder
- Pelvic organ prolapse
- Persistent genital arousal disorder
- Sexual arousal disorder
- Sexual aversion disorder
- Sexual pain disorder
- Vaginismus
- Vulvovaginitis

Sexually Transmitted Infections
Protozoa
- Trichomoniasis

Viruses
- Cytomegalovirus
- Hepatitis A and hepatitis B
- Herpes simplex virus 1 and 2 (HSV)
- HIV
- Human papillomavirus (HPV)

Bacteria
- Chancroid
- *Chlamydia*
- Genital mycoplasmas
- Gonorrhea
- Group B *Streptococcus*
- Syphilis

Other Exemplars
- Intimate partner violence
- Sexual violence
- Intersex

 ACCESS EXEMPLAR LINKS IN YOUR GIDDENS EBOOK

CLINICAL EXEMPLARS

Any number of exemplars could be chosen to effectively illustrate the concept of human sexuality. Those presented in Box 21.2 address a continuum of concerns that have a significant impact on a person's sexual health and well-being across the lifespan.

Featured Exemplars
Erectile Dysfunction
ED is estimated to affect 18 to 30 million men in the United States; it is believed to be an underreported disease process as a result of embarrassment, shame, and lack of understanding of the condition. ED affects men of all ages and can be chronic or transient in nature. ED is positively correlated with age, cardiovascular conditions, risk factors, physical inactivity, alcohol use, smoking, and obesity; these conditions impact vascular perfusion, which is necessary for penile erection. For some men, there is an associated alteration in body image, self-concept, and self-esteem, all of which can be negatively impacted by a perceived loss of manhood.[42]

Menopause
Menopause is associated with the cessation of ovulation. The age of onset is variable, with the average age at 51 years. Common symptoms include hot flashes, night sweats, impaired sleep, headaches, changes in memory, loss of sexual desire, urinary concerns, mood alterations, and dryness of skin and vaginal tissues.[43] In addition to managing symptoms, issues to be addressed include nutrition, bone health, heart disease prevention, weight management, hormonal balance, and cancer screening, along with psychosocial concerns of relationships, retirement, and available community support systems. Nurses have the ability to provide accurate information to patients regarding the physiology of menopause and its effect on sexuality.[36]

Pelvic Organ Prolapse
Symptoms of sexual dysfunction and altered body image often coexist with prolapse of the female reproductive organs (uterus, cystocele, and rectocele). Approximately 50% of women experience some degree of prolapse by the time they reach the age of 40 years.[44] Intercourse may be painful or embarrassing and associated with fecal or urinary incontinence. Conservative management includes lifestyle changes—such as losing weight, avoiding constipation, and reducing high-impact exercise (e.g., running)—and pelvic muscle floor training (Kegel exercises),[44] although surgical intervention may be necessary for advanced cases.

Intimate Partner Violence
IPV is a serious, preventable public health issue that affects millions of Americans. The CDC defines IPV as

actual or threatened physical, sexual, psychological, emotional, or stalking abuse by an intimate partner. An intimate partner can be a current or former spouse or nonmarital partner, such as a boyfriend, girlfriend, or dating partner. Intimate partners can be of the same or opposite sex.[45]

It is clearly documented that IPV during adolescence is associated with negative biopsychosocial health effects, poor school performance, and a predisposition for sexual ill-being and problems in future relationships throughout life.[45]

Sexual Violence
Sexual violence is a public health issue throughout the world and is detrimental to the sexual well-being of an individual, a family, and a community. The CDC defines sexual violence as "a sexual act committed against someone without that persons' freely given consent."[46] Sexual violence includes child sexual abuse, intimate partner violence, incest, drug-facilitated sexual assault, sexual harassment, sexual exploitation, stalking, voyeurism, exhibitionism, frottage, and unwanted exposure to pornography.

Intersex

Intersex represents a group of conditions in which an infant's external genitals do not appear distinctly male or female or the external genitalia may not match the internal sex organs or genetic sex of the infant. This condition is confusing and distressing for families, as well as challenging for the healthcare team, which may have limited experience with and understanding of the condition. Medical care includes chromosomal analysis, endocrine studies, and radiologic studies to assist in guiding gender assignment. Physiological complications of the condition of intersex include infertility and an increased risk of certain types of cancer.[46,47]

CASE STUDY

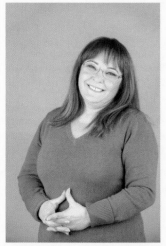

Case Presentation

Anna Garner is a 44-year-old married white female who has an appointment to see her nurse practitioner (NP) for her annual examination. As part of her annual physical, Anna will be having a pelvic examination, including a Papanicolaou test, to screen for cervical cancer. Anna has three teenage daughters, all born by spontaneous vaginal delivery. Several years ago, Anna returned to work full-time at a rather sedentary job. Anna has found her weight to be increasing during these past few years and is now carrying 160 pounds at 5 feet, 4 inches tall. Throughout the years, Anna and her NP have developed a trusting and therapeutic relationship. As part of the history-taking process, the NP asks Anna if there have been any changes in the past year related to the sexual relationship that she has with her partner. Anna appears somewhat embarrassed; however, with some encouragement, she goes on to explain that in the past she and her husband have always enjoyed intercourse two or three times a week and that this is a very important part of their marriage. Anna states that for the past 9 or 10 months, she has begun to "lose urine" during intercourse. Sometimes this occurs during foreplay, and on other occasions it will happen during orgasm. Anna reports that she often interrupts their sexual activity to go to the bathroom. Recently, she has been finding excuses to avoid sex altogether and is concerned that she is driving her husband away. The NP explains to Anna that this condition is referred to as "stress or coital incontinence" and may be the result of childbearing, aging, and her recent weight gain. Education is provided regarding the necessity for urodynamic evaluation and the possible treatment modalities available. Anna is instructed on how to perform Kegel exercises. The NP reassures Anna that although this condition is neither uncommon nor life-threatening, if left untreated it may result in other unanticipated symptomatology, including depression, loss of self-esteem, altered body image, worsening of incontinence, reduced social interaction, and decreased sexual interest and activity. Anna is very reassured by this education and agrees to the treatment plan.

Case Analysis Questions

1. What risk factors does Anna have for impairment in sexual health?
2. Review Fig. 21.3. Which concepts are associated with Anna's case? What other interrelated concepts are evident?

From bbevren/iStock/Thinkstock.

🌿 ACCESS EXEMPLAR LINKS IN YOUR GIDDENS EBOOK

REFERENCES

1. World Health Organization. (2006). *Defining sexual health: Report of a technical consultation on sexual health, Jan 28–31, 2001.* Geneva, Geneva: World Health Organization.
2. Online Etymology Dictionary. (2018). *Sex.* Retrieved from http://www.etymonline.com/index.php?allowed_in_frame=0&search=sex&searchmode=none.
3. Office of the Surgeon General. (2001). *The Surgeon General's call to action to promote sexual health.* Rockville, MD, Office of the Surgeon General; and Centers for Disease Control and Prevention.
4. Center for Disease Control and Prevention. (2018). *Sexual Health.* Retrieved from http://www.cdc.gov/sexualhealth/Default.html.
5. Merriam–Webster. (n.d). *Well-being.* Retrieved from http://www.merriam-webster.com/dictionary/well-being.
6. Merriam–Webster. (n.d). *Ill-being.* Retrieved from http://www.merriam-webster.com/dictionary/ill-being.
7. Masters, W. H., & Johnson, V. E. (1966). *Human sexual response.* Boston: Little, Brown.
8. Bancroft, J. (2002). Biological factors in human sexuality. *Journal of Sex Research, 30*(1), 15–21.
9. Basson, R., Leiblum, S., Brotto, L., et al. (2003). Definitions of women's sexual dysfunction reconsidered: Advocating expansion and revision. *J Psychosom Obstet Gynecol, 24,* 221–229.
10. Merck. (2018). *Merck manuals: Sexual dysfunction: Overview of male sexual function.* Retrieved from http://www.merckmanuals.com/professional/genitourinary-disorders/male-sexual-dysfunction/overview-of-male-sexual-function.
11. Oswalt, S. B., Evans, S., & Drott, A. (2016). Beyond alphabet soup: Helping college health professionals understand sexual fluidity. *Journal of American College Health, 64*(6), 502–508.
12. Bancroft, J. (Ed.), (2003). *Sexual development in childhood.* Bloomington, IN: Indiana University Press.
13. Kneisl, C. R., & Trigoboff, E. (2013). *Contemporary psychiatric–mental health nursing* (3rd ed.). New York: Pearson.
14. Kleinplatz, P. J., & Menard, A. D. (2007). Building blocks toward optimal sexuality: Constructing a conceptual model. *Family J, 15,* 72–78.
15. Herdman, T. H. (2008). *North American Nursing Diagnosis Association: NANDA-I nursing diagnoses: Definitions & classification, 2009–2011.* Oxford: Wiley–Blackwell.
16. Berman, J. R. (2005). Physiology of female sexual function and dysfunction. *Int J Impotence Res, 17,* S44–S51.
17. Sobczak, J. A. (2009). Female sexual dysfunction: Knowledge development and practice implications. *Perspectives in Psychiatric Care, 45*(3), 161–172.
18. Kann, L., McManus, T., Harris, W. A., et al.. (2017). *Youth Risk Behavior Surveillance – United States.* Retrieved from https://www.cdc.gov/mmwr/volumes/67/ss/ss6708a1.htm.
19. Sedgh, G., Finer, L. B., Bankole, A., et al. (2015). Adolescent pregnancy, birth and abortion rates across countries: Levels and trends. *Journal of Adolescent Health, 56*(2), 223–230.

20. Ailey, S. H., Marks, B. A., Crisp, C., et al. (2003). Promoting sexuality across the lifespan for individuals with intellectual and developmental disabilities. *The Nursing Clinics of North America, 38,* 229–252.

21. Lowdermilk, D. L., Perry, S. E., Cashion, K., et al. (Eds.), (2012). *Maternity & women's health care* (10th ed.). St Louis: Mosby.

22. Dowshein, N., & Garofalo, R. (2009). Optimizing primary care for LGBTQ youth. *Contemporary Pediatrics, 26*(10).

23. Brown, R. T., & Brown, J. D. (2006). Adolescent sexuality. *Prim Care Clin Office Pract, 33,* 373–390.

24. Sanders, S. A., Reece, M., Herbenick, D., et al. (2010). Condom use during most recent vaginal intercourse event among a probability sample of adults in the United States. *The Journal of Sexual Medicine, 7*(Suppl. 5), 362–373.

25. Fenton, K. A. (2010). Time for change: Rethinking and reframing sexual health in the United States. *The Journal of Sexual Medicine, 7*(Suppl. 5), 250–252.

26. Herbenick, D., Reece, M., Schick, V., et al. (2010). An event-level analysis of the sexual characteristics and composition among adults ages 18 to 59: Results from a national probability sample in the United States. *The Journal of Sexual Medicine, 7*(Suppl. 5), 346–361.

27. Gott, M., Galena, E., Hinchliff, S., et al. (2004). "Opening a can of worms": GP and practice nurse barriers to talking about sexual health in primary care. *Family Practice, 21,* 528–536.

28. Hoekstra, T., Lesman-Leegte, I., Couperus, M. F., et al. (2012). What keeps nurses from the sexual counseling of patients with heart failure? *Heart and Lung: The Journal of Critical Care, 41*(5), 492–499.

29. Palmer, H. (1998). Exploring sexuality and sexual health in nursing. *Professional Nurse, 14*(1), 15–17.

30. Reynolds, K. E., & Magnan, M. A. (2005). Nursing attitudes and beliefs toward human sexuality. *Clin Nurse Specialist, 19*(5), 255–259.

31. Zillotto, G. C., & Marcolan, J. F. (2013). Perception of nursing professionals on sexuality in people with mental disorders. *Acta Paul Enferm, 26*(1), 86–92.

32. Ayaz, S. (2013). Sexuality and nursing process: A literature review. *Sexuality Disability, 31,* 3–12.

33. Shifren, J. L., Johannes, C. B., Monz, B. U., et al. (2008). Help-seeking behavior of women with self-reported distressing sexual problems. *J Women's Health, 18*(4), 461–468.

34. Centers for Disease Control and Prevention. (2018). *A guide to taking a sexual history.* Retrieved from http://www.cdc.gov/std/treatment/sexualhistory.pdf.

35. Quigley, B. H., Palm, M. L., & Bickley, L. (2012). *Bates' nursing guide to physical examination and history taking.* Philadelphia: Wolters Kluwer.

36. Ignatavicius, D. D., & Workman, M. L. (2016). *Medical–surgical nursing* (8th ed.). St Louis: Elsevier.

37. Robinson, S. J., Stellatu, A., Stephens, J., et al. (2013). On the road to well-being: The development of a communication framework for sexual health. *Public Health Reports, 128,* 43–52.

38. Centers for Disease Control and Prevention. *2015 STD treatment guidelines.* Retrieved from http://www.cdc.gov/std/tg2015.

39. U.S. Preventive Services Task Force. (2014). *USPSTF recommendations for STI screening.* (Updated 2018). Retrieved from http://www.uspreventiveservicestaskforce.org/Page/Name/uspstf-recommendations-for-sti-screening.

40. U.S. Preventive Services Task Force. (2013). *Intimate partner violence and abuse of elderly and vulnerable adults: Screening.* Retrieved from http://www.uspreventiveservicestaskforce.org/Page/Topic/recommendation-summary/intimate-partner-violence-and-abuse-of-elderly-and-vulnerable-adults-screening.

41. McCoy, K., & Jones, N. (2012). *Is COPD ruining your sex life?* Retrieved from http://www.everydayhealth.com/copd/copd-and-your-sex-life.aspx.

42. Corretti, G., & Baldi, I. (2007). The relationship between anxiety disorders and sexual dysfunction. *Psychiatric Times.*

43. Selvin, E., Burnett, A., & Platz, E. (2007). Prevalence and risk factors for erectile dysfunction in the U.S. *The American Journal of Medicine, 120*(2), 151–157.

44. Northrup, C. (2012). *The wisdom of menopause: Creating physical and emotional health and healing during the change.* rev ed. New York: Random House.

45. Richardson, K., Hagen, S., Glazener, C., et al. (2009). The role of nurses in the management of women with pelvic organ prolapse. *British Journal of Nursing (Mark Allen Publishing), 18*(5), 294–296, 298–300.

46. Centers for Disease Control and Prevention. (2015). *Intimate partner violence.* Retrieved from http://www.cdc.gov/ViolencePrevention/intimatepartnerviolence.

47. Sanders, C., Carter, B., & Goodacre, L. (2012). Parents need to protect: Influences, risks, and tensions for parents of pre-pubertal children born with ambiguous genitalia. *Journal of Clinical Nursing, 21,* 3315–3323.

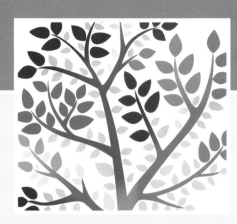

Immunity

Carolyn E. Sabo

The ability of the human body to sustain health within the environment requires multiple protective mechanisms. One of the most complex protective mechanisms is the immune response. When immune processes are functioning optimally, the body has the ability to mount an efficient defense in response to the invasion of foreign substances. Such a response is critical to maintaining health. It is reasonable, then, to conclude that multiple health problems occur in the absence of a normal immune response. Although this concept presentation describes the concept of immunity from the perspective of both normal and abnormal functioning, the primary focus is on that of abnormal function because of the multitude of health-related problems that result.

DEFINITION

Immunity is commonly defined as a physiological process that provides an individual with protection or defense from disease. It is a characteristic that allows one to be resistant to a particular disease or condition; the term is derived from the Latin word *immunis*, meaning exempt.[1] Immunity is accomplished through the actions of the immune system, which is a body-wide, complex, interrelated group of cells, tissues, and organs that work within a dynamic communication network to protect the body from attacks by foreign antigens, typically proteins. These foreign antigens may include microorganisms (bacteria, viruses, parasites, or fungi), but they may also be proteins found in pollens; foods; bee, snake, or spider venom; vaccines; transfusions; and transplanted tissues.[2] As noted previously, this concept includes abnormal function leading to health problems. For the purpose of this concept presentation, a broader definition of immunity is used: *the normal physiological response to microorganisms and proteins as well as conditions associated with an inadequate or excessive immune response.*

Additional terms are used to differentiate the type of immunity protection. *Innate immunity* (also referred to as *natural* or *native*) is the immunity present at birth; it provides nonspecific response not considered antigen specific. *Acquired immunity* refers to immunity protection that is gained after birth either actively or passively. *Active acquired immunity* develops after the introduction of a foreign antigen resulting in the formation of antibodies or sensitized T lymphocytes. For example, active immunity may be obtained artificially through the immune response to an immunization, or it may be obtained naturally through the immune response to exposure to infectious pathogens such as varicella–zoster virus. *Passive acquired immunity* occurs by the introduction of preformed antibodies—either from an artificial route, such as a transfusion of immunoglobulin (Ig), or from a natural route, such as from a mother to her fetus through placental blood transference or through colostrum transfer during breastfeeding.[3–5]

SCOPE

The complexity of immunity often makes it a difficult topic to fully understand from a traditional presentation. From a conceptual perspective, it is useful to think about what this concept represents from a very broad view and consider the context of patient-related issues. The scope of immunity and related immunity problems are described as optimal and abnormal responses (Fig. 22.1). An optimal response represents an immune system that protects the body from the invasion of microorganisms, removes dead and damaged tissue and cells, and recognizes and removes cell mutations. Abnormal function includes a suppressed immune response and exaggerated immune response.[2]

To the far left of the immune response spectrum (see Fig. 22.1) is a hypo- or suppressed immune response. Individuals who have suppressed immune responses are referred to as immunocompromised or are considered to be in a state of immunodeficiency. Individuals with suppressed immune responses are at significant risk for infection, or if immunosuppression occurs over time, they are at risk for cancer because of the loss or removal of mutating cells.[2,6,7]

To the far right of the immune response spectrum (see Fig. 22.1) is a hyperimmune or exaggerated immune response. Hyperimmune responses range among allergic reactions, cytotoxic reactions, and autoimmune reactions. A critical component of the immune system is its ability to differentiate between "self" and "non-self." When this recognition fails, the immune system may begin attacking host cells in an exaggerated immune response. This process leads to the development of autoimmune diseases and disorders.[2,5–7]

NORMAL PHYSIOLOGICAL PROCESS

The immune response involves the following three primary protective functions:
1. Protects the body from invasion of microorganisms and other antigens
2. Removes dead or damaged tissue and cells
3. Recognizes and removes cell mutations that have demonstrated abnormal cell growth and development

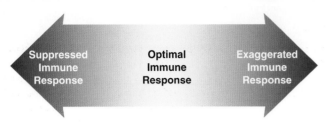

FIGURE 22.1 Scope of Immunity Concept.

To accomplish these functions, the immune system reacts with three lines of defense. The first line of defense is the skin boundary surfaces, including mucous membranes, enzymes, natural microbial flora, and complement proteins. The second line of defense is accomplished by the activities of phagocytes, natural killer T lymphocytes, granulocytes, and macrophages providing innate, nonspecific immunity. Finally, the third line of defense comes from antibodies derived from B lymphocytes and the T lymphocytes resulting from learned or acquired specific immunity.[2,5–7]

Recognition of the "self" and recognition of foreign proteins are the hallmarks of a properly functioning immune system. The individual must be able to differentiate between host and foreign proteins in order to respond appropriately. With the invasion of foreign proteins, a protective response is needed; failure to respond appropriately (immunosuppression or immunodeficiency) results in infection or disease. Likewise, the body must maintain the ability to recognize host proteins and not initiate an immune response. When this recognition fails, the immune system launches an attack on host cells (autoimmune response) or initiates a hyperactive immune response (hyperimmune response).

Major Histocompatibility Complex Proteins

Surface proteins called major histocompatibility complex (MHC) proteins are divided into two classes, with class I being found on all cells and class II on specialized cells. MHC proteins function, in part, to differentiate cells of the self/host from foreign proteins. Substances that are "nonself" are capable of initiating an immune response. A foreign antigen may be a whole cell, a virus, a bacterium, an MHC marker protein, or a small portion of a larger foreign protein. Epitopes are the markers on foreign antigens that cause the immune response in individuals.[3] The MHC provides what has been termed a "scaffold" that presents the foreign antigen to the immune cells. The empty MHC scaffold, also termed a self-marker scaffold, of a foreign cell from a donor organ may be introduced into the host during a transplant. These MHC self-marker scaffolds are the individual's tissue type or human leukocyte antigen.[2,3]

Organs Comprising the Immune System

Organs of the immune system are spread throughout the body. They are termed lymphoid organs and include the bone marrow, thymus gland, spleen, tonsils, adenoids, and appendix. From these organs, the lymphocytes are formed, grow, mature, and released into the body. The body's lymphatic system provides the network by which organs of the immune system are connected. The blood also provides a connection among the organs and provides the route for lymphocyte movement throughout the body.

Origin of Cells in an Immune Response

A variety of components work together to provide an immune response. All cells in the immune system are derived from stem cells in the bone marrow and begin as either myeloid progenitor or lymphoid progenitor cells. Myeloid progenitors include neutrophils, monocytes (which become macrophages in body tissues), eosinophils, basophils, and mast cells. Lymphoid progenitor cells include B lymphocytes (which become plasma or memory B cells), mature T lymphocytes, and natural killer cells.[2,6–8]

B and T Lymphocytes

During fetal development, B and T lymphocytes are produced in large numbers. All immune cells begin as immature stem cells in the bone marrow and grow into specific immune cell types such as B or T lymphocytes and phagocytes. Preprocessing and maturation of the B lymphocytes occur in the liver during mid-fetal life and in the bone marrow during late fetal life and after birth. Maturation of T lymphocytes occurs in the thymus gland. This process is called generation of clonal diversity. As a person is challenged by the presence of foreign antigens during life, *specificity* of lymphocytes to a specific antigen emerges—a process termed *clonal selection*.[2,6] On re-exposure to the same antigen, the person will have a more rapid and efficient immune response, indicating a *memory* capacity for the immune system.

Antibody Production

Antibodies are secreted by B lymphocytes. Antibodies or immunoglobulins are formed after a B lymphocyte encounters and engulfs an antigen and then interacts with helper T lymphocytes; the B lymphocyte then begins producing identical copies of a specific antibody. Researchers have identified nine classes of antibodies or immunoglobulins (four forms of IgG, two forms of IgA, and one form each of IgE, IgM, and IgD). Immunoglobulins are found in various concentrations at different sites throughout the body:[2,3,6]

- IgG: Primary immunoglobulin in the blood (80% to 85% of circulating immunoglobulins); may enter tissue spaces; selectively crosses the placenta; coats antigen for more effective and efficient presentation for an immune response; binds to macrophages and neutrophils for increased phagocytosis
- IgD: Found within the cell membrane of B lymphocytes
- IgE: Responsible for allergy symptoms and increases in the presence of parasitic worms; normally found in trace amounts
- IgA: Protects entrances to the body; found in high concentrations in body fluids (tears, saliva, and secretions of the respiratory and gastrointestinal tracts)
- IgM: Remains in the blood and efficiently kills bacteria; largest of the immunoglobulins; first antibody produced with an initial (primary) immune response

Phagocytes

Phagocytes are found throughout the body and are usually responsible for recognizing and ingesting foreign antigens as they enter the body. Macrophages and neutrophils are the primary phagocytic cells responsible for this first line of defense during an immune response. Macrophages are the primary defensive cells against antigen entry to the body, when awaiting the need for phagocytic activity, large numbers of macrophages are stored in connective tissue, the spleen and liver, and the lining of the gastrointestinal and respiratory tracts. Neutrophils remain circulating in the blood.[2,3,6]

Phagocytosis is the process of ingesting cellular material and involves the ability of phagocytes to be selective in recognizing cells that must be ingested and discarded. Healthy cells of the self tend to be smooth and covered with a smooth protein coat that normally functioning phagocytes tend to ignore. Antibody–antigen complexes have rougher surfaces and are particularly susceptible to phagocytic functioning. Although both neutrophils and macrophages are phagocytes, in an immune response, the macrophages are more effective than neutrophils.[2]

Complement System

The complement system works to enhance the immune response and to help rid the body of antibody–antigen complexes. The complement system is composed of 25 major proteins that circulate in an inactive form in the blood and are engaged in a cascade of interactions when the first protein molecule (C1) encounters an antigen–antibody complex. The complement cascade is also responsible for the dilation and ultimate leaking of fluid from the vascular system, leading to the redness and swelling during the inflammatory process that are associated with an immune response.[2,3,6,8]

Lymphocyte Function in an Immune Response

A general overview of immune system development and maturation leading to an immune response to a foreign antigen is presented in Fig. 22.2.

B Lymphocyte Response

McCance and colleagues[6] differentiate immunoglobulins as all molecules that have specificity to an antigen and an antibody as one particular set of immunoglobulins with specificity against a known antigen. Immunoglobulin, or antibody, is a glycoprotein produced by B lymphocyte plasma cells in response to the presentation of an antigen. Plasma cells are B lymphocytes that have differentiated into plasma cells and memory cells from exposure to an antigen. The major classes of immunoglobulins and areas of focus in an immune response have been previously identified. Immunoglobulins are primarily responsible for the body's response to invading bacteria and viruses and provide the humoral immunity component of an immune response.[2]

T Lymphocyte Response

T lymphocytes undergo differentiation on exposure to a foreign antigen, developing into subtypes of cells that may directly attack the antigen or stimulate the activation of other leukocytes. Cytotoxic T lymphocytes attack and kill antigens directly, with preference for viruses or mutated cells that have become cancerous. This type of innate immunity is termed cellular or cell-mediated immunity.[3,6–8]

Several types of T lymphocytes (or T cells) may be classified into three primary groups: helper T cells, cytotoxic T cells, and suppressor T cells. Helper T cells (CD4 cells) comprise approximately 75% of all T lymphocytes. They help in the functions of the immune system by regulating most of the system's functions via the protein mediators, lymphokines. They help direct and encourage other T cells and also help to activate B lymphocytes. Cytotoxic T cells, also termed *killer cells*, directly kill foreign antigens and may kill cells of the self. Suppressor T cells suppress the function of both helper and cytotoxic T cells in order to prevent hyperimmune responses.[6]

Complement System Response

The 25 primary proteins of the complement system contribute to an immune response by amplifying and increasing the efficiency and efficacy of the other components of the immune system. The complement system also contributes to the inflammatory response. The primary activities resulting from activation of the complement cascade include increasing bacterial susceptibility to phagocytosis, lysing some types of bacteria and foreign antigens, producing chemotactic substances, increasing vascular permeability, and increasing smooth muscle contraction.[9]

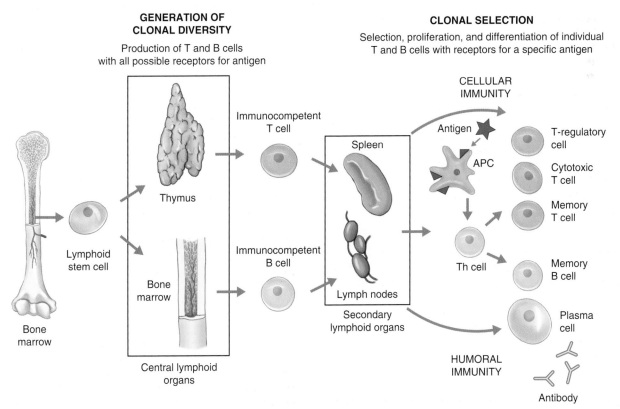

FIGURE 22.2 Overview of Immune Response. (From McCance KL, Huether SE, Brashers VL, et al. [2014]. *Pathophysiology: The biologic basis for disease in adults and children* [7th ed.]. St Louis: Mosby.)

Dendritic Cell Function in an Immune Response

Dendritic cells are potent cells in asserting control from initiation to termination of the immune response. Dendritic cells have a "sentinel" function throughout the body as they look for foreign antigens and alert lymphocytes to the presence of injury or infection. They are also considered *antigen-presenting cells*; they bind to antigens and then process and present them to both B and T lymphocytes in an immune response. They have been found to directly activate helper and killer T cells and present cancer cells to cytotoxic T cells, which respond by killing mutant cells.[10]

Age-Related Normal Differences

Age-related changes within the immune system occur throughout the lifespan. In utero, the immune system is accepting of maternal alloantigens and remains immature at birth. The cells responsible for innate immunity include neutrophils, monocytes, macrophages, and dendritic cells, though these responses are weaker and the cells immature until infancy. Pathways to activate complement are weak because of a significantly lower concentration of required component cells for activation and response. The immune system progressively matures during infancy and is supported by exposure to antigens (e.g., bacteria or virus) and vaccinations during childhood. Pregnancy presents an immune challenge whereby the fetus is able to mount only a minimal response to the mother and the mother's immune system tolerates the fetus without rejecting it, in the absence of externally introduced immunosuppression.

Immunity and immune responses decline with advancing age, predisposing the elderly to higher risk of acute bacterial or viral infections, and a diminished immune response leading to more serious complications. The reduced immune response also accounts for a lessened efficacy of vaccinations. An increased prevalence of autoimmune diseases also results from a concurrent failure to recognize self-antigens in the elderly.

VARIATIONS AND CONTEXT

Problems associated with immunity may occur in individuals across the lifespan with a range of impact from minor symptoms such as a runny nose to life-threatening consequences. Variations may occur as a result of diminished or exaggerated immune functioning or responses to autoimmune situations in which the immune system is attacking the "self."

Suppressed Immune Response

An inadequately functioning immune system leaves the individual immunocompromised. Immunodeficiency is either classified as primary or secondary.

Primary immunodeficiency (PI) is a situation in which the entire immune defense system is inadequate and the individual is missing some, if not all, of the components necessary for a complete immune response. The National Institutes of Health (NIH) has identified more than 200 different types of immunodeficiencies.[11,12] Ten warning signs of PI were also identified by the NIH, with PI suspected if two or more of the signs are evident. The 10 warning signs include the following: four or more new ear infections within 1 year; two or more serious sinus infections within 1 year; two or more months of taking antibiotics with little effect; two or more pneumonias within 1 year; failure of an infant to gain weight or grow normally; recurrent, deep skin, or organ abscesses; persistent thrush in mouth or fungal infection on skin; need for intravenous antibiotics to clear infections; two or more deep-seated infections, including septicemia; and a family history of PI. Common variable immunodeficiency is one of the most prevalent PI diseases and is manifest with a defect in antibody formation following a defect in B lymphocytes that interferes with the ability of the cells to differentiate into plasma (antibody-producing) cells.[13]

Secondary immunodeficiency is a loss of immune functioning (in a person with previously normal immune function) as a result of an illness or treatment. A depressed immune system may be created with medication in order to avoid rejection of transplanted tissue, or it may be induced as a result of treatment for various types of cancer. In the treatment of some types of leukemia, destruction of the bone marrow is necessary before healthy stem cells can be reintroduced allowing for the reestablishment of a healthy immune system. Throughout the treatment process, the immune system is partially destroyed, leaving the individual immunocompromised. Conversely, some cancers, such as multiple myeloma, Hodgkin disease, and non-Hodgkin lymphoma, may directly lead to immune system dysfunction and immunocompromise.

Exaggerated Immune Response

An exaggerated immune response will generally be classified as one of four classes of hypersensitivity disorders: type I, IgE-mediated or atopic ("allergic"); type II, tissue-specific or cytotoxic; type III, immune complex-mediated; and type IV, cell-mediated or delayed hypersensitivity. Hypersensitivity may be defined as "an abnormal condition characterized by an exaggerated response of the immune system to an antigen … hypersensitivity reaction is inappropriate and excessive."[1] The pathology associated with hypersensitivity reactions is summarized in Table 22.1.

Exaggerated immune responses may be localized or they may affect all body systems. A bee sting may cause a localized type I allergic reaction or it may cause a systemic anaphylactic reaction. Systemic anaphylactic reactions caused by a number of foreign antigens are also considered type I hypersensitivity reactions. Type II tissue-specific reactions may lead to myasthenia gravis, hyperacute graft rejection with transplanted

TABLE 22.1 Immunologic Mechanisms of Tissue Destruction

Type	Name	Rate of Development	Class of Antibody Involved	Principal Effector Cells Involved	Complement Participation	Examples of Disorders
I	IgE-mediated reaction	Immediate	IgE	Mast cells	No	Seasonal allergic rhinitis
II	Tissue-specific reaction	Immediate	IgG IgM	Macrophages in tissues	Frequently	Autoimmune thrombocytopenic purpura, Graves disease, autoimmune hemolytic anemia
III	Immune complex–mediated reaction	Immediate	IgG IgM	Neutrophils	Yes	Systemic lupus erythematosus
IV	Cell-mediated reaction	Delayed	None	Lymphocytes, macrophages	No	Contact sensitivity to poison ivy and metals (jewelry)

Ig, Immunoglobulin.
From McCance, K. L., Huether, S. E., Brashers, V. L., et al. (2014). *Pathophysiology: The biologic basis for disease in adults and children* (7th ed.). St Louis: Mosby.

tissues, or autoimmune-based hemolytic anemia. Type III immune complex-mediated responses are the basis for rheumatoid arthritis or systemic lupus erythematosus (SLE). Type IV cell-mediated responses are seen with transplant rejection or poison ivy allergic responses.[6,7,14]

In cases of exaggerated immune response, the individual may be damaged or otherwise harmed by a response that is supposed to be protective or curative as is seen in the presence of anaphylaxis. Autoimmune responses may result in the development of type 1 diabetes mellitus, SLE, or rheumatoid arthritis.

CONSEQUENCES

Consequences of Immunosuppression

A number of serious health problems develop for the immunocompromised individual. Some problems include an increase in the incidence of infection by bacteria and viruses, the development of superinfections such as methicillin-resistant *Staphylococcus aureus* (MRSA) or *Clostridium difficile* (*C. difficile* or *C. diff.*), or the development of treatment-resistant fungal infections secondary to antibiotic treatment for primary bacterial infections.[15,16] In situations in which a suppressed immune response is evident, the individual may not be able to mount a sufficient response to avoid or repair a diseased body organ or system. For example, cancer, particularly in the elderly, has been associated with an immunocompromised state and a diminished ability to recognize and destroy mutant cells.

Consequences of an Exaggerated Immune Response

Multisystem or single system disease may result from an initiating hypersensitivity response. Cardiovascular diseases may emerge as a consequence of autoimmune disorders such as Graves disease or SLE. Renal failure may result from chronic glomerulonephritis or polycystic kidney disease. HIV disease weakens the immune system, and a variety of opportunistic diseases and infections will ultimately result.

Autoimmune disorders occur when the immune system attacks and destroys healthy cells following a breakdown of what has been termed "self-tolerance." With more than 80 autoimmune disorders already identified, an individual may have more than one autoimmune disorder simultaneously.[17] This type of immune disorder is associated with three potential outcomes: destruction of one or more types of body tissues, abnormal organ growth, or changes in organ function. The degree of destruction and functional loss varies dramatically and depends on the type of immune disorder, age, overall physical and nutritional health, and treatment. Some of the more commonly occurring autoimmune diseases include rheumatoid arthritis, SLE, muscular sclerosis, Graves disease, and diabetes mellitus. Genetic predisposition is an important factor in the development of autoimmune diseases, with manifestation of the disease often associated with some type of environmental trigger, such as bacterial or viral infections, or physiological or environmental stressors.[2,6,18]

RISK FACTORS

People from all age, socioeconomic, and racial/ethnic groups can potentially have impaired immune systems. However, some population groups and individuals are at greater risk than others. Risk factors for suppressed and exaggerated immune function are presented separately in the following sections.

Suppressed Immune Response
Age
In the very young, the immune system is immature with inadequate lymphocyte function—particularly T lymphocyte deficiency. Newborns rely on immune protection from the mother through placental blood transfer and from the high levels of immunoglobulin found in colostrum during breastfeeding. During the next few months, maternal antibodies are slowly destroyed, with the rate of catabolism exceeding the rate of newborn immunoglobulin production. This mild hypogammaglobulinemia contributes to the increased risk of infection in the newborn.

In the elderly, loss of immune effectiveness occurs in part because of the physiological aging and shrinking of the thymus gland, leaving it at approximately 15% of its maximum size by middle age and decreasing the ability of T lymphocytes to mature in the gland over time.[19] Research has also demonstrated that elderly people have fewer T lymphocytes, produce fewer immunoglobulins, experience a delayed and diminished hypersensitivity response, and demonstrate an increase in autoantibodies.[2,6,19] B lymphocyte function is diminished secondary to a decrease in circulating memory cells that evolve after approximately 60 years of age.

Nonimmunized State

Individuals who are not immunized are susceptible to a number of infections, including rubella, measles, mumps, tetanus, diphtheria, and hepatitis. Many of these diseases can be fatal to the very young, the elderly, or those who are immunocompromised as a result of disease processes or their treatment and other environmental factors.

Environmental Factors

Environmental factors such as poor nutrition, exposure to pollutants (including tobacco smoke) or heavy metals, and other stressors may depress immune functioning.[6,12,20] Unsafe sanitary conditions, food and water contamination, and poor hand hygiene also contribute to disease transmission and are particularly dangerous to the very young or elderly and those with other chronic illnesses. Some of these situations are easily remedied by the individual, whereas others require more of a community-focused attention to solving the problem.

Chronic Illnesses

Depressed immune function can develop as a result of chronic illness or treatments for medical conditions. In addition to primary immunodeficiency conditions that directly impair the immune system (e.g., HIV), many chronic conditions (e.g., diabetes mellitus, chronic obstructive pulmonary disease, malnutrition, and cancer) also lead to reductions in immune function as a secondary consequence to the disease or its treatment.

Medical Treatments

Medical treatments may be implemented specifically to inhibit a normal immune response or an autoimmune response, or they may lead to immunosuppression as a consequence of the treatment. For instance, in the case of tissue graft or tissue/organ transplantation, medication is administered to induce a state of immunosuppression so that the body does not mount a normal immune response and cause rejection of the graft tissue. Conversely, pharmacologic treatments for autoimmune hypersensitivity reactions, such as SLE or multiple sclerosis, include treatment regimens that inhibit the immune response. Immunosuppression is a common side effect of cancer treatment. The stress associated with many medical treatments, both psychological and physical, places an added burden on the immune system and may leave the individual vulnerable to illness.

Genetics

An individual's genetic base, overall health, and history of exposure to potential antigens influence immune functioning.[21] A number of genetic diseases may lead to depressed or absent functioning of parts or all of the immune system. As a group, complement deficiencies are comparatively rare, and their prevalence varies, depending on the specific deficiency and the age of a person. Another immune deficiency, common variable immunodeficiency, is one of the most prevalent primary immunodeficiency diseases, with an estimated 1 case per 25,000 to 50,000 depending on the population of interest.[22,23] Allergies to food or environmental stimuli and type 1 diabetes mellitus are also considered a type of immune dysfunction. The incidence of those diseases is widespread in both children and adults of all ethnic origins, with variations depending on geography and ethnicity.

High-Risk Behaviors and Substance Abuse

A number of high-risk behaviors have been associated with the development of a dysfunctional immune system. Transmission of HIV and hepatitis virus may be directly related to high-risk sexual behaviors and sharing needles among intravenous drug abusers. According to Boule and colleagues,[24] excessive alcohol consumption leads to compromised immunity (innate and acquired), dysfunction of components of the immune system, and increased risk of infection.

Pregnancy

Immunity is influenced by pregnancy, creating a situation in which the mother is immunocompromised. The developing fetus exists in what has been termed a "privileged" immunity environment in which fetal antigens from the father do not stimulate an immune response and rejection of the graft created by the fetus–placenta connection and the mother. The placental barrier between mother and fetus is open to communication between mother and fetal cells. It has been found that fetal cells may remain in the mother's tissues for long periods of time, creating a situation termed *microchimerism* or a mixing of cells of different origins. A microchimerism may also be created in the fetus, and research is investigating the role that this may play in the development of autoimmune diseases.[6]

Exaggerated Immune Response
Gender, Race, and Ethnicity

Some hypersensitivity disorders have higher incidence and prevalence by virtue of gender, race, or ethnicity. For example, SLE occurs more often in women than in men by a 10:1 ratio, African Americans are eight times more likely than white non-Hispanics to contract the disease, and Asians have a higher incidence and more severe organ damage than individuals of European heritage.[6]

Genetics

Genetics is often responsible for the formation of an exaggerated immune response. An exaggerated reaction may be minor and serve more as an annoyance, such as seen with some environmental or food allergies, or may lead to destruction of normal tissue, loss of organ function, or death. In some cases, the genetic basis for the development of hyperimmune disorders requires that the gene or chromosome be carried by both parents (or sometimes only one parent), and some disorders require an environmental or physiologic trigger (e.g., hormonal changes seen in puberty) in addition to the predisposition to a hyperimmune disorder created by genetics.

Environmental or Medication Exposure

Environmental or medication exposure to a foreign antigen may elicit an exaggerated immune response. Foods, drugs, pollens, dust, molds, bee venom, vaccines, or serum may all evoke hypersensitivity reactions (types I, II, or III), and some may evoke more than one type of hypersensitivity.[2,5,6] In general, these hypersensitivity reactions do not occur on first exposure to the foreign antigen but, rather, on reexposure.

However, genetic predisposition, exposure by the mother during fetal development, or other contributing factors may cause an exaggerated response on first presentation of the pathogen. In many cases, individuals who manifest an allergic type of exaggerated response to one type of pathogen (e.g., pollen) will demonstrate a similar reaction to other antigens in the same or similar class.

Medication exposure may act similarly to environmental exposure in inducing an exaggerated response. Some individuals report an allergic type of exaggerated reaction on first exposure to some medications (e.g., penicillin). In some individuals, a previously expressed exaggerated immune response may be amplified further in the presence of specific medications. For example, cancer treatment that includes the use of monoclonal antibodies has triggered exaggerated hypersensitivity reactions in some patients even though a milder reaction to the same pathogen was experienced in the past.

ASSESSMENT

Assessment of immune response and dysfunction begins with a thorough health history and physical examination. Basic laboratory and diagnostic testing procedures are followed with more specific tests depending on the individual's history and current presenting symptoms. Genetic testing may also be important to confirm a diagnosis, to determine appropriate counseling concerning the person's prognosis, or to make reproduction recommendations.

History

The health history is useful to determine a patient's risk for an altered immune response and to determine if symptoms are described that link to problems with the immune system. The history should include current and past medical problems including treatments, especially the presence of conditions associated with immune problems (see Box 22.1 later in the chapter). The patient should be asked about allergies to substances, including the response that occurs with exposure. Also included are current medications taken by the patient and the vaccination history. Ask questions related to general health status including energy levels, nutritional status including normal dietary intake, and recent changes in weight and wound healing. Associated health topics of concern include health problems during pregnancy, conditions causing significant or consistent psychological stress, exposure to environmental agents or stressors, physical trauma, and a history of exposure to microorganisms that may cause immunosuppression (Epstein-Barr virus, HIV, cytomegalovirus, herpes simplex virus type 6, hepatitis B virus, etc.).

Examination Findings

Examination findings indicative of immune status are presented from the perspective of normal (optimal) immune functioning, suppressed immune functioning, and exaggerated immune functioning.

Clinical Findings Indicative of Optimal Immune Functioning

Clinical indicators of optimal immune functioning reveal an individual who generally appears well and is well nourished. Vital signs are within normal parameters for age; lymph nodes are soft, movable, and nontender (although lymph nodes are often not palpable among older adults). Wounds that may be present are healing within a time frame normal for the type of wound.

Clinical Findings: Suppressed Immune Function

Clinical indicators of suppressed immune functioning may be mild or widespread, and they may be indicative of impending immune system failure. Vital signs may or may not be within normal parameters for age depending on the amount of suppression and the degree of host immunocompromise. The individual may not appear to be well nourished, may present with weight loss or wasting syndrome, and may complain of generalized fatigue or malaise. Impaired wound healing is present, and with advanced immune system suppression, opportunistic infections and diseases may also be present. Inflammation and infection within the central nervous system may cause a change in cognitive functioning or depression. The presence of seizure activity or changes in motor behavior should also be determined. Should the individual present with clinical manifestations indicating significant immunocompromise, a more thorough evaluation related to specific opportunistic infections and diseases would be appropriate.

Clinical Findings: Exaggerated Immune Function

Clinical findings associated with an allergic response may vary from typical mild symptoms (sneezing, watery eyes, and nasal congestion) to severe responses (rashes, swelling, and shock syndrome). Allergic resposnes may produce a minor decrease in quality of life or can be life-threatening.

Clinical manifestations of autoimmune disorders are often vague and less obvious while often affecting multiple organ systems. Symptoms may become more apparent when system function is impaired. For example, cardiovascular symptoms may include pericarditis, congestive heart failure, pulmonary or peripheral edema, and anemia. Renal symptoms will range from no symptoms to glomerulonephritis and from acute to chronic renal failure and end-stage renal disease. Musculoskeletal manifestations can include joint pain or the inability to control movements, including walking, as seen with multiple sclerosis. Some autoimmune disorders have classic findings. For example, a subtle butterfly rash across the nose and cheeks is a common finding associated with SLE.

Diagnostic Tests
Primary Testing

Laboratory and diagnostic testing begins with basic blood tests to determine red blood cell and white blood cell counts with differential evaluation. A fluorescent antinuclear antibody test is standard in the evaluation of potential autoimmune diseases. Screening tests—C-reactive protein (CRP) and erythrocyte sedimentation rate (ESR)—may also be completed. CRP is used to determine inflammation in the body and not to diagnose a specific immune dysfunction. It may also be used to follow the progress of and response to treatment for diseases such as rheumatoid arthritis, SLE, and other autoimmune disorders. An ESR is useful in monitoring inflammatory or cancerous diseases, rheumatoid arthritis and other autoimmune diseases, and tuberculosis.[25]

Allergy Testing

Allergy testing is often important in diagnosis, and it may necessitate a skin test, an allergen-specific immunoglobulin (IgE) blood test, or both. Skin testing helps determine allergens to which the individual is sensitive, and the IgE blood test measures the amount of IgE in the blood—higher levels are associated with a more severe allergic response. Circulating blood levels of IgM and IgA may also be measured.

Advanced or Disease-Specific Testing

More specific blood testing includes cytogenic analysis to detect chromosomal instability, indicative of chromosomal disorders; DNA analysis to detect genetic mutations; and enzyme-linked immunosorbent assay (ELISA) to determine blood levels of IgG subclasses and diagnose IgG deficiency. T lymphocyte levels and proliferative response to antigen introduction testing aids in determining T cell capacity in an immune

response and provides another avenue for information. Rheumatoid factor is a blood test to determine the presence of antibodies against immunoglobulins and is evaluated in combination with other blood tests on the immune system.[25] The ELISA and confirmatory Western blot tests are done to confirm the presence of antibodies to HIV infection. The TORCH antibody panel searches for the presence of antibodies to toxoplasmosis, rubella, cytomegalovirus, and herpes simplex.[25] Complement system testing is done to determine the presence of deficiencies or abnormalities in complement proteins, addressing both quality and activity of the proteins. Deficiencies contribute to increased incidence and severity of infections and autoimmune dysfunction.

Tests of Organ Function

Tests are often performed to aid in assessing specific organ function or to monitor the effectiveness of treatment regimens. These tests include hemoglobin A_{1c} levels in diabetes mellitus management, hepatic function tests, and thyroid screening panels. In most cases, serial laboratory testing is recommended to assess both progression of disease and effectiveness of treatment strategies.

CLINICAL MANAGEMENT

The clinical management of individuals with immunosuppression or hyperimmune conditions varies widely depending on the type of condition, severity, and attribute variables such as age, health status, and underlying medical conditions. Such variables must be considered when making clinical management decisions.

Primary Prevention

The cornerstone of primary prevention for immune system disorders is based on recommended vaccinations across the lifespan. The Centers for Disease Control (CDC) Advisory Committee on Immunization Practices has established recommended vaccination schedules for children, adolescents, and adults, in addition to a "catch-up" schedule.[26,27] Schedules and updates are easily found on the CDC website. Primary prevention also includes reduction of modifiable risk factors noted previously. This includes avoiding high-risk behaviors, minimizing exposure to environmental triggers, eating a proper diet, and engaging in regular exercise. Research has demonstrated that achieving the daily recommended doses of vitamins and minerals contributes to a properly functioning immune system. Ongoing research addressing the role of vitamins A and D in protecting and supporting the immune response may serve a valuable contribution to many medical treatment regimens in addition to their dietary usefulness for health maintenance.

Secondary Prevention (Screening)

Secondary prevention focuses on screenings for the presence or emergence of immune system disorders. There are few screenings specifically directed at immune system dysfunction for the general public. However, some screenings (e.g., HIV screening) are recommended for high-risk groups. Advances in genomic testing may prove useful in developing screening tests for more diseases affecting the immune system in the future.

Collaborative Interventions

Collaborative treatment strategies vary depending on whether the immune dysfunction is one of deficiency or an exaggerated response. Thus interventions may range from supporting an inadequate immune response to diminishing the consequences of an exaggerated response. An overview of selected clinical management strategies for the treatment of immune system diseases or dysfunction is provided in Table 22.2.

TABLE 22.2   Interventions in the Clinical Management of Immune Dysfunction

Management of Clinical Manifestations	Clinical Outcomes
Suppressed Immune Response	
Infection	Normal gastrointestinal transit time
Clinical management of infection and opportunistic diseases is typically an important part of clinical care; interventions and clinical outcomes are discussed in Concept 24, Infection	Resolution of infection
Gastrointestinal dysfunction	Adequate hydration
Pharmacologic treatment of diarrhea, candidiasis, and fluid and electrolyte loss	Adequate nutrition
Skin disorders	Resolution of skin rash
Pharmacologic treatment of skin rash	Restoration of adequate nutrition, body weight, and BMI
Nutrition	
Multiple vitamin and mineral supplements	
Dietary supplements such as Ensure or equivalent	
Evaluation of weight and BMI	
Exaggerated Immune Response	
Anaphylaxis	Adequate ventilation
Support of airway, breathing, and circulation: Subcutaneous epinephrine if type 1 reaction; other bronchodilators; intubation and ventilator support, circulatory volume expanders, and vasopressors to maintain blood pressure and circulating volume	Restoration of blood pressure and pulse to pre-reaction normal levels
Pharmacotherapy: Epinephrine and bronchodilators as described previously	Adequate urine output indicating adequate circulatory volume
Education: Avoiding contact with pathogen initiating anaphylactic response; proper use of an EpiPen for self-administration of epinephrine	Modulation of hypersensitivity responses
Immunosuppression	Management of pain experience
Pharmacotherapy: Corticosteroids, chemotherapeutic agents, NSAIDs, immunomodulators	Maintenance of joint and muscle mobility; self-care for ADLs where possible; restoration or maintenance of adequate levels of physical activity
Pain management	
Pharmacotherapy: NSAIDs, corticosteroids	
Hypothermia or hyperthermia treatments as appropriate	
Maintenance of mobility and physical activity	

ADLs, Activities of daily living; *BMI*, body mass index; *NSAIDs*, nonsteroidal antiinflammatory drugs.

INTERRELATED CONCEPTS

The concept of immunity is closely related to the concepts of **Inflammation** and **Infection**. Overlap among these concepts exists in the areas of pathology, laboratory and diagnostic tests, clinical manifestations, nursing interventions, and clinical outcomes. A discussion of the concepts inflammation and infection is found in Concept 23, Inflammation, and Concept 24, Infection, respectively. **Tissue Integrity** is also closely aligned to immunity because an impairment in tissue integrity will cause an immune response and may lead to both inflammation and infection. As a concept, **Stress and Coping** is linked to Immunity because the stress response may initiate an immune response and may lead to immune dysfunction. Stress may also lead to an alteration in **Glucose Regulation**. Resultant elevated blood glucose levels can exaggerate both inflammation and infection situations. Both inadequate **Nutrition** and extreme or prolonged **Fatigue** are stressors to the body, either of which may cause the individual to become immunocompromised or cause the individual to have an exaggerated preexisting immune response. These concepts were previously discussed as methods by which an individual may become immunocompromised. Interrelationships are shown in Fig. 22.3.

CLINICAL EXEMPLARS

Examples of diseases that may develop with immune system diseases represent cases of B or T lymphocyte dysfunction, hypersensitivity reactions, complement dysfunction, or dysfunction of more than one component. Many examples have been introduced throughout this concept presentation. Box 22.1 provides a brief overview of some of the more common diseases that may lead to immunocompromise.

When considering an immune response, it is most important to remember that the response is a complex interaction between a foreign antigen and a wide variety of differing cells and is also dependent on genetic, environmental, and overall health parameters that are unique to each individual. The presence and progress of immune responses and the development of immunocompromise are unique to each individual and require a thorough review of health history, presenting symptoms, and laboratory and diagnostic data when determining nursing care strategies.

Featured Exemplars
Hodgkin and Non-Hodgkin Lymphoma

Hodgkin and non-Hodgkin lymphoma are types of cancer that originate in the lymphatic system and represent a suppressed immune state. Non-Hodgkin lymphoma is more common than Hodgkin lymphoma, and it may arise from either the B cells or the T cells. Symptoms for both types of lymphoma include swollen lymph nodes in the neck, axilla, or groin; abdominal pain; persistent fatigue; fever and chills; night sweats; and weight loss. Most people diagnosed with non-Hodgkin lymphoma have no obvious risk factors. Some factors that may increase the risk include medications that suppress the immune system, infection with selected bacteria or viruses, pesticides, or older age (>60 years).[28]

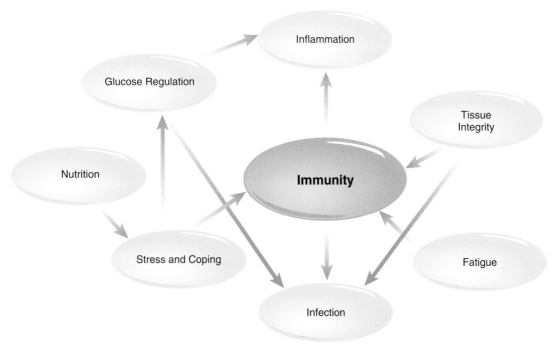

FIGURE 22.3 Immunity and Interrelated Concepts.

BOX 22.1   EXEMPLARS OF INEFFECTIVE IMMUNITY

Suppressed Immune Response
- Classic complement pathway deficiency
- Deficiencies of immunoglobulin A, G, D, or M
- DiGeorge syndrome
- HIV
- Hodgkin and non-Hodgkin lymphoma
- Plasma cell disorders
- Primary immunodeficiency
- Severe combined immunodeficiency

Exaggerated Immune Response
Allergic Responses
- Allergic reaction
- Allergic rhinitis
- Anaphylaxis
- Asthma

Autoimmune Responses
- Autoimmune thrombocytopenic purpura
- Crohn disease
- Diabetes mellitus (type 1, insulin-dependent)
- Glomerulonephritis
- Graves disease
- Multiple sclerosis
- Myasthenia gravis
- Rheumatoid arthritis
- Systemic lupus erythematosus
- Ulcerative colitis

HIV Disease

Infection with the retrovirus, HIV, leads primarily to destruction of CD4[+] T cells, leaving the person with an immune deficiency and a diminishing ability to fight other opportunistic diseases and infections. CH4[+] or "helper" T cells are critical in the overall functioning of the immune response by signaling other cells in the immune system to perform their designated function. HIV-mediated destruction of lymph nodes and lymph organs also contributes to immune system dysfunction. Ultimately, CD4[+] destruction results in the development of AIDS, the third and final stage of HIV disease.[29,30]

Anaphylaxis

Anaphylaxis is an extreme, exaggerated allergic response to foods, medication, stinging insects, and exercise. Anaphylaxis may involve a few or multiple body organs or systems, with symptoms ranging from non-life-threatening (sneezing, hives, itching, and diarrhea) to life-threatening with restriction of breathing and circulation. Symptoms can occur from minutes to hours after exposure to the allergen, with the reaction being one of three types: single reaction occurring immediately after exposure, double reaction with the first reaction minutes to hours after exposure and a second reaction 8 to 72 hours after the first reaction, and a single long-lasting reaction that may last hours to days.[31]

Allergic Rhinitis

Allergic rhinitis, commonly referred to as "hay fever" or "pollen allergy," may also be associated with food allergies, atopic dermatitis (eczema), or asthma. Allergic rhinitis is common in all age groups and in approximately 10% of children younger than age 18 years. The condition is often seasonal, and symptoms typically include inflammation of the nasal passages, resulting in a runny nose, sneezing, congestion of the nose, and itchy, red, watery eyes. Hyposensitization by injection of a diluted form of the antigen may be a necessary part of the treatment regimen.[1,32]

Systemic Lupus Erythematosus

SLE is a chronic, inflammatory autoimmune disease, with no cure, that affects multiple body organs and systems, including joints, skin, kidneys, blood cells, brain, heart, and lungs. The most obvious sign of SLE is a butterfly-shaped facial rash that spreads across the cheeks and bridge of the nose. This rash is present in most, but not all, cases of SLE. As an autoimmune disease with an exaggerated response, cells of the immune system begin to attack cells of the "self," damaging or destroying multiple organs with periods of flare and remission.[33]

Type 1 Diabetes Mellitus

Type 1 diabetes mellitus, another autoimmune disease, typically manifests in young people, although it can occur in adults, presenting with hyperglycemia as a result of the β cells in the pancreas either not producing or not producing enough insulin because the immune system has attacked and destroyed the insulin-producing cells. Heredity plays a major role in determining susceptibility to β cell destruction. The most common presenting symptoms include hyperglycemia, polydipsia, polyuria, and metabolic acidosis. If uncontrolled, chronic high glucose levels lead to damage to the vascular and microvascular system, peripheral neuropathy, kidney damage, and hypertension.[34]

Multiple Sclerosis

Multiple sclerosis is a neurologic disease that ranges from being relatively benign to overwhelmingly disabling as the immune system attacks the nerve-insulating myelin sheaths and disrupts communication between nerves and muscles. The first symptoms generally occur between the ages of 20 and 40 years and include a combination of blurred vision, blindness in one eye, muscle weakness, balance or coordination impairment, paresthesias, numbness or tingling, speech impediments, dizziness, or hearing loss. Over time, many people experience cognitive impairment, difficulty with concentration or memory, poor judgment, and depression. Although there is no cure, some medications are demonstrating promise in reducing the number of exacerbations and slowing the progression of physical disability.[35]

CASE STUDY

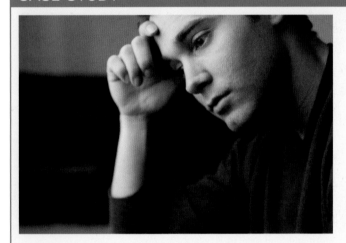

Case Presentation

Jonathan Eckert is a 22-year-old white male who has been involved in a number of high-risk sexual behaviors. Three months ago, he developed a 4-day course of fever and chills, malaise, lethargy, night sweats, diarrhea, and anorexia. He believed he had acquired the flu (influenza) and self-medicated with acetaminophen, vitamin C, and increased fluid intake. He became increasingly concerned about his health because he had friends who were infected with HIV, so he contacted his primary care provider to obtain a blood screening test for HIV and hepatitis B and C.

Jonathan's screening test for hepatitis B and C was negative, and the HIV screening tests—ELISA and confirmatory Western blot—both returned positive for HIV infection. Additional laboratory testing was done to assess his red blood cell count, white blood cell count with differential, and CD4 and CD8 lymphocyte counts (lymphocyte immunophenotyping). All of his blood tests were within the normal range. Serologic testing for hepatitis B and C was negative, skin testing for tuberculosis returned negative, and a chest x-ray was unremarkable.

Jonathan was given information on the need to maintain a healthy lifestyle with appropriate nutrition; physical activity; stress management; avoidance of cigarettes and other forms of tobacco; maintenance of appropriate vaccinations, including an annual influenza vaccination; and adherence to safer sexual practices to avoid reinfection with a potentially more virulent strain of the virus and transmission of the virus to others. He was given information on community support groups and a referral to a care provider specializing in HIV/AIDS care. Research on the advantages of early treatment, following HIV exposure and seroconversion, were discussed with him. Although he demonstrated an understanding of the information, ongoing health education is recommended.

Case Analysis Questions

1. How would you describe Johnathan's current infection status?
2. Consider the immune response. How has John's immune system responded to the pathogen invasion?

From Fuse/Thinkstock.

ACCESS EXEMPLAR LINKS IN YOUR GIDDENS EBOOK

REFERENCES

1. Mosby. (2016). *Mosby's dictionary of medicine, nursing, and health professions* (10th ed.). St Louis: Mosby.
2. Hall, J. E. (2016). *Guyton and Hall Textbook of medical physiology* (13th ed.). Philadelphia: Elsevier.
3. National Institutes of Health: *Immune system*, 2014. Retrieved from https://www.niaid.nih.gov/research/immunesystem.
4. Centers for Disease Control and Prevention: *Immunity types*, 2017. Retrieved from http://www.cdc.gov/vaccines/vac-gen/immunity-types.htm.
5. National Institutes of Health, & National, U. S. *Library of Medicine: Immune response*, 2018. Retrieved from https://medlineplus.gov/ency/article/000821.htm.
6. McCance, K. L., Huether, S. E., Brashers, V., et al. (Eds.), (2014). *Pathophysiology: The biologic basis of disease in adults and children* (7th ed.). St. Louis: Elsevier Mosby.
7. Gasteiger, G., Ataide, M., & Kastenmuller, W. (2016). Lymph node – an organ for T-cell activation and pathogen defense. *Immunological Reviews*, 271(1), 200–220.
8. Dimeloe, S., Burgener, A. V., Grahlert, J., & Hess, C. (2016). T-cell metabolism governing activation, proliferation and differentiation; a modular view. *Immunology*, 150(1), 35–44.

9. Lubbers, R., van Essen, M. F., van Kooten, C., & Trouw, L. A. (2017). Production of complement components by cells of the immune system. *Clinical and Experimental Immunology, 188*(2), 183–194.

10. Steinman, R.: *Introduction to dendritic cells*, 2015. Retrieved from http://lab.rockefeller.edu/steinman.

11. National Institutes of Health, U.S. National Library of Medicine: *Immune system and disorders*, 2018. Retrieved from https://medlineplus.gov/immunesystemanddisorders.html.

12. National Institutes of Health, U.S. National Library of Medicine: *Immunodeficiency disorders*, 2018. Retrieved from https://medlineplus.gov/ency/article/000818.

13. Genetic & Rare Diseases Information Center, National Center for Advancing Translational Sciences, National Institutes of Health: *Common variable immunodeficiency*, 2016. Retrieved from https://rarediseases.info.nih.gov/diseases/6140/common-variable-immunodeficiency.

14. Marcalino de Silva, E. Z., Jamur, M. C., & Oliver, C. (2014). Mast cell function, a new version of an old cell, 2014. *Journal of Histochem Cytochem, 62*(10), 698–738.

15. Mayo Clinic: *MRSA Infection*, 2015. Retrieved from https://www.mayoclinic.org/diseases-conditions/mrsa/symptoms-causes/syc-20375336.

16. Schaffler, H., & Breitruck, A. (2018). Clostridium difficile – from colonization to infection. *Frontiers in Microbiology, 9*, doi:10.3389/fmicb.2018.00646. Article 646.

17. National Library of Medicine, National Institutes of Health: *Autoimmune Diseases*, 2018. Retrieved from https://medlineplus.gov/autoimmunediseases.html.

18. National Institutes of Health, National Institute of Allergy and Infectious Diseases: *Immune system: Immune tolerance*, 2014. Retrieved from http://www.niaid.nih.gov/research/immune-tolerance.

19. National Institutes of Health, U.S. National Library of Medicine: *Aging changes in immunity*, 2018. Retrieved from http://medlineplus.gov/ency/article/004008.htm.

20. U.S. National Library of Medicine, National Institutes of Health: *Aging changes in organs, tissues, and cells*, 2018. Retrieved from https://medlineplus.gov/ency/article/004012.htm.

21. van Sluijs, L., Pijlman, G. P., & Kammenga, J. E. (2017). Why do individuals differ in viral susceptibility? A story told by model organisms. *Viruses, 9*(10), 284. doi:10.3390/v9100284.

22. U.S. National Library of Medicine, National Institutes of Health: *Immunodeficiency Disorders*, 2018. Retrieved from https://medlineplus.gov/ency/article/000818.htm.

23. U.S. National Library of Medicine, National Institutes of Health: *Immune System and Disorders*, 2018. Retrieved from https://medlineplus.gov/immunesystemanddisorders.html.

24. Boule, L. A., Ju, C., Agudelo, M., et al. *Summary of the 2016 Alcohol and Immunology Research Interest Group (AIRIG) meeting*, 2018. doi:10.1016/j.alcohol.2017.005. Retrieved from https://reader.elsevier.com/reader/sd/46599CE56264CDF96327493F1C955C914319FC699F317F6C4DE28D2DF7053C48A4F60A3919A321A9565EAB8C0AD60081.

25. Pagana, K. D., Pagana, T. J., & Pagana, J. (2017). *Mosby's diagnostic and laboratory test reference* (13th ed.). St Louis: Mosby.

26. Centers for Disease Control and Prevention: *Children and Adolescents Immunization and Catch-up Schedule*, 2018. Retrieved from https://www.cdc.gov/vaccines/schedules/downloads/child/0-18yrs-child-combined-schedule.pdf.

27. Centers for Disease Control and Prevention: *Adult Immunization Schedule*, 2018. Retrieved from https://www.cdc.gov/vaccines/schedules/downloads/adult/adult-combined-schedule.pdf.

28. U.S. National Library of Medicine, National Institutes of Health: *Lymphoma*, 2018. Retrieved from https://medlineplus.gov/lymphoma.html#.

29. National Institutes of Health, *National Institute of Allergy and Infectious Diseases: HIV/AIDS*, 2018. Retrieved from https://www.niaid.nih.gov/diseases-conditions/hivaids.

30. Centers for Disease Control and Prevention: *HIV basics*, 2018. Retrieved from https://www.cdc.gov/hiv/basics/index.html.

31. Mayo Clinic: *Anaphylaxis*, 2018. Retrieved from https://www.mayoclinic.org/diseases-conditions/anaphylaxis/symptoms-causes/syc-20351468.

32. American College of Allergy, Asthma, and Immunology: *Allergic rhinitis*, 2018. Retrieved from https://acaai.org/allergies/types/hay-fever-rhinitis.

33. Mayo Clinic: *Lupus*, 2017. Retrieved from https://www.mayoclinic.org/diseases-conditions/lupus/symptoms-causes/syc-20365789.

34. National Institutes of Health, National Institute of Diabetes and Digestive and Kidney Diseases: *Diabetes overview*, 2016. Retrieved from https://www.niddk.nih.gov/health-information/diabetes/overview/all-content.

35. National Institute of Neurological Disorders and Stroke, National Institutes of Health: *Multiple sclerosis: hope through research*, 2017. Retrieved from https://www.ninds.nih.gov/Disorders/Patient-Caregiver-Education/Hope-Through-Research/Multiple-Sclerosis-Hope-Through-Research.

Inflammation

Carolyn E. Sabo

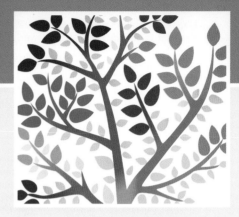

Inflammation is a normal and expected physiologic response to cellular injury. The response is protective in that it provides an opportunity for the body to heal and repair the injury. This biophysical concept is foundational to patient care across the lifespan.

DEFINITION

The term *inflammation* is derived from the Latin *inflammare*—to set on fire. As a concept, *inflammation* is defined as *an immunologic defense against tissue injury, infection, or allergy*. The Centers for Disease Control and Prevention (CDC) has defined inflammation as "the body's reaction to injury, irritation, or infection characterized by redness, swelling, warmth, and/or pain; caused by accumulation of immune cells and substances around the injury or infection."[1] Inflammation is a protective process initiated to minimize or remove the pathologic agent or stimulus triggering the inflammation, and to promote healing. Although inflammation is always present with infection, inflammation may also occur in the absence of infection. Inflammation is the body's physiologic response to injury—not the agent causing the injury as is seen with infection. The inflammatory process is very similar regardless of the cause of cellular injury; however, there is variability in the degree of response depending on the severity and scope of injury and the physiologic capacity of the affected individual.[2–4]

SCOPE

The scope of inflammation ranges from no inflammation to active inflammation. Active inflammation is classified as acute, chronic, or repair/restorative (Fig. 23.1). The scope also reflects an inflammation as localized or systemic.

An initial injury leading to an inflammatory response may be from various sources, including mechanical trauma (e.g., laceration, splinter, and crushing); thermal, electrical, or chemical injury; radiation damage; or biological assault (viral, bacterial, or fungal infections). Acute inflammation is the immediate response to tissue injury and is short in duration (minutes to days). The role of an acute inflammatory response is to eradicate the harmful stimuli from the body and to initiate repair. Inflammation that continues for weeks to years after the initial injury is termed chronic; tissue is repeatedly being destroyed and repaired, thus impairing healing. Localized chronic inflammation results in the formation of a granuloma—an accumulation of macrophages, fibroblasts, and collagen—as seen with untreated *Mycobacterium tuberculosis*. Systemic chronic inflammation may result from many diseases or may be the consequence of disease processes, including autoimmune diseases such as the inflammatory bowel diseases ulcerative colitis (UC) and Crohn disease. Chronic inflammation may be a complication of the inflammatory process, or it may be a consequence of disease, as seen in rheumatoid arthritis (RA).[1–5]

NORMAL PHYSIOLOGIC PROCESS

The functioning of the immune system and the primary activities of an immune response, both acute and chronic, were presented in Concept 22, Immunity. An inflammatory response is often directly linked to the activities of the immune system, demonstrating an overlap and interplay of physiologic processes between the two (immune and inflammatory) providing protection to the host. Also, it has been noted that an inflammatory process has two primary functions directed at a positive outcome for the individual: (1) restitution of normal functioning cells following injury, or (2) fibrous repair when functional cells cannot be restored.

Inflammation is a process involving white blood cells (WBCs) and a number of different chemicals that serve to protect the body against invading pathogens or cellular/tissue trauma. WBCs are attracted to an area of inflammation by chemotaxis. Chemotaxis is a complex process involving more than a dozen different chemicals whose release is initiated by stimuli that may generally be classified into four categories: (1) bacterial or viral exotoxins, (2) degenerative by-products of inflammation, (3) products of complement system activation, and (4) reactive products of plasma clotting in the inflamed area.

Proinflammatory hormones are mediating factors in the inflammatory response and are critical to the effective implementation of the response. There are three major hormone groups: prostaglandins, cytokines, and histamines. In general, the proinflammatory hormones increase blood flow to the injured area, increase vascular membrane permeability, activate various components of an immune response (including the complement system of proteins), attract leukocytes to the area of injury, promote angiogenesis, stimulate growth of connective tissue, and cause fever.[3] Specific actions of selected proinflammatory, mediating hormones are listed in Table 23.1.

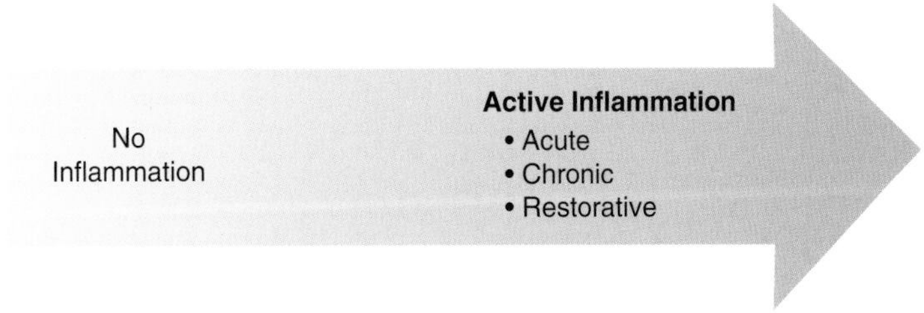

FIGURE 23.1 Scope of Inflammation.

TABLE 23.1 Effects of Proinflammatory Mediators

Proinflammatory Factor	Source	Effect on Inflammatory Response
Prostaglandins	Phospholipids from mast cell and other cell membranes; derived from arachidonic acid in cell membrane	Mediate late stages of acute inflammatory response
Leukotrienes		Increase vasodilation
		Increase vascular permeability
		Active in anaphylactic hypersensitivity reactions
Bradykinins	Plasma protein	Increase vascular permeability
	Kinins	Increase vasodilation
		Responsible for pain production
Complement proteins	Macrophages	Primarily from proteins C3a, C4a, and C5a: initiate chemotaxis of neutrophils and macrophages
	Liver endothelium	Activate mast cells and basophils to release histamine, heparin, and other chemicals
		Result in increased blood flow, increased vascular permeability, and leaking of plasma proteins to extracellular fluid
Histamine	Mast cells	Mediates early acute inflammatory response
Serotonin	Basophils	Increases vasodilation
		Increases vascular permeability
IL-1	Macrophages	Promotes T lymphocyte proliferation and differentiation
	Neutrophils	Promotes release of acute-phase inflammatory proteins
	B lymphocytes	Promotes neutrophil adhesion to endothelial cell walls
	Dendritic cells	Promotes development of fever
	Other antigen-presenting cells	
IL-8	T lymphocytes	Chemotaxic factor for neutrophils
	Monocytes (blood)	Chemotaxic factor for T lymphocytes
	Macrophages (tissue)	
IL-17	Helper T lymphocytes (Th17 cells)	Increases chemotaxis of neutrophils
		Increases chemotaxis of macrophages
		Increases epithelial cell chemokine production
Platelet-activating factor	Platelets	Promotes secretion of chemical mediators
		Promotes vasodilation and increased permeability
		Activates neutrophils
Transforming growth factor-β	T lymphocytes	Inhibits T and B lymphocyte activity
	Activated macrophages	Chemotaxic factor for macrophages
	Fibroblasts	Increases macrophage IL-1 production
		Inhibits macrophages
TNF-α	Activated macrocytes	Promotes cellular proliferation
	Selected lymphocytes	Increases phagocytosis
		Increases leukocytosis
		Induces fever
		Promotes neutrophil adhesion to endothelial cell walls
		Toxic to some tumor cells

Adapted from O'Toole, M.T. (editor), (2016). *Mosby: Mosby's dictionary of medicine, nursing, and health professions* (10th ed.). St Louis: Mosby; Hall, J. E. (2016). *Textbook of medical physiology* (13th ed.). Philadelphia: Saunders; and McCance, K. L., Huether, S. E., Brashers, V. L., & Rote, N. S. (Eds.). (2014). *Pathophysiology: The biologic basis for disease in adults and children* (7th ed.). St Louis: Mosby.

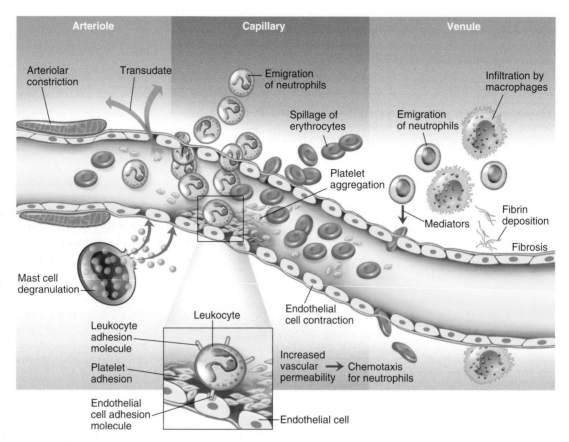

FIGURE 23.2 Acute Inflammation Response. (From McCance, K. L., Huether, S. E., Brashers, V. L., & Rote, N. S. [Eds.]. [2014]. *Pathophysiology: The biologic basis for disease in adults and children* [7th ed.]. St Louis: Mosby.)

Acute Inflammation

The pathologic processes associated with acute inflammation are complex but sequential, as shown in Fig. 23.2. They involve a constant interaction with various components of the immune system and are regulated by feedback systems. The primary steps in an acute inflammatory response have the following sequence:

1. Injury to, or death of, tissue and release of chemical mediators
2. Vasodilation and increased blood flow to the small vessels surrounding the area of injury
3. Swelling and partial retraction or separation of activated endothelial cells
4. Increased vascular permeability and leakage of water, salts, fibrinogen (later becoming fibrin), and other small plasma proteins into the surrounding tissue
5. "Walling off" of the area from surrounding tissues to delay the spread of the pathogen and toxic products from the pathogen
6. Margination and migration of polymorphonucleocytes, monocytes, lymphocytes, and macrophages (later) to the endothelial cell walls and out of the vascular system to the area of injury; margination of endothelial cell walls by neutrophils is possible because of the increased level of cellular adhesiveness created by activation of the endothelial cell.
7. Exudates exiting the vascular system fill spaces left by damaged, necrotic tissue
8. Movement of glucose and oxygen to the area in support of removal of necrotic tissue and cellular repair
9. Release of nitric oxide and prostacyclin, endothelin, thromboxane A_2, angiotensin II, growth factor, and chemokines from activated endothelial cells

Neutrophils are of significant importance in an acute inflammatory response. Movement of neutrophils is mediated by several chemotaxic factors that arise from the area of tissue damage. The chemotaxic factors bind to the surface of the neutrophils and cause them to release additional factors, resulting in pathogen breakdown from lysosomal cytoplasmic enzymes. The neutrophils are also directly involved in phagocytosis after they bind to antibodies already connected to the antigen. In preparation for the neutrophil, opsonization has occurred with either the antibody or the complement proteins; then neutrophil lysosomal granules can be released to begin phagocytosis. Note that during the process of phagocytosis, reactive oxygen species (ROS) are created by the neutrophils and macrophages. ROS bind with the lysosomes to help kill the invading pathogen.[6–8]

Neutrophil blood counts increase four- to fivefold within a few hours after the onset of acute severe inflammation, making more neutrophils available to continue the inflammatory response. Neutrophils comprise the primary WBC component of exudate created during an acute inflammatory response to bacterial invasion. Band cells, or immature neutrophils, also may be present in the blood to achieve the increased numbers of neutrophils required of the severe response. The bone marrow will also significantly increase production of both granulocytes and monocytes; however, it takes 3 or 4 days before these cells are mature and ready to leave the bone marrow.[2]

Lymphocytes are most prominent in inflammatory responses to viral antigens. They are also important in combination with monocytes and macrophages in situations of chronic inflammation. Eosinophils are most evident in inflammatory responses to parasitic infections and in association with allergic hypersensitivity immune reactions. Mast cells and basophils release histamine, which contributes to the increased vascular permeability seen in an inflammatory response.[2,9]

An acute inflammatory response may last minutes to days, with the majority of activity taking place in the first 12 to 24 hours after tissue injury. The response may be localized or systemic. Localized inflammatory responses begin when damaged tissue or invading organisms activate the immune system. Complement system proteins and cytokines begin a cascading sequence of events that lead to the classic signs and symptoms associated with the immune response. Autoimmune reactions may cause systemic activation of the inflammatory response with the body being attacked by its own cells. In most people, the inflammatory response may last up to 5 days while invading pathogens are destroyed, phagocytosis of antigens and necrotic tissue occurs, and fibroblasts begin the process of tissue healing.

Chronic Inflammation

Macrophages are critical in a chronic inflammatory response. They release tissue thromboplastin to facilitate hemostasis and to promote fibroblast activity. They are instrumental in removing necrotic tissue and foreign pathogen material from the area of injury (debridement), allowing for repair and healing. Macrophages and lymphocytes will comprise the majority of the WBCs found in the exudate during a chronic inflammatory response. Unfortunately, when inflammation is chronic, healing processes may be interrupted by reinjury or renewed inflammation and immune system activity with the inflammatory cycle being reactivated.

Chronic inflammation may also be subclinical, manifesting with elevated levels of nonspecific blood markers such as C-reactive protein (CRP) or an increased erythrocyte sedimentation rate (ESR) with no obvious overt symptoms. A WBC scan, or inflammatory scan, may be required to identify areas of inflammation. Low-grade chronic inflammation has been associated with systemic manifestations including body aches and pains, frequent infections, diarrhea, dry eyes, and shortness of breath.[9–11]

Regardless of whether the inflammation is acute or chronic, a number of systemic manifestations result. Localized symptoms depend on the degree of injury and the resistance of the host to injury. Systemic responses include neutrophilia, fever, malaise, loss of appetite, and muscle catabolism. The liver will respond by releasing a number of proteins, called acute phase proteins, that include complement system proteins, clotting factors, and protease inhibitors. The acute phase proteins also stimulate an increase in the level of fibrinogen, promoting hemostasis. CRP and serum amyloid are also released by the liver. CRP assists in opsonization of the foreign pathogen to facilitate phagocytosis.[2,3,7]

Age-Related Differences

A number of age-related differences in an inflammatory response occur similarly to those seen in the discussion of Concept 22, Immunity. Neonates typically have reduced inflammatory responses to bacteria or virus. This is due to a combination of decreased numbers of granulocytes, particularly neutrophils, and monocytes with an associated decreased chemotaxic ability of those cells. Neonates also have substantially depressed complement responses due to insufficient numbers of complement components, predominantly those of the alternate pathway. Like immune responses, this is a transient deficiency with maturation of the inflammatory response evident as the neonate grows to adulthood.[2,3]

The older adult is increasingly more susceptible to impaired inflammation and wound healing. Older adults also tend to have diminished inflammatory responses associated with chronic illnesses, including cardiovascular disease and diabetes mellitus. The aging skin barrier leads to a loss of protection with diminished collagen and subcutaneous fat, while age-related atrophy of capillary beds can lead to tissue hypoxia and slowed wound healing.[2,3]

VARIATIONS AND CONTEXT

Variations in inflammation may occur in individuals across the lifespan, with a range of impact from minor symptoms such as mild redness of the skin to life-threatening consequences. Variations may occur as a result of an acute or a chronic inflammatory response or an autoimmune response. An acute inflammatory response following tissue insult or injury may evolve into a chronic condition, as demonstrated by the development of chronic sinusitis or cirrhosis following an acute inflammatory response to an antigen with continued tissue damage. An acute response may lead to additional tissue injury beyond the initial insult. For example, if inadequately treated, a mildly sprained ankle with tendon or ligament damage may lead to additional tissue injury and cellular death if postinjury swelling is not controlled. Chronic cirrhosis may also be the result of an acute infection with hepatitis C virus. Autoimmune diseases may also manifest with chronic inflammation, as is seen with rheumatoid arthritis.

CONSEQUENCES

Although inflammation has significant physiologic benefit, negative consequences are also possible and may include an overly severe immune response to stimuli resulting in additional tissue damage or an inadequate response leading to infection or chronic inflammation and illness.[2] Spinal cord injuries are an example of one type of trauma in which the inflammatory response may cause significant additional tissue damage if swelling to the damaged region is not controlled. The physiologic response to injury that an inflammatory response provides—in this case with increased blood flow, increased vascular permeability, and the movement of exudate to the damaged tissue—may cause additional compression-based trauma to an already damaged spinal cord.

Excessive stimulation of the inflammatory response and the development of chronic inflammation also may be a consequence of hypersensitivity reactions by the immune system, including allergies and autoimmune diseases such as asthma, rheumatoid arthritis, multiple sclerosis, and systemic lupus erythematosus. In these diseases, an initial immune response and resultant inflammatory response trigger a sequence of cyclic physiologic responses that result in a pathologic disease process.

Systemic pathology may also result from an inflammatory response. Systemic inflammatory response syndrome may emerge as a consequence of a variety of underlying pathologic conditions. A similar pathology presents with minor differences, depending on the initiating etiology. The syndrome follows a 3-stage process as Stage I presents with increased cytokine production, cellular inflammatory response, localized vasodilation, swelling, pain, increased heat production, loss of function, and leukocyte migration to the site. Stage II involves growth factor stimulation and increased macrophages and platelets to the region with the need for proinflammatory mediators to control the response. Stage III produces a systemic reaction and end-organ dysfunction if homeostasis has not been restored.[11] Multisystem organ failure associated with sepsis or septic shock invokes both a strong immune response and a strong inflammatory response. One of the negative consequences of inflammatory activity in the presence of shock is that inflammatory mediators instigate the activation of coagulation inhibitors of fibrinolysis and may cause diffuse endovascular injury, organ dysfunction, or death. Widespread inflammation may also lead to hypovolemia, pleural effusion, respiratory distress, renal failure, and death.[12–14]

Chronic inflammation has been linked to a number of systemic diseases or diseases with systemic consequences if the affected individual is compromised. For example, recent studies have examined the role of inflammation in coronary artery calcification, a critical component in the development of coronary atherosclerosis. Dubin and colleagues presented ongoing results of the Chronic Renal Insufficiency Cohort Study (CRIC) demonstrating relationships among chronic renal disease and inflammation, cardiovascular diseases, and identification of high-risk subgroups. The relationship between chronic renal disease, the proinflammatory state that exists in individuals with this disease, and the need to mediate the inflammatory process to prevent consequential tissue damage.[15] Chronic inflammation is also correlated to chronic diseases including Crohn disease, ulcerative colitis, anemia, neurologic disorders, and renal dysfunction. Similarly, interrelationships among autoimmune diseases such as asthma and diabetes mellitus, cancer, and inflammation are no longer considered theoretical.[2,15–17]

RISK FACTORS

Populations at Risk

Individuals of all ages, genders, ethnic and socioeconomic groups, geographic locations, and prior health histories are susceptible to an acute or chronic inflammatory process. Age plays a role in the development of more severe inflammatory responses. For the very young, an immature immune system may lead to a more severe inflammatory response because the immune system is unable to control a minor pathogen, and infection may be severe. For the elderly, the immune system becomes less able to respond to foreign pathogens, resulting in a stronger inflammatory response than might have been encountered earlier in life. Those who are uninsured or underinsured are at increased risk because they may not have access to sufficient or early healthcare intervention, and a comparatively simple inflammatory response to injury may escalate to one with more severe injury or to a chronic inflammatory state.[2,3,7,9]

Individual Risk Factors

Individual risk factors for an inflammatory response include the presence of autoimmune diseases and allergies, exposure to pathogens with or without resultant infection, and being very young or elderly with a compromised immune system. Genetics plays a role in the emergence of chronic inflammatory processes because many autoimmune diseases have a genetic basis for predisposition and involve an inflammatory response. Certain chronic disease processes, such as atherosclerosis, rheumatoid arthritis, diabetes mellitus, and cancer, may lead to or be the result of chronic inflammation. Research is also underway to evaluate the role of obesity, and vitamin D and magnesium deficiency, in the development of chronic inflammation.[18]

Any process that weakens the immune system increases the potential for what might have been a mild inflammatory response to develop into an acute severe inflammation or chronic inflammatory process.[2,3,7] The absence of effective hand hygiene procedures, the sharing of personal hygiene or grooming material and equipment, poor sanitation, poor nutrition, and living or congregating in tight spaces with large numbers of people increase the risk for infection and accompanying inflammation. Within the healthcare system, inadequate use of standard precautions increases the individual's risk for infection, with a resulting inflammatory response. Environmental factors, such as pollution and smoking, or exposure to repeated trauma, also increase the risk of stimulating an inflammatory response.

TABLE 23.2 Clinical Manifestations of Inflammation	
Local Manifestations	**Systemic Manifestations**
Swelling	Fever
Pain	Leukocytosis
Heat	Increase in plasma proteins
Redness	Malaise
Exudate	Fatigue
Serous exudate	
Fibrinous exudate	
Purulent exudate	
Hemorrhagic exudate	

ASSESSMENT

As with any other pathologic process, the basis and extent of disease must be assessed in order to guide appropriate treatment interventions to either eradicate or manage inflammation, whether acute or chronic. Assessment of an individual for the presence of inflammation includes asking appropriate questions to elicit a history, and conducting a physical examination. In addition, laboratory and diagnostic testing aids in the diagnosis. Common clinical findings associated with inflammation are featured in Table 23.2.

History

The history should be focused on determining the nature of the inflammatory trigger (e.g., recent injury and exposure to allergens and infectious agents), the patient's physiologic ability to respond, and determining the risk for an ineffective inflammatory response. The nurse should also inquire about the presence of symptoms commonly associated with inflammation, including swelling, pain, and fatigue. It is also important to determine the duration of the inflammatory process and the treatment measures, if any, that have already been initiated.

Examination Findings

Several classic findings are associated with inflammation. Obvious trauma or minor wounds will likely appear red, be warm to the touch, and be associated with some degree of pain. Swelling may be present with or without an open wound, such as would be seen with a strained or sprained joint. Drainage or pus may be evident from a laceration or other injury in which the skin or mucosal surface has been broken. Any time an infection is evident, some degree of inflammation will also be present. Inflammation associated with an immune response, but without external trauma, will present with some combination of swelling, pain, fever, and decreased or absent functioning of the tissue or organ. Severe inflammation may be associated with shock syndrome or multiorgan failure, significant hyperthermia, seizure, coma, or death.

Diagnostic Tests

Laboratory testing and diagnostic data collection will be determined by the clinical presentation of the individual, the evidence of obvious trauma, the likelihood of exposure to infection-causing pathogens, and the patient's health history particularly related to immune dysfunction or deficiency, or a history of any chronic illnesses.

Blood Tests

Blood testing for WBC count with differential white blood cell count is helpful in determining if neutrophil, lymphocyte, or macrophage cell counts are elevated, indicating bacterial or viral infection, and acute or chronic inflammation. CRP and ESR blood testing are nonspecific tests that will confirm the presence of inflammation but not the location or cause. Various serologic tests for viruses or antibodies against pathogens, such as hepatitis, HIV, Epstein–Barr virus, severe acute respiratory syndrome, herpes simplex, syphilis, methicillin-resistant *Staphylococcus aureus*, *Clostridium difficile*, and *Helicobacter pylori*, will be helpful in determining the cause of inflammation and will guide treatment regimens to eradicate or control infection and minimize damage from inflammation.[7]

Radiographic and Other Testing

Computerized (or computed) tomography (CT) scan, magnetic resonance imaging, proton emission tomography scans, or colonoscopy are useful in determining the location and extent of inflammation within the body.

CLINICAL MANAGEMENT

Primary Prevention

Preventing inflammation is directed at reducing risk for injury and infection. Although many injuries occur as a result of accidents with an associated inflammatory response being unavoidable, some precautions can be taken. Following appropriate hand hygiene precautions can significantly decrease the risk of pathogen transmission between people, thus reducing the potential for an inflammatory response. Using designated safety equipment when involved in sports or other physical activity can also minimize the incidence of injury. In addition, being aware of food and water safety standards and any issues that may arise from contamination can prevent the transmission of pathogens and avoid potential inflammation associated with an immune response.

Secondary Prevention (Screening)

There are no routine screening procedures for inflammation, making primary prevention strategies critical in reducing the incidence and severity of inflammatory responses.

Collaborative Interventions

The clinical management of inflammation is directed at mediating the inflammatory process to promote repair and healing and to avoid an excessive inflammatory response that may lead to further tissue injury. Some general guidelines to treatment can be made depending on the cause of the inflammation. If inflammation is due to infection, the underlying cause of the infection must be eradicated. If inflammation is due to a hypersensitivity-type immune response (e.g., allergies, asthma, or autoimmune diseases) the management of inflammation must be combined with the management of the immune response and the pathologic consequence of immune dysfunction (e.g., diabetes mellitus, inflammatory bowel syndrome, rheumatoid arthritis, or muscular sclerosis). If inflammation is due to an uncomplicated strain or sprain, the standard treatment regimen of *rest*, *ice*, *compression*, and *elevation* (RICE) combined with nonsteroidal antiinflammatory drugs (NSAIDs) will help with both pain management and moderating the inflammatory response.

Chronic inflammatory responses to disease require careful monitoring to prevent or slow the process of tissue damage that may result in organ failure. Treatment of the underlying cause of the disease, support for ongoing tissue function, and prevention of organ or limb dysfunction or deformity are all important areas of clinical management. Sometimes treatment is aimed at finding alternative routes to achieve physiologic outcomes (e.g., providing insulin to the individual with type 1 diabetes mellitus), replacing endogenous insulin that is no longer being manufactured in the pancreas.

Rest, Ice, Compression, and Elevation

Rest, ice, compression, and elevation (referred to as RICE) represents a set of activities directed at minimizing the swelling associated with a sprain or strain. As described previously, swelling of the tissues immediately surrounding an area of injury is a part of the normal inflammatory response. By minimizing swelling, the injured tissue and surrounding tissue will be protected from additional damage resulting from the swelling itself. The first 24 to 48 hours after the injury is the critical period when RICE measures will be most beneficial. Typically, icing the sprain or strain for 10 minutes at a time every 2 or 3 hours is indicated. However, leaving the ice in place for a longer period of time may cause additional tissue damage. Compression of the damaged area also helps to minimize swelling; the compression wrap must be snug but not so tight as to impede circulation (be alert to fingers or toes becoming cool, tingling, or turning blue in color). Whenever possible, elevation of the injured area above the level of the heart is useful to help minimize swelling.

Immobilization Devices

Immobilization devices, such as splints or slings, contribute to the ability to rest the injured area. Wheelchairs, walkers, or crutches also may be useful in minimizing weight bearing to an injured extremity. If bed rest is indicated, leg exercises or pneumatic compression devices should be considered to protect against thrombus formation in the legs.

Pharmacologic Agents

Pharmacologic intervention options are diverse and depend on the cause of inflammation. Three major goals of treatment include reducing inflammation, managing fever, and providing pain relief. For this reason, many pharmacologic agents prescribed for the treatment of inflammation have one or more of these properties.

Steroidal agents. Glucocorticoids (e.g., prednisone) are steroids used to suppress the immune system and thus suppress an inflammatory response. They are particularly effective in reducing the swelling and pain that accompany inflammation. Steroids such as prednisone are used in a wide range of inflammatory conditions—from swelling secondary to trauma to inflammation found in allergies and autoimmune diseases such as rheumatoid arthritis or systemic lupus erythematosus.[19]

Nonsteroidal antiinflammatory drugs. NSAIDs, such as ibuprofen or naproxen, are important in the management of pain, fever, and inflammation. These medications may be found as over-the-counter products, or they may be combined with narcotics (e.g., hydrocodone or oxycodone) and require a prescription. Significant inflammation may require the use of cyclooxygenase (COX) inhibitors. COX-1 is produced by all tissues and promotes a number of protective functions. COX-2 is produced primarily at sites of tissue injury and acts to mediate inflammation and to sensitize receptors to painful stimuli. It is also found in the brain, where it helps to mediate fever and assist the brain in pain perception. Inhibition of COX-2 is important in treating an inflammatory response because the medication triggers processes that lead to the suppression of inflammation, the control of pain, and the reduction of fever. First-generation NSAIDs inhibited both COX-1 and COX-2, and newer-generation NSAIDs (e.g., celecoxib) are able to inhibit COX-2 only.[19]

Recombinant DNA and monoclonal antibodies. Recombinant DNA and monoclonal antibody development have produced an entirely new line of pharmacologic treatment for inflammation. Interleukin-1 (IL-1) antagonists inactivate IL-1 receptors, whereas tumor necrosis factor-α (TNF-α) inhibitors prevent IL-1 from producing its inflammatory actions but leave the individual more susceptible to infection. Recombinant protein C helps the body dissolve microvascular clots formed during inflammation, and although infliximab (Remicade) is a TNF inhibitor, it has been key to more recent treatments of lymphoma, rheumatoid arthritis, and inflammatory bowel diseases.[19]

Antipyretics. Fever is a common physiologic response to an inflammation. For this reason, antipyretics are often administered for fever management. Antipyretic agents, such as acetaminophen, aspirin, and NSAIDs (described previously), reduce fever by inhibiting cyclooxygenase. These are often administered in combination with opioid analgesic agents.

Analgesics. Nonopioid analgesic agents, such as acetaminophen or aspirin, are the most common type of analgesic used for pain relief caused by inflammation. NSAIDs are also considered analgesics because a reduction in inflammation tends to also relieve associated pain. Opioid analgesic agents are used when inflammatory pain is severe.

Antimicrobials. Antibiotics, antivirals, and other antimicrobials are important in treating the underlying cause of infection leading to inflammation. Antimicrobials encompass a wide variety of medications that are required to treat diseases associated with immune and inflammatory responses. These are discussed further in Concept 24, Infection.

INTERRELATED CONCEPTS

Several concepts featured in this textbook are interrelated to inflammation (Fig. 23.3).

Immunity and Infection are probably the most closely related concepts. Many of the pathophysiologic processes associated with inflammation are also found in both immunity and infection, with pathology from one process overlapping those of the other two processes or with one process triggering another. This can be seen with hypersensitivity reactions of the immune system triggering an inflammatory response, or infection stimulating an inflammatory response.

Tissue Integrity is at risk in an inflammatory response, as is impaired mobility and pain associated with an initial injury and with the consequences (swelling) of an inflammatory response. Thermoregulation may be influenced by inflammation depending on the severity of the response to tissue injury. Gas Exchange may be insufficient in the presence of inflammation-induced pleural effusion. Hemostasis alterations in the form of microvascular clotting leads to impaired Perfusion as a consequence of inflammation, particularly if the condition is chronic.

Both Fatigue and Stress and Coping are often associated with injury and recovery from an acute inflammatory response or may be prolonged during the chronic inflammation from an autoimmune hypersensitivity reaction.

CLINICAL EXEMPLARS

Exemplars for the concept of inflammation are presented in Box 23.1. These examples are divided into conditions that represent acute inflammation, chronic inflammation, or inflammation based on the presence of an autoimmune hypersensitivity response. Note that overlap often occurs between acute and chronic inflammation, with chronic inflammatory conditions having acute exacerbations and acute inflammatory responses developing into chronic conditions. Thus, some artificial division among the three types of inflammation is unavoidable. It is beyond the scope of this concept to provide details for each of these exemplars, but some of the most common are briefly described here. Additional information about these exemplars can be easily found in a variety of nursing textbooks.

Featured Exemplars
Bronchitis

Bronchitis is inflammation of the bronchial tubes and may begin as an acute irritation and progress to chronic infection. Bronchitis is commonly seen after the introduction of a cold virus or other respiratory infection. Acute bronchitis typically presents with symptoms such as

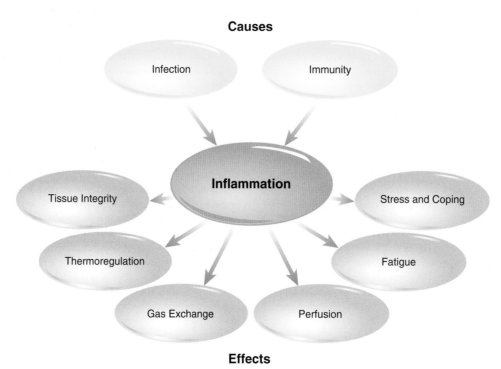

Causes

Infection   Immunity

Inflammation

Tissue Integrity   Stress and Coping

Thermoregulation   Fatigue

Gas Exchange   Perfusion

Effects

FIGURE 23.3 Inflammation and Interrelated Concepts.

BOX 23.1 EXEMPLARS OF INFLAMMATION

Acute Inflammation
- Acute infection (bacterial, viral, fungal, parasitic)
- Bronchitis
- Burn
- Bursitis
- Foreign body injury
- Insect bite or sting
- Joint sprain or strain
- Nephritis
- Rheumatic fever
- Tendonitis
- Traumatic injury

Chronic Inflammation
- Atherosclerosis
- Chronic infection
- Chronic obstructive pulmonary disease
- Cirrhosis
- Diverticulitis
- Fibromyalgia
- Gingivitis
- Inflammatory bowel disease
- Myocarditis
- Osteoarthritis
- Psoriasis
- Vasculitis

Autoimmune-Based Inflammation
- Asthma
- Crohn disease
- Goodpasture syndrome
- Graves disease
- Multiple sclerosis
- Myasthenia gravis
- Rheumatoid arthritis
- Systemic lupus erythematosus

ACCESS EXEMPLAR LINKS IN YOUR GIDDENS EBOOK

and include nausea or vomiting, abdominal cramps and diarrhea, or a low-grade fever. The course of the inflammation is usually self-limiting, but it may require more aggressive treatment if symptoms persist for more than 2 days. Dehydration is a common manifestation and can be life-threatening if undetected and untreated.[20,21]

Atherosclerosis

Atherosclerosis is a disease characterized by the buildup of plaque on the intimal layer of arteries and represents a chronic inflammatory process. Plaque is made up of fat, cholesterol, calcium, and other substances that harden and narrow the lumen of arteries over time. Arterosclerosis can affect every artery in the body, including those in the heart, peripheral arteries, brain, and kidneys. Atherosclerosis of the coronary arteries leads to coronary artery disease and myocardial infarction, whereas atherosclerosis of the carotid arteries may lead to stroke. Chronic kidney disease and end-stage renal disease or kidney failure are consequences of atherosclerosis of the renal arteries.[7,22]

Cirrhosis

Cirrhosis is a disease state that results from the destruction of healthy liver tissue and replacement with scar tissue. Chronic cirrhosis may evolve from an acute injury or be the result of chronic liver tissue insult. The scar tissue may block blood flow through the liver or cause the transformation of sufficient healthy functioning cells to scarred cells and nonfunctional tissue, and the liver is not able to sufficiently provide the metabolic support to maintain homeostasis. Cirrhosis results in disturbance of many systems because of the diminished ability of the liver to produce clotting factors, immune factors, and bile, and to remove the waste products of metabolism and medications.[7,23]

Asthma

Asthma represents an autoimmune-based inflammation. The National Asthma Education and Prevention Program Expert Panel defined asthma as "a common chronic disorder of the airways that is complex and characterized by variable and recurring symptoms, airflow obstruction, bronchial hyperresponsiveness, and an underlying inflammation. The interaction of these features determines the clinical manifestations and severity of asthma."[24] Airway inflammation leads to airway obstruction and the development of bronchoconstriction, airway hyperresponsiveness to stimuli, and airway edema with hypersecretion of mucus. Asthma may be caused by innate immunity, genetics, exposure to tobacco smoke, or environmental factors (e.g., airborne antigens or viral infections).[25]

Rheumatoid Arthritis

Rheumatoid arthritis (RA) is an autoimmune disease that causes inflammation in the joints and is characterized by periods of "flares" and "remission." Although the exact cause of RA is unclear, research has demonstrated links among genetics, the environment, and some hormones. There is no cure for RA, but it has been documented to flare and then go into complete remission with no long-term sequelae. Treatment involves pain management, control of joint swelling, and retention of joint function. Recent research is directed at immunotherapies to restore immune tolerance of the "self" and the critical immunopathogenic pathways seen in RA.[26]

cough, increased production of thick mucus that may be clear or discolored, shortness of breath, fever and chills, and chest tightness on inspiration. The cough associated with acute bronchitis may persist for days or weeks after resolution of the initial infection. Should chronic bronchitis develop over time, it would be considered a chronic obstructive pulmonary disease.[6,7]

Gastroenteritis

Gastroenteritis is inflammation of the stomach and intestines. It may be caused by a variety of viruses, contaminated water or food, or as a side effect of medications; in infants it may present with the introduction of allergens within new foods. Symptoms generally last for a few days

CASE STUDY

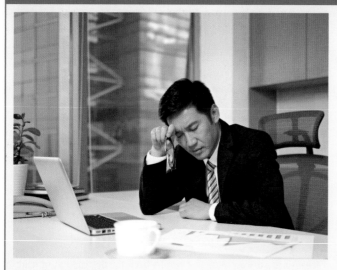

Case Presentation

Chris Shomni is a 40-year-old male in a stressful, professional position. He was recently diagnosed with ulcerative colitis (UC) after developing abdominal pain and cramping and bloody diarrhea intermittently (although more frequently recently) during the past several weeks. He has lost 10 pounds in the past 4 weeks and has complained of nausea and fatigue. A colonoscopy demonstrated the presence of significant inflammation and ulcers in the colon and rectum. No strictures, perforations, or areas of paralysis of the colon were noted. Biopsy and further evaluation of the colonoscopy confirmed the presence of UC and ruled out Crohn disease. He has no family history of inflammatory bowel disease. Assessment of the skin revealed the presence of erythema nodosum lesions, which are characteristic of UC. Laboratory testing further identified the presence of lowered red blood cell (RBC) and hemoglobin levels, elevated platelet count, and normal white blood cell count. Serum total protein and albumin levels were low.

From imtmphoto/iStock/Thinkstock.

Diagnosis of UC was made, with complications of anemia and hypoalbuminemia. Mr. Shomni was also demonstrating impaired nutrition as a result of impaired nutrient absorption, and diarrhea and anemia secondary to inflammation of the bowel and loss of fluid, protein, and RBCs. Pain from inflammation and abdominal cramping was present but not significant, and he was at risk for fluid volume deficiency. It was determined that the bowel needed to be rested, that bowel resection surgery was not indicated at this time, and that inflammation must be reduced. Mr. Shomni was admitted to the hospital to begin treatment for inflammation, rest the bowel, reduce his diarrhea, and balance his fluid and electrolyte levels.

The overall goals of treatment for Mr. Shomni included controlling colon inflammation, ensuring adequate nutrition and hydration, and relieving pain and diarrhea. With control of inflammation and diarrhea, it is expected that the anemia and hypoalbuminemia will resolve. Pharmacologic intervention included aminosalicylates containing 5-aminosalicylic acid (5-ASA) to control inflammation. Corticosteroids to reduce inflammation will only be used if Mr. Shomni has an exacerbation of his UC and his disease becomes severe and nonresponsive to 5-ASA. If Mr. Shomni does not respond sufficiently to the 5-ASA or corticosteroids, then immunomodulators (e.g., 6-mercaptopurine) or monoclonal antibodies (e.g., infliximab) may have to be introduced in the future. With chronic inflammatory bowel disease, at some point in his life Mr. Shomni may need to have surgery for a colostomy or ileostomy because tissue damage to the intestinal tract may be so severe that it no longer functions.

Mr. Shomni was discharged after 3 days with new medications and instructions to avoid enteric and time-released medications; an understanding of dietary changes to include specifically prescribed bacterial probiotic cultures; strategies for stress reduction; and actions to be taken should signs and symptoms of an inflamed or infected bowel be evident.

Case Analysis Questions

1. Consider Fig. 23.1. Where does this case fit on the scope of inflammation?
2. What are the primary treatment options represented in this case?

 ACCESS EXEMPLAR LINKS IN YOUR GIDDENS EBOOK

REFERENCES

1. Centers for Disease Control and Prevention (2014). *Inflammation.* Retrieved from https://www2a.cdc.gov/nip/isd/ycts/mod1/scripts/glossary.asp?item=inflammation.
2. Hall, J. E. (2016). *Textbook of medical physiology* (13rd ed.). Philadelphia: Elsevier.
3. McCance, K. L., Huether, S. E., Brashers, V. L., et al. (Eds.), (2014). *Pathophysiology: The biological basis for disease in adults and children* (7th ed.). St Louis: Mosby.
4. Kimball's Biology Pages (2013). *Inflammation.* Retrieved from http://www.biology-pages.info/I/Inflammation.html.
5. Mosby. (2016). *Mosby's dictionary of medicine, nursing, and health professions* (10th ed.). St Louis: Mosby.
6. Kimball's Biology Pages (2015). *ROS.* Retrieved from http://www.biology-pages.info/R/ROS.html.
7. Pagana, K. D., Pagana, T. J., & Pagana, J. (2017). *Mosby's diagnostic and laboratory test reference* (13rd ed.). St Louis: Mosby.
8. Humpath.com (n.d.). *Acute inflammation.* Retrieved from http://www.humpath.com/spip.php?article3575.
9. Humpath.com (n.d.). *Chronic inflammation.* Retrieved from http://www.humpath.com/spip.php?article3576.
10. American Heart Association (2017). *Inflammation and heart disease.* Retrieved from http://www.heart.org/HEARTORG/Conditions/Inflammation-and-Heart-Disease_UCM_432150_Article.jsp#.WymbM1VKipo.
11. Kaplan, L. J. (2018). *Systemic inflammatory response syndrome.* Retrieved from https://emedicine.medscape.com/article/168943-overview.
12. U.S. National Library of Medicine, National Institutes of Health (2016). *Sepsis.* Retrieved from https://medlineplus.gov/sepsis.html.
13. U.S. National Library of Medicine, National Institutes of Health (2017). *Septic shock.* Retrieved from https://medlineplus.gov/ency/article/000668.htm.
14. U.S. National Library of Medicine, National Institutes of Health (2018). *Anemia of chronic disease.* Retrieved from https://medlineplus.gov/ency/article/000565.htm.
15. National Institutes of Health, National Institute of Neurological Disorders and Stroke (2018). *Chronic inflammatory demyelinating polyneuropathy (CIDP).* Retrieved from https://www.ninds.nih.gov/Disorders/All-Disorders/Chronic-Inflammatory-Demyelinating-Polyneuropathy-CIDP-Information-Page.
16. National Institutes of Health, National Institute of Diabetes and Digestive and Kidney Diseases (2017). *Chron's disease.* Retrieved from https://www.niddk.nih.gov/health-information/digestive-diseases/crohns-disease/all-content.
17. Dubin, R. F., Deo, R., Bansal, N., et al. (2017). Associations of conventional echocardiographic measures with incident heart failure and

mortality: The chronic renal insufficiency cohort. *Clinical Journal of the American Society of Nephrology, 12*(1), 60–68.

18. National Institutes of Health, National Cancer Institute (2015). *Chronic inflammation*. Retrieved from https://www.cancer.gov/about-cancer/causes-prevention/risk/chronic-inflammation.

19. Adams, M., Holland, N., & Urban, C. (2017). *Pharmacology for nurses: A pathophysiologic approach* (5th ed.). Boston: Pearson.

20. Mayo Clinic (2018). *Gastritis*. Retrieved from https://www.mayoclinic.org/diseases-conditions/gastritis/symptoms-causes/syc-20355807.

21. Mayo Clinic (2014). *Viral Gastroenteritis*. Retrieved from https://www.mayoclinic.org/diseases-conditions/viral-gastroenteritis/symptoms-causes/syc-20378847.

22. National Institutes of Health, National Heart, Lung, and Blood Institute (n.d.). *Atherosclerosis*. Retrieved from https://www.nhlbi.nih.gov/health-topics/atherosclerosis.

23. National Institutes of Health, National Institute of Diabetes and Digestive and Kidney Diseases (2018). *Cirrhosis*. Retrieved from https://www.niddk.nih.gov/health-information/liver-disease/cirrhosis/all-content.

24. National Heart, Lung, and Blood Institute, National Institutes of Health (2007). *Guidelines for the diagnosis and management of asthma: Expert panel report 3*. Retrieved from https://www.nhlbi.nih.gov/files/docs/guidelines/asthgdln.pdf.

25. National Institutes of Health, National Heart, Lung, and Blood Institute (2012). *Asthma care quick reference: diagnosing and managing asthma*. Retrieved from https://www.nhlbi.nih.gov/sites/default/files/media/docs/asthma_qrg_0_0.pdf.

26. National Institutes of Health, National Institute of Arthritis and Musculoskeletal and Skin Diseases (2017). *Rheumatoid arthritis*. Retrieved from https://www.niams.nih.gov/health-topics/rheumatoid-arthritis.

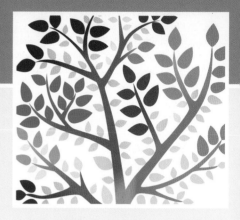

CONCEPT

24

Infection

Carolyn E. Sabo

Microorganisms are found throughout the environment. As a consequence, humans are constantly exposed to a multitude of microorganisms at any moment. Although many microorganisms do not pose a health threat to humans, some cause human disease and are known as pathogens. Our bodies are constantly confronted with pathogens in the forms of bacteria, viruses, parasites, or fungi. These pathogens are routinely found on the skin; the mucous membranes; the linings of the respiratory, gastrointestinal, and urinary tracts; and the mouth and eyes.[1] Typically, an individual's immune system is able to rid the body of pathogens without developing an infection. An infection occurs when a susceptible host is invaded by a pathogen that multiplies and causes disease. This concept presentation provides an overview of the infection concept, including identifying individuals most at risk, recognizing signs and symptoms of infection, and understanding ways to treat or manage an infection.

DEFINITION

For the purposes of this concept presentation, infection is defined as *the invasion and multiplication of microorganisms in body tissues, which may be clinically unapparent or result in local cellular injury due to competitive metabolism, toxins, intracellular replication, or antigen–antibody response.* Several additional terms are important to understand. When an infection occurs, it may be *acute* (resolving in a few days or weeks) or *chronic* (an infection that typically lasts longer than 12 weeks and in some cases is noncurable). Terms are also used to describe the extent of spread in the body. A *localized infection* is limited to a specific body area. *Disseminated* is a term used to describe a spread of infection from an initial site to other areas of the body. The term *systemic* is used to describe an infection that affects the body as a whole or has spread throughout the body. *Sepsis*, a common type of systemic infection, is the presence of pathogens in the blood or other tissues throughout the body.

Two additional terms that are significant to the concept of infection are epidemic and pandemic. The term *epidemic* is used to describe a situation in which there are more cases of an infectious disease than is normal for the population or geographic area. A *pandemic* is a worldwide epidemic of a disease.[2] The global nature of our modern world presents challenges because people with asymptomatic infections can travel from home to virtually anywhere in the world in less than 24 hours. Professional conferences, worldwide sporting events, and gatherings for various types of entertainment can bring large numbers of people together

from all over the world. They are often transported to and from the events in confined airplanes and participate in events in close proximity of others. Exposure to infection can lead to the spread of disease before returning to their homes.

SCOPE

Infections may be categorized in several ways, including on the basis of the multiple variables involved such as mode of transmission, trajectory of illness, and body systems affected. The most common way to categorize and discuss infections is based on the classification of the causative microorganism (Fig. 24.1).

The most common microorganisms initiating an infection are bacteria, viruses, fungi, and parasites or protozoa. Table 24.1 identifies common pathogens for each of these microorganism categories. The type of invading organism influences the immune response. B lymphocytes and T lymphocytes take "leadership" roles depending on whether it is a bacterial or viral invasion, the complement system is always present to enhance the immune response, and dendritic cells will help to modulate the immune response.[1,3]

Bacterial Infections

Bacteria are one-celled organisms without a true nucleus or cellular organelles. They synthesize deoxyribonucleic acid (DNA), ribonucleic acid (RNA), and proteins and can reproduce independently, but they require a host for a suitable environment for multiplication. Bacteria cause cellular injury by releasing toxins that are either exotoxins (enzymes released by gram-positive bacteria into the host) or endotoxins (part of the bacterial cell wall of gram-negative bacteria that can cause damage to the host even if the bacteria are dead). Diseases caused by bacterial invasion depend on the type of bacterial pathogen and the area of the body that is primarily invaded.[4,5]

Viral Infections

A virus is a pathogen with a nucleic acid within a protein shell and requires invasion of a host for replication. An invading virus may immediately cause disease or may remain relatively dormant for years. The virus causes cellular injury by blocking its genetically prescribed protein synthesis processes and using the cell's metabolic processes for the reproduction of the virus. Diseases develop as a result of interference of normal cellular functioning of the host, with destruction of the virus by the immune system also requiring death of the host cell.[4,5]

TABLE 24.1   Common Pathogens

Bacteria	Virus	Fungus	Parasite or Protozoa
Methicillin-resistant *Staphylococcus aureus*	HIV	Tinea pedis	Giardiasis
Clostridium difficile	Hepatitis A, B, C, or E virus	Candidiasis	Trichinosis
Vancomycin-resistant *Enterococci*	Human papillomavirus	Histoplasmosis	Toxoplasmosis
Streptococcus pyogenes (group A)	Ebola virus	Lobomycosis	Malaria
Corynebacterium diphtheria	Hantavirus	Cryptococcosis	Ascariasis
Escherichia coli	SARS-associated coronavirus	Aspergillosis	Pediculosis
Mycobacterium tuberculosis	Respiratory syncytial virus	Coccidioidomycosis	Cryptosporidiosis
Pseudomonas aeruginosa			*Pneumocystis jirovecii* pneumonia
Neisseria gonorrhoeae			
Clostridium tetani			

SARS, Severe acute respiratory syndrome.

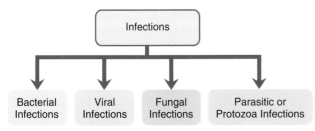

FIGURE 24.1 Scope of Infection.

Fungal Infections

A fungus is a microorganism belonging to the kingdom Fungi, which includes yeasts, molds, and mushrooms. They may grow as single cells (yeasts) or as multicellular filamentous colonies (molds or mushrooms). In an otherwise healthy individual, fungi do not cause disease and are contained by the body's natural flora. Fungi causing disease are termed fungi imperfecti, and in the immunocompromised individual they can result in infections that lead to death.[4,5] Other fungal infections, such as tinea pedis (athlete's foot) or ringworm, may also develop in the individual with a competent immune system.

Protozoa/Parasitic Infections

Protozoa include a subcategory termed parasitic protozoa and, with few exceptions, generally infect individuals with compromised immune responses. They are typically found in dead material in water and soil and are spread by the fecal–oral route by ingesting food or water that is contaminated with the parasitic spores or cysts. Disease may develop in an otherwise healthy individual when the spores invade organs and stimulate an immune response, interfering with normal functioning of the organ system.[4,5]

Other Types of Infections

Sometimes an infection will develop that begins as one type and after an additional pathogen is introduced, a secondary infection occurs. Fungal infections may develop when treatment for a bacterial infection decimates the body's natural flora, or bacterial infections may arise while a debilitated body is treated for a viral infection. When considering bacterial infections, some bacteria are always pathogenic, are never part of the normal flora, but may cause subclinical infection (*Mycobacterium tuberculosis*); some bacteria are part of the normal flora but can become pathogenic (*Escherichia coli*); some are part of the normal

flora but can cause infection if they reach deep tissues, perhaps by surgery (*Staphylococcus epidermidis*); and some bacteria are part of the normal flora and become pathogenic when the individual is immuno-compromised (*Acinetobacter*).[4,5]

An increase in morbidity and mortality secondary to infections has been seen from the emergence of previously unknown infections and the reemergence of infections that were considered controlled in various areas of the world.[4] As these infections manifest, globalization of travel and increased ease of introducing new infections into a geographic area have contributed to changes in morbidity and mortality.

Healthcare-acquired and community-acquired infections have emerged as a significant public health concern. Although methicillin-resistant *Staphylococcus aureus* (MRSA), *Clostridium difficile* (C. diff.), and vancomycin-resistant *Enterococci* (VRE) are debilitating healthcare-acquired diseases, community-acquired MRSA is even more prevalent in some areas.[6] Hospitals and other healthcare centers have been proactive in providing alcohol-based solutions for hand hygiene in both patient care rooms and public areas, but this same attention to infection prevention has not translated nearly as extensively to sporting arenas, areas where children gather for sporting and other group events, restaurants, food stores and other shopping facilities, movie theaters, and other group activity locales.[7-10]

NORMAL PHYSIOLOGICAL PROCESS

Pathogens may be highly virulent and able to cause disease when small numbers invade the body. Other pathogens are weakly virulent and able to cause disease only when an excess number invade the body or the host body is already weakened by disease, malnutrition, excessive fatigue, or other stresses. Opportunistic infections cause disease when the host immune system is severely compromised, such as seen in HIV infection leading to AIDS.

Some diseases are communicable before symptoms are evident in the carrier (herpes simplex virus, varicella–zoster virus, human papillomavirus, influenza, or poliomyelitis), whereas others remain communicable after initial symptoms have subsided (HIV and Epstein–Barr virus). Some infections remain dormant within the host and may resurface as the same or as a different disease; an example is the varicella–zoster virus (VZV), which first presents as chickenpox and later may manifest as shingles.[11] The "iceberg" concept of infectious disease has also emerged. This concept postulates that there are three levels of infection: (1) The vast majority of a population may, at any given time, carry an infection wherein they are asymptomatic or undiagnosed. This group is thought to be the largest section of individuals—the part of

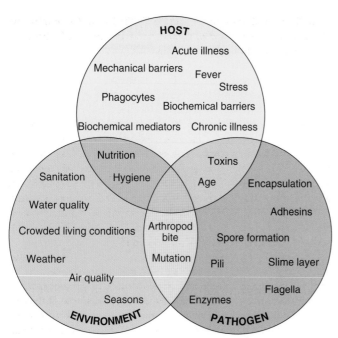

FIGURE 24.2 Process of Infection: Interactions of Host, Pathogens, and the Environment. (Modified from Copstead, L. C., & Banasik, J. L. [2013]. *Pathophysiology* [5th ed.]. St Louis: Saunders.)

the iceberg that is underwater. (2) A smaller population group presents with an infection that manifests as a less severe, symptomatic disease. (3) The smallest group presents with classical, clinical symptoms of disease, and is at the very tip of the iceberg. Epidemiology is important in the study of infection because it is concerned with the manner in which a disease spreads through groups or a population, and with the application of this information to the control of health problems.[5]

Infection Process

An infection involves an interface with a person, the environment, and a pathogen (Fig. 24.2). The process of infection requires the following six elements, all of which must be present for the infection to develop: pathogen, susceptible host, reservoir, portal of exit (from the reservoir), mode of transmission, and portal of entry (to the susceptible host). The reservoir is anywhere the pathogen may live and multiply, either in the body or on objects within the environment contaminated with the organism (e.g., door handles, stagnant water, and healthcare equipment). Portals of exit for a pathogen include urine or feces, saliva, blood, skin, or the gastrointestinal tract. Portals of entry include broken skin, intimate sexual contact, mouth, respiratory tract, gastrointestinal tract, and contaminated food or water. The spread of infection is dependent on a reliable mode of transmission.

Pathogen Invasion

When a pathogen invades the body, a number of immune system responses are initiated to minimize tissue and organ damage. B lymphocytes are activated to differentiate into plasma cells for the production of antibodies and memory cells in preparation for a future re-exposure. T lymphocytes directly kill the invading organism, secreting lymphokines that attract and stimulate the activity of macrophages. Macrophages and monocytes initiate phagocytosis. The complement system is activated to enhance the entire immune response. Some tissue damage will occur as a result of endotoxins released by the pathogen that kill host cells, neurotoxins that affect nerve impulse transmission,

or enterotoxins that damage cells of the gastrointestinal tract. The physiological effect of endotoxins may be mild (fever, chills, weakness, and malaise) or severe (shock syndrome or disseminated intravascular coagulation). Some injuries leading to infection will also manifest with swelling and tenderness at the site, drainage from a wound, or red streaks on the skin leading away from the injury. These manifestations are associated with an inflammatory response.[1]

Infections remain a significant cause of morbidity and mortality as a result of the emergence of antibiotic-resistant bacteria, the development of infections that have become resistant to multiple antibiotics, and the occurrence of both infections that had previously been controlled and newly discovered infections. Some bacteria are able to adapt, with the ability to produce toxins and extracellular enzymes that destroy phagocytic cells, coat part of an antibody to prevent its activation of the complement system, or degrade and suppress an immune response.[4] Exotoxins released by bacteria may act locally at the site of infection or enter the blood and produce symptoms throughout the body. Symptoms associated with the release of exotoxins from various pathogens include profuse diarrhea (cholera), spastic paralysis (tetanus), phagocyte death (gangrene), and prevention of nerve impulse transmission (botulism). Severe exotoxin release may cause septic shock syndrome, which, if not controlled rapidly, can lead to death.

Age-Related Differences

Variations in the body's response to infection are evident in pregnant women, infants and young children, and the elderly as a result of either an immature immune system or a compromised immune system. Infants and young children may have a diminished response to an invading pathogen (i.e., bacteria or virus) resulting in increased susceptibility to infection. Older adults with diminished immune response may have a muted inflammatory response to infection. For example, an older adult may have limited purulent drainage or pus within an infected wound, or they could be afebrile in the presence of an infection (i.e., urinary tract infection). Older adults may instead present with symptoms such as dizziness, confusion, anorexia, or fatigue. The presence of comorbidities (diabetes, cancer, kidney disease), particularly in the elderly, may also alter the body's response to infection.

VARIATIONS AND CONTEXT

Infections vary by severity, location, host response to treatment, and potential for debilitating consequences or sequela. Variations such as these can affect individuals of any age, gender, ethnicity, socioeconomic status, geographic location, or prior health history. Infections may occur singularly or in combination, such as bacterial infections superimposed on an existing viral infection (e.g., *Streptococcus pneumoniae* following infection with a cold virus), a new viral infection occurring secondary to an existing viral infection (e.g., cytomegalovirus and HIV), or a fungal infection developed during treatment for a bacterial infection (e.g., development of *Candida albicans* following antibiotic administration). Infections also may be mild and self-limiting, as is often observed when an infection develops in a simple cut or abrasion requiring first-aid treatment, or the infection may be life-threatening, as is the case with systemic septicemia requiring hospitalization.

CONSEQUENCES

Infections that are severe, poorly responsive to therapy, or initially untreated may challenge the body's restorative and compensatory responses. This can potentially lead to the development of septic shock syndrome and multiorgan dysfunction syndrome (MODS) – also known as multisystem organ failure (MSOF). Symptoms of MODS may include hypotension, tachycardia, tachypnea, oliguria or anuria, hypoxia, hypercapnia, seizures, or coma. The pathologic processes leading from uncontrolled infection or septicemia to multisystem failure and the symptoms just identified involve a complex interaction among a number of body systems. A bacterial infection is described as the foundation for this potential progression.

Unresponsive or Untreated Infection

When a bacterial pathogen invades the body and initiates an immune response, lymphocytes (to produce antibodies), the complement system, and phagocytes will respond aggressively. Following invasion, bacteria will cause cellular injury by the release of exotoxins or endotoxins—or both—into the host and initiate an inflammatory response. Exotoxins released during bacterial growth damage host cells, as do endotoxins released after bacterial cell death. In some cases, a combination of the relative virulence of the bacteria and the immunocompromised status of the host may allow for the bacterial infection to overwhelm the immune system and cause significant host damage before the mounting of an effective defense against the bacteria. When this happens, the host will initiate compensatory actions to support vital functions, but these actions will eventually fail without supportive treatments, leading to the death of the host.

Vascular, Renal, and Nervous System Compensation

An inflammatory response to the invading bacteria will initiate the host defense mechanisms. This response will trigger a complement system response and all of the activities inherent in that type of response. Vascular permeability will increase and allow for the shift of fluid from the intravascular compartment to the extravascular/extracellular spaces in the tissues, leading to hypovolemia and hypotension. The nervous system will attempt to compensate for the hypotension with peripheral vascular constriction and shunting of blood from nonessential to essential organs such as the brain, heart, and lungs. Acute systemic hypoperfusion may ensue and result in increased heart rate and cardiac contractility in an effort to maintain the cardiac output. In this early period, inadequate tissue perfusion may have caused organ damage despite a hyperdynamic cardiovascular state.

The renal system will initially attempt to compensate by creating a vasodilatory response of the glomeruli in an attempt to maintain an internal degree of pressure to continue filtration. Continued hypoperfusion of the kidneys leads to decreased urine output to retain cardiovascular volume, resulting in oliguria or anuria. Peripheral vasoconstriction may lead to increased cardiac ventricular preload. Should the myocardium become compromised, an increase in ventricular afterload may challenge the pulmonary vascular system with excess fluid that the ventricles cannot eject.

Respiratory Compensation

The respiratory system will attempt to compensate for inadequate tissue perfusion (oxygenation) or hypoxemia by increasing the rate of respiration. This process may well be hampered by cardiovascular decompensation, leading to decreased cardiac output and resultant fluid accumulation and pulmonary edema. Inadequate tissue perfusion (hypoxia) and hypercapnia will result, leading to central nervous system decompensation as evidenced by an early change in mental status progressing to seizures, stupor, and coma.

Multisystem Failure

In severe cases without effective treatment, bacterial invasion may lead to the development of septic shock syndrome with MODS. Eventually, the consequences of inadequate tissue perfusion, overextended compensatory mechanisms, and host cell damage will result in irreversible organ failure and death of the host.[4,12] Fig. 24.3 provides an overview of the primary pathologic processes and consequences of a bacterial infection leading to septic shock syndrome.

RISK FACTORS

Populations at Risk

Infectious diseases may cause health concerns for all individuals regardless of age, ethnicity, gender, socioeconomic status, geographic location, or prior health history. However, there are risk factors linked to some population groups based on age, socioeconomic status, and geographic location. Of the 10 leading causes of infant death in the United States, bacterial sepsis ranks ninth, and disorders related to short gestation and low birth weight rank third. Because an infant's immune system is immature at birth, any additional stress, such as low birth weight, further places the infant at risk for infection.[13–15]

The growing population of individuals of low socioeconomic status has increased the risk of infection for several reasons. Those who are uninsured or underinsured may be at risk for the consequences of absent or insufficient preventive health care. For example, if the cost of vaccinations is too expensive or the ability to access clinics where free vaccinations may be provided is not available, both children and adults can be at risk for acquiring infections from which they should be protected. Furthermore, this same population may not have the resources available to travel for preventive healthcare screenings or treatments for infection; purchase medicines; or buy food and food supplements that may contribute to health maintenance, disease prevention, and more rapid recovery from infections and other illnesses. Meanwhile, the prevalence of some diseases and infections is increasing in specific age or ethnic groups (HIV) or in geographic locations worldwide (cholera and malaria), all of which influence the prevalence of infection in the United States.

Individual Risk Factors

Individual risk factors for infection are influenced by a number of variables. The immune status of the host is a very important risk factor, as is the type, frequency, and dose of exposure to microorganisms.

Compromised Host Because of Immunodeficiency

Individual risk factors for infection include being very young or elderly because these individuals have immune systems that are immature or become less responsive and efficient with age. Those who are immunocompromised are also at increased risk for infection. An immunocompromised state may develop as a result of genetic factors (primary immunodeficiency), malnutrition, preexisting infection with other pathogens (e.g., HIV or Epstein–Barr virus), acute or chronic psychological or environmental stress, use of medications that induce immunosuppression, and the presence of or treatment for cancer. These processes associated with immunodeficiency were discussed in Concept 22, Immunity.

Compromised Host Because of Chronic Disease

Chronic illness and associated treatments increase the risk for infection. In the United States, infections accounted for 4 of the top 10 leading causes of adult deaths in 2015, including chronic lower respiratory tract diseases, influenza and pneumonia, and nephritis.[15] Diseases such as diabetes mellitus, inflammatory disorders, cancers, and hepatic or respiratory disorders challenge the immune system and increase individual vulnerability to infection. Pathologic changes within these body systems may alter the structural integrity of the system and create an environment conducive to infection, while treatment regimens are imposed that may also increase the risk of infection. Treatment strategies requiring

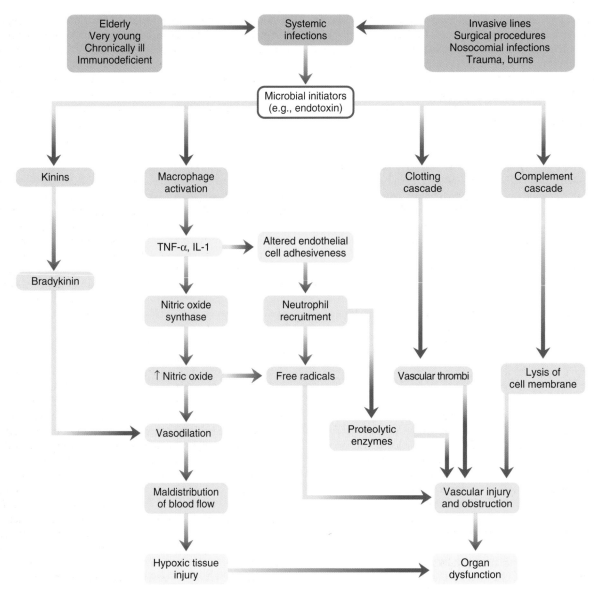

FIGURE 24.3 Pathophysiological Process of Septic Shock. *IL-1*, Interleukin-1; *TNF-α*, tumor necrosis factor-α. (Modified from Copstead, L. C., & Banasik, J. L. [2013]. *Pathophysiology* [5th ed.]. St Louis: Saunders.)

the introduction of invasive lines (parenteral or other catheters), immunosuppressive medications (corticosteroids), antibiotics or antivirals, surgery, or intubation and mechanical ventilation all expose the body to avenues of entry for pathogenic organisms. In association with chronic illness-derived immunosuppression, required treatment regimens may only serve to enhance the risk of individual infection.

Environmental Conditions

Exposure to unsafe sanitary conditions may also make an individual vulnerable to a multitude of pathogens. These pathogens may directly cause infection or challenge the immune system and increase the potential for infection upon future introduction of other microorganisms. Crowded living conditions increase the likelihood of the spread of disease and may contribute to less than optimal sanitation, both of which increase the potential for infection. Other environmental factors influence the individual's susceptibility to infection and include the presence or absence of clean food and water, conditions involving food preparation, and sufficiency of air ventilation.

ASSESSMENT

History

A health history includes questions to assess an individual's risk for infection, recognize symptoms associated with infection, and appreciate factors associated with a presenting infection. Questions include the incidence of injury, known exposure to pathogens, and a history of prior infections. Current or immediate past treatment for cancer, recent surgical procedures, the presence of autoimmune or immunodeficiency disease, and the use of immunosuppressant medication regimens also must also be assessed. Travel should also be evaluated, particularly outside of the United States or to underdeveloped areas of the world that may expose the individual to pathogens in air, food, and water or to pathogens that are generally not found in the United States, such as smallpox. Other avenues of inquiry may include assessing incidences of interaction with larger groups of people, such as attending entertainment or sporting events where the close proximity of others may facilitate the transmission of infectious pathogens.

Symptoms of infection are those verbalized by the patient and are often caused by the inflammatory response to infection, such as pain, swelling, or redness (see Concept 23, Inflammation); other clinical manifestations may be those associated with the effect of the infectious process on the body system. Specific symptoms are often influenced by the affected organ, such as a cough with an infection of the respiratory system. Some symptoms are a result of generalized stress to the host, such as fatigue or malaise.

Examination Findings

Physical examination findings of particular importance in assessing for the presence of infection include fever, swelling, chills, malaise, redness or drainage in or around a wound, pain, and respiratory congestion. In general, clinical manifestations associated with infection parallel those of inflammation. Should infection with *C. diff.* or parasites be suspected, the presence of watery diarrhea, loss of appetite, nausea, and abdominal pain or tenderness should also be evaluated because these symptoms may be indicative of infection with these pathogens.

Diagnostic Tests

Laboratory and diagnostic studies are foundational to the diagnostic process for infections. Laboratory studies may be done on any type of body fluid or tissue and can confirm the presence of infection. Radiographic diagnostic tests provide additional information to understand the location and extent of infections.

Laboratory Tests

Complete blood count. The complete blood count with a white blood cell (WBC) differential count is one of the most critical laboratory tests to evaluate the presence of infection. Elevated levels of B and T lymphocytes, neutrophils, and monocytes are indicative of infection, particularly a bacterial or viral infection. Neutrophil counts are significantly elevated with bacterial infections and may lead to an increase in the number of band cells (immature neutrophils) when an infection is acute. Parasitic infections may result in an increase in the number of basophils and eosinophils; however, these two WBCs are not elevated in the presence of bacterial or viral infections.

Culture and sensitivity. A culture and sensitivity (C&S) test is done to identify the invading pathogen and to determine the antimicrobial most likely to be effective in treatment. This test can be done on any body fluid, tissue, or exudates and is critical in the management of infections. Some of the most common specimens for C&S are obtained from the genitourinary tract (urine culture), respiratory tract (sputum culture), oropharynx (throat culture), blood, wounds, and spinal fluid. Specimens may also be obtained from within the body during invasive procedures or surgeries, or from invasive equipment such as intravenous lines, feeding tubes, endotracheal tubes, and indwelling urinary catheters. Nurses are often responsible for the collection of specimens for C&S; correct collection procedures must be followed to avoid sample contamination leading to incorrect pathogen identification. Details of collection procedures are typically outlined in textbooks about laboratory and diagnostic procedures.

Other laboratory tests. Several other blood and body fluid screening tests are used to determine the presence of or evaluate an infection. These include C-reactive protein, erythrocyte sedimentation rate (ESR), and various serologic tests for the detection of a virus or antibodies against pathogens such as hepatitis, HIV, Epstein–Barr virus, severe acute respiratory syndrome (SARS), herpes simplex virus, syphilis, MRSA, *C. diff.*, and *Helicobacter pylori.*[16]

Radiographic Tests

Radiographic tests typically do not lead to an affirmative diagnosis of infection by themselves because this requires confirmation through clinical pathology analysis (gained through laboratory testing). Radiographic tests are useful in visualizing certain body tissues to gain insight to the possibility of an infection (if not yet diagnosed) and/or the extent and scope of some confirmed infections. Chest x-rays, computerized tomography (CT) scan, magnetic resonance imaging scans, positron emission tomography scans, and indium (indium-111) scans are examples of radiographic testing procedures that are useful in identifying areas of infection and inflammation within the body.[16]

CLINICAL MANAGEMENT

Success in the prevention and treatment of infections has progressed dramatically during the past century with the introduction of antibiotics, the modernization of sanitation practices, the development of public health initiatives, and the spread of immunization programs. Morbidity and mortality rates for many infections have decreased substantially, with some infections being nearly eradicated worldwide. In the United States, smallpox vaccinations are no longer recommended and poliomyelitis is nearly eradicated with widespread vaccination protocols. Progress is being made in the development of vaccines for other diseases such as HIV, and a combined vaccination for smallpox and anthrax is being investigated.[4,17,18]

Success gained in the prevention and treatment of infections must also be tempered by the following facts: (1) some community- or hospital-acquired bacterial infections are now difficult to treat because of emerging antibiotic resistance (e.g., MRSA and VRE), (2) the prevalence of hospital-acquired infections is increasing in the form of both MRSA and *C. diff.*, (3) tuberculosis remains one of the world's leading causes of death, and (4) foodborne and waterborne bacteria (*Salmonella* and *Campylobacter*) continue to cause debilitating diarrheal disease throughout the world. Following Alexander Fleming's discovery of penicillin in 1928, 85 years of using increasingly more potent antimicrobials has resulted in bacteria and viruses that are resistant to even the most potent weapons in our arsenal. The National Institute of Allergy and Infectious Diseases (NIAID) issued a statement of concern about the increasingly difficult process of disease management given the microbial resistance that has emerged against some of the most powerful antimicrobials. NIAID particularly expressed concern related to treating staphylococcal infection, tuberculosis, influenza, gonorrhea, *Candida* infection, and malaria.[4,6,18,19]

Effective methods of protecting individuals and populations from exposure to infectious pathogens is well documented. However, lack of or incomplete implementation infection control measures, including standard precautions, has led to the reemergence of many diseases thought to be eradicated or significantly diminished. Antibiotic resistance, including multiple antibiotic resistant pathogen strains, has emerged as a significant consequence to their use from over-prescribing/ overuse or lack of completing a treatment regimen. Increasing development of new antibiotics, alternative forms of treatment, and new vaccinations for more pathogens is underway.[4] Continued research to find more powerful antimicrobials, while teaching the population about the consequences of overuse or inappropriate use of antimicrobials, will challenge healthcare providers and researchers for years to come.

Primary Prevention

Primary prevention involves a wide variety of infection control measures. Infection control has been defined by the World Health Organization as measures aimed at the protection of those who might be vulnerable to acquiring an infection, including both individuals residing in the community and persons receiving care for healthcare problems within a wide variety of settings. The basic tenant of infection control is identified as *hygiene* and encompasses such topics as patient safety, infection control and prevention in health care, injection safety, and food safety.[10,20]

Hand Hygiene and Standard Precautions

Following basic hand hygiene principles and adhering to Standard Precautions are the most effective methods of blocking transmission of infection in community and healthcare settings. The Centers for Disease Control and Prevention (CDC) has published guidelines for infection control and hand hygiene within healthcare settings, as well as guidelines related to healthcare-associated infections. The guidelines are updated periodically and serve as excellent resources for ensuring adherence to infection control principles.[10]

The following are some recommendations for infection control proposed by the CDC: Keep hands clean by washing thoroughly with soap and water (for at least 20 seconds) or using an alcohol-based hand rub (for at least 15 seconds; not as effective if hands are visibly dirty or greasy), keep cuts and scrapes clean and covered with a bandage until healed, avoid contact with other people's wounds and bandages, and refrain from sharing personal items such as towels or razors. In athletic settings, participants should shower immediately after participation and before using whirlpools. Uniforms should be washed and dried after each use. In healthcare settings, prevention of infection requires following accepted principles of hand hygiene, Standard Precautions, and contact precautions. Visitors should follow hand hygiene principles and avoid touching wound dressings, catheters, or wound sites of an infected person.[10,20]

Immunizations

Another significant primary prevention measure is the administration of vaccinations. Worldwide, healthcare organizations have demonstrated various levels of success in providing vaccinations in an effort to eradicate some of the more devastating infectious diseases, such as polio and smallpox.[21,22] Standard vaccinations in the U.S. arsenal to control the spread of disease through prevention of initial infection include those for human papillomavirus (HPV); hepatitis A and hepatitis B; varicella; measles, mumps, and rubella (MMR); influenza (annual); pneumococcus; tetanus, diphtheria, pertussis (Td/Tdap); and polio. Research continues worldwide to discover an effective vaccine for HIV.[17] Vaccinations are recommended for individuals across the lifespan; specific vaccination schedules are readily available from the CDC website (https://www.cdc.gov/vaccines/schedules).

Secondary Prevention (Screening)

Secondary prevention through disease screening is less effective in controlling infection, but represents an opportunity to identify an infection with the intent for earlier treatment and for reducing transmission.

The areas of screening most strongly supported are those for the identification of sexually transmitted diseases such as bacterial infections (*Chlamydia trachomatis*, *Neisseria gonorrhoeae*, or group B *Streptococci*), viral pathogens (HIV, herpes simplex virus, hepatitis virus, or HPV), fungal pathogens (*Candida albicans*), or protozoa (*Giardia lamblia*). Pap smears for sexually active women can be used as screening tools not only for cancer cells but also for the presence of HPV.

Collaborative Interventions

The management of infections requires both treatment of the infectious process itself and support for the affected body systems. The goal of treatment is to eradicate the infection, prevent secondary infections, and limit damage to the body. Many interventions are related to supporting affected body systems. The following infection control measures are critical for a rapid recovery and are universal in that they apply to infection treatment regardless of the system involved: know and follow the principles of effective hand hygiene; clean and disinfect environmental surfaces; and avoid close contact with infected individuals or crowded conditions in which bacterial or viral infections may be easily disseminated.

CLINICAL NURSING SKILLS FOR INFECTION

- Hand hygiene
- Personal protective equipment
  - Gloves
  - Mask
  - Protective eyewear
  - Gown
  - Cap
- Isolation precautions
- Sterility
- Collecting specimens for culture
- Medication administration
- Patient and family teaching/education

Antimicrobials

Interventions in the treatment of various infections begin with the use of antibiotics, antivirals, and other antimicrobials. The laboratory and diagnostic testing identified previously helps to direct the healthcare provider to the appropriate antimicrobial. Instructing the infected individual to complete the full course of antimicrobial therapy helps to avoid a secondary infection or re-emergence of infection because of inadequate initial treatment.

Antibiotic agents. There are several classifications of antibiotics based on bacterial spectrum and activity (bactericidal or bacteriostatic). Spectrum refers to the number of organisms affected by the antibiotic (i.e., broad-spectrum or narrow-spectrum antibiotic). Activity refers to the way in which the antibiotic kills bacteria. Bactericidal agents attack and kill the bacteria directly, whereas bacteriostatic agents interfere with replication of the pathogen. The common classifications of antibiotics are presented in Table 24.2. Antibiotics within a structural class generally have similar patterns of effectiveness, toxicity, and allergic potential.

Antiviral agents. Like antibiotics, antiviral agents either kill viruses or suppress their replication, preventing their ability to multiply and reproduce. These agents are primarily used to minimize the severity of illness by limiting the viral spread. Common classifications of antiviral agents are presented in Table 24.2.

TABLE 24.2   Classification of Antibiotic and Antiviral Agents

Antibiotics	Antiviral Agents
Penicillin	Adamantane
Cephalosporins	Antiviral chemokine receptor agonist
• First generation	Antiviral interferon
• Second generation	Neuraminidase inhibitors
• Third generation	Nonnucleoside reverse-transcriptase
• Fourth generation	inhibitors
Fluoroquinolones	Nucleoside reverse-transcriptase
Tetracyclines	inhibitors
Macrolides	Protease inhibitors
Aminoglycosides	Purine nucleosides

Antifungal agents. Antifungal agents kill fungal organisms. Because there are various types of fungi that cause infection, multiple classifications of antifungal agents are available and include polyenes, imidazoles, triazoles, thiazoles, allylamines, and echinocandins.

Nutrition and Fluids

Replacement of fluids and electrolytes (oral or parenteral) is critical in the presence of fever, vomiting, or diarrhea. Adequate rest and nutrition provide the body with the energy needed for optimal functioning of the immune system and resolution of infection. Allowing time for rest and ensuring adequate fluids and nutritional intake are equally important.

INTERRELATED CONCEPTS

The concept of infection is closely aligned with several concepts featured in this textbook. These interrelated concepts are presented in Fig. 24.4.

Immunity is critical in providing a level of surveillance for early identification of pathogen entry into the body. The immune system is the first line of defense against infection and the body's primary method of response to an invading organism. Inflammation is part of the body's response to a foreign antigen, with many of the symptoms of infection being those of the body's inflammatory response (redness, swelling, and pain). Tissue Integrity is critical to avoiding infection, with the skin being the largest component of the immune system. Intact tissues are less vulnerable to pathogen entry and form natural barriers to infection. As noted previously, the concept Stress and Coping is linked because stress challenges the immune system and makes it more vulnerable to damage, less able to respond effectively and efficiently to pathogen invasion, and more difficult for the body to respond to treatment for an infection. Finally, maintaining adequate Nutrition and rest is also necessary for the body to respond to active infection treatment regimens and to support the work of an immune response.

CLINICAL EXEMPLARS

Table 24.1 identifies examples of common pathogens that cause infection. A variety of infections have been presented as recurring, emerging, resistant, and global. Box 24.1 presents some of the more commonly occurring infections by body systems. Some of the most common or important exemplars briefly described in the section that follows.

Featured Exemplars

Pneumonia

Pneumonia is an infection in the lungs that may range from mild to severe and occurs in people of any age, gender, or ethnicity. Worldwide, it is the leading cause of death in children younger than age 5 years.[23] A person's potential for developing pneumonia is diminished with proper hand hygiene and by disinfecting regularly touched surfaces, being a nonsmoker, not having underlying diseases such as diabetes mellitus or heart disease, and being vaccinated with the pneumonia vaccine. Pneumonia symptoms include chest tightness, shortness of breath, difficulty breathing, cough, and fever, and the disease is treated with antibiotics and antiviral drugs.[23]

Conjunctivitis

Commonly called "pink eye," conjunctivitis is characterized by redness and swelling of the conjunctiva, thick discharge from the eye with crusting on the eyelids or lashes, and itchy, inflamed eyes. Pain is not typically associated with the infection. Conjunctivitis is common in children and adults, and easily spread from one person to another. When one child in a family is diagnosed with conjunctivitis, all children are commonly treated as a prophylactic measure. In the newborn, conjunctivitis occurring within the first 3 weeks of life is often caused by gonococcal or chlamydial infections of the mother and, if left untreated, may lead to blindness.[24]

Otitis Media

Otitis media may be classified into one of three types: acute otitis media (AOM), otitis media with effusion (OME), and otitis externa (Swimmer's ear). Guidelines require differentiation of OME and AOM, and the patient's age, to determine appropriate antibiotic use. AOM is usually painful and often requires treatment with antibiotics. Other symptoms include redness of the tympanic membrane, pus, and fever. AOM may also be a consequence of other infections such as measles, mumps, or pneumonia. OME is a buildup of fluid in the middle ear without symptoms of infection and is often caused by viral upper respiratory infections and allergies, generally resolving on its own. Swimmer's ear is an infection of the ear and outer ear canal. Treatment with antibiotics is usually required.[25]

Hepatitis

Hepatitis is inflammation of the liver and generally refers to one of three viral causative agents: hepatitis A virus (HAV), hepatitis B virus

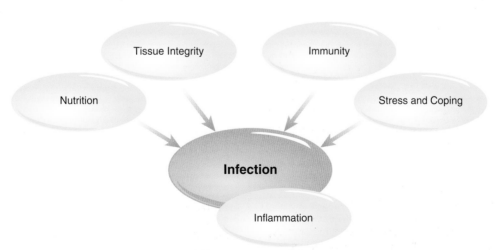

FIGURE 24.4 Infection and Interrelated Concepts.

BOX 24.1   EXEMPLARS OF INFECTION

Neurologic
- Encephalitis
- Meningitis

Respiratory
- Pneumonia
- Respiratory syncytial virus

Cardiovascular
- Endocarditis
- Myocarditis

Eyes
- Conjunctivitis

Ears
- Otitis media

Skin
- Cellulitis
- Methicillin-resistant *Staphylococcus aureus*
- Pressure ulcers
- Surgical wounds

Gastrointestinal
- *Clostridium difficile*
- Gastroenteritis
- Hepatitis
- Tapeworm

Genitourinary
- Cystitis
- Pyelonephritis
- Urinary tract infection

Reproductive
- *Candida albicans*
- *Chlamydia trachomatis*
- Group B *Streptococci*
- Herpes simplex virus
- Human papillomavirus
- *Neisseria gonorrhoeae*

Systemic
- HIV
- Measles
- Mumps
- Sepsis

🌱 **ACCESS EXEMPLAR LINKS IN YOUR GIDDENS EBOOK**

(HBV), and hepatitis C virus (HCV). It is the leading cause of liver cancer and the most common cause of liver transplantation. The CDC estimates that only 50% of HAV, 15.4% of HBV, and 7.2% of HCV cases are diagnosed and reported. Since 1990, effective vaccination strategies have led to a decrease in the incidence of acute HBV; however, the incidence of acute HCV has been on the rise: a 3.5-fold increase in cases from 2010 to 2016. Furthermore, significant underreporting of HBV and HCV is acknowledged due to asymptomatic infections. Acute onset of symptoms is discrete and includes nausea and vomiting, fever, malaise, dark urine, and jaundice. Ascites develops later in disease progression.[26]

Human Papillomavirus

HPV is the most common sexually transmitted infection, with more than 40 types, and is typically passed through genital contact during vaginal, anal, or oral sex. Symptoms may develop years after exposure and may lead to genital warts and cancer. HPV tests can be used to screen for cervical cancer. A vaccination is available to men and women against the types of HPV that most often lead to cancer, and is recommended between the ages of 9 and 14 years with a second dose 6 months after the first. HPV is so common that the CDC estimates that most sexually active men and women will get at least one type of HPV sometime in their life.[27]

CASE STUDY

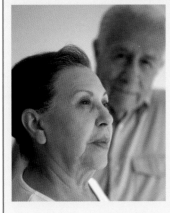

Case Presentation

Mrs. Bovier is a 72-year-old woman who recently spent 5 days in hospital for pneumonia, where she received intravenous antibiotics and respiratory therapy. She was discharged 1 week ago and has been at home with her elderly husband, who assists in her care. She has arthritis and typically is not very physically active.

Mrs. Bovier returned to her primary care provider for a checkup and complained of increasing difficulty breathing, headache, and coughing up yellowish-colored sputum. On examination, she was found to have a low-grade fever; chest auscultation revealed areas of atelectasis; oxygen saturation (PaO_2) was 91%; and she was diaphoretic. A sputum specimen was obtained for culture and sensitivity that later revealed the presence of methicillin-resistant *Staphylococcus aureus* (MRSA). Chest x-ray confirmed pulmonary congestion and atelectasis. Laboratory analysis showed an elevated white blood cell count, the presence of band cells (immature neutrophils), and an elevated erythrocyte sedimentation rate.

Mrs. Bovier was again hospitalized because of the severity of her respiratory distress; the need for intravenous antibiotics to manage the MRSA pulmonary infection; pulmonary therapy to assist in resolving her pulmonary congestion; and the need for contact isolation because of her recurrent pneumonia and MRSA infection. Mrs. Bovier's age and lack of physical activity are complications that may influence MRSA treatment, requiring a more watchful course of initial therapy.

Hospital care for Mrs. Bovier included instruction in methods to improve the productivity of her cough, humidified oxygen to assist with loosening secretions while improving ventilation, and respiratory therapy to help with expectoration and to facilitate lung expansion and air exchange. She received intravenous vancomycin, mucolytic agents, a bronchodilator, and expectorants to treat her pulmonary disease and assist in breathing.

On discharge, Mrs. Bovier received instructions in the proper technique for effective hand hygiene; the importance of avoiding large crowds of people as well as areas where people are smoking, to diminish her exposure to irritating respiratory stimuli; and the need to increase her physical activity, including frequent ambulation in her home, to help stimulate deep breathing and avoid peripheral vascular clot formation. She demonstrated understanding of her medication regimens and the need to maintain adequate food and fluid intake to support her immune system and to provide energy while healing. The need for rest to promote healing was also emphasized. Finally, Mrs. Bovier was instructed on the warning signs of recurring pulmonary disease or dysfunction.

Case Analysis Questions

1. What risk factors does Mrs. Bovier have that put her at risk for the development of MRSA?
2. What clinical findings did Mrs. Bovier have consistent with the concept of infection?

From Medioimages/Photodisc/Thinkstock.

ACCESS EXEMPLAR LINKS IN YOUR GIDDENS EBOOK

REFERENCES

1. Hall, J. C. (2016). *Textbook of medical physiology* (13th ed.). Philadelphia: Elsevier.
2. Mosby. (2013). *Mosby's dictionary of medicine, nursing, and health professions* (10th ed.). St Louis: Mosby.
3. National Institutes of Health. (2014). *Immune system.* Retrieved from https://www.niaid.nih.gov/research/immunesystem.
4. McCance, K. L., Huether, S. E., Brashers, V. L., et al. (Eds.), (2014). *Pathophysiology: The biological basis for disease in adults and children* (7th ed.). St Louis: Mosby.
5. Venes, D. (Ed.), (2017). *Taber's cyclopedic medical dictionary* (23rd ed.). Philadelphia: Davis.
6. Schaffler, H., & Breitruck, A. (2018). *Clostridium difficile – from colonization to infection. Frontiers in Microbiology, 9,* doi:10.3389/fmicb.2018.00646. Article 646.
7. Centers for Disease Control and Prevention. (2018). *Healthcare-associated infections.* Retrieved from https://www.cdc.gov/hai/.
8. Centers for Disease Control and Prevention. (2016). *MDRO prevention and control.* Retrieved from https://www.cdc.gov/infectioncontrol/guidelines/mdro/prevention-control.html#.
9. Centers for Disease Control and Prevention. (2018). *Methicillin-resistant Staphylococcus aureus (MRSA).* Retrieved from https://www.cdc.gov/mrsa/.
10. Centers for Disease Control and Prevention. (2017). *Hand hygiene in healthcare settings: Healthcare providers.* Retrieved from https://www.cdc.gov/handhygiene/providers/index.html.
11. Centers for Disease Control and Prevention. (2016). *Chickenpox (varicella): For health care professionals.* Retrieved from https://www.cdc.gov/chickenpox/hcp/index.html.
12. Copstead, L. C., & Banasik, J. L. (2013). *Pathophysiology* (5th ed.). St Louis: Saunders.
13. National Institutes of Health, U.S. National Library of Medicine. (2018). *Aging changes in immunity.* Retrieved from http://medlineplus.gov/ency/article/004008.htm.
14. U.S. National Library of Medicine, National Institutes of Health. (2018). *Aging changes in organs, tissues, and cells.* Retrieved from https://medlineplus.gov/ency/article/004012.htm.
15. Murphy, S. L., Xu, J., Kochanek, K. D., et al. (2017). *National vital statistics reports: Deaths: Final data for 2015.* Retrieved from https://www.cdc.gov/nchs/data/nvsr/nvsr66/nvsr66_06.pdf.
16. Pagana, K. D., Pagana, T. J., & Pagana, J. (2017). *Mosby's diagnostic and laboratory test reference* (13th ed.). St Louis: Mosby.
17. National Institutes of Health, National Allergy and Infectious Diseases Institute. (2018). *HIV vaccine development.* Retrieved from https://www.niaid.nih.gov/diseases-conditions/hiv-vaccine-development.
18. National Institutes of Health, National Allergy and Infectious Diseases Institute. (2018). *NIH statement on HIV vaccine awareness day, May 18, 2018.* Retrieved from https://www.niaid.nih.gov/news-events/nih-statement-hiv-vaccine-awareness-day-may-18-2018.
19. National Institutes of Health, National Institute of Allergy and Infectious Diseases. (2016). *Antimicrobial (drug) resistance.* Retrieved from https://www.niaid.nih.gov/research/antimicrobial-resistance.
20. Siegel, J. D., Rhinehart, E., Jackson, M., et al. (2017 update). *2007 Guideline for isolation precautions: Preventing transmission of infectious agents in healthcare settings.* Retrieved from https://www.cdc.gov/infectioncontrol/pdf/guidelines/isolation/.
21. Centers for Disease Control and Prevention. (2018). *Smallpox: For clinicians.* Retrieved from https://www.cdc.gov/smallpox/clinicians/.
22. Centers for Disease Control and Prevention. (2017). *Global health: What is polio.* Retrieved from https://www.cdc.gov/polio/about/index.htm.
23. Centers for Disease Control and Prevention. (2017). *Pneumonia.* Retrieved from https://www.cdc.gov/pneumonia/.
24. Centers for Disease Control and Prevention. (2017). *Conjunctivitis (pink eye).* Retrieved from https://www.cdc.gov/conjunctivitis/.
25. Mayo Clinic. (2018). *Ear infection (middle ear).* Retrieved from https://www.mayoclinic.org/diseases-conditions/ear-infections/symptoms-causes/syc-20351616?p=1.
26. Centers for Disease Control and Prevention. (2018). *Surveillance for viral hepatitis—United States, 2016.* Retrieved from https://www.cdc.gov/hepatitis/statistics/2016surveillance/commentary.htm.
27. Meites, E., Kempe, A., & Markowitz, L. E. (2016). Use of a 2-dose schedule for human papillomavirus vaccination—updated recommendations of the advisory committee on immunization practices. *MMWR. Morbidity and Mortality Weekly Report, 65*(49), 1405–1408.

CONCEPT
25

Mobility

Jean Giddens

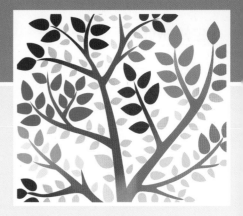

The 10-month-old baby taking his first steps, the 6-year-old girl riding a bicycle, the high school athlete "dunking" the basketball, the newly married couple dancing at their wedding, the 40-year-old neighbor walking his dog, and the 76-year-old grandmother knitting a scarf demonstrate various examples of mobility accomplished through functions of the musculoskeletal and nervous systems. As a basic physiological process, mobility is required for optimal health. Changes in mobility can significantly affect biophysical health, psychosocial health, and functional status. Nurses should be familiar with interventions to promote optimal mobility, prevent situations leading to immobility, and minimize complications when immobility occurs.

DEFINITION

Mobility refers to purposeful physical movement, including gross simple movements, fine complex movements, and coordination. Mobility is dependent on the synchronized efforts of the musculoskeletal and nervous systems as well as adequate oxygenation, perfusion, and cognition. Specifically, mobility requires adequate energy, adequate muscle strength, underlying skeletal stability, joint function, and neuromuscular coordination to carry out the desired movement. For the purposes of this concept presentation, mobility is defined as a *"state or quality of being mobile or movable."*[1, p.1479] There are many variations on the term *mobility* seen throughout the literature that are worth mentioning. The term *immobility* refers to an inability to move. *Impaired physical mobility* describes a state in which a person has a limitation in physical movement but is not immobile. Impaired physical mobility, as defined by the North American Nursing Diagnosis Association (NANDA), is a "limitation in independent, purposeful movement of the body or of one or more extremities."[2, p.219] NANDA further differentiates impaired physical mobility by multiple types including impaired bed mobility, impaired wheelchair mobility, impaired standing, impaired transfer ability, and impaired walking.[2] Although immobility is typically considered a negative state, there are times when immobility or immobilization is therapeutic. For example, the immobilization of a shoulder if it has been dislocated provides desired rest, recovery, and comfort.

The term *deconditioned* is used to describe a loss of physical fitness. This applies not only to an athlete who fails to maintain an optimal level of training but also to an individual who does not maintain optimal physical activity. In the context of health care, this term applies to patients who experience extended immobility (e.g., following prolonged bed rest), resulting in an overall deconditioned state of the musculoskeletal

and cardiopulmonary systems. This is particularly a problem among older adults. Another similar term, *the disuse syndrome*, first proposed more than 30 years ago by Bortz, describes the predictable adverse effect on body tissues and functions associated with sedentary lifestyle and inactivity.[3] Identifying characteristics of the disuse syndrome, as defined by Bortz, included cardiovascular vulnerability, obesity, musculoskeletal fragility, depression, and premature aging.

SCOPE

The scope of mobility as a concept ranges on a continuum from full mobility to partial mobility (also referred to as impaired mobility) and complete immobility (Fig. 25.1). Mobility can be considered on a micro or macro perspective. Mobility and immobility may refer to a particular part of the body (e.g., an arm or a leg), or they can refer to the entire body. Thus, mobility and immobility are not mutually exclusive; for example, a patient with an immobilized extremity can be mobile. Also, because mobility is on a continuum, a change in mobility may be temporary.

NORMAL PHYSIOLOGICAL PROCESS

Optimal mobility relies on bones, joints, articular cartilage, tendons and ligaments, skeletal muscle, and the mechanics of muscle contraction. Underlying these functions is an intact neurologic system whereby signals for all movement are communicated to and from the brain through nerve impulses.

Neurologic System

All movement is coordinated by the brain through a complex process of sensing internal and external data signals, integrating these data signals, and responding by triggering motor activity. The motor cortex in the frontal lobe of the brain is responsible for voluntary motor activity through a series of nerve impulses sent from the brain, through the spinal cord and peripheral nerves, to the target muscle. The cerebellum, located at the base of the brain, coordinates movement, equilibrium, muscle tone, and proprioception.

Musculoskeletal System
Bones

The skeleton has three overarching roles relating to mobility: It acts as the structural foundation for the body and as leverage to move body

FIGURE 25.1 Scope of Mobility as a Concept.

parts, supports and protects tissues and internal organs, and provides attachment sites for muscles and ligaments. Bones also serve as a storage center for calcium and as a production center for red blood cells within the bone marrow.[4] The human body has 206 bones classified into two groups: the axial skeleton (bones that comprise the skull, thorax, and spinal column) and the appendicular skeleton (bones that comprise the upper and lower extremities).

All structures designed for use over time require ongoing maintenance and intermittent repair. The same is true for the skeletal system. Remodeling is a term that describes an ongoing maintenance of bone tissue through a process in which new bone tissue replaces existing bone tissue in bone-remodeling units.[5] The remodeling process also provides the mechanism to repair injured bones (e.g., a fracture). Remodeling requires adequate nutrition, hormonal regulation, and blood supply. The severity of the bone injury and the availability of remodeling elements influence the rate or speed at which injured bone heals.

Joints

Bones come together at joints. Joints provide stability to bones and allow skeletal movement. Mobility is impacted by the degree of joint freedom; joints allow for skeletal positioning to carry out the desired action. The various types of movement provided by joints include flexion, extension, rotation, adduction, abduction, supination, and pronation. Some of the most common problems associated with mobility arise as a result of joint pain and/or changes in joint function.

Three classifications of joints (based on stability and movement) include synarthrosis joints (nonmovable), amphiarthrosis joints (slightly movable), and diarthrosis joints (freely movable).[5] Joints are also classified by structure. Fibrous joints serve to hold bones together in place with connective tissue. For example, the tibia and fibula are held together by a fibrous ligament. Cartilaginous joints feature cartilage material that holds the joint together and provides some movement. For example, ribs are attached and held to the sternum by cartilaginous material, allowing movement for the process of breathing but providing chest stability required for the breathing process. Joints that allow the most movement are also the most complex. Synovial joints have multiple elements, including a joint capsule, synovial membrane, joint cavity, synovial fluid, and articular cartilage. Articular cartilage acts as a cushion by distributing joint loads over a wide area, thereby reducing prolonged compression of articulating bones within the joint. Without cartilage, significant friction and pain result from joint movement.

Muscles

Skeletal muscle differs from other types of muscle in the body in many ways, but one of the most important differences is that it is under voluntary control.[1] Optimal skeletal muscle function depends on the following five factors: nerve impulses reaching the muscle, muscle fibers' response to nerve stimulus, proprioception, mechanical load, and joint mobility. Impairment of any one of these factors negatively impacts purposeful movement.

Nerve impulses reach skeletal muscle from the spinal cord and peripheral nerves via motor neurons. The motor neurons innervate a group of muscle fibers known as the motor or muscle unit. There are many different types of muscle fibers within a muscle unit depending on the function and type of responsiveness required. Muscles that maintain body posture do not have the same need for quick responsiveness as do the ocular muscles, for example, but are less sensitive to fatigue.

Muscle movement occurs in response to nerve stimulation of the muscle fibers triggering muscle contraction. On a cellular level, the functional units of muscle contraction are myofibrils. Movement occurs in a reciprocal manner among muscle groups. If one group contracts, another group must relax. For example, flexion of the elbow to move the forearm up requires contraction of the biceps muscles and relaxation of the triceps muscles; likewise, extension of the elbow joint requires contraction of the triceps muscles and relaxation of the biceps muscles. If both are contracted at the same time, no movement occurs.

Proprioception is the mechanism that provides a sense of position and movement; this process allows for accuracy in the degree of movement with muscle contraction. Mechanical load of movement is associated with having adequate strength within the muscle group to carry out the desired task. For example, most humans would struggle to pick up a 250-pound object and walk 50 feet with it. However, such a feat is entirely possible for individuals who are well conditioned for this.

Age-Related Differences

Significant changes to the musculoskeletal system occur throughout infancy and childhood as a function of growth and development. The appendicular skeleton (extremities) grows faster than the axial skeleton (head, thorax, and spine)—partly because the appendicular skeleton is disproportionately shorter than the axial skeleton. Throughout infancy, childhood, and adolescence, bones change in composition, grow in length and diameter, and undergo changes in rotation and alignment. Similarly, the size and composition of muscles undergo changes as a result of physical growth and development throughout childhood, and they are a major factor in weight gain during adolescence.[5,6]

A number of musculoskeletal changes occur with aging. In the spinal column, a thinning of vertebral disks, shortening of the spinal column, and onset of kyphosis with spinal column compression occur. Bone density decreases and becomes brittle (particularly in females), leaving older adults more susceptible to fracture. Cartilage becomes rigid and fragile, and there is a loss of resilience and elasticity of ligaments. Muscle mass and tone reduce significantly in late adult years. Cumulatively, these changes result in mobility impairment attributable to reduced range of motion and pain in joints, reduced muscle strength, and increased risk for bone fracture.[4]

VARIATIONS AND CONTEXT

Variations in mobility are seen among individuals across the lifespan with multiple causative factors and a wide range of degree of impact and duration. Changes in mobility can be temporary, long term, or permanent, and are influenced by general health status, with specific conditions associated with the neurologic or musculoskeletal system (Fig. 25.2). Restrictions in mobility may also be indicated following a medical procedure or diagnostic test.

An individual's general health status has significant influence on mobility. Many conditions lead to changes in mobility, including acute illness or injury (e.g., influenza or fracture), debilitating chronic conditions (particularly cardiovascular and pulmonary conditions leading to fatigue), and conditions involving end-of-life care (e.g., cancer or dementia). Conditions that specifically lead to mobility impairment include neurologic (including the brain, the spinal cord, and the peripheral nerves), musculoskeletal (bones, joints, and muscles), or a combination of both (neuromuscular conditions). Conditions in these

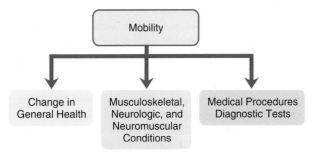

FIGURE 25.2 Categories Leading to a Change in Mobility.

TABLE 25.1	Consequences of Immobility
System Affected	Physiological Effect and Potential Complications
Cardiovascular system	Reduced cardiac capacity
	Decreased cardiac output
	Orthostatic hypotension
	Venous stasis
	Deep vein thrombosis
Respiratory system	Recued lung expansion
	Atelectasis
	Pooling of respiratory secretions
Musculoskeletal system	Reduction in muscle mass and atrophy
	Contracture of joints
	Bone demineralization
Integumentary system	Skin breakdown
Gastrointestinal system	Reduced peristaltic motility
	Constipation
Urinary system	Renal calculi
	Urinary stasis
	Infection

three categories can be caused by congenital defects, genetic conditions, injury, inflammation, infection, autoimmune disorders, and neoplasms. Medical procedures (e.g., surgery) and diagnostic tests may require temporary restrictions on mobility to reduce complications.

CONSEQUENCES

Attaining and/or maintaining mobility is paramount to health. The human body was designed to move; thus, when movement is limited, consequences occur. The degree of consequence is largely dependent on the degree of mobility impairment and length of time the impairment exists. As a general rule, the greater the extent and length of time, the greater the physiological consequences. A state of complete immobility has a significant impact on the entire body; literally all body systems are affected (Table 25.1).

Cardiovascular Complications

Cardiovascular complications occur both with central and with peripheral perfusion. A lack of physical activity results in reduced cardiac capacity. According to one study, a 15% reduction in muscle mass will occur after 12 weeks of complete immobility.[7] This translates to reduced force of cardiac contraction and a reduction in cardiac output. The loss of endurance and the deconditioned state present challenges when the resumption of physical activity is desired.

Problems also occur within the vascular system. Decreased efficiency of orthostatic neurovascular reflexes and diminished vasopressor mechanism cause orthostatic hypotension intolerance when an individual attempts to attain an upright position because of blood pooling in the extremities.[5] Adequate perfusion and venous return depend on skeletal muscle contraction and frequent changes in body position. Because muscular contraction (particularly in the legs) facilitates venous return, venous stasis occurs during periods of inactivity. Slowed blood flow provides an opportunity for the formation of blood clots. Deep vein thrombosis is a relatively common complication associated with immobility.

Respiratory Complications

Physical activity is associated with full lung expansion, particularly among those engaging in exercise. Immobility contributes to reduced lung expansion and eventually leads to atelectasis (an airless state of the alveoli) and reduced capacity for gas exchange. Pooling of respiratory secretions, coupled with a reduced cough effort, places the immobilized patient at risk for stasis pneumonia.

Musculoskeletal Complications

Muscle tone, joint movement, and maintenance of bone density require active skeletal contraction and weight bearing. Skeletal muscle adapts to nonuse by reducing mass. Thus, prolonged immobility leads to

significant reductions in muscle mass and atrophy; in fact, an average loss of 25% muscle mass occurs with permanent immobility.[7] The lack of activity leads to contracture in the joint, primarily as a result of muscle shortening. Muscle atrophy and joint contraction are particularly concerning because together these negatively affect functional ability.

The lack of weight bearing leads to bone demineralization and calcium loss from the skeletal system. The degree of bone demineralization and calcium depletion is related to the severity and duration of immobility as well as the degree of weight-bearing ability. Over time, osteoporosis can develop in response to immobility.

Integument System

Sustained pressure on the skin reduces perfusion to the tissues. A reduced flow of oxygenated blood causes hypoxemia of the tissues and increases the risk for skin breakdown. Individuals who lack the ability to move in bed have increased risk not only because of pressure but also because of shearing forces that often accompany certain positions or occur during transfers. These problems are further exacerbated if the patient has a poor nutritional status and is incontinent. Development of pressure ulcers commonly results.

Gastrointestinal Complications

Constipation is a frequently reported complication of immobility for several reasons. First, not being able to assume an optimal upright position makes having a bowel movement more challenging; for many people, relying on the assistance of others to have a bowel movement is embarrassing and may lead to reluctance in acting on the urge. From a physiological standpoint, the gastrointestinal tract slows during states of immobility, resulting in reduced peristaltic motility. Constipation, reduced appetite, and anorexia negatively impact nutritional status.

Urinary Complications

Immobility leads to three common problems that occur within the urinary system: renal calculi, urinary stasis, and infection. Renal calculi result from stasis of urine in the renal pelvis and because of increased circulating serum calcium levels (as a result of bone reabsorption mentioned previously). The bladder loses tone, making it difficult to completely empty the bladder, particularly in a lying position for voiding. This often results in urinary tract infection because the presence of urinary stasis provides an optimal environment for the growth of bacteria.

Psychological Effects

Acute and chronic psychological conditions that result from immobility include boredom, depression, feelings of helplessness/hopelessness, grieving, anxiety, anger, disturbed body image, and decreased verbal and nonverbal communication. Individuals who are unable to work or are even unable to meet basic activities of daily living often experience a loss of self-worth or value associated with the role change. Social isolation and mood disturbances are common.

Psychological effects of immobility are especially concerning among children. For children, physical activity is integral to daily activity. Not only is it essential for physical growth and development but also it is central to expression, communication, and making sense of the world around them. Immobilization can interfere with intellectual and psychomotor function. Emotional responses range from anger and aggressive behavior to passive quiet demeanor and withdrawal. Developmental regression is common. Children often become less communicative and may experience depression; in some cases, hallucinations occur.[6]

RISK FACTORS

Populations at Risk

All individuals are potentially at risk for altered mobility regardless of age, ethnicity, race, or socioeconomic status. Because of the effects of aging, the population group at greatest risk for impaired mobility is older adults. These changes predispose older individuals to a greater incidence of falls and greater challenges regaining full mobility following a period of impaired mobility. An estimated 90% of hip fractures are a result of falling; 76% of hip fractures occur among elderly women.[8]

Individual Risk Factors

Individual risk factors for changes in mobility are often attributed to acute and chronic conditions, chronic pain, and injury/trauma. Specifically, individuals with orthopedic injury, congenital deformities, neurologic disorders, strokes, head injury, spinal injury or deformities, nutritional deficiencies, cardiopulmonary conditions, and end-stage cancer are particularly susceptible. Side effects and adverse effects of many medications (e.g., corticosteroids and chemotherapy) and medical treatments can also affect mobility. Substance use disorders are more prevalent in major trauma patients than the general population[9] also representing risk for mobility impairment.

ASSESSMENT

History

The history, as it relates to the concept of mobility, includes general health information (past health history, medications, and surgery/treatments) and social history (lifestyle, employment, family assessment, and activities of daily living) as a starting point.[10] In addition, the history includes an investigation of specific symptoms experienced by the patient. Areas of questions specific for mobility include the following:
- Presence of pain with movement
- Recent changes in mobility or problems with balance
- Presence of fatigue
- Recent falls
- Recent changes in ability to complete activity of daily living

Examination Findings

Objective data regarding the assessment of the musculoskeletal system include an assessment of gait and body posture; joints; size, symmetry, and strength of muscles; and range of motion of joints.[10] Pediatric assessment also involves observation of motor activities as related to developmental milestones.[6]

Expected findings include erect posture and symmetry of extremities. Gait should be smooth, coordinated, and balanced. The spine should be straight with expected curvatures. Muscles and joints should be assessed for size, symmetry, strength, range of motion, and stability. Comparisons are made between right and left sides.[10] Assessment of muscle strength is done utilizing a muscle strength scale (0 = no detection of muscular contraction; 5 = full muscle strength). Findings considered abnormal include observed deformity of bone or joint, edema, ecchymosis, localized warmth and redness, a loss of function, numbness, guarding (due to pain), and limitations in movement or mobility. Further information related to conducting an assessment of the musculoskeletal system can be found in physical assessment textbooks.

Diagnostic Tests

Many diagnostic tests are used to evaluate musculoskeletal disorders. These are briefly described next.

Radiographic Diagnostics
- *X-ray:* evaluates the integrity of bones and joints and is the most common radiographic test used to diagnose fractures.
- *Computed tomography scan:* identifies soft tissue and bony abnormalities and evaluates musculoskeletal trauma.
- *Magnetic resonance imaging:* uses radio waves and magnetic fields to provide an image of soft tissue. This is used most efficiently to evaluate soft tissues, such as a vertebral disk, tumor, ligaments, and cartilage.[11]
- *Myelogram:* a radiographic study of the spinal cord and nerve root using a contrast dye. This is particularly useful in the evaluation of individuals with back pain.
- *Arthrography (arthrogram):* visualization of a joint by the injection of a radiopaque substance into the joint cavity, allowing for the evaluation of bones, cartilage, and ligaments. This is most commonly performed on the knee and shoulder joints, but it also can be done on hips, ankles, and wrists.[11]
- *Bone mineral density:* a diagnostic test used to determine the core mineral content and the density of bone. This test is used for the diagnosis of osteoporosis and osteopenia.
- *Bone scan:* evaluates the bone uptake of a radionuclide material; the uptake is related to the metabolism of the bone. The primary indication of this test is to detect metastatic cancer in the bone,[11] but it is also used to evaluate avascular necrosis or unexplained bone pain.

Other Diagnostic Tests
- *Arthroscopy:* a procedure that allows direct visualization of the interior of a joint through an endoscope. This procedure is most commonly performed on the knee, but it can be done on other joints as well.
- *Electromyography:* an evaluation of electrical activity generated within the muscle. This is used to determine the quality of neuromuscular innervation.
- *Laboratory tests:* used to provide various types of information about the functional state of muscles, bones, or joints. Types of tests include blood tests (e.g., alkaline phosphatase, calcium, phosphorus, uric acid, creatine kinase, blood urea nitrogen, creatinine, and myoglobinuria), analysis of joint fluids, mod pathologic analysis of biopsied tissue (e.g., a muscle biopsy or bone biopsy).

CLINICAL MANAGEMENT

Primary Prevention

Regular physical activity is associated with multiple health benefits and is foundational to primary prevention measures.[12,13] Prevention of problems associated with mobility is relatively simple—that is, maintaining the highest level of regular physical activity possible along with optimal nutrition, keeping an ideal body weight, and getting adequate rest. Taking measures to prevent injury and trauma are also considered primary prevention strategies.

Nutrition, as a primary prevention strategy, links to musculoskeletal development. During infancy, childhood, and adolescence, adequate protein and calcium in the diet are critical for the musculoskeletal development described previously. Adequate calcium intake is also necessary to prevent osteoporosis among older individuals. Maintaining a healthy body weight prevents excessive joint strain and is associated with fewer problems with back pain. Falls represent one of the most common mobility problems among older adults; thus, fall prevention is an important aspect of primary prevention. Strategies include participating in regular physical activity (to maintain muscle strength and balance), making the environment safer (e.g., avoiding hazards, using hand rails, wearing sturdy shoes with nonslip soles, and having adequate lighting), and optimizing vision.[8]

Secondary Prevention (Screening)

The primary areas to highlight related to mobility and screening are osteoporosis, mobility screening, and fall risk assessment. For osteoporosis screening, the U.S. Preventive Services Task Force (USPSTF) recommends screening women age 65 years or older for osteoporosis with bone measurement testing to prevent osteoporotic fractures.[14] Among postmenopausal women under 65, screening is recommended for those with increased risk of osteoporosis. In younger women who have increased fracture risk, dual-energy x-ray absorptiometry (DXA) of the hip and spine is the recommended method to measure bone density. There is no recommendation for the screening interval. Furthermore, USPSTF concludes that evidence is insufficient to recommend screening for men.[14]

A large number of mobility and fall risk assessment screening tools are available. Scott and colleagues reviewed 38 different fall and mobility assessment tests for use among older adults and concluded that most are reliable. However, they were unable to conclude whether one screening test was better than another because of the wide range of settings for use.[15] A recent study evaluating tools for assessing fall risk in the elderly concluded that two assessment tools used together (as opposed to using a single tool) provide a better evaluation of fall risk among older adults.[16] One of the most common screening tests is the Timed Get Up and Go test, which measures mobility in people who are able to walk on their own (assistive devices allowed).[17] Another common screening is the Performance-Oriented Mobility Assessment test,[18] which aids in the identification of gait and balance impairments. Mobility scales, such as the Greenville Early Mobility Scale, are used in inpatient settings to track the status and progress of a patient's mobility, thus enhancing the effectiveness of mobility interventions among interdisciplinary teams.[19]

Collaborative Interventions

Numerous interventions for the care of individuals with limitations in mobility exist and are usually presented based on the underlying medical condition or diagnosis. Interventions specific for a health condition associated with changes or loss in mobility often overlap. From a conceptual perspective, a general discussion of interventions delivered by various members of the healthcare team that address mobility impairments includes several categories, such as care of the immobilized patient, exercise therapy, pharmacologic agents, surgical interventions, immobilization, and assistive devices.

Patients with impaired mobility are at risk for injury when interventions are not carried out properly. Likewise, healthcare workers caring for patients with mobility impairment are at risk for occupational injury—often caused by manually moving a patient. National standards for safe patient handling and mobility, released by the American Nurses Association in 2013, are designed to improve the safety of patients and healthcare workers. The standards were developed by an interprofessional working group and are intended to provide a blueprint to adopt a safe patient handling and mobility program that can be adapted to any healthcare setting and with any patient population. Included in the standards are establishing a culture of safety, education and training; the application of ergonomic principles in the care environment; patient-centered assessment; and the integration of safe patient handling technology in the care environment.[20]

CLINICAL NURSING SKILLS FOR MOBILITY

- Assessment
  - General assessment
  - Mobility assessment
- Patient handling/transfers
- Positioning
- Range-of-motion exercises
- Continuous passive motion
- Sequential compression device and elastic stockings
- Ambulation
- Assistive devices
  - Cane
  - Crutches
  - Walker
  - Wheelchair
- Patient-handling technology
  - Mats
  - Slings
  - Lifts
- Traction
- Heat and cold therapy
- Immobilization devices
- Medication administration

Care of Immobilized Patient

An important overarching principle to emphasize is the need for early mobility. Early mobility requires a cultural mindset among interdisciplinary teams to overcome challenges and barriers associated with patient mobility. A study assessing barriers to early mobility among patients in an intensive care unit found that about 50% of barriers were patient-related factors (excessive sedation or delirium, morbid obesity, and multiple invasive devices) while a variety of care delivery factors represented other barriers including structural, intensive care unit culture, and process-related barriers such as fragmented care, availability of adequate equipment, time constraints, adequate number of providers, and concerns for patient safety.[21]

Many nursing interventions are incorporated into care for the immobilized patient, regardless of the underlying condition. Progressive mobility refers to the application of a mobility plan involving a series of gradual progressive interventions and activities that include positioning, turning, continuous lateral rotation therapy (CLRT), range-of-motion exercise, head elevation, tilt table, chair position, dangling, and ambulation. The patient should be positioned with appropriate *body alignment*. This is important to prevent injury to extremities and joints and is critical to prevent pulmonary complications. For example, pillows are commonly used to support the body alignment of a patient placed in a Sims position. The patient should be *repositioned* at least once every 2 hours. Principles of safe patient handling should be applied when patients are moved for repositioning. The patient dependent on caregivers for positioning is at significant risk for skin breakdown because of prolonged pressure over bony prominences. Thus, *skin care* is a priority for immobilized patients; the skin should be kept clean, dry, and protected to prevent skin breakdown. The skin is regularly monitored and examined for evidence of adequate circulation.

Because immobilized patients are at risk for stasis pneumonia, coughing and deep breathing are part of the standard treatment plan. Patients with adequate cognition are encouraged to use an incentive spirometer every hour to maintain ventilator capacity. Rotational bed therapy and CLRT have been shown to reduce the incidence of pneumonia among patients receiving mechanical ventilation in intensive care settings.[22,23]

Bed exercises should be encouraged to the extent possible to minimize atrophy and maintain joint movement. Many types of exercise can be done, including flexion and extension of the foot to promote venous blood return and to prevent venous stasis. If a patient has a trapeze bar over the bed, pull-up exercise should be encouraged if he or she is able. Range-of-motion (ROM) exercise is critical to promote circulation and to minimize complications to the joints. Active ROM is performed by the patient; assisted ROM involves a patient doing most of the exercise but under the guidance/assistance of a health professional. Passive ROM involves the nurse taking each affected joint through the full range of motion. It is important not to force the joints past the point of resistance. If tolerated, patients should be encouraged to stand at the side of the bed to promote weight bearing. Doing this a few times a day for a few minutes helps to reduce bone demineralization.

Exercise Therapy

Exercise therapy is a cornerstone intervention in the management of individuals with mobility impairment. The overall goal of exercise therapy is rehabilitative (relieving symptoms and/or improving/restoring ROM, strength, and balance) or preventive. Several forms of exercise therapy exist, including the following: Exercise Therapy: Ambulation; Exercise Therapy: Joint Mobility; Exercise Therapy: Stretching; and Exercise Therapy: Balance. Specific examples of exercise therapy include ROM exercises mentioned previously, stretching, weight lifting, water exercise, and gait training. Specific exercise therapy interventions are planned, structured, and repetitive; these are customized to address the needs of each patient. Exercise therapy is performed by nurses, occupational therapists, and physical therapists in acute care, community-based, and home care settings.

Pharmacologic Agents

Many of the drugs used to treat mobility problems are for the relief of pain or inflammation or to treat underlying conditions. It is beyond the scope of this concept presentation to describe each drug separately, but general categories are briefly presented.

Anti-inflammatory agents. Inflammation is a common primary or secondary finding among conditions leading to changes in mobility, from an underlying autoimmune condition to a traumatic injury. Oral antiinflammatory agents, such as corticosteroids and nonsteroidal anti-inflammatory drugs (NSAIDs), are by far the most commonly used agents. Corticosteroid injections into a joint space (such as ankle, knee, hip, wrist, elbow, shoulder, and spine) may be effective in reducing inflammation (and subsequently pain) associated with a number of conditions. However, because repeated corticosteroid injections might cause damage to cartilage, the number of injections into a joint is typically limited. Another group of agents used to reduce inflammation are the immunomodulators. These function to weaken or modulate the activity of the immune system, thereby decreasing the inflammatory response.

Analgesics. Although a reduction in inflammation provides some relief of discomfort associated with inflammation, analgesic agents are an important component of drug therapy. Agents that are specific for analgesia include opioids (e.g., morphine), NSAIDs, and aspirin.

Muscle relaxants. Several medications are used to provide relief from discomfort associated with skeletal muscle spasms. These agents act as central nervous system depressants and reduce nerve transmission to skeletal muscles, thus promoting muscle relaxation. The most common indication for muscle relaxants is for acute, non-specific low back pain. Common agents include baclofen, chlorazoxazone, carisoprodol, cyclobenaprine, dantrolene, and tizanidine.

Supplements. In addition to adequate dietary intake, nutritional supplementation with vitamin D and calcium is a useful prevention and treatment measure for osteoporosis, particularly for postmenopausal women. Bisphosphonates are antiresorptive agents that slow or stop the reabsorption of calcium from the bone, resulting in maintained or increased bone density and strength. These agents are used to treat osteoporosis.

Surgical Interventions

Many conditions that affect mobility are treated with surgical intervention. Surgical intervention can be either curative or palliative, depending on the underlying cause.[24] Examples of surgical interventions related to mobility/immobility include arthroscopic procedures, open and/or closed reduction of a fracture with or without external and/or internal fixation, amputation, synovectomy, osteotomy, debridement, arthroplasty, arthrodesis, diskectomy, and spinal fusion. Specific details about these procedures can be found in medical–surgical textbooks.

Immobilization

Following an injury or surgery, immobilization of a joint or bone is often necessary to provide stability and hold the appendage in place so that healing can occur. Following a fracture, for example, bone remodeling takes several weeks before the fracture is stable. Immobilization is necessary to enhance the healing process, to protect the bone from further injury, and to provide comfort to the patient. Common examples of immobile devices include casts, splints, abductor pillows, shoulder restraints, braces, and traction. Assessment to verify adequate perfusion (the presence of pulse and/or rapid capillary refill in nail beds), movement, and sensation is critical. Another indication for immobilization is to prevent injury. For example, for all patients with suspected spinal injury, spinal immobilization is routinely applied in the prehospital setting by strapping the patient on a backboard and using a cervical collar to prevent head rotation.

Assistive Devices and Patient Handling Technology

Assistive devices are objects to provide assistance with a task. Many types of assistive devices are commonly used in patient care, including assistive devices for ambulation and for activities of daily living. Common assistive devices to enhance mobility include canes, crutches, walkers, wheelchairs, grabbing/reaching devices, power-operated vehicles, prostheses.[25] Patients must be taught to use these devices correctly to avoid injury.

Patient handling technology refers to a variety of equipment in the care environment designed to assist with the handling and movement of patients. Examples include transfer mats, slings, and lifts. Education and training on indications and use of these devises, including assessment and decision algorithms for equipment selection, are essential to ensure the safety of the patient and the healthcare providers.

Other Therapies

Transcutaneous electric nerve stimulation. Transcutaneous electric nerve stimulation (TENS) is a therapeutic intervention involving low-voltage electrical current for the relief of pain. Electrodes are placed on the patient's skin near the area of pain; the electrical current creates electrical impulses that travel along the nerve fiber, which is thought to send a signal to the brain that blocks pain signals. TENS is often used for the treatment of joint pain such as osteoarthritis (OA), tendinitis, back pain, and neck pain.

Thermotherapy. Another common collaborative intervention is thermotherapy. Heat therapy involves the application of moist or dry heat (heating pad, warm water bottle, warm bath) to the skin surface. The heat causes a dilation of blood vessels that promotes blood flow and helps to relax muscles that are tight. It is particularly effective for symptomatic relief muscle pain and inflammation (e.g., osteoarthritis, strains, tendonitis, pain or spasms in the back or neck), but is not indicated for a new injury or open wound. Cold therapy involves the application of a cold compress (or immersion in cold water) to an area of inflammation. It causes vasoconstriction of underlying blood vessels to reduce inflammation and is most effective for recent injuries (e.g., a pulled muscle, muscle strain, or sprain). Cold therapy should not be used on an open wound or with vascular disease or injury, and is not generally recommended for low back pain.

INTERRELATED CONCEPTS

Mobility links to numerous concepts. Those considered most important are shown in Fig. 25.3 and discussed further.

Individuals who have inadequate **Gas Exchange** may experience reduced mobility because of excessive fatigue. Immobile patients are at risk of developing complications associated with gas exchange, such as stasis pneumonia due to reduced lung expansion. The brain controls movement, coordination, and balance. Thus, optimal mobility is dependent on an intact neurologic system. Individuals who have problems associated with **Intracranial Regulation** may become immobile as a result of unsteadiness, imbalance, or the inability to initiate or execute purposeful movement to the arms, legs, or trunk. Individuals who are immobile may be unable to purchase, prepare, and/or consume adequate **Nutrition**; likewise, individuals with inadequate nutrition may have decreased mobility because of excessive fatigue. Malnutrition can lead to muscle wasting and bone loss. In addition, individuals experiencing extended immobility often experience reduced appetite. **Pain** (acute or chronic) may interfere with mobility. For example, an individual with chronic pain associated with cancer or back pain may experience changes in mobility as a pain management strategy. Likewise, some conditions that are directly associated with immobility (e.g., a fracture) are very painful. Individuals who have impaired **Perfusion** are less able to be mobile because of reduced oxygenated blood reaching peripheral tissues. Among individuals who are immobile, perfusion is less effective because of reduced venous return (which increases the risk for venous clots) and because of extended pressure on tissue. Immobility is a significant risk factor for impaired **Tissue Integrity**. Extended pressure on bony prominences reduces the perfusion of oxygenated blood (especially on the sacrum, hips, elbows, and heel), and skin sheering from movement and transfers may occur, particularly with extended immobility. Individuals who are immobile may have changes to their pattern of **Elimination** or be at risk of experiencing problems such as constipation or urinary retention. This often leads to discomfort and reduced appetite that could negatively affect nutritional intake.

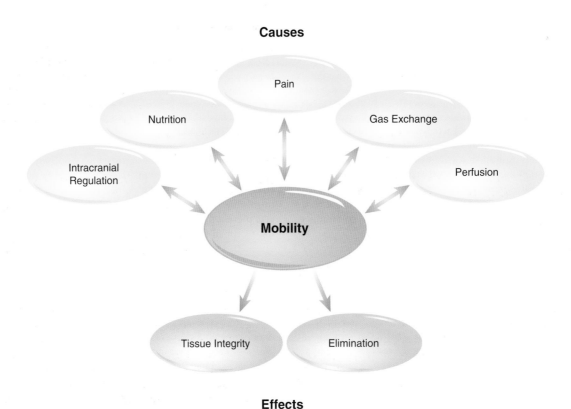

FIGURE 25.3 Cause-and-Effect Model: Mobility and Interrelated Concepts.

BOX 25.1 EXEMPLARS OF IMPAIRED MOBILITY

Congenital Defects
- Club foot
- Developmental dysplasia of the hip
- Metatarsus adductus
- Spina bifida
- Syndactyly

Skeletal Conditions
- Amputation
- Fracture
- Fibrosarcoma
- Osteochondroma
- Osteosarcoma
- Osteomalacia
- Osteomyelitis
- Osteoporosis
- Osteogenesis imperfecta
- Rickets

Muscle Conditions
- Disuse atrophy
- Fibromyalgia
- Myotonia
- Myositis
- Rhabdomyoma
- Rhabdomyosarcoma

Back and Spine Conditions
- Spinal cord injury
- Herniated disk
- Intervertebral disk disease
- Low back pain (acute/chronic)
- Scoliosis
- Spinal stenosis

Neuromuscular Dysfunction
- Amyotrophic lateral sclerosis
- Cerebral palsy
- Guillain–Barré syndrome
- Huntington disease
- Multiple sclerosis
- Muscular dystrophy
- Myasthenia gravis
- Parkinson disease

Joint and Connective Tissue Conditions
- Sprains
- Tendonitis
- Joint dislocation
- Osteoarthritis
- Rheumatoid arthritis
- Juvenile idiopathic arthritis
- Gout

 ACCESS EXEMPLAR LINKS IN YOUR GIDDENS EBOOK

CLINICAL EXEMPLARS

Many clinical exemplars related to mobility and impaired mobility exist and are seen in all population groups. The following featured exemplars provide a brief explanation of classic conditions causing immobility. Detailed explanations and the nursing care for these conditions are presented in medical–surgical, pediatric, and gerontology resources. Box 25.1 presents additional common exemplars across the lifespan.

Featured Exemplars
Osteoarthritis

OA is caused by gradual degenerative changes of the joint (cartilage, joint lining, ligaments, and bone), usually affecting weight-bearing joints (hips, knees, and vertebra) and hands. These changes lead to pain, swelling, and reduced mobility of the joint. It most commonly affects middle-aged and older adults, and typically begins after age 40 years; OA is estimated to affect 33% of adults older than age 65 years.[26]

Rheumatoid Arthritis

Rheumatoid arthritis (RA) is a systemic autoimmune condition with genetic predisposition that creates an inflammatory process in the synovial membrane of the joints and other body tissues. Over time, the joint inflammation leads to erosion of the membrane and cartilage, causing pain, swelling, and joint deformity; significant impairment in mobility can result. Affecting less than 1% of the general population, RA is most common among women and individuals older than age 60 years.[27]

Juvenile Idiopathic Arthritis

Juvenile idiopathic arthritis (JIA) represents a group of diseases characterized by chronic inflammation of joints from autoimmune conditions. Depending on severity and duration, JIA can cause significant disability, with joint deformity, mobility impairments, and physical disability. It affects children younger than age 16 years, with a peak onset between ages 1 and 2; girls are affected at a rate twice that of boys. It is estimated that 294,000 children under the age of 18 have JIA; fortunately, many children and adolescents afflicted with this condition often experience remission.[28]

Bone Fracture

Bone fracture refers to a partial or complete disruption in the bone structure. Interruption of bone structure leads to a reduction or loss in movement and pain. Although fractures are usually the result of traumatic injury, spontaneous fractures can occur in the presence of bone disease (e.g., osteoporosis or a neoplasm). Fractures occur at any age, but they are unusual during infancy. Most fractures occur in children and adolescents and adults older than age 65 years (wrist and hip fractures as a result of falls).

Parkinson Disease

Parkinson disease (PD) is a neurologic disorder associated with a loss of dopamine production in the brain. This disorder leads to changes in mobility resulting from muscular tremor, rigidity of the extremities and trunk, slowness of movement, and impaired coordination and balance. Mobility impairment increases with disease progression. Typically, PD affects adults older than age 50 years, with a higher incidence among men than women.

Spinal Cord Injury

Spinal cord injury (SCI) is an injury to the spinal cord that runs through the spinal column. Depending on the degree of injury, SCI may result in temporary or permanent neurologic impairment and mobility. The primary cause of SCI is traumatic injury from motor vehicle accidents, falls, sports, or personal violence. SCI can occur at any age, but males between the ages of 15 and 40 years account for the highest percentage of those affected.[29]

Low Back Pain

Low back pain is one of the most common conditions affecting mobility; nearly all individuals experience low back pain at some point during their life. Back pain generally is caused by muscle, bone, or nerve irritation from a variety of conditions, including muscle strain or spasm, degenerative conditions (e.g., arthritis, stenosis, or intervertebral disc disease), and trauma; it is also a common symptom in late-term pregnancy. Severe back pain can be debilitating and can significantly impair mobility. Back pain can occur in all age groups, but it is most common between ages 30 and 50 years.

CASE STUDY

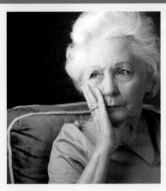

Case Presentation

Mrs. Lydia Martin, an 88-year-old widow, lives alone independently in her single-story home. During the middle of the night, Mrs. Martin fell in her home while walking to the bathroom. Unable to get up, she crawled to reach her phone and dialed 911. She was transported to the emergency department and underwent diagnostic tests including hip and femur x-ray and computed tomography, which confirmed a left femoral neck fracture. Her past medical history includes anxiety, osteoporosis, arthritis, and cataracts.

Mrs. Martin underwent an open reduction internal fixation procedure. Following surgery, she had a compression dressing with ice to the left hip, a Foley catheter, antiembolism stockings, a sequential compression device, and an order to use the incentive spirometer every hour while awake. Her medications included hydrocodone bitartrate 7.5 mg/acetaminophen 750 mg (Vicodin ES) two tabs by mouth every 4 hours as needed for pain and enoxaparin (Lovenox) 40 mg daily subcutaneously.

The day after surgery, the physical therapist began to work with Mrs. Martin; the goal of the session was to get her out of bed to a chair. During the attempted transfer, Mrs. Martin's surgical site was painful, and her Foley catheter was pulled, causing pelvic pain. She screamed in pain and refused to continue the process. Mrs. Martin was anxious and fearful of pain and became worried that she would never walk again and would end up in a nursing home. She was unwilling to move and declined physical therapy over the next 3 days. Mrs. Martin became constipated and lost her appetite. She also developed a stage 2 pressure ulcer over her sacrum. Eventually, on post-op day 4, Mrs. Martin agreed to work with the physical therapist. By this time, she experienced significant weakness and fatigue and was unable to move independently. Mrs. Martin was later transferred to a rehabilitation center to continue regaining her mobility.

Case Analysis Questions

1. Did Mrs. Martin have any risk factors prior to her injury? If so, what were they?
2. What complications emerged as a result of Mrs. Martin's immobility?
3. How do the collaborative interventions help to improve her mobility?

From Stockbyte/Digital Vision/Thinkstock.

 ACCESS EXEMPLAR LINKS IN YOUR GIDDENS EBOOK

REFERENCES

1. Venes, D. (Ed.), (2013). *Taber's cyclopedic medical dictionary* (22th ed.). Philadelphia: Davis.
2. Herdman, T. H., & Kamitsuru, S. (2018). *Nursing diagnoses definitions and classifications 2018-2020* (11th ed.). New York: Thieme.
3. Bortz, W. M. (1984). The disuse syndrome. *The Western Journal of Medicine, 141*(5), 691–694.
4. Banasik, J. L., & Copstead, L. C. (2019). *Pathophysiology* (6th ed.). St Louis: Elsevier.
5. McCance, K. L., & Huether, S. E. (2019). *Pathophysiology: The biologic basis for disease in adults and children* (8th ed.). St Louis: Elsevier.
6. Hockenberry, M. J., Rodgers, C. C., & Wilson, D. (2017). *Wong's essentials of pediatric nursing* (10th ed.). St Louis: Mosby.
7. Hill, J. (2008). Cardiac plasticity: Mechanisms of disease. *The New England Journal of Medicine, 358*(13), 1370–1380.
8. Centers for Disease Control and Prevention. *Hip fractures among older adults,* 2016. Retrieved from http://www.cdc.gov/homeandrecreationalsafety/falls/adulthipfx.html.
9. Nguyen, T. Q., Simpson, P. M., & Gabbe, B. J. (2017). The prevalence of pre-existing mental health, drug and alcohol conditions in major trauma patients. *Australian Health Review, 41*(3), 283–290.
10. Wilson, S., & Giddens, J. (2017). *Health assessment for nursing practice* (6th ed.). St Louis: Elsevier.
11. Pagana, K. D., & Pagana, T. J. (2018). *Mosby's manual of diagnostic and laboratory tests* (6th ed.). St Louis: Elsevier.
12. Office of Disease Prevention and Health Promotion. *Healthy People 2030.* Retrieved from https://www.healthypeople.gov/2020/About-Healthy-People/Development-Healthy-People-2030/Framework.
13. Pender, N., Murdaugh, C., & Parsons, M. A. (2015). *Health promotion in nursing practice* (7th ed.). Upper Saddle River, NJ: Pearson.
14. U.S. Preventive Services Task Force. *Final Update Summary: Osteoporosis to Prevent Fractures: Screening.* U.S. Preventive Services Task Force. June 2018. Retrieved from https://www.uspreventiveservicestaskforce.org/Page/Document/UpdateSummaryFinal/osteoporosis-screening1.
15. Scott, V., Votova, K., Scanlan, A., et al. (2007). Multifactorial and functional mobility assessment tools for fall risk among older adults in community, home-support, long-term and acute care settings. *Age Aging, 36*(2), 130–139.
16. Park, S. H. (2018). Tools for assessing fall risk in the elderly: A systematic review and meta-analysis. *Aging Clinical and Experimental Research, 30*(1), 1–16.
17. Wall, J. C., Bell, B. S., Campbell, S., et al. (2000). The timed get-up-and-go test revisited: Measurement of component tasks. *Journal of Rehabilitation Research and Development, 37*(1), 109–111.
18. Tinetti, M. E. (1986). Performance-oriented assessment of mobility problems in elderly patients. *Journal of the American Geriatrics Society, 34*(2), 119–126.
19. Czaplijski, T., Marshburnm, D., Hobs, T., et al. (2014). Creating a culture of mobility: An interdisciplinary approach for hospitalized patients. *Hospital Topics, 92*(3), 74–79.
20. American Nurses Association. (2013). *Safe patient handling and mobility: Interprofessional national standards across the care continuum.* Washington, DC: Author.
21. Dubb, R., Nydahl, P., Hermes, C., et al. (2016). Barriers and strategies for early mobilization of patients in intensive care units. *Annuals of the American Thoracic Society, 13*(5), 724–730.
22. Goldhill, D. R., Imhoff, M., McLean, B., et al. (2007). Rotational bed therapy to prevent and treat respiratory complications: A review and meta-analysis. *American Journal of Critical Care, 16*(1), 50–61.
23. Wanless, S., & Matthew, A. (2011). Continuous lateral rotation therapy—A review. *Nursing in Critical Care, 12*(1), 28–35.
24. Lewis, S. L., Bucher, L., Heitkemper, M., et al. (2017). *Medical–surgical nursing: Assessment and management of clinical problems* (10th ed.). St Louis: Elsevier.

25. Olatinwo, O. M. (2012). Assistive devices for independence in the elderly: A case series. *Clinical Geriatrics, 20*(12). Retrieved from https://www.consultant360.com/articles/assistive-devices-independence-elderly-case-series//0/1.

26. Centers for Disease Control and Prevention. *Arthritis*, 2018. Retrieved from https://www.cdc.gov/arthritis/basics/osteoarthritis.htm.

27. Center for Disease Control and Prevention. *Rheumatoid Arthritis*, 2018. Retrieved from https://www.cdc.gov/arthritis/basics/rheumatoid-arthritis.html.

28. National Institute of Health. *Juvenile Arthritis*, 2015. Retrieved from https://www.niams.nih.gov/health-topics/juvenile-arthritis.

29. National Spinal Cord Injury Statistical Center. *Spinal cord injury facts and figures at a glance*, 2017. Retrieved from https://www.nscisc.uab.edu/Public/Facts%20and%20Figures%20-%202017.pdf.

Tissue Integrity

Debra Hagler

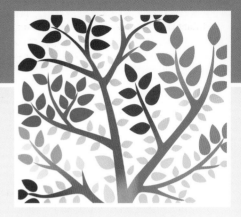

The skin supports critical life functions including management of temperature, conservation of fluid, and protection from infection.[1] Nurses play a pivotal role in helping persons of all ages to maintain healthy skin and tissue. When an individual experiences disruption of tissue integrity, nurses contribute independently and collaboratively to manage the care.

DEFINITION

Tissues are organized groups of cells with common functions. Of the four types of tissues—muscle, neural, connective, and epithelial—the concept of tissue integrity is most closely aligned with epithelial tissue. The term *impaired skin integrity* is specifically focused on damage to the epidermal and dermal layers of epithelial tissue, but deep damage to skin integrity is associated with disruption of underlying tissues. For the purposes of this concept presentation, tissue integrity is defined as *the state of structurally intact and physiologically functioning epithelial tissues, such as the integument (including the skin and subcutaneous tissue) and mucous membranes.* The term *impaired tissue integrity* reflects varying levels of damage to one or more of those groups of cells.[2,3]

SCOPE

The concept of tissue integrity ranges from an intact state serving as the body's protective barrier to some level of disrupted or impaired surface. Disrupted tissue integrity ranges from superficial or partial-thickness injury of the epidermis to deep or full-thickness injury of the dermis and deeper tissues (Fig. 26.1). Individuals at all points across the lifespan experience disruptions to tissue integrity.

NORMAL PHYSIOLOGICAL PROCESS

The skin is the largest organ of the body. Epithelial cells join to cover nearly every internal and external surface of the body, providing protection from the external environment, absorption of needed substances, secretion into body cavities, and excretion of wastes. The skin, as an external surface, protects other tissues and organs from mechanical trauma, fluid loss, chemical disruption, and infectious organisms. The nerves in the skin layer provide a safety mechanism as sensations of pain, temperature, and touch inform a person about the environment and reveal the need to take actions that prevent or limit damage to the body. The integument is made up of the two layers commonly known

as skin—the epidermis and the dermis—and the underlying subcutaneous or fat tissue (Fig. 26.2). Sweat glands and the small muscles in the dermal layer that control piloerection (goosebumps) help to maintain body temperature within a fairly narrow range despite air temperature changes. Subcutaneous tissue, under the dermal layer, contains fat cells and additional sweat glands that assist in temperature regulation.

Mucous membranes are epithelial tissues continuous with the skin that line the eyelids, nose and mouth, ears, genital area, urethra, and anus. Some but not all mucous membranes secrete thick, slippery mucus that helps to protect the body from infection.[1]

Age-Related Differences
Infants, Children, and Adolescents

Skin texture and function change over the course of the lifespan. Infants have thinner, more permeable skin with less subcutaneous fat than older children and adults, which leads to a greater potential for fluid loss and less effective temperature regulation. The skin texture of infants and young children is smooth and dry. Apocrine glands are nonfunctional until puberty. Adolescents experience increased apocrine sweat glands and sebaceous gland activity, resulting in more oily skin and acne.[4]

Older Adults

Several changes to the skin occur as a result of the aging process. The skin becomes thin, with a decrease in strength, moisture, and elasticity. A decrease in underlying supportive structures such as lean muscle mass and subcutaneous fat often results in skin wrinkling or hanging loosely over other tissues. A diminished perception of pain may prevent early recognition of injury, and reduced arterial and venous blood flow to the tissues not only make skin more prone to injury but also may result in slow wound healing when a disruption of skin occurs. In addition, the growth of hair and nails slows with aging, and a decrease in sebaceous gland activity can result in rough, dry, itchy skin.[4] The aging process of skin is partly influenced by genetics and race, but it is also largely associated with environmental exposure—particularly to sun and wind.[1]

VARIATIONS AND CONTEXT

Six major categories of impaired tissue integrity are trauma/injury, loss of perfusion, immunological reaction, infections and infestations, thermal or radiation injury, and lesions. Within each of these categories, partial- or full-thickness injury can occur.

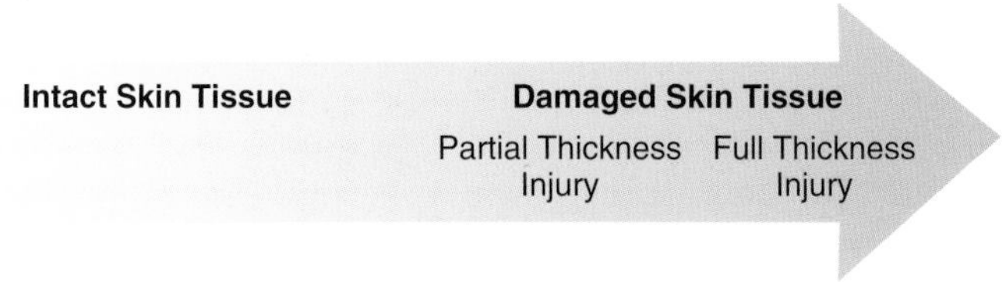

Intact Skin Tissue → **Damaged Skin Tissue**
Partial Thickness Injury   Full Thickness Injury

FIGURE 26.1 Scope of Tissue Integrity. Tissue integrity ranges from intact skin to partial-thickness injury and full-thickness injury.

Trauma/Injury

Tissue trauma or injury includes intentional and unintentional damage that can range from a superficial abrasion or scrape to a deep wound penetrating the skin and subcutaneous layers, with possible extension to muscle, internal organs, and bone. In areas where there is little or no subcutaneous tissue (e.g., the back of the hand, top of the foot, or skull), a relatively minor blunt or penetrating injury may extend directly through the skin layers to the muscle or bone. A surgical incision is an example of an intentional injury to the skin, inflicted to reach deeper structures for a therapeutic purpose.

Loss of Perfusion

All tissue requires a continuous supply of oxygenated blood. The skin is relatively tolerant of poor circulation compared with other organs; in times of shock, it even survives a temporary shunting of oxygenated blood away from the skin to protect the perfusion of other organs, such

as the heart and brain. However, prolonged poor perfusion or a shorter period of no perfusion can lead to tissue necrosis. Examples of impaired tissue integrity from chronic poor perfusion include ulcerations, necrosis, and loss of digits. Examples of short-term or temporary disruption of perfusion to tissue caused by unrelieved pressure are pressure ulcers/pressure injuries. Tissue damage may be caused by a number of factors, including excessive pressure, but a dermal ulcer is not necessarily caused by pressure alone.[5]

Immunologic Reaction

The skin is a visible indicator of an allergic response to a foreign substance, and the presence of redness, rash, or hives is a common way in which allergies are first noted. Common substances that lead to skin irritation and/or local allergic response are soaps, detergents, cleaning products, fragrances, and metals such as nickel, silver, and copper.[1] In addition, many common skin disruptions, such as psoriasis, are thought to be chronic immune responses to unknown antigens. In rare cases, a hypersensitivity response to a medication can cause extensive tissue sloughing. Severe hypersensitivity disorders such as Stevens-Johnson syndrome or toxic epidermal necrolysis involve large areas of epidermal tissue sloughing with a high risk for life-threatening fluid loss, hypothermia, and infection.[1]

Infections and Infestations

Acute skin infections are the most common dermatological conditions seen during emergency department visits in the United States.[6] Skin and mucous membrane infections can be the result of bacteria, fungi, or viruses. Live arthropods can cause tissue disruption by burrowing

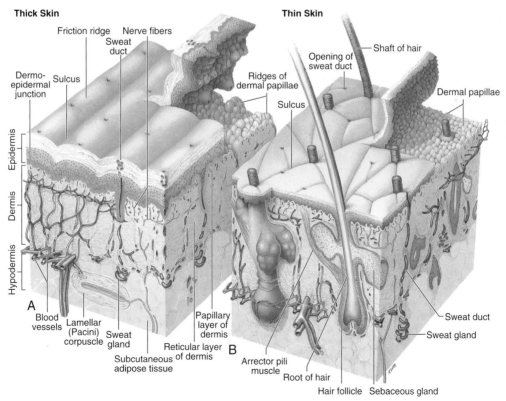

FIGURE 26.2 Diagram of Skin Structure. (A) Thick skin, found on surfaces of the palms and soles of the feet. (B) Thin skin, found on most surface areas of the body. In each diagram, the epidermis is raised at one corner to reveal the papillae of the dermis. (From Patton, K. T., & Thibodeau, G. A. [2016]. *Anatomy and physiology* [9th ed.]. St. Louis: Mosby.)

under the skin or attaching to skin structures such as hair shafts. Tissue damage from infestation and the resulting scratching behavior increase the risk of secondary infection.

Bacterial Infection

Bacteria that are normally present on the skin generally cause no harm, but pathogenic bacteria can cause superficial or deep infection. A small abrasion or lesion can provide a portal for opportunistic or pathogenic infectious organisms to infect deeper tissues. Superficial skin infections involve only the dermis, but deeper bacterial infection causes cellulitis, an inflammation of the subcutaneous tissues and potentially also muscle tissues. Impetigo, caused by staphylococci or β-hemolytic streptococci, is the most common superficial bacterial infection, and it spreads easily among small children on contact. A common bacterial infection of the skin seen in adolescents is acne vulgaris.

Fungal Infections

The fungi that cause superficial fungal infections live on the dead skin cells of the epidermis. *Candida albicans* and other *Candida* species thrive in warm, moist areas of the skin and mucous membranes, particularly the mouth, vagina, and skin folds. In the absence of the bacterial protection of normal flora on the skin or mucous membranes, *Candida* grow more readily. It is common for a person to experience a fungal infection with *Candida* after a course of antibiotics for a bacterial infection has decreased the normal protective flora and allowed *Candida* to flourish. *Tinea* refers to a group of diseases caused by a fungus; these conditions vary with skin sites and the types of fungal species, such as tinea capitis on the head and tinea pedis (athlete's foot) on the feet.[1]

Viral Infections

Several viruses cause disruptions in skin integrity. A common form of skin virus is the verruca, or wart. Although warts most commonly occur on the skin of the hands and feet, they can also be found on the genitalia. Herpes simplex virus (HSV) can infect the skin and mucous membranes; HSV type 1 (HSV-1) is more common on the face and mouth, whereas HSV-2 is more common on the genital mucosa.[1]

Infestations

The skin can be infested with live arthropods such as mites and lice. The scabies mite burrows into the epidermis and lays eggs. Mites are transmitted person-to-person or through infested sheets or clothing, where they can live for up to 2 days. Lice most commonly infect the body, head, or pubic hair. Lice lay eggs along the hair shafts and are transmitted by personal contact, clothing and bedding, and shared hair care items or hats.[1]

Thermal or Radiation Injury

Thermal and radiation injuries to the skin range from the common sunburn to extensive scald burns and radiation burns. Sunburn appears after the epidermis has been exposed to excessive ultraviolet (UV) radiation. It appears as redness and inflammation and may extend to blistering—with chills, fever, and pain—followed by peeling skin. Burns resulting from a scald with hot liquids or contact with flame and/or heated items cause a series of chemical and mechanical events at the tissue level. Radiation therapy, used to treat some forms of cancer, requires careful monitoring and skin care to prevent burns.

The initial tissue response to burns is inflammation and vasoconstriction; edema at the site of a burn can last for several days. Later, fibroblasts produce the proteins collagen and elastin, which restore some structure and elasticity to the wound. Macrophages remove bacteria and foreign substances to clean the wound. New vascular networks form and new epithelial cells grow and cover the open area from the burn wound edges to the center as the wound begins to contract.[7]

Lesions

Lesions can range from benign skin growths and vascular lesions to invasive malignant tumors. The most common types of skin cancers are melanoma, basal cell carcinoma, and squamous cell carcinoma.[8] Benign skin growths may be of concern if they cause pressure on or displacement of other structures or change the person's appearance in a distressing way.

Expected Physiological Process for Wound Healing

Tissue injuries and wounds heal by processes of primary, secondary, or tertiary intention. Healing by primary intention occurs when wound margins are well approximated, as in a sutured surgical incision or a simple laceration; it takes place more rapidly than the other types of healing. Healing by secondary intention occurs when wounds such as ulcerations have distant edges and granulation tissue gradually fills the gap to close the wound. Healing by tertiary intention occurs when a wound is sutured closed much later, resulting in more scarring than that which occurs for wounds closed with primary intention. Tertiary closure is used when a wound must stay open until infection or wound contamination is resolved; later, the clean wound is sutured to facilitate continued healing.

There are three phases of wound healing: inflammatory, granulation, and maturation. The inflammatory phase lasts 3 to 5 days, while blood clots form at the site of injury and platelets release growth factors to begin the healing process. A matrix of cells and debris forms at the site and is later removed by macrophages. During the granulation phase, new vessels and collagen structures are formed, resulting in a very vascular pink wound. White blood cells continue to remove debris, while the epithelium begins to grow from the edges toward the center of the wound. The maturation phase of collagen fiber remodeling and scar contraction may continue for months or years.[7]

CONSEQUENCES

When tissue integrity is impaired, a number of body functions are affected, including thermoregulation, elimination, fluid and electrolyte balance, protection from infection, safety, comfort/pain, and body image. The skin normally regulates body temperature within a narrow range through the constriction or relaxation of piloerector muscles, vasodilation or vasoconstriction of vessels in the dermis, and the production of sweat. In the absence of intact skin and underlying tissue, such as an overwhelming burn surface, the ability to regulate body heat and prevent excess fluid loss is impaired, requiring external maintenance of temperature and massive fluid replacement. Whether the skin is disrupted by a small abrasion or a massive wound, that loss of the skin as a barrier means that underlying structures are no longer protected from the environment's infectious and chemical dangers. Even a small open wound can provide a portal that could lead to an overwhelming infection if the person is immunocompromised or the infectious agent is particularly virulent. Loss of deep structures such as nerve endings prevents normal sensation, which provides cues about the environment and helps promote safety during movement. Because the skin has many sensory nerve endings, particularly over the hands and face, injuries and lesions can be painful. Skin conditions are often highly visible to the individual and others, potentially affecting body image and provoking psychological distress about one's physical appearance.[7]

RISK FACTORS

Age-Related Risks

Some risk factors for skin disruptions are related to age or developmental level. For example, diaper rash is a common rash among infants and toddlers; likewise, this age group is at risk for injuries to the skin and mucosa secondary to uncertain mobilization, the affinity for placing various objects in the mouth, and the inability to protect oneself from environmental dangers. Communicable skin infections such as impetigo are more commonly transmitted where there is frequent skin-to-skin contact, as in child care centers or on playgrounds. School-age children may experience frequent minor tissue injuries such as abrasions, bruises, and small lacerations that can occur during active play. Thermal and scald burns are among the most common types of injuries in children under 16 years of age.[9]

The changes to skin associated with aging are actually a result of sun and environmental damage over a long period of time, leading to a wrinkled and leathery appearance. Exposure of the skin to sun over an extended period of years increases the risk of skin cancers.[8] Older adults are also more prone to skin tears that can occur with minimal contact or pressure as a result of the skin's thin, fragile texture.[4]

Individual Risk Factors

Many individual risk factors for tissue disruption are associated with underlying health conditions. Health conditions associated with poor peripheral perfusion, malnutrition, obesity, fluid deficit or excess, impaired physical mobility, and immunosuppression increase the risk of tissue disruption. In addition, exposure to chemical irritants, radiation, excessively hot or cold temperatures, and mechanical damage may cause a loss of tissue integrity. Individuals who have undergone medical treatments, surgical procedures, or invasive procedures have disruptions to skin and tissue integrity as a result of those procedures.

Genetics

A number of inherited skin disorders are associated with an underlying metabolic condition or a chronic condition that affects many body systems. Examples of inheritable skin conditions include ichthyosis vulgaris, xeroderma pigmentosa, albinism, epidermolysis, ectodermal dysplasia, and incontinentia pigmenti.

Skin Cancer Risk

Basal cell skin cancer usually occurs in areas that have been exposed to the sun, such as the face, and is the most common skin cancer in light-skinned persons. Squamous cell skin cancer is usually found in areas less exposed to the sun, such as the legs or feet, and is the most common type of skin cancer in dark-skinned persons. Melanoma is a virulent and potentially life-threatening form of skin cancer that has a good prognosis if detected early. It begins in the pigment cells or melanocytes, can grow on any skin surface, and is found most commonly in men on the head, neck, and torso. In women, melanoma is more commonly found on the torso or the lower legs. Although rare in people with dark skin, when it does develop, melanoma is found under the nails and on the palms and soles. Fair-skinned men and women older than 65 years of age, persons with atypical moles, and those with more than 50 moles are at substantially increased risk for melanoma. Other risk factors for skin cancer include family history and a considerable history of sun exposure and sunburns.[10]

Pressure Injury Risk

A pressure injury is defined as "localized damage to the skin and underlying soft tissue usually over a bony prominence or related to a medical or other device. The injury can present as intact skin or an open ulcer and may be painful. The injury occurs as a result of intense and/or prolonged pressure or pressure in combination with shear."[11] Risk factors for pressure injuries include impaired cognition or sensory perception, immobility, friction and shearing, poor nutrition, impaired perfusion or oxygenation, impaired sensation, incontinence, and/or moisture. Certain medical conditions (many of which are associated with these risk factors) are also associated with increased risk (Box 26.1).

ASSESSMENT

Assessment of the skin involves taking a history, conducting a skin examination, and performing diagnostic testing.

History

The health history begins with questions related to past and current conditions, medications, known allergies, and family history. Medications may cause rashes through an allergic reaction, a side effect, or by inducing hypersensitivity to sunlight. Box 26.2 lists specific information about tissue integrity to discuss during the health history.

Examination Findings
Inspection

Examination of the skin starts with inspection, which includes color and the presence of lesions. Normal adult skin is a consistent color,

---

BOX 26.1   Common Conditions Associated with Pressure Injury or Dermal Ulcer Development

- Spinal cord injury
- Stroke or traumatic brain injury
- Musculoskeletal trauma/fracture
- Neuromuscular disorders
- Rheumatoid arthritis
- Alzheimer disease
- Heart failure
- Peripheral artery disease
- Chronic obstructive pulmonary disease
- Diabetes (types 1 and 2)

BOX 26.2   Health History Related to Tissue Integrity

- Previous history of skin disease
- Change in pigmentation
- Change in mole
- Change in nails
- Hair loss
- Excessive dryness or moisture
- Pruritus
- Excessive bruising
- Rash or lesion
- Self-care behaviors
- Medications
- Environmental or occupational hazards

From Jarvis, C. L. (2020). *Physical examination and health assessment* (8th ed.). Philadelphia: Saunders.

ranging from light pink to olive tones and deep brown, with relatively darker shades in areas of sun exposure. Oral and eye mucosa may appear pale pink to darker pink, red, or brown. Skin findings may vary by natural skin color; for example, cyanosis may appear as a blue-gray color in light-skinned persons, whereas it appears as an ashen gray color in dark-skinned persons and is particularly visible in the nail beds and mucosa. The more visible areas for identifying generalized changes in skin color for a dark-skinned person are those with the least pigmentation, particularly the subglossal mucosa, the buccal mucosa, the palpebral conjunctiva, and sclera.[4]

There is a wide range of types of skin lesions, including both normal variations and lesions that indicate possible disease. A bright light, a ruler, and a magnifying glass are helpful tools for skin inspection. Describe the location, size, shape, color, elevation, consistency, and pattern of lesions. Also, describe the grouping of multiple lesions in rings, lines, or diffusely scattered arrangements and the color, odor, and consistency of any exudates.[4]

Palpation

The skin should be smooth and intact, with an even surface and minimal perspiration or oiliness except after exercise or heat exposure. There should be no dryness, peeling, or cracking, although there may be calluses over the hands, feet, elbows, and knees. Skin folds should not be excessively moist or macerated. Skin mobility and turgor are assessed by picking up and slightly pinching the skin on the forearm or under the clavicle. The skin should move easily when lifted and should return to place immediately when released. Checking for skin turgor using the older adult's hand may give a false impression of dehydration, so turgor should be checked in the forearm or under the clavicle instead. The loss of subcutaneous tissue in the hands causes an appearance of skin tenting even when hydration is normal.[4]

Wound Assessment

Wounds may be caused by direct or indirect tissue injury. Assess the wound location, size, shape, and color as well as the color, odor, and consistency of any drainage or exudate. Redness of the surrounding tissue, foul odor, or purulent drainage may indicate wound infection.

A surgical wound may be left open to the air or covered with a dressing to protect the wound site and absorb drainage. Covered wounds should be carefully assessed when the wound is exposed during dressing changes. Describe the amount and character of any wound drainage.[7]

Assessment of dermal pressure injuries. Pressure injuries, a specific type of wound, are assessed for size and depth, as well as for level of tissue injury. Pressure injuries are classified by four stages, presented in Box 26.3. If the ulcer is covered with eschar,—a dry scab covering—it will not be possible to determine the stage of the wound. The eschar may have to be removed through pharmacological, mechanical, or surgical debridement to allow for the wound's accurate assessment and promote healing.[5]

Diagnostic Tests

Only a few common diagnostic tests are linked to the concept of tissue integrity:

- *Patch testing*: This is a test used to identify specific allergens causing contact dermatitis. One or many potential allergens can be tested simultaneously by applying a small amount of the substance to a marked area of the skin, usually on the back.
- *Wound cultures*: Cultures identify the organisms causing infection. Because some bacteria are present on healthy skin, normal skin flora may be identified in wound cultures along with any pathogenic bacteria.

BOX 26.3   Pressure Injury Stages from the National Pressure Ulcer Advisory Panel

Stage 1: Nonblanchable Erythema

Intact skin with a localized area of nonblanchable erythema, which may appear differently in darkly pigmented skin. Presence of blanchable erythema or changes in sensation, temperature, or firmness may precede visual changes. Color changes do not include purple or maroon discoloration; these may indicate deep tissue pressure injury (DTPI).

Stage 2: Partial Thickness

Partial-thickness loss of skin with exposed dermis. The wound bed is viable, pink or red, moist, and may also present as an intact or ruptured serum-filled blister. Adipose (fat) is not visible and deeper tissue is not visible. Granulation tissue, slough, and eschar, are not present. These injuries commonly result from adverse microclimate and shear in the skin over the pelvis and shear in the heel.

Stage 3: Full-thickness Skin Loss

Full-thickness skin loss in which adipose (fat) is visible in the ulcer and granulation tissue and epibole (rolled wound edges) is often present. Slough and/or eschar may be visible. The depth of tissue damage varies by anatomical location; areas of significant adiposity can develop deep wounds. Undermining and tunneling may occur. Fascia, muscle, tendon, ligament, cartilage, or bone is not exposed. If slough or eschar obscures the extent of tissue loss, this is an unstageable pressure injury.

Stage 4: Full-thickness Tissue Loss

Full-thickness skin and tissue loss with exposed or directly palpable fascia, muscle, tendon, ligament, cartilage, or bone in the ulcer. Slough and/or eschar may be visible. Epibole (rolled edges), undermining, and/or tunneling often occur. Depth varies by anatomical location. If slough or eschar obscures the extent of tissue loss, this is an unstageable pressure injury.

Unstageable Pressure Injury: Obscured full-thickness skin and tissue loss

Full-thickness skin and tissue loss in which the extent of tissue damage within the ulcer cannot be confirmed because it is obscured by slough or eschar. If slough or eschar is removed, a stage 3 or 4 pressure injury will be revealed. Stable eschar (i.e., dry, adherent, intact, without erythema or fluctuance) on ischemic limb or heels should not be softened or removed.

Deep Tissue Pressure Injury (DTPI): Persistent nonblanchable deep red, maroon, or purple discoloration

Intact or nonintact skin with localized area of persistent nonblanchable deep red, maroon, and/or purple discoloration or epidermal separation revealing a dark wound bed or blood-filled blister. Pain and temperature change often precede skin color changes. Discoloration may appear differently in darkly pigmented skin. This injury results from intense and/or prolonged pressure and shear forces at the bone-muscle interface. The wound may evolve rapidly to reveal the actual extent of tissue injury or may resolve without tissue loss. If necrotic tissue, subcutaneous tissue, granulation tissue, fascia, muscle, or other underlying structures are visible, this indicates a full-thickness pressure injury (unstageable, stage 3 or 4). Do not use DTPI to describe vascular, traumatic, neuropathic, or dermatologic conditions.

From National Pressure Ulcer Advisory Panel: NPUAP Pressure Injury Stages. (2016). Copyright NPUAP, used with permission. Retrieved from http://www.npuap.org/resources/educational-and-clinical-resources/npuap-pressure-injury-stages/

- *Tissue biopsy*: Various types of biopsies—such as punch, incision, excision, and shave—are conducted for pathological evaluation of tissue when skin lesions are suspected to be malignant. The type and depth of biopsy are based on the lesion and the location.
- *Woods lamp*: Use of a Woods lamp (black light) or immunofluorescence enhances inspection with magnification and special lighting. It is used to identify the presence of infectious organisms and proteins.[7]

CLINICAL MANAGEMENT

Primary Prevention

Primary prevention measures guard against the development of disease. Primary measures to prevent disrupted tissue integrity include hygiene, nutrition, and protection from excessive sun exposure or other environmental hazards.

General Skin Hygiene

Basic skin hygiene prevents many common skin irritations and infections. Infants and toddlers need frequent cleansing of the hands and face to remove food residue and frequent perineal care to prevent irritation from urine and stool. During adolescence, sebaceous and sweat glands become more active; therefore more frequent bathing becomes necessary to reduce body odors and oils. In older adults, sebaceous and sweat glands become less active again and skin loses some of its moisture and elasticity. Older adults may find that a complete daily bath with soap can cause excessively dry skin; therefore they may prefer to bathe less frequently and use a gentle moisturizing cleanser.

Hygiene practices are often linked to cultural norms and rituals. Although in North America it is common to bathe or shower daily and to use deodorant, people of a variety of cultures may prefer to bathe less frequently or not bathe at all when they are ill or after childbirth.[12]

Nutrition

Adequate protein, calories, minerals, vitamins, and hydration are needed for maintenance of healthy skin. In the chronic absence of adequate nutrition, skin becomes dry and flaky, hair appears dull, and subcutaneous fat disappears. Even a short period of poor nutrition, such as being unable to eat before and after surgery, can damage tissue integrity and delay wound healing.[7]

Sun Exposure

Box 26.4 lists National Cancer Institute recommendations for skin cancer prevention through protection from sun exposure. Population-based interventions designed to increase sun-protective behaviors in recreational settings include offering culturally relevant educational materials and reminders at the entrances to the setting; providing sun-safety training for—and role modeling by—lifeguards, aquatic instructors, recreation staff, parents, and children; increasing the availability of shaded areas; and having sunscreen readily available.[13]

Burn Prevention

Hot-water temperature in the home should be set at a maximum of 120°F to avoid scald burns. Smoke alarms should be installed and maintained. Electrical cords should be inspected regularly and frayed cords not be plugged in.

Infants and toddlers are at particular risk for burns. Advise parents not to carry an infant and hot liquids or foods at the same time. Milk and formula should not be heated in the microwave oven because the uneven temperatures can scald the infant's mouth. Young children should be kept away from hot oven doors, irons, wall heaters and grills, electrical cords, and cups or dishes of hot food. Older children should be taught stovetop and microwave oven safety.[14] Those with decreased temperature sensation, such as the elderly and individuals with peripheral neuropathy, should test bath water with a thermometer before stepping in.

Pressure Injury and Dermal Ulcer Prevention

Prevention of pressure injuries and dermal ulcers requires an initial assessment and daily reevaluation and documentation for inpatients at risk of ulcer development using a tool such as the Braden Scale for Predicting Pressure Sore Risk.[15] The Braden scale consists of six subscales based on common causes of dermal ulcers: sensory perception, moisture, activity, mobility, nutrition, and friction and shear. Adults scoring less than 18 of 23 possible points on the Braden scale are considered at risk for dermal ulcers. The scale is often completed as part of a healthcare facility's admission assessment and periodic reassessment. Persons found to be at higher risk should have more intensive preventive measures instituted. Those at risk in home settings can be taught to assess their own skin with the assistance of family members or caregivers. Preventive interventions include minimizing or eliminating friction and shear (e.g., sliding on sheets), minimizing pressure through frequent repositioning and use of pressure-relieving devices, managing moisture on skin surfaces, and maintaining adequate nutrition and hydration.[5]

Secondary Prevention (Screening)

Malignant melanoma is a particularly virulent type of skin cancer, but early detection and treatment improves the outcome. The mnemonic ABCDE can be used to remember the early signs of melanoma during a skin assessment; it can also be taught to patients to guide their own comprehensive monthly skin self-assessments:[8]

- *Asymmetry:* The shape of one half does not match that of the other half.
- *Border* that is irregular: The edges are often ragged, notched, or blurred in outline. The pigment may spread into the surrounding skin.
- *Color* that is uneven: Shades of black, brown, and tan may be present. Areas of white, gray, red, pink, or blue may also be seen.
- *Diameter:* There is a change in size, usually an increase. Melanomas can be tiny, but most are larger than the size of a pea (larger than 6 mm or approximately $\frac{1}{4}$ in.).
- *Evolving:* The mole has changed during the past few weeks or months.

Collaborative Interventions
Pharmacotherapy

Medications for skin disorders include topical and oral or parenteral antibiotics, steroids, topical moisturizers, and anticancer agents or immunosuppressive chemotherapy.

BOX 26.4 Recommendations for Protection from Sun Exposure

- Avoid outdoor activities during the middle of the day. The sun's rays are the strongest between 10 AM and 4 PM. When you must be outdoors, seek shade.
- Protect yourself from the sun's rays reflected by sand, water, snow, ice, and pavement. The sun's rays can go through light clothing, windshields, windows, and clouds.
- Wear long sleeves and long pants. Tightly woven fabrics are best.
- Wear a hat with a wide brim all around that shades your face, neck, and ears. Keep in mind that baseball caps and some sun visors protect only parts of your skin.
- Wear sunglasses that absorb ultraviolet (UV) radiation to protect the skin around your eyes.
- Sunscreen lotions may help to prevent some skin cancers. It is important to use a broad-spectrum sunscreen lotion that filters both *ultraviolet B* and *ultraviolet A radiation*. Apply sunscreen lotions to uncovered skin 30 min before going outside, and apply again every 2 h or after swimming or sweating. However, you still need to avoid the sun during the middle of the day and wear clothing to protect your skin.

From National Cancer Institute. (2017). *Skin Cancer Prevention (PDQ®)—Patient Version*. Bethesda, MD: National Institutes of Health. Retrieved from https://www.cancer.gov/types/skin/patient/skin-prevention-pdq#section/_16.

Antibiotics. When a specific organism is identified through culture, topical or parenteral antibiotics may be prescribed. Common fungal infections such as athlete's foot may be treated with over-the-counter antifungal creams or sprays. When arthropod infestations appear in the skin, an antibiotic is commonly administered in shampoo or lotion form and applied to the affected area.

Steroids. Topical steroids are often used to treat allergic dermatitis and the irritating symptom of pruritus (itching). Oral or parenteral steroids may be used when urticaria (hives) manifests on the skin, indicating a systemic allergic reaction.

Emollients. Lotions, creams, and ointments may be used to retain moisture in the skin or as a base for other medications. Gels and powders are used when excessive moisture is present.

Chemotherapy agents. When skin lesions are malignant, cancer chemotherapy and systemic adjunct therapy may be used.[8]

CLINICAL NURSING SKILLS FOR TISSUE INTEGRITY

- Assessment
- Skin hygiene
- Wound care
- Medication administration
- Patient teaching

Wound Care

Cleansing. The goal of wound cleansing is to promote wound healing by removing debris and excessive exudates. Shallow wounds that appear healthy are generally cleaned with mild soap and water, and deeper but healthy wounds are cleaned gently with normal saline. Harsh solutions such as diluted bleach, acetic acid, or hydrogen peroxide can break down the cell walls of the newly formed tissues, so those solutions are reserved for use in heavily contaminated wounds.

Dressings. Wounds may be mechanically protected to promote healing in a moist but not soggy environment using a simple adhesive bandage or more complex dressings. Dry dressings are used to absorb excessive exudates, whereas moist dressings are used to maintain a slightly damp environment to promote tissue repair. Nonadherent dressings are useful when the wound drainage is slight and may dry between dressing changes, causing the dressing to stick to the fragile wound surface and thus disrupt the wound during dressing removal. Occlusive and semiocclusive dressings are used for clean wounds that have minimal drainage but need to be protected from environmental pathogens, such as a central intravenous catheter puncture site. Hydrocolloid, hydrogel, and alginate dressings are used to absorb exudates while maintaining a therapeutically moist wound surface to promote healing. Vacuum-assisted closure systems are special dressings for complex wounds attached to a device that maintains negative pressure at the wound surface, aiding in removal of large amounts of exudates.[7]

Phototherapy

Some skin disorders, such as psoriasis and atopic dermatitis, respond to controlled phototherapy with UV light. Protection from excessive UV exposure is important to prevent tissue damage.[16]

Surgical Treatment

Excisions—scalpel or laser. Surgical removal is indicated for benign lesions such as deep plantar surface warts unresponsive to other therapy and malignant lesions such as squamous, basal cell, and melanoma skin cancers. Surgical excision of primary melanoma includes not only removal of the lesion but also that of an additional margin around the lesion to ensure the eradication of malignant cells.[8]

Debridement. Wounds covered with a dry, leathery eschar may not heal until the eschar has been removed. Surgical debridement enables rapid removal of the eschar and debris, whereas debridement using topical collagenase or wet-to-dry dressings is done slowly over a longer period of time. Collagenase ointment breaks down the peptide bonds in necrotic ulcers or burn wound tissues without damaging the healthy tissue.[7]

Skin grafts. When extensive damage is associated with large or deep burns, wound excision and skin grafting are required to cover and heal the wounds. Grafts may be taken from other areas of the person's skin or from living or nonliving donors; porcine grafts may also be used. In addition to grafts, skin substitutes and bioengineered skin coverings are available.[7]

Nutrition

Tissue maintenance and repair is dependent on adequate nutrition. Protein and vitamins A and C are particularly critical for collagen synthesis in wound healing. In the absence of adequate nutrition, wound healing is delayed and infection is more likely. Early enteral or parenteral nutrition is important to consider for patients at risk.[7]

INTERRELATED CONCEPTS

Multiple concepts have a close interrelationship with tissue integrity. Adequate **Perfusion** with oxygen- and nutrient-enriched blood (**Gas Exchange**) promotes tissue integrity; in the absence of oxygen or sufficient **Nutrition**, the tissues can be suffocated and/or starved, leading to atrophy or necrosis. Adequate **Sensory Perception** and **Mobility** provide the stimulus and action needed to prevent prolonged pressure from limiting the perfusion to a specific tissue area. The nerves of the skin provide feedback about temperature and pressure that serve as a safety mechanism for the person negotiating the environment. Unrelieved pressure on a body tissue eventually causes injury.

In the presence of tissue integrity, the skin functions to maintain balance of **Fluid and Electrolytes** and has a role in **Thermoregulation**. Production of sweat, which includes both water and electrolytes, serves to cool the excessive body temperatures that could lead to organ damage, and it also serves to remove wastes. Altered **Elimination** through urinary or bowel incontinence can also contribute to impairment of tissue integrity through skin contact with caustic excretions. A loss of tissue integrity often results in **Pain** because the skin is laden with sensory nerve endings reactive to the irritation of the local damage. The skin and mucous membranes provide a barrier to most organisms and many toxic substances in the environment. A break in the barrier that is provided by intact skin and mucous membranes provides a portal for **Infection** with environmental organisms. These interrelationships are depicted in Fig. 26.3.

CLINICAL EXEMPLARS

There are a large number of clinical exemplars related to tissue integrity. Box 26.5 presents common clinical conditions associated with tissue integrity impairment by categories noted previously: trauma/injury, loss of perfusion, immunologic conditions, infections, thermal/radiation injuries, and lesions. In this section, several exemplars are featured because of their importance or frequency seen in practice. Also, a case study is presented illustrating the concept in a specific clinical context.

Causes

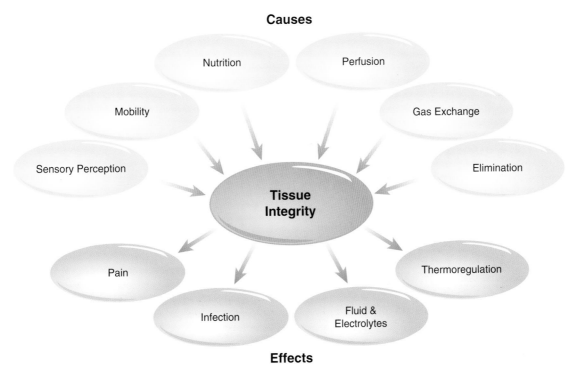

Effects

FIGURE 26.3 Tissue Integrity and Interrelated Concepts. This is a cause-and-effect model showing the concepts that impact tissue integrity and those concepts that are negatively impacted when tissue integrity is disrupted.

Featured Exemplars

The following featured exemplars provide a brief explanation of common conditions causing impaired tissue integrity. For detailed explanations and suggested nursing care for these conditions, consult specific medical-surgical, pediatric, and gerontology resources.

Abrasion/Laceration

Abrasions and lacerations are superficial traumatic injuries to the epidermis, dermis, and subcutaneous layers or to mucous membranes. Superficial injuries to highly vascular areas such as the scalp and oral mucosa may bleed extensively. The major risk of epidermal and dermal injury is the loss of a protective barrier, increasing the possibility of infection by contact with pathogens.

Pressure Injury/Pressure Ulcer

Unrelieved pressure can disrupt perfusion and oxygenation to tissue cells, leading to tissue necrosis of varying depths from superficial to bone-deep. Individuals who have decreased sensation or mobility are at greater risk for pressure injuries. The recognition of risk factors (see Box 26.1) and prevention are critical for reducing the prevalence of pressure ulcers.[5]

Psoriasis

Psoriasis is a recurrent inflammatory skin disease that affects an estimated 125 million people worldwide.[16] Individuals most commonly develop psoriasis between ages 15 and 35 years. Although most cases involve mild silvery scales and redness over a small percentage of the body, individuals with severe psoriasis and extensive lesions may feel isolated and withdraw from social contact. Up to one-third of those with psoriasis also have psoriatic arthritis, a painful joint inflammation.[16]

Bacterial Infection: Cellulitis

Cellulitis is inflammation of the skin and subcutaneous tissues, often caused by *Staphylococcus aureus* or streptococcal infection following a break in skin integrity such as a minor laceration or surgical incision. A hot, tender, reddened area of local infection develops at the site of injury. The individual may experience generalized responses to infection, such as fever and malaise.[7]

Fungal Infection: Tinea Pedis (Athlete's Foot)

Tinea pedis, a fungal infection of the foot, causes scaling and maceration between the toes and may cause red scales and blisters across the plantar surface. Tinea pedis is contagious and commonly acquired in shared facilities such as locker rooms or dormitory showers. Treatment includes the administration of an antifungal agent.[7]

Sunburn

Sunburn can range from a mild redness to blistering or deep tissue damage. The following increase the risk of sunburn: direct exposure of the skin to the sun; use of tanning booths or sunlamps; being near snow, water, or at high altitude. Sunburn and recurrent thermal damage to the skin is a risk factor for skin cancers.[14]

Malignant Melanoma

Malignant melanoma, a malignant tumor that develops from melanin-producing skin and mucosal cells, is the most common cause of skin cancer deaths. The risk of death from melanoma is greatest for people who have light-colored hair, eyes, and skin. White individuals are 10 times more likely than African Americans to die of melanoma. Individuals should consult a healthcare provider immediately if moles or lesions show a sudden or progressive change in size, shape, or color. Melanoma cells can metastasize to other organs.[8]

BOX 26.5   EXEMPLARS OF IMPAIRED TISSUE INTEGRITY

Trauma/Injury
- Abrasion
- Blister
- Chemical irritant
- Ecchymosis
- Hematoma
- Laceration
- Surgical incision

Loss of Perfusion
- Dermal ulcer
- Pressure injury
- Diabetic foot ulcer

Immunologic Disorders
- Atopic dermatitis
- Psoriasis

- Scleroderma
- Stevens-Johnson syndrome
- Systemic lupus erythematosus
- Toxic epidermal necrolysis

Bacterial Infection
- Cellulitis
- Impetigo

Fungal Infection
- Tinea pedis (athlete's foot)
- Vaginitis

Viral Infection
- HSV-1 (usually oropharyngeal)
- HSV-2 (usually genital)
- Verruca (warts)

Infestations
- Lice
- Scabies

Thermal/Radiation
- Burns
- Frostbite
- Radiation burns
- Sunburn

Lesions
- Basal cell carcinoma
- Benign tumors
- Malignant melanoma
- Squamous cell carcinoma

HSV, Herpes simplex virus.

 ACCESS EXEMPLAR LINKS IN YOUR GIDDENS EBOOK

CASE STUDY

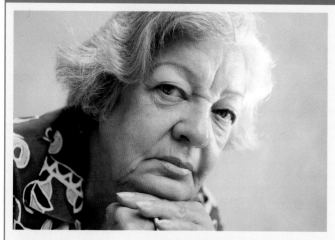

Case Presentation

Mrs. Ramona Garcia, 76 years old, is admitted to a medical respiratory unit with pneumonia after 4 days of increasing difficulty breathing, fever, dehydration, and a productive cough with purulent sputum. She reports that she has had very little sleep, explaining that she has been trying to sleep in a chair because she cannot breathe well lying down. She also mentions that she has had very little to eat during the past several days due to a poor appetite and fatigue.

When Mrs. Garcia's breathing becomes comfortable enough for her to be turned briefly for a full skin assessment, the nurse notes a 4-cm red area on the buttock over the left ischial tuberosity that does not blanch to pressure. Recognizing the reddened area as a stage I dermal ulcer, the nurse collaborates with the patient, family, and health team on a plan to prevent further tissue breakdown, including frequent movement and positioning, adequate nutrition, hygiene to prevent the collection of moisture from sweat or urine—which could lead to skin maceration—and the use of pressure-relieving devices.

Case Analysis Questions

1. What physiological and environmental factors increased Mrs. Garcia's risk for dermal ulcer?
2. What does "Stage I dermal ulcer" mean, and where does this fall in the scope of this concept?
3. Review the interrelated concepts presented in this chapter. Which apply to Mrs. Garcia?

From diego cervo/iStock/Thinkstock.

 ACCESS EXEMPLAR LINKS IN YOUR GIDDENS EBOOK

REFERENCES

1. Huether, S. E., McCance, K. L., Brashers, V. L., & Rote, N. S. (2017). *Understanding pathophysiology* (6th ed.). St Louis: Elsevier.
2. Carpenito-Moyet, L. J. (2017). *Nursing diagnosis: Application to clinical practice* (15th ed.). Philadelphia: Wolters Kluwer.
3. Mosby. (2017). *Mosby's dictionary of medicine, nursing & health professions* (10th ed.). St. Louis: Elsevier.
4. Wilson, S., & Giddens, J. (2017). *Health assessment for nursing practice* (6th ed.). St Louis: Mosby.
5. Wound, Ostomy and Continence Nurses Society (WOCN). (2016). *Guideline for prevention and management of pressure ulcers (injuries)*. Mt. Laurel (NJ): WOCN.
6. Gupta, M. A., Vujcic, B., & Gupta, A. K. (2017). Dermatologic disorders that are associated with emergency department visits in the US: Results from a nationally representative US sample. *Journal of the American Academy of Dermatology, 76*(6), AB94.
7. Lewis, S. L., Bucher, L., Heitkemper, M., et al. (Eds.), (2017). *Medical–surgical nursing: Assessment and management of clinical problems* (10th ed.). St Louis: Mosby.
8. American Cancer Society. (2018). *Melanoma skin cancer*. Retrieved from: http://www.cancer.org/cancer/skincancer-melanoma/index.
9. Yin, S. (2017). Chemical and common burns in children. *Clinical Pediatrics, 56*(5_suppl), 8S–12S.
10. Bibbins-Domingo, K., et al. (2016). Screening for skin cancer: US Preventive Services Task Force recommendation statement. *JAMA: The Journal of the American Medical Association, 316*(4), 429–435.
11. Edsberg, L. E., et al. (2016). Revised National Pressure Ulcer Advisory Panel pressure injury staging system: Revised pressure injury staging

system. *Journal of Wound, Ostomy, and Continence Nursing, 43*(6), 585–597.

12. Potter, P. A., Perry, A. G., Stockert, P., et al. (2015). *Basic nursing* (8th ed.). St Louis: Mosby.

13. Guide to Community Preventive Services. (2017). *Skin Cancer: Interventions in Outdoor Recreational and Tourism Settings.* Retrieved from: https://www.thecommunityguide.org/findings/skin-cancer-interventions-outdoor-recreational-and-tourism-settings.

14. American Academy of Pediatrics. (2017). *Burn treatment & prevention tips for families.* Retrieved from: http://www.healthychildren.org/English/health-issues/injuries-emergencies/Pages/Treating-and-Preventing-Burns.aspx.

15. Bergstrom, N., Braden, B. J., Laguzza, A., et al. (1987). The Braden scale for predicting pressure sore risk. *Nursing Research, 36*(4), 205–210.

16. National Psoriasis Foundation. (n.d.). *About psoriasis.* Retrieved from: https://psoriasis.org/about-psoriasis.

CONCEPT
27

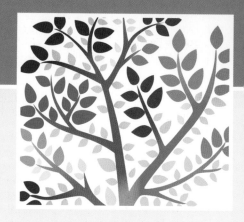

Sensory Perception

Beth S. Hopkins

Sensory perception represents a complex physiological process that allows humans to interact efficiently with the environment. The five senses provide the basis for social interactions, communication, and learning. Sensory perception also provides a level of protection, enabling individuals to detect and react to dangers within the environment. Impairment in any of the five senses can lead to significant challenges that negatively affect development, health, and well-being with potentially significant consequences. This concept presentation provides an overview of sensory perception, including ways to recognize those most at risk for impairment and appropriate interventions when impairment occurs.

DEFINITION

To describe the concept of sensory perception, it is important first to define both sensation and perception. *Sensation* is the ability to perceive stimulation through one's sensory organs, such as the nose, ears, and eyes. This stimulation can be internal, from within the body, or external, from outside the body, and includes feelings of pain, temperature, and light. External stimuli are commonly received and processed through the five senses: vision, hearing, taste, smell, and touch. *Perception* is defined as the process by which we receive, organize, and interpret sensation. Sensory perception can then be defined as *the ability to receive sensory input and, through various physiological processes in the body, translate the stimulus or data into meaningful information.*[1]

SCOPE

Both sensation and perception occur within various body systems and through a complex interaction of both sensory receptors and the nervous system. For persons to interact fully with the environment in which they live, it is important that these systems be as functional as possible. This concept represents five senses:

- Vision
- Hearing
- Taste
- Smell
- Touch

With each of these senses, the level of function ranges from optimal functioning to impairment (Fig. 27.1). For the purposes of this concept presentation, impairment of sensory perception includes altered function

or perceptual ability but does not include psychiatric symptoms such as hallucinations (auditory, visual, tactile) or psychosis.

NORMAL PHYSIOLOGICAL PROCESS

Vision

Vision requires functioning of the visual system, which includes the eyes; surrounding optic muscles; and cranial nerves II (optic), III (oculomotor), IV (trochlear), V (trigeminal), and VI (abducens). The eyelid, conjunctiva, lacrimal gland, and eye muscles all comprise the external eye, which helps to regulate and control the visual input as well as protect the eye, aid with tear production, and move the eye when desired. The internal eye consists of three separate layers: the outer sclera and cornea; the middle layer, which houses the choroid, ciliary body, and iris; and the innermost layer, which is the retina.[2] The iris allows light to enter the eye and regulates the amount of light entering the eye at any given time. The lens bends entering light rays so that they can properly fall on the retina. The ciliary body, which consists of ciliary muscles, is fed by the choroid, a highly vascular structure (Fig. 27.2). The innermost area of the eye is the retina, which transforms light impulses into electrical impulses that are transmitted to the optic nerve. The optic nerve, in turn, communicates with the brain to produce vision.[2] Cranial nerves II to VI all have important roles in eye function (Table 27.1).

Hearing

Hearing involves the peripheral and central auditory systems. The peripheral system comprises the external, middle, and inner ear and is concerned with hearing and processing sound. The external ear includes the auricle and external auditory canal and functions primarily to collect and transmit sound to the tympanic membrane and to protect the inner ear (Fig. 27.3).[3]

The middle ear is an air-filled space that is located in the temporal bone. It is connected to the throat/nasopharynx by the eustachian tube, whose primary function is to equalize air pressure on both sides of the eardrum. The eustachian tube opens to allow airflow when one is chewing and swallowing. Vibrations of the tympanic membrane (or eardrum), which separates the external ear from the middle ear, cause the auditory ossicles to further amplify the sound waves and transmit these airborne waves to the fluid-filled inner ear.

The inner ear consists of a bony labyrinth surrounding a membrane. Within this structure is the cochlea, closely connected to hearing ability,

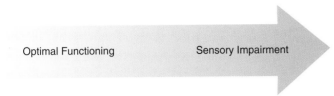

FIGURE 27.1 Scope of Sensory Perception. The scope of sensory perception ranges from optimal functioning to impairment of vision, hearing, taste, smell, and tactile perception.

and the vestibular system, which helps to control balance.[4] Sound waves stimulate this series of actions, and once these waves reach the inner ear, the hair cells or sensory receptor cells of the cochlea pick up the vibrations. These cochlear cells, by means of a complex series of mechanical wave activities, innervate impulses that are carried by nerve fibers to cranial nerve VIII (the vestibulocochlear nerve) to the brain—where the cerebellum receives the signals and helps to maintain a sense of balance—and then further, reaching the auditory area of the temporal lobe for hearing.[5]

Taste

A person's gustatory system, or sense of taste, involves various cranial nerves and is directly related to the ability of the mouth and tongue to detect the chemicals—also referred to as tastants—in the foods that we eat. These taste signals are initiated by chemical stimulation of the taste buds, located primarily on the surface of the tongue and in the pharynx. Sensory receptor stimulation—conducted via cranial nerves VII, IX, and X—is then transmitted to the nucleus of the solitary tract in the medulla of the brain and also sent to other areas within the brain. Messages about smell converge here, along with visceral sensory fibers from the esophagus, stomach, intestines, and liver, allowing taste and odor signals to initiate digestive activity.[6]

Smell

The sense of smell is controlled primarily by cranial nerve I (the olfactory nerve) and plays a critical role in controlling the desire to eat and maintain a healthy nutritional state.[6] Smell depends on sensory receptors located in the mucous membranes of the upper and posterior

parts of the nasal cavity that respond to airborne chemicals. These chemicals bond to the ciliary receptors in the nose, which trigger a series of reactions that eventually lead to signals traveling along the olfactory nerve to the brain. The brain then processes this information and makes a determination as to the type of smell. It is estimated that in healthy young adults approximately 10,000 different chemicals can be identified by smell.[6]

Touch

The perception of sensation originates in the sensory receptors throughout the body; by means of complex travel pathways it ultimately converges in the somatosensory cortex. This somatic organization allows for the precise localization of signals related to fine and crude touch, vibration, pressure, temperature, itch, and pain.[7]

Age-Related Differences
Infants and Children

Significant changes occur during growth and development in early infancy that primarily affect visual acuity and hearing perception. Although the eyes are physically developed by the eighth month in utero, making the fetus capable of opening its eyes, the development of gross visual ability to recognize objects, perform purposeful eye movement, and color recognition primarily occurs during the first year of life. The 1-year-old typically has developed 20/50 vision or is able to see at 20 feet what an individual with normal vision can see at approximately 50 feet. Most research suggests that visual acuity progressively improves in early childhood, reaching 20/30 or better by age 5 years, as is generally required for passing mandatory state vision standards upon entry into primary school.[8,9] The ear structures and the ability to hear sounds are developed during the early part of embryonic life; thus, hearing is fully developed at birth. Infants have the ability to detect a few distinct odors, such as the smell of the mother's milk; however, refined taste discrimination is limited until infants reach approximately 3 months of age.[10] Infants also have a well-developed sense of touch and are able to respond to peripheral tactile stimulation at birth.[10] This ability to distinguish tactile stimulation develops rapidly from a tight hand grasp at 1 month of age to pincer grasp, holding a cup, and walking steadily by 1 year of age.

Older Adults

Research illustrates that a decline in sensory function occurs with aging. This is increasingly prevalent among the older population and is believed to be due in part to prescribed treatments for other age-related conditions

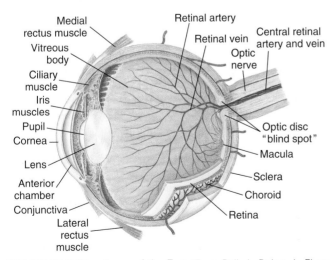

FIGURE 27.2 Structures of the Eye. (From Ball, J., Dains, J., Flynn, J., Solomon, B., Stewart R. [2015]. *Seidel's guide to physical examination* [8th ed.]. St Louis: Mosby.)

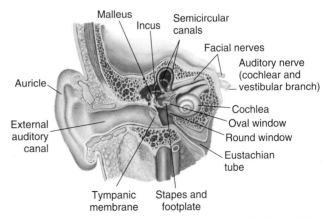

FIGURE 27.3 Structures of the Ear. (From Ball, J., Dains, J., Flynn, J., Solomon, B., Stewart R. [2015]. *Seidel's guide to physical examination* [8th ed.]. St Louis: Mosby.)

TABLE 27.1   Cranial Nerves and Their Function

Cranial Nerve	Function
I: Olfactory	Smell reception and interpretation
II: Optic	Visual acuity and visual fields
III: Oculomotor	Raising eyelids, extraocular movements, and papillary constriction
IV: Trochlear	Downward and inward eye movement
V: Trigeminal	Jaw opening and closing; sensation to eye, forehead, nose, mouth, teeth, ear, and face
VI: Abducens	Eye movement laterally
VII: Facial	Controls most facial expressions; taste with anterior two-thirds of tongue; excretion of tears and saliva
VIII: Acoustic	Hearing and equilibrium
IX: Glossopharyngeal	Swallowing and speaking; sensation of nasopharynx, gag reflex, and taste to posterior third of tongue; secretion of salivary glands and carotid reflex; certain speech sounds and swallowing
X: Vagus	Sensation behind ear and portion of external ear canal; secretion of digestive enzymes; peristalsis; carotid reflex; heart, respiratory, and digestive processes
XI: Spinal accessory	Turning one's head and shrugging one's shoulders
XII: Hypoglossal	Tongue movement, speech, and swallowing

Modified from Ball, J., Dains, J., Flynn, J., Solomon, B., Stewart R. (2015). *Seidel's guide to physical examination* (8th ed.). St Louis: Mosby.

(e.g., medications used for treatment of cardiovascular disease).[11] The National Social Life, Health, and Aging Project began a major research study in 2005 that is exploring the health and social factors of older Americans as they age. This is the first national study attempting to provide a comprehensive assessment of sensory function among older adults. The study has examined more than 3000 people ages 57 to 85 years, and the data show declines in all five senses within this population.[12]

Age-related changes in vision begin in the fourth decade, when reduced elasticity of the lens occurs, making it difficult to focus on near objects (presbyopia).[13] Age-related hearing loss (presbycusis) is caused by changes in the inner ear or in the nerve pathways from the inner ear to the brain. This results in a decreased ability to hear and process sound, although the degree of hearing loss is variable.[14] Another physiological change with aging is reduced olfactory epithelium along with a decreased number of nasal ciliary receptors available to assist in sending olfactory signals to the brain. Not only is the ability to smell decreased with aging but so is the ability to distinguish between various smells.[6] Reduced sense of smell typically begins at approximately age 60 years, with increasing loss into the seventies and eighties. A study of more than 90 people ages 45 to 84 years showed olfactory impairment in approximately 25% of the subjects, and impairment increased with age in both genders.[15] It is unknown why one's sense of taste tends to decline with age. It is thought to be related to both the decrease in olfaction and potential chewing problems due to tooth loss.[16] Furthermore, decreased levels of certain hormones, such as testosterone, in the older adult population can contribute to a decrease in cell growth, including taste cells located in the taste buds. The decrease in the number of taste cells thus leads to a decrease in the sense of taste.[6] Evidence suggests that aging and dementia-related diseases such, as Alzheimer disease and Parkinson disease, can lead to a decline in the detection and recognition of smells.[17]

Tactile thresholds (perception of touch) tend to increase with aging. An example of this is a delay in the process of sensing a wrinkled sheet under the back or a slight prick from a small needle, thus resulting in potential injuries. In addition, certain tests that measure the ability to assess tactile sensation tend to show a decline in function that corresponds with aging—a decline of 1% per year between the ages of 20 and 80 years.[18] Sensation at the fingertips and toes declines faster, especially with heat and cold, which can lead to problems with burns and potential frostbite in the older adult population.[6] A study comparing sensation thresholds of older (mean age 93 years) and younger (mean age 28 years) subjects found that older subjects required two to more than five times the tactile stimulation required by the younger group.[19]

VARIATIONS AND CONTEXT

A number of problems and conditions are represented by this concept and are grouped by problems with vision, hearing, smell, taste, and tactile perception. Common to all senses, conditions affecting sensory perception can be primary or secondary problems, representing both acute and chronic change, caused by congenital abnormalities, primary and chronic conditions, treatment-related negative effects, and acute injury.

Problems with Vision

Problems with vision are seen across the lifespan. Although most individuals experience changes in vision associated with the normal aging process (previously discussed), there are many medical conditions that affect vision. Poor vision is defined as best-corrected visual acuity of less than 20/40 in the better-seeing eye, and blindness is considered corrected visual acuity of 20/200 in the better-seeing eye. Visual problems can occur as primary eye disorders (e.g., cataracts, glaucoma, retinal detachment, and macular degeneration), as secondary disorders caused by systemic chronic conditions such as diabetes or hypertension (diabetic retinopathy), or due to congenital abnormalities (e.g., a congenital cataract).[20] As of 2010, blindness affected more than 1 million Americans, and an additional 12 million are visually impaired. This number is predicted to double by 2030 because of the increasing epidemics of diabetes and other chronic diseases as well as the rapidly aging population.

Ocular infection in the first few weeks of life is increasingly more common among newborns, often caused by previously untreated maternal-induced infection by *Neisseria gonorrhoeae* and/or *Chlamydia*. Younger children are at risk for eye injury from accidental blunt trauma and chemical burns caused by household cleaners. Insult or injury to the eye at any age may result in visual impairment or permanent blindness. Eye malignancies, although rare, can have devastating effects. Choroidal melanoma is the most common intraocular cancer in adults and often has metastasized by the time it is detected.[21] Retinoblastoma, the second leading cause of intraocular cancer, is found in children between the ages of 14 months and 3 years.[21]

Problems with Hearing

Hearing impairment is among the most prevalent chronic health conditions in the population older than 65 years of age, resulting in substantially reduced quality of life.[22] Problems with hearing result from a disruption in the mechanisms required for the transmission of sound and/or nerve impulse within the ears. Sensorineural hearing loss, the most prevalent type of hearing loss, occurs when there is disruption in the afferent nerves necessary to transmit impulses. Conductive hearing loss results when there is disruption in the transmission of sound or vibration in the outer ear canal and middle ear structures. Some individuals may experience some degree of both types of hearing loss, described as a mixed hearing loss. Many subtypes of sensorineural hearing loss exist, including congenital hearing loss, genetic hearing loss, noise-induced hearing loss, presbycusis, sudden sensorineural hearing loss, and autoimmune hearing disorders.[22] Conductive hearing loss can be a result of cerumen impaction in the ear canal or the more serious consequence of an acute ear infection leading to a tympanic membrane perforation or rupture. Hearing loss at birth or congenital hearing loss occurs in 1 to 6 per 1000 newborns, of which 50% is suspected to be genetic related and 25% is nongenetic in origin.[23] Other genetic syndromes (such as Down and Alport syndromes) are often associated with hearing loss.[24]

Problems with Taste and Smell

Multiple factors influence the perception of smell and taste across the lifespan. These changes can be sudden and temporary when associated with an acute viral upper respiratory infection or long-term changes when associated with the untoward effects of chemotherapeutic cancer-related treatment.[6,11] Some chronic conditions of adulthood, such as dementias, strongly correlate with loss of smell.[11] Among infants and children, problems with taste and smell are usually associated with direct injury or trauma to the olfactory ciliary receptor sensory and neural pathways, or they are associated with congenital abnormalities.

Problems with Tactile Sensation

Acute injury or trauma to the head, spinal cord, or peripheral appendages may result in disruption of sensory perception. Nontraumatic changes associated with the sense of touch are most common and are frequently caused by the progression of comorbid disease. Normal aging affects touch, as is experienced with the other senses as well. Studies indicate that it is likely that both central nervous processing of stimuli and a peripheral component contribute to diminishing touch sensation as people age.[24]

CONSEQUENCES

Impaired sensory perception can lead to a number of consequences, depending on the type, extent, and number of impairments and also adjustments made to the impairment. Sensory-perceptual impairments share many of the same types of consequences, including a reduced overall quality of life. There is significant risk for many types of injury as a result of impairments in sensory perception (such as falls, burns, cold, or pressure) and the inability to smell or taste spoiled food or to smell toxic gases or smoke. Impaired vision and hearing can contribute to significant developmental delay and learning disabilities among infants and children and a loss of functional ability for adults. Psychosocial consequences can include difficulty establishing vocations, impaired interpersonal relationships, social isolation, depression, anxiety, and loss of self-worth. Another consequence less easily measured is the financial burden many of these impairments represent—both in direct cost of treatments and assistive devices and in the loss of income if the impairment represents an inability to work.

RISK FACTORS

All individuals—regardless of age, gender, ethnicity, or socioeconomic status—are at risk for disturbances in sensation and perception. However, there are certain populations and individual factors associated with increased risk.

Populations at Risk

The elderly population comprises those at the highest risk as a result of changes in sensory perceptual functioning associated with the aging

process (previously described). There are no significant population risk factors accountable to race/ethnicity, gender, or socioeconomic status associated with a decline in sensory perception in older adults.[25] Visual acuity begins to decline in the fourth decade of life, and by the sixth decade most individuals will experience some degree of declining visual acuity.[21] Hearing loss related to aging affects an estimated 50% of individuals older than age 75 years of age.[25]

Individual Risk Factors

Significant individual risk factors include genetic predisposition, adverse effects of medications, chronic medical conditions, lifestyle choices, and occupation.

Congenital Conditions and Genetics

If not detected early in life, congenital conditions that may result in detrimental long-term effects on an infant's visual perception include congenital glaucoma, congenital cataracts, and retinoblastoma (intraocular malignancy).[21] Congenital hearing loss is commonly the result of congenital malformations in the structure or functional components of the auditory system, although more than half of infants born with hearing loss have no significant risk factors.[26] Hearing loss at birth may be associated with maternal infection during pregnancy (e.g., measles) or family history of childhood hearing loss. Additional risk factors for congenital hearing loss include history of meningitis, low Apgar score, intensive care unit admission, and elevated bilirubin.[21]

Adverse Reactions and Side Effects of Medications

Changes in sensory perception are a common side effect or adverse effect of many medications, particularly when taken for a long time, as with chronic illness (Table 27.2). Visual disturbances are among the most common undesirable side effects associated with medication therapy. Examples include blurred vision, papillary constriction, retinal toxicity, halo effects, and dry eyes.[6] Ototoxicity, another potential adverse effect due to medication, can result in permanent or temporary inner ear problems that can affect hearing, balance, and speech. This represents one of the main preventable causes of deafness.[27]

Many drugs also affect both taste and smell. In fact, medications (especially chemotherapeutic agents) are the most common cause of

TABLE 27.2 Common Medications that Can Affect Sensation and Perception

Drug Classification	Possible Side Effects
Antihistamines (loratadine, diphenhydramine)	Blurred vision, dry mouth
Antihypertensives (β blockers, calcium channel blockers, ACE inhibitors)	Blurred vision, alterations in taste and smell
Miotic eye drops (pilocarpine, carbachol)	Changes in vision, increase in nearsightedness, blurred vision
Antiseizure drugs (topiramate, acetazolamide)	Numbness in hands and feet, dry mouth, tinnitus (ringing in ears), blurred vision, eye pain, metallic taste
Diuretics (furosemide)	Hearing loss, tinnitus, alterations in taste and smell
Chemotherapeutic drugs	Alterations in taste and smell, paresthesia
Antibiotics	Alterations in taste and smell, ototoxicity

ACE, Angiotensin-converting enzyme.

taste disturbances.[28] It is often reported that up to half of all cancer patients experience changes in their taste and/or smell perception.[29,30] Alterations in taste and smell that are considered severe are associated with poor nutrient intake, reduced food enjoyment, and reduced quality of life.[31] Other drugs that cause taste disturbances include antimicrobial drugs, antivirals, antihypertensives, calcium channel blockers, and diuretics. If it is possible for the medication to be discontinued, the person's sense of smell and taste is often restored; however, some medications induce long-term changes in taste and smell and occasionally cause permanent loss.[31]

Paresthesia can also be caused by various medications, including select antineoplastic agents. Certain anticonvulsants can cause paresthesia in the hands, feet, face, and lips, which does not tend to improve until the medication is discontinued.

Acute Injury

Accidental and nonaccidental trauma to the eye in childhood is common. Ocular damage is dependent on the type of impact, with high-velocity impacts often causing extensive damage. Nonaccidental inflicted neurotrauma (formerly known as shaken baby syndrome) occurs in an estimated 1300 abused children annually, resulting in death within the first few days in approximately 20% of cases from the head trauma sustained.[21] Among children who survive, many develop traumatic retinoschisis as a result of retinal damage.

Chronic Medical Conditions

A number of medical conditions place an individual at risk for sensory perception impairment as a matter of the disease sequelae. Some of the most common medical conditions leading to such impairments are presented in Box 27.1.

Brain tumors, cancers, head injuries, infectious diseases, stroke, and some cardiovascular diseases, such as hypertension, are risk factors for visual and auditory problems.[6] Sinus and upper respiratory tract infections, seasonal allergies, and also dental problems can alter both the sense of smell and the sense of taste. In addition, nasal polyps and exposure to certain environmental chemicals can cause disturbances in both smell and taste.

A cerebrovascular accident (CVA) or stroke can affect many aspects of sensation and perception. Alterations in taste sensation, balance issues, and visual disturbances can result from a stroke depending on the area of the brain affected. Children and adults with autism report sensory disturbances such as insensitivity to pain as well as unusual sensory responses to visual, auditory, tactile, and olfactory stimulation. Although many children with developmental delays have sensory impairments, these problems tend to be more prevalent in children with autism.[32]

Lifestyle Choices and Occupation

Certain lifestyle choices can increase the risk of sensory and perceptual alterations. Smoking creates an increased risk for alterations in both smell and taste primarily because it damages the taste receptors on the tongue and sensory receptors in the nose. However, when a smoker who experiences a decreased sense of smell and taste stops smoking, both senses typically return to their proper level of functioning.[33] Individuals exposed to loud noise at work or during recreation activities are at risk for hearing deficit because such loud vibrations damage the small hair-like cells in the inner ear. This loss can be spontaneous or may occur over time, typically when the sound is at or above 85 decibels. Once damage has occurred, it is typically irreversible.[34] Individuals who work where flying debris is commonly present (such as miners and steelworkers), and those who work with certain chemicals are at high risk for eye injuries, especially when they are not wearing protective equipment.

BOX 27.1   Medical Conditions or Treatments Leading to Changes in Sensory Perception

Vision
- Retinopathy of prematurity
- Diabetes and hypertension-induced retinopathy
- Eye infection
- Foreign body of eye
- Corneal abrasion
- Traumatic eye injury
- Optic neuropathy and increased intraocular pressure

Auditory
- Acute suppurative otitis media
- Otitis media with effusion
- Tympanic membrane perforation
- Traumatic ear injury
- Foreign body

Olfactory
- Sinus and other upper respiratory infections
- Brain injury or trauma
- Parkinson disease
- Alzheimer disease
- Medications and chemical exposure
- Head and neck radiation
- Growths or tumors of nasal cavity

Gustatory
- Head and neck surgery
- Radiation to head and neck
- Head injury
- Oral abscess and other dental problems
- Brain
- Exposure to chemicals and medication
- Burning mouth syndrome

Somatosensory
- Systemic sclerosis
- Raynaud syndrome
- Cerebrovascular accident or stroke
- Third-degree burns
- Spinal cord injury
- Peripheral vascular disease

ASSESSMENT

A comprehensive health assessment is essential to determining current health status, identifying present health risks, predicting future health risks, and identifying appropriate health-promoting activities. An assessment includes conducting a history and examination as well as diagnostic testing when sensory perceptual conditions are suspected.

History and Physical Examination

When performing any type of physical assessment, a thorough health history (including past medical, surgical, family, and social history) is taken. For infants, it is important to ask about prenatal and maternal history. Because of the potential for adverse effects with medications, a list of all medications (prescription and over-the-counter) used by the patient should be included. Health history questions should also specifically ask about sensory perceptual symptoms/problems for each of the categorical areas. A physical examination, particularly related to symptoms, is crucial. Common symptoms that suggest impairments are described for each category.

Vision

Ask the patient about changes in vision (blurred vision, difficulty seeing close up and/or far away), peripheral visual changes, and eye pain. For the infant and toddler, ask caregivers if tracking of the eyes has been observed when the child is watching movement and to ensure that the eyes have been observed moving in synchrony.

Examination of the eyes starts by inspecting external eye structures—including the eyebrows, eyelashes, and eyelids—paying attention to symmetry, size, and extension. In addition, the nurse should palpate both the eyelid and the eye and inspect the conjunctiva—the thin membrane that covers the inner eyelid and sclera—closely for redness and irritation. The sclera should be predominantly white, and the lens should be transparent.

Visual acuity (a measure of how well a person sees) is also included in the examination. Infants and young children are challenging to test for visual acuity; however, it is essential to do a thorough penlight examination of the cornea. At approximately 6 months of age, the cover test is helpful to screen for possible visual loss. Once a child reaches 3 years of age, visual testing is achieved using the Snellen letter chart. Visual acuity is recorded as a fraction in which the numerator shows the distance that the patient was from the chart, typically 20 feet, and the denominator represents the distance that the average eye can read that same line of the chart.[2] For example, 20/60 means a patient can see clearly at 20 feet what the average eye sees at 60 feet.

Eye movement is typically controlled by cranial nerves III, IV, and VI and by six extraocular muscles. It is tested by having the patient follow the examiner's finger, keeping the head stationary as the finger moves through the six cardinal fields of gaze.[2] A person's inability to follow through all the fields can indicate a host of visual disorders. Nystagmus—a rapid, involuntary movement of the eye—can often be detected during this part of the visual assessment.

The internal eye exam allows for visualization of the optic disc, arteries, veins, and retina. This is done using an ophthalmoscope and often following dilation of the pupils, although this is not always necessary. Some unexpected findings include hemorrhages, optic disc swelling (referred to as papilledema), or cotton-wool spots, which are poorly defined yellow areas on the retina and often related to damage of the nerve fibers.[2] Pupils should be checked for response to light in both the adult and the pediatric population.

Hearing

Difficulty hearing, tinnitus, and ear pain are common symptoms that prompt a patient to have the auditory system evaluated by a healthcare professional. For the pediatric population, frequent problems with otitis media are common and can include symptoms such as ear drainage, pain, and fever.

Inspection of the outer portion of the ear (also known as the auricle or pinna), includes noting symmetry, size, shape, and possible discharge. Inspection of the inner ear is performed using an otoscope. The nurse should look for cerumen (earwax), noting its color and any odor if present.[2] The tympanic membrane (see Fig. 27.3) should be translucent, with a pearly, gray color. Abnormal findings include a bulging or retracted tympanic membrane (or eardrum) and/or perforations of the tympanic membrane. Evaluation of hearing is usually done by assessing the patient's ability to hear during general conversation. If a hearing deficit is suspected, further diagnostic studies are indicated.

Taste

The most common complaint associated with the sense of taste is a lack of one. Most patients who think they have a taste disorder actually have a problem with smell.[35] Obtaining a complete list of current medications is especially important, because many medications can cause alterations in taste.

Inspect the tongue and oral cavity, searching for any abnormalities such as an atrophied tongue or a tongue that does not appear red and moist.[2] Overgrowth of yeast or ulcerations or nodules should be noted. However, patients with taste disturbances often have normal-appearing, well-functioning tongues. Several validated taste tests[36] are available; however, they are may be costly to obtain and time-consuming to perform. Thus, before doing further testing, it is prudent to ensure that a patient has a good sense of smell.

Smell

Assessing the sense of smell is first done by obtaining a detailed history, including medications the patient is taking, and assessing for recent upper respiratory tract complaints such as sinus infections, allergies, and nasal polyps. Examination includes inspection of the nose, searching for abnormalities such as nasal discharge or blockages, and evaluation of the color and size of the nasal passages. If discharge is observed, the nurse should note the color, consistency, odor, and amount. Nasal breathing is assessed by pinching one naris or one nostril and asking the patient to breathe in and out with his or her mouth closed, alternating nostrils. Breathing through each unobstructed side of the nasal passage should be quiet and effortless.[2]

Touch

Touch and balance are largely regulated by the body's neurologic system. Alterations in perception can often manifest as balance disturbances. Balance is routinely tested by the Romberg test, which involves asking patients to stand with their feet together and arms at their sides with their eyes first open and then closed. Some slight swaying is normal, but the patient should be able to stand still for the most part. The nurse should also observe the patient's gait for abnormal findings, such as shuffling, staggering, and asymmetric stride.

Evaluation of sensory function is accomplished by having the patient identify stimuli affecting the major peripheral nerves, including the hands, arms, feet, legs, and abdomen. Cranial nerve VII, the trigeminal nerve, is most closely associated with sensory function. The patient should be able to correctly identify if a stimulus feels sharp or dull and the location of the sensation. In addition, the patient should be able to properly differentiate temperature (hot/cold), indicate the location of the stimulus, including the correct side of the body that is being stimulated.[2] Monofilament testing is a common way to assess for peripheral neuropathies that cause decreased sensation to the extremities. Monofilaments are single-fiber nylon threads that are placed on the patient's skin, typically on the feet. An abnormal finding is that the patient will not be able to detect the presence of the filament.[37]

Diagnostic Tests

After a basic history and a physical assessment have been completed, occasionally further diagnostic testing is warranted. This is described by sensory classification.

Vision

Some common visual diagnostic tests include evaluating peripheral vision by testing visual fields with automated perimetry. A patient looks straight ahead into a device with a concave dome while small flashes of light are shown sporadically in all visual fields. The patient then pushes a button every time he or she sees a light. Decreased visual field acuity could be indicative of glaucoma, optic nerve damage, and other visual problems. Another example is noncontact tonometry, or the puff-of-air test. This involves an eye's resistance to a puff of air from a small handheld jet, which calculates a range of intraocular pressure (IOP). Elevations in IOP can be indicative of glaucoma. Radiographic examinations of the brain may be indicated if a tumor is suspected of causing visual disturbances.

Hearing

If hearing loss is suspected, a referral to a licensed audiologist is often done for further testing. A pure-tone air conduction audiometric test determines the faintest tones a person can hear at selected frequencies ranging from low to high. Earphones are usually worn so that information can be obtained for each ear separately.[38] Other common screening methods used often with infants are otoacoustic emissions (OAEs) and auditory brain stem responses (ABRs). OAEs are sounds from the inner ear after the cochlea has been stimulated by a sound; these are measured by using a small probe in the ear canal. Those with hearing loss do not produce such sounds. The ABR test is performed by placing electrodes on the head to record brain wave activity in response to sounds.[38]

CLINICAL MANAGEMENT

Primary Prevention

Many measures exist to prevent injury and disease to the eyes, ears, mouth, and nose. Basic measures to protect the eyes and ears include the use of protective devices; patient education related to these practices is essential. Safety goggles are recommended for selected sporting activities and work activities in which small particles (e.g., sawdust, wood chips, metal pieces, and vegetation debris) are present in the air. More than 2000 workers in the United States receive medical treatment each year because of eye injuries that occur on the job.[39] The use of earplugs or other ear protection is also a requirement in many work settings involving loud machinery and is suggested for other activities such as attending loud concerts. Wearing a helmet when riding a bicycle, skiing, or participating in contact sports can prevent brain injury—another cause of sensory disturbances.

Primary prevention extends beyond wearing protective devices. Newborns receive erythromycin eye ointment in their eyes at the time of birth to help reduce the chance of the mother passing on certain sexually transmitted diseases. Reinforcing the importance of proper oral hygiene to prevent diseases of the mouth is essential to reducing the risk for changes in ability to discriminate taste or smell.

Secondary Prevention (Screening)

Screening tests are common for vision and hearing. There are no routine screenings to evaluate the sense of smell or taste. Screening for sensory function is often performed as part of the physical assessment.

Vision

Vision screens are recommended across the lifespan. Starting in the newborn period, a pediatric eye evaluation is recommended at each well-child visit. Eye evaluations for children up to 3 years of age should occur at all well-child checkups and include history, assessment, external inspection of the eyes and lids, ocular motility assessment, pupil examination, and red reflex examination.[40] After age 3 years, the evaluation should also include age-appropriate visual acuity measurement and an attempt at ophthalmoscopy. Any abnormal findings would warrant a referral to a pediatric ophthalmologist.

Adults up to 40 years of age should receive an eye exam at least every 2 years.[41] The same recommendation is applicable for middle-aged adults, those up to age 60 years; however, special attention should be paid to individuals with chronic conditions such as diabetes, heart disease, and hypertension, who would then be considered to be high risk for the development of visual problems. In addition, this is the time frame in which presbyopia often begins to develop.

For adults older than age 60 years, yearly eye exams are recommended to screen for simple vision loss related to aging as well as age-related eye disorders such as glaucoma and macular degenerative disease.[41] Eye examination with dilation and careful inspection can often diagnose these problems, but tonometry is necessary when considering glaucoma, a disease in which fluid pressure in the eye is consistently elevated, causing damage to the optic nerve and leading to loss of vision. Tonometry involves the use of a covered probe to gently touch the corneal surface several times to record the average intraocular pressure. The cornea is anesthetized first with eye drops before the pressures are measured. Normal IOP is 10 to 22 mm Hg, and pressures greater than 22 mm Hg are considered abnormal. Those with ongoing pressures greater than 27 mm Hg are at a higher risk of glaucoma.[4]

Hearing

Screening for hearing is recommended for all neonates by 1 month of age; if abnormal, they should be repeated by 3 months of age.[26] Hearing tests are usually done within 48 hours of birth in the hospital setting. Infants who fail the hearing test are referred to their local Early Hearing Detection and Intervention program for follow-up. However, sometimes the failure is due to external ear canal vernix or middle ear fluid resulting in temporary hearing loss.[42] The two common screening methods used with infants are OAEs and ABRs, which have already been discussed. Outer and inner ear inspection, with the use of an otoscope, is typically done at each well-child visit; for adults, however, otoscopic inspection is usually completed only when the patient reports a hearing problem.

Collaborative Interventions: Vision

For many visual problems, especially those associated with decreased visual acuity, corrective lenses (glasses and contact lenses) are a relatively easy and inexpensive treatment.

Surgery

There are a number of surgical procedures performed to treat conditions of the eye. Laser-assisted in situ keratomileusis (LASIK) is a surgical procedure that involves cutting a small flap in the cornea and then retracting the flap. Pulses from a computer-controlled laser then remove small parts of the cornea, permanently reshaping its surface. The reshaped cornea can better focus light onto the eye and onto the retina, allowing for improved vision.[43] The most common treatment for a cataract is the surgical removal of the lens. Laser surgery may be indicated for some patients with macular degeneration.[31] Microsurgical and laser procedures are also available to treat many other visual disorders and are being done more frequently.[44]

Pharmacotherapy

Certain visual disorders can be initially treated with β-adrenergic eye drops, which decrease the production of aqueous humor. Other types of eye drops prescribed include prostaglandin analogues, adrenergic agonists, and carbonic anhydrase inhibitors. Oral forms of carbonic anhydrase inhibitors can also be prescribed. Individuals with macular degeneration may have the option of injectable drug treatments and photodynamic therapy.[45] Other common forms of ophthalmic pharmacotherapy include the use of antibiotic, steroidal, and analgesic agents.

Collaborative Interventions: Hearing

Surgery

For recurrent otitis media in children, unresolved by the use of an antimicrobial, surgical intervention may become necessary. A myringotomy involves a small incision made in the tympanic membrane, removal of fluid, and the insertion of a small tube. This surgery is typically done as an outpatient procedure under general anesthesia.[46]

Cochlear implants are devices that are surgically implanted to provide direct electrical stimulation to the auditory nerve. Children as young as 2 years of age and adults with profound hearing loss may have success with these implants. Although a cochlear implant may not restore hearing, it may allow for the perception of sound.[7]

Adaptive Methods

Adaptive methods provide additional options for hearing and vision problems and include braille, guide dogs, sign language, closed-caption television, assistive listening, and newer technologies. As previously mentioned, if a person is experiencing sensory loss from medication therapy, it is likely that discontinuing the therapy may result in the deficit being restored.

Collaborative Interventions: Smell and Taste

Individuals with disorders of the nose, sinuses, and mouth that affect taste and smell may require surgical intervention or the use of medication therapy to improve or restore sensory perception.

Surgery

Surgical removal of nasal polyps, chronically inflamed sinus tissue, and retained secretions is performed to restore a normal sense of smell. Oral and dental surgical procedures to remove diseased tissue or teeth aim to restore normal flora and function.

Pharmacotherapy

The use of an intranasal corticosteroid spray is recommended to reduce or eliminate inflammation in the nasal and sinus passages. Further use of medications such as antihistamines is effective for the treatment and control of allergic rhinitis, which often causes chronic sinus congestion and polyposis.

Adaptive Methods

Avoidance measures to reduce or eliminate environmental chemicals and toxins and/or allergens with the use of masks and filtration systems are advised, furthering the preservation of the sense of smell and taste.

Collaborative Interventions: Touch

Loss of the sense of touch is most often associated with comorbid disease; therefore treatment with surgery and/or medications are aimed at controlling or eliminating the underlying cause.

Adaptive Methods

For individuals with an impaired sense of touch, the use of adaptive devices aimed at ensuring safety in the home and injury prevention is imperative. This can be achieved in many ways, from setting the hot water heater to a lower temperature to prevent unintentional burns to the wearing of proper footwear to prevent trauma to the feet when walking and gain better balance control. Protecting the fingertips during cold temperatures is imperative for individuals with Raynaud syndrome and other peripheral vascular problems to prevent frostbite.

CLINICAL NURSING SKILLS FOR SENSORY PERCEPTION

- Assessment
  - General assessment
  - Assessment of senses
- Irrigation of eye and ear
- Medication administration
- Oral hygiene demonstration/teaching
- Prevention strategies for occupational and recreational exposure to hazards
  - Eye protection
  - Hearing protection
  - Other proper protective equipment
- Foreign body removal
- Age-appropriate teaching strategies for safety in the home (e.g., childproof cupboard locks and hot water heater setting)
- Assistive devices
  - Hearing aid
  - Eyewear
  - Cane/walker/wheelchair
  - Prosthetics (e.g., eye and lower limb)

INTERRELATED CONCEPTS

As previously mentioned, the concept of Sensory Perception is interrelated with several other concepts discussed in this textbook, but especially Intracranial Regulation, Pain, Mobility, Nutrition, Development, and Functional Ability (Fig. 27.4).

The brain is an amazing organ with more than 100 billion cells that regulate sensory input and output. For this reason, Intracranial Regulation is highly interrelated to this concept. This is most notable in the presence of brain disturbances, when presenting symptoms are seen with changes in sensory function. Pain is a sensation that most people do not want to experience; however, sometimes pain is necessary to provide the brain with the signals needed to cause action to remove the pain source. Certain disorders, especially neurologic disorders, have the potential to alter sensation and perception, thus affecting Mobility. For example, when a person has suffered a neurologic impairment such as a CVA, or stroke, mobility is often impaired due to paralysis and paresthesia of an arm or leg.

The inability to taste and smell reduces the desire to eat because these senses have a vital role in initiating the digestive process. Failure to consume sufficient quantities and types of food can lead to Nutrition impairment. For example, patients undergoing chemotherapy often experience taste disturbances that decrease their desire for food, leading to nutritional deficiencies.

Development can be significantly affected among children with limitations in hearing and vision. Such problems can lead to delays in speech, language, and communication skills. Adaptation to special methods of communication must begin early in life to ensure progression throughout this critical developmental period to avoid isolation, reduced academic achievement, and poor self-concept.[47] Among adults, Functional Ability may be impeded when an individual experiences either diminished or complete loss of sensory perception. Adequate sensory perception allows humans to interact efficiently within the environment and provides the basis for social interactions, communication, and learning. Impairment at any age or stage of life can have detrimental effects on the ability to enjoy human interaction and impacts quality of life and well-being. As individuals age, age-related decline in hearing and vision occurs, often leading to depression, anxiety, and social isolation.[48]

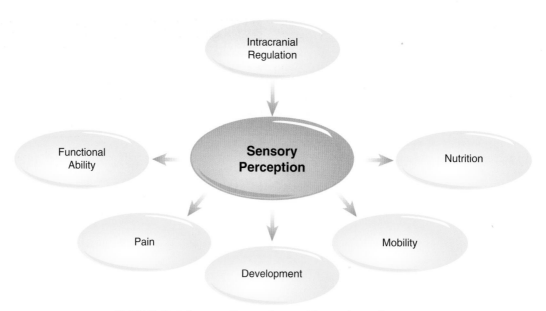

FIGURE 27.4 Sensory Perception and Interrelated Concepts.

CLINICAL EXEMPLARS

The concept of sensory perception represents the five senses; therefore, a multitude of exemplars exist. Box 27.2 details several exemplars that may occur across the lifespan. Note that an overlap of one or more acute and/or chronic conditions affecting sensory perception often occurs in one's lifetime. Detailed explanations and the nursing care for these conditions are presented in a variety of medical–surgical, pediatric, and gerontology resources. Brief explanations of several classic conditions are described next.

Featured Exemplars
Presbycusis
Age-related hearing loss, called presbycusis, is typically sensorineural (caused by pathologic changes in the inner ear or in the nerve pathways from the inner ear to the brain) and refers to a decrease in the ability to hear and process sound that is associated with aging and cannot be explained by the patient's genetic history, other diseases, or injury to the auditory system.[14] Presbycusis is present in approximately 35% of individuals 65 to 75 years of age; it is present in 50% of individuals older than age 75 years.[25]

Otitis Media
Otitis media is the second most common illness diagnosed in children. Children younger than 7 years of age are particularly vulnerable because of their immature immune system, and this illness is further complicated by poorly functioning eustachian tubes. Persistent or prolonged otitis media can lead to repeated use of antimicrobial therapy, conductive hearing loss, and associated developmental delay in speech and language. It can also cause disseminated infection, disruption of the tympanic membrane, and the requirement for surgery.[49]

Nasal Polyps
Nasal polyps are known to be associated with several immunologic conditions, infection, and aspirin sensitivity. Although the etiology for the development of nasal polyposis is unclear, the condition appears to be directly related to chronic inflammation in the nose and nasal passages. Patients with nasal polyps frequently experience significant

changes in their ability to smell, often leading to partial (hyposmia) or complete loss of smell (anosmia). The presence of nasal polyps is also associated with exacerbation of asthma, or poorly controlled asthma. Treatment is generally with the use of oral or intranasal corticosteroids. Treatment of severe nasal polyposis is often surgical, although recurrence is common.[50]

Meniere Disease
Meniere disease is characterized by episodic unilateral temporary hearing loss often accompanied by ringing (tinnitus) and a sensation of ear fullness or congestion in the affected ear as well as severe dizziness (vertigo). Patients often experience these symptoms in clusters of varying severity and duration with interspersed complete remission. Meniere disease is thought to be caused by a dysfunction of the endolymphatic system in the inner ear, resulting in interference with balance and hearing. Because there is no cure, treatment is focused on symptom control, with low-sodium diet, diuretic therapy, vestibular suppressant, cognitive therapy, pulse pressure treatment, and, in rare cases, ear surgery.[17]

Raynaud Syndrome
Raynaud syndrome is caused by vasospasms of distal arteries and arterioles, resulting in limitation of blood supply, causing the skin to turn white (pallor) and then blue (cyanosis). Patients will experience numbness, prickly feeling, stinging pain, and coldness of the hands and feet, which are generally triggered by a sudden exposure to cold temperature. Raynaud syndrome is more common in individuals who reside in colder climates and occurs more frequently in women. Treatment is primarily cold avoidance, wearing protective clothing, tobacco avoidance, and, if needed, medications to dilate blood vessels and promote circulation.[21]

Chemotherapy-Induced Alteration in Taste
It is reported that nearly three-fourths of patients who receive chemotherapy experience alterations in taste.[29] These changes can range from a sweet, sour, or bitter taste in the mouth to complete loss of taste perception. Patients also often experience inflammation of the oral mucosa (stomatitis), oral thrush, dry mouth, and other changes associated with cancer treatment. Changes in taste perception occur in approximately

BOX 27.2 EXEMPLARS OF IMPAIRED SENSORY PERCEPTION

Congenital Exemplars
- Deafness
- Cleft palate/lip
- Structural ear anomalies
- Congenital cataracts
- Retinopathy of prematurity

Visual Exemplars
- Amblyopia
- Blindness
- Presbyopia
- Cataract
- Retinal detachment
- Macular degenerative disease
- Glaucoma

Auditory Exemplars
- Sensorineural hearing loss
- Conductive hearing loss
- Mixed hearing loss
- Neoplasm and cholesteatoma
- Meniere disease

Gustatory Exemplars
- Ageusia
- Hypogeusia
- Dysgeusia
- Burning mouth syndrome

Olfactory Exemplars
- Anosmia
- Hyposmia
- Parosmia
- Phantosmia
- Tobacco use disorder

Somatosensory Exemplars
- Peripheral neuropathy
- Peripheral artery disease
- Raynaud syndrome
- Systemic sclerosis

ACCESS EXEMPLAR LINKS IN YOUR GIDDENS EBOOK

50% of patients receiving chemotherapy and may result in food aversion, subsequent weight loss, and malnutrition.[29] Diminished quality of life and social isolation may occur as a result, further challenging the resolve of the cancer patient.

Diabetic Retinopathy

Diabetic retinopathy is the leading cause of blindness among adults in America.[22] The effects of diabetic retinopathy are often already present in patients diagnosed with type 2 diabetes at age 30 years or older.[22] Diabetic retinopathy is the result of changes to the blood vessels of the retina that occur over time. Patients are often unaware of these changes during the early stages of development; however, as the damage becomes more extensive, vision loss ensues. Prevention is the primary focus of care with good control of blood sugar levels. In addition, surgical procedures such as laser treatment and vitrectomy to control bleeding of the damaged retina and restore sight may be used.

CASE STUDY

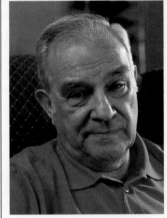

Case Presentation
Mr. Robert Holton, 74 years old and retired, spent his entire working career as a self-employed carpenter. He has a 22-year history of type 2 diabetes; he also has hypertension and emphysema. He is an active smoker (52-pack-year smoking history), although he has attempted to stop smoking on several occasions. He wears a hearing aid in each ear because of hearing loss as a result of working around machinery for many years.

Robert presents for a routine 3-month visit with the nurse practitioner accompanied by his wife. Mrs. Holton reports that Robert's feet smell very bad, but he does not seem to notice the odor. The nurse practitioner removes Robert's shoes and socks; a large infected foot ulcer is observed on the bottom of the foot. Robert is surprised that he was unaware of the wound. When asked about other changes, Robert does not respond. Mrs. Holton reports that he recently failed his visual acuity test for driver's license renewal and now must depend on her for transportation. She adds that he has become increasingly withdrawn over the past 6 months and does little to communicate with her or others; he is also not interested in leaving the house. She asks the nurse practitioner if he is depressed.

Case Analysis Questions
1. What risk factors are present in this case that relate to the concept?
2. What sensory and perception impairments are exemplified in this case?
3. Review Fig. 27.4. Which interrelated concepts apply to this case? Are there other interrelated concepts that apply to this case?

From Juanmonino/iStock/Thinkstock.

ACCESS EXEMPLAR LINKS IN YOUR GIDDENS EBOOK

REFERENCES

1. Day, A. (2008). Sensation, perception, and cognition. In R. Daniels (Ed.), *Nursing fundamentals: Caring and clinical decision making.* Florence, KY: Delmar Cengage Learning.
2. Seidel, H., Dains, J., Flynn, J., et al. (2015). *Mosby's guide to physical examination.* St Louis: Elsevier.
3. Centers for Disease Control and Prevention. (2017). *Blindness and Visual Impairment.* Retrieved from https://www.cdc.gov/healthcommunication/toolstemplates/entertainmented/tips/Blindness.html.
4. Lewis, S. (2017). Assessment of visual and auditory systems. In S. Lewis, L. Bucher, M. Heitkemper, et al. (Eds.), *Medical–surgical nursing: Assessment and management of clinical problems* (10th ed.). St Louis: Elsevier.
5. Banasik, J. L. (2018). *Pathophysiology* (6th ed.). St. Louis: Saunders.
6. Schiffman, S. S. (2007). Critical illness and changes in sensory perception. *The Proceedings of the Nutrition Society, 66,* 331–345.
7. American Speech Language Hearing Association. (n.d.). *Cochlear implants.* Retrieved from http://www.asha.org/public/hearing/Cochlear-Implant.
8. Burns, C. E., Dunn, A. M., Brady, M. A., et al. (2013). *Pediatric primary care* (5th ed.). Philadelphia: Saunders.

9. The University of the State of New York. (2011). *The State Education Department Student Support Service Team: School vision screening guidelines*. Retrieved from http://www.p12.nysed.gov/sss/schoolhealth/ schoolhealthservices/VisionScreeningGuidelines2011.pdf.

10. Wilson, S., & Giddens, J. (2017). *Health assessment for nursing practice* (6th ed.). St. Louis: Elsevier.

11. Institute of Medicine (U.S.). (2010). *Food Forum: Providing healthy and safe foods as we age:* Workshop summary. Washington, DC: National Academies Press.

12. Schumm, L., McClintock, M., Williams, S., et al. (2009). Assessment of sensory function in the national social life, health, and aging project. *The Journals of Gerontology. Series B, Psychological Sciences and Social Sciences, 64*, i76.

13. Taffet, G. E. (2017). *Normal Aging*. Retrieved from https:// www.uptodate.com/home.

14. Bance, M. (2007). Hearing and aging. *Canadian Medical Association Journal, 176*, 925.

15. Murphy, C., Schubert, C., Cruickshanks, K., et al. (2007). Prevalence of olfactory impairment in older adults. *JAMA: The Journal of the American Medical Association, 288*, 2307.

16. Boyce, J., & Shone, G. (2006). Effects of ageing on smell and taste. *Postgraduate Medical Journal, 82*, 239.

17. Lalwani, A. K. (2004). *Diagnosis & treatment in otolaryngology—Head & neck surgery*. New York: McGraw-Hill.

18. Wickremaratchi, M., & Llewelyn, J. (2005). Effects of ageing on touch. *Postgraduate Medical Journal, 82*, 301.

19. Craig, J., Rhodes, R., Busey, T., et al. (2010). Aging and tactile temporal order. *Attention Percept Psychophys, 72*, 226.

20. Sharts-Hopko, N. (2010). Lifestyle strategies for the prevention of vision loss. *Holistic Nursing Practice, 24*, 284.

21. Rakel, R. E., & Rakel, D. P. (2016). *Textbook of family medicine* (9th ed.). Philadelphia: Saunders.

22. Harris, L. L., & Huntoon, M. B. (2008). *Core curriculum for otorhinolaryngology and head–neck nursing* (2nd ed.). New Smyrna Beach, FL: Society of Otorhinolaryngology and Head–Neck Nurses.

23. American Speech Language Hearing Association. (n.d.). *Hearing loss at birth (congenital hearing loss)*. Retrieved from https://www.asha.org/ public/hearing/Congenital-Hearing-Loss/.

24. Wickremaratchi, M. M., & Llewelyn, J. G. (2006). Effects of ageing on touch. *Postgraduate Medical Journal, 82*(967), 301–304.

25. Freedman, V., Martin, L., & Schoeni, R. (2002). Recent trends in disability & functioning in older adults in the United States. *Journal of the American Medical Association, 228*(24), 3137–3146.

26. U.S. Preventive Services Task Force. (2008). *Clinical summary: Hearing loss in newborns*. Retrieved from http://www.uspreventiveservicestaskforce. org/Page/Topic/recommendation-summary/hearing-loss-in-newborns- screening.

27. Yorgason, J., Fayad, J., & Kalinec, F. (2006). Understanding drug ototoxicity: Molecular insights for prevention and clinical management. *Expert Opinion on Drug Safety, 5*, 383.

28. Madnani, N., & Khan, K. (2010). Doc, I can't taste my food! *Indian J Dermatol Venerol Leprol, 76*, 296.

29. OncoLink. (2018). *Taste changes during cancer therapy*. Retrieved from https://www.oncolink.org/treatment-binder.

30. Hutton, J., Baracos, V., & Wismer, W. (2007). Chemosensory dysfunction is a primary factor in the evolution of declining nutritional status and quality of life in patients with advanced cancer. *Journal of Pain and Symptom Management, 33*, 156.

31. Doty, R., & Bromley, S. (2004). Effects of drugs on olfaction and taste. *Otolaryngologic Clinics of North America, 37*, 1229.

32. Leekam, S., Nieto, C., Libby, S., et al. (2007). Describing the sensory abnormalities of children and adults with autism. *Journal of Autism and Developmental Disorders, 37*, 894.

33. Vennemann, M., Hummel, T., & Berger, K. (2008). The association between smoking and smell and taste impairment in the general population. *Journal of Neurology, 255*, 1121.

34. National Institute on Deafness and Other Communication Disorders. (2014). *Noise-induced hearing loss*. Retrieved from http:// www.nidcd.nih.gov/health/hearing/pages/noise.aspx.

35. National Institute on Deafness and Other Communication Disorders. (2017). *Taste Disorders*. Retrieved from https://www.nidcd.nih.gov/health/ taste-disorders.

36. American Academy of Otolaryngology-Head and Neck Surgery. (2018). *Smell and Taste*. Retrieved from https://www.entnet.org//content/ smell-taste.

37. Dros, J., Wewerinke, A., Bindels, P., et al. (2009). Accuracy of the monofilament testing to diagnose peripheral neuropathy: A systematic review. *Annals of Family Medicine, 7*, 556.

38. American Speech Language Hearing Association. (n.d.). *Hearing screening and testing*. Retrieved from http://www.asha.org/public/hearing/ Hearing-Testing.

39. National Eye Institute. (2012). *Occupational Eye Safety*. Retrieved from https://www.nei.nih.gov/faqs/resources-occupational-eye-safety.

40. American Academy of Pediatrics. (2003). Eye examination in infants, children, and young adults by pediatricians. *Pediatrics, 111*, 902.

41. American Optometric Association. (n.d.). *Comprehensive eye and vision examination*. Retrieved from http://www.aoa.org/patients-and-public/ caring-for-your-vision/comprehensive-eye-and-vision-examination?sso=y.

42. Doyle, K. J., Burggraaff, B., Fujikawa, S., et al. (1997). Neonatal hearing screening with otoscopy, auditory brain stem response, and otoacoustic emissions. *Otolaryngology–Head and Neck Surgery : Official Journal of American Academy of Otolaryngology-Head and Neck Surgery, 116*, 597–603.

43. U. S. Department of Health and Human Services. (2018). *Lasik*. Retrieved from http://www.fda.gov/MedicalDevices/ProductsandMedicalProcedures/ SurgeryandLifeSupport/LASIK/default.htm.

44. Dahl, A. (2015). *Glaucoma*. Retrieved from http://www.medicinenet.com/ glaucoma/article.htm.

45. Mayo Clinic. (2018). *Retinal Diseases*. Retrieved from https:// www.mayoclinic.org/diseases-conditions/retinal-diseases/ symptoms-causes/syc-20355825.

46. Cunha, J. (2018). *Ear tubes*. Retrieved from http://www.medicinenet.com/ ear_tubes/article.htm.

47. American Speech–Language–Hearing Association. (2018). *Effects of hearing loss on development*. Retrieved from http://www.asha.org/public/ hearing/Effects-of-Hearing-Loss-on-Development.

48. Heine, C., & Browning, C. J. (2002). Communication and psychosocial consequences of sensory loss in older adults: Overview and rehabilitation directions. *Disability & Rehabilitation, 24*(15), 763–773.

49. Rosenfeld, R. M., Schwartz, S. R., Pynnonen, M. A., et al. (2013). Clinical practice guideline: Tympanostomy tubes in children. *Otolaryngology– Head and Neck Surgery : Official Journal of American Academy of Otolaryngology-Head and Neck Surgery, 149*(Suppl. 1), S1–S35.

50. Newton, J. R., & Ah-See, K. W. (2008). A review of nasal polyposis. *Therapeutics and Clinical Risk Management, 4*(2), 507–512.

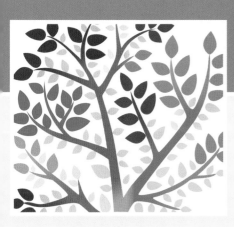

Pain

Angela Renee Starkweather

Across the lifespan, pain is one of the most common reasons people seek health care, a frequent reason for taking medication, and a major cause of disability.[1] In the United States, common chronic pain conditions affect more than 100 million people and cost more than $560 billion annually in direct medical treatment and lost productivity.[2] Although the field of pain management has experienced rapid growth in technology and research during the past several years, pain continues to be undertreated across care settings. Aligned with ethical standards for healthcare professionals regarding the provision of measures to minimize pain and suffering, adequate assessment and management of pain is viewed as a human right.[3] As healthcare professionals who provide 24-hour presence 7 days a week, nurses play an important role in the management of pain and can be instrumental in ensuring their patients receive the best possible pain relief available.

DEFINITION

The International Association for the Study of Pain defines pain as "an unpleasant sensory and emotional experience associated with actual or potential tissue damage, or described in terms of such damage."[4,p.209] This definition describes pain as a complex phenomenon with multiple components that impact a person's psychosocial and physical functioning. The accepted clinical definition of pain, which was proposed by Margo McCaffery in 1968, is accepted worldwide and reinforces that pain is a highly personal and subjective experience: "Pain is whatever the experiencing person says it is, existing whenever he says it does."[5,p.8] This is why all accepted guidelines consider the patient's report to be the most reliable indicator of pain.[6]

SCOPE

Pain is a universal experience, although each person may experience pain in a different way. Conceptually, pain is a multidimensional symptom that can influence virtually every aspect of a person's life—the physical, psychological, emotional, social, and spiritual realms. The scope of pain as a concept may be viewed as a normal physiological response to tissue injury or as a pathological symptom associated with a disease process or alteration of the somatosensory system. Normally, pain serves as a protective mechanism that is meant to alert the brain to potential or actual bodily harm or tissue damage, such as pain that results from an ankle sprain or fractured limb. However, pain that persists after the usual time for healing to take place serves no useful purpose and is viewed as pathologic. The concept of pain also ranges across several descriptive continuums, including location, intensity, frequency, and duration. In terms of location, pain may be well localized such as in a joint, or widespread, occurring all over the body. The intensity continuum of pain ranges from none to minimal, moderate, and severe pain (Fig. 28.1). The frequency of pain may be intermittent, occurring every few minutes, hourly, or daily with episodes of no pain, or it may be constant without any breaks at all. Pain may be acute, such as pain that occurs directly after an injury and that dissipates with time as the injury heals. However, pain can also be chronic when it is associated with a disease process or when it persists after injury, and may last for months, years, or a lifetime.

NORMAL PHYSIOLOGICAL PROCESS

The sensations that we experience in our body are orchestrated by an eloquent network of cells, fibers, and organs, known as the somatosensory system, which receives, transmits, and interprets sensory information. Specialized sensory receptor cells carry specific types of sensory information (vision, hearing, touch, heat/cold, proprioception, and pain) along different anatomical pathways depending on the information carried.[7] The cells of free nerve endings in the skin and peripheral organs that are somatosensory receptors for the sensation of pain are known as nociceptors. Nociceptors are found in all tissues except the central nervous system (CNS). Tissue injury activates nociceptors to transmit pain information through the somatosensory system, a process known as nociception. When the brain receives and interprets the information as an unpleasant painful sensation, it is known as nociceptive pain, which is a protective mechanism to alert the brain to potential or actual tissue damage.[5] Although nociceptive pain requires the occurrence of nociception, nociception does not always result in nociceptive pain. The brain has a powerful influence on how we perceive sensory information and may filter or block pain information from awareness, or change our perception of the sensory information.[8] First proposed in 1965 by Melzack and Wall, the gate control theory is considered to be one of the most influential theories of pain because of its focus on a neural basis of pain.[9] The gate control theory asserts that nonnoxious input can close the "gate" to the CNS, thereby preventing painful input from reaching the brain. In this manner, nonpainful stimulation is able to suppress pain. Since that time, it has become well-recognized that pain is a complex condition involving numerous areas of the brain and is influenced by emotional, cognitive, and environmental elements.

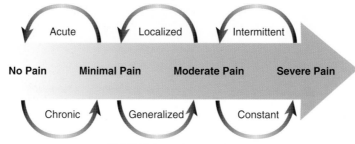

FIGURE 28.1 Scope of Pain.

Neurological System

Pain is a conscious experience that requires an awareness of sensations via an intact CNS to receive sensory information and interpret the information as an unpleasant and painful sensation. Nociception, or the response of the sensory nervous system to potentially damaging mechanical, thermal, or chemical stimuli, is a physiologic process, whereas pain is a subjective experience. The mechanisms that lead to the perception of nociceptive pain are described here and illustrated in Fig. 28.2.

Transduction

Tissue damage results in the release of chemical mediators from damaged cells that activate nociceptors. These chemical mediators include prostaglandins, bradykinin, serotonin, substance P, and histamine.[10] When the chemical mediators attach to the membrane of the nociceptor, this can result in the opening of sodium channels that activate the nociceptor and cause the generation of an action potential.

Transmission

The action potential subsequently moves from the site of nociceptor activation along specialized afferent nerve fibers that carry pain impulses, known as Aδ and C fibers, to the spinal cord. Aδ fibers are thinly myelinated sensory fibers that send pain impulses faster than unmyelinated C fibers. Due to the myelin covering the Aδ fibers, they are capable of transmitting sharp, stabbing pain sensations, whereas C fibers transmit aching burning-type pain sensations. Substance P and other neurotransmitters allow the action potential to proceed across the cleft to the dorsal horn of the spinal cord, where it ascends the spinothalamic tract to the thalamus and midbrain.

Perception

Fibers from the thalamus send the nociceptive message to the somatosensory cortex, frontal and parietal lobe, as well as the limbic system, where pain is perceived and interpreted based on past experience, beliefs, attitudes, and meaning.

Modulation

Activation of the midbrain results in the release of substances such as endorphins, enkephalins, serotonin, and dynorphin from neurons that descend to the lower areas of the brain and spinal cord, stimulating the release of endogenous opioids that inhibit transmission of pain impulses at the dorsal horn.

Age-Related Differences

The mechanisms of nociceptive pain are normally present at birth and remain functional throughout the adult lifespan. The presence of acute pain remains approximately the same across the adult lifespan; however, there is an age-related increase in the prevalence of chronic pain, which affects more than 50% of older persons living in the community and greater than 80% of nursing home residents.[11] Although chronic pain is prevalent among older adults, it is not a normal part of aging.[12] Clinical studies have shown that elderly individuals are more vulnerable to chronic pain and that the ability to tolerate severe pain decreases with age.[2]

VARIATIONS AND CONTEXT

Acute and Chronic Pain

Pain is usually described as being *acute* or *chronic (persistent)*.[4] Acute pain is of sudden onset and is typically clearly linked to a specific event injury or illness. For example, tissue damage as a result of surgery, trauma, or burns produces acute pain, which is expected to be relatively short-lived and to diminish with normal healing. However, there may be variations in the intensity, frequency, and duration of pain between individuals after having the same surgical procedure or injury. This is why the subjective report of pain is so important; the experience of pain is highly individualized. However, when referring to acute pain, it is expected to dissipate with time along with the normal healing process.

In contrast, chronic pain is defined as pain lasting more than 3 months and may last for years.[4] Chronic pain may result from underlying medical conditions (pathology), such as cancer pain from tumor growth or osteoarthritis pain from joint degeneration. Chronic pain may also develop from an injury, medical treatment, inflammation, or unknown causes that alter the somatosensory system, in the periphery, spinal cord, or brain. As an advancement from the gate control theory which describes the origins of pain, the neuromatrix theory posits that pain is the output of the neural network that is "genetically determined and modified by sensory experience" throughout life.[13] This theory has promoted new thinking about chronic pain conditions, such as fibromyalgia, that do not have an obvious cause but are associated with changes in the CNS. Chronic pain can persist throughout a person's lifespan and varies in intensity, frequency, and duration. In addition, patients may experience both acute and chronic pain, such as when a patient with chronic cancer pain experiences acute pain after undergoing a painful procedure related to cancer treatment.

Pain Classification

Pain is most often classified by its inferred mechanism as being either *nociceptive pain* or *neuropathic pain*.[4] Nociceptive pain refers to normal functioning of the somatosensory system in response to noxious stimuli (tissue injury) that is perceived as being painful. Simply stated, nociception means "normal" pain transmission. Normal transduction of pain sensation by nociceptors is also known as eudynic pain. Examples of nociceptive pain include pain from a sunburn, surgery, or trauma. Patients often describe this type of pain as "aching," "cramping," or "throbbing." Nociceptive pain may also be categorized as somatic or visceral. Somatic pain is characterized as sharp pain that is well localized to a specific area of injury. Visceral pain arises from within the body cavity, most commonly the thorax, abdomen, and pelvis. Pain receptors in the visceral cavities respond to stretching, swelling, and

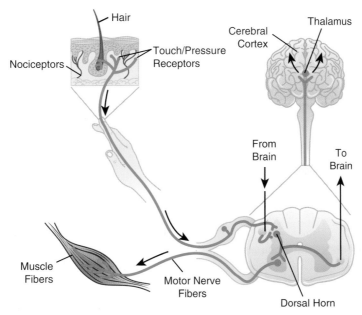

FIGURE 28.2 Pain Pathways from the Periphery to the Brain and Back.

oxygen deprivation, and the pain may radiate to other locations in the back or chest.

Although the normal mechanisms of nociceptive pain occur from stimulation of nociceptors, pain may also occur as neuropathic pain, which results from a pathology or disease of the somatosensory system.[4] Simply stated, neuropathic pain is pathologic. Examples of neuropathic pain include postherpetic neuralgia, diabetic neuropathy, phantom pain, complex regional pain syndrome, trigeminal neuralgia, and poststroke pain syndrome. Patients with neuropathic pain use very distinctive words to describe their pain, such as "burning," "sharp," and "shooting." Other forms of neuropathic pain are described by the mechanism involved. Sympathetically mediated pain is accompanied by evidence of edema, changes in skin blood flow, and abnormal sensations such as allodynia, hyperalgesia, and hyperpathia. Deafferentation pain is chronic and results from the loss of afferent input to the CNS. The pain may arise in the periphery from a peripheral nerve avulsion or in the CNS from spinal cord lesions or multiple sclerosis. Neuralgia pain is lancinating and associated with nerve damage or irritation along the distribution of a single nerve. Central pain arises from a lesion in the CNS, usually involving the spinothalamic cortical pathways, such as a thalamic infarct. The pain is usually constant with a burning, electrical quality. It is exacerbated by activity, and hyperesthesia and hyperpathia and/or allodynia are usually present.

Some patients have a combination of nociceptive and neuropathic pain. For example, a patient may have nociceptive pain as a result of a peripheral tumor that is growing and activates nociceptors around actual tissue damage; if the tumor is pressing against a nerve plexus, the patient may also report radiating sharp and shooting neuropathic pain. Some painful conditions and syndromes are not easily categorized and are thought to be unique with multiple underlying and poorly understood mechanisms. These are referred to as *mixed pain syndromes* and include fibromyalgia and some low back and myofascial pain.

CONSEQUENCES

Pain triggers a number of physiological and psychosocial responses and can produce a cascade of harmful effects in all body systems.

Physiologic Consequences

The stress response causes the endocrine system to release excessive amounts of hormones, such as cortisol, catecholamines, and glucagon. Insulin and testosterone levels decrease.[14] Increased endocrine activity in turn initiates a number of metabolic processes, particularly accelerated carbohydrate, protein, and fat destruction (catabolism), which can result in weight loss, tachycardia, increased respiratory rate, shock, and even death.[15] The immune system is also affected by pain, as demonstrated by research showing a link between unrelieved pain and a higher incidence of nosocomial infections[16] and increased tumor growth.[17,18]

Unrelieved pain impacts the respiratory system, causing small tidal volumes and decreases in functional lung capacity, which can lead to pneumonia, atelectasis, and an increased need for mechanical ventilation.[19,20] Effects on the cardiovascular system include increased postoperative blood loss[21] and hypercoagulation,[22] which can lead to myocardial infarction and stroke. Increased heart rate and blood pressure are autonomic responses to acute pain.

Pain can affect a patient's level of physical functioning. When pain is experienced with movement or mobility, the patient may associate the movement with pain. In this situation, it is very important for patients to understand that nonuse of the affected area and immobility can lead to muscle atrophy and joint contraction, which further promotes pain and impairs physical functioning. Sympathetic nervous system activation caused by acute pain decreases the release of digestive enzymes in the gastrointestinal tract and slows peristalsis. When mobility is not restored after surgery or trauma, this can further impair gastrointestinal function.[23] In turn, many opioid medications used to treat pain can cause constipation, making it necessary to have routine stool softeners along with the opioid medications. The use of opioids, even when prescribed and taken as directed, can lead to abuse, misuse and addiction in some people.[24] Vigilant screening and assessment of substance use disorders and follow-up of patients on opioids is necessary to ensure that addiction is properly managed.

Psychosocial Consequences

Along with the array of physical consequences that can develop due to pain, chronic pain in particular may be associated with significant psychological and social consequences, including fear, anger, depression, anxiety, and reduced ability to maintain relationships, engage in normal activities, and continue to work.[2] Pain that does not dissipate with normal healing, and pain that is undertreated or untreated, can have a negative impact on nearly every aspect of a person's life and result in psychological and social consequences. Psychosocial consequences of pain treatment with opioids can include opioid use disorder, characterized by an overwhelming urge to use opioids even when they are no longer medically necessary to treat pain.[24] Addiction can affect every aspect of a person's life, including their relationships, employment, and economic status.

RISK FACTORS

With rare exception, everyone experiences pain at some point during the course of their lifetime. However, some population groups and individuals are at higher risk of experiencing severe or unrelieved pain than others.

Populations at Risk
Infants and Children

Neonates are at risk for pain, primarily from procedures such as heel sticks, venipuncture, and circumcision.[2] Critically ill infants are at very high risk for pain due to the high number of procedures performed. In the neonatal intensive care unit, sick neonates are commonly exposed to numerous painful procedures, including endotracheal intubation and suctioning, insertion of chest tubes, and arterial and venous punctures.[2] Infants, toddlers, and developmentally preverbal children do not have the cognitive skills to report and describe pain; thus other indicators besides self-report must be used to recognize and treat pain.

Older Adults

Although not all older adults experience pain, the incidence of pain increases with age, placing this population at higher risk for pain than younger individuals.[11] Pain has been shown to be very common in the older adult in the inpatient acute care setting and in the outpatient setting, such as nursing homes.[12] This is in large part because older adults suffer many of the conditions associated with pain, including musculoskeletal disorders such as degenerative spine conditions and arthritis. They are frequent recipients of surgical procedures and at increased risk of injury from falls and trauma, all of which can result in pain.[11] Some pain syndromes, such as postherpetic neuralgia, poststroke pain, and diabetic neuropathy, are more prevalent in the older population.[12] Cancer is more common in older adults than in younger adults, and as many as 80% of cancer patients experience pain as a consequence of the disease process, as well as its treatment. The older adult is at high risk for undertreatment of pain as well. Many are reluctant or unable to report their pain because of illness or cognitive impairment.[8] Research shows that clinicians fail to provide adequate analgesia based on the misconception that analgesics are not needed or fears that analgesics may cause adverse effects, such as confusion and respiratory depression.[12]

Other Population Groups

Other risk factors for pain or undertreatment of pain include sex, race, and ethnicity.[25] Across settings, women report a higher prevalence of chronic pain than men, which may relate to the various chronic pain syndromes that occur exclusively or predominantly in women, such as endometriosis and fibromyalgia. In experimental studies, women report lower pain thresholds (the amount of stimulus at which pain begins to be felt) and less tolerance for pain (the maximum level of pain that a person can tolerate).[2] Such gender differences are linked in part to hormone levels. Social factors that have an influence on access to pain treatments include income, education, and geographic location. Cultural and/or religious convictions may pose a barrier to reporting pain. In addition, as a population group, military veterans have increased vulnerability to pain due to the high risk of combat-related injury or trauma.[2]

Individual Risk Factors

A number of individual risk factors exist that place individuals at greater risk for experiencing pain, or risk for having insufficient pain relief, including communication barriers, genetic predisposition, cognitive impairment, substance use, individuals who have sustained significant injury, and those suffering from conditions that are known to cause pain.

Communication Barriers

Regardless of age, anyone who cannot report pain is at risk for undertreatment of pain. These individuals are referred to as *nonverbal* and include infants, toddlers, the cognitively impaired, and anesthetized, critically ill, comatose, and imminently dying patients. Patients who speak a different language may not understand the questions asked by healthcare providers and may lack the ability to adequately describe their pain experience. Furthermore, they may exhibit behavioral responses to pain differently, and these cues may be missed or misinterpreted by nurses from different cultural backgrounds.

Cognitive Impairment or Developmental Disability

The prevalence and burden of pain is higher in cognitively impaired or developmentally disabled children and adults compared to healthy individuals. Although a majority of individuals with cognitive impairment or developmental disability are verbal and can use a self-report pain assessment tool, behavioral pain tools should be used as well for initial and ongoing assessments.

Mental Health Conditions

Patients with a history or current use of illicit substances may be perceived as trying to obtain pain medication as part of their addiction. However, individuals with addictive disease also experience pain, and their report of pain should be addressed through multimodal therapies.[2] Mental illness is a common comorbidity with chronic pain.[2] A preexisting psychiatric illness may affect pain severity. In addition, patients with chronic pain may develop depression or anxiety disorders, particularly when they feel powerless or view their condition as hopeless. When patients present with mental illness and pain, both conditions should be addressed.

Injury or Conditions Associated with Pain

Some of the most obvious risk factors for pain are traumatic injury, critical illness, surgical procedures, or other conditions associated with pain. Acute and chronic medical conditions that are classically associated with severe pain include fractures, cluster headaches, passing kidney stones, trigeminal neuralgia, pancreatitis, shingles, herniated disc, and late stages of cancer. Critically ill patients of all ages experience a significant amount of pain from underlying painful pathologic conditions and the repetitive painful procedures to which they are exposed during the course of care.[15,19] Research has shown that the most painful procedure in the intensive care unit is turning,[20,21] which underscores the high prevalence of pain in the critical care setting.

ASSESSMENT

In a national agenda for improving pain assessment and management, The Joint Commission emphasized the need for frequent assessment and reassessment of pain.[2] More recently, the U.S. Department of Health and Human Services (DHHS), and Centers for Disease Control and Prevention (CDC) published recommendations for assessment and management of pain along with guidelines for opioid prescribing, which include routine assessment for actual or potential substance use disorders.[26,27] Precise and systematic assessment is required to determine the areas affected by pain, likely contributing factors, and most effective treatment plan for patients who present with pain. In addition, the location and description of pain can serve as a diagnostic clue to underlying pathology. The past medical history should be obtained, including relevant health conditions that may affect pain, past surgeries and injuries, psychiatric illnesses and chemical dependence, and prior problems with pain and treatment outcomes. Current stressors that the patient is facing can also help to identify psychosocial issues affecting the pain. The health of family members and family history of pain or illness should be obtained.

Conducting a Pain Assessment

The gold standard of pain assessment is the patient's subjective report of the pain experience.[4–6] A thorough pain assessment is obtained by asking the patient a number of questions, and it serves as the foundation for effective pain management. It is used to establish the initial treatment plan and determine when changes are needed.[6] The components of a comprehensive pain assessment are presented here.

Location(s) of Pain

Ask the patient to point to the area(s) of pain on the body.

Intensity

Ask the patient to rate the intensity of pain using a reliable and valid pain assessment tool. A number of scales in several language translations have been evaluated and made available for use in clinical practice and for educational purposes.[6] The following scales are most commonly used:

- *Numeric rating scale (NRS):* The NRS is most often presented as a horizontal 0- to 10-point scale, with word anchors of "no pain" at one end of the scale, "moderate pain" in the middle of the scale, and "worst possible pain" at the end of the scale.
- *Faces Pain Scale–Revised (FPS-R):* The FPS-R has six faces to make it consistent with other scales using the 0 to 10 metric. The faces range from a neutral facial expression to one of intense pain and are numbered 0, 2, 4, 6, 8, and 10. Patients are asked to choose the face that best describes their pain. The FPS-R is valid and reliable for use in children and adults, including cognitively intact and impaired elders.[28] Although young children may be able to select a face on a faces scale, they are unable to optimally quantify pain (identify a number) until approximately 8 years of age.[29]
- *Wong–Baker FACES Pain Rating Scale:* The FACES scale consists of six cartoon faces with word descriptors, ranging from a smiling face on the left for "no pain (no hurt)" to a frowning, tearful face on the right for "worst pain (hurts worst)." The faces are most commonly numbered using a 0, 2, 4, 6, 8, 10 metric; however, 0 to 5 can also be used. Patients are asked to choose the face that best describes their pain. The FACES scale is used in adults and children as young as age 3 years.[30]
- *Verbal descriptor scale (VDS):* A VDS uses a series of different words or phrases to describe the intensity of pain, such as "no pain," "mild pain," "moderate pain," "severe pain," "very severe pain," and "worst possible pain." The patient is asked to select the phrase that best describes his or her pain intensity. The scale can be presented horizontally or vertically and can be helpful for patients with difficulty using a numeric scale.[31]

Quality

Ask the patient to describe how the pain feels. Descriptors such as "burning" or "shooting" may identify the presence of neuropathic pain.

Onset and Duration

Ask the patient when the pain started, what activities he or she was performing when it began, as well as whether it is constant or intermittent.

Alleviating and Relieving Factors

Ask the patient what makes the pain better and what makes it worse. The answers help to determine which pain medications and nonpharmacologic interventions are effective and which are not.

Effect of Pain on Function and Quality of Life

Ask the patient to describe medication side effects (e.g., constipation, nausea, and sedation) and difficulty sleeping or eating. Assess for comorbidities, such as anxiety and depression. It is particularly important to ask patients with chronic pain how pain has affected their lives; ask what they could do before the pain began that they can no longer do, or what they want to do but cannot do because of the pain.

Comfort–Function (Pain) Goal

Discuss the expectation of functional goal achievement. For example, tell surgical patients that they will need to deep breathe, cough, turn, and ambulate or participate in physical therapy after surgery. Patients with chronic pain can be asked to identify their unique functional or quality-of-life goals, such as being able to work, walk the dog, or garden. Ask the patient to identify (using a 0 to 10 scale) a level of pain that will allow accomplishment of the identified functional or quality-of-life goals with reasonable ease. A realistic goal for most patients is 2 or 3, and pain intensity ratings that are consistently above the goal warrant further evaluation and consideration of an intervention and possible adjustment of the treatment plan.[6]

Breakthrough Pain

An important part of the pain assessment is to determine whether the patient is experiencing *breakthrough pain* and if its treatment is effective. Breakthrough pain (also called *pain flare*) is a transitory exacerbation of pain in a patient who has relatively stable and adequately controlled baseline pain.[8] When breakthrough pain is brief and precipitated by a voluntary action, such as movement, it is referred to as *incident pain.* Another type of breakthrough pain called *idiopathic pain* is not associated with any known cause and often lasts longer than incident pain. Episodes of pain that occur before the next analgesic dose is due are called *end-of-dose failure pain.* A fast-onset, short-acting formulation of a first-line analgesic, such as morphine, oxycodone, hydromorphone, or fentanyl, is used to manage breakthrough pain. Analgesic doses or the frequency of their administration is adjusted as needed to minimize the occurrence of breakthrough pain.[8]

Reassessment

Following initiation of the pain management plan, pain is reassessed and documented on a regular basis as a way to evaluate the effectiveness of the treatments. At a minimum, pain should be reassessed with each new report of pain and before and after the administration of analgesics.[32] The frequency of reassessment depends on the stability of the patient's pain and is guided by institutional policy. For example, in the acute care hospital setting, reassessment may be necessary as often as every 10 minutes when pain is unstable during the titration phase (gradual increases in dose to establish analgesia) and every 8 hours in patients with stable pain. Findings that warrant further evaluation or notification of the prescriber include pain ratings that continue to be higher than the patient's comfort–function goal, a change in the location or quality of pain, and the development of medication-induced side effects that do not respond to treatment. Nurse monitoring of side effects is essential to ensure patient safety during analgesic administration. Life-threatening opioid-induced respiratory depression is the most serious of the opioid side effects; however, nurses can be key to preventing this complication by performing systematic assessments of their patients' sedation levels.[8] Less opioid is required to produce sedation than to produce respiratory depression, a characteristic that makes sedation a particularly sensitive indicator of impending respiratory depression. Gradual increases in sedation level warrant prompt reduction of opioid dose and increased frequency of nurse monitoring until the patient demonstrates an acceptable level of sedation.[33]

Challenges in Assessment

Many patients are unable to provide a report of their pain because they are cognitively impaired or too young (infants and small children) to use customary self-report pain assessment tools. Other patients who present challenges in pain assessment are the critically ill (intubated and unresponsive) and those who are receiving neuromuscular blocking agents or are sedated from anesthetics and other drugs given during surgery. All of these patients are collectively referred to as "nonverbal" patients.[34]

When patients are unable to report pain using traditional methods, an alternative approach based on the Hierarchy of Importance of Pain Measures is recommended.[6,34,35] The key components of the hierarchy are to (1) attempt to obtain self-report, (2) consider underlying pathology or conditions and procedures that might be painful (e.g., surgery), (3) observe behaviors, (4) evaluate physiological indicators, and (5) conduct an analgesic trial.

Diagnostic Tests

Diagnostic tests, such as x-rays, computed tomography, magnetic resonance imaging, or ultrasound, may be used to examine the areas of pain to identify a potential etiology. However, these should not delay appropriate treatment of pain.

CLINICAL MANAGEMENT

For most of the health and illness concepts presented in this text, clinical management includes all phases of health promotion, including primary and secondary prevention. However, for the concept of pain, the relevant focus of clinical management involves interventions to treat pain.

Collaborative Interventions
Pharmacologic Strategies

Because pain is a complex phenomenon involving multiple underlying mechanisms, a multimodal regimen, which combines drugs with different underlying mechanisms, is often indicated. This allows lower doses of each of the drugs in the treatment plan, thereby reducing the potential for adverse effects[11,36] and can result in comparable or greater pain relief than can be achieved with any single analgesic.[11] Guidelines recommend the use of multimodal analgesia for all types of pain.[36–38] In addition, every patient encounter provides an opportunity to assess for substance abuse disorders and reevaluate the need for prescription analgesics.[27]

   Analgesics. There are three major analgesic groups:
- Nonopioid analgesics
- Opioid analgesics
- Adjuvant analgesics

Fig. 28.3 shows the first-line analgesics in each group.

Nonopioid analgesics are appropriate alone for mild to some moderate nociceptive-type pain and are added to opioid analgesics as part of a multimodal analgesic regimen for more severe nociceptive pain.[10,39] For example, unless contraindicated, all surgical patients should routinely be given acetaminophen and a nonsteroidal antiinflammatory drug (NSAID) in scheduled doses throughout the postoperative course. Opioid analgesics are added to the treatment plan to manage moderate to severe postoperative pain. A local anesthetic is sometimes administered

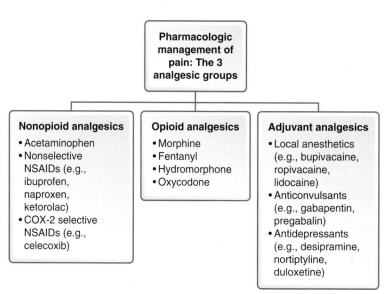

FIGURE 28.3 Pharmacologic Management of Pain. This figure shows the three analgesic groups and examples of first-line options within each group. *COX,* Cyclooxygenase; *NSAIDs,* nonsteroidal antiinflammatory drugs.

epidurally or by continuous peripheral nerve block. An anticonvulsant may be added to the treatment plan as well to control severe pain or prevent a chronic postsurgical pain syndrome, such as postthoracotomy or postmastectomy pain.[39]

Anticonvulsants and antidepressants are first-line analgesics for neuropathic pain.[40] These analgesics require a period of several days to weeks of dose titration to determine efficacy and safety and to achieve adequate pain control. Lidocaine patch 5% is used for well-localized peripheral neuropathic types of pain, such as postherpetic neuralgia (shingles-related pain). Long-term opioid therapy can be effective for improving function in some individuals with chronic pain, however, the risks of opioid addiction or overdose should be discussed with the patient and family, with appropriate monitoring in place to identify and treat substance abuse dsorders.[11,27] It is not unusual to find a multimodal pain treatment regimen for a person with neuropathic pain that includes an antidepressant, anticonvulsant, local anesthetic, and an analgesic.

Routes of administration. A variety of routes of administration is used to deliver analgesics. A principle of pain management is to use the oral route of administration whenever feasible.[11] All of the first-line analgesics used to manage pain are available in short-acting and long-acting formulations. For patients who have continuous pain in the hospital setting, a long-acting analgesic, such as modified-release oral morphine, oxycodone, hydromorphone, or transdermal fentanyl, is used to treat the persistent baseline pain. A fast-onset, short-acting analgesic (usually the same drug as the long-acting) is used to treat breakthrough pain if it occurs.[11]

When the oral route is not possible, other routes of administration are used, including intravenous (IV), subcutaneous, transdermal, and rectal. Opioids are often given by IV patient-controlled analgesia (PCA). Patients who use PCA must be able to understand the relationships between pain, pushing the PCA button, and pain relief. They must also be able to cognitively and physically use the PCA equipment.[11] Other routes for pain administration include intraspinal analgesia and continuous peripheral nerve block infusions with or without PCA capability. Nurses play a key and extensive role in the successful management of these therapies, and the American Society for Pain Management Nursing (http://aspmn.org) provides guidelines for care.[37] As more information is gathered regarding how genetic factors influence the metabolism of medications used to treat pain and the side effects produced, a more patient-centered pain management approach may be used.[36]

For patients with pain who are being discharged or treated in the outpatient setting, nonpharmacologic and nonopioid therapies are preferred and it is important to establish treatment goals, discuss the risks and benefits of opioid use, and discuss patient and provider responsibilities if opioids are prescribed.[26,27] Prior to providing an opioid prescription, the state's prescription drug monitoring program should be checked to identify any recent or overlapping opioid prescriptions. Along with a thorough medical and social history and physical exam to evaluate the risk of opioid use disorder, urine toxicology may be used to assess for substance use. As with all opioids, avoid concurrent prescriptions of benzodiazepines to reduce the risk of opioid overdose, and ensure that the patient is prescribed immediate release (not long-acting) formulations at the lowest effective dose and at no greater quantity than needed—typically for less than 3 to 7 days for those initiating opioid therapy.[26,27] Patients who are identified as having opioid use disorder should be offered appropriate treatment with buprenorphine or methadone, or referred for treatment of substance use disorder.

Invasive or Surgical Strategies

Regional anesthetic strategies for pain management include epidural steroid injections to treat radicular pain, joint injections, nerve blocks, and implantation of intrathecal analgesic delivery systems. More invasive measures may include spinal cord stimulators, rhizotomy or neurectomy, nerve decompression, and joint replacement therapies. These invasive procedures are typically performed after other treatment modalities have failed to provide pain relief.

Nonpharmacologic Strategies

Nonpharmacologic strategies encompass a wide variety of nondrug treatments that may contribute to comfort and pain relief. These include the body-based (physical) modalities, such as massage, acupuncture, and application of heat and cold, and the mind–body methods, such as guided imagery, relaxation breathing, and meditation. In addition, psychological therapies such as cognitive–behavioral therapy, biofeedback, and hypnosis may be used along with other strategies to help manage pain. There are also biologically based therapies, which involve the use of herbs and vitamins, and energy therapies such as reiki and tai chi.[38]

Nonpharmacologic methods may be effective alone for mild to some moderate-intensity pain and are used to complement, but not replace, pharmacologic therapies for more severe pain.[41] The effectiveness of nonpharmacologic methods can be unpredictable, and although not all have been shown to relieve pain, they offer many benefits (such as facilitating relaxation and reducing stress) to patients with pain.[38–41] Many patients find that the use of nonpharmacologic methods helps them cope better with their pain and feel greater control over the pain experience.[42] The following list provides examples of nonpharmacologic measures that are noninvasive and relatively easy to incorporate into daily clinical practice. They can be used individually or in combination with other nondrug therapies:

- Proper body alignment achieved through proper *positioning* and regular repositioning can help prevent or relieve pain. Pillows can be used to maintain the position and support the patient's back and extremities.[43]
- Thermal measures such as the *application of localized, superficial heat and cooling* may relieve pain and provide comfort by decreasing sensitivity to pain and muscle spasms, and alleviating joint and muscle aches. The two measures are often used interchangeably.[42]
- *Mind–body therapies* are designed to enhance the mind's capacity to affect bodily function and symptoms[40] and include music therapy, distraction techniques, meditation, prayer, hypnosis, guided imagery, relaxation techniques, and pet therapy.[42,44]

CLINICAL NURSING SKILLS FOR PAIN

- Pain assessment
- Nonpharmacologic pain management
- Massage
- Splinting
- Relaxation and guided imagery
- Distraction
- Pharmacologic pain management
- Oral medications
- Intravenous medications
- Epidural analgesia
- Patient-controlled analgesia
- Local anesthesia

INTERRELATED CONCEPTS

Pain is connected to numerous concepts, with those considered more relevant listed here. These are presented in Fig. 28.4.

The expression and interpretation of pain varies widely across cultural groups, thus **Culture** is an important interrelated concept. Having

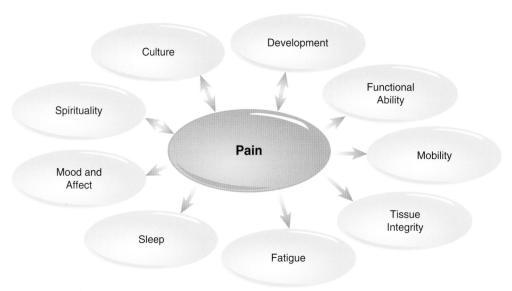

FIGURE 28.4 Pain and Interrelated Concepts.

an awareness of such differences is critical for nurses so that an accurate pain assessment can be conducted and appropriate pain interventions can be implemented. The expression of pain may also be influenced by one's Spirituality. A person may be more accepting and tolerant of pain, gained through spiritual strength. An individual's level of Development impacts how pain is interpreted by the individual and the ability of that individual to communicate his or her pain. Nociceptive pain is typically associated with altered Tissue Integrity. Acute pain associated with compromised tissue integrity is expected to dissipate with the normal healing process. Mobility is an important interrelated concept because severe pain can be immobilizing to individuals, and, in fact, some of the most disturbing effects of unrelieved pain are seen in the musculoskeletal system with impaired muscle, skeletal, or joint function. Inadequately managed pain can affect Functional Ability. This is often seen in the postoperative setting where the patient's ability to ambulate and participate in important physical therapy activities[45] prolongs recovery,[46,47] and is associated with a higher incidence of complications including long-term disability.[48] In the outpatient setting, individuals with poorly managed chronic pain report inability to complete even the simplest of activities of daily living, which can result in loss of independence and greater reliance on family, friends, and the healthcare system.[49,50] Patients with poorly managed chronic pain frequently report Sleep disturbances,[51] and sleep disturbances can contribute to increased pain perception, as well as a reduced ability to cope with pain. Pain also leads to Fatigue, particularly when sleep is impaired. Increased levels of fatigue along with pain can further impair mobility and functional ability. Pain also affects Mood and Affect. Patients with severe pain are more likely to rate their general health as poor,[52] and describe having suicidal thoughts. Research has even shown that severe chronic pain is associated with increased mortality, independent of sociodemographic factors such as income, age, and gender.[53]

CLINICAL EXEMPLARS

As mentioned previously, most individuals experience pain across the lifespan and in many different ways. Thus, the nurse will encounter multiple situations that will require pain assessment and interventions. A discussion of each situation is beyond the scope of this concept analysis; however, Box 28.1 presents the most common pain conditions in the context of the major categories of pain.

Featured Exemplars
Osteoarthritis Pain

Osteoarthritis is a condition that causes the cartilage in a joint to become stiff and lose elasticity. As this occurs, the cartilage can wear away, causing tendons and ligaments to stretch and bones to rub against one another, resulting in pain. Osteoarthritis commonly affects the hands as well as weight-bearing joints and is more frequent in women than in men. Osteoarthritis pain is an example of nociceptive, somatic pain.

Trigeminal Neuralgia

Also known as tic douloureux, trigeminal neuralgia is a form of neuropathic pain arising from the trigeminal (fifth) cranial nerve. It causes extreme, sporadic burning or shocklike facial pain that can last seconds to minutes per episode. The intensity of pain can be physically and mentally incapacitating.

Postherpetic Neuralgia

Another type of neuropathic pain is postherpetic neuralgia, which develops after a case of shingles caused by the herpes zoster virus. Typically, thin blisters associated with shingles disappear within a few weeks, but when the pain continues after the blisters have disappeared, the burning pain is known as postherpetic neuralgia. The incidence of postherpetic neuralgia increases with age.

Poststroke Pain

More than half of all stroke survivors report some form of poststroke pain. It can occur immediately following a stroke or weeks to months afterwards and may affect any area of the body. Patients typically describe burning pain or unpleasant and painful "pins-and-needles" sensation.

Complex Regional Pain Syndrome

Complex regional pain syndrome (CRPS) is a form of neuropathic pain that affects one of the limbs (arm, leg, hand, or foot) after an injury or trauma of the limb. CRPS is characterized by prolonged or excessive pain and mild to dramatic changes in skin color, temperature, and swelling of the affected area. It is more frequent in women.

Fibromyalgia

Fibromyalgia is a mixed pain disorder that is associated with widespread musculoskeletal pain, fatigue, sleep disturbances, and cognitive and

BOX 28.1   EXEMPLARS OF PAIN

Nociceptive Pain
Somatic Pain
- Ankylosing spondylitis
- Cancer pain (tumor growth) and pain associated with bony metastases
- Labor pain (cervical changes and uterine contractions)
- Osteoarthritis pain
- Osteoporosis pain
- Pain of Ehlers–Danlos syndrome
- Rheumatoid arthritis pain
- Surgical trauma/postoperative pain
- Pain from traumatic injuries
  - Wounds
  - Burns
  - Fractures
  - Deep tissue bruising

Visceral Pain
- Crohn disease
- Irritable bowel syndrome
- Organ-involved cancer pain
- Pancreatitis
- Ulcerative colitis

Neuropathic Pain
Centrally Generated Pain
- Complex regional pain syndrome
- Pain following spinal cord injury
- Phantom pain as a result of peripheral nerve damage
- Poststroke pain

Peripherally Generated Pain
- Alcohol–nutritional neuropathy
- Diabetic neuropathy
- Nerve root compression, nerve entrapment
- Pain of Guillain–Barré syndrome
- Postherpetic neuralgia
- Some types of neck, shoulder, and back pain
- Trigeminal neuralgia

Mixed Pain
- Fibromyalgia
- Myofascial pain
- Pain associated with HIV
- Pain associated with Lyme disease
- Some headaches
- Some types of neck, shoulder, and back pain

ACCESS EXEMPLAR LINKS IN YOUR GIDDENS EBOOK

mood disorders. Symptoms often begin after physical trauma, surgery, infection, or significant psychological stress and accumulate over time. Fibromyalgia is more common in women.

Phantom Pain

Phantom pain feels like it is coming from a body part that is no longer there.[2] Although phantom pain most often develops after removal of an arm or a leg, with up to 75% of patients developing pain within the first few days after limb amputation, it can also occur after removal of other body parts. Many factors are thought to influence the risk of phantom pain, particularly pre-amputation pain and genetic factors; however, phantom pain is thought to originate in the brain. Multimodal therapies are often required to reduce pain, although most patients experience a decrease in pain over time.

CASE STUDY

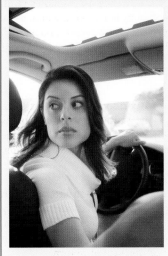

Case Presentation

Jenny Alvers is a 38-year-old otherwise healthy female who has been admitted directly to the intensive care unit (ICU) after an automobile accident and emergency abdominal surgery. In addition to surgery, she has deep face, neck, and chest lacerations and contusions. Jenny is on a ventilator and somewhat disoriented and restless with elevated blood pressure and heart rate. She is unable to provide a report of pain, but based on her pathologic condition, the nurse assumes that Jenny has pain and consults with the surgeon about orders for a continuous IV opioid infusion. Knowing that Jenny will be subjected to painful procedures such as endotracheal suctioning and wound care during her stay in the ICU, the nurse also requests supplemental IV opioid doses to administer prophylactically. Jenny's sister reported that Jenny has no allergies but experienced severe nausea when she was given IV morphine following an appendectomy 3 years ago. The surgeon prescribes an IV infusion of hydromorphone at a dosage appropriate for an adult with moderate to severe pain and supplemental IV hydromorphone bolus doses every hour as needed. Scheduled doses of IV acetaminophen and IV ibuprofen are also ordered.

The nurse suspects that Jenny's restlessness could be related to unrelieved pain and therefore administers an IV hydromorphone loading dose before initiating the infusion. Infusions of IV ibuprofen followed by IV acetaminophen are also administered. An aqua pad circulating cool water is placed over Jenny's chest to provide additional analgesia. The nurse reduces the external stimuli in the room as much as possible and provides Jenny with calm reassurance and orientation while caring for her. Within 45 minutes of these interventions, Jenny is no longer restless, her vital signs are within normal limits and stable, and she appears to be resting comfortably.

Case Analysis Questions

1. What factors place Jenny at high risk for inadequate pain relief?
2. What methods should be used now, and in the future, to assess Jenny's pain?
3. What type of pain is Jenny most likely experiencing? How does this information affect treatment decisions?

From Siri Stafford/Digital Vision/Thinkstock

ACCESS EXEMPLAR LINKS IN YOUR GIDDENS EBOOK

REFERENCES

1. Nicholas, M. K. (2015). Expanding patients' access to help in managing their chronic pain. *IASP. Pain Clinical Updates, 23*, 1–8.
2. Institute of Medicine. (2011). *Relieving pain in America: A blueprint for transforming prevention, care, education and research.* Washington, DC: National Academies Press.
3. International Association for the Study of Pain. (2014). *Desirable characteristics of national pain strategies.* Washington, DC: IASP Press.
4. International Association for the Study of Pain. (1994). Part III: Pain terms, a current list with definitions and notes on usage. In H. Mersky & N. Bogduk (Eds.), *Classification of chronic pain* (2nd ed., pp. 209–214). Seattle: IASP Press.
5. McCaffery, M. (1968). *Nursing practice theories related to cognition, bodily pain, and man–environment interactions.* Los Angeles: University of California.
6. McCaffery, M., Herr, K., & Pasero, C. (2011). Assessment. In C. Pasero & M. McCaffery (Eds.), *Pain assessment and pharmacologic management* (pp. 13–176). St Louis: Mosby.
7. Haines, D. E. (2012). *Fundamental neuroscience for basic and clinical applications* (4th ed.). New York: Saunders.
8. Pasero, C., & Portenoy, R. K. (2011). Neurophysiology of pain and analgesia and the pathophysiology of neuropathic pain. In C. Pasero & M. McCaffery (Eds.), *Pain assessment and pharmacologic management* (pp. 1–12). St Louis: Mosby.
9. Moayedi, M., & Davis, K. D. (2013). Theories of pain: From specificity to gate control. *Journal of Neurophysiology, 109*(1), 5–12.
10. Starkweather, A. R., & Pair, V. E. (2013). Decoding the role of epigenetics and genomics in pain management. *Pain Management Nursing, 14,* 358–367.
11. American Geriatrics Society. (2009). Pharmacological management of persistent pain in older persons. *Journal of the American Geriatrics Society, 57,* 1331–1346.
12. Herr, K. (2010). Pain in older adult: An imperative across all health care settings. *Pain Management Nursing, 11*(2), S1–S10.
13. Melzack, R. (2005). Evolution of the neuromatrix theory of pain. *Pain Practice, 5,* 85–94.
14. Grace, P. M., Hutchinson, M. R., Maier, S. F., et al. (2014). Pathological pain and the neuroimmune interface. *Nature Reviews. Immunology, 14,* 217–231.
15. Cata, J. P., Bauer, M., Sokari, T., et al. (2013). Effects of surgery, general anesthesia, and perioperative epidural analgesia on the immune function of patients with non-small cell lung cancer. *Journal of Clinical Anesthesia, 25*(4), 255–262.
16. Kaye, A. D., Patel, N., Bueno, F. R., et al. (2014). Effect of opiates, anesthetic techniques and other perioperative factors on surgical cancer patients. *The Ochsner Journal, 14*(2), 216–228.
17. Pei, L., Tan, G., Wang, L., et al. (2014). Comparison of combined general–epidural anesthesia with general anesthesia effects on survival and cancer recurrence: A meta-analysis of retrospective and prospective studies. *PLoS ONE, 9*(12), e114667.
18. Verma, V., Sheikh, Z., & Ahmed, A. S. (2014). Nociception and role of immune system in pain. *Acta Neurologica Belgica, 12*(1), 120–128.
19. Erb, J., Orr, E., Mercer, D., et al. (2008). Interactions between pulmonary performance and movement-evoked pain in the immediate postsurgical period: Implications for perioperative research and treatment. *Regional Anesthesia and Pain Medicine, 33*(4), 312–319.
20. Panretou, V., Toufektzian, L., Siafaka, I., et al. (2012). Postoperative pulmonary function after open abdominal aortic aneurysm repair in patient with chronic obstructive pulmonary disease: Epidural versus intravenous analgesia. *Annals of Vascular Surgery, 26*(2), 149–155.
21. Guay, J. (2006). Postoperative pain significantly influences postoperative blood loss in patients undergoing total knee replacement. *Pain Medicine (Malden, Mass.), 7*(6), 476–482.
22. Bigeleisen, P. E., & Goehner, N. (2015). Novel approaches in pain management in cardiac surgery. *Current Opinion in Anaesthesiology, 28*(1), 89–94.
23. Vincent, H. K., Adams, M. C., Vincent, K. R., et al. (2013). Musculoskeletal pain, fear avoidance behaviors, and functional decline in obesity: Potential interventions to manage pain and maintain function. *Regional Anesthesia and Pain Medicine, 38,* 481–491.
24. Substance Abuse and Mental Health Services Administration. (2018). *Prescription drug misuse and abuse.* Rockville, MD: SAMHSA.
25. Barr, D. A. (2008). *Health disparities in the United States: Social class, race, ethnicity and health.* Baltimore, MD: Johns Hopkins University Press.
26. U.S. Department of Health and Human Services. (2016). *National pain strategy: a comprehensive population health-level strategy for pain.* Washington, D. C.: U.S. Department of Health and Human Services.
27. Dowell, D., Haegerich, T. M., & Chou, R. (2016). CDC guideline for prescribing opioids for chronic pain — United States, 2016. *MMWR. Recommendations and Reports: Morbidity and Mortality Weekly Report. Recommendations and Reports, 65*(1), 1–49.
28. Ware, L., Epps, D. E., Herr, K., et al. (2006). Evaluation of the revised faces pain scale, verbal descriptor scale, numeric rating scale and Iowa pain thermometer in older minority adults. *Pain Management Nursing, 71,* 117–125.
29. Spagrud, L. J., Piira, T., & Von Baeyer, C. L. (2003). Children's self-report of pain intensity: The Faces Pain Scale–Revised. *The American Journal of Nursing, 103*(12), 62–64.
30. Herr, K. A., Spratt, K. F., Mobily, P. R., et al. (2004). Pain intensity assessment in older adults: Use of experimental pain to compare psychometric properties and usability of selected pain scales with younger adults. *The Clinical Journal of Pain, 20,* 207–219.
31. Miaskowski, C., Cleary, J., Burney, R., et al. (2005). *Guideline for the management of cancer pain in adults and children.* Glenview, IL: American Pain Society.
32. Pasero, C. (2009). Assessment of sedation during opioid administration for pain management. *Journal of Perianesthesia Nursing, 24*(3), 186–190.
33. Nisbet, A. T., & Mooney-Cotter, F. (2009). Selected scales for reporting opioid-induced sedation. *Pain Management Nursing, 10*(3), 154–164.
34. Herr, K., Coyne, P. J., McCaffery, M., et al. (2011). Pain assessment in the patient unable to self-report: Position statement with clinical practice recommendations. *Pain Management Nursing, 12*(4), 230–250.
35. Pasero, C. (2009). Challenges in pain assessment. *Journal of Perianesthesia Nursing, 24*(1), 50–54.
36. Pasero, C., Quinn, T. E., Portenoy, R. K., et al. (2011). Opioid analgesics. In C. Pasero & M. McCaffery (Eds.), *Pain assessment and pharmacologic management* (pp. 277–622). St Louis: Mosby.
37. Ashburn, M. A., Caplan, R. A., Carr, D. B., et al. (2004). Practice guidelines for acute pain management in the perioperative setting: An updated report by the American Society of Anesthesiologists task force on acute pain management. *Anesthesiology, 100*(6), 1573–1581.
38. Dworkin, R. H., O'Connor, A. B., Backonja, M., et al. (2007). Pharmacologic management of neuropathic pain: Evidence-based recommendations. *Pain, 132*(3), 237–251.
39. National Heart, Lung and Blood Institute. (2014). Managing chronic complications of sickle cell disease. In *Evidence-based management of sickle cell disease* (pp. 55–70). Bethesda, MD: Author.
40. Pasero, C., Polomano, R. C., & Portenoy, R. K. (2011). Adjuvant analgesics. In C. Pasero & M. McCaffery (Eds.), *Pain assessment and pharmacologic management* (pp. 623–818). St Louis: Mosby.
41. Pasero, C., Portenoy, R. K., & McCaffery, M. (2011). Nonopioid analgesics. In C. Pasero & M. McCaffery (Eds.), *Pain assessment and pharmacologic management* (pp. 177–276). St Louis: Mosby.
42. Gatlin, C. G., & Schulmeister, L. (2007). When medication is not enough: Nonpharmacologic management of pain. *Clinical Journal of Oncology Nursing, 11,* 699.
43. Allred, K. D., Byers, J., & Sole, M. L. (2010). The effect of music on postoperative pain and anxiety. *Pain Management Nursing, 11,* 15.
44. National Center for Complementary and Integrative Health. (2015). *Complementary, Alternative, or Integrative Health: What's in a Name?* Retrieved from https://nccih.nih.gov/health/integrative-health.

45. Morrison, R. S., Magaziner, J., McLaughlin, M. A., et al. (2003). The impact of post-operative pain on outcomes following hip fracture. *Pain, 103*, 303–311.

46. Kehlet, H., & Wilmore, D. W. (2008). Evidence-based surgical care and the evolution of fast-track surgery. *Annals of Surgery, 248*(2), 189–198.

47. Pavlin, D. J., Chen, C., Penaloza, D. A., et al. (2002). Pain as a factor complicating recovery and discharge after ambulatory surgery. *Anesthesia and Analgesia, 95*(3), 627–634.

48. Pavlin, D. J., Chen, C., Penaloza, D. A., et al. (2004). A survey of pain and other symptoms that affect the recovery process after discharge from an ambulatory surgery unit. *Journal of Clinical Anesthesia, 16*(3), 200–206.

49. Rudy, T. E., & Lieber, S. J. (2005). Functional assessment of older adults with chronic pain. In S. J. Gibson & D. K. Weiner (Eds.), *Pain in older persons* (pp. 153–173). Seattle: IASP Press.

50. Simmonds, M. J., Novey, D., & Sandoval, R. (2005). The differential influence of pain and fatigue on physical performance and health status in ambulatory patients with human immunodeficiency virus. *The Clinical Journal of Pain, 21*(3), 200–206.

51. Turk, D. C., & Cohen, M. J. M. (2010). Sleep as a marker in the effective management of chronic osteoarthritis pain with opioid analgesics. *Seminars in Arthritis and Rheumatism, 39*(6), 477–490.

52. Mantyselka, P. T., Turunen, J. H. O., Ahonen, R. S., et al. (2003). Chronic pain and poor self-rated health. *JAMA: The Journal of the American Medical Association, 290*(18), 2435–2442.

53. Torrance, N., Elliott, A. M., Lee, A. J., et al. (2010). Severe chronic pain is associated with increased 10 year mortality: A cohort record linkage study. *European Journal of Pain, 14*, 380–386.

CONCEPT
29

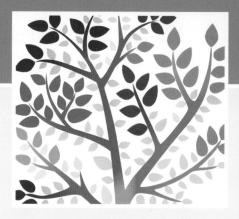

Fatigue

Katherine Fletcher

Fatigue is a common symptom reported by people seeking health care. It is experienced by individuals across the lifespan and populations.[1] If fatigue is left unchecked, it can significantly impact a person's school or work performance and impact family and social relationships. Fatigue can become so pervasive in a person's life that it can impair their ability to physically and emotionally care for themselves, resulting in a decreased quality of life.[2] Despite its pervasive nature and prevalence, fatigue has traditionally failed to elicit the same level of attention from healthcare professionals as symptoms such as pain.[3] As such, the scientific knowledge of fatigue, pathogenesis, techniques for assessment, and treatment are not as well developed. Nurses can play a pivotal role in early recognition of this detrimental problem and initiation of care management strategies to mitigate its effects.[2]

DEFINITION

Many authors have tried to define the true nature of fatigue, but there is no widely accepted definition. For the purposes of this concept presentation, fatigue is defined as a "distressing, persistent, subjective sense of physical, emotional, and/or cognitive tiredness or exhaustion … that is not proportional to recent activity and interferes with usual functioning."[4,pFT-1] This definition highlights the subjective nature of the concept that makes it so difficult to detect, as well as the interference it can cause in daily life. This definition also describes fatigue in a broader manner, indicating that it is a multidimensional concept which affects the physical, psychological, and/or cognitive aspects of the person's life. Lou[5] suggests that fatigue has two defining characteristics:

1. A perception of generalized weakness, resulting in inability to initiate certain activities. The described weakness is not proportional to the amount of recent activity.
2. Easy physical fatigability that reduces capacity to maintain performance, and/or easy mental (cognitive and emotional) fatigability in that there is a lack of motivation to engage in an activity, or has difficulty with concentration and memory to start or complete an activity.

The definition and defining characteristics allow the nurse to recognize fatigue more easily in the assessment process.

SCOPE

The scope of fatigue is presented on a continuum of having vitality and energy with no fatigue at one end to a feeling of exhaustion at the other end (Fig. 29.1). A continuum is a useful representation of this symptom because it is not fixed and is highly variable. The scope considers two factors—the intensity and frequency of symptoms. The degree or intensity of fatigue experience varies in all individuals, in part due to the underlying health status but also based on how the symptoms are interpreted and expressed. The frequency of fatigue is influenced by underlying health status and includes those who rarely experience fatigue and those who experience fatigue on a regular basis. The intensity and frequency of fatigue influence the effect the symptom has on the individual's functional ability.[6] Moderate fatigue to exhaustion makes completion of daily activities a significant challenge and is less likely to be relieved by rest when compared to mild fatigue.

NORMAL PHYSIOLOGICAL PROCESS

Fatigue can be considered an expected symptom experienced by healthy individuals, but it is not considered a normal or expected finding when fatigue is persistent or severe. Individuals in a healthy state have the mental and physical strength to initiate and sustain actions to take care of life needs. This inner strength and the ability to maintain performance support a positive outlook that motivates the person to psychologically stay focused to achieve goals. Healthy individuals experience fatigue intermittently when they have overexerted themselves physically and/or mentally; in these situations, fatigue serves as a useful physiological signal as the need to rest.[7] In healthy individuals, fatigue is relieved by physical, emotional, and/or cognitive rest.

VARIATIONS AND CONTEXT

When fatigue is persistent and impairs normal life functioning, it is considered a health problem. For fatigue to be recognized as a significant health problem, it needs to be a prominent symptom for at least 2 consecutive weeks.

Classifications of Fatigue

Most sources describe two general classifications of fatigue which are physiological and pathological (Fig. 29.2). *Physiological fatigue* occurs when there is an imbalance between physical, cognitive, and emotional activity, with the restorative actions such as sleep and diet.[8] There is no underlying medical problem with physiologic fatigue. *Pathological fatigue* is the fatigue that is associated with mental or physical diseases. This type of fatigue is caused by an underlying medical condition or

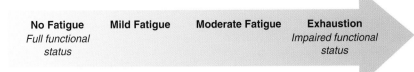

No Fatigue
Full functional status

Mild Fatigue

Moderate Fatigue

Exhaustion
Impaired functional status

FIGURE 29.1 Scope of Fatigue as a Concept.

treatment and may be resolved or decreased if the underlying problem is addressed.

Mental health conditions leading to pathological fatigue include psychological or psychiatric disorders. Other causes of fatigue are further delineated as originating from neurologic or nonneurologic causes. Neurologic origins include conditions that cause fatigue through the spinal or supraspinal avenues (central fatigue) or through the muscles (peripheral fatigue). Nonneurologic fatigue is associated with dysfunction within body systems (i.e., renal or immunologic), infections, malignancy, and/or medical treatments.[8] Fatigue can be further categorized as temporary or chronic depending on its duration. Although there is not total agreement about the duration, many define chronic fatigue as persisting greater than 6 months.[8] About 30% of those with chronic pathological fatigue have no identifiable etiology to their fatigue.[9] A severe and debilitating fatigue condition, chronic fatigue syndrome/myalgic encephalomyelitis (CFS/ME) is also known as Systemic Exertion Intolerance Disease (SEID). Regardless of the term used, diagnostic criteria are presented in Box 29.1.

Causes of Fatigue

Although fatigue is associated with many conditions, the actual pathogenesis remains uncertain. Physiological studies have defined the causes of neurologic fatigue as occurring at the central and/or peripheral level. There has been promising research demonstrated in this arena.[10] Peripheral fatigue results from a physiologic process within the muscle that impairs contraction. This can be caused by a number of things—including a loss of electrical conduction, impaired calcium levels, or buildup of waste products—which affects muscle performance. However, central fatigue is associated with changes in the synaptic concentration of neurotransmitters (e.g., serotonin), increased cortisol levels, or accumulation of inflammatory products within the central nervous system (CNS) which affects exercise performance

and muscle function. The symptoms of central fatigue can include lack of motivation, poor mood, impaired cognitive ability, and the perception that the person is working harder than they really are.[11] It is thought the basal ganglia and suprachiasmatic nucleus of the brain are involved in this process and it is mediated by a complex interaction of neurotransmitters and immune factors.[12,13] Research into cancer-related fatigue has demonstrated that those experiencing severe fatigue had increased proinflammatory cytokines produced either by the tumor or tissue damage from chemotherapy or radiation therapy. It is believed that cancer-related fatigue could be attributed to those increased inflammatory products.[12]

CONSEQUENCES

Fatigue can cause significant changes in a person's life that result in the loss of a job, loss of relationships, and inability to care for oneself. Over time, when confronted with persistent fatigue, the person will base their routines on a certain level of fatigue that is consistently present. Individuals with fatigue will eliminate leisure activities to leave more energy for basic activities of daily living, which often decreases their quality of life.[14] Quality of life is affected and further losses can lead to significant psychological consequences, particularly depression. Although fatigue does not cause death or organ failure, mortality from suicide is higher in patients with chronic idiopathic fatigue than in the general population.[15] Chronic fatigue is resistant to treatment and the course of the disease is variable. About 22% to 60% of patients achieve a moderate to full recovery at 1 year. Fewer than half of these persons return to work.[16]

RISK FACTORS

All individuals are potentially at risk for fatigue, regardless of age, gender, race, or ethnicity. Specific risk factors for chronic fatigue are linked to underlying causes of the condition.

Populations at Risk
Older Adults

Fatigue perception and fatigability increase with age.[7] The elderly are at greatest risk for experiencing fatigue due to physiological changes associated with aging and the fact that many elderly have underlying conditions contributing to fatigue.[7] Middle-aged adults between ages 40 and 50 years are the most common group to experience chronic fatigue.[16] Although fatigue is reported by all age groups, researchers found that younger adults reported fatigue more frequently than older adults.[17] The researchers suggested that older adults may attribute the fatigue to other conditions they have or to their advanced age and thus may not view it as abnormal. Young adults, on the other hand, with heavy responsibilities of balancing career, marriage, and childbearing, may view this same fatigue as a significant change in their lifestyle.

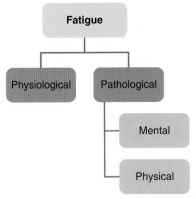

FIGURE 29.2 Classifications of Fatigue.

BOX 29.1   Diagnostic Criteria for Chronic Fatigue Syndrome/Myalgic Encephalomyelitis

1. A substantial reduction or impairment in the ability to engage in pre-illness levels of occupational, educational, social, or personal activities, that persists for more than 6 months and is accompanied by fatigue, which is often profound, is of new or definite onset (not lifelong), is not the result of ongoing excessive exertion, and is not substantially alleviated by rest, **and**
2. Post-exertional malaise, **and**
3. Unrefreshing sleep
4. At least one of the two following manifestations is also required:
   - Cognitive impairment **or**
   - Orthostatic intolerance

From Institute of Medicine. (2015). *Beyond myalgic encephalomyelitis/chronic fatigue syndrome, redefining an illness.* Washington DC: National Academy of Sciences.

Women

Women are more likely than men to experience fatigue; however, some researchers believe that data might be skewed because it is socially more acceptable for women to express unpleasant symptoms.[9] During childhood, diagnosis of CFS is equally weighted in the genders. However after puberty, females are two to three times more likely to be diagnosed with CFS.[18]

Individual Risk Factors
Genetic Predisposition

Preliminary evidence suggests that variations in inflammation-related genes may increase risks for fatigue. Although this area needs more study, findings suggest a genetic predisposition to fatigue and should be considered a general risk factor.[12]

Underlying Conditions

Many individuals experiencing fatigue have an underlying health condition. Fatigue is a common feature of many illnesses, such as neurologic disease, malignancy, hematologic disease, CFS, and autoimmune disease (e.g., systemic lupus erythematosus); heart, liver, thyroid, or kidney disease; and many infections. A hematologic condition such as anemia, in which there is a loss or decreased production of red blood cells, represents an example of fatigue due to physical disease. The resultant fatigue would be accentuated if the anemia occurred during a short period of time. Fatigue is highly correlated with mental health conditions as well. Fatigue is nearly always reported in people with depression. Researchers have found that exposure to childhood stress, including abuse or neglect is also associated with increased risk for fatigue.[19] It is estimated that medical or psychiatric diagnoses explain the fatigue in approximately 70% of patients with chronic fatigue.[9]

Treatment-Related Factors

Many cases of fatigue are attributable to medical treatments for other conditions. For example, β-blockers, a gold standard in the treatment of heart failure, have at times made patients' fatigue worsen. β-Blockers have been shown to increase free fatty acids and glycogenolysis, which lead to insufficient nutrient supply and thus increase fatigue.[20] Fatigue is a common side effect associated with many medications (e.g., sedative–hypnotics, antidepressants, muscle relaxants, opioids, antihypertensives, antihistamines, and many types of antibiotics). Psychoactive substances such as alcohol, nicotine, and caffeine can also result in fatigue,

especially during periods of withdrawal. Therapy for cancer, such as radiation and chemotherapy, kills rapidly proliferating cells. This therapy can cause anemia, resulting in decreased tissue oxygenation and fatigue.[21]

Nutritional Status

Proper nutrition is necessary to provide the body with essential nutrients for optimal functioning. Individuals with nutritional deficiencies, particularly protein–calorie malnutrition, are at risk for experiencing fatigue due to inadequate energy sources. Because nutritional deficiencies accompany many chronic conditions, the fatigue symptoms may be attributed to both or either.

Lifestyle Choices

A person's lifestyle choices have a significant impact on fatigue. Physiological fatigue can be induced by exercising excessively, consuming a poor diet, excessive alcohol consumption, not sleeping, or working excessively. People with a history of working nights or rotating shifts are also at risk. A disruption of the circadian rhythm may make individuals feel tired when they need to be awake and/or interfere with sleeping, thus causing fatigue.[22]

ASSESSMENT
History

Because fatigue is a subjective experience, the best assessment should be focused on the patient's report about his or her fatigue experience.[23] Use open-ended questions that encourage the patient to describe the fatigue in his or her own words. The patient's personal experience of fatigue must be understood so that an appropriate plan of care can be formulated. The examination of fatigue from this perspective can assist the nurse in planning specific interventions to ameliorate the effects of a person's fatigue experience. The following are components of a comprehensive history of fatigue:

- *Personal description of the fatigue:* Fatigue is a subjective experience so it will be a different experience for each person. Most patients experiencing fatigue will describe their fatigue as the inability to complete specific activities because of a lack of energy or stamina. However, patients with depression describe their fatigue more globally and express that they are unable to do anything.[24]
- *Onset and course:* Ask the patient if the fatigue occurred suddenly or appeared more gradually. Also review the patient's medical history to evaluate if the patient has any potential risk factors that occurred at approximately the time of the onset of fatigue. Asking questions about the course of the fatigue will help determine if the fatigue has remained approximately the same, worsened, or improved.
- *Duration and daily pattern:* Ask the patient about the length of time he or she has experienced the fatigue. This will provide information to determine if the problem is acute or chronic. Fatigue, as a symptom, is not a static entity and may change daily, so it is also important to determine the usual daily pattern of the fatigue. This will help clarify the patient's usual fatigue pattern and identify when it worsens.
- *Factors that alleviate or exacerbate:* Ask the patient what makes the fatigue worse or better to tailor patient-centered interventions. There may be symptoms of other conditions that are contributing to the fatigue. For this reason, it is important to assess the existence of pain, sleep pattern disturbance, and poor nutrition. Assessing for interrelated concepts could help the nurse identify other contributing factors. For example, assessing the effect of rest/sleep on fatigue will help to detect if the fatigue is caused by a physical or mental illness. Generally, fatigue that worsens with activity and lessens with

rest suggests a physical disorder. Fatigue that is constantly present, does not lessen with rest, and has only occasional bursts of energy may indicate a psychological disorder.[25] There are always exceptions to this generalization in that individuals with CFS will experience unrefreshing sleep regardless of how long they sleep.

- *Impact on daily life:* Ask the patient how the fatigue affects activities of daily living (such as his or her ability to work, socialize, participate in family activities, and libido) as well as what accommodations the patient/family has made to adjust. Keeping an activity and rest journal may help to discover the patient's personal limits.
- *Other physical, emotional, and cognitive symptoms that accompany the fatigue:* Studies of fatigue indicate that there is a strong positive correlation among fatigue, depression, and perceived stress.[26] Ask the patient about depression and stress to rule out these disorders.

Many self-report scales have been developed, but they often overlap with other symptoms and/or do not capture all the features of this multidimensional concept.[27] Table 29.1 presents reliable and valid

TABLE 29.1 Self-Report Instruments to Measure Fatigue

Instrument	Dimensions Assessed/Target Population
Brief Fatigue Inventory (BFI)	Measures amount of fatigue but hard to distinguish between mild and moderate types and activities affected by fatigue. Used with adults having Parkinson disease or cancer.
Child Fatigue Scale (CFS)	Assesses the multidimensional aspects of fatigue in children. Used with children experiencing cancer.
Fatigue Severity Scale (FSS)	Measures severity, how fatigue interfered with certain activities over the previous week. Used with adults having multiple sclerosis or lupus.
Fatigue Symptom Inventory	Measures severity, frequency, diurnal variation, and interference with daily functioning. Used with adults experiencing cancer.
Multidimensional Fatigue Inventory (MFI)	Measures general, physical, and mental fatigue; reduced motivation; and reduced activity. Used with various adult populations, including those with cancer, chronic fatigue syndrome, or COPD.
Multidimensional Assessment of Fatigue (MAF)	Measures severity, distress, degree of interference in activities of daily living, timing (frequency of occurrence and changeability). Used with adults with arthritis, cancer, or COPD.
Modified Fatigue Impact Scale (MFIS)	Shorter version of the full Fatigue Impact Scale; Measures the impact of fatigue over the previous 4 weeks on physical, cognitive, and psychosocial functioning. Used for adults with MS.
Piper Fatigue Scale	Measures fatigue in four dimensions: sensory, behavioral/severity, affective meaning, and cognitive/mood. Used with adults having cancer, myocardial infarction, or HIV.
Visual Analog Scale of Fatigue	Represents severity of physical and mental fatigue over last 24 h. Used with adults having neuromuscular disease, cancer, or end-stage renal disease. Adaptable to children.

COPD, Chronic obstructive pulmonary disease; *HIV*, human immunodeficiency virus.

instruments commonly used to measure the concept of fatigue. It is also important to use an age-appropriate instrument; there are fewer instruments that are appropriate for children.

Examination Findings

The history can guide appropriate focused physical assessment and diagnostic tests to rule out underlying diseases. Recognition of pathological causes of fatigue is important so that the life-altering effects of fatigue can be diminished by appropriately treating this disease.

Inspection

Observe the individual's general appearance. Is the individual alert? Is he or she displaying any psychomotor agitation or impairment? Take note of the individual's personal grooming. Poor alertness, psychomotor impairment or agitation, and poor grooming could be evidence that the patient is experiencing a mood and affect disorder such as depression. If the patient's grooming appears unkempt, it could also indicate that the fatigue is affecting the patient's self-care. Look at the patient's posture. Does he or she appear slumped? Is the patient's gait appropriate? Observe the patient's skin. Is the skin pale, suggesting anemia?

Palpation and Auscultation

Palpation is indicated to assess for the presence of lymphadenopathy, thyroid nodules, or goiter. These findings could indicate the need to test further for cancer, thyroid disease, or infection. Examine muscle appearance, strength against resistance, deep tendon reflexes, and sensory and cranial nerve action to assess the neuromuscular system. Some neuromuscular diseases can decrease muscular bulk, tone, and strength, which increases the patient's risk for fatigue. Auscultation of the heart and lungs helps to identify underlying pulmonary or cardiac conditions that may be contributing factors.

Diagnostic Tests

There are no specific diagnostic markers for fatigue. Diagnostic testing is primarily completed to rule out underlying diseases. Common laboratory tests include thyroid function tests, complete blood cell count with differential (to rule out anemia and infection), chemistry profile (to rule out electrolyte imbalances and alteration in glucose levels), tests of liver and renal function, human immunodeficiency virus (HIV) antibody, erythrocyte sedimentation rate (inflammatory disease), urinalysis (urinary infection and renal impairment), and a pregnancy test in women of childbearing age. If peripheral fatigue is suspected, an electromyography could be performed to test muscle performance. A transmagnetic stimulation (TMS), magnetic resonance imaging (MRI), and magnetic resonance spectroscopy could be completed to determine if brain problems are causing the fatigue. Some health professionals use performance-based testing to determine if a patient experiences fatigue with difficult physical or cognitive activities. Researchers have found that measurement of muscular or cognitive fatigue through performance tests does not correlate with the individual's perception of the amount of fatigue they experience.[26]

CLINICAL MANAGEMENT

Primary Prevention

Primary prevention refers to purposeful activities to prevent disease. In the case of fatigue, basic primary prevention measures are associated with following a healthy lifestyle—good nutrition, exercise, getting adequate sleep, and managing stress. In addition, the nurse can advocate for patients and families with fatigue risk so they can obtain resources needed to prevent fatigue. Patient teaching designed for an individual with risk factors can be considered primary prevention because it will allow them to take measures to avoid fatigue. For example, women experiencing excessive menstrual flow can be advised to increase dietary intake of iron or iron supplements to avoid developing iron deficiency anemia, which is a common cause of fatigue.

Secondary Prevention (Screening)

Secondary prevention refers to screening efforts for early detection of disease. Because fatigue is a symptom associated with multiple health conditions, there are no population-wide screening efforts for fatigue. However, nurses can screen patients who are identified as being at risk for fatigue by asking additional questions during an interview or using a fatigue screening tool (see Table 29.1).

Collaborative Interventions

Collaborative interventions are geared toward assisting the patient who is experiencing fatigue to accomplish the activities of daily living, return to work, maintain interpersonal relationships, and perform some form of daily exercise. To accomplish these goals, the interprofessional team must first manage the fatigue associated with poor lifestyle choices or disease. The team can also utilize other treatment strategies, such as exercise/rest therapy, pharmacological treatment, psychological care, and complementary therapies, to help the patient meet health goals.

Manage Physiological Fatigue

It is important for an individual to balance nutrition, sleep, stress, and psychological coping skills. For example, every individual should get an adequate amount of sleep. The amount of sleep considered "adequate" varies with different age groups, but it is usually 7 or 8 hours per night for adults, 9 hours for adolescents, and 11 or 12 hours for toddlers. When helping patients with sleep hygiene, discourage oversleeping because it will increase fatigue. Patient teaching in the areas of nutrition and stress management is another intervention geared toward minimizing contributory factors for fatigue.

Manage Secondary Fatigue

Because many people have fatigue caused by underlying health conditions, optimal management of the conditions helps to reduce fatigue. For example, teaching a patient with iron deficiency anemia about nutrition therapy could include taking iron supplements and eating iron-rich foods, such as lean meat, liver, shellfish, beans, and enriched cereal.

Exercise and Rest Therapy

Exercise can often help relieve the effects of fatigue, especially more short-lived, acute forms of fatigue.[28] Usual exercise should include stretching and aerobic exercise such as walking for 30 minutes on a daily basis. The exercise should be tailored to the individual but it is usually recommended to get 150 minutes of moderate intensity aerobic activity in a week.[6,29,30] More research needs to be completed on the type, intensity, and duration of physical exercise most beneficial in reducing different degrees of fatigue.[20] Graded exercise therapy, a structured exercise regimen, may be more appropriate therapy for those who are more deconditioned. It is important for the person to maintain activities yet pace themselves by listening to their bodies to avoid overexertion, which can not only be detrimental to the body, but can also add to the fatigue.[31,32] Teaching the patient to self-monitor their fatigue levels to balance rest and activity will help them prioritize based on their pattern of fatigue.[20] Motivating children and adolescents to adhere to exercise regimens has been found to be difficult so it is important to involve parents to increase adherence.[33]

Planned rest breaks throughout the day can also be a benefit to the patient. Naps should be short and limited to less than 1 hour. The

BOX 29.2   Energy Conservation Strategies

- Plan the day to balance work and rest times. Plan work around times of the day when fatigue is least. Include rest periods in the day or rest at least an hour. Rest during fatiguing activities that take 30 min or longer.
- Communicate needs for assistance to family members or willing helpers. Delegate part or all of an activity to that person.
- Analyze and modify activities to reduce energy expenditures. Conserve energy so it can be consumed doing something that the person really enjoys. Simplify activities so they require less energy. Eliminate part or all of an activity that is difficult. Modify frequency or expected outcomes of an activity. Adjust priorities for energy expenditure.
- Organize self ahead of time to avoid rushing.
- Organize work spaces. Assess height of work surfaces. Avoid working above head—better to keep items at waist level. Organize work centers so that equipment is within easy reach. Position equipment, furniture, or supplies for easy access; arrange household activities on one floor.
- Use adaptive equipment, gadgets, or energy-saving devices.
- Use body efficiently. Use larger muscles, bend knees, and sit whenever possible.

Adapted from Blikman, L. J., Huissede, B. M., Kooijmans, H., Stam, H. J., Bussmann, J. B., & van Meeteren, J. (2013). Effectiveness of energy conservation treatment in reducing fatigue in multiple sclerosis: A systematic review and meta-analysis. *Archives of Physical Medicine and Rehabilitation, 94*(7), 1360–1376.

best time for naps is early afternoon because fatigue in most patients worsens as the day progresses.[4] Energy conservation activities are also a valuable asset to avoid fatigue (Box 29.2). Energy conservation activities implies that the patient would focus on saving as much energy as possible to spend when participating in activities that are meaningful to them.[34] When delegating some responsibilities to others, patients are often afraid of becoming a burden, but it is important to use those who volunteer to do chores when the patient does not have the energy to do it.[31]

For CFS patients, exercise might make the fatigue worse. This is called "post-exertional malaise," and it occurs approximately 12 to 48 hours after exercise and remains for days or weeks. Pacing the exercises by balancing rest and activity will help avoid post-exertional malaise.[35] A carefully structured program of graded exercise therapy is recommended for patients with CFS. This exercise is supervised exercise that begins gradually and builds to a moderate daily amount of exercise to build stamina and prevent increased fatigue.[16]

Pharmacologic Agents

Agents aimed at treating underlying conditions. Several pharmacologic agents may be used in the treatment of fatigue, with a focus on treating underlying diseases linked to the fatigue. For example, thyroxine may be administered to patients experiencing fatigue associated with hypothyroidism. Thyroxine, a synthetic hormone, will increase the basal metabolic rate to normal, resulting in a reduction of fatigue. As another example, antidepressants are often administered to those experiencing depression. Because fatigue often coexists with depression, an improvement in depression may alleviate the symptoms of fatigue. If depression is not treated, then it is unlikely that the fatigue will respond to other therapies. These are but two examples of many pharmacologic agents that improve fatigue through the treatment of the underlying condition.

Agents for treatment of fatigue. With continued physiological exploration of the cause of fatigue, researchers hope to find targeted therapy for treatment. Recent cancer research has identified biomarkers that could be used to target treatments to remediate cancer-related fatigue.[36] For example, those experiencing pathological fatigue believed to be related to inflammatory cells, are currently in clinical trials using anti-inflammatory agents such as infliximab.[10] Other types of agents are utilized to specifically treat fatigue, but their exact mechanisms of action are unknown. These medications are typically indicated for treatment of CFS. CNS stimulants such as methylphenidate (Ritalin), modafinil (Provigil), and caffeine can help. However, this group of drugs can cause headaches, restlessness, insomnia, and dry mouth. Recommendations are to use these medications with more advanced disease or for short-term use.[37] In fact, it has been found that the overuse of caffeine may actually make the fatigue worse.

Psychoeducational Interventions

Most patients who experience chronic fatigue state that they believe their fatigue is misunderstood by healthcare professionals. Many healthcare providers mistake serious fatigue for a mental health condition or consider it to be all in the individual's imagination. This perceived lack of concern causes patients with fatigue extreme frustration because they have difficulty getting a diagnosis and treatment for this problem.[38] As healthcare providers, it is important to validate with patients that fatigue is a genuine problem and that it exists as they say it does. Nurses need to acknowledge that it is a subjective experience like pain and can significantly impact an individual's quality of life. Establishing a therapeutic relationship between the patient and the healthcare team could be instrumental in supporting the patient during this experience. Through this relationship, nurses can support the patient's feelings of control, which can help to lessen the patient's fatigue. Psychoeducational interventions usually incorporate anticipatory guidance about patterns of fatigue and tailored recommendations for self-management of the fatigue.[28] Activities designed to distract the patient (e.g., games, music, reading) may be helpful at decreasing fatigue, but the mechanisms behind this strategy are unknown.

Studies of cancer patients indicate that psychosocial support, individualized counseling, and spiritual care have fatigue-reduction effects.[11] With CFS and multiple sclerosis, cognitive–behavioral therapy (CBT) has been beneficial in treatment.[39] CBT uses a series of sessions designed to help patients become aware of the stressors that make their symptoms worse and alter their beliefs and behaviors that might delay recovery.

Complementary Therapy

Although the evidence has not been clearly established, many complementary therapies such as yoga, meditation, progressive muscle relaxation, and American ginseng may be effective in managing fatigue. These therapies are often recommended as supplementary to other established interventions for fatigue.[28,40] The benefit of many other therapies such as acupuncture, acupressure, massage, and aromatherapy are also inconclusive; however, patients may find these useful.

INTERRELATED CONCEPTS

The concept of fatigue is closely interrelated with many concepts presented in this textbook (Fig. 29.3). Mood and Affect, Nutrition, and Pain are shown with bidirectional arrows because of the interrelated cause and effect on fatigue. With each of these concepts, fatigue is a prime symptom of many of their exemplars and can also increase the risk for fatigue. Depression is an example of this phenomenon. Fatigue is listed as one of the diagnostic criteria for depression,[41] an exemplar of mood and affect. In addition, fatigue can cause the individual to experience many losses, and this could lead to depression. Gas Exchange, Perfusion, Cellular Regulation, Sleep, and Stress and Coping are contributors to fatigue. Also, fatigue can significantly affect the concepts of Mobility, Cognition, and Functional Ability, shown as ovals with an arrow pointing toward those concepts in Fig. 29.3. If an individual is significantly exhausted, his or her ability to think, mobilize, and perform normal daily activities becomes impaired.

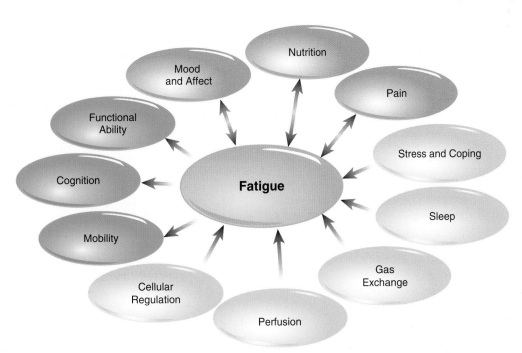

FIGURE 29.3 Fatigue and Interrelated Concepts.

BOX 29.3 EXEMPLARS OF FATIGUE

Physiological Fatigue
- Protein–calorie malnutrition
- Excessive physical activity
- Sleep deprivation
- Excessive caffeine or alcohol use
- Dehydration
- Pregnancy

Pathological Fatigue
Mental
- Depression
- Psychosis
- Addiction

Physical, Nonneurologic
- Infection (mononucleosis, influenza, pneumonia)
- Immunologic (HIV infection)

- Rheumatologic (systemic lupus erythematosus, rheumatoid arthritis)
- Hematologic (anemia)
- Cardiac (heart failure)
- Endocrinologic (hypothyroidism, diabetes type 1 and type 2)
- Pulmonary (COPD, asthma)
- Renal (acute renal failure, chronic renal failure)
- Malignancy (cancer)
- Treatment-related (chemotherapy, radiation therapy, surgery, medications)
- Chronic fatigue syndrome (CFS)/systemic exertion intolerance disease (SEID)

Physical, Neurologic
- Central—spinal/supraspinal (traumatic brain injury, stroke, amyotrophic lateral sclerosis, multiple sclerosis, Parkinson disease)
- Peripheral—nerve/neuromuscular transmission/muscle (neuromuscular disorder, muscle ischemia)

🌿 **ACCESS EXEMPLAR LINKS IN YOUR GIDDENS EBOOK**

CLINICAL EXEMPLARS

Featured Exemplars

Many exemplars related to fatigue exist in the clinical arena and are seen in all areas of the population. The following featured exemplars demonstrate conditions that can cause physiological and pathological fatigue. Box 29.3 presents additional common exemplars across the lifespan.

Cancer-Related Fatigue

Many cancer patients experience some level of fatigue during their course of treatment, and approximately one-third will have persistent fatigue for a number of years post treatment.[42] Prevalence rates for fatigue in cancer patients range from 15% to 96%, depending on the type of treatment, the stage of the cancer, and the method for measuring the fatigue. Cancer-related fatigue is thought to be a result of pro-inflammatory cytokines, hypothalamic-pituitary-adrenal dysregulation, circadian rhythm desynchronization, skeletal muscle wasting, and/or genetic dysregulation. However, evidence is limited to support any of these mechanisms.[4] The National Comprehensive Cancer Network (NCCN) has developed an algorithm to assess and treat fatigue in those patients experiencing cancer,[4] and fatigue has been added to the ICD-10 diagnosis list to ensure a standardized diagnosis in research and practice settings.[3]

Diabetes

Diabetes is a condition in which abnormally high levels of sugar remain in the bloodstream instead of entering the body's cells where it would be converted into energy. This results in the body tissues such as the muscles not receiving the needed nutrition to function appropriately despite the person having enough to eat. Without appropriate nutrition, the individual will experience fatigue. Fatigue is one of the presenting symptoms in both type 1 and type 2 diabetes.[43]

Mononucleosis

Mononucleosis is characterized by the symptoms of fatigue, sore throat, fever, generalized lymphadenopathy, and splenomegaly. These symptoms vary greatly in type, severity, and duration. Patients will typically complain of difficulty maintaining their usual level of activity. The prognosis for recovery from the disease is good. The acute symptoms of the disease will last 10 days to 6 weeks after exposure and may persist for several months.[43]

Pregnancy

Pregnancy is diagnosed by examining presumptive, probable, and positive indicators. One of the presumptive indicators of pregnancy is the subjective symptom of fatigue.[44] This symptom is particularly challenging during the first trimester, during which the pregnant woman will spend much time sleeping secondary to this increased fatigue. The exact cause of this fatigue is unknown, but it is believed that it might be caused by increasing levels of estrogen, progesterone, and human chorionic gonadotropin (hCG), and the psychological/physical adaptations to the pregnancy.

Chronic Obstructive Pulmonary Disease

Chronic obstructive pulmonary disease (COPD) is a chronic condition associated with airway obstruction making it difficult to move air out of the lungs, leading to dyspnea and hypoxemia. A significant amount of energy is utilized by the patient just for the work of breathing. With COPD, a person has a decline in lung function, which can result in decreased exercise tolerance. Over time, patients may also experience decreased muscle strength from deconditioning. The patient with COPD experiences decreased endurance due to fatigue, dyspnea, and an imbalance between oxygen supply and demand, and can lead to a reduced ability to accomplish activities of daily living.[45]

CASE STUDY

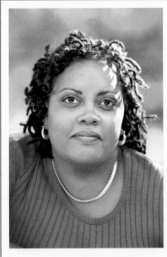

Case Presentation

Helen Morris is a 55-year-old female who lives with her husband in a suburban community. She is the senior managing editor for a major newspaper. She presents to a healthcare clinic with the complaint of "getting the flu and cold" for the second time in 3 months and reports "feeling exhausted" and having to "drag herself into work." On the weekends, she describes spending most of her time resting so that she can go back to work on Monday. She adds, "The rest does not last long because by Wednesday I feel exhausted again. My life has become limited—all I can do is to go to work." She states that when she is at the office, by the afternoon she is exhausted and her muscles ache. She states, "Sometimes I am so tired I cannot even think well enough to complete my work." She states that she has tried to eat better and stopped drinking anything with caffeine, but it has not seemed to make her fatigue any better. She describes the fatigue as

starting approximately 6 months ago. The fatigue worsens with any activity. She expresses frustration at being unable to do the things she enjoys, and she wants to find the cause.

Her history reveals anemia with pregnancy, but otherwise she has had no health problems, nor does she take any prescribed medications. She says she sleeps but does not feel rested when she wakes up. She denies weight loss or gain, polyuria, polydipsia, or cold intolerance. Her social history is negative for the use of alcohol, relationship problems, or situational stress. She denies having symptoms of depression.

On examination, the patient is alert and well groomed. Her skin is race appropriate, not pale or jaundiced. She is afebrile, and her vital signs are within normal limits. The heart, lung, musculoskeletal, and neurologic exam yields normal results. She has no lymphadenopathy. She reports going through menopause and having no menstruation for 2 years. Her hemoglobin is 11.2 mg/dL, and total serum iron is 150 mcg/L. Her thyroid-stimulating hormone, kidney, and liver enzymes are within normal limits.

Case Analysis Questions

1. In what ways does this case exemplify chronic fatigue?
2. What factors make this situation consistent with CFS?
3. What kind of collaborative interventions would be helpful to increase the quality of life for Helen Morris?

From Stockbyte/Thinkstock.

 ACCESS EXEMPLAR LINKS IN YOUR GIDDENS EBOOK

REFERENCES

1. Barroso, J., & Voss, J. G. (2013). Fatigue in HIV and AIDS: An analysis of evidence. *The Journal of the Association of Nurses in AIDS Care, 24*(1), S5–S14.
2. Patterson, E., Wan, Y. W. T., & Sidani, S. (2013). Nonpharmacological nursing interventions for the management of patient fatigue: A literature review. *Journal of Clinical Nursing, 22*, 2668–2678.
3. Curt, G. A., Breitbart, W., Cella, D., et al. (2000). Impact of cancer-related fatigue on the lives of patients: New findings from the fatigue coalition. *The Oncologist, 5*, 353–360.
4. National Comprehensive Cancer Network (NCCN). (2018). *Cancer-Related Fatigue Version 2.* https://www.nccn.org.
5. Lou, J. S. (2012). Techniques in assessing fatigue in neuromuscular diseases. *Physical Medicine and Rehabilitation Dlinics of North America, 23*(1), 11–22.
6. Kirshbaum, M. (2010). Cancer-related fatigue: A review of nursing interventions. *British Journal of Community Nursing, 15*, 214–219.
7. Al-Mulla, M. R., Sepulveda, F., & Colley, M. (2011). A review of non-invasive techniques to detect and predict localised muscle fatigue. *Sensors, 11*(4), 3545–3594.
8. Finsterer, J., & Mahjoub, S. Z. (2013). Fatigue in healthy and diseased individuals. *The American Journal of Hospice & Palliative Care, 31*(5), 562–575.
9. Goldenberg, D. L. (2016). *Chronic Widespread Pain: Lessons Learned from Fibromyalgia and related disorders.* eBook PPM Practical Pain Management, 16(10).
10. Davis, M. P., & Walsh, D. (2010). Mechanisms of Fatigue. *The Journal of Supportive Oncology, 8*(4), 164–174.
11. Neefjes, E. C. W., van der Vorst, D. L., Blauwhoff-Buskermolen, S., et al. (2013). Aiming for a better understanding and management of cancer-related fatigue. *The Oncologist, 18*, 1135–1143.
12. Bower, J. E. (2014). Cancer-related fatigue: Mechanisms, risk factors, & treatments. *Nature Reviews. Clinical Oncology, 11*(10), 597–609.

13. Dantzer, R., Heijnen, C. J., Kavelaars, A., et al. (2014). The neuroimmune basis of fatigue. *Trends in Neurosciences, 37*(1), 39–46.
14. Stout, K., & Finlayson, M. (2011). Fatigue management in chronic illness. *Occupational Therapy Practice, 16*(1), 16–26.
15. Smith, W., Noonan, C., & Buchwald, D. (2006). Mortality in a cohort of chronically fatigue patients. *Psychological Medicine, 35*, 1301.
16. Karakashian, A. L., & Schub, T. (2018). *Chronic Fatigue syndrome.* CINAHL Information systems: Glendale, CA.
17. Gambert, S. R. (2013). "Why do I always feel tired?" Evaluating older patients reporting fatigue. *Consultant, 53*(11), 1–6.
18. Crawley, E. (2018). Pediatric chronic fatigue syndrome: Current perspectives. *Public Health, Medicine, and Therapeutics, 20*(2), 27–33.
19. Bower, J. E., Crosswell, A. D., & Slavich, G. M. (2014). Childhood adversity and cumulative life stress: Risk factors for cancer-related fatigue. *Clinical Psychological Science, 2*(1), 108–115.
20. Kendall, M. (1990). Do we need a new classification of beta-blockers? *Journal of Human Hypertension, 4*, 27–29.
21. Koornstra, R. H. T., Peters, M., Donofrio, S., et al. (2014). Management of fatigue in patients with cancer-a practical overview. *Cancer Treatment Reviews, 40*, 791–799.
22. Davy, J. (2014). Good sleep, good health, good performance. It's obvious, or is it? The importance of education programmes in general fatigue management. *Journal of the Ergonomics Society of South Africa, 26*(1), 64–73.
23. Berger, A. M., Mooney, K., Alvarez-Perez, A., et al. (2015). Cancer-related fatigue, version 2.2015: Clinical practice guidelines in oncology. *Journal of the National Comprehensive Cancer Network, 13*(8), 1012–1039.
24. Rosenthal, T., Majeroni, B., Pretorius, R., et al. (2008). Fatigue: An overview. *American Family Physician, 78*(10), 1173–1179.
25. Wasserman, M. R. (2018). *Fatigue. Merck Manual.* Kenilworth, NJ: Merck Sharp & Dohme.
26. Lyon, D., McCain, N., Elswick, R., et al. (2014). Biobehavioral examination of fatigue across populations: Report from a P30 Center of Excellence. *Nursing Outlook, 62*, 322–331.
27. Lee, K., Dziadkowiec, O., & Meek, P. (2014). A systems science approach to fatigue management in research and health care. *Nursing Outlook, 62*, 313–321.

28. Mitchell, S. A., Hoffman, A. J., Clark, J. C., et al. (2014). Putting evidence into practice: An update of evidence-based interventions for cancer-related fatigue during and following treatment. *Clinical Journal of Oncology Nursing, 18*(6), 38–58.

29. Wang, Y. J., Boehmke, M., Wu, Y. W. B., et al. (2011). Effects of 6 week walking program on Taiwanese women newly diagnosed with early-stage breast cancer. *Cancer Nursing, 34*(2), E1–E13.

30. Yeo, T. P., Burrell, S. A., Sauter, P. K., et al. (2012). A progressive postresection walking program significantly improves fatigue and health-related quality of life in pancreas and periampullary cancer patients. *Journal of the American College of Surgeons, 214*(4), 463–475.

31. Picariello, F., Moss-Morris, R., Macdougall, I. C., et al. (2018). 'It's when you are doing too much you feel tired': A qualitative exploration of fatigue in end-stage kidney disease. *British Journal of Health Psychology, 23*, 311–333.

32. Smith, M. E. B., Haney, E., McDonagh, M., et al. (2015). Treatment of myalgic encephalomyelitis/chronic fatigue syndrome: A systematic review for the National Institutes of Health Pathways to Prevention Workshop. *Annals of Internal Medicine, 162*(12), 841–850.

33. Yeh, C. H., Man Wai, J. P., Lin, U. S., et al. (2011). A pilot study to examine the feasibility and effects of a home-based aerobic program on reducing fatigue in children with acute lymphoblastic leukemia. *Cancer Nursing, 34*(1), 3–12.

34. Finlayson, M., & Preissner, K. (2012). Outcome moderators of a fatigue management program for people with multiple sclerosis. *The American Journal of Occupational Therapy, 66*(20), 187–197.

35. Center for Disease Control. (2018). *Myalgic Encephalomyelitis/Chronic Fatigue Syndrome*. Retrieved from https://www.cdc.gov/me-cfs.

36. Black, D. S., Cole, S. W., Christodoulou, G., et al. (2018). Genomic mechanisms of fatigue in survivors of colorectal cancer. *Cancer, 14*, 2637–2644.

37. Minton, O., Richardson, A., Sharpe, M., et al. (2011). Psychostimulants for management of cancer-related fatigue: A systematic review and meta-analysis. *Journal of Pain and Symptom Management, 41*(4), 761–767.

38. Committee on the Diagnostic Criteria for Myalgic Encephalomyelitis/Chronic Fatigue Syndrome. (2015). *Beyond myalgic encephalomyelitis/Chronic fatigue syndrome: redefining an illness*. Institute of Medicine of the National Academies: Washington D.C.

39. Larun, L., Brurberg, K. G., Odgaard-Jenson, J., et al. (2017). *Exercise therapy for chronic fatigue syndrome (Review). Cochrane Library*. Wiley & Sons.

40. Finnegan-John, J., Molassiotis, A., Richardson, A., et al. (2013). A systematic review of complementary and alternative medicine interventions for the management of cancer-related fatigue. *Integrative Cancer Therapies, 12*(4), 276–290.

41. American Psychiatric Association. (2013). *Diagnostic and statistical manual of mental disorders* (5th ed.). Arlington, VA: APA.

42. Wang, X. S., Zhao, F., Fisch, M. J., et al. (2014). Prevalence and characteristics of moderate to severe fatigue: A multicenter study in cancer patients and survivors. *Cancer, 120*(3), 425–432.

43. Hockenberry, M., & Wilson, D. (2015). *Wong's nursing care of infants and children* (10th ed.). St Louis: Mosby.

44. Loudermilk, D. L., Perry, S. E., Cashion, M. C., et al. (2016). *Maternity & women's health* (11th ed.). St Louis: Mosby.

45. Ignatavicius, D., & Workman, M. (2018). *Medical–surgical nursing: Patient-centered collaborative care* (9th ed.). St Louis: Saunders.

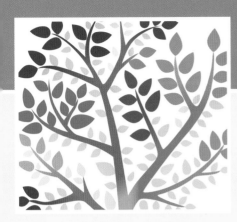

Stress and Coping

Lynne Buchanan

Stress is a common topic in society. The term stress is frequently used to describe a feeling of pressure or emotional strain from life's demands, perceived events, and stimulus.[1] Because all people experience stress, it is considered a normal physiological process associated with regulation and homeostasis. Coping represents an individual's response to stress. Individual responses to stress vary because what is perceived as a stressful situation to one person may not be perceived in the same way by another. Coping responses are actions taken to minimize or reduce the stressor to get back to a state of homeostasis, well-being, and health. The experience of stress involves cognitive appraisal, perception, physiological and psychological manifestations, feelings, and symptoms.[2] Coping actions are part of the experience and in the perfect scenario are applied appropriately to the level and severity of stress.[2–5] Although humans are resilient, there is a finite capacity for responding to and managing stress. Those who exceed the capacity to cope with stress are at risk for disease and disability.[6] This concept presentation focuses on physiologic and psychologic stressors, the consequences of stress, and the process of coping.

DEFINITION

The word "stress" has existed since the 14th century with a meaning of hardship, adversity, or affliction. In the early 20th century, Walter Cannon first described the stimulus and response (fight or flight) to the perception of a physical or emotional threat.[7] Hans Selye brought the concept of a general adaptation syndrome to popular society by proposing a reaction theory that stress is the sum of all the effects of factors that act on the body, with both pleasant and unpleasant stressors being equally important.[8] Although early experiments supported various species responding in a stereotypical reaction to events such as infection, trauma, nervous strain, heat, cold, or fatigue, continuing work demonstrated that there was not always a precise uniform response.[8–10] Later theorists proposed stress as an appraisal process with a defined series of steps. The foundation for contemporary perspectives evolved with stress characterized as a response, interaction, and outcome.[2,4] A commonly accepted view is that stress is a series of reactions to external and internal demands with the full reaction determined by the duration, severity, resources, and coping actions taken, whereas coping is an action directed toward change through conscious or unconscious thoughts and behaviors to avoid harm and restore balance.[6]

Lazarus and Folkman laid the foundation of the contemporary view of stress and coping through their transactional theory.[2] The conceptualization is based on their research and is viewed as a person-environment interaction, cognitive appraisal for level of threat, harm, or taxing of resources, and coping action to reduce or manage threat. Coping is most effective if there is a matching between threat level and the individual's ability to adapt and change a situation within the available coping resources, skills, and abilities.[2–5] For the purposes of this concept presentation, stress and coping as a concept is defined as *a continual process that starts with an event that is experienced by the individual, perceived through intact information processing channels, appraised for scope and meaning, assessed as neutral, manageable, or threatening within current capacity of coping skills, resources, and abilities, ending ideally in a positive outcome of homeostasis and feeling of well-being.*

SCOPE

The scope of stress and coping is shown in Fig. 30.1 on a continuum of stress-neutral, challenge-manageable, and threat-not manageable (severe). Stress-neutral represents typical day-to-day stress and is well within existing coping resources to manage. Challenge-manageable stress represents a person who is faced with moderate to greater stress and necessitates use of existing and potentially new resources and coping actions to effectively reduce, eliminate, or manage stress. In situations resulting in severe stress (stress-not manageable), the stress threat exceeds coping capacity leading to a state of exhaustion of resources. Outside assistance and resources are needed.

This concept presentation primarily focuses on the way a stressor impacts the individual, specifically on the internal localized context (cells, organs, or body systems). However, stress and coping can also be viewed within a family or community.[11] This includes how an event affects the family or community and the resources that are available to family members within their community. Schools, teachers, counselors, parks, recreation, and healthcare provider access are important resources that vary within communities. Family resources refer to the ability of family members to respond when individual members are faced with challenges.[11] Communities have a capacity to respond using available resources and will do so effectively if resources are appropriate for the duration and severity and do not exceed capacity. Stress and coping can also be considered at the macro level. For example, an environmental event such as a natural disaster or a terroristic attack has implications on a society. Although there are societal outcomes, each individual within the population involved will respond based on his or her own perception of the event and the personal impact it has for him or her.

NORMAL PHYSIOLOGICAL PROCESS

Stress is a normal aspect of the human experience. In most cases, day-to-day stress is managed successfully; the individual maintains homeostasis and the stress minimally impacts or interrupts daily life activities. The optimal stress/coping action relies on intact, functioning body systems. Stress triggers a physiologic response involving the nervous, endocrine, and immune systems which affect other body systems including the cardiovascular, respiratory, renal, gastrointestinal, and reproductive systems as well as have an effect on psychological well-being.

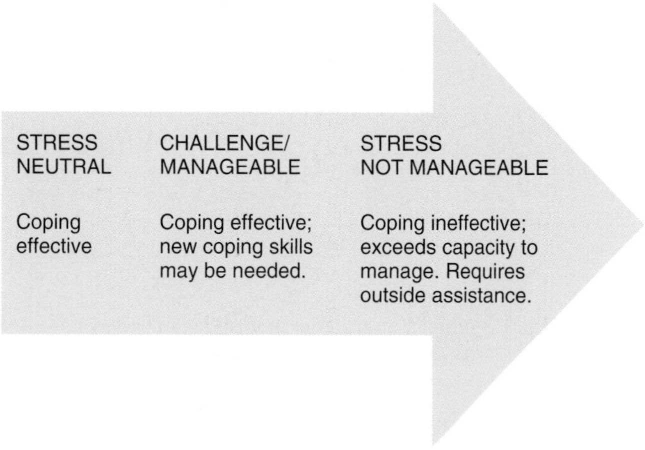

Neuroendocrine Response

Perceived events or demands cause an anticipatory response beginning in the limbic system. If the stressor is perceived as minor, subtle physiological, psychological, and behavioral processes compensate for the stressor. The individual may not be aware these processes are occurring and are being managed.[6]

When a stressor is perceived as a more serious threat, a stress response is initiated by the nervous and endocrine systems, particularly the hypothalamus, sympathetic nervous system (SNS), the pituitary gland, and the adrenal gland. These systems synchronize a complex series of reactions leading to a coordinated response, directing energy for adaptation (Fig. 30.2).

The hypothalamus secretes corticotropin-releasing factor (CRF), which activates the SNS, the anterior pituitary, and the posterior pituitary. Activation of the SNS causes the release of catecholamines (norepinephrine, epinephrine, and dopamine). Norepinephrine is released throughout the brain, triggering neural pathways for sensory information and stimulating arousal, vigilance, anxiety, and labile emotions.[6,12] The physiological response (known as the *fight-or-flight response*) is due to the release of catecholamines epinephrine and norepinephrine. Specifically, these hormones lead to increased heart rate, blood pressure, and cardiac output; dilation of bronchial airways; pupil dilation; increased

STRESS NEUTRAL	CHALLENGE/ MANAGEABLE	STRESS NOT MANAGEABLE
Coping effective	Coping effective; new coping skills may be needed.	Coping ineffective; exceeds capacity to manage. Requires outside assistance.

FIGURE 30.1 Scope of Stress and Coping.

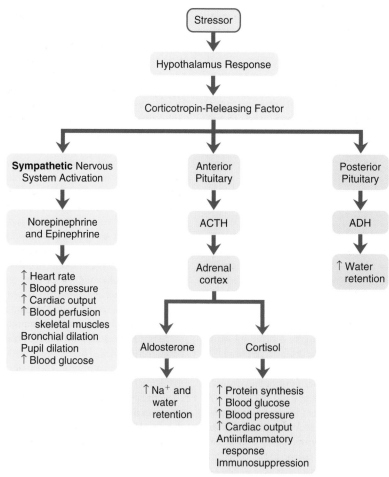

FIGURE 30.2 Physiology of Alarm Response Sympathetic Nervous System Effects. *ACTH,* adrenocorticotropic hormone; *ADH,* antidiuretic hormone.

blood flow to the skeletal muscles; and increased blood glucose. There is a concomitant decrease in blood flow to nonessential organs (e.g., the digestive system).

At the same time, CRF stimulates the anterior and posterior pituitary gland to release several hormones, including antidiuretic hormone, prolactin, growth hormone, and adrenocorticotropic hormone (ACTH). ACTH triggers the secretion of cortisol and aldosterone from the adrenal cortex. The activation of the adrenal cortex during the stress response leads to the secretion of cortisol, a glucocorticoid. Cortisol mobilizes cellular metabolism, particularly glucose and protein metabolism. The net effect is increased blood glucose (through gluconeogenesis and inhibition of glucose update and oxidation in selected body cells) and increasing amino acids (through catabolic effects of muscle). In elevated levels, cortisol also has a role in the immune response, including immunosuppressive and antiinflammatory effects.

When the stressor and threat is eliminated, or when the individual appraises an event as neutral or challenge and within their capacity to manage, the alarm response is halted. Sustained stress, however, has a negative impact on organs, body systems, and health and well-being.[6] A prolonged or chronic situation involving a heightened stress response which is not adequately managed through effective coping exhausts capacity and the ability to maintain homeostasis. Physical, psychological, and behavioral manifestations lead to overt stress symptoms.[6,12]

Age-Related Differences

Because the stress response is based on a neuroendocrine response, there are few discernable differences in the physiologic stress response across the lifespan. Age-related differences are primarily associated with cognitive appraisal of events that determine if a situation is a threat or not. Cognitive appraisal and coping strategies are associated with cognitive development and life experiences.

VARIATIONS AND CONTEXT

There are variations in stress and coping responses seen across the lifespan, especially when stress is severe and/or prolonged. These variations include the sources and type of stress, and how the stress is perceived, as interpreted through a cognitive appraisal. Individual variables such as age, developmental level, maturation, environment, life experiences, and the individual's general mental and physical health status impact the cognitive appraisal.

Sources of Stress
Physiological Stressors
Physiological stress refers to a stressor that originates as a physiological trigger and usually is specifically associated with an injury or illness (Table 30.1). Some acute physiological stressors are life-threatening states such as trauma, acute myocardial infarction, or acute renal failure. An acute stress response is immediate, often intense, and necessary for survival. Chronic physiological stress can lead to debilitating disease.

Psychological/Emotional Stressors
Psychological and emotional stressors are more common stressors encountered on a regular basis and generate a state of unpleasant arousal. Common stressors include occupational pressures, academic pressures, major life events (both positive and negative), financial stress, or bereavement (see Table 30.1). According to a 2017 survey conducted by the American Psychological Association, the most common sources of stress among Americans include the future of our nation (63%), finances (62%), work (61%), politics (57%), and violence and crime (51%). With regards to concerns of the future of our nation, the most common causes of concerns include the economy, health care, government distrust

TABLE 30.1	Sources of Stress
Physiological Stressors	**Psychological/Emotional Stressors**
• Autoimmune disorders	• Birth of child
• Cancer	• Caregiving
• Chronic obstructive pulmonary disease	• Change in health status
• Dementia	• Death of close family member or friend
• Diabetes	• Diagnosis of terminal illness
• Organ failure (such as heart, renal, or respiratory failure)	• Divorce
	• Environmental emergencies
	• Failing an examination
• Myocardial infarction	• Finances
• Acute and chronic pain	• National events
• Traumatic injury	• Loss of job
	• Marriage
	• Moral distress
	• Moving
	• Parenting
	• Politics
	• Physical disability
	• Relationship problems
	• Social unrest
	• Spiritual distress
	• Violence

and scandals, hate crimes, international conflicts, concerns over terrorist attacks, Social Security, and taxes.[13]

Psychological stress can be acute or chronic. An event in which danger is perceived (such as fleeing from a house fire or reacting to an automobile accident) or an emotionally traumatic event (such as the unexpected death of a close friend or family member) triggers an acute stress response. Chronic emotional stress is a long-term state associated with psychosocial stressors such as difficult relationships, ongoing occupational stress, or financial stress.

Types of Stress
In general, unhealthy stress is categorized as acute stress, episodic acute stress, and chronic stress. The source of all three types of stress can be physiological or psychological/emotional (discussed previously):

- *Acute stress:* Acute stress is, by far, the most common type of stress and typically occurs for a short period of time. It usually occurs in reaction to a real or perceived demand, threat, or pressure. Resolution of the stressor leads to elimination of the stress response.
- *Episodic acute stress:* Episodic stress is often described as "self-inflicted" stress or in regular chaos and is common among type A personalities. This often occurs by taking on unrealistic assignments beyond what is typically or reasonably expected. These individuals may always be in a hurry and irritable. Constant worry is another form of episodic acute stress.
- *Chronic stress:* This type of stress represents a perpetual or sustained demand, threat, or pressure that is harmful to health because it wears on individuals continuously. It can stem from long-term stressors such as chronic occupational stress, relationship stress, and financial stress. Chronic stress is often associated with a loss of hope that the situation can improve.

Cognitive Appraisal
One variation in the stress response is the individual's cognitive assessment (appraisal) of the situation and perceived threat level. This is a

complex, nonlinear process because of the multiple variables involved. The cognitive appraisal represents the process of sorting out information to derive meaning and is the underlying factor in how an individual will respond.[14] Cognitive appraisal occurs in two phases. The primary appraisal is an initial evaluation for harm to self or to a loved one's well-being, self-esteem, or personal values. The secondary appraisal involves the evaluation of resources available to overcome, reduce, or eliminate the stressor and determines to what extent the problem is controllable. Several variables such as level of education, past life experiences, current coping style, values, expectations, beliefs, self-efficacy, worldviews, and engagement affect the cognitive appraisal process.

CONSEQUENCES

Although short-term stress is a normal physiological response, the effect of chronic stress on health is profound. Chronic stress results in the continuous activation of the nervous system and eventually produces negative outcomes across multiple body systems leading to a number of chronic health conditions.[6,12]

- **Central nervous system:** Chronic stress affects cognitive function, including headaches, nervousness, irritability, problems with decision-making, insomnia, memory problems, confusion, anxiety disorders, and depression. Prolonged release of corticosteroids can also lead to stress-induced damage to the hippocampus, which can affect long-term memory.
- **Cardiovascular system:** Chronic stress results in excessive activation of the SNS and in long-term exposure to catecholamines. This increases heart rate and blood pressure and can lead to cardiovascular disease such as hypertension, atherosclerosis, cardiac arrhythmias, myocardial infarction, or stroke. Furthermore, individuals with pre-existing cardiovascular disease are particularly at risk for exacerbation of the condition if exposed to prolonged stress.
- **Immune system:** Excessive and long-term exposure to cortisol has been shown to decrease white blood cells, leading to stress-induced immunosuppression placing the individual at greater risk for bacterial and viral infections, and cancer. There also appears to be a correlation between stress and immune-based conditions such as rheumatoid arthritis, multiple sclerosis, asthma, and cancer, although specific details of this relationship are unclear.
- **Musculoskeletal system:** The stress response is associated with muscle tension as a way to protect against injury. Chronic stress can result in an overly taut muscle over a long period of time, leading to pain and discomfort, particularly in the head, neck, and shoulders. Protracted muscle tension of both the head and the neck are two contributors to tension and migraine headache. Nervous tics may also develop with chronic stress because of muscle tension.
- **Gastrointestinal system:** Individuals under chronic stress may experience a number of gastrointestinal problems associated with excessive excretion of catecholamines and cortisol. Gastritis, ulcerative colitis, irritable colon, and diarrhea have been linked to chronic stress, as have obesity and eating disorders.
- **Integumentary system:** The hair, skin, and nails may be affected by chronic stress. Elevated stress over time may cause excessive hair loss. There may be skin problems that are exacerbated by stress, including acne, eczema, and psoriasis. There may also be stress-related ulcers in the mouth from dry mouth and cold sores.
- **Sexuality and reproduction system:** Chronic stress affects reproductive health in both men and women. In men, reduced sex drive, reduced testosterone production, reduced sperm production, maturation, erectile dysfunction, and impotence occur. Among women, excessive stress may be associated with menstrual cycle disorders and dysmenorrhea, as well as exacerbation of menstrual symptoms (cramping, fluid retention and bloating, and irritability) or menopausal symptoms (irritability, mood swings, and hot flashes).

RISK FACTORS

Populations at Risk

Individuals across all population groups are at risk for physical and psychological stress. Serious psychological distress is recognized throughout our society and according to the 2014 National Health Interview Survey, an estimated 3.1% of adults older than age 18 years experienced a serious psychological event that required a coping action in the previous 30 days.[15] This was found to be highest among middle-aged adults in the 45- to 64-year-old age group, Hispanics, and women. The three populations that report the greatest level of general stress are lower-income Americans, young adults (particularly those with children), and women. These groups often also have fewer resources available to them or less developed coping abilities.

Infants and Children

Research on children's perception of stress is based on age and developmental stages and the child's level of self-efficacy and control. Self-efficacy and control are learned over time. An infant is not able to cope with stressors of hunger, pain, or fear due to inability in motor and cognitive functioning which has not developed. As they mature, they start to learn coping skills. Children who live in an environment of chaos and loss of autonomy may not learn effective coping responses and could be at risk as they enter school.[16] A child in a dysfunctional home may learn ineffective ways of coping with the demands put on them. Younger children with hospitalizations may be at higher risk for ineffective coping.[17]

Adolescents

Adolescence is a time of psychosocial, emotional, cognitive, and moral development during a period when teens are also being given more freedom to make decisions including driving a car and going out with friends. The hormonal interaction among the hypothalamus, pituitary, and gonads is increased. Adolescents are focused on body image and changes to their bodies may be disturbing. They are at risk for ineffective coping especially if there are not strong family dynamics and social supports in place.[18] Adolescence is characterized by a shift in cognitive abilities to formal operations and more formalized abstract thinking ability. Adolescence is a risky time and because the brain is not fully formed and critical thinking skills are still developing, they are at high risk to choose ineffective coping responses during stress. Adolescents who lack adequate coping skills and social support are at higher risk for speeding, substance abuse, sexual encounters, depression, and suicide.[18]

Older Adults

Although older adults have the advantage of a lifetime of coping experiences, a disadvantage for many is that social support may decrease and their circle of friends and experiences becomes smaller, especially if they experience physical and psychological changes. These physical and psychological changes impact resilience as health conditions effect immune and other body systems. Mobility and cognition can change to a degree of causing inaccurate appraisal of events and ineffective coping actions. They may utilize ineffective coping that is not matched to the level and duration required. Older adults may also use more coping methods of withdrawal and succumb to emotional coping strategies that may not be appropriate.[19]

Individual Risk Factors

Risk for Psychological Stress

There are many sources of psychological stress on individuals. Some of the most common situations placing individuals at risk for stress include problems with interpersonal relationships, strained family relationships, financial strain, occupational stress, and food insecurity to name a few.[20] Other sources of increased risk of stress are in individuals with health conditions or who are in care-giving roles, for example for a loved one with dementia or terminal illness.[21]

Risk for Physiologic Stress

Individuals with a significant injury or illness are at risk for experiencing a stress response. Examples are those who are in life-threatening states such as traumatic injury, cardiovascular compromise, or organ failure or chronic conditions such as cancer, infections, or chronic pain.

ASSESSMENT

Nurses learn about an individual's perceived stressors and coping responses through a detailed history and examination. The priority of assessment should be an evaluation of signs and symptoms of stress and the association to disease. Stress signs and symptoms and disease pathologies manifest in a variety of ways and vary in severity. Stress can be evaluated using assessment tools that capture the physiological, cognitive, psychological/emotional, and behavioral signs and symptoms and coping responses. Nurses should recognize individuals who are experiencing a challenging or threatening stress response so that appropriate interventions can be initiated. There are reliable questionnaires for assessing stress symptoms and coping actions. There are assessments for tobacco, alcohol, substance abuse, and depression that may also be appropriate.

History

When conducting a history, the nurse queries about the past and current state of health (past medical history, current conditions, and current medications), family history, psychosocial history, and stress symptoms associated with body systems. Clues about the presence of stress are often identified in the psychosocial component of the history. Specifically, ask about mental health problems and past or current conditions or life events associated with psychological stress, such as a death, loss of job, or illness. Also ask about demands and recent life events. Common symptoms of stress include irritability, nervousness or anxiousness, fatigue, feeling overwhelmed, or feeling depressed or sad. Ask about unexplained abdominal pain or indigestion, headaches, insomnia, fatigue, restlessness, lack of concentration, dizziness, excessive sweating, sweaty palms, back pain, tight shoulders or neck, skin eruptions, hair loss, hyperventilation, palpitations, and tightening of the chest. A number of tools are available to further assist with assessment in relation to context (Box 30.1). Perhaps the most widely recognized tool is the Holmes Life Events Scale[22] which can be easily administered and scored by nurses in clinic settings.

The history should also include data regarding the individual's appraisal of the stressor, and should learn what coping strategies have been used—both effective and ineffective methods. A nurse might ask the question, "What is the meaning of this event for you?" Recall that the meaning or perception is developed from several factors including past experiences, internal needs, external needs, ability to acknowledge the problem, cognitive abilities, values, expectations, culture, social supports, and their perceived control over the situation.

It is also important to ask the individual how he or she has coped with stressful events in the past. For example, did this person seek support from another person? Did he or she turn to alcohol or other substances? Additionally, learning the individual's perception of the effectiveness of these coping behaviors helps to gain insight into the strengths and/or weaknesses of the individual's coping patterns. It is particularly important to determine if the patient is relying on problem-based or emotion-based coping strategies. Specific questions about coping assessment tools may be helpful.

BOX 30.1   Coping Measurement Instruments

- Miller Behavioral Style Scale
- Mainz Coping Inventory
- Brief Cope Inventory (BCI)
- Billings and Moos Coping Measures
- Ways of Coping Questionnaire (WCQ)
- Coping Strategy Indicator (CSI)
- Life Events and Coping Inventory (LECI) (children)
- Adolescent Coping Orientation for Problem Experiences Inventory (A-COPE) (adolescents)
- Life Situations Inventory (LSI) (middle and older adult)
- Stress and Coping Process Questionnaire (SCPQ)
- Coping Inventory for Stressful Situations (CISS)

Examination

Examination findings associated with stress are usually consistent with sympathetic nervous system activation. In the acute phase, these signs may include elevated heart rate, irregular heart rate, elevated blood pressure, increased respiratory rate and depth, excessive sweating, dilated pupils, and muscle tension. Such findings may not be as evident when stress is chronic. Assessment in cardiac, respiratory, musculoskeletal, and neurological systems should be done to look for stress-related pathologies and also for acute manifestations of stress overload. For example, auscultation may reveal heart palpitations and increased heart rate, and blood pressure monitoring may show hypertension. An assessment of cognitive functioning is also appropriate as part of the examination. General observations such as personal appearance, grooming, facial expressions, and affect aid the nurse in determining cognitive ability (which affects the ability for effective coping).[23] Findings associated with poor coping behaviors include anger, anxiousness, sadness, or hopelessness. Evidence of adequate coping behavior includes insight and engagement with the primary appraisal and the development of a coping plan. Willingness to use coping strategies or problem-solving techniques is also consistent with positive coping.

CLINICAL MANAGEMENT

Nurses in all areas of practice should be able to recognize stress in patients (and their families) and help them identify high-risk stressors. The aim of clinical management is to implement effective strategies that reduce the stress. Further, nurses help patients support the foundation of effective coping strategies and also assist the patient in finding new resources, building self-efficacy, and reinforcing or guiding development of new ways for coping. An organizing framework for the concept of stress and coping that nurses can use in their practice is shown in Fig. 30.3. This framework starts with an event and ends with an outcome. In the framework, there are antecedents that include individual characteristics, family, community, and environment. The personal appraisal and reappraisal assist the individual in focusing the scope of the experience and determining the magnitude of the stressor. Psychological and physiological stress responses occur and based on the appraisal or magnitude of them appropriate coping actions are taken.

Antecedents

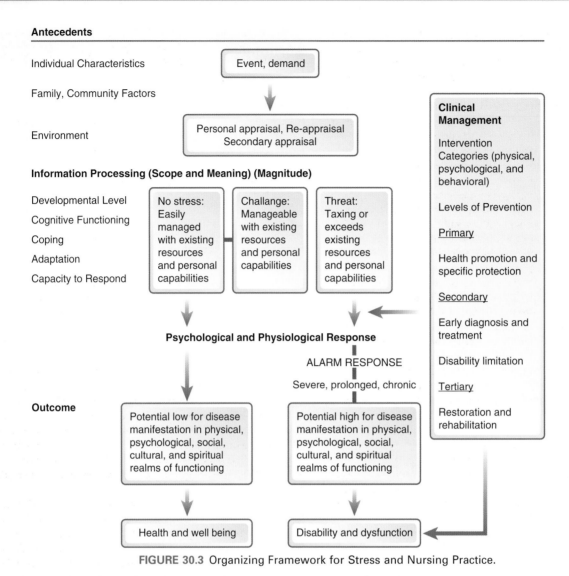

FIGURE 30.3 Organizing Framework for Stress and Nursing Practice.

Primary Prevention

Primary prevention focuses on preventing illness as a result of stress. Thus, the goal is to promote effective coping, health, and well-being. Primary prevention settings that focus on wellness and prevention of stress-related disease and disability include the workplace, schools, senior centers, community wellness centers, primary healthcare clinics, and medical homes. Maintaining good health and proper nutrition, exercising regularly, sustaining positive personal relationships and social support networks, and preserving positive self-esteem are all common primary prevention strategies for stress and coping. Health education for stress prevention is aimed at helping the individual to understand the components of a healthy lifestyle and the relationship of chronic stress and disease, and to learn effective preventative coping strategies that can be used when needed.

Secondary Prevention (Screening)

There are currently no national recommendations for stress screening for general or designated populations. However, there are recommendations for certain situations that are related to mental health conditions that are often linked to ineffective or maladaptive coping such as substance abuse and depression. A number of stress screening tools are available for use in clinical practice; some of these are presented in Box 30.1.

Collaborative Interventions

The goal of clinical management for an individual experiencing stress is to restore the individual to optimal function. Specific interventions are geared toward reducing the actual or perceived threats (if possible), and reinforcement of perceived control over the stressor by adopting positive coping strategies. For patients experiencing acute stress associated with a life-threatening physiologic insult (such as trauma, shock, or sepsis) interventions are geared toward stabilizing the patient. The collaborative interventions discussed in this section focus on measures to assist individuals who are physiologically stable, but at risk for illness or injury due to acute or chronic stress. Nurses have a role in helping patients adapt positive coping strategies and discouraging or redirecting the individual from maladaptive coping strategies.

Categories of Coping Strategies

Coping strategies fall into three broad categories: problem-focused, emotion-focused, and meaning-focused coping.[4,5] Although individuals typically apply a combination of coping strategies as a response to stress, problem-focused coping tends to be more effective than emotion-focused or meaning-focused coping.[24]

Problem-focused coping. Problem-focused coping involves generating solutions to reduce or eliminate the identified stressors. A cognitive appraisal of the situation is done (including if the stressor is one that has been faced before or is a new type of stressor) and then action is taken to manage or change the situation or circumstance associated with the stressor. The coping action is aimed at eliminating or reducing harm from the stressor. For example, a woman is experiencing significant stress at work due to multiple competing projects with similar deadlines and she knows she is unable to meet all the obligations. A problem-focused coping strategy might be to schedule a meeting within her department to develop a plan for additional support and resources so all projects can be completed, or negotiate alternative deadlines.

Emotion-focused coping. Emotion-focused coping emphasizes the regulation of emotional response (such as anger, fear, or anxiety) that occurs in a given situation. Actions are directed at maintaining emotional control through self-regulating thinking and behavior. An example is going for a run, talking with a friend about how one is feeling, and journaling. No attempt is made to change the stressor—rather the focus is on controlling the emotional response to the stressor.

Meaning-focused coping. In meaning-focused coping, the individual draws on values, beliefs, and goals to modify the personal interpretation and response to a problem. The foundation of meaning-focused coping is cultural beliefs, values, ethical foundations, education, and life experiences with a goal of confronting feelings and biases.[5] In meaning-focused coping, the action taken is to start a conversation with a reliable individual (friend or professional) to make meaning of the situation in order to understand one's responses and personal biases and find ways to reframe or modify the personal interpretation and response.

Common Positive Coping Strategies

Effective coping involves positive behavior change or adaptation to address the underlying stressor. Coping strategies that can effectively help manage stress to the benefit of an individual's health are referred to as positive coping strategies. The effectiveness of strategies is highly individualized—and most people apply more than one. Ideally the coping strategies are matched to the severity, duration, situation, and context of the stressor. If coping has been successful in the past and there is similarity of circumstances use of similar coping action is more likely to result in a positive outcome.[14] The most common coping mechanisms include listening to music, exercise, praying, meditation, and yoga.[13] Table 30.2 presents many common positive coping strategies. A few are described further below.

Education. Education regarding the situation and alternative coping measures is a powerful tool to increase self-efficacy and control.[14] For example, the cancer patient who is educated about treatment alternatives and is given a choice of treatment will feel more in control of the situation and stress will be reduced.

Social support. Social support represents a group of strategies that involve gaining support from others. Social support leverages the power of relationships with a network of close friends, family members, community groups, spiritual groups, and support groups organized by specific problems, such as cancer survivors support groups. Having the support of others assists with appraisal, self-regulation of emotions, and feeling of confidence and strength[25,26] and helps to build resilience. Nurses can assist by providing information about resources and support groups in the local community or helping to develop these resources if they are not present.

Exercise. Exercise is a very powerful coping strategy that includes a variety of activities that lead to aerobic movement. Exercise can be implemented in various settings, including a hospital, community center, or home. Exercise should be individualized but can include any cardiovascular–aerobic activity, including walking, running, swimming, and cycling. The benefits of exercise include relief of tension, reduction of stress, relaxation, and enhanced sense of well-being.[24,25] About half of Americans engage in exercise to cope with stress.[13]

TABLE 30.2 Positive and Maladaptive Coping	
Positive Coping Strategies	**Maladaptive Coping Behaviors**
• Art therapy	• Avoidance coping
• Counseling	• Attacking or bullying
• Distraction and diversion activities	• Compartmentalizing
• Education	• Denial
• Massage	• Dependency
• Meditation	• Displacement
• Music therapy	• Dissociation
• Physical activity	• Emotional outbursts
• Praying	• Excessive eating
• Relaxation techniques	• Regression
• Social support	• Rationalization
• Spiritual resources	• Self-harm
• Yoga	• Sensitization
	• Social isolation/withdrawal
	• Substance use
	• Violence

Therapeutic lifestyle change. A therapeutic lifestyle change (TLC) collaborative intervention is aimed at promoting adaptation, coping, and support to promote positive changes that lead to checking of stress or of decreasing severity levels. The collaboration involves exercise, dietary, and counseling professionals who work with the nurse to develop a TLC treatment plan. Topics and skills include self-talk; muscle relaxation; exercise; and dietary approaches avoiding tobacco, alcohol, and drugs. TLC incorporates aspects of motivational interviewing to motivate individuals to change.[25]

Music therapy. Another positive coping strategy is music therapy. Music (particularly slow, quiet classical music) can have a physiologically relaxing effect through the reduction of heart rate, blood pressure, and reduction of stress hormones. Stress reduction through music therapy has been demonstrated in a number of settings and population groups. It helps to reduce stress in disabled children, reduce anxiety in patients in the perioperative environment, reduce depression and increase self-esteem among older adults, and reduce emotional distress among cancer patients.[27]

Relaxation strategies. Relaxation strategies are among the most effective coping strategies for stress management. The goal of relaxation strategies is to achieve a relaxation response—that is a state of physiologic and psychologic rest. Specifically, the relaxation response results in a reduction in SNS activity which leads to reductions in heart rate, respiratory rate, blood pressure, muscle tension, and a state of reduced brain activity. There are many types of relaxation strategies. Some of the more common relaxation strategies include imagery, massage, music therapy, meditation, relaxation breathing, yoga, Tai Chi, and Qigong.[24,28]

Complementary and alternative therapies. Another group of interventions effective for stress reduction includes complementary and alternative medicine strategies. Strategies listed as possibly effective for relieving stress include acupuncture, herbals/botanicals, and aromatherapy.[29]

Ineffective and Maladaptive Coping Responses

Collaborative care also includes the identification of maladaptive coping responses with the intent to redirect the patient toward positive coping responses. Ineffective and maladaptive coping behaviors are those that do not adequately address the underlying problem. An ineffective coping response occurs when an appropriate coping mechanism is used, but may be insufficient for the severity of the stressor. For example, an individual who is experiencing serious financial strain can take a course on personal finance (a positive strategy) but the gains made in education alone may not be sufficient to overcome significant debt.

Maladaptive coping responses include those that ignore the underlying cause of the stressor, and many actually lead to other problems. Common maladaptive coping responses include the use or abuse of alcohol and other substances, smoking, excessive eating, denial, withdrawal, or avoidance. According to the 2017 National Stress survey, 14% of adult respondents reported smoking as a coping mechanism.[13] Maladaptive behaviors may increase the risk for negative outcomes. For example, in one study among glaucoma patients, denial was associated with worse visual field mean deviation compared to those who adopted positive coping strategies.[30] Although avoidance, as a coping strategy, can be somewhat useful in specific situations that are perceived as short term and uncontrollable, long-term avoidance can lead to increased emotional distress, longer recovery times, less effective problem solving, and other maladaptive responses.[25,31] Table 30.2 presents many other maladaptive coping responses.

Pharmacologic Agents

Although there are no medications used to prevent stress or treat stress directly, many types of medications are used in the management of stress, particularly conditions that coexist or are caused by stress. Drugs that act on the central and peripheral nervous systems, such as anxiolytics and hypnotics, antidepressants, antianxiety agents, psychotherapeutics, muscle relaxants, antimigraine agents, and narcotic pain medications, may be used. Selective serotonin reuptake inhibitors and tricyclic antidepressants may be used for individuals with chronic stress and depression. Some of the most common drugs are for relief of muscle tension and pain associated with stress.[32]

INTERRELATED CONCEPTS

The concept of stress and coping has multiple interrelated concepts featured in this textbook and shown in Fig. 30.4. **Anxiety** is closely aligned with stress because this is a typical feeling when pressure occurs. Anxiety can be useful for mobilizing resources to cope with the stressor or can lead to overt mental health illnesses when the stressor is severe and/or sustained.

Functional Ability and **Family Dynamics** are shown as interrelated concepts because these are often associated with stressors. Many of life's most significant stressors are generated from problems managing life's events and challenges with relationships. Another key interrelated concept is the health and illness concept of **Cognition**. Adequate cognitive skills are needed in order to perform an appraisal of an event because of the need to accurately process information. Chronic stress, as discussed earlier, can lead to cognitive impairment. Many other consequences of chronic stress are represented by the concepts **Mood and Affect**, **Perfusion**, **Sexuality**, **Sleep**, and **Immunity**.

CLINICAL EXEMPLARS

Clinical exemplars of stress are presented in Box 30.2 and represent conditions that can result from chronic stress. Stress disorders that

> ### BOX 30.2   EXEMPLARS OF STRESS-RELATED DISORDERS
>
> - Acne
> - Anxiety disorders
> - Autoimmune disorders
> - Cardiac arrhythmias
> - Coronary artery disease
> - Depression
> - Dysmenorrhea
> - Dyspepsia
> - Eating disorders
> - Eczema
> - Erectile dysfunction
> - Fatigue
> - Fibromyalgia
> - Hypertension
> - Immunodeficiency
> - Insomnia
> - Irritable bowel syndrome
> - Low back pain
> - Stroke
> - Tension headache

ACCESS EXEMPLAR LINKS IN YOUR GIDDENS EBOOK

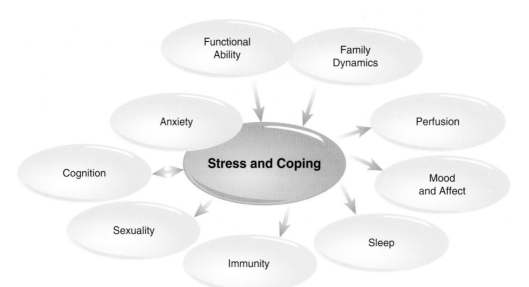

FIGURE 30.4 Interrelated Concepts of Stress and Coping.

result from or are exacerbated by chronic stress are due to sustained exposure to catecholamines. A number of variables affect the onset and severity of the stress-related disorder and include the type of stressor, the perception of the stressor, coping skills, and length and severity of the stress. A few classic and common exemplars are discussed briefly in the following section.

Featured Exemplars
Anxiety Disorders

Anxiety is an adaptive response to stress that ranges from mild anxiety to panic disorder. Anxiety can be acute or chronic—consistent with the stressor involved. Anxiety affects individuals across the lifespan and represents the most common of mental health disorders among pediatric, adolescent, and adult populations. Individuals who develop anxiety disorders tend to have impairments in social, family, and occupational relationships. Effective coping exemplars include problem-focused and emotion-focused strategies.[25]

Tension Headache

Tension headaches are the most common type of headache among adults and are associated with moderate to severe stress causing prolonged muscle tension. It is described as a bilateral, dull, bandlike, or pressing pain that builds up gradually and has a prolonged duration. Tension headaches can occur periodically or for several days in a row, lasting from 30 minutes to days. This type of headache is worsened by noise and light. The severity of symptoms tends to be positively correlated with the frequency of occurrence. Effective coping includes progressive muscle relaxation, meditation, and exercise.[25]

Hypertension

Hypertension is a chronic elevation of blood pressure. This is one of the most common manifestations of stress related to catecholamine effect on the sympathetic nervous system. Catecholamines cause peripheral vasoconstriction and an increased rate and force of cardiac contraction, leading to the elevation of blood pressure. Hypertension is most commonly diagnosed among adults, although hypertension among young adults and children is on the rise. Effective coping includes the relaxation response, meditation, and nutrition counseling.[12,25]

Insomnia

Insomnia represents a group of disorders associated with a disruption of sleep. Acute and chronic stress is one of the leading causes of insomnia. Insomnia is described as the inability to fall asleep or stay asleep. The effects include daytime sleepiness, generalized fatigue, irritability, and cognitive problems. Chronic insomnia is associated with multiple health-related conditions. Insomnia can affect individuals of all ages, but it is more commonly associated with adults and older adults. Effective coping exemplars include meditation and progressive muscle relaxation.[24,29]

Irritable Bowel Syndrome

Irritable bowel syndrome (IBS) refers to a group of symptoms associated with discomfort in the large intestine, including cramping pain, bloating, gas, diarrhea, and/or constipation. Because there is no identified pathology, IBS is not considered a disease but, rather, a functional syndrome with no known cause. However, stress has been identified as a common trigger of IBS. It affects an estimated 20% of the population at one or more times during their lifetime. IBS can occur at any age, but it most commonly affects adults and older adults and affects women more often than men. Effective coping includes meditation, exercise, and progressive muscle relaxation.[25]

Eczema

Eczema is a chronic condition associated with chronic inflammation of the skin. It presents as erythema, scaling, itching, and weeping sores. This condition is thought to be an autoimmune condition that is exacerbated by stress. In other words, eczema is not caused by stress, but the condition is made worse by stress. It occurs among individuals of all ages and affects men and women equally. Effective coping examples include meditation and exercise.[25]

CASE STUDY

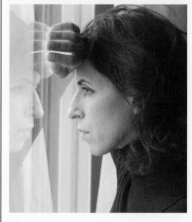

Case Presentation

Jennifer Williams is a 43-year-old recently divorced female who has two teenage daughters aged 18 and 16 years. She is employed full-time as an office assistant and regularly has difficulty making ends meet financially. Her 16-year-old daughter is 7 months pregnant. Jennifer's ex-husband is an alcoholic and is involved with her daughters but cannot be relied on for financial assistance. She lives in an older home in a low-income neighborhood. Her aging and widowed mother, who lives a few blocks away, is in the early stages of Alzheimer's disease and needs regular assistance. Ms. Williams is the main caregiver for her mother.

A number of recent events have been challenging for Jennifer. Her pregnant daughter recently broke up with her boyfriend and Jennifer knows she will be largely supporting and raising her grandchild. She also recently had an intense argument with her oldest daughter about attending college—something she supports but cannot afford. In addition to all of these issues, Jennifer's mother fell and broke her arm. She is now trying to meet the increasing care her mother needs.

All these events have been weighing heavily on Jennifer's mind. She is feeling highly anxious and is experiencing difficulty sleeping. She has had intermittent diarrhea and has become highly irritable, leading to arguments at work with her coworkers. Jennifer also began experiencing headaches. Fearing she had something seriously wrong with her (like a brain tumor), she went to an urgent care clinic. After a brief visit focusing on her headache, she was told not to worry because she was "only experiencing a tension headache" and was a little hypertensive, and she was advised to see her primary care physician. Jennifer was relieved to learn she did not have a brain tumor, but she has no intention of seeing another physician for the headaches. She does not want to spend any more money on herself.

Case Analysis Questions

1. In what ways is Jennifer at risk for poor health outcomes due to her situation?
2. How should the nurse assess Jennifer's coping capacity?
3. What strategies could be implemented to enhance Jennifer's coping effectiveness?

From MariaDubova/iStock/Thinkstock

CASE STUDY

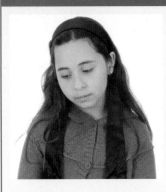

Case Presentation

Carlie Wendell is a 10-year-old female who has recently been diagnosed with diabetes. She has no history of any major illnesses. Carlie lives with her single mother and four younger siblings in a small apartment. Her mother is unemployed and the family has very limited resources. When the nurse meets with Carlie and her mother, Carlie appears angry and tearful. Carlie's mother tells the nurse her daughter did this to herself because she eats too much candy. Carlie appears withdrawn and tearful. The mother also mentions that she already knows how to "give the shots" because her own father had diabetes and was "in and out of the hospital a lot before he died." Carlie cries out in fear about having shots every day. Although Carlie's mother is present, she lacks full engagement in the discussion. She tells the nurse she cannot afford the medications needed to take care of Carlie's problem.

Case Analysis Questions

1. What risk factors does Carlie have for ineffective coping?
2. What information is presented that suggests Carlie's mother has ineffective coping?

♠ ACCESS EXEMPLAR LINKS IN YOUR GIDDENS EBOOK

REFERENCES

1. American Psychological Association. (2015). *Stress in America: Paying with our health.* Retrieved from http://apa.org/news/press/releases/stress/2014/stress-report.pdf.
2. Lazarus, R. S., & Folkman, S. (1984). *Stress, appraisal and coping.* New York: Springer.
3. Lazarus, R. S., & Lazarus, B. N. (1994). Passion and reason: *Making sense of our emotions.* New York: Oxford University Press.
4. Folkman, S., Lazarus, R., Dunkel-Schetter, C., et al. (1986). Dynamics of a stressful encounter: Cognitive appraisal, coping, and encounter outcomes. *Journal of Personality and Social Psychology, 50*(5), 992–1003.
5. Folkman, S., & Moskowitz, J. (2004). Coping: Pitfalls and promise. *Psychology (Savannah, Ga.), 55*(1), 745–774.
6. McCance, K., Huether, S., Brashers, V., & Rote, M. S. (2019). *The biologic basis for disease in adults and children* (8th ed.). St Louis: Mosby.
7. Cannon, W. (1915). *Bodily changes in pain, hunger, fear and rage: An account of recent researches into the function of emotional excitement.* New York: Appleton.
8. Selye, H. (1946). The general adaptation syndrome and the diseases of adaptation. *The Journal of Clinical Endocrinology and Metabolism, 6,* 117.
9. Selye, H. (1965). Stress syndrome. *The American Journal of Nursing, 65*(3), 97–99.
10. Selye, H. (1975). Confusion and controversy in the stress field. *Journal of Human Stress, 1,* 37–44.
11. Edelman, C., Kudzma, E., & Mandle, C. (Eds.), (2014). Health Promotion and the community. In *Health promotion throughout the life span* (8th ed.). St Louis: Elsevier.
12. Lewis, S. L., & Bonner, P. N. (2017). Stress and stress management. In S. L. Lewis, L. Bucher, M. M. Heitkemper, & M. M. Harding (Eds.), *Medical surgical nursing* (10th ed.). St. Louis: Elsevier.
13. American Psychological Association. (2017). *Stress in America: The state of our nation.* Retrieved from: https://www.apa.org/news/press/releases/stress/2017/state-nation.pdf.
14. Mitrousi, S., Travlos, A., Koukia, E., et al. (2013). Theoretical approaches to coping. *International Journal of Caring Sciences, 6*(2), 131–137.
15. Schiller, J., Ward, B., Freeman, G., et al. (2014). *National Health Interview Survey, Early Release Program.* National Center for Health Statistics. Retrieved from http://www.cdc.gov/nchs/nhis.htm.
16. Skinner, E., & Wellborn, J. (1997). Children's coping in the academic domain. *International Journal of Behavioral Development, 13,* 157–176.
17. Small, L. (2002). Early predictors of poor coping outcomes in children following intensive care hospitalization and stressful medical encounters. *Pediatric Nursing, 28*(4), 393–401.
18. Garcia, C. (2010). Conceptualization and measurement of coping during adolescence: A review of the literature. *Journal of Nursing Scholarship: An Official Publication of Sigma Theta Tau International Honor Society of Nursing / Sigma Theta Tau, 42*(2), 166–185.
19. Nery de Souza-Talarioc, J., Correâ Chaves, E., Nitrini, R., et al. (2008). Stress and coping in older people with Alzheimer's disease. *Journal of Clinical Nursing, 18,* 457–465.
20. Web, M. D. (2018). *Common Causes of Stress.* Retrieved from https://www.webmd.com/balance/guide/causes-of-stress#1.
21. Damianakis, T., Wilson, K., & Marziali, E. (2018). Family caregiver support groups: Spiritual reflections' impact on stress management. *Aging & Mental Health, 22*(1), 70–76.
22. Holmes, T. H., & Rahe, R. H. (1967). Social readjustment rating scale. *Journal of Psychosomatic Research, 11,* 213–218.
23. Wilson, S., & Giddens, J. (2017). *Health assessment for nursing practice* (6th ed.). St. Louis: Elsevier.
24. Seward, B. L. S. (2018). *Managing stress: Principles and strategies for health and well-being* (9th ed.). Burlington MA: Jones & Bartlett.
25. Horowitz, J. A. (2014). Stress management. In C. Edelman, E. Kudzma, & C. Mandle (Eds.), *Health promotion throughout the life span* (8th ed.). St Louis: Elsevier.
26. Van Woerden, H. C., Pooertinga, W., Bronserting, K., et al. (2011). The relationship of different sources of social support and civic participation with self-rated health. *Journal of Public Mental Health, 10,* 126–139.
27. Collingwood, J. (2018). The power of music to reduce stress. *Psych Central.* Retrieved from https://psychcentral.com/lib/the-power-of-music-to-reduce-stress/.
28. Kim, S. D. (2014). Effects of yogic exercise on life stress and blood glucose levels in nursing students. *Journal of Physical Therapy Science, 26*(12), 2003–2006.
29. Kudzma, E., & Brunton, J. (2014). Complementary and alternative strategies. In C. Edelman, E. Kudzma, & C. Mandle (Eds.), *Health promotion throughout the life span* (8th ed.). St Louis: Elsevier.
30. Freeman, E. E., Lesk, M. R., Harasymowycz, P., et al. (2016). Maladaptive coping strategies and glaucoma progression. *Medicine, 95*(25), 1–5.
31. Suls, J., & Fletcher, B. (1985). The relative efficacy of avoidant and nonavoidant coping strategies: A meta-analysis. *Health Psychology, 4*(3), 249–288.
32. Karch, A. M. (2017). *Focus on nursing pharmacology* (7th ed.). Philadelphia: Wolters Kluwer.

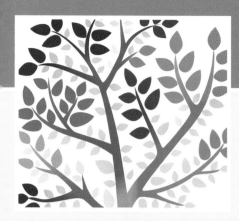

Mood and Affect

Richard A. Pessagno

Mood and affect is a psychosocial concept that underlies all other concepts in the significant impact it has on health outcomes.[1] The purpose of this concept presentation is to enable the generalist practice nurse to have an understanding of mood and affect, develop an awareness of the expected variability or range of the mood spectrum, and recognize affective instability so that these patients can be managed safely and referred to advanced practitioners for evaluation and treatment of any possible mood spectrum disorders.

DEFINITION

The term *mood* is defined as *the way a person feels,* and the term *affect* is defined as *the observable response a person has to his or her own feelings.*[2] The term *euthymia* is used to describe normal, healthy fluctuations in mood. The *mood spectrum* is a continuum of all possible moods that any person may experience. *Mood spectrum disorders* disrupt the individual's ability to function normally, and individuals with mood spectrum disorders are at increased risk for many problems, such as health status impairment, addiction, and potential for violence.[1,3] These disorders should only be diagnosed by qualified advance practice nurses or physicians who have expertise and training in diagnosing medical or psychiatric related problems. Diagnosing a mood spectrum disorder is not within the scope of practice for the nurse generalist.

Because mood is a subjective experience of feelings, and affect is an objective reflection of feelings, the evaluation and description of mood is often done in terms of affect,[1] and generalist practice nurses are qualified and expected to assess affect. In particular, nurses must be able to recognize unstable affective states known as *affective instability.*[3] Signs of affective instability, such as crying, rage, euphoria, and blunting, indicate the need for further assessment because such individuals may have a mood disorder. *Functional status* describes the individual's ability to perform activities of daily living and to realistically solve problems of daily living;[4] it is used as one indicator to determine the severity of a mood spectrum disorder.

SCOPE

From the simplest perspective, the scope of mood and affect can be thought of in terms of being low or depressive range, normal range, and elevated range. There is considerable evidence to support a conceptual model of mood and affect in a single spectrum possible affective states.[3] Normal mood, or euthymia, actually represents a *range*

of expected mood cycles—normal happiness and normal sadness—and is shown in the middle of the spectrum in Fig. 31.1; the curvy line illustrates normal euthymic mood cycling. The amplitude and frequency of euthymic mood cycles may be normally regular or irregular and vary from one person to another.[3]

The low end of the mood spectrum represents mild to moderate to severe melancholy. On the other end of the mood spectrum is mild to moderate to severe mania. As the mood cycles out of the euthymic range in either direction, the functional status decreases proportionately. In extreme mood states such as severe mania or severe melancholy, the individual may be completely disabled and experience symptoms of acute confusion such as hallucinations and/or delusions. Fig. 31.1 illustrates the full scope of the mood spectrum from extreme melancholy to extreme mania in language consistent with the current generalist nurse paradigm and scope of practice.

NORMAL PHYSIOLOGICAL PROCESS

Regulation of mood is complex and poorly understood, as it involves the integration of multiple brain functions and processes. Mood regulation depends on optimal function of neurons, neurotransmitters, and optimal coordination of several parts of the brain, including the prefrontal cortex, anterior cingulate cortex, and the limbic system. Changes to the function and/or coordination of any of these areas can dramatically impact mood regulation.

Neurotransmitters are chemicals that serve to transmit nerve signals from neuron to neuron and to different parts of the brain, such as the limbic system and prefrontal cortex. Neurotransmitters (especially dopamine, norepinephrine, and serotonin) have a powerful role in mood regulation by regulating appetite, sleep, thought, emotion, mood, learning, memory, motivation, and concentration. Excessive or insufficient levels of neurotransmitters are associated with mood disorders and other mental health conditions.

The prefrontal cortex and the anterior cingulate cortex are responsible for judgment, decision-making, problem solving, feelings, and emotional responses.[3] The left half of the prefrontal cortex is involved with the establishment of positive feelings and the right half with negative feelings. The prefrontal cortex also has an indirect role in controlling mood by moderating feelings generated in the limbic structures and having an effect on neurotransmitter release. The limbic system is the area of the brain that is most directly involved in regulation of emotion, particularly the thalamus, amygdala, hippocampus, and cingulate gyrus.

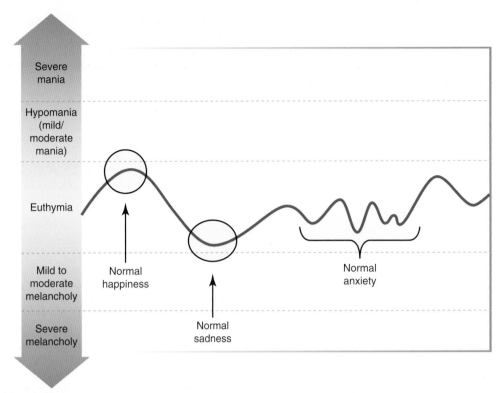

FIGURE 31.1 Unitary Model of Affect (shown here in euthymic range). The left sidebar shows the scope of affect from severe melancholy at the lower end to severe mania at the top end. The green line depicts normal mood as it cycles within the euthymic range from happiness to sadness and back to happiness. (Adapted from MacKinnon, D. F., & Pies, R. [2006]. Affective instability as rapid cycling: theoretical and clinical implications for borderline personality and bipolar spectrum disorders. *Bipolar Disorder, 8*(1), 1–14.)

The amygdala is a limbic structure that is involved with memories, learning to fear events, and persistent negative thoughts. The hippocampus has a role in the creation and storage of new memories, and it also has a role in a major mood circuit known as the hypothalamic–pituitary–adrenal axis.[3]

Age-Related Differences in Emotional Regulation

Emotional regulation evolves throughout life and is closely linked with growth and development. This section briefly describes the evolution of emotional regulation.[3]

Infants and Children

There is a lack of agreement regarding at what point mood is experienced by infants. Mood can only be surmised based on what is observed. Initially, this is limited to facial expressions and behavior and is influenced by an increasing awareness of the environment. For example, infants initially smile beginning at approximately 6 weeks of age, often in response to a parent's smile; this response becomes more diverse as the child experiences positive feelings regarding things he or she sees and experiences. Thus, an infant's expression of emotion is largely regulated by the degree of physical comfort and by cues from adults.

Emotional understanding emerges in toddlers as language, cognitive, and social development. Emotional regulation is thought to be associated with the child's ability to recognize the emotions of others and to mimic the behaviors he or she has observed and/or experienced. For example, toddlers will attempt to alleviate the distress of another by caressing or hugging. Preschool children continue to develop emotional regulation skills primarily based on observations of their parents or

primary caregivers. An internalization of cultural norms regarding how they are expected to behave when they are feeling a certain way also becomes more developed.

The ability to self-regulate emotion becomes more evident during the middle childhood years. At this age, children understand the variety of verbal and nonverbal responses available for the expression of feelings. School-age children may be more willing to express feelings of sadness or anger toward a parent than toward a peer, and they develop an understanding of emotional states of others and the complexity of context in which they occur.

Adolescents

Adolescents typically have developed an array of skills to regulate their emotions and are highly aware of social circumstances related to emotional regulation. Evidence suggests that adolescents experience more variability in mood states and affect compared to adults. It is unclear if these differences are due to physiological changes such as hormonal imbalances or differences in emotional reactivity or emotional regulation.[5]

Older Adults

Mood regulation in older adults is generally physiologically consistent with what was previously described. However, despite the fact that older adults experience physical and cognitive decline, they often report higher levels of well-being (less negative affect and increased positive affect) and are more responsive to positive emotions compared to younger adults. It is thought that this difference can be explained by the fact that older adults activate emotional regulation processes to compensate for any negative stimuli they may experience.[6]

VARIATIONS AND CONTEXT

Conceptually, mood spectrum disorders occur when the mood cycles downward from the euthymic range into affective states seen as melancholy or when the mood cycles upward from the euthymic range into hypomania or severe mania. There are a large number of medical/psychiatric conditions with diagnostic criteria derived using medical reasoning in the fifth edition of the *Diagnostic and Statistical Manual of Mental Disorders (DSM-5)*.[7] In medical psychiatry, these conditions are grouped dichotomously as disorders in either the depressive spectrum or the manic spectrum. *Depression* and *mania* are medical/psychiatric diagnostic terms used to indicate the extreme poles of the mood spectrum disorders.[7] Although this dichotomous model is weakened by recent evidence supporting a unitary model of mood spectrum disorders,[3] it provides an excellent source for exemplars of the concept. There is a mixed state depression diagnosis that does not fit neatly in the depressive or the manic column because it contains features of both, and it provides useful borderline characteristics for concept analysis purposes. Suicide or suicidal behaviors in general may also be useful for analysis as exemplars.

Depressive Spectrum

Conceptually, depression is characterized by such overwhelming sadness and despair that one feels drained of energy. An individual suffering from depression may feel so sad and empty that he or she becomes incapacitated by a loss of the will to live, and suicidal thoughts may prevail. Caution should be exercised in the use of the word "depression" to avoid misunderstandings for two reasons. First, the word "depression" is commonly misused to describe normal euthymic sadness when there is little or no loss of functional status. Second, depression is a medical/psychiatric diagnostic term, and the clinical psychiatric use of the word "depression" has a variety of diagnostic applications. For clarity, the undiagnosed mood state characterized by sadness, despair, and loss of functional status is best referred to as *melancholy*.

Mania Spectrum

Individuals with *mania* are recognizable in the nursing paradigm by the presence of euphoric or agitated affective states, and they often suffer from varying degrees of *perceptual disturbances* as well, such as racing thoughts, grandiose delusions, difficulty concentrating, impulsivity, and lack of insight. Consequently, individuals with mania experience impaired functional status, and behavior associated with mania may be reckless and dangerous.

Another term used as a defining characteristic for some medical/psychiatric diagnoses is *hypomania*. Nurses are expected to be able to recognize hypomania as an unstable affective state. Hypomanic affective states are expansive or agitated and possibly euphoric but to a less severe degree than in mania and with less impairment. Although the individual with hypomania experiences racing thoughts and agitation or euphoria, perceptual disturbances are much less likely in hypomania. To facilitate the assessment of affective instability in the generalist nurse conceptual paradigm, the presence of perceptual disturbances is used to distinguish mania from hypomania.

CONSEQUENCES

The consequences of mood disturbances are significant from both a physical and a social perspective. Patients with mood spectrum disorders are high users of medical care, and the incidence of mood spectrum disorders is increased in general medical care patients.[8] Various neuroimaging studies of mood spectrum disorders demonstrate reduced blood flow and abnormal phosphorus metabolism in the cerebral cortex and especially the prefrontal cortex.[9] The activity of various neurotransmitters is also disturbed in mood spectrum disorders, particularly the levels of dopamine, norepinephrine, and serotonin. This is why medical interventions are aimed at restoring neurotransmitter balance.

Interpersonal relationships and productivity may be greatly limited by functional status impairment during mood spectrum disorders. Psychosocial variables such as negative life events, personality traits, and individual cognitive styles are associated with mood spectrum disorders.[3]

The most ominous consequence, of course, is the increased potential for suicide. Probably because of increased energy levels, patients on the manic or hypomanic pole of the mood spectrum are at a higher risk for suicide than are those with low energy at the melancholic pole.

RISK FACTORS

Fluctuations within the euthymic range occur normally and even daily among all populations and across the lifespan. However, although anyone may experience mood spectrum disorders, there are known risk factors. A landmark, broad-based assessment of mood spectrum disorders in the United States was the National Comorbidity Survey Replication (NCS-R) study conducted from 2001 to 2003; this study, based on 9282 interviews, provides a basis for understanding risk factors.[8]

Populations at Risk

According to the NCS-R, the 12-month prevalence of clinically significant depression in the general population was 6.6%, and the lifetime prevalence was 16.2%. The rate of depression among women is two or three times higher than that in men, and the first episode of depression for either gender usually occurs during adolescence or early adulthood. The incidence of depression peaks bimodally, occurring with the highest frequency during the late 20s/early 30s and again during the late 60s.

Individual Risk Factors

Individual risk factors for depression are stress, early trauma, neglect, abuse, family history, comorbid medical and psychiatric disorders, and personality disorders. Comorbid anxiety or substance-related disorders prevail in 75% to 80% of those with depression, and 22% of adults report comorbid substance dependence. Among those who reported no psychological distress, only 7% reported substance dependence.[8]

ASSESSMENT

Although generalist practice nurses are not qualified to diagnose mood spectrum disorders, they should be able to recognize affective instability as an outward manifestation of a possible mood spectrum disorder. Affective instability may present as any combination of agitation, sadness, elation, or blunting. Blunting is particularly difficult to recognize because it may not be noticeable immediately; blunting is an absence or diminished presence of any affect, and this should be considered a sign of affective instability. Speech may be monotone during blunting, and responses may be unusually brief. Blunting must not be overlooked because it may mask dangerously unstable affect.

The combined interaction between mood, energy, and cognition results in what is called affect;[3] therefore the recognition of affective instability is facilitated by an analysis of mood, energy, and cognition. The defining characteristics for the mood and affect concept in this analysis are derived from the diverse presentations of affective instability that result from the various problematic ways that mood, energy, and cognition interact. The defining characteristics are persistent mood disturbance, functional impairment, and disturbed vegetative functioning (sleep, appetite, and energy). To facilitate assessment, each of these characteristics is discussed individually.

Persistent Mood Disturbance

The assessment of mood is based on the patient's self-report. Occasionally, nurses will infer mood from affect, but this can be misleading because affect is not always congruous with mood. For example, individuals may laugh and cry simultaneously. In any case, persistent mood disturbance may include sadness, melancholy, irritability, lack of interest in normal activities (anhedonia), euphoria, elation, rage, or the lack of any ability to feel emotions at all. Moods should fluctuate normally in the full range of euthymia, but moods should not fluctuate so rapidly or to such extremes or for so long that functional status is disrupted.

The important point that underlies this defining characteristic is the idea of persistence. Anyone will normally experience sadness, irritability, and even euphoria or rage occasionally. However, daily, persistent melancholic feelings for longer than 2 weeks or persistent manic feelings for more than 4 days endorse a nursing assessment of persistent affective instability.[7] To illustrate useful reasoning in the recognition of persistent mania and hypomania by nurses, the fieldworkers who administered the face-to-face questionnaires during the NCS-R study were trained to ask the following:

> Some people have periods lasting several days or longer when they feel much more excited and full of energy than usual. Their minds go too fast. They talk a lot. They are very restless or unable to sit still and they sometimes do things that are unusual for them, such as driving too fast or spending too much money. Have you ever had a period like this lasting several days or longer? … Or have you ever had a period lasting several days or longer when most of the time you were so irritable that you started arguments, shouted at people, or hit people?[10]

Functional Impairment

A useful way to assess functional impairment is to think of it as the inability to realistically solve ordinary problems of daily living.[4] Functional status may also be known as *functional ability*, although *functional ability* refers more specifically to the *capacity* of an individual to perform ADLs, whereas functional *status* refers to the individual's actual performance of the ADLs, which may not utilize his or her total functional capacity.[4] Functional impairment is closely linked to disturbed vegetative functioning.

Disturbed Vegetative Functioning

Vegetative functioning refers to the individual's appetite, sleep, and energy level. Some clinicians may evaluate sexual energy or changes in sexual desire (libido) as a separate measure of vegetative functioning. During a melancholic period, the patient typically exhibits reduced energy level, increased sleep, decreased appetite, and decreased interest in sex. Atypically, individuals with melancholy may overeat, may become more sexual, or may be too agitated to sleep—this is known as mixed state depression in the medical/psychiatric paradigm.[11]

Nurses may be confused to hear that the aforementioned increased appetite, hypersexuality, agitation, and insomnia present in the so-called mixed state depression diagnoses are also vegetative functioning characteristics in mania and/or hypomania. In fact, there is some debate in the medical/psychiatric paradigm regarding differentiation between mixed state depression diagnoses and the various bipolar diagnoses.[11] Although interesting, this debate is not very relevant in the nursing process, and nurses are advised to focus on assessing for the defining characteristics of mood and affect while avoiding speculation about possible medical/psychiatric diagnoses.

Mental Status Assessment

The mental status assessment is well within the nursing scope of practice and important in analyzing the defining characteristics for the mood and affect concept. In the same way that a nurse should generally be aware of any patient's pulse rate and character, respiratory rate and character, blood pressure, temperature, and pain, the nurse should also know the following elements of mental status assessment: general appearance, motor activity, mood, affect, speech, and alertness and orientation.[10]

The assessment and continuous monitoring of mental status enables the nurse to accurately assess cognitive status and functional status. Instruments such as the Mini-Mental State Exam, the Neecham Confusion Scale, and the Confusion Assessment Method Instrument permit the nurse to quantifiably measure mental status for particular situations, such as monitoring changes during or between shifts, day to day, or over the long term.[12] However, although these instruments can be very useful, they are not replacements for the continuous monitoring and documentation of the patient's mental status that makes it a sixth vital sign.

A complete discussion of the mental status examination is beyond the scope of this concept presentation, but sources are readily available that provide details of this part of the assessment. It is helpful to remember that the assessment of information processing lies at the heart of the mental status assessment. That is, assessing the patient's ability to process information is the purpose of the mental status assessment. Specifically, the following combine to form a clinical impression of the patient's total information processing ability and thereby form a basis for clinical management: the patient's appearance; motor functioning; speech and speech content; cognitive processes such as perception, judgment, insight, and memory; and alertness and orientation.

CLINICAL MANAGEMENT

An effective and easily remembered way for nurses to translate data from the mental status assessment to clinical management is by analyzing it in the context of affect and the three main components of affect: mood, energy, and cognition. Fig. 31.2 illustrates these components and the normal cycling of euthymia into an unstable melancholy and then back into euthymia. Note that during the unstable period illustrated in Fig. 31.2, the individual displays a melancholic mood (*green line*) with reduced energy (*red line*) but increased cognition (*blue line*). Behaviorally, this individual would struggle with persistent sadness and low energy but agitated thoughts that disturbed his or her sleep. For individuals with affective instability, one or more of the three affective components will cycle out of euthymia in either direction, causing a variety of behavioral responses. By studying Fig. 31.2, one can picture different affective (behavioral) manifestations. What makes the assessment of disorders associated with affective instability so challenging is that each affective component may cycle at different rates and extremes. Different combinations of affective components will have quite different manifestations. Also, when components occur simultaneously at the extremes, the disabling effects are increased.

Primary Prevention

Primary prevention measures for mood spectrum disorders are not well established, and efforts toward prevention focus on societal egalitarian interventions such as reduction in poverty, racism, violence, and stress.[2] According to systematic reviews,[2] programs that target prevention of mood disorders have been shown to reduce the severity of symptoms, but these programs tend to be early interventions rather than true prevention programs. Similar systematic reviews of universal prevention programs showed them to be ineffective.

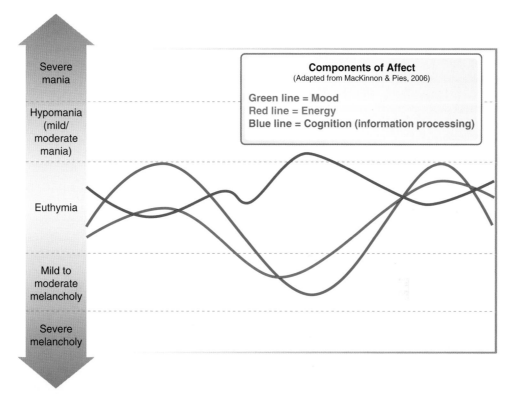

FIGURE 31.2 Components of Affect. *Green line*, Mood; *red line*, energy; *blue line*, cognition (information processing). (Adapted from MacKinnon, D. F., & Pies, R. [2006]. Affective instability as rapid cycling: theoretical and clinical implications for borderline personality and bipolar spectrum disorders. *Bipolar Disorder, 8*(1), 1–14.)

Secondary Prevention (Screening)

Secondary prevention or screening efforts are aimed at early detection of mood spectrum disorders with the hope of preventing serious consequences, and there is compelling evidence to support mood disorder screening.[2] The U.S. Preventive Services Task Force (USPSTF) recommends the routine screening of adults for mood disorders in primary care.[13] The USPSTF further recommends that healthcare providers "remain alert" for mood spectrum disorders in children and adolescents, and that systems should be established to handle the diagnosis, treatment, and follow-up care for individuals who do screen positive for mood spectrum disorders. According to the USPSTF, the following two questions may be as effective as longer screening measures: "Over the past 2 weeks, have you ever felt down, depressed, or hopeless?" and "Have you felt little interest or pleasure in doing things?"[12]

Screening instruments do not diagnose mood spectrum disorders; instead, they measure the severity of associated symptoms.[13] By measuring the severity of symptoms associated with mood spectrum disorders, screening instruments assist clinicians to assess acuity and treatment effectiveness. There are numerous screening instruments validated for use at different times in the lifespan and appropriate for varying levels of cognition. Whatever instrument is used, it is important to realize that simple screening questions detect only approximately half of patients with mood spectrum disorders.[14] For this reason, it is recommended that nurses do not completely rely on screening instruments but, rather, use their assessment skills to detect affective instability followed by an assessment of functional status and potential for violence when indicated. It is noteworthy that diminished functional status may appear vaguely as somatic symptoms and vegetative complaints such as fatigue, sleep disturbance, pain, altered interest in sexual activity, or other persistent vague complaints.[12]

Collaborative Care

The generalist practice nurse who is proficient in the assessment of affective instability plays a key role in detecting mood spectrum disorders and providing patients with opportunities for preventing deterioration in functional status. The most extreme outcome the nurse may prevent is death or disability by a suicide attempt. The evidence supports the idea that when mood spectrum deterioration is prevented in an individual, he or she stands a good chance of living a long, happy, and productive life.

This point is illustrated in an ex post facto review of interviews with individuals prevented from jumping off the Golden Gate Bridge between 1937 and 1978.[15] During that period, 625 people are known to have died of suicide there, and perhaps another 200 possible deaths may have occurred unseen at night or in bad weather. Dr. Seiden carefully followed the 515 "attempters" who were restrained from leaping off the bridge. Of those who were prevented from suicide by jumping off the bridge, there were higher rates of violent death, but approximately 90% of those prevented from suicide did not die later by violent death. Other data from this study interpreted by Dr. Seiden enabled him to form the following conclusions:[15]

1. The chances are good that a person prevented from suicide will live a long and satisfying life. Ending one's life by suicide overlooks what might have happened—good feelings and good that could have been done.

2. Suicidal people should not be left to handle these emotions on their own. They should receive psychosocial help immediately, with at least 6 months of close support.

3. No matter how intense at the moment, the desire to die is temporary in almost all circumstances, negating the notion that "suicide is a choice."

4. Therapy, medication, relatives, friends, and groups all offer hope.

Individuals suffering from mood spectrum disorders are known to be slow in seeking treatment. Because the generalist nurse is quite likely to be the first clinician to detect the possibility of a mood spectrum disorder, it is imperative that the nurse is also able to discuss with the patient treatment options and reasonable expectations for treatment outcomes. In this way, the nurse may exert a substantial influence in convincing the patient to seek care. This influence is done most effectively with communication techniques called *motivational interviewing*.[16] Although additional training is helpful, motivational interviewing techniques lie within the generalist nurse scope of practice, and the effectiveness of motivational interviewing for mood spectrum disorders and suicidal ideation has been established.[16] Motivational interviewing was first developed to motivate individuals suffering from addictions to pursue change, and so it is further discussed in Concept 35, Addiction.

In addition to motivational interviewing, collaborative care for mood spectrum disorders consists of psychotherapy and/or pharmacotherapy and/or brain and vagus nerve stimulation therapies (e.g., electroconvulsive therapy). Collaborative care also includes managing emergent situations (potential for suicide and/or other violence) among individuals suffering from affective instability. Each of these areas of interventions is discussed next. The nursing role in collaborative care may include case management activities when functional status impairment persists.

Psychotherapy Options

There are many different types of psychotherapy, and no particular therapy has been found to be more effective than any other.[17] Compared to pharmacotherapy, there are fewer well-designed clinical trials of psychotherapy "because of the lack of a 'placebo therapy' condition."[17] However, there is sufficient evidence, including randomized controlled trials, to conclude that long-term outcomes of pharmacotherapy versus psychotherapy are similar.[17] Relapse rates appear to be lower in psychotherapy following termination of treatment. Psychotherapy has been found to take approximately 8 weeks for a 50% remission rate, 26 weeks for a 75% remission rate, and 52 weeks for an 80% remission rate.[18]

Because a person's thoughts and beliefs have been found to affect mood, cognitive therapy attempts to change thoughts and beliefs as needed to be more adaptive and healthy. In comparison, behavioral therapy is aimed at changing patterns of behavior that are repeated over time with the same negative results. Cognitive and behavioral therapy is a combined approach that has been found to be effective in numerous applications that share the characteristic of repetitive dysfunctional patterns.[18] Interpersonal therapy focuses on communication patterns and the way the patient relates to others. Grief issues respond well to interpersonal therapy, and the patient is provided the opportunity to learn ways to express such uncomfortable feelings. Variations of this modality have been demonstrated to be effective in managing bipolar spectrum disorders.[18] Family-focused therapy includes family members in a therapeutic process aimed at problem solving and managing conflict in ways that produce positive outcomes. All these therapeutic approaches are known to adapt well to the treatment of mood disorders in children and adolescents.[18]

Play therapy is an approach for children and adolescents in which a variety of toys and games are used to establish rapport so that the child may better express him- or herself. Toys and games may also be used for children who lack the cognitive and language abilities of expression. Sand tray therapy is a variant of play therapy in which the individual places objects provided by the therapist but selected by the individual in a sand tray. The therapist then interprets the meaning of the objects and their placement to better understand the conflict present for the individual. Other therapeutic modalities include light therapy, art therapy, and animal-assisted therapies, each with its own applications. Light therapy is used to treat seasonal affect disorder, a mood disorder that

---

BOX 31.1   Pharmacotherapy for Mood Spectrum Disorders

Antidepressants
- Selective serotonin reuptake inhibitors (SSRIs)
- Serotonin–norepinephrine reuptake inhibitors (SNRIs)
- Tricyclic antidepressants (TCAs)
- Norepinephrine–dopamine reuptake inhibiters (NDRIs)
- Monoamine oxidase inhibitors (MAOIs)

Mood Stabilizers
- Lithium
- Antiepileptic drugs (AEDs)
- Second-generation antipsychotic medications

---

tends to occur during the winter months when there is less light. For some individuals, decreasing light is associated with melancholy. Animal therapies are often used in the recovery from psychological trauma, and art therapies may help with psychological self-healing.[18]

Pharmacotherapy for Mood Spectrum Disorders

The main drug categories used in the treatment of mood spectrum disorders are antidepressants and mood stabilizers; antianxiety agents (anxiolytics) are also used (Box 31.1). In general, antidepressants are prescribed to treat patients diagnosed with depression and mood stabilizers are used to treat diagnoses associated with mania and hypomania such as the various bipolar diagnoses.[7] Subcategories of antidepressants include the selective serotonin reuptake inhibitors (SSRIs), the norepinephrine–dopamine reuptake inhibiters (NDRIs), the tricyclic antidepressants (TCAs), the serotonin–norepinephrine reuptake inhibitors (SNRIs), and the monoamine oxidase inhibitors (MAOIs). The mood stabilizers are either lithium or antiepileptic drugs (AEDs), and numerous second-generation antipsychotic medications also have been approved as mood stabilizers.

Antidepressants. Many factors affect the choice of antidepressant medications, with remission or partial remission dependent on the particular neurochemical imbalance. The current first-line choice for the treatment of depression is the SSRI category because positive response rates are excellent and this category has the best rates of adherence as a result of its lower incidence of adverse effects.[17] SSRIs may be prescribed by primary care providers, as over 60% of all psychotropic medications are prescribed by these providers. If depression is complicated by anxiety, the anxiety may dissipate once the antidepressant medication takes effect. The patient may notice a reduction in symptoms during the first 2 to 3 weeks but full effect can take at least 4 weeks, and sometimes as long as 6 to 8 weeks depending on medication dose adjustments. During this period, anxiety may temporarily be treated with an anxiolytic, but persistent agitation may be treated with an atypical second-generation antipsychotic agent or mood stabilizer. Individual responses to any pharmacotherapy are highly variable. To achieve a positive response, the dose might need to be increased after the initial 2 weeks based on the specific medication and the patient's tolerance to the medication; it is not unusual for medications to take 6 to 8 weeks to achieve a full response.

The dual-action antidepressants known as SNRIs affect serotonin and norepinephrine levels, and these are also used in some cases of depression that has not responded to treatment as well, known as refractory depression.[17] SNRIs can also be effective in the treatment of patients who have anxiety disorders or depression that is accompanied by anxiety symptoms. For many years, the TCA antidepressants were the standard choice in the treatment of depression, and they are still used occasionally; however, because of their multiple adverse effects, TCAs are rarely or never used as first-line choices.[17] Overdose of TCA medications can be lethal, so compliance and risk for suicide must be carefully evaluated before initiating medications from this category.

The MAOI antidepressants have also been demonstrated to be effective in the treatment of refractory depression, but they are typically not used as first-line treatment because of concerns about potentially fatal interactions (hypertensive crisis) between MAOI medications and foods containing tyramine. Tyramine occurs widely in foods, especially "spoiled" (fermented) or pickled foods. Foods to be avoided include many meats, chocolate, alcoholic beverages, cheese, tofu, beans, pineapples, plums, raspberries, figs, and nuts.

It is not unusual for patients to experience some mild side effects when SSRI medications are initiated or when the dosage is increased.[19] These side effects should subside within a few weeks and include insomnia, abdominal discomfort, dry mouth, and mild headaches. However, there is some potential for any antidepressant medication, including the safer SSRI category, to produce a dangerous condition known as *serotonin toxicity*.[19] Serotonin toxicity may occur abruptly, and initial presentation includes tachycardia, shivering, diaphoresis, dilated pupils, myoclonus (intermittent tremor or twitching), and hyperreflexia. Hyperthermia is common during serotonin toxicity, and temperatures may reach as dangerously high as 106°F (41°C). Serotonin toxicity is treated with serotonin blockade drugs such as chlorpromazine or cyproheptadine.

Patients should be instructed not to abruptly discontinue antidepressant medications because this may result in anticholinergic rebound symptoms known as SSRI withdrawal syndrome (also known as SSRI discontinuation syndrome). In SSRI withdrawal syndrome, the individual experiences flulike symptoms such as headache, diarrhea, nausea, vomiting, chills, dizziness, fatigue, insomnia, agitation, impaired concentration, and vivid dreams. Symptoms last from 1 to 7 weeks and may be dangerous if there is an increased presence of suicidal ideation.

Mood stabilizers. For many years, lithium and AEDs have been the two main types of pharmacologic agents used as mood stabilizers. In recent years, increasing numbers of second-generation antipsychotic drugs have been approved and used for this purpose. The presumed action of lithium is through the regulation of the neurotransmitter glutamate. Kidney and thyroid function should be established before initiation of lithium therapy, and it is important to note that lithium has a very narrow therapeutic blood range of between 0.8 and 1.4 mEq/L. The toxic range begins at 1.5 mEq/L and may even overlap the therapeutic range, making dosage calculations difficult.

Patients taking lithium should be taught to recognize early signs of lithium toxicity, including diarrhea, vomiting, drowsiness, muscular weakness, and lack of coordination. Severe symptoms include ataxia (failure or irregularity of muscle action), giddiness, tinnitus (ringing in the ears), blurred vision, and a large output of dilute urine. Long-term side effects include thirst, frequent urination, tremors, diarrhea, weight gain, and edema. The cause of weight gain is not definitely known, and it may even be due to an increased consumption of caloric beverages for thirst.[19] Patients taking lithium should be instructed to maintain a steady fluid and electrolyte balance through dietary sources because lithium is lost during perspiration, affecting its narrow therapeutic range. Lithium should not be taken by pregnant or breast-feeding women. Antiepileptic medications such as carbamazepine, valproic acid/valproate, and lamotrigine are often used as mood stabilizers, but risk is substantial because AED overdose may be lethal.[19] Hepatic and renal functioning tests should be implemented prior to initiation of AED therapy and intermittently during treatment to detect and prevent long-term renal or hepatic damage.[19]

Brain Stimulation Therapy

The brain stimulation therapies are used primarily for treatment-resistant mood disorders that have failed to respond to other therapies.[18] During electroconvulsive therapy, the patient is sedated with a general anesthetic and a seizure lasting less than 1 minute is induced with electricity through electrodes placed at precise locations. It is not known exactly how brain stimulation works to relieve depression, but a general course of treatment is three sessions per week for 4 weeks. Common side effects include headaches, nausea, muscle aches, and occasional loss of memory. Magnetic pulses may be used instead of electricity in a brain stimulation therapy called repetitive transcranial magnetic stimulation.[18] Nursing management of patients who undergo brain stimulation therapies is identical to preoperative and postoperative nursing care of patients who are administered a general anesthetic. Nurses should perform teaching before the procedure so the patient will know what to expect. After the procedure, nurses should monitor the airway and mental status and assist the patient by orienting him or her to person, place, time, and situation as in any postoperative procedure.

Managing the Potential for Suicide and Other Violent Potential

The generalist nurse who suspects the possibility of a mood spectrum disorder should first assess for emergency situations. It should be considered an emergency when patients are at risk for suicide or violence; these patients should not be left alone. Any patient who presents with decreased functional status and affective instability should be evaluated for suicidal ideation. If there is any doubt regarding the severity of affective instability, functional status, or suicidal ideation, the nurse should order continuous observation and refer the patient for an immediate, full evaluation. Fig. 31.3 demonstrates affective states associated with varying levels of suicide risk and potential for violence. In this figure, the individual reflects a persistently low mood, as depicted by the green line. On the left side of the figure, cognition and energy are declining, so despite the low mood, he or she will tend to lack the energy and cognitive ability necessary to plan and carry out a suicidal act.

Comparatively, in the center of Fig. 31.3, the individual's energy and cognition begin to cycle upward, increasing the risk of suicide. This condition may sometimes occur on initiation of antidepressant medications. On the far right side of the figure, the mood is very low, whereas energy and cognition are very high. The individual has a low, suicidal mood with sufficient energy and cognitive ability to plan and execute a suicidal act or other acts of violence. This person is unlikely to perceive reality accurately, and if mood were elevated here, then the individual would be manic and out of control—at risk for dangerous and reckless behaviors such as gambling, violence, and promiscuity. Such individuals are likely to have hallucinations and/or delusions.

Minimum standards of practice by the generalist nurse for managing the potential for suicide and other violence are not well established. It is recommended that the minimum standard for the generalist nurse in any setting is to assess for violence potential, and when the potential for violence is endorsed, the patient should be assessed for acuity. This is done by asking the patient if he or she has been thinking about suicide or if he or she has any other thoughts of violence. The nurse should remember that talking about frightening thought content is known to provide relief for the patient.[20] It has been consistently demonstrated that talking about suicidal feelings does not increase the likelihood of acting on those feelings at any age.

The sudden appearance of unexplained euthymia in a person who has shown persistent affective instability may be an ominous sign of an impending suicidal act. In such cases, the appearance of euthymia results from the relief of making the decision to commit suicide. This

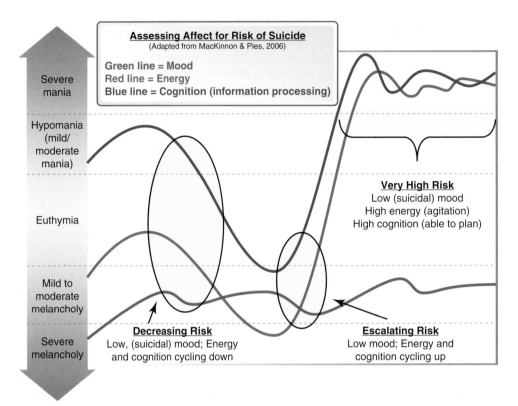

FIGURE 31.3 **Assessing Affect for Risk of Suicide.** *Green line*, Mood; *red line*, energy; *blue line*, cognition (information processing). (Adapted from MacKinnon, D. F., & Pies, R. [2006]. Affective instability as rapid cycling: theoretical and clinical implications for borderline personality and bipolar spectrum disorders. *Bipolar Disorder, 8*(1), 1–14.)

decision may be accompanied by gift giving and acts of farewell. Not all suicides are predictable, especially impulsive suicide, but nurses who include assessment strategies discussed in this section will be more effective at recognizing possible mood spectrum disorders, initiating immediate interventions, and referring such patients to collaborative care. Other strategies include noting suicidal situations such as loss.[20] Loss may include the death of a loved one (including pets), separation, illness, employment status, and self-esteem. Behavioral signals may warn of suicidal ideation, including writing or creating art about death; giving away prized possessions; and joking about death, dying, suicide, or leaving.[20]

INTERRELATED CONCEPTS

A number of concepts in this textbook are connected to mood and affect in some way. Three concepts are specifically worth mentioning and are shown in Fig. 31.4. Like mood and affect, **Addiction** and **Cognition** share impairment in **Functional Ability** as a defining characteristic. That is, any individual experiencing affective instability, addictions, or confusion will also experience functional ability impairment. The affective disturbance may assume a variety of presentations, such as crying, rage, euphoria, or even flatness during loss of contact with reality, which is typical of confused states whether chronic or acute. Whatever the presentation, the standard of care should be to assess for any deficit in functional status and from that assessment proceed to establish a nursing diagnosis based on the presence or absence of other defining characteristics. For example, functional ability may be impaired by addiction, or it can be caused by confusion; it can also be caused by a mood spectrum disorder. Only by a thorough assessment can the nurse differentiate underlying etiologies.

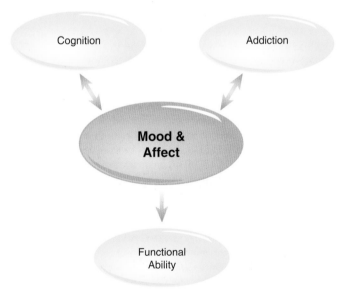

FIGURE 31.4 Interrelated Concepts of Mood and Affect Include Addiction, Cognition, and Functional Ability.

CLINICAL EXEMPLARS

There are a large number of medical psychiatric conditions with diagnostic criteria (medical defining characteristics) derived using the medical reasoning in the *DSM-5*. These medically defined conditions provide useful exemplars for this concept. In medical psychiatry, these conditions are traditionally grouped dichotomously as disorders in either

BOX 31.2 EXEMPLARS OF MOOD AND AFFECT

Depressive Disorders
- Disruptive mood dysregulation disorder
- Major depressive disorder
- Persistent depressive disorder
- Postpartum depression
- Premenstrual dysphoric disorder
- Psychotic depression
- Situational depression
- Suicide

Manic Disorders
- Bipolar I
- Bipolar II
- Cyclothymia
- Suicide

🌿 **ACCESS EXEMPLAR LINKS IN YOUR GIDDENS EBOOK**

the depressive spectrum or the manic spectrum, but the unitary model of affect is more relevant to generalist nursing practice (Box 31.2).[21]

Featured Exemplars
Major Depressive Disorder

As one of the most common mental health conditions, major depressive disorder is characterized by severe depressive mood symptoms that interfere with functional status, employment, and/or relationships that last for at least a 2-week period of time. This disorder can occur as a single episode, but more likely it occurs several times. This condition affects more than 6% of adults and 3% of adolescents in the United States each year. The average age of onset is 33 years; the populations at greatest risk are non-Hispanic whites and women.[8]

Persistent Depressive Disorder

Persistent depressive disorder (formerly known as dysthymic depressive disorder) differs from major depressive disorder in that the condition is chronic. Symptoms occur most of the day nearly every day for more than 2 years for adults or 1 year for children or adolescents. Symptom-free intervals last no longer than 2 months. Disqualifiers for use of this diagnosis include evidence of manic or hypomanic episodes during the first 2 years of symptoms, and the symptoms cannot be due to the direct use of substances (drugs and alcohol) or a medical condition.[8]

Disruptive Mood Dysregulation Disorder

Disruptive mood dysregulation disorder is applied to children and adolescents who have a persistent or angry mood most of the day nearly every day with intermittent recurrent severe temper outbursts or episodes of explosive rage. The intensity and duration of the outbursts are out of proportion to the situation and must occur in at least two settings (e.g., home and school). The time of diagnosis should occur between ages 6 and 18 years, and the onset of symptoms must appear before age 10 years; not more than 3 months can pass without symptoms.[7]

Bipolar I Disorder

Although the cause is not well understood, bipolar I disorder is thought to be caused by an imbalance of neurotransmitters and is characterized by extreme mood swings—both lowering of mood and exaggerated elevation of mood.. There are several categories of this diagnosis, including manic, depressive, and mixed. Nearly 2.5 million adults in the United States have bipolar I disorder. The median age of onset is 18 years.[8]

Bipolar II Disorder

Like bipolar I, bipolar II disorder is also characterized by mood swings but is considered less severe. The main difference is a less exaggerated elevation of mood or "lesser mania" compared to bipolar I. This condition does not lead to life-threatening consequences, nor does psychosis occur. The median age of onset is 20 years, with a higher prevalence of bipolar II disorder among women.[8]

CASE STUDY

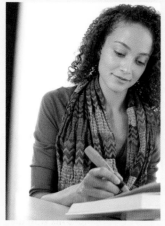

Case Presentation

Daniela Diaz is a 30-year-old computer engineer whose mood is typically euthymic with an affect that is consistent with this mood. Her cognition, energy level, and mood are mostly consistent throughout the entire day. Recently Ms. Diaz has been experiencing challenges at work. Daniela's boss informed her that the quality of her work has been slipping, that she is behind on her current project, and that the quality of the project needs to improve. Because Daniela has a great deal at stake and feels at risk, she has been ruminating about the project. She has recently had problems sleeping, leading to fatigue and excessive tiredness during the day. She feels "down" and has a hard time concentrating at work. On the day of her final project presentation to management, she has a great deal of energy with her mind racing. She has a hard time calming herself and is noticeably anxious during the presentation. The following day, Daniela is given feedback from her boss and learns that the management team considered the project presentation very poor and she did not meet their expectations. She knows her upcoming performance evaluation will reflect this poor performance and is concerned about her job. Over the next month, her mood deteriorates and she experiences overwhelming sadness and lacks energy. She has periods of uncontrollable crying and makes statements that she is worthless. She continues to ruminate about her job; her continued worried thoughts contribute further to insomnia and she experiences agitation that fluctuates widely from lethargy to agitation.

Case Analysis Questions

1. In what way does this case represent exogenous factors in affective instability?
2. Refer to Fig. 31.2. How does Ms. Diaz's case reflect the components of affect as shown?

🍃 **ACCESS EXEMPLAR LINKS IN YOUR GIDDENS EBOOK**

REFERENCES

1. Hofman, S. G., Sawyer, A. T., Fang, A., et al. (2012). Emotion dysregulation model of mood and anxiety disorders. *Depression and Anxiety, 29*(5), 409–416.

2. Venes, D. (Ed.), (2017). *Taber's cyclopedic medical dictionary.* Philadelphia: Davis.

3. Renaud, S. M., & Zacchia, C. (2012). Toward a definition of affective instability. *Harvard Review of Psychiatry, 20*(6), 298–308.

4. Evans, S. J., Sayers, M., Mitnitski, A., & Rockwood, K. (2014). The risk of adverse outcomes in hospitalized older patients in relation to a frailty index based on a comprehensive geriatric assessment. *Age and Ageing, 43*(1), 127–132.

5. Ahmed, S. P., Bittencourt-Hewitt, A., & Sebastian, C. (2015). Neurocognitive bases of emotion regulation development in adolescent. *Developmental Cognitive Neuroscience, 15*(10), 11–15.

6. Smith, J. L., & Hollinger-Smith, L. (2015). Savoring, resilience, and psychological well-being in older adults. *Aging and Mental Health, 12*(3), 192–200.

7. American Psychiatric Association. (2013). *Diagnostic and statistical manual of mental disorders* (5th ed.). Arlington, VA: American Psychiatric Publishing.

8. Kessler, R. C., Petukhova, M., Sampson, N. A., et al. (2012). Twelve-month and lifetime prevalence and lifetime morbid risk of anxiety and mood disorders in the United States. *International Journal of Methods in Psychiatric Research, 21*(3), 169–184.

9. Harper, D. G., Jensen, J. E., Ravichandran, C., et al. (2014). Tissue-specific differences in brain phosphodiesters in late-life major depression. *The American Journal of Geriatric Psychiatry, 22*(5), 499–509.

10. National Institute of Mental Health. (2017). *Symptoms of depression.* Retrieved from https://www.nimh.nih.gov/health/topics/depression/index.shtml#part_145397.

11. Angst, J., Cui, L., Swendsen, J., et al. (2010). Major depressive disorder with subthreshold bipolarity in the National Comorbidity Survey Replication. *The American Journal of Psychiatry, 167*(10), 1194–1201.

12. Registered Nurses Association of Ontario. (2010). *Screening for delirium, dementia and depression in older adults 2010 supplement,* Toronto, Ontario, Canada, Author.

13. Sui, A. L. (2016). US Preventive Services Task Force: Screening for depression in adults US prevention service task force recommendation statement. *Journal of the American Medical Association, 315*(4), 380–387.

14. National Institute of Mental Health. (n.d). *Real men. Real depression. Men and depression: Screening and treatment in primary care settings.* Retrieved from https://www.nimh.nih.gov/health/topics/men-and-mental-health/men-and-depression/nimhs-real-men-real-depression-campaign.shtml.

15. Seiden, R. (1978). Where are they now? A follow-up study of suicide attempters from the Golden Gate Bridge. *Suicide and Life-Threatening Behavior, 8*(4), 203–216.

16. Berger, B. A., & Villaume, W. A. (2013). *Motivational interviewing for healthcare professionals.* Washington, DC: American Pharmaceutical Association.

17. Bschor, T., & Kilarski, L. L. (2016). Are antidepressants effective? A debate on the efficacy for the depressed adult. *Expert Review of Neurotherapeutics, 16*(4), 367–374.

18. National Institute of Mental Health. (2016). *Brain Stimulation Therapies.* Retrieved from http://www.nimh.nih.gov/health/topics/brain-stimulation-therapies/brain-stimulation-therapies.shtml.

19. Gutierrez, M. A., & Lam, J. L. (2017). Psychobiology and pharmacology. In M. J. Halter (Ed.), *Varcoarolis' foundation of psychiatric mental health nursing: A clinical approach* (8th ed., pp. 36–59). Philadelphia.

20. Grund, F. J. L. (2017). Suicidal and nonsuicidal self-injury. In M. J. Halter (Ed.), *Varcoarolis; foundation of psychiatric mental health nursing: A clinical approach* (8th ed., pp. 474–489). Philadelphia.

21. Marwaha, S., He, Z., Broomer, M., & Singh, S. P. (2014). How is affective instability defined and measured? a systematic review. *Psychological Medicine, 44*(9), 1793–1808.

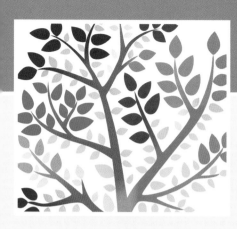

CONCEPT

32

Anxiety

Sean P. Convoy

Anxiety is an adaptive response to stress that is ubiquitous across the lifespan. Anxiety is a subjective experience that can be measured objectively through physiologic and psychological dimensions. As an adaptive response, anxiety has and continues to serve an evolutionary purpose. Early humans spent most of their time hunting, gathering, and maintaining shelter. Survival was predicated on the ability to address basic needs and simultaneously remain vigilant to potential threat. Upon exposure to threat, humans relied on their evolutionary ability to rapidly translate sensory information into a cascade of internal biochemical responses that heightened awareness and generated the necessary energy to either fight or retreat. Although modern humans have fewer threats to contend with, their biochemical temperament has not appreciably changed. Simply stated, human prehistoric brains defined by "fight or flight" operating in present day society can be conceptualized as anxiety.

Anxiety can be episodic or chronic, mild or severe, adaptive or functionally impairing, a symptom or a disorder. The nurse who understands the concept of anxiety is in a unique position to assess and meaningfully deliver care that has the potential to reduce illness, promote wellness, and instill self-efficacy.

DEFINITION

Several definitions of anxiety are found within the literature. While studying animals under stress, Cannon conceptualized the "fight-or-flight response" or the physiologic reaction that occurs in response to perceived threat.[1] This observation influenced many of the definitions of anxiety that followed. Peplau defined anxiety as a "response to a psychic threat" and codified it along a continuum that is discernable through the lenses of *observation, focus,* and *learning ability.*[2] Freud initially conceptualized anxiety as a "physiologic buildup of libidinal energy" but later redefined it as a "feeling of impeding danger that can be based on objective, neurotic or moral threats."[3,p.61] Barlow and Cerney defined anxiety as a "diffuse state characterized by an unpleasant affective experience marked by a significant degree of apprehension about the potential appearance of future aversive or harmful events."[4,p.1] Beck proposed that anxiety is the product of "biased information processing of stimuli, which results in a systematic distortion of the person's thinking and construction of his or her experiences."[5,p.xvi] A psychobiologic definition of anxiety would invariably involve a complex interaction of neuroanatomic activation coupled with neurotransmitter activation and sensitivity that manifests above a clinical threshold as a constellation of symptoms. Each definition shares common themes involving both the perception of threat and a subsequent reaction. For the purpose of this concept presentation, anxiety is defined as *a subjectively distressful experience activated by the perception of threat, which has both a potential psychological and physiologic etiology and expression.*

SCOPE

Simply conceptualized, anxiety exists along a continuum (Fig. 32.1) comparable with Peplau's model ranging from mild anxiety to moderate anxiety, severe anxiety, and panic.[2] This is considered a continuum because the level of anxiety any individual experiences at any given time fluctuates. It is widely accepted that in the mild to moderate form, anxiety can actually be beneficial because it promotes learning, motivation, and heightens awareness. In more severe or chronic forms, anxiety can be debilitating because it restricts cognitive capability and degrades functioning (Table 32.1). In that regard, anxiety is analogous to rainfall because it is needed regularly to promote growth but not so often that one risks drowning.

NORMAL PHYSIOLOGIC PROCESS

Anxiety is the product of a number of complex physiologic and psychological processes best presented through the flight-or-flight response, the general adaptation syndrome, genotype, and neurophysiology.

Fight-or-Flight Response

During the fight-or-flight response, the sympathetic division of the autonomic nervous system interacts with the adrenal cortex to release adrenalin, which causes the heart to speed up and circulate blood faster, the lungs to dilate to increase the oxygen-carrying capacity of the blood, the liver to release stored glucose for a quick infusion of energy, the pupils to dilate for improved visual acuity, and the stomach to inhibit peristalsis as a means to conserve energy.[1] Secondary to these organ system changes, there are observable signs of the fight-or-flight response that include tachycardia, disambiguation, bladder relaxation, tremors, blushing, xerostomia, delayed digestion, and hyperacusis. If the experience is both infrequent and of short duration, the human body has the endogenous capacity to downregulate and return to homeostasis.

General Adaptation Syndrome

Building on Cannon's research, Hans Selye's general adaptation syndrome is relevant to our conceptual discussion of anxiety.[6] The *general*

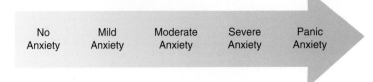

FIGURE 32.1 Scope of Anxiety.

TABLE 32.1	Peplau's Four Levels of Anxiety		
Mild Anxiety	**Moderate Anxiety**	**Severe Anxiety**	**Panic Anxiety**
• Sharp senses	• Narrowed perceptional field	• Concentration progressively narrowed	• Complete lack of focus
• Increased motivation	• Less alert	• Severe impairment of attention	• Tendency to misperceive environment
• Heightened awareness	• Decreased concentration	• Severe cognitive impairment	• Marked change in baseline behavior
• Enhanced learning	• Decreased problem solving	• Physical symptoms	• Marked functional impairment
• Optimal functioning	• Muscular tension	• Emotional symptoms	• Emotional and behavioral dysregulation
	• Restlessness		

adaptation syndrome model establishes that an event (or *stressor*) that threatens an organism's well-being leads to a predictably staged process of bodily response:

- *Stage 1—Alarm*: Upon perceiving the stressor, the body reacts with an autonomic response that activates the sympathetic nervous system (see Fight-or-Flight Response), thus mobilizing the body's resources to respond to the perceived stressor.
- *Stage 2—Resistance*: The parasympathetic nervous system attenuates the reaction, returning many physiologic functions to homeostasis while other functions remain hyperactive, ensuring that the body remains alert and ready to respond.
- *Stage 3—Exhaustion*: If the nature of the stressor is sufficiently intense or of a protracted nature, it may exceed the body's capacity to compensate, thus exposing susceptibility to disease and death.

Genotype

A relevant variable to the discussion of anxiety includes genotype (or genetic makeup). As an individual blueprint for development, one's genotype drives the division of every cell that splits and diversifies within one's body. The development of vital neuroanatomy, neural circuits, and neurotransmitter systems within the brain is genotypically directed. Changes in genotypic expression set the stage for potential vulnerability to stress and anxiety. Although there is no one single gene complicit, the evidence suggests a number of possible gene variations (single nucleotide polymorphism, or SNP) may explain the range of vulnerability that is seen. Changes in genomic expression represent the antecedent element of vulnerability. Genotype cannot be underestimated because it contextualizes why some appear to be more or less vulnerable, or resilient, to stress than others.

Brain Structure and Neurochemistry

Although the field of neuroscience is not yet so advanced to declaratively implicate all of the brain structures, neural circuits, neurotransmitter systems, and gene variations associated with anxiety, it has made considerable progress. Critical structures within the limbic system, such as the thalamus, hypothalamus, cingulate gyrus, amygdala, hippocampus, and basal ganglia appear to play a central role in anxiety. Likewise, critical neurotransmitters and hormones such as serotonin, norepinephrine, γ-amino butyric acid (GABA), dopamine, and thyroid hormone are also central to anxiety.

The state of the science is able to trace certain symptoms of anxiety back to certain neural circuits and neurotransmitter systems. For example, anxiety-based symptoms such as panic and phobia are linked to a malfunction within the amygdala-centered neural circuit that integrates the amygdala, orbitofrontal cortex, and anterior cingulate cortex, along with a number of different neurotransmitters systems (e.g., serotonin, norepinephrine, GABA, glutamate, and corticotropin-releasing factors).[7] Similarly, the symptom of worry can be traced back to a malfunction within a neural circuit incorporating the cortico-striatal-thalamo-cortical circuit and its unique constellation of neurotransmitter systems (e.g., serotonin, GABA, dopamine, norepinephrine, and glutamate).[7]

Age-Related Differences

The evidence assessing age-related differences in anxiety is mixed. The symptom of worry appears to play a less prominent role in the presentation of anxiety, suggesting older adults experience anxiety differently than younger adults.[8] A reasonable argument can be made that, although anxiety occurs across the lifespan, critical windows of vulnerability for certain expressions of anxiety exist. Likewise, an argument can also be made to suggest that the perceptual experience of anxiety changes over the lifespan.

VARIATIONS AND CONTEXT

The concept of anxiety can be symptomatically expressed a number of ways, as shown in Fig. 32.2. A visual representation of anxiety, based on symptom duration, symptom intensity, and functional impairment, is shown in Fig. 32.3. Anxiety must be of a sufficient intensity, duration, and degree of functional impairment to be clinically recognizable. That point of observable recognition is defined as the *clinical threshold*. *Clinical perception* is defined as the nurse's ability to recognize anxiety-based symptoms. The novice or advanced beginner nurse may possess a sufficient understanding of anxiety to recognize overt symptoms such as a panic attack or an obsessive-compulsive behavior. Through experience, the proficient nurse is potentially able to widen his or her clinical perception to recognize subtler symptoms of anxiety. The expert nurse understands the concept of anxiety and its symptomatic expression so well that he or she is sometimes able to perceive anxiety below the clinical threshold.

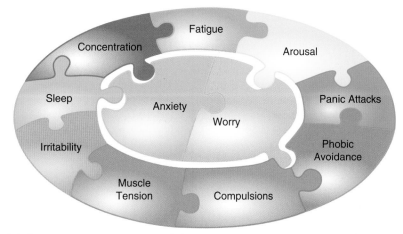

FIGURE 32.2 Symptomatic Expressions of Anxiety. (Redrawn from Stahl, S. M. [2013]. *Stahl's essential psychopharmacology* [4th ed.]. Cambridge, UK: Cambridge University Press.)

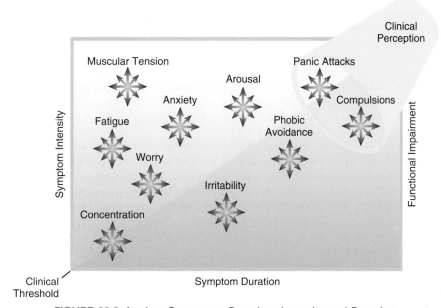

FIGURE 32.3 Anxiety Symptoms Based on Intensity and Duration.

The clinical opportunity for the nurse lies in the ability to understand anxiety and all of its symptomatic expressions, overt and subtle. Being able to recognize the earlier, subtler symptoms can create new opportunities that exist below the clinical threshold. Such opportunities can dramatically influence the trajectory of care, health, and wellness.

CONSEQUENCES

If the physiologic consequences of anxiety are dependent on symptom duration, symptom intensity, and degree of functional impairment, one can reasonably conclude that the physiologic consequences of anxiety are variable. The general adaptation syndrome establishes that certain stressors are powerful enough to result in exhaustion and subsequent physiologic consequence. The physiologic realization of alarm, resistance, and exhaustion is varied. This variation is influenced by endogenous (or genotype), exogenous (or environment), and the dynamic interaction between endogenous and exogenous (or epigenetic) sources.

Physiologic consequences of anxiety link back to the deleterious effect of chronic sympathetic activation on renal, cardiovascular, endocrine, gastrointestinal, immune, neurologic, and psychiatric systems. Recent research has provided additional evidence associating anxiety disorders with future projected risk for medical morbidity, specifically cerebrovascular, atherosclerosis, ischemic heart, gastrointestinal, hypertensive, respiratory, and genitourinary system diseases.[9,10]

Advances in psychoneuroimmunology (or the study of interactions between psychological, neurologic, and immune systems) have established that the mind and body have equal potential to both influence and be influenced by the other. The symptomatic manifestations and potential consequences of anxiety are both psychological and physiologic in nature.

RISK FACTORS

Research associated with risk factor determinations for anxiety has largely been performed in relation to clinical diagnosis. Many anxiety disorders appear to also be influenced by different environmental, temperament, and genetic variables.[11]

Populations at Risk

Anxiety disorders represent the most prevalent subgroup of mental illness in the United States, with a 12-month prevalence rate of 18.1% and 25.1% for adults and children, respectively.[12] Average age of onset is 11 years. Demographically, women are 60% more likely than men to manifest clinically significant anxiety.[11] Whites appear to be more vulnerable to anxiety compared with their black or Hispanic counterparts. Age prevalence appears to peek in middle adulthood (30s to 50s).[13] A systematic review of research linking socioeconomic status (SES) among youth with anxiety reveals that lower SES is associated with higher rates of depressed mood and anxiety.[14]

Individual Risk Factors

Individual risk factors for anxiety exist within four potentially inter-related domains of temperament, environmental, genetic, and physiologic. Although the desire to weigh risk factors linearly might be enticing, our evolving understanding of the science suggests the relationship among these variables is anything but rectilinear. The experienced nurse dynamically considers all four domains.

Temperament

Temperament refers to the way a person typically responds to external events both emotionally and behaviorally.[15] Research identifies nine different temperamental traits of children (i.e., activity level, distractibility, intensity, regularity, sensory threshold, approach/withdrawal, adaptability, persistence, and mood). Temperament shapes how an individual will interact with society and also how society will likely interact with the individual. Kagan et al. concluded that babies are born with an established temperament, of which approximately 20% are born with a predisposition to anxiety.[16] Temperament is a potential risk factor for anxiety with selective mutism, specific phobia, social anxiety disorder, panic disorder, agoraphobia, and generalized anxiety disorder (GAD).[14]

Environmental

Environmental factors are linked to certain clinical manifestations of anxiety. For example, separation anxiety disorder centers on a stress event defined by loss, death, or profound change. Parental social inhibition may serve as a role model for selective mutism among children. A number of environmental factors appear to influence the development of phobias, including parental overprotectiveness, parental loss or separation, and physical or sexual abuse. Childhood maltreatment and adversity during childhood appear to be risk factors for social anxiety disorder. Physical and sexual abuse appear to be more common among those with panic disorder than other anxiety disorders. Stressful life events during early childhood appear to be a risk factor for agoraphobia.[13]

Genetics

Heritable evidence associated with anxiety continues to evolve. Separation anxiety disorder research established a 73% heritability rate among a sample of 6-year-old twins.[13] There is some early evidence demonstrating genetic susceptibility to zoophobia among patients with first-degree relatives who possess the same condition.[13] Those traits that predispose individuals to social anxiety disorder (e.g., behavioral inhibition) are strongly influenced by genetics. A number of gene variations have been implicated in increasing the vulnerability to panic attacks and panic disorder.[17,18] Agoraphobia has the strongest and most specific genetic linkage and a heritability rate of 61%.[19] Meta-analytical integrations of family and twin studies calculated an odds ratio recurrence of 6.1 and a genetic heritability rate of 31.6% with the same predisposing genes across sexes for GAD.[20]

BOX 32.1   Conditions Commonly Associated with Anxiety

- Cancer
- Chronic obstructive pulmonary disease
- Asthma
- Heart disease
- Diabetes
- Drug or alcohol withdrawal
- Thyroid disease (hyperthyroidism or hypothyroidism)
- Pheochromocytoma
- Chronic infections
- Vestibular dysfunction
- Irritable bowel syndrome

Physiologic

Researchers have identified a limited number of physiologic variables that can also serve as risk factors for anxiety. For reasons not yet understood, children with separation anxiety disorder display particularly enhanced sensitivity to respiratory stimulation with CO_2-enriched air.[21] Likewise, individuals with blood injection injury phobias demonstrate a unique propensity to vasovagal syncope in the presence of the phobic stimulus.[22] In addition, a number of medical conditions have the potential to independently promote anxiety and anxiety-based symptoms (Box 32.1).

ASSESSMENT

Individuals with time-limited, mild to moderate anxiety may appear asymptomatic or merely distracted during a nursing assessment. The proficient or expert nurse may be able to perceive more subtle signs of anxiety, such as impaired concentration, distractibility, and talkativeness, whereas the novice or advanced beginner is usually only sensitized to the more overt signs of anxiety, such as panic or compulsive behavior. Regardless of proficiency level, assessment for anxiety requires the collection of a history, physical assessment, and mental status examination (MSE) (Box 32.2).

History

Prior to collecting a history, meaningful effort must be put into establishing a therapeutic rapport. Perfunctorily asking a list of rote questions involving extraordinarily sensitive medical history without building rapport is at best ill advised and at worst unprofessional. The goal of the history is to obtain vital and time-sensitive health information that has the potential to immediately and significantly influence the trajectory of care.

When collecting history, be advised that not every individual understands or even acknowledges terms such as "anxiety" or "panic." Although some individuals may have experienced clinically significant and functionally impairing anxiety-based symptoms for years, they will not necessarily understand or convey the symptom experience the way the nurse does. Consequently, the nurse is advised to strip away psychological terminology when communicating with patients. As opposed to asking, "Do you experience anxiety?" the nurse can alternatively ask, "Do you find yourself worrying a lot and feel unable to control it?" Instead of asking, "Do you ruminate?" the nurse can alternatively ask, "Do you find it hard to shut off your mind from overthinking?" A good exercise prior to assessing a patient for anxiety is to review the symptomatic expressions of anxiety (see Fig. 32.2) and develop more user-friendly, nonclinical terms for the identified symptoms. Somatic symptoms often require a systematic measure of assessment to improve

BOX 32.2   Nursing Assessment of Anxiety

Medical History
- Risk factor identification
- Mental health history
- Substance use history
- Current medical problems
- Familial medical history
- Trauma exposure

Physical Examination
- Vital signs
- Auscultation of heart and lungs
- Palpation of thyroid
- Cranial nerve assessment
- Blood and urine studies

Mental Status Examination
- Appearance
- Attitude
- Behavior
- Mood and affect
- Speech
- Thought process
- Thought content
- Perceptions
- Cognition
- Insight
- Judgment

reliability. For this reason, using scaled questions such as "On a scale of 1 to 10, with 1 being no distress and 10 being severe distress, how is your worry today?" becomes a way to operationalize subjective data in a meaningful way.

Physical Assessment

Understanding human physiology, the competent nurse can reasonably anticipate many of the physical manifestations of anxiety. Autonomic activation can manifest in hypertension, tachycardia, tachypnea, diaphoresis, ataxia, tremulousness, gastrointestinal distress, and muscular tension. Although many of these physical findings are sensitive to anxiety, they are by no means specific to anxiety. Making a determination of anxiety should never be done until other high-risk medical explanations (e.g., myocardial infarction, embolism, and stroke) have been ruled out. Serial evaluation of physical symptoms is vital to determine both functioning and response to treatment.

A well-executed mental status examination (MSE) is another objective data point that can meaningfully quantify anxiety. As established in Box 32.2, the MSE systematically evaluates a number of variables (e.g., distractibility, psychomotor agitation, tremulousness, rapid rate of speech, confusion, perseverated thought, and impaired short-term memory) that are potentially sensitive to anxiety.

Diagnostic Tests and Screening Measures

There is no specific test or study that can definitively rule anxiety in or out. However, there are a number of studies worthy of discussion. Laboratory studies (complete blood count, comprehensive metabolic profile, arterial blood gas, thyroid function test, spinal fluid analysis, urinalysis, and urine drug screen), radiologic studies (computerized tomography), or procedural studies (electrocardiogram, stress test, or electroencephalogram) often provide vital findings that contextualize suspected anxiety-based symptoms. Sometimes the only way to rule in anxiety is to first rule out all other medical explanations.

Evidence-based screening tools are also available to assess for anxiety across the lifespan. The fifth edition of the *Diagnostic and Statistical Manual of Mental Disorders (DSM-5)* has implemented a cross-cutting symptoms measure, for both children and adults, that also has general value as a crude psychiatric assessment.[12] The Beck Anxiety Inventory for Youth (BYI),[23] Spence Children's Anxiety Scale (SCAS),[24] and Revised Children's Manifest Anxiety Scale (RCMAS-2)[24] are all well-established screening tools for children and adolescents. The Hamilton Anxiety Scale,[25] Beck Anxiety Inventory (BAI),[26] Generalized Anxiety Disorder–7 Item (GAD-7),[27] and Post-traumatic Stress Disorder Checklist (PCL-5)[28] are all well-researched tools for adults.

CLINICAL MANAGEMENT

Primary Prevention

Primary prevention seeks to deter injury or illness via risk reduction. This is done by education, altering risk behaviors, decreasing exposure, and enhancing resistance to those agents that promote anxiety. Prevention measures used to target anxiety-based disorders are growing in both frequency and scope.[29-32] Our developing understanding of neuroscience suggests that the psychobiologic damage of mental illness commonly precedes symptomatic expression. Consequently, prevention measures are vital.

Primary prevention targeting anxiety theoretically begins during pregnancy by promoting the health, wellness, and functioning of the pregnant mother and associated family support system. Mental health–focused well visits across the lifespan conducted by informed healthcare professionals are integral to risk recognition. Therein, a thorough family history that quantifies mental illness is critical. Resources and investment into strengthening family functioning and stability can serve as a protective measure against anxiety.

Secondary Prevention

Secondary prevention involves screening for the early detection of an illness. There are no population-based screening recommendations for anxiety, although screening tools (previously discussed) are available to use if symptoms have been recognized. Maintaining an awareness of and monitoring for symptoms and functional impairment allows for early identification and treatment.

Collaborative Management

Anxiety is commonly recognized as one of the most treatable psychiatric conditions. Because psychiatric illness is etiologically multifactorial and requires multimodal responses, it is uncommon that one treatment approach alone effectively and definitively treat anxiety. More often, a combination of therapies is associated with the best results. It is also important to distinguish between treatment and symptom management. Psychotropic interventions have great potential to manage symptoms, and psychotherapeutic interventions alongside psychotropic interventions have the greatest potential to treat the disorder.

Pharmacotherapy

Dating back to the mid-1950s, antianxiety agents such as meprobamate, otherwise known as "mother's little helper," quickly found a lucrative market in American society, with an estimated 36 million prescriptions filled in the first decade of its existence. In the 1960s, benzodiazepines (BZDs) became the prescribed drug of choice for anxiety. Although BZDs continue to dominate the pharmaceutical market, a number of other agents have expanded treatment options during the past few decades.

β-Adrenergic receptor antagonists. Considering Fig. 32.3, some individuals only episodically or situationally experience anxiety above the clinical threshold. In those instances, there may be an indication for a psychotropic agent that can be used as needed. β-Adrenergic antagonists or β-blockers (e.g., propranolol, metoprolol, clonidine, and atenolol) have been used to treat varied expressions of anxiety (e.g., performance anxiety, traumatic nightmares, and extrapyramidal side effects of antipsychotic medications) for decades.[33,34] β-Blockers work by binding the β-adrenergic receptor and subsequently blocking the effects of epinephrine and norepinephrine, consequently (and temporarily) blocking the physiologic manifestations of anxiety. Although β-blockers are generally well tolerated, they can result in postural hypotension, dizziness, and bradycardia.[35]

Benzodiazepines. BZDs are a commonly used antianxiety agent prescribed on a scheduled and as-needed basis. BZDs (e.g., lorazepam, alprazolam, clonazepam, and diazepam) enhance the effect of the neurotransmitter GABA, which is known to inhibit or calm nerve activity, and are exceptionally effective for the short-term management of anxiety symptoms. Unfortunately, BZDs are also highly addictive agents that pose serious risk for complicated, potentially life-threatening withdrawal. They also pose risk for central nervous system sedation and rebound anxiety. A meta-analysis evaluated the risk of BZD use and dementia risk, yielding a 78% higher risk for dementia among those who regularly use BZDs compared with those who did not.[36] It is for these reasons that the long-term scheduled use of a BZA is ill-advised.

Nonbenzodiazepine antianxiety agents. Buspirone is a serotonin$_{1A}$ partial agonist that diminishes serotonin activity postsynaptically, consequently delivering anxiolytic actions with less central nervous system sedation. Hydroxyzine is an antihistaminergic agent that blocks histamine$_1$ receptors, consequently prompting sedation. Each agent may be able to provide some degree of symptomatic relief of anxiety but will likely be of less utility if the patient has already been sensitized to the effects of a BZD.

Antidepressant agents. Although antidepressant agents have historically been used to treat symptoms of depression, a commonality between depression and anxiety is serotonin and norepinephrine (or monoamine) dysregulation. Consequently, there are currently a number of antidepressants on the market that hold a U.S. Food and Drug Administration (FDA) indication for the treatment of anxiety:

- *Tricyclic antidepressants (TCAs)*: TCAs influence a number of different neurotransmitter receptors potentially relevant to anxiety. Doxepin is the only drug in this group that has an FDA indication for the treatment of anxiety. Although effective, this is considered third- and fourth-tier treatment choice due to its significant side effects, potential for suicidal thinking and lethality if used as an overdose agent.
- *Monoamine oxidase inhibitors (MAOIs)*: MAOIs (e.g., isocarboxazid, phenelzine sulfate, tranylcypromine sulfate, and selegiline) inhibit the activity of monoamine oxidase enzymes, obstructing the breakdown of monoamine neurotransmitters and hence increasing monoamine availability. Phenelzine sulfate is effective in treating symptoms associated with social anxiety,[37,38] but it is considered a second- or third-tier choice compared with the newer agents that boast fewer side effects.
- *Selective serotonin reuptake inhibitors (SSRIs)*: SSRIs (e.g., fluoxetine, paroxetine, sertraline, citalopram, and escitalopram) inhibit the reuptake of the neurotransmitter serotonin presynaptically, thus increasing the availability of serotonin postsynaptically. SSRIs indicated for anxiety disorders include fluoxetine, paroxetine, sertraline, and escitalopram. SSRIs are generally well-tolerated agents but demonstrate an increased risk for a life-threatening condition (serotonin syndrome) when combined with other agents that agonize serotonin. Abrupt discontinuation of SSRIs can lead to discontinuation syndrome.
- *Serotonin-norepinephrine reuptake inhibitors (SNRIs)*: Like their SSRI counterparts, SNRIs (e.g., venlafaxine, duloxetine, and desvenlafaxine) block the presynaptic reuptake of both serotonin and norepinephrine, thus increasing the availability of both neurotransmitters postsynaptically. The SNRIs indicated for anxiety include venlafaxine (for panic disorder, social anxiety disorder, and GAD) and duloxetine (for GAD). Like SSRIs, abrupt discontinuation of SNRIs can lead to discontinuation syndrome.

Psychotherapy

A number of different psychotherapeutic modalities have demonstrated efficacy in treating clinically significant anxiety.

Psychoeducation. Psychoeducation is a modality of care that provides patients and their support systems with basic instruction on a wide array of topics, including diagnosis, treatment, risk management, health promotion, illness prevention, and anticipatory guidance. A meta-analysis published in 2009 established that brief passive psychoeducational interventions can reduce symptoms.[39] Although not as stimulating as other forms of therapy, psychoeducation is a foundational resource that is vital to all treatment, especially anxiety. Psychoeducation is the hallmark of nursing and the nursing profession.

Cognitive-behavioral therapy. Of all the recognized psychotherapies, cognitive-behavioral therapy (CBT) has the largest evidentiary base supporting its utility for the treatment of anxiety. CBT is based on the notion that how one perceives and processes sensory stimuli has a direct bearing on the reaction one has to that situation. CBT uses a systematic process of Socratic questioning to expose cognitive distortions and core beliefs. Once identified, the therapist and patient collaborate in a process of initially recognizing and neutralizing and later modifying those cognitive distortions and core beliefs. The result of this process is the alleviation of anxiety.

Prolonged exposure therapy. Prolonged exposure (PE) is a specialized form of psychotherapy that targets anxiety born of trauma by systematically exposing patients to their own trauma via a structured process of education, breathing, retraining, and real-world (or in vivo) and imaginal exposure. Conceptually, the goal of PE is to take patients back to their index trauma and systematically expose them to those sensory aspects of the trauma, thereby changing the subsequent reaction to the sensory trigger henceforth.

Cognitive processing therapy. Cognitive processing therapy (CPT) is a manualized form of cognitive therapy that also targets anxiety born of trauma.[40–42] CPT (1) provides psychoeducation about trauma symptoms and its etiology, (2) heightens awareness of one's own thoughts and feeling associated with the trauma, and (3) teaches skills for managing distressing thoughts and feelings about the trauma. It ultimately aspires to understand how beliefs associated with safety, trust, control, self-esteem, other people, and relationships have changed.

Mindfulness-based cognitive therapy. Traditional CBT teaches the patient to challenge his or her own cognitive distortions, whereas mindfulness-based cognitive behavioral therapy (MBCT) teaches the patient to reconceptualize cognitive distortions as a transient experience that is a predictable part of the human experience. MBCT has established efficacy with numerous anxiety disorders.[43] MBCT aspires to teach the patient how to develop the skill of nonjudgmental awareness of his or her own thoughts and feelings because doing so delimits the symptomatic experience of anxiety that commonly follows.

Eye movement desensitization and reprocessing. Eye movement desensitization and reprocessing psychotherapy is a nontraditional manualized form of psychotherapy that aspires to process traumatic memories while simultaneously focusing on other sensory stimuli (e.g., sounds, hand taps, and/or eye movements). Although the therapeutic mechanism of action still eludes researchers, the evidence of its benefit has steadily grown.[44,45]

Other therapies. A number of other therapies (e.g., animal-assisted therapy, lifestyle modification, and complementary and alternative medicine) have shown evidence of benefit for a number of anxiety-based conditions. Animal-assisted therapy is building an evidentiary base as a complimentary treatment for trauma.[46–48] Likewise, a number of complementary and alternative medicine methods (e.g., supplements, botanical remedies, meditation and spiritual practices, acupuncture, and dietary practices) appear to also demonstrate benefit in the treatment of anxiety-based disorders.[49–52] Although there are a number of supplements (e.g., kava kava, valerian root, and St. John's wort) on the market that boast efficacy in treating anxiety, these agents are not subject

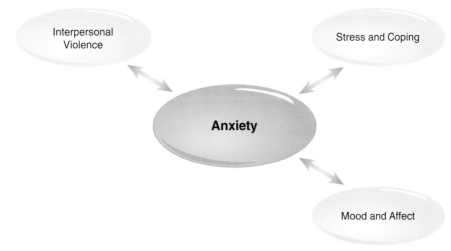

FIGURE 32.4 Anxiety and Interrelated Concepts.

to the rigorous scrutiny of a governing body such as the FDA to ensure quality control. Consequently, there are demonstrated risks associated with combining supplements with psychotropic medications.

INTERRELATED CONCEPTS

There are several interrelated concepts that potentially demonstrate a linkage with anxiety (Fig. 32.4), including Stress and Coping, Mood and Affect, and Interpersonal Violence. Stress and Coping is an interrelated concept because individuals with clinically significant anxiety are by definition in stress overload. It logically follows that if stress can exacerbate anxiety, so too can anxiety make one more vulnerable to stress. Coping is the response to stress and is linked to anxiety particularly if coping skills are ineffective to resolve the stress. Mood and Affect comprise the subjective (mood) and objective (affect) manifestation of stress, coping, and anxiety. Lastly, Interpersonal Violence is defined as a set of overt behaviors that have the potential to place both the patient and others at risk. Therein, we can establish interpersonal violence as one of many potential expressions of stress, coping, and anxiety.

CLINICAL EXEMPLARS

There are a number of exemplars of anxiety that represent established medical diagnoses (Box 32.3). It is beyond the scope of this text to provide detailed information on each of these exemplars, but a brief explanation of some of the most common exemplars is presented in the section that follows. For detailed information and nursing care for each of these exemplars, consult a psychiatric—mental health nursing textbook.

Featured Exemplars
Simple Phobia
A simple phobia is characterized as an intense fearful reaction to an object or situation. The reaction is disproportionate and excessive and goes against rational thinking. Examples of common simple phobia "triggers" include fear of insects, heights, water, or closed spaces. When exposed to the object or situation, the individual typically has a paniclike experience and a subsequent strong urge to avoid or eliminate the situation. Some individuals develop simple phobias as a result of a physical or psychological traumatic exposure, such as being bitten by

a dog prompting cynophobia or being trapped in a closed space prompting cleithrophobia.

Social Phobia
Social phobia refers to a type of anxiety characterized by extreme fear of situations involving social interactions in public settings. Examples include attending social events, eating in public, speaking in public, and using public bathrooms. An individual with social phobia often seeks ways to avoid social situations. When faced with an event, the individual will often experience anxiety nearing panic leading up to, during, and following a social situation.

Panic Disorder
A panic disorder occurs when an individual experiences a constellation of anxiety-based symptoms that approximate panic. Panic triggers include a fear of an impending disaster or fear of losing control in the absence of an actual threat. These recurrent panic events can interfere with one's life to the point that they become disabling. Common physical symptoms include a racing or pounding heart, chest pain, difficulty breathing, sweating, weakness, and dizziness. Panic disorders affect approximately 6 million Americans, occur twice as often in females as in males, and most often develop in adolescents or adults.

Generalized Anxiety Disorder
A GAD is described as generalized worry (and often an inability to control worry) accompanied by uncomfortable symptoms of anxiety that can near the level of panic. The nature of the worry typically involves varied aspects of the individual's life and would be considered disproportionate or excessive by other people's standards. Examples include worries related to completing tasks on time, worrying about performance, and worrying about family members.

Obsessive-Compulsive Disorder
Obsessive-compulsive disorder (OCD) is a psychological state characterized by obsessive thoughts that manifest as compulsive behavior. Common examples include a need to repeatedly wash hands, check things, repeat an action, count things, a preoccupation with symmetry, and hoarding. The inability to fulfill the ritual is commonly associated with profound anxiety. An individual with OCD spends excessive time engaged in the repetitious thoughts or behaviors, which interfere with the individual's daily life.

BOX 32.3   EXEMPLARS OF ANXIETY

Depressive Disorders
- Major depressive disorder with anxious distress

Anxiety Disorders
- Separation anxiety disorder
- Selective mutism
- Specific phobia
- Social anxiety disorder
- Panic disorder
- Agoraphobia
- Generalized anxiety disorder
- Substance/medication-induced anxiety disorder
- Anxiety disorder due to another medical condition
- Unspecified anxiety disorder

Obsessive-Compulsive and Related Disorders
- Obsessive-compulsive disorder
- Body dysmorphic disorder
- Hoarding disorder
- Trichotillomania

- Excoriation disorder
- Substance/medication-induced obsessive-compulsive and related disorder
- Obsessive-compulsive and related disorder due to another medical condition
- Unspecified obsessive-compulsive and related disorder

Trauma and Stressor-Related Disorders
- Reactive attachment disorder
- Disinhibited social engagement disorder
- Posttraumatic stress disorder
- Acute stress disorder
- Adjustment disorder with anxiety
- Unspecified trauma- and stressor-related disorder

Substance Use Disorders
- Substance-induced anxiety disorder

Personality Disorders (Cluster C)
- Avoidant personality disorder
- Dependent personality disorder
- Obsessive-compulsive personality disorder

ACCESS EXEMPLAR LINKS IN YOUR GIDDENS EBOOK

CASE STUDY

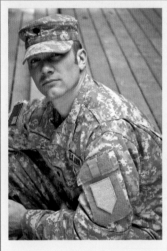

Case Presentation
Roger is a Reserve Army Sergeant with 18 years of military service and three operational deployments. Roger has significant family history for both anxiety and alcohol dependence. Roger's first deployment was unremarkable because he saw no direct combat and reported only limited stress associated with geographic separation from his family. His second deployment to was markedly different because he participated in more than 100 supply runs during a peak period of military conflict. He incurred three improvised explosive device attacks, two small arms fire exchanges with the enemy resulting in two confirmed kills, and perpetual risk of mortar attack. Two of his close friends died of injuries, with one dying in his arms (this event represents the index trauma).

In the months that followed return from the deployment, Roger avoided all reminders of his experiences during the deployment and began to consume excessive amounts of alcohol to facilitate sleep. His marriage disintegrated, he alienated his support systems, and his work performance declined resulting in missed opportunities for promotion.

During his third deployment he began to experience intrusive recollections of the deaths of his friends from the previous deployment with flashbacks and nightmares. Each time he put on his Kevlar in anticipation of going outside the safe zone, he would experience disabling panic. His inability to avoid triggers of his trauma made it impossible to continue in a combat zone. He developed a plan to kill himself by leaving the safe zone without support with the intent to kill as many insurgents as he could before they killed him. After informing his chaplain of his plans, Roger was medically evacuated back to the United States.

Case Analysis Questions
1. What risk factors does Rodger have for anxiety?
2. Referring to the four levels of anxiety (Table 32.1), what category does Roger fall in during his third deployment?
3. What collaborative interventions are most likely going to help Rodger?

From Shelly Perry/iStock/Thinkstock

 ACCESS EXEMPLAR LINKS IN YOUR GIDDENS EBOOK

REFERENCES

1. Cannon, W. (1929). *Bodily changes in pain, hunger, fear and rage.* New York: Appleton-Century-Crofts.
2. Peplau, H. E. (1952). *Interpersonal relations in nursing, a conceptual frame of reference for psychodynamic nursing.* New York: Putnam.
3. Hall, C. S. (1954). *A primer of Freudian psychology.* Cleveland, OH: World Publishing.
4. Barlow, D. H., & Cerny, J. A. (1988). *Psychological treatment of panic.* New York: Guilford Press.
5. Beck, A. T., Emery, G., & Greenberg, R. L. (2005). *Anxiety disorders and phobias: A cognitive perspective* (15th anniversary ed.). Cambridge, MA: Basic Books.
6. Selye, H. (1976). *Stress in health and disease.* Boston: Butterworths.
7. Stahl, S. M. (2014). *Stahl's essential psychopharmacology: The prescriber's guide* (5th ed.). Cambridge, UK: Cambridge University Press.
8. Brenes, G. A. (2006). Age differences in the presentation of anxiety. *Aging and Mental Health, 10*(3), 298–302.
9. Bowen, R. C., Senthilselvan, A., & Barale, A. (2000). Physical illness as an outcome of chronic anxiety disorders. *Canadian Journal of Psychiatry. Revue Canadienne de Psychiatrie, 45*(5), 459–464.
10. Harter, M. C., Conway, K. P., & Merikangas, K. R. (2003). Associations between anxiety disorders and physical illness. *European Archives of Psychiatry and Clinical Neuroscience, 253*(6), 313–320.
11. American Psychiatric Association. (2013). *Diagnostic and statistical manual of mental disorders* (5th ed.). Arlington, VA: American Psychiatric Publishing.

12. Stucky, K. J., Kirkwood, M. W., & Donders, J. (2014). *Clinical neuropsychology study guide and board review*. Oxford, UK: Oxford University Press.

13. The National Institute of Mental Health: *Anxiety disorders*, 2014. Retrieved from http://www.nimh.nih.gov/health/publications/anxiety-disorders/index.shtml?rf=57640.

14. Lemstra, M., Neudorf, C., D'Arcy, C., et al. (2008). A systematic review of depressed mood and anxiety by SES in youth aged 10–15 years. *Canadian Journal of Public Health*, 99(2), 125–129.

15. Medina, J. J. (2010). The genetics of temperament: An update. *Psychiatric Times*. Retrieved from http://www.psychiatrictimes.com/articles/genetics-temperament%E2%80%94-update.

16. Kagan, J., Snidman, N., Kahn, V., et al. (2007). The preservation of two infant temperaments into adolescence. *Monographs of the Society for Research in Child Development*, 72(2), 1–91.

17. Domschke, K., Tidow, N., Schrempf, M., et al. (2013). Epigenetic signature of panic disorder: A role of glutamate decarboxylase 1 (GAD1) DNA hypomethylation? *Progress in Neuro-Psychopharmacology and Biological Psychiatry*, 46, 189–196.

18. Judd, F. K., Burrows, G. D., & Hay, D. A. (1987). Panic disorder: Evidence for genetic vulnerability. *The Australian and New Zealand Journal of Psychiatry*, 21(2), 197–208.

19. Kendler, K. S., Karkowski, L. M., & Prescott, C. A. (1999). Fears and phobias: Reliability and heritability. *Psychological Medicine*, 29(3), 539–553.

20. Gottschalk, M. G., & Domschke, K. (2017). Genetics of generalized anxiety disorder and related traits. *Dialogues in Clinical Neuroscience*, 19(2), 159–168.

21. Pine, D. S., Klein, R. G., Coplan, J. D., et al. (2000). Differential carbon dioxide sensitivity in childhood anxiety disorders and nonill comparison group. *Archives of General Psychiatry*, 57(10), 960–967.

22. Sarlo, M., Buodo, G., Munafo, M., et al. (2008). Cardiovascular dynamics in blood phobia: Evidence for a key role of sympathetic activity in vulnerability to syncope. *Psychophysiology*, 45(6), 1038–1045.

23. Steer, R. A., Kumar, G., Ranieri, W. F., et al. (1995). Use of the Beck Anxiety Inventory with adolescent psychiatric outpatients. *Psychological Reports*, 76(2), 459–465.

24. Essau, C. A., Muris, P., & Ederer, E. M. (2002). Reliability and validity of the Spence Children's Anxiety Scale and the Screen for Child Anxiety Related Emotional Disorders in German children. *Journal of Behavior Therapy and Experimental Psychiatry*, 33(1), 1–18.

25. Maier, W., Buller, R., Philipp, M., et al. (1988). The Hamilton Anxiety Scale: Reliability, validity and sensitivity to change in anxiety and depressive disorders. *Journal of Affective Disorders*, 14(1), 61–68.

26. Osman, A., Kopper, B. A., Barrios, F. X., et al. (1997). The Beck Anxiety Inventory: Reexamination of factor structure and psychometric properties. *Journal of Clinical Psychology*, 53(1), 7–14.

27. Beard, C., & Bjorgvinsson, T. (2014). Beyond generalized anxiety disorder: Psychometric properties of the GAD-7 in a heterogeneous psychiatric sample. *Journal of Anxiety Disorders*, 28(6), 547–552.

28. Demirchyan, A., Goenjian, A. K., & Khachadourian, V. (2015). Factor structure and psychometric properties of the posttraumatic stress disorder (PTSD) checklist and DSM-5 PTSD symptom set in a long-term postearthquake cohort in Armenia. *Assessment*, 22(5), 594–606.

29. Christensen, H., Batterham, P., Mackinnon, A., et al. (2014). Prevention of generalized anxiety disorder using a web intervention, iChill: Randomized controlled trial. *Journal of Medical Internet Research*, 16(9), e199.

30. Corrieri, S., Heider, D., Conrad, I., et al. (2014). School-based prevention programs for depression and anxiety in adolescence: A systematic review. *Health Promotion International*, 29(3), 427–441.

31. Johnstone, J., Rooney, R. M., Hassan, S., et al. (2014). Prevention of depression and anxiety symptoms in adolescents: 42 and 54 months follow-up of the Aussie Optimism Program–Positive Thinking Skills. *Frontiers in Psychology*, 5, 364.

32. Stallard, P., Taylor, G., Anderson, R., et al. (2014). The prevention of anxiety in children through school-based interventions: Study protocol for a 24-month follow-up of the PACES project. *Trials*, 15, 77.

33. Bachmann, S., Muller-Werdan, U., Huber, M., et al. (2011). Positive impact of the beta-blocker celiprolol on panic, anxiety, and cardiovascular parameters in patients with mitral valve prolapse syndrome. *Journal of Clinical Psychopharmacology*, 31(6), 783–785.

34. Chaturvedi, S. K. (1985). Metoprolol, a new selective beta-blocker in anxiety neurosis. *Psychopharmacology*, 85(4), 488.

35. *Epocrates I: Drug search*, 2014. Retrieved from https://online.epocrates.com/noFrame.

36. Islam, M. M., et al. (2016). Benzodiazepine use and risk of dementia in the elderly population: A systematic review and meta-analysis. *Neuroepidemiology*, 47(3–4), 181–191.

37. Aarre, T. F. (2003). Phenelzine efficacy in refractory social anxiety disorder: A case series. *Nordic Journal of Psychiatry*, 57(4), 313–315.

38. Blanco, C., Heimberg, R. G., Schneier, F. R., et al. (2010). A placebo-controlled trial of phenelzine, cognitive behavioral group therapy, and their combination for social anxiety disorder. *Archives of General Psychiatry*, 67(3), 286–295.

39. Donker, T., Griffiths, K. M., Cuijpers, P., et al. (2009). Psychoeducation for depression, anxiety and psychological distress: A meta-analysis. *BMC Medicine*, 7, 79.

40. Holliday, R., Link-Malcolm, J., Morris, E. E., et al. (2014). Effects of cognitive processing therapy on PTSD-related negative cognitions in veterans with military sexual trauma. *Military Medicine*, 179(10), 1077–1082.

41. Nixon, R. D. (2012). Cognitive processing therapy versus supportive counseling for acute stress disorder following assault: A randomized pilot trial. *Behavior Therapy*, 43(4), 825–836.

42. Walter, K. H., Varkovitzky, R. L., Owens, G. P., et al. (2014). Cognitive processing therapy for veterans with posttraumatic stress disorder: A comparison between outpatient and residential treatment. *Journal of Consulting and Clinical Psychology*, 82(4), 551–561.

43. Hofmann, S. G., Sawyer, A. T., Witt, A. A., et al. (2010). The effect of mindfulness-based therapy on anxiety and depression: A meta-analytic review. *Journal of Consulting and Clinical Psychology*, 78(2), 169–183.

44. Chen, Y. R., Hung, K. W., Tsai, J. C., et al. (2014). Efficacy of eye-movement desensitization and reprocessing for patients with posttraumatic-stress disorder: A meta-analysis of randomized controlled trials. *PLoS ONE*, 9(8), e103676.

45. McGuire, T. M., Lee, C. W., & Drummond, P. D. (2014). Potential of eye movement desensitization and reprocessing therapy in the treatment of post-traumatic stress disorder. *Psychology Research and Behavior Management*, 7, 273–283.

46. Beck, C. E., Gonzales, F., Jr., Sells, C. H., et al. (2012). The effects of animal-assisted therapy on wounded warriors in an occupational therapy life skills program. *U.S. Army Medical Department Journal*, 38–45.

47. Berget, B., & Braastad, B. O. (2011). Animal-assisted therapy with farm animals for persons with psychiatric disorders. *Annali Dell'istituto Superiore Di Sanita*, 47(4), 384–390.

48. Rossetti, J., & King, C. (2010). Use of animal-assisted therapy with psychiatric patients. *Journal of Psychosocial Nursing and Mental Health Services*, 48(11), 44–48.

49. Bazzan, A. J., Zabrecky, G., Monti, D. A., et al. (2014). Current evidence regarding the management of mood and anxiety disorders using complementary and alternative medicine. *Expert Review of Neurotherapeutics*, 14(4), 411–423.

50. Bystritsky, A., Hovav, S., Sherbourne, C., et al. (2012). Use of complementary and alternative medicine in a large sample of anxiety patients. *Psychosomatics*, 53(3), 266–272.

51. Ekor, M., Adeyemi, O. S., & Otuechere, C. A. (2013). Management of anxiety and sleep disorders: Role of complementary and alternative medicine and challenges of integration with conventional orthodox care. *Chinese Journal of Integrative Medicine*, 19(1), 5–14.

52. McPherson, F., & McGraw, L. (2013). Treating generalized anxiety disorder using complementary and alternative medicine. *Alternative Therapies in Health and Medicine*, 19(5), 45–50.

Cognition

Jean Giddens

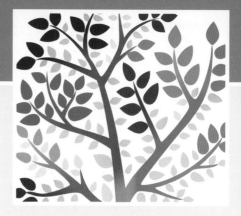

The ability to think has long been considered a defining characteristic of what it means to be human. Attesting to this are the words of the French philosopher Rene Descartes, who said "Cogito, ergo sum," which translates to "I think, therefore I am." Thus the understanding of cognition, a term derived from the Latin verb "to think," is essential to understanding human behavior in health and in disease.

The study of cognition is multidisciplinary in scope with involvement and contributions from psychologists, philosophers, linguists, artificial intelligence scientists, and neuroscientists.[1] Two fields exclusively dedicated to the study of cognition are cognitive psychology and cognitive neuroscience. Cognitive psychology is committed to the study of cognition from an information processing perspective.[1] Cognitive neuroscience is the combined study of the mind and brain.[2]

DEFINITION

Cognition is a comprehensive term used to refer to all the processes involved in human thought.[1] These processes relate to the reception of sensory input, its processing, its storage, its retrieval, and its use.[2] For the purposes of this concept presentation, cognition is defined as *the mental action or process of acquiring knowledge and understanding through thought, experience, and the senses*.[3] Six domains of cognitive function include perceptual motor function, language, learning and memory, social cognition, complex attention, and executive function.[4] Three related terms—perception, memory, and executive function—are also described here for further clarification. *Perception* is the interpretation of the environment and is dependent on the acuity of sensory input. A related construct is awareness or consciousness, which refers to the ability to perceive or be sensitive to stimuli in the environment and respond to them. Attention is a focus on a particular area of conscious content. It implies selection as well as the ability to direct cognitive effort.[2]

Memory broadly refers to the retention and recall of past experiences and learning. It is not a single, unified mental ability but rather a series of different neural subsystems, each of which has a unique localization in the brain. These different subsystems support different types of memory—namely declarative episodic memory, declarative semantic memory, immediate memory, working memory, and procedural memory. Declarative memory refers to the ability to consciously learn and recall information. When the information relates to specific events, the terminology used is declarative episodic memory. This is distinct from declarative semantic memory, which refers to memory of knowledge, words, and facts.[5] Declarative memory provides for long-term storage of large amounts of information. Immediate memory or "attention span" allows memory of very small amounts of information, such as a series of six or seven digits, for a very short time.[5] Working memory allows a small amount of information (approximately four chunks or meaningful units) to be actively maintained and manipulated for a short period of time. Procedural memory refers to the retention and retrieval of motor skills. It requires extensive training and provides for long-term storage of a moderate amount of information. Related to memory is visuospatial cognition, which is the capacity to comprehend, retain, and use visual representations and their spatial relationships.[6]

Executive function refers to the higher thinking processes that allow for flexibility, adaptability, and goal directedness. Executive function determines the contents of consciousness, supervises voluntary activity, and is future-oriented.[2]

SCOPE

At the most basic level, cognition may be described as intact or impaired. Intact cognition means that an individual exhibits cognitive behaviors that are considered to be within the range of normal for age and culture. The scope of cognition is shown on a continuum because the level of cognition is not a matter of "all or none"; it can change over time, and if cognitive impairment is present, the degree of impairment can be mild to severe (Fig. 33.1).

Higher-order cognitive function is characterized by learning, comprehension, insight problem solving, reasoning, decision making, creativity, and metacognition. Basic cognitive functioning includes perception, pattern recognition, and attention. Impaired cognition signifies an observable or measurable disturbance in one or more of the cognitive processes resulting from an abnormality within the brain or a factor interfering with normal brain function.

Among individuals with impaired cognition, there is variability related to the degree of impairment because of a number of influencing variables. In addition to considering the degree of impairment, cognitive changes can also be considered from a time perspective—that is, a temporary state or a chronic (permanent) state. Depending on the underlying cause, chronic states of impaired cognition can remain stable or can be associated with steady decline over time.

Higher Order Cognitive Function   Basic Order Cognitive Function   Cognitive Impairment
Mild - Moderate - Severe

FIGURE 33.1 Scope of Cognition Ranges From Higher-Order Cognitive Functioning to Cognitive Impairment.

NORMAL PHYSIOLOGIC PROCESS

One of the most distinctive features of humans, compared with other forms of life, is advanced cognitive abilities. In the absence of injury or disease, cognitive development occurs throughout life, with the most significant changes from infancy through adolescence. Less dramatic development and maintenance of cognition occurs during adulthood.

There are four major units of the human brain: cerebrum, diencephalon, brain stem, and cerebellum (Fig. 33.2A). The brain is responsible for multiple processes, including those that involve purposeful thought and responses and those that are automated and occur without purposeful thought (e.g., breathing, heart rate, reflexes, hormonal control, temperature regulation, and sensory regulation).

Most cognitive tasks occur in the cerebrum, which is divided into two hemispheres (right and left); each hemisphere has four lobes (frontal lobe, parietal lobe, temporal lobe, and occipital lobe) (see Fig. 33.2B). Another key area of the brain that supports cognitive processing is the limbic system, which is a structure that overlaps the cerebrum and diencephalon. The ability to reason, function intellectually, express personality, and purposefully interact with the external environment is a result of a highly advanced brain. The cerebral cortex is primarily responsible for carrying out such functions, in which highly sophisticated neurons and neurotransmitters deliver information through complex networks. The brain is continually involved in receiving internal and external data signals. These signals are integrated and interpreted, which then triggers a sensory or motor response. This process is continuous and automatic.

Cognitive thought requires the ability to take in data signals and actively think about (integrate) and act on the information. Data signals that represent important information are transferred to memory. The hippocampus (a part of the limbic system) plays a significant role in committing information to long-term memory. Anatomic areas that have been identified as playing a key role in specific cognitive functions are presented in Table 33.1.[2,7] Optimal brain function depends on the continuous perfusion of oxygenated and nutrient-rich blood. Decreases in oxygen and glucose supply, as well as electrolyte and acid–base imbalances, significantly impair cognitive function.

Age-Related Differences
Infants and Children

Significant cognitive development occurs during infancy and childhood. Although the brain stem and spinal cord are fully developed (and needed to sustain extrauterine life), the limbic system and cerebral cortex are in undeveloped states at birth. Thus newborn infant behavior (e.g.,

TABLE 33.1   Cognitive Function and Associated Anatomic Location in the Brain

Cognitive Function	Anatomic Location
Memory	
Declarative episodic memory	Hippocampus, medial thalamus
Declarative semantic memory	Temporoparietal association cortices
Immediate memory/attention	Primary auditory or visual cortex
Working memory	Lateral frontal cortex
Procedural memory	Basal ganglia, association neocortices
Language	
Receptive language function	Auditory association areas: posterior superior temporoparietal supramarginal gyrus
Expressive language function	Lateral inferior posterior frontal lobes
Visuospatial Cognition	
	Occipital lobe, inferior temporal and posterior parietal lobes
Executive Function	
	Network of brain regions anchored by prefrontal and anterior lobe neocortex

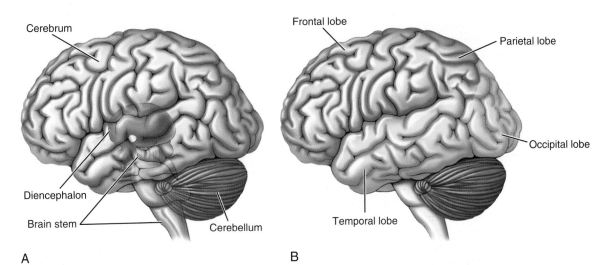

FIGURE 33.2 Brain Structures. (A) Four main areas of the brain. (B) Lobes of the cerebrum. (Modified from Herlihy, B. [2014]. *The human body in health and illness* [5th ed.]. St Louis: Saunders.)

sleeping, crying, feeding, sucking, kicking, and other reflexive behaviors) is controlled by the lower brain. The process of cognitive development from infancy throughout childhood has been described by many—perhaps most notable is Piaget.[8] According to Piaget, cognitive development is an orderly and sequential process that occurs in four stages: sensorimotor (birth to age 2 years), preoperational (ages 2 to 7 years), concrete operational (ages 7 to 11 years), and formal operational (age 11 years and older). (Piaget's theory of cognitive development is presented in Concept 1, Development.)

From a physiologic perspective, three primary changes occur that influence the developing brain: increase in brain mass, neuronal-synaptic connections, and myelination. The growth of the brain and development of cognitive processing occur throughout infancy and childhood. The brain itself triples in weight during the first year, representing the single greatest change in brain size after birth. Along with an increase in brain mass, the number of neurons in the brain increases until approximately age 2 years. A massive explosion of neuronal-synaptic connections develops after birth and continues throughout childhood and adolescence, fueling the progression of cognitive developmental milestones. The connections occur in different regions of the cerebral cortex (e.g., sensory cortex, temporal lobes, and frontal lobes) during this time, which explains the various milestone achievements typically seen at different stages of development. Another physiologic change is myelination of the neurons. Myelination occurs with the formation of a myelin sheath around nerve fibers needed for efficient neurotransmission of signals between neurons within the brain. This has a direct impact on cognitive development. Although infants are born with very little myelination, the process of myelination occurs throughout childhood and continues well into young adulthood, allowing for more complex or advanced thought with aging.

Older Adults

The size and weight of the brain and number of neurons decrease with aging. The reduction in and atrophy of neurons results in less efficient neurotransmission and a slowing of neural responses. However, these normal physiologic changes with aging are not necessarily associated with a loss of cognitive function. In other words, cognitive impairment or intellectual loss is not a part of normal aging; rather, it is indicative of disease.[7] Throughout life, humans have the ability to continue to learn. The ability to retain cognitive function is often associated with brain "exercise"—meaning that regular purposeful thought is correlated to cognitive function, particularly among the oldest of older adults. A decline in memory is associated with aging, but the extent and degree are highly variable. Committing new information (particularly complex information) to memory is less efficient in older adults, but the majority of memory functioning remains intact.[9] This is especially true when older adults are in familiar situations and doing things they have done before.

VARIATIONS AND CONTEXT

Cognitive impairment refers to deficits in intellectual functioning. It is estimated that more than 16 million people in the United States have some degree of cognitive impairment.[10] A wide range of categories for cognitive impairment exists. For the purposes of this concept presentation, the following categories are used: delirium, neurocognitive disorders (NCDs), cognitive impairment (not dementia), focal cognitive disorders, intellectual disabilities, and learning disabilities (Fig. 33.3).

Delirium

Delirium is a state of disturbed consciousness and altered cognition with a rapid onset occurring over hours or a few days. During a delirious state, the individual experiences a dulled awareness of the environment

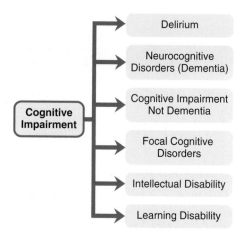

FIGURE 33.3 Categories of Cognitive Impairment.

and a reduced ability to focus, sustain, and shift attention. Memory and judgment are impaired, and disorientation may occur. Speech is rapid, rambling, and/or incoherent. Sudden, intense emotional swings, hallucinations, vivid dreams, and delusions may also occur. Restlessness is common, although in some cases activity may be reduced.

Delirium is the most frequent complication of hospitalization in the elderly population. A number of underlying conditions can lead to delirium such as dehydration, electrolyte imbalances, fever, hypoxia, sleep deprivation, adverse effect of medications, and illicit drug use, to name a few. It may also be the initial symptom of life-threatening problems such as pneumonia, urosepsis, or myocardial infarction. Delirium is usually reversible with prompt treatment of the underlying problem and management of related predisposing factors.[11,12]

Neurocognitive Disorders

NCDs refer to a group of disorders better known as dementia. The commonality within these disorders is an acquired and progressive deterioration of all cognitive functions (with little or no disturbance of consciousness or perception), including impairment in memory, judgment, calculation ability, attention span, and abstract thinking. These impairments develop over a period of months to years. Primary dementia is irreversible and not secondary to another disease. Secondary dementia occurs as a result of another disease process.[12] It has long been known that the incidence of dementia is associated with advanced age. However, the prevalence of dementia among older adults over age 65 declined from 11.6% to 8.8% between 2000 and 2012, possibly associated with increased educational attainment.[13]

There are many types of dementia that are classified as etiologic subtypes of NCDs.[4] These subtypes include Alzheimer disease (AD), Parkinson disease, human immunodeficiency virus (HIV) infection, frontotemporal, Lewy body type, traumatic brain injury, vascular, substance induced, Huntington disease, prion disease, and other medical conditions. Each of these subtypes is classified as major or minor, depending on the degree of cognitive decline and functional ability.[4]

Cognitive Impairment, Not Dementia

Individuals with mild cognitive impairment, also known as cognitive impairment, not dementia (CIND), demonstrate a greater reduction of cognitive function than expected for an individual's age and education, but it does not interfere with functional ability. This is in itself not a medical diagnosis but rather a recognized state between normal cognitive function and true cognitive impairment. Individuals with mild cognitive impairment are at higher risk of progressing to dementia compared to the general population.[14,15]

Focal Cognitive Disorders

Focal cognitive disorders, unlike delirium and dementia, affect a single area of cognitive function. The area involved may be memory, language, visuospatial ability, or executive function.[7] These disorders may be associated with an NCD or may be seen independently. For example, one focal cognitive disorder involving memory is an amnestic disorder characterized by a significant decline in the ability to learn and recall new information and to recall previously learned material. This leads to impaired social and occupational function.[12]

Intellectual Disability

Intellectual disability refers to limitations of cognitive functioning and below-average intelligence (IQ score <70), in addition to limitations in conceptual skills, social skills, and activities of daily living.[16] Intellectual disability differs from NCDs in that the cognitive processing never fully develops and the symptoms are identified before age 18 years. Intellectual disability is described as mild (IQ scores of 55 to 70, representing 85% of the population with intellectual disability), moderate (IQ scores of 40 to 55, representing 10% of the population with intellectual disability), severe (IQ scores of 25 to 40), or profound (IQ scores <25).[17] Common intellectual disabilities include chromosomal abnormalities (e.g., Down syndrome), genetic/inherited conditions (e.g., fragile X syndrome and Tay-Sachs), and other conditions that damage the developing brain (e.g., exposure to toxins, malnourishment, and cerebral anoxia).

Learning Disability

Learning disabilities represent another category of impaired cognition. Often identified during childhood, there exists a challenge in taking data signals in and then processing the information received. Learning disorders occur among individuals having average or above-average intelligence, which is an important distinction compared to intellectual disability. Like intellectual disabilities, the severity of impairment ranges from mild to profound and can involve one or more areas of learning, including speaking, listening, reading (skills and comprehension), writing, and mathematics (calculation and reasoning).[17]

CONSEQUENCES

The consequences of cognitive impairment can be devastating for the affected person and for family and friends. Cognitive impairment places an individual at significant risk for a number of adverse physical, psychological, and social outcomes. Individuals with cognitive impairment are at higher risk for injury due to falls (particularly those with dementia) and other injuries within the environment due to the lack of accurate perceptions, risk recognition, and/or lack of capacity for an appropriate response to dangerous situations. Impaired cognition also complicates disease management, making optimal health management a challenge.[12] Cognitive impairment is associated with a higher incidence of hospitalization and long-term care. Advanced forms of cognitive impairment affect functional ability, the patient's capacity for independent living, and normal social interaction. The need for assistive services can range from help with some of the instrumental activities of daily living to constant supervision and complete care. Financial hardship and caregiver burden can result.

RISK FACTORS

Preventative interventions aimed at modifiable risk factors and risk recognition are an essential strategy with cognitively impaired patients. Early identification of cognitive impairment is also essential. There are many different types of cognitive impairment and many causes of each, with a wide array of risk factors, not all of which apply to every case.

Populations at Risk

Individuals across all population groups are potentially at risk for developing cognitive impairment. Results of several studies indicate that a primary risk factor for cognitive impairment is advancing age.[14] Moreover, the primary age group at risk is the elderly population.[18] No differences in impairment have been found across populations based on race, ethnicity, or gender; however, correlated risk factors among women and men differ.

Significant risk factors found for women are overall poor health status, dependency, lack of social support, and insomnia. Risk factors specific to men include a history of stroke or diabetes.[14]

Although the primary population at risk is the elderly, a number of pediatric risk factors exist in prenatal, perinatal, and postnatal periods, including genetic syndromes, toxicity and metabolic conditions, maternal disease, events during labor leading to hypoxic ischemic injury, and brain malformation.[19]

Individual Risk Factors

Many individual risk factors are associated with impaired cognition. The most common factors are personal behaviors, environmental exposures, congenital or genetic conditions, and other health-related conditions.

Personal Behaviors

Personal behaviors that predispose to impaired cognition are those related to chemical exposure and risk of traumatic injury to the brain. Specific examples of high-risk behaviors include substance abuse (e.g., alcohol, amphetamines, cannabis, cocaine, hallucinogens, inhalants, opioids, phencyclidine, sedatives, hypnotics, and anxiolytics); participation in high-risk activities that could result in traumatic brain injury; and omission of basic safety measures, such as wearing a helmet (e.g., skiing, cycling, motorcycle riding, and rock climbing) or wearing a seat belt (or seat restraint for children) when riding in vehicles. Accidental injuries associated with work, recreation, or violence in the absence of high-risk behaviors can also lead to brain injury and cognitive impairment.

Environmental Exposures

Environmental exposures to toxic substances can negatively impair cognitive function. Despite changes in environmental regulations, lead exposure continues to be a problem due to the presence of lead in the soil and dust, as well as old lead-based paint. Lead exposure among young children is particularly concerning because the developing brain is especially vulnerable. Other chemical agents, such as pesticides, can also negatively impair cognitive function.[20]

Congenital and Genetic Conditions

The term congenital means "present at birth"; genetic conditions differ in that the genetic problem exists at birth, but the condition may or may not be present at birth, manifesting later in life. Many congenital and genetic conditions are associated with impaired cognition. Some are related to maternal conditions (e.g., fetal alcohol syndrome [FAS] or cocaine or methamphetamine exposure), and some are caused by birth injuries (e.g., cerebral palsy). Cognitive impairment also results from many chromosomal abnormalities (e.g., Down syndrome or fragile X syndrome) or other genetic conditions evident in infancy (e.g., phenylketonuria and galactosemia)[21] or those that emerge later in life (e.g., Huntington disease, in which mental deterioration begins typically in the fourth decade of life).

Physical Disability and Reduced Mobility

There appears to be a relationship between physical disability and a decline in cognitive function. In a study of older adults, Rajan and colleagues found that cognitive function declines faster following disability in basic and instrumental activities of daily living.[22] In fact, slow gait is considered a predictor of cognitive decline.[22–24]

Health Conditions

Many health conditions can lead to temporary or long-term impairments in cognition. Fluid and electrolyte imbalance, systemic or intracranial infection, fever, pain, hypoglycemia, and anoxia can cause delirium that is reversible with treatment of the precipitating cause. Stroke and intracranial tumor can cause irreversible long-term amnestic and other cognitive impairments. Many chronic conditions, such as cardiovascular disease,[25] chronic pulmonary disease, and depression, have also been found to be significant risk factors for cognitive impairment in both men and women. Individuals with type 2 diabetes have been shown to have cognitive impairment due to poor disease management.[26]

Changes in cognition may occur as an adverse effect of medical treatments and medications. This is a particular risk among the elderly population because of decreased physiologic reserve, decline in hepatic and renal function, altered metabolism, the presence of chronic disease, and multiple drug regimens. Psychoactive drugs are particularly notorious—these agents can cause delirium or cognitive decline. Examples include sedative-hypnotics (especially the long-acting benzodiazepines flurazepam and diazepam), narcotics (especially meperidine), anticholinergics (e.g., antihistamines, antispasmodics, heterocyclic antidepressants, neuroleptics, and antiparkinsonians), digitalis glycosides, antidysrhythmics (e.g., quinine and procainamide), and antihypertensives such as β-blockers. H_2-antagonists, nonsteroidal antiinflammatory drugs, corticosteroids, and anticonvulsants, as well as over-the-counter sleep aids, cold and sinus medications, and antinausea and acid reflux preparations, can also lead to changes in cognition. Chemotherapy, used to kill cancer cells, has been shown to impair normal brain function—a long-term consequence referred to as chemo-brain.[27]

ASSESSMENT

Characteristics of normal cognitive status vary with the individual's stage of development. In infants and young children, expected cognitive development is indicated by achievement of developmental milestones and tasks, with specialized age-appropriate tests of development used when indicated to determine developmental delays (see Concept 1, Development). During the remaining life span, identification of new problems with cognition relies primarily on routine observations by healthcare providers, patient self-report, and report of family or others.

History
Adults

Assessment of cognitive functioning occurs as part of the health history. It begins with assessment of consciousness because unless the patient is fully aware of self and the environment, other cognitive assessments may not be valid. The nurse observes the patient for wakefulness, alertness, and appropriate responses to introductions and to the environment as the health history interview is begun. The patient's speech pattern and content are noted, and memory, logic, and judgment are assessed while the interview progresses.[28] Questions related to cognition included in the interview relate to history of intracranial disease or trauma; substance abuse; use of medications that can impair cognition; environmental or occupational exposure to hazards such as lead or insecticides; the presence of symptoms such as difficulty in forming words or saying what

is meant, headache, behavior changes, or seizures suggestive of a brain disorder; unexplained emotional or behavioral changes; and any noticed change in memory or mental function. If any abnormalities are noted, a more specific cognitive assessment is performed. A family member who can assist with the history helps to provide greater understanding of the patient's cognitive level prior to hospitalization.

Infants and Children

Parents should be asked about prenatal and birth history, in addition to a three-generation family health history (to establish familial syndromes).[28] Intellectual disability may have an association with the pregnancy or birth process. Having an understanding of developmental tasks met and those not met provide helpful clues regarding impairment.

Examination

A mental status assessment forms the basis for cognitive assessment and includes general appearance, behavior, and cognitive functions.

General Appearance

Observation of general appearance often provides initial clues to an individual's cognitive functioning. The posture and body movements should be relaxed, coordinated, and smooth. Slumped posture, slow movements while walking, and dragging feet may be indicative of dementia. Observe the patient's dress and overall hygiene, and consider if it is appropriate for the weather, setting, gender, and age. Individuals with cognitive impairment may present with inappropriate dress and/or poor hygiene.

Behavior

Assess the level of consciousness. The expected finding is an individual who is awake, alert, and aware of the environment. Abnormal findings include lethargy, obtunded, stupor, or confusion.

Facial expressions should be appropriate and consistent with the situation. Flat expressions could be associated with dementia. Note the quality of speech. Expected findings include effortless conversation that is fluent, articulate, and of moderate pace. Individuals with impaired cognition may have trouble recalling words, blocking, distorted speech, disconnected sentences, or loose associations. Confabulation (the fabrication of events to fill in memory gaps) may also be demonstrated.

Assessment of Cognitive Function

Formal assessment of cognition goes further to include a test of orientation to person, place, and time and also attention, memory, judgment, insight, spatial perception, calculation, abstract reasoning, thought process, and content. Orientation is usually established during the course of the interview by asking the patient to state his or her name, provide date of birth, state address, etc. Typically, a patient is considered orientated if he or she is aware of the date, time, and location. The Mini-Mental State Exam (MMSE) is one of the most common standardized cognitive assessment tools used across care settings to screen for dementia and delirium, to detect cognitive impairment occurring during illness, and to monitor response to treatment. The test consists of 11 cognitive tasks that cover the categories of time orientation, place orientation, immediate recall, short-term memory recall, serial 7s, reading, writing, drawing, and verbal/motor comprehension. The test takes 5 to 10 minutes and is simple to administer. The lower the score (out of a total of 30), the more severe the impairment. Individuals who score less than 27 should be referred for further evaluation.[29] Another simple cognitive assessment tool for memory impairment is the Three Words Three Shapes test. It involves recall of three words written down by the patient followed by three shapes drawn by the patient. Kiral

BOX 33.1   Common Cognitive Assessment Tools

Global Cognitive Performance

- *Mini-Mental State Examination (MMSE)*: A 30-item, 10-minute questionnaire to measure cognitive impairment and progression of disease.
- *Severe Impairment Battery (SIB)*: Used with significantly cognitively impaired patients to assess lower levels of cognitive function; in other words, provides differentiating clarity among individuals who score less than 12 on the MMSE.

Executive Functioning

- *Controlled Oral Word Association Test (COWAT)*: Assesses ability to generate a list of as many words starting with a designated letter as possible in 1 min. Tests attention, thought process, judgment, aphasia and memory, ability to adhere to a set of rules to assess attention, thought process, and judgment.
- *Behavioral Dyscontrol Scale (BDS)*: Nine-item screening test to evaluate the capacity of an older adult related to independent functioning. The tool evaluates motor control processes and insight regarding accuracy of performance.

Motor Speed

- *Hand Tapping Test*: Used to evaluate motor speed and involves tapping the hands. Slowed tapping speed is associated with cognitive impairment.

Episodic Memory

- *Three Words Three Shapes Test*: Measures memory, recall, and recognition using verbal and nonverbal information.
- *Fuld Object Memory Evaluation*: Tests for recognition, memory, and learning in older adults. Ten objects in a bag are presented to individuals who are asked to identify the objects by touch (stereognosis) and then allowed to see if they were correct. After a few minutes, they are asked to recall the things in the bag.

Cognitive Impairment

- *Global Deterioration Rating Scale (GDRS)*: Behavioral rating scale assessment for three phases of cognitive impairment: forgetfulness, confusion, and dementia.

and colleagues found that use of the MMSE and Three Words Three Shapes test was effective for early detection of memory impairment among individuals in a community-based setting.[30] For delirium, a short screening test called the Confusion Assessment Method (CAM) (CAM-ICU for patients who are unable to speak as a result of intubation) is used.

Several assessment tools are available for use in clinical practice that assess various aspects of cognitive skills; some of these are listed in Box 33.1. Regardless of the tests used, adults should be able to evaluate and respond appropriately in situations requiring judgment; demonstrate a realistic insight into self; state the abstract meaning of a metaphor appropriate to their culture; and exhibit logical, coherent, and goal-directed thought processes based on reality.[31] Adults with normal cognition have an attention span and calculation ability adequate to complete a task such as counting backwards from 100 by subtracting 7 each time. Short-term memory allows functions such as repeating a list of three words after 5 minutes of another conversation. Long-term memory allows for correctly responding to questions about events occurring 24 hours or more in the past.

Adults with intact cognitive processes also exhibit spatial perception sufficient to allow copying of a simple shape without difficulty and identify right and left sides of the body. Observable behaviors associated with altered cognition have been well documented, named, and defined. Terms used to describe abnormal cognitive findings are presented in Table 33.2.[2,6] Cognitive assessment of infants and children also includes behavioral, cognitive, and psychosocial development. This is presented in Concept 1, Development.

Diagnostic Tests

There are no laboratory tests that diagnose cognitive impairment, although laboratory tests are critical in determining the presence of associated disease or contributing factors. For example, a laboratory test can detect an electrolyte imbalance, which may be the underlying cause associated with an acute state of confusion. Brain imaging techniques such as magnetic resonance imaging and positron emission tomography scans can identify some brain abnormalities such as intracranial tumors, infarcts associated with vascular dementia, and frontotemporal lobe atrophy. However, their usefulness is limited in the majority of cases of cognitive impairment. Formal neuropsychometric testing by a neuropsychologist is needed for the identification of mild cases of cognitive impairment. Such testing uses more detailed standardized tests of memory and advanced methods of determining visuospatial function, which can identify impairments missed by standard clinical evaluation tests.[6]

CLINICAL MANAGEMENT

Nursing practice has four major dimensions of concern relative to an individual's cognitive status: recognition of risk for impaired cognition, cognitive assessment, the planning and delivery of individualized care appropriate to level of cognitive ability, and evaluation of outcomes.

Primary Prevention

Promoting a healthy lifestyle—including optimal nutrition, exercise, social activity, regular medical care to prevent and/or manage chronic diseases, avoidance of substance abuse (especially during pregnancy), and other high-risk behaviors—through teaching and community programs is basic to prevention across the spectrum of cognitive impairment. It is essential for healthy pregnancies, growth and development into adulthood, healthy aging, and decreasing vulnerability to delirium and vascular dementia.

Genetic counseling is another primary prevention strategy related to risk for disorders characterized by impaired cognition. This ranges from pregnancy risks associated with advanced maternal age (e.g., Down syndrome) to available genetic testing for inherited disorders (e.g., Huntington disease) that could affect decisions about having children.

Primary prevention specific to delirium involves educating healthcare providers about changes in practice that can decrease vulnerability to the disorder. Practices that constitute risk factors for delirium, such as use of sleeping medications, use of urinary catheters, and immobilization, need to be identified along with alternative methods of care.

Secondary Prevention (Screening)

Secondary prevention, or screening, refers to periodic assessment of specified population groups to detect early onset of a condition. Several screening tests to assess cognitive function were presented in the Assessment Section and Box 33.1. According to the U.S. Preventive Services Task Force,[32] the current evidence is insufficient to recommend for or against routine screening of cognitive impairment in older adults. Likewise, no routine screening tests are recommended for early detection of intellectual disability.

TABLE 33.2   Common Cognitive Functional Abnormalities and Definitions

Cognitive Area	Abnormality	Definition
Memory	Anterograde amnesia	Loss of ability to learn and recall new information on an ongoing basis
	Retrograde amnesia	Impaired ability to retrieve information from the past
Language	Aphasia	Language impairment at the conceptual level; may have difficulty with production or comprehension of language or both
	Wernicke aphasia	Impaired comprehension of both written and verbal language, even understanding single words; speech fluent and person is unaware that words used are incorrect
	Broca aphasia	Impaired language expression characterized by nonfluent, labored speech; comprehension of language intact
	Global aphasia	Both language reception and expression are impaired
	Anomia	Impaired ability to name places or objects; may have difficulty with sentence repetition, although comprehension and expression abilities are basically intact
Visuospatial	Alexia	Impaired reading ability
	Agraphia	Inability to write
	Agnosia	Impaired ability to recognize objects or persons through sensory stimuli; may be visual, tactile, auditory, olfactory, or gustatory
	Object agnosia	Impaired ability to recognize visual forms
	Prosopagnosia	Impaired ability to recognize faces
	Simultanagnosia	Impaired ability to integrate complex visual scenes
	Apraxia	Inability to perform purposeful movements or manipulate objects, although sensory and motor ability is intact
	Constructional apraxia	Inability to reproduce figures on paper
	Ideomotor apraxia	Inability to translate an idea into action
	Hemispatial (unilateral) neglect	Inability to process and perceive stimuli on one side of the body or the environment despite intact senses; results in a deficit in attention and awareness to the affected side
Calculation	Dyscalculia	Inability to perform calculations correctly
Abstract reasoning	Conceptual concreteness	Inability to describe in abstractions, generalize, or apply principles
Thought process and content	Flight of ideas	Topic of speech changes within a sentence
	Confabulation	Making up answers without regard to facts
	Circumstantiality	Indirect speech characterized by countless details and explanations with resultant prolonged time to reach point
	Echolalia	Involuntary repetition of a word or sentence spoken by someone else
	Clanging	Use of meaningless, rhyming words
	Blocking	Unconscious interruption in the train of thought manifested as a sudden obstruction to the spontaneous flow of speech
	Pressured speech	Frantic, energetic, jumbled speech; speech trying to keep up with thoughts
	Word salad	Meaningless mixture of words or phrases

Collaborative Interventions

Cognition is a consideration in virtually all areas of health care and for all members of the healthcare team. It is a critical element in communicating with the patient and in the determination of care.[12] It is also critical to discharge planning from acute care facilities and is one determinant of need for home care services or placement in a long-term care facility.

The focus of treatment varies, depending on the underlying cause of the cognitive impairment. Clearly, the management of a child with intellectual disability differs from the focus of care for an older adult with dementia. In some cases the treatment of a precipitating trauma or disease is possible, but in many cases of cognitive impairment, the disease process is not well understood and no treatments or only treatments with limited effectiveness are available. However, several underlying principles apply to all individuals with intellectual impairment. For example, regardless of the cause, management of the patient with cognitive impairment involves a multidisciplinary effort. Depending on the type and cause of the impairment, one or more of the following services may be required: nursing, medicine, physical therapy, occupational therapy, psychological intervention, individual and/or family counseling, nutritional consulting, speech and language services, audiology services, home health or homemaker assistance community services such as day care, caregiver support groups, and assistive technologies.

General Management Strategies

Promoting adequate rest, sleep, fluid intake, nutrition, elimination, pain control, and comfort are essential elements of care for persons with cognitive impairment. Also of great importance is ensuring an appropriate level of environmental stimulation. Excessive stimulation can create agitation and confusion, whereas a lack of stimulation can result in sensory deprivation effects and withdrawal. If behavior is a problem, attempts should be made to identify and manage environmental triggers while avoiding the use of physical and pharmacologic restraints.[12]

Virtually all patients with cognitive impairment benefit from predictable routines, consistent caregivers, simple instructions, eye contact, and the presence of familiar people and objects. If needed, sensory aids such as eyeglasses and hearing aids should be used consistently to maximize accurate sensory input. To the extent possible, patients should be involved in self-care and decision making even if the latter is limited to deciding which of two shirts to wear or whether to drink milk or juice. Verbal reorientation to time and place should be provided if needed, and a clock and calendar should be within easy vision. For patients with delirium or who are otherwise agitated, a private room, soft music, relaxation tapes, or massage can be helpful.

Safety is a priority concern for all patients with cognitive impairment. Precise interventions needed vary with the person's age, developmental status, and degree of impairment. Patients should not drive, use machinery, or handle firearms, and the environment should be kept free of potential hazards. Supervision is generally needed with activities such as cooking or taking medications. If the patient wanders, an identification tag or bracelet should be worn or, if appropriate, a wander guard device should be used.

Pharmacologic Agents

In the management of patients with cognitive impairment, pharmacologic agents primarily treat associated diseases and control behavioral alterations such as sleeplessness, anxiety, agitation, and depression.[33] However, for patients with AD, pharmacologic therapy is aimed at maintaining cognitive function and slowing disease progression by regulating neurotransmitters in the brain. The two classes of drugs used in the treatment of AD are the cholinesterase inhibitors and a glutamate receptor antagonist. The three cholinesterase inhibitors approved by the U.S. Food and Drug Administration for the treatment of AD are donepezil (Aricept), rivastigmine (Exelon), and galantamine (Razadyne). All three of these drugs have been shown to help maintain memory, thinking, and speaking skills for a few months to a few years in *some* patients with mild to moderate AD; donepezil also is used in severe AD. The glutamate receptor antagonist memantine (Namenda) has been shown to delay functional decline in moderate to severe disease.[33]

Family and Caregiver Support

Engaging family members or significant others in goal setting and care planning is an essential component of care. Advanced planning is encouraged, and caregiver needs for education and support should be recognized and addressed. Information about support groups, respite options, day care, and other community services is provided. Parents of a child born with intellectual disability require a great deal of support, particularly when they learn their child will have lifelong special needs. Caregivers of individuals with intellectual disability and dementia should be referred to support groups and other community resources.

INTERRELATED CONCEPTS

Because cognition depends on the interplay of multiple elements within the physical, psychological, and social dimensions and because it allows for purposeful interaction with the environment, a multitude of concepts can be identified as influencing and/or being influenced by it. Fig. 33.4 depicts the most prominent of these interrelationships. The physiologically focused concepts of Glucose Regulation, Mobility, Nutrition, Gas Exchange, Perfusion, Intracranial Regulation, Fluid and Electrolytes, and Acid–Base Balance have a clearly reciprocal relationship with cognition. These concepts are represented in Fig. 33.4 by the ovals surrounding the upper half of the cognition conception and double-headed arrows because of their mutual interaction with it. The concepts of Functional Ability and Development are shown at the very bottom of the figure, with arrows pointing from cognition to them because of the primarily unidirectional relationship of these concepts.

CLINICAL EXEMPLARS

Exemplars of impaired cognition are classified into categories described previously in this chapter and include delirium, NCDs, focal cognitive disorders, intellectual disability, and learning disability; these are presented in Box 33.2. Although it is beyond the scope of this textbook to present each of these exemplars in detail, brief descriptions of the most important exemplars are featured here. Refer to other resources, particularly a pediatric and geriatric textbook, for a more comprehensive presentation of these conditions.

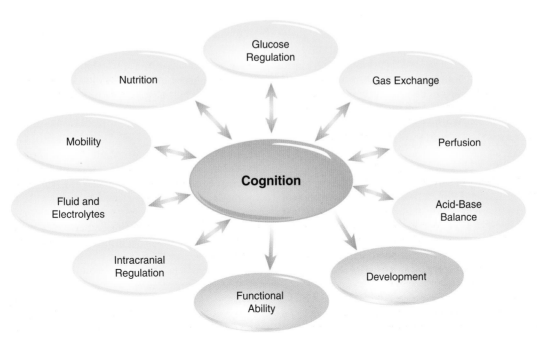

FIGURE 33.4 Cognition and Interrelated Concepts.

BOX 33.2   EXEMPLARS OF IMPAIRED COGNITION

Neurocognitive Disorders
- Alzheimer disease
- Vascular neurocognitive disorder (NCD)
- Frontotemporal NCD
- Lewy body dementia
- Parkinson disease
- Human immunodeficiency virus–associated NCD
- Huntington disease
- Prion disease
- Traumatic brain injury
- Substance-induced NCD
- NCD due to other medical conditions

Cognitive Impairment, Not Dementia
- Mild cognitive disorder
- Postconcussion syndrome

Focal Cognitive Disorders
- Amnesia
- Aphasia

Intellectual Disability
- Down syndrome
- Fragile X syndrome
- Prader-Willi syndrome
- Galactosemia
- Hunter syndrome
- Phenylketonuria
- Rett syndrome
- Tay-Sachs disease
- Fetal alcohol syndrome
- Congenital hypothyroidism

Learning Disability
- Dyslexia
- Dyscalculia
- Dysgraphia
- Dyspraxia

 ACCESS EXEMPLAR LINKS IN YOUR GIDDENS EBOOK

Featured Exemplars

Delirium

Delirium is a state of disturbed consciousness and altered cognition. Three categories of delirium exist: hyperactive delirium, hypoactive delirium, and mixed. Delirium is caused by a number of variables. Some of the most common causes include pharmacologic agents (particularly when four or more pharmacologic agents are given in combination), metabolic dysfunction, dehydration, electrolyte imbalance, hypoglycemia, renal impairment, urinary retention, fecal impaction, hypoxia, acute illness, infection, and trauma.

Alzheimer Disease

AD is the most common form of dementia among individuals older than age 65 years, and it is the sixth leading cause of death among adults aged 18 years or older. Estimates vary, but experts suggest that up to 5 million Americans aged 65 years or older have AD, and this number is expected to double by 2050.[34] It is thought that AD is caused by a combination of tau protein clumps that form inside neurons and amyloid plaques that form in spaces between brain cells, leading to neuronal dysfunction and death. Symptoms include a combination of deficits, including loss of memory, language skills, visual perception, focus, attention, reasoning skills, and functional ability.[4]

Lewy Body Dementia

The third most common form of dementia, Dementia with Lewy bodies (DLB), is a type of synucleinopathy characterized by the formation of balloon-like protein structures inside the neurons. Early symptoms, which can appear as long as a decade before dementia occurs, include loss of smell, visual hallucinations, and difficulty sleeping; these symptoms are often attributed to other causes. Once dementia occurs, symptoms of DLB are similar to those of AD, and parkinsonian signs and symptoms are often noted.

Vascular Dementia

Vascular dementia, also known as vascular cognitive impairment (VCI), is the second most common type of neurocognitive impairment. VCI results from damage to cerebral blood vessels; thus it represents a number of underlying conditions. Vessel damage can be associated with stroke or other conditions affecting the vasculature, such as diabetes, hypertension, and plaque formation from hyperlipidemia. Reduced or loss of perfusion leads to death of neurons affected. The risk for VCI parallels risk for stroke—in fact, stroke is the greatest risk factor. VCI has a higher mortality rate compared with AD because of the coexistence of underlying vascular disease; VCI is also associated with greater limitations in activities of daily living compared with AD.[35]

Fetal Alcohol Syndrome

FAS is a disorder that leads to intellectual disability and is estimated to affect 0.2 to 1.5 infants for every 1000 live births.[36] FAS is caused by maternal alcohol intake; because alcohol crosses the placenta, the fetus is exposed to alcohol and this can lead to disruption of fetal development. Children with FAS have growth deficits, distinctive facial features, and central nervous system (CNS) abnormalities. Because alcohol affects CNS development, individuals with FAS often have problems with one or more of the following: learning, memory, attention, communication, vision, and hearing.

Down Syndrome

Down syndrome is the most common type of chromosomal abnormality. Down syndrome is usually caused by an extra chromosome 21 (referred to as trisomy 21), although in a few cases it may be caused by translocation of chromosomes 15, 21, or 22. The distinctive features of Down syndrome lead to identification and diagnosis at birth. This condition is associated with intellectual disability (ranging in severity from mild to profound) and many other physical conditions, especially congenital heart malformations. The prevalence of Down syndrome is approximately 1 in 700 births; with a sharp rise as the mother's age increases, particularly after age 35 years.[37]

CASE STUDY

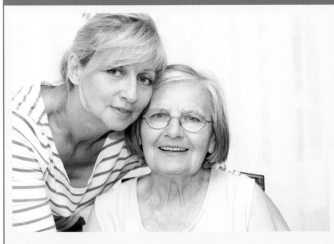

Case Presentation

As part of a community health awareness event, a community health nurse has presented a program on problems associated with aging and their management; the nurse is available for meetings with individuals who have questions or concerns. One of the persons requesting a meeting was a middle-aged woman named Karen, who expressed concern regarding her mother's condition and asked for guidance. Karen explained that her 79-year-old mother, Ruby Long, lives with Karen and has become increasingly difficult to manage during the past 8 to 10 months. Karen states that her mother has become lax in her hygiene, is

very forgetful of details of recent events, seems to be focused only on herself and unconcerned with anyone else's needs, is unwilling to try new things or go new places, and has lost interest in activities that she formally enjoyed. Karen also tells the nurse that her mother sometimes makes what appear to be poor decisions, has trouble managing money, and becomes very upset if any mistakes are mentioned. Upon further questioning, the nurse learns that Ruby Long has hypertension (for which she takes a diuretic), osteoporosis, and has spinal stenosis which often causes back pain. She wears eyeglasses (last eye exam 2 years ago) and has difficulty hearing (but does not use a hearing aid). Ruby has a family physician; her last visit was approximately 1 year ago. Karen tells the nurse that her grandparents and two aunts on her mother's side had dementia, although she is not exactly sure exactly what caused dementia in her relatives.

The nurse encourages Karen to arrange for Ruby to have a complete physical examination to rule out a physical cause of the behaviors and to determine the presence of any comorbidities, including a hearing and vision examination (to determine if the observed problems are resulting from changes in sensory perception). The nurse stresses the importance of maintaining a safe environment for Ruby.

Case Analysis Questions

1. What risk factors for impaired cognition are present for Ruby Long?
2. Consider the scope of cognition. Based on what you know from the case, where does Ruby Long fit on the continuum?
3. Consider the suggestions made by the nurse. What else might be offered to Karen?

From BakiBG/iStock/Thinkstock.

ACCESS EXEMPLAR LINKS IN YOUR GIDDENS EBOOK

REFERENCES

1. Wiley, J., & Jee, B. D. (2011). Cognition: Overview and recent trends. In V. G. Aukrust (Ed.), *Learning and cognition in education*. New York: Academic Press.
2. Baars, B. J., & Gage, N. M. (2010). *Cognition, brain and consciousness: Introduction to cognitive neuroscience* (2nd ed.). New York: Academic Press.
3. Oxford Dictionaries. (2018). *Cognition*. Retrieved from http://www.oxforddictionaries.com/us/definition/american_english/cognition.
4. American Psychiatric Association. (2013). *Diagnostic and statistical manual of mental disorders* (5th ed.). Arlington, VA: American Psychiatric Publishing.
5. Magnussen, S., & Brennan, T. (2010). Memory. In B. J. Baars & N. M. Gage (Eds.), *Cognition, brain and consciousness. Introduction to cognitive neuroscience* (2nd ed.). New York: Academic Press.
6. Aminoff, M. J. (2008). Regional cerebral dysfunction: Higher mental functions. In L. Goldman & D. Ausiello (Eds.), *Cecil medicine* (23rd ed., pp. 2262–2266). Philadelphia: Saunders.
7. Goldman, L., & Schafer, M. (Eds.), (2016). *Cecil medicine* (25th ed.). Philadelphia: Elsevier.
8. Piget, J. (1969). *The theory of stages in cognitive development*. New York: McGraw-Hill.
9. Perrot, A., Bherer, L., & Messier, J. (2012). Preserved special memory for reaching to remembered three-dimensional targets in aging. *Experimental Aging Research*, 38(5), 511–536.
10. Centers for Disease Control and Prevention. (2011). *Cognitive impairment: A call for action, now!* Retrieved from http://www.cdc.gov/aging/pdf/cognitive_impairment/cogImp_poilicy_final.pdf.
11. Inouye, S. K. (2012). Delirium and other mental status problems in the older patient. In L. Goldman & M. Schafer (Eds.), *Cecil medicine* (24th ed.). Philadelphia: Saunders.
12. Halter, M. J. (2018). *Varcarolis' foundations of psychiatric mental health nursing: A clinical approach* (8th ed.). Philadelphia: Saunders.
13. Langa, K. M., Larson, E. B., Crimmins, E. M., et al. (2017). A comparison of the prevalence of dementia in the United States in 2000 and 2012. *JAMA Internal Medicine*, 177(1), 51–58.
14. Plassman, B., Langa, K., McCammon, R., et al. (2011). Incidence of dementia and cognitive impairment, not dementia in the United States. *Annals of Neurology*, 70(3), 418–426.
15. Hugo, J., & Ganguli, M. (2014). Dementia and cognitive impairment: Epidemiology, diagnosis and treatment. *Clinics in Geriatric Medicine*, 30(3), 421–442.
16. Mefford, H. C., Batshaw, M. L., & Hoffman, E. P. (2012). Genomics, intellectual disability and autism. *The New England Journal of Medicine*, 366(8), 733–743.
17. Learning Disabilities Association. (2018). *Types of learning disabilities*. Retrieved from https://ldaamerica.org/types-of-learning-disabilities/.
18. Davey, A., Dai, T., & Woodard, J. (2013). Profiles of cognitive function in a population-based sample of centenarians using factor mixed analysis. *Experimental Aging Research*, 39(2), 125–144.
19. Schofield, D. W. (2016). *Cognitive deficits: Overview, diagnosis, risk factors, and etiology*. Retrieved from https://emedicine.medscape.com/article/917629-overview.
20. Yan, D., Zhang, Y., Lie, L., & Yan, H. (2016). Pesticide exposure and risk of Alzheimer's disease: A systematic review and meta-analysis. *Scientific Reports*, 6, doi:10.1038/srep32222. Retrieved from https://www.nature.com/articles/srep32222.pdf.
21. Hockenberry, M. J., Rodgers, C., & Wilson, D. W. (2017). *Wong's essentials of pediatric nursing* (10th ed.). St Louis: Elsevier.

22. Rajan, K. B., Hebert, L. E., Scherr, P. A., et al. (2013). Disability in basic and instrumental activities of daily living is associated with faster rate of decline in cognitive function of older adults. *The Journals of Gerontology. Series A, Biological Sciences and Medical Sciences, 68*(5), 624–630.

23. Mielke, M., Roberts, R., Savica, R., et al. (2013). Assessing the temporal relationship between cognition and gait: Slow gait predicts cognitive decline in the Mayo Clinic study of aging. *The Journals of Gerontology. Series A, Biological Sciences and Medical Sciences, 68*(8), 929–937.

24. Holtzer, R., Wang, C., Lipton, R., et al. (2012). The protective effects of executive functions and episodic memory on gait speed decline in aging defined in the context of cognitive reserve. *Journal of the American Geriatrics Society, 60*(11), 2093–2098.

25. Ganguli, M., Fu, B., Snitz, B. E., et al. (2013). Mild cognitive impairment: Incidence and vascular risk factors in a population-based cohort. *Neurology, 80*(23), 2112–2120.

26. Tran, D., Baxter, J., Hamman, R. F., et al. (2014). Impairment of executive cognitive control in type 2 diabetes, and its effects on health-related behavior and use of health services. *Journal of Behavioral Medicine, 37*(3), 414–422.

27. Mayo Clinic. (n.d.). *Chemo brain.* Retrieved from http://www.mayoclinic.org/diseases-conditions/chemo-brain/basics/definition/con-20033864.

28. Wilson, S., & Giddens, J. (2017). *Health assessment for nursing practice* (6th ed.). St Louis: Elsevier.

29. Creavin, S. T., et al. (2016). *Mini-mental State Examination for the detection of dementia in people aged over 65.* Cochrane. Retrieved from http://www.cochrane.org/CD011145/DEMENTIA_mini-mental-state-examination-mmse-detection-dementia-people-aged-over-65.

30. Kiral, K., Ozge, A., Sungur, M., et al. (2013). Detection of memory impairment in a community-based system: A collaborative study. *Health and Social Work, 38*(2), 89–96.

31. Lin, J., O'Connor, E., Rossom, R., et al. (2013). Screening for cognitive impairment in older adults: A systematic review for the U.S. Preventative Services Task Force. *Annals of Internal Medicine, 159*(9), 601–612.

32. U.S. Preventive Services Task Force. (2014). *Cognitive impairment in older adults: Screening.* Retrieved from http://www.uspreventiveservicestaskforce.org/Page/Topic/recommendation-summary/cognitive-impairment-in-older-adults-screening?ds=1&s=.

33. Lewis, S. (2017). Dementia and Delirium. In S. Lewis, et al. (Eds.), *Medical surgical nursing: Assessment and management of clinical problems* (10th ed.). St Louis: Elsevier.

34. National Institutes of Health. (2017). *The dementias: Hope through research,* NIH Publication No. 17-NS-2252. Retrieved from https://catalog.ninds.nih.gov/pubstatic//17-NS-2252/17-NS-2252.pdf.

35. Gure, T. R., Kabeto, M. U., Plassman, B. L., et al. (2010). Differences in functional impairment across subtypes of dementia. *The Journals of Gerontology. Series A, Biological Sciences and Medical Sciences, 65A*(4), 434–441.

36. Centers for Disease Control and Prevention. (2017). *Fetal alcohol spectrum disorders (FASDs).* Retrieved from http://www.cdc.gov/ncbddd/fasd/index.html.

37. Centers for Disease Control and Prevention. (2017). *Down syndrome: Data and statistics.* Retrieved from http://www.cdc.gov/ncbddd/birthdefects/downsyndrome/data.html.

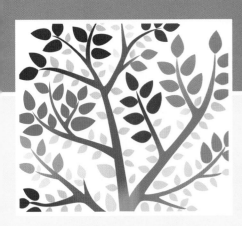

Psychosis

Sean P. Convoy

M uch like many other psychiatric experiences, psychosis has been misjudged, misunderstood, and mislabeled for centuries. Society's relative lack of understanding of psychosis produces rich soil from which stigma and social injustice have traditionally grown. The purpose of this concept presentation is to introduce the basic elements of psychosis for application into nursing practice, with a secondary intent to strip away commonly held misperceptions and illuminate the evidence so that the nurse is better able to understand psychosis and those it affects.

DEFINITION

Although psychosis has not appreciably changed over the centuries, human understanding and subsequent definition of it have changed considerably. One of the oldest medical references, published in 1500 BC, the Egyptian Ebers Papyrus, spoke generally to what would later be referred to as psychosis in a chapter titled "The Book of Hearts," crudely defining it as a "madness" born of "poison, demons, fecal matter and blood trouble."[1] During the Middle Ages, the treatment of those with psychosis was undistinguished from that of criminals, commonly involving physical punishment and torture. When torture did not "cure" the psychosis, witchcraft was then conveniently suspected.[2]

The term *psychosis* was formally coined in 1845 and synonymously linked with terms such as *mental handicap* and *psychopathy*.[3] Although the present-day understanding and tolerance of psychosis have unquestionably improved, society's persisting fear and misunderstanding of it continue to complicate an already complex condition.

The *Diagnostic and Statistical Manual of Mental Disorders*, fifth edition (DSM-5), currently defines psychosis as abnormalities in five different symptomatic domains: delusions, hallucinations, disorganized thought, disorganized or abnormal motor behavior, and negative symptoms.[4] A psychobiological definition of psychosis would implicate dopamine and glutamate dysregulation between the limbic system and prefrontal cortex. Stephen Stahl defines psychosis as a syndrome associated with many different disorders in which a "person's mental capacity, affective response, and capacity to recognize reality, communicate, and relate to others is impaired."[5] Each definition provides a unique but arguably incomplete description of this complex state. For the purpose of this concept presentation, *psychosis* is defined as *a syndrome of neurocognitive symptoms that impairs cognitive capacity, leading to deficits of perception, functioning, and social relatedness.*

SCOPE

The scope of psychosis exists along a continuum ranging from absence of psychosis to severe psychosis (Fig. 34.1). Between the extremes there exists a line of demarcation where the symptoms are of a sufficient intensity, duration, and degree of functional impairment to be considered clinically significant. Symptoms that exist below this threshold are consequently referred to as subclinical. Like most health states, psychosis is not static. Rather, psychosis is best conceptualized in the form of a distinct episode of clinically significant symptoms. The frequency of psychotic episodes is contingent on the etiology of the psychosis. Psychosis can be acute in onset and relatively short in duration, as can be seen with a delirium or substance-induced psychotic episode. Likewise, psychosis can be chronic, as can be seen with schizophrenia or schizoaffective disorder.

NORMAL PHYSIOLOGIC PROCESS

Under no circumstances should the symptoms associated with psychosis be considered "normal" or acceptable. Regardless of etiology, the duration of untreated psychosis is associated with poor outcomes.[6]

Normal physiology is defined by the absence (or reduced number) of vulnerability gene mutations that influence the development of critical neural pathways in the brain. In other words, in the absence of critical gene variations, the critical neural circuits in the brain develop and mature. Thus the brain is better able to regulate dopamine, leading to optimal dopaminergic neurotransmission between critical neural circuits that span the distance between the limbic system and prefrontal cortex.[7] The normal regulation of dopamine within the mesocortical and mesolimbic pathways of the brain would reflect the absence of psychosis.

VARIATIONS AND CONTEXT

Etiologies of Psychosis

Psychosis can manifest from varied etiologies and can be categorized as either primary or secondary in origin.[8] *Primary* psychosis has a psychiatric etiology, as can be seen in schizophrenia, schizoaffective disorder, and, in some instances, other psychiatric illnesses. *Secondary* psychosis has an organic etiology, as can be seen in acute substance intoxication, delirium, or dementia. Primary and secondary forms of psychosis are not mutually exclusive; not only do they coexist but, in some instances, they can also potentiate one another. Absent a primary source of

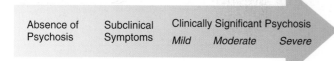

FIGURE 34.1 Scope of Concept. The concept of psychosis ranges from an absence of psychosis to severe psychosis.

psychosis, individuals who manifest secondary psychosis have greater potential to recover from a psychotic episode without clinically significant sequelae. Those with a primary etiology of psychosis are more likely to manifest subsequent episodes of psychosis due to the predisposing genomic variations and subsequent compromises of the neural circuit that subsume the condition.

Primary Psychosis

Schizophrenia spectrum and other psychotic disorders. Within the classification of "Schizophrenia Spectrum and Other Psychotic Disorders," psychosis is the principal symptom of interest. Clinical disorders in this category include delusional disorder, schizophreniform disorder, schizophrenia, schizoaffective disorder, catatonia, and brief psychotic disorder.[4] Under the heading of brief psychotic disorder, there are specifiers associated with postpartum onset. As a primary etiology of psychosis, the schizophrenia spectrum and other psychotic disorders reflect greater potential for long-term disability due to their genomic and neurodevelopmental etiology. Schizophrenia is a diagnosis of exclusion in that all other possible (typically medical) explanations must first be ruled out.

Other psychiatric illnesses. Other psychiatric illnesses can also manifest psychotic symptoms or episodes. Disorders such as bipolar I disorder and major depressive disorder have the potential to manifest symptoms of psychosis.[4] More than half of those diagnosed with bipolar disorder will experience psychosis at some time in their lives.[9] Psychosis associated with bipolar disorder is commonly an acute presentation that has potential to subside but is commonly associated with poor outcomes.[10] Among the depressive disorders, psychosis is exclusively associated with the most severe expressions of clinical depression and occurs in 14% to 20% of those who are clinically depressed.[11] Psychotic episodes that manifest in the context of a depressive disorder are more commonly acute in presentation and typically have high rates of recovery with treatment.

Psychotic symptoms are not explicitly seen within the personality disorders. However, personality disorders can be comorbid with a number of conditions that have the potential to manifest psychosis. For example, personality disorders have a 13.4% comorbidity rate with major depressive disorders, 8.1% with bipolar spectrum disorders, 10.9% with alcohol use disorder, and 5.6% with substance use disorders.[12] Consequently the presentation of psychosis (e.g., acute or chronic) is typically dependent on the comorbid condition and not the personality disorder.

Secondary Psychosis

Toxic psychosis. Toxic psychosis is the product of an underlying and untreated medical issue. Delirium is an example of toxic psychosis. Psychosis associated with delirium is typically rapid in onset and defined by a hallmark sign of dramatic fluctuations in mental status. Between 10% and 30% of medically ill inpatients and 80% of terminally ill patients exhibit delirium.[7] Medically treating a secondary source of psychosis as one would a primary source of psychosis will not resolve

the psychosis and actually increases the relative risk that the underlying medical illness will further deteriorate. Provided that the healthcare team isolates and treats the underlying medical issue, there is a reasonable expectation of complete resolution of the psychosis.

Dementia. Dementia is one of many neurocognitive disorders that have potential to manifest psychosis. Dementia can be the product of multiple etiologies, including Alzheimer disease, the presence of Lewy bodies, vascular disorders, HIV, prion disease, Parkinson disease, traumatic brain injury, and Huntington disease.[4] A slow but progressive manifestation of psychotic symptoms within the context of a suspected neurocognitive disorder is more consistent with a dementing condition and requires specialty consultation.

Medical illness. Numerous medical conditions can, given the right circumstances, manifest symptoms of psychosis. Patients can manifest psychosis secondary to endocrinopathies (e.g., adrenal or thyroid disorders), metabolic disorders (e.g., porphyria and Wilson disease), nutritional and vitamin deficiencies (e.g., vitamins A, D, and B_{12}; magnesium and zinc deficiencies), central nervous system disorders (e.g., cerebrovascular accident, epilepsy, and hydrocephalus), degenerative disorders (e.g., Friedreich ataxia), autoimmune disorders (e.g., multiple sclerosis and paraneoplastic syndrome), infections (e.g., encephalitis, neurosyphilis, Lyme disease, and sarcoidosis), space-occupying lesions (e.g., congenital vascular malformations and tuberous sclerosis), and chromosomal abnormalities (e.g., Klinefelter and fragile X syndromes).[8] When recognized, this secondary source of psychosis will commonly be classified as a Psychotic Disorder Due to Another Medical Condition. Owing to the diverse etiologies, the presentation of psychosis is varied in expression but more commonly resolves in accordance with the associated illness state.

Toxins, drugs, and medications. Psychosis can also be a product of numerous toxins, drugs, and medications. This form of psychotic expression is typically most challenging to identify causally. When recognized, this secondary source of psychosis will commonly be classified as a Substance/Medication-Induced Psychotic Disorder.[4] Toxins known to potentially induce psychosis include but are not limited to carbon monoxide, organophosphates, and heavy metals such as arsenic, magnesium, mercury, and thallium.[8] Possible drugs that can induce psychosis include synthetic cannabis (or Spice), synthetic cathinones (or bath salts), alcohol, cocaine, methamphetamine (or crystal meth), psychotomimetic drugs (or LSD), cannabis (or marijuana), and anabolic steroids. Likewise, certain prescribed medications also demonstrate an elevated risk for psychosis as a side effect, including sedative-hypnotic agents, amphetamines, anticholinergic agents, antiseizure agents, corticosteroids, and mefloquine. Depending on the substance used, psychosis can potentially go unrecognized and consequently be insufficiently treated. Unless the patient has a preexisting psychotic condition, psychosis that manifests within the context of a toxin or substance will typically be acute in onset with a high rate of recovery after the substance has been eliminated from the system.

Symptomatic Variations of Psychosis

The presence of psychosis suggests progressively compromised neural circuits. Psychiatric (or primary) etiologies of psychosis typically reflect epigenetically mediated compromise of the neural circuit long before symptoms eclipse the clinical threshold. Some secondary causes of psychosis (e.g., those caused by drugs, toxins, and medical illness) are not necessarily associated with a progressive compromise of the neural circuit; hence we can see variations in symptoms.

A number of symptoms can be expressed in a state of psychosis. Classic symptoms are described in Box 34.1. A conceptual or symptomatic representation of psychosis is presented in Fig. 34.2. Symptoms must be of sufficient intensity, duration, and degree of functional

BOX 34.1   Symptomatic Domains of Psychosis

- *Delusions*: Fixed beliefs that are not amenable to change in light of conflicting evidence
- *Hallucinations*: Perception-like experiences that occur without an external stimulus
- *Disorganized thinking*: Most commonly inferred from speech, defined by derailment, loose associations, tangentiality, and incoherence
- *Disorganized/abnormal motor behavior*: Markedly abnormal behavior ranging from agitation to catatonia that is commonly situationally incongruent
- *Negative symptoms*: Alogia, affective blunting, asociality, anhedonia, and avolition

TABLE 34.1   Physiologic Sequelae of Psychosis and Treatment

Pharmacotherapy Related	Behaviorally Related
• Extrapyramidal side effects	• Activity intolerance
• Hyperglycemia	• Obesity
• Dyslipidemia	• Substance use
• Hypertension	• Violence-related risk
• Hepatotoxicity	• Infectious disease exposure
• Immune compromise	• Vitamin deficiency
• Lens opacities (cataracts)	

Data from Keks, N. A., & Hope, J. (2007). Long-term management of people with psychotic disorders in the community, Australian Prescriber. *An Indepedent Review*, *30*(2), 44–46.

impairment to be recognizable as such. That point of observable recognition is defined as the *clinical threshold*.

CONSEQUENCES

Physiologic Consequences

Regardless of the underlying cause, untreated psychosis is associated with poor outcomes.[6] Untreated, psychosis reflects a persisting neurotoxic state that has the potential to further degrade neural pathways over time,[13] which may explain why dementia occurs twice as often among those diagnosed with schizophrenia.[14] The physiologic consequences of psychosis are largely dependent on etiology and those variables that influence symptom duration, symptom intensity, and functional impairment.

Untreated psychosis has the potential to cause dementia; thus, a determination of consequences follows the trajectory of both the etiology and symptoms. Much as a compromised nuclear power plant cannot control its core reactor temperature, the consequence of unregulated neural circuits is the release of inflammatory markers that further degrades the circuit.[15] Consequently the early and decisive treatment of psychosis is critical.

Although the degradation of neural circuits is the primary consequence of psychosis, a number of secondary consequences are also worth mentioning (Table 34.1). Ironically, many of the secondary consequences are associated with treatment. Although the use of antipsychotic medications has revolutionized the treatment of psychosis, antipsychotic agents are not without risk. Long-term use of antipsychotic medications is associated with elevated risk of drug-induced movement disorders; metabolic syndrome; and cardiovascular, hepatic, and immune system problems.

Psychosocial Consequences

Behaviorally related consequences are influenced by both the symptomatic expression of psychosis and its treatment. Psychotic symptoms, coupled with the sedating effects of many of the antipsychotic agents, can commonly lead to decreased activity and weight gain.[16,17] The comorbidity of psychosis and substance abuse is well documented; nearly half of those diagnosed with a schizophrenia spectrum disorder have either alcohol or illicit substance dependence, and more than 70% are nicotine-dependent.[18] Also concerning, individuals with persisting psychosis typically shun and are shunned by society. This reality brings with it major implications in terms of employment, housing, and one's ability to attend to basic needs. The seriously mentally ill population is subsequently more vulnerable to violence, infectious disease, and malnutrition.[19]

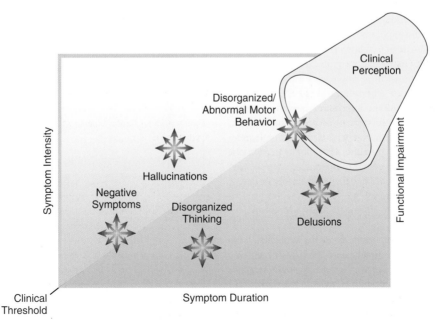

FIGURE 34.2 Symptomatic Expressions of Psychosis Below and Above the Clinical Threshold.

RISK FACTORS

All individuals are potentially susceptible to psychosis regardless of age, gender, race, and/or ethnicity. There are no conclusive factors for psychosis in general; however, family history for psychosis, past psychotic episodes, substance use, stress intolerance, ineffective coping skills, and preexisting psychiatric illness are common variables among those who manifest psychosis. A large body of research exists on risk factors associated with schizophrenia; for this reason, the following discussion of risk factors is presented from this perspective. The determination of risk factors reflects both genetic and environmental influences.

Populations at Risk

Schulz et al. identified that children with a premorbid intelligence quotient (IQ) in the learning disability range demonstrate a statistically significant risk for schizophrenia.[20] Likewise, Werner et al. determined that lower individual- and community-level socioeconomic status at the time of birth are associated with an increased risk for schizophrenia.[21] Interestingly, the prevalence of schizophrenia has also been correlated with population density in cities with populations exceeding 1 million.[7]

Individual Risk Factors

Individual risk factors for psychosis exist within four potentially interrelated domains of temperament, environment, genetics, and physiology.

Temperament

Research has established that those with a preexisting personality disorder appear to be more vulnerable to brief psychotic disorder. An increased risk of schizophrenia may also be associated with asociality.[22]

Environmental

Environmental risk factors for schizophrenia spectrum disorder appear to be clustered temporally by early life (e.g., obstetric complication, season of birth, prenatal/postnatal infection, maternal malnutrition, and maternal stress), childhood (e.g., adverse childrearing, child abuse, and head injury), and later life (e.g., drug abuse, migration/ethnicity, urbanization, social adversity, and life events).[23]

Genetic

The research suggests that schizophrenia currently has the strongest demonstrated genetic linkage among the known psychiatric disorders. Gene variants or single nucleotide polymorphisms (SNPs) increase the relative risk for the development of psychosis through the subsequent degradation of developing key neural pathways in the brain over time. Although psychosis is not defined by a single gene variant, there is evidence that both the number of gene variations (or SNPs) and the temporal sequence of those variations in relation to environmental stress can increase the relative risk for psychosis. Recent research has established that specific gene mutations associated with chromosomes 1, 6, 8, 12, 13, and 22 demonstrate an increased vulnerability to psychotic disorders.[5] The concordance rate for a schizophrenia spectrum disorder is 48% among monozygotic twins, 17% among fraternal twins, 9% among siblings, and 6% among parents.[24]

Physiologic

In terms of potential biomarkers, some research establishes that decreased cortical gray matter may also be associated with increased risk for schizophrenia spectrum disorder.[25] Currently there is active research on many fronts seeking to establish reliable biomarkers for schizophrenia. There is also strong evidence that sleep deprivation has the potential to induce psychotic states.[26] Further still, Davison et al. (2018) recently conducted a systematic review looking for metabolite biomarkers associated with schizophrenia, finding metabolite signatures associated with reduced levels of polyunsaturated fatty acids, vitamin E and creatine, and elevated levels of lipid peroxidation metabolites and glutamate.[27]

ASSESSMENT

Assessment for psychosis requires the systematic collection of a history, physical assessment, mental status examination, and diagnostic testing (Box 34.2). As mentioned previously, psychosis is associated with progressively compromised neural circuits; for this reason, the symptoms are progressive and evolve over time. Many subclinical symptoms appear before the patient is overtly psychotic (see Fig. 34.2); thus early recognition requires a critical eye. To the casual observer, individuals with subclinical symptoms of psychosis may appear odd, socially awkward, or easily distracted. The proficient or expert nurse is better able to perceive subtle signs of psychosis, such as hallucinations and negative symptoms, whereas the novice or advanced beginner is usually sensitized only to the more overt signs of psychosis, such as delusional and disorganized behavior.[28] The expert nurse understands the concept of psychosis and its symptomatic expression so well that he or she is sometimes able to perceive psychosis below the clinical threshold.

History

The goal of the history is to obtain vital and time-sensitive health information that has the potential to immediately and significantly influence the trajectory of care. Cognitive impairment and diminished reality

---

BOX 34.2   Nursing Assessment of Psychosis

History
- Risk factors
- Personal medical history
- Mental health history
- Substance use
- Perinatal trauma
- Developmental history
- Family history
- Trauma exposure
- Culture and beliefs

Physical Examination
- Vital signs
- Cranial nerve assessment
- Mental status examination
  - Appearance
  - Attitude
  - Behavior
  - Mood and affect
  - Speech
  - Thought process
  - Thought content
  - Perceptions
  - Cognition
  - Insight
  - Judgment

Diagnostic Tests
- Laboratory tests
- Imaging

testing commonly complicate history taking with a patient experiencing psychosis. Thus efforts to obtain collateral information from friends, family, coworkers, and past healthcare professionals are vital. A complete health history includes subjective data from the patient and (when available) a collateral source. Questions should be straightforward, concrete, and open-ended. The nurse should afford the patient with suspected psychotic symptoms additional time to answer questions. Patients with psychosis commonly experience paranoia, which makes rapport building very important.

Patients who are experiencing psychosis often lack awareness of their own medical condition or disability. This is referred to as a state of anosognosia. Consequently, using clinical terms such as *hallucination*, *delusion*, *paranoia*, and *catatonia* with a patient experiencing psychosis is contraindicated. Develop questions using nonclinical terms as part of the interview. For example, as opposed to asking, "Are you experiencing hallucinations?" ask, "Do you ever see or hear things that other people can't see or hear?" Instead of asking, "Are you delusional?" nonjudgmentally ask the patient about those beliefs that he or she feels strongly about and assess the nature of those beliefs in relation to reality. As opposed to asking, "Do you feel paranoid a lot?" ask, "Are you influenced strongly by the beliefs of others?"

Physical Assessment

Physical manifestations of psychosis follow etiology. If the etiology of psychosis is medically or chemically induced, any number of physical symptoms may be present. For example, a psychotic patient under the influence of a psychoactive stimulant would also demonstrate those symptoms associated with psychoactive stimulant intoxication or withdrawal (e.g., mydriasis, bruxism, nonintentional tremor, elevated blood pressure, tachypnea, and hyperthermia). Alternatively, a psychotic patient with a comorbid history of dementia would also manifest symptoms associated with dementia (e.g., memory loss, impaired judgment, impaired abstract reasoning, impaired communication skills, and disorientation). Regardless of etiology, a mental status examination is used to assess symptoms.

Diagnostic Tests

Although there are currently no diagnostic tests that definitively rule in or out psychosis, a number of tests are available that can aid the nurse in differentiating between the primary and secondary etiologies of psychosis. Laboratory studies such as a complete blood count, chemistry panel (Chem18), thyroid function test, rapid plasma reagin, dexamethasone suppression test, HIV test, heavy metals panel, urinalysis, urine drug screen, urine culture and sensitivity, computed tomography, and magnetic resonance imaging can rule out a number of potential organic etiologies.[7]

CLINICAL MANAGEMENT

Clinical management of psychosis is principally dependent on etiology. If the nature of the psychosis is secondary, the healthcare team must treat the underlying cause of the psychosis while simultaneously managing the symptoms of psychosis. In instances in which psychosis does not have a secondary cause, a number of treatment options are available. For the purposes of this section, clinical management focuses on the primary etiology of psychosis.

Primary Prevention

Understanding that psychosis is born of both genomic and environmental variables, primary prevention targeting the genomic influence would focus on prepregnancy genetic counseling. Alternatively, primary prevention targeting environmental influences requires a reconsideration

---

BOX 34.3 Pharmacologic Agents for the Treatment of Psychosis

First-Generation Antipsychotics
- Haloperidol (Haldol)
- Fluphenazine (Prolixin)
- Thiothixene (Navane)
- Trifluoperazine (Stelazine)
- Perphenazine (Trilofon)
- Chlorpromazine (Thorazine)
- Thioridazine (Mellaril)
- Loxapine (Loxitane)

First-Generation Antipsychotic Long-Acting Injectables
- Haloperidol decaonate (Haldol Decanoate)

Second-Generation Antipsychotics
- Clozapine (Clozaril)
- Olanzapine (Zyprexa)
- Risperidone (Risperdal)
- Quetiapine (Seroquel)
- Aripiprazole (Abilify)
- Paliperidone (Invega)
- Ziprasidone (Geodon)
- Asenapine (Saphris)
- Iloperidone (Fanapt)
- Paliperidone (Invega)
- Lurasidone (Latuda)
- Pimavanserin (Nuplazid)
- Brexpiprazole (Rexulti)
- Cariprazine (Vraylar)

Second-Generation Antipsychotic Long-Acting Injectables
- Aripiprazole lauroxil (Aristida)
- Aripiprazole (Abilify Maintena)
- Paliperidone palmitate (Invega Sustenna)
- Paliperidone palmitate (Invega Trinza)
- Risperidone (Risperdal Consta)
- Olanzapine (Zyprexa Relprevv)
- Olanzapine (Zyprexa Zydis)

Anticholinergic Agents
- Benzotropine (Cogentin)
- Bromocriptine (Parlodel)
- Trihexyphenidyl (Artane)
- Diphenhydramine (Benadryl)

---

of previously discussed environmental risk factors (e.g., obstetric complication, maternal health, malnutrition and stress, stable parenting, and injury prevention).

Secondary Prevention (Screening)

The focus of secondary prevention as it relates to psychosis involves screening individuals with a family history and monitoring for subclinical symptoms. A number of evidence-based screening instruments may aid in diagnosis, including the Brief Psychiatric Rating Scale (BRPS),[29] the Positive and Negative Syndrome Scale (PANSS),[30] the Minnesota Multiphasic Personality Inventory–2 (MMPI-2),[31] and the DSM-V's Level I Cross-Cutting Symptoms Measure.[4]

Available evidence indicates that early intervention within the prodromal phase (the period in which subtle symptoms of psychosis begin to rise to the level of clinical significance) is associated with the best possible outcome. In that regard, the proficient or expert nurse who is able to discern symptoms at or below the clinical threshold is in a particularly unique position to positively influence the trajectory of care.

Collaborative Interventions

The clinical management of psychosis is subdivided into four classifications: pharmacologic (Box 34.3), nonpharmacologic, lifestyle modification, and community integration. Although nearly half of those with a schizophrenia spectrum disorder do not receive care, those who do typically do not receive comprehensive care. The National Institute of Mental Health funded the Schizophrenia Patient Outcomes Research Team (PORT) to develop and disseminate evidence-based recommendations for the treatment of schizophrenia.[32] The results of the PORT study recommended an individualized, multimodal approach to care involving interventions from all four classifications.

Pharmacotherapy

First-generation antipsychotics. Most first-generation antipsychotics are no longer considered first-tier choices for the treatment of psychosis; however, they are still seen in community-based and forensic settings throughout the country. First-generation antipsychotics (see Box 34.3) reduce the transmission of dopamine at the D_2 receptor site of four key dopaminergic pathways in the brain. Their ability to target the positive symptoms associated with a schizophrenia spectrum disorder is well established. Regrettably, they are not as effective with negative symptoms. Additionally, they are also known for significant side effects—including anticholinergic high-risk extrapyramidal side effects (EPSs), sedation, and weight gain—that have historically led to medication adherence problems.

Second-generation antipsychotics. Second-generation antipsychotic agents (see Box 34.3) also target positive symptoms of psychosis with their D_2 antagonism; in addition, they target negative symptoms with their $5\text{-}HT_{2a}$ antagonism and (for certain agents) $5\text{-}HT_{1a}$ agonism.[33] Their tendency to more loosely bind to targeted receptor sites result in a lower risk for EPSs. Although the second-generation antipsychotics are considered first-line choices for the treatment of psychosis and have a lower risk for EPSs, they have a markedly increased risk for metabolic disorders such as dyslipidemia, diabetes, and weight gain if used for long periods of time.

Anticholinergic agents. Anticholinergic agents (see Box 34.3) are used to treat EPSs resulting from the use of antipsychotic medication. EPSs can occur because of excessive D_2 binding within the nigrostriatal pathway. Because certain forms of EPSs are considered medical emergencies (e.g., acute pharyngeal dystonia) and potentially permanent (e.g., tardive dyskinesia), anticholinergic agents can be delivered orally, intramuscularly, or intravenously to target EPSs.

Nonpharmacologic Therapies

Social skills training. Psychosis, by its very definition, has the potential to slowly and progressively dissolve interpersonal relational skills. The acquisition and maintenance of social skills can be seen as a bridge to long-term symptom management. Social skills training (SST) is typically done in a homogeneous group format and teaches individuals about verbal, nonverbal, and paraverbal communication.[34] Assertiveness training is also an element of SST, as is social cue interpretation.

Family-focused therapy. Tailored to families influenced by schizophrenia spectrum disorder, family-focused therapy (FFT) educates the family on the nature of psychosis, its symptoms, and common management strategies. Research has established that FFT improves medication adherence, reduces the rate of relapse, and reduces psychiatric readmission rates.[35-37]

Cognitive-behavioral therapy for psychosis. Cognitive-behavioral therapy is premised on the notion that how one perceives and interprets sensory stimuli has a direct bearing on the reaction one has to that situation. Upon initial consideration, this form of therapy would seem contraindicated for an individual struggling with psychosis. It is important to note that an individual with a schizophrenia spectrum disorder is not perpetually psychotic and can go months or even years without psychotic symptoms. Evidence suggests that cognitive-behavioral therapy for individuals with a history of schizophrenia who are not currently experiencing psychosis can improve medication adherence, insight, and social functioning.[38]

Cognitive enhancement therapy. Cognitive enhancement therapy employs elements of cognitive-behavioral therapy with social skills training for symptomatically stable individuals with severe mental illness.

Delivered via computer-based training and group-based activities, cognitive enhancement therapy focuses on improving mental stamina, active information processing, and learning how to negotiate unrehearsed social challenges.[39]

Electroconvulsive therapy. Electroconvulsive therapy (ECT) is a medical procedure in which electrical currents are passed through the brain with the intent to trigger seizure activity, which has the potential to cause changes in brain chemistry and subsequently influence psychotic symptoms. ECT has great efficacy in treating catatonia but poses a risk for cognitive and memory side effects.[40] Depending on the severity of symptoms, 6 to 12 rounds of ECT commonly demonstrate improvement in target symptoms with the potential for longitudinal maintenance sessions thereafter.

Lifestyle Modification

Lifestyle modification addresses behaviors that have the potential to either improve or worsen one's condition. Most second-generation antipsychotics pose an increased risk for weight gain and impaired glucose tolerance.[41] For this reason, lifestyle modification approaches are a critical element in the long-term management of psychotic disorders and, if implemented in a group-based format, can also reinforce social skills development.[42]

Serial health monitoring. Second-generation antipsychotic agents have greatly improved the management of positive and negative symptoms. Research suggests that a second-generation antipsychotic metabolic monitoring process that serially assesses abdominal obesity, triglycerides, high-density lipoprotein cholesterol, blood pressure, and fasting glucose has the potential to mitigate some degree of the risk associated with the long-term use of these agents.[43]

Case management. Case management employs a team of healthcare workers to serve as a liaison between the patient and the community to maximize patient autonomy without compromising patient health and well-being. Assertive community treatment (ACT) is a popular model that includes a team consisting of a case manager, primary care provider, mental health provider, and nurse and in which care is decentralized away from the traditional brick-and-mortar environment and accessible 24 hours a day. ACT has proven to be both clinically and fiscally efficacious.[44-46]

Vocational therapy. Vocational therapy is a process that individualizes resources for those with functional, psychological, developmental, or cognitive impairments; it is intended to overcome barriers to accessing, maintaining, or returning to employment. In individuals with a schizophrenia spectrum disorder, vocational therapy has been shown to improve cognitive and negative symptoms,[47] clinical outcomes,[48] and social functioning.[49]

INTERRELATED CONCEPTS

Multiple concepts are clearly interrelated to the concept of psychosis (Fig. 34.3). Incorporating several key psychosocial concepts and professional nursing concepts is essential to improving health outcomes when caring for psychotic patients. Health Policy is important in the context of regulations that oversee the delivery of mental health care in the United States. The concepts of Ethics and Health Care Law relate to ensuring appropriate use of restrictive treatment interventions (i.e., seclusion, sedation, and restraints). In terms of psychiatric commitment, the legal concepts of habeas corpus and justification for involuntary treatment must be respected. Communication is a key concept because this represents an important skill needed to establish therapeutic relationships with psychotic patients. The concept of Patient Education is linked to the instructional treatment of protocols, disease processes, and pharmacologic interventions. Collaboration is essential for effective

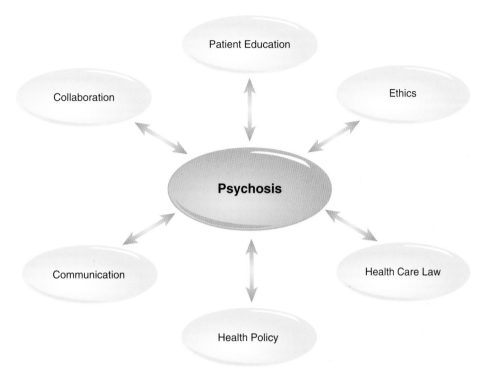

FIGURE 34.3 Psychosis and Interrelated Concepts.

treatment and includes the interprofessional team to optimize specialty-related patient outcomes.

CLINICAL EXEMPLARS

As already established, psychosis can manifest from multiple etiologies. Box 34.4 presents common exemplars associated with psychosis. A comprehensive description and explanation of each exemplar is beyond the scope of this text; here, however, some of the most common exemplars are featured, with a short description. The psychiatric/mental health references offer more detailed information about each of these conditions.

Featured Exemplars
Schizophrenia
Schizophrenia is a severe mental illness defined by a constellation of positive symptoms (e.g., hallucinations, delusions, disorganized speech and behavior, catatonia, and agitation), which commonly distance society from the patient; it also comprises negative symptoms (e.g., alogia, affective blunting, asociality, anhedonia, and avolition) that frequently distance the patient from society. Schizophrenia commonly manifests insidiously between late adolescence and early adulthood with a prodromal phase and requires lifelong management to control psychotic episodes. In addition to psychotherapy, treatment typically involves the use of antipsychotic agents.

Major Depressive Disorder, Severe with Psychotic Features
Major Depressive Disorder, Severe with Psychotic Features is defined by a primary constellation of major depressive symptoms with a symptomatic overlay of psychotic features. Psychosis seen within the context of this condition is episodic in nature but nonetheless a poor prognostic indicator. In addition to psychotherapy, treatment for a severe major depressive disorder with psychotic features requires antidepressant and antipsychotic agents to control target symptoms.

Delirium
Delirium is defined by rapid changes in brain function and cognitive capacity that occur within the context of a co-occurring physical condition. Symptoms can manifest as disturbance in attention, cognition, and behavior.[4] Consequently psychosis or psychotic behavior can result from a delirium state. A cardinal symptom of delirium is defined by a waxing and waning of mental status. Delirium is considered a medical emergency. Common sources of delirium can be substance withdrawal, severe electrolyte abnormality, systemic infection, poor nutrition or dehydration, multiple co-occurring medical problems, and polypharmacy. Treatment follows the underlying etiology of the delirium state.

Major Neurocognitive Disorder
Major neurocognitive disorder is defined by a demonstrable cognitive decline from a previous level of performance as seen within different cognitive domains.[4] Consequently psychosis or psychotic behavior can also result from a progressing neurocognitive disorder. The onset of symptoms with a major neurocognitive disorder is slow and progressive and not defined by the waxing and waning of mental status. Most etiologies of a major neurocognitive disorder are not typically reversible but can be slowed with different forms of pharmacotherapy and rehabilitation.

Substance/Medication-Induced Psychotic Disorder
Substance/medication-induced psychotic disorder is a time-limited manifestation of psychotic symptoms triggered by the ingestion of a substance or medication known to promote psychosis. Psychotic symptoms typically have a rapid onset with no evidence of prodrome

BOX 34.4 EXEMPLARS OF PSYCHOSIS

Schizophrenia Spectrum and Other Psychotic Disorders
- Schizotypal personality disorder
- Delusional disorder
- Brief psychotic disorder
- Schizophreniform disorder
- Schizophrenia
- Schizoaffective disorder
- Substance/medication-induced psychotic disorder
- Psychotic disorder due to a general medical condition
- Catatonia associated with another mental condition
- Catatonic disorder due to another medical condition
- Unspecified catatonia
- Other specified schizophrenia spectrum disorder and other psychotic disorder
- Unspecified schizophrenia spectrum and other psychotic disorder

Bipolar and Related Disorders
- Bipolar I disorder with psychotic features
- Substance/medication-induced bipolar and related disorder
- Bipolar and related disorder due to another medical condition

Depressive Disorders
- Major depressive disorder with psychotic features
- Substance/medication-induced depressive disorder
- Depressive disorder due to another medical condition

Substance-Induced Disorders
- Substance intoxication and withdrawal

Neurocognitive Disorders
- Delirium
- Major neurocognitive disorder
- Substance/medication-induced major neurocognitive disorder

Personality Disorders
- Cluster A personality disorders

🌸 **ACCESS EXEMPLAR LINKS IN YOUR GIDDENS EBOOK**

and commonly dissipate after the substance has sufficiently degraded within the body. Long-term use of some agents (e.g., marijuana, cocaine, methamphetamine) can lead to an increased risk for chronic psychosis.[50–52]

Brief Psychotic Disorder with Postpartum Onset

Brief psychotic disorder with postpartum onset is rare (0.890 to 2.6 in 1,000 women).[53] However, when it presents, it commonly does so within the first month following childbirth and can manifest with both positive and negative symptoms. Although medically treated, as in the case of any other expression of psychosis, confounding variables are associated with the potential risks associated with breastfeeding while on antipsychotic medications as well as impaired mother-child bonding. Postpartum psychosis may be a manifestation of either a bourgeoning schizophrenia spectrum or bipolar spectrum disorder activated by the marked hormonal shifts associated with pregnancy.[54]

CASE STUDY

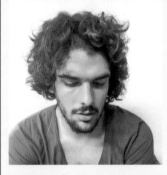

Case Presentation

Ethan is 21 years old, unemployed, and homeless. He was readmitted to the state hospital after a serious suicidal gesture when he attempted to walk into oncoming traffic on the highway. Prior to this most recent admission, Ethan's established diagnosis was *schizophrenia, first episode, currently in partial remission*, and *nicotine dependence*. Ethan has a significant family history of psychosis, both his biological brother and father having been diagnosed with schizophrenia prior to the age of 20 years. His father completed suicide at age 30 years, and his brother is currently incarcerated. Ethan's mother is alcohol-dependent and her support has historically been unreliable. Ethan's first break of psychosis occurred at age 18 years during his first 6 months at college. His prodromal period was more prominent for negative symptoms (e.g., alogia, affective blunting, asociality, anhedonia, and avolition), with positive symptoms (e.g., audiovisual hallucinations and disorganized speech and behavior) surfacing much later and remitting much more quickly with treatment. Ethan was initially prescribed risperidone and achieved remission of all positive symptoms and

some portion of his negative symptoms after 3 months of treatment, with two hospitalizations and an eventual transition to a long-acting injectable form of risperidone (Risperdal Consta). A review of his outpatient record indicates that his negative symptoms have tidaled around the clinical threshold during the past 3 years and he has been struggling with suicidal thoughts for the better part of the past 6 months. The persistent nature of his depressive symptoms prompts a diagnostic reconsideration of *schizoaffective disorder, multiple episodes, depressive type*. During this hospitalization, Ethan's positive symptoms again quickly resolved, but his negative symptoms persisted, prompting the decision to add an antidepressant (Prozac) to his medication plan. Upon stabilization, Ethan was transferred to a partial hospitalization program, where cognitive enhancement therapy, art therapy, nutritional counseling, case management, and vocational rehabilitation were provided. With this augmented plan of care, Ethan was able to get remarkably better control of his negative symptoms and is now currently working part-time in a bookstore and considering reenrolling in a local community college.

Case Analysis Questions

1. What risk factors are evident in Ethan's case that might be contributing to Ethan's condition?
2. Which clinical findings in Ethan's case are consistent with psychosis?
3. What are the potential benefits of cognitive enhancement therapy for Ethan?

From veronica89/iStock/Thinkstock.

ACCESS EXEMPLAR LINKS IN YOUR GIDDENS EBOOK

REFERENCES

1. Juhas, D. (2013). Throughout history, defining schizophrenia has remained a challenge. *Scientific American*, *24*(1).
2. Mandal, A. *Psychosis history*. Retrieved from: http://www.news-medical.net, 2014.
3. Beer, M. D. (1996). Psychosis: A history of the concept. *Comprehensive Psychiatry*, *37*(4), 273–291.
4. American Psychiatric Association. (2013). *Diagnostic and statistical manual of mental disorders* (5th ed.). Arlington, VA: American Psychiatric Publishing.
5. Stahl, S. M. (2014). *Stahl's essential psychopharmacology: The prescriber's guide* (5th ed.). Cambridge, UK: Cambridge University Press.
6. Penttila, M., Jaaskelainen, E., Hirvonen, N., et al. (2014). Duration of untreated psychosis as predictor of long-term outcome in schizophrenia: Systematic review and meta-analysis. *The British Journal of Psychiatry: The Journal of Mental Science*, *205*(2), 88–94.
7. Sadock, B. J., Sadock, V. A., & Ruiz, P. (2014). *Kaplan & Sadock's synopsis of psychiatry: Behavioral sciences/clinical psychiatry* (11th ed.). Philadelphia: Wolters Kluwer.
8. Freudenreich, O. (2012). Differential diagnosis of psychotic symptoms: Medical "mimics.". *Psychiatric Times*, *27*(12).
9. Keck, P. E., Jr., McElroy, S. L., Havens, J. R., et al. (2003). Psychosis in bipolar disorder: Phenomenology and impact on morbidity and course of illness. *Comprehensive Psychiatry*, *44*(4), 263–269.
10. Harrow, M., Grossman, L. S., Herbener, E. S., et al. (2000). Ten-year outcome: Patients with schizoaffective disorders, schizophrenia, affective disorders and mood-incongruent psychotic symptoms. *The British Journal of Psychiatry: The Journal of Mental Science*, *177*(5), 421–426.
11. Meyers, B. S. (2014). Psychotic depression: Underrecognized, undertreated—and dangerous. *Psychiatric Times*, *31*(7).
12. Lenzenweger, M. F., Lane, M. C., Loranger, A. W., et al. (2007). *DSM-IV* personality disorders in the National Comorbidity Survey Replication. *Biological Psychiatry*, *62*(6), 553–564.
13. McGlashan, T. H. (2006). Schizophrenia in translation: Is active psychosis neurotoxic? *Schizophrenia Bulletin*, *32*(4), 609–613.
14. Hendrie, H. C., Tu, W., Tabbey, R., et al. (2014). Health outcomes and cost of care among older adults with schizophrenia: A 10-year study using medical records across the continuum of care. *The American Journal of Geriatric Psychiatry*, *22*(5), 427–436.
15. Fillman, S. G., Cloonan, N., Catts, V. S., et al. (2013). Increased inflammatory markers identified in the dorsolateral prefrontal cortex of individuals with schizophrenia. *Molecular Psychiatry*, *18*(2), 206–214.
16. Bonfioli, E., Berti, L., Goss, C., et al. (2012). Health promotion lifestyle interventions for weight management in psychosis: A systematic review and meta-analysis of randomised controlled trials. *BMC Psychiatry*, *12*, 78.
17. Faulkner, G., & Cohn, T. A. (2006). Pharmacologic and nonpharmacologic strategies for weight gain and metabolic disturbance in patients treated with antipsychotic medications. *Canadian Journal of Psychiatry. Revue Canadienne de Psychiatrie*, *51*(8), 502–511.
18. Winklbaur, B., Ebner, N., Sachs, G., et al. (2006). Substance abuse in patients with schizophrenia. *Dialogues in Clinical Neuroscience*, *8*(1), 37–43.
19. Foster, A., Gable, J., & Buckley, J. (2012). Homelessness in schizophrenia. *The Psychiatric Clinics of North America*, *35*(3), 717–734.
20. Schulz, J., Sundin, J., Leask, S., et al. (2014). Risk of adult schizophrenia and its relationship to childhood IQ in the 1958 British birth cohort. *Schizophrenia Bulletin*, *40*(1), 143–151.
21. Werner, S., Malaspina, D., & Rabinowitz, J. (2007). Socioeconomic status at birth is associated with risk of schizophrenia: Population-based multilevel study. *Schizophrenia Bulletin*, *33*(6), 1373–1378.
22. Smith, M. J., Cloninger, C. R., Harms, M. P., et al. (2009). Temperament and character as schizophrenia-related endophenotypes in non-psychotic siblings. *Schizophrenia Research*, *104*(1–3), 198–205.
23. Dean, K., & Murray, R. M. (2005). Environmental risk factors for psychosis. *Dialogues in Clinical Neuroscience*, *7*(1), 69–80.
24. Heckers, S. (2005). 2009: Who is at risk for a psychotic disorder? *Schizophrenia Bulletin*, *35*(5), 847–850.
25. National Alliance on Mental Illness. *First episodes of psychosis*. Retrieved from: http://www.nami.org/Template.cfm?Section=First_Episode, 2014.
26. Petrovsky, N., Ettinger, U., Hill, A., et al. (2014). Sleep deprivation disrupts prepulse inhibition and induces psychosis-like symptoms in healthy humans. *The Journal of Neuroscience: The Official Journal of the Society for Neuroscience*, *34*(27), 9134–9140.
27. Davison, J., et al. (2017). A systematic review of metabolite biomarkers of schizophrenia. *Schizophrenia Research*, *195*, 32–50.
28. Benner, P. E. (1984). *From novice to expert: Excellence and power in clinical nursing practice*. Menlo Park, CA: Addison-Wesley.
29. McGorry, P. D., Goodwin, R. J., & Stuart, G. W. (1988). The development, use, and reliability of the brief psychiatric rating scale (nursing modification)—An assessment procedure for the nursing team in clinical and research settings. *Comprehensive Psychiatry*, *29*(6), 575–587.
30. Kay, S. R., Fiszbein, A., & Opler, L. A. (1987). The Positive and Negative Syndrome Scale (PANSS) for schizophrenia. *Schizophrenia Bulletin*, *13*(2), 261–276.
31. Butcher, J. N. (2001). *MMPI-2: Minnesota Multiphasic Personality Inventory-2: Manual for administration, scoring, and interpretation* (rev ed.). Minneapolis, MN: University of Minnesota Press.
32. Kreyenbuhl, J., Buchanan, R. W., Dickerson, F. B., Schizophrenia Patient Outcomes Research team, et al. (2010). The Schizophrenia Patient Outcomes Research Team (PORT): Updated treatment recommendations 2009. *Schizophrenia Bulletin*, *36*(1), 94–103.
33. Stahl, S. M. (2013). *Stahl's essential psychopharmacology: Neuroscientific basis and practical application* (4th ed.). Cambridge, UK: Cambridge University Press.
34. Hofmann, S. G., & Tompson, M. C. (2002). *Treating chronic and severe mental disorders: A handbook of empirically supported interventions*. New York: Guilford.
35. Bressi, C., Manenti, S., Frongia, P., et al. (2008). Systemic family therapy in schizophrenia: A randomized clinical trial of effectiveness. *Psychotherapy and Psychosomatics*, *77*(1), 43–49.
36. O'Brien, M. P., Miklowitz, D. J., Candan, K. A., et al. (2014). A randomized trial of family focused therapy with populations at clinical high risk for psychosis: Effects on interactional behavior. *Journal of Consulting and Clinical Psychology*, *82*(1), 90–101.
37. Simon, G. E. (2003). Family focused psychoeducational therapy decreases relapse and rehospitalisation in people with a manic episode and bipolar disorder. *Evidence-Based Mental Health*, *6*(4), 114.
38. Velligan, D. I., Tai, S., Roberts, D. L., et al. (2015). A randomized controlled trial comparing cognitive behavior therapy, cognitive adaptation training, their combination and treatment as usual in chronic schizophrenia. *Schizophrenia Bulletin*, *41*(3), 597–603.
39. Hogarty, G. E., Flesher, S., Ulrich, R., et al. (2004). Cognitive enhancement therapy for schizophrenia: Effects of a 2-year randomized trial on cognition and behavior. *Archives of General Psychiatry*, *61*(9), 866–876.
40. Kellner, C. H. (2013). ECT and catatonia: Out of the shadows. *Psychiatric Times*, *30*(12).
41. Fontaine, K. R., Heo, M., Harrigan, E. P., et al. (2001). Estimating the consequences of anti-psychotic induced weight gain on health and mortality rate. *Psychiatry Research*, *101*(3), 277–288.
42. Rosenbaum, S., Watkins, A., Teasdale, S., et al. (2015). Aerobic exercise capacity: An important correlate of psychosocial function in first episode psychosis. *Acta Psychiatrica Scandinavica*, *131*(3), 234.
43. Grundmann, M. (2014). Kacirova I, Urinovska R: Therapeutic drug monitoring of atypical antipsychotic drugs. *Acta Pharmaceutica (Zagreb, Croatia)*, *64*(4), 387–401.
44. Karow, A., Reimer, J., Konig, H. H., et al. (2012). Cost-effectiveness of 12-month therapeutic assertive community treatment as part of integrated care versus standard care in patients with schizophrenia treated with quetiapine immediate release (ACCESS trial). *The Journal of Clinical Psychiatry*, *73*(3), e402–e408.

45. Lambert, M., Bock, T., Schottle, D., et al. (2010). Assertive community treatment as part of integrated care versus standard care: A 12-month trial in patients with first- and multiple-episode schizophrenia spectrum disorders treated with quetiapine immediate release (ACCESS trial). *The Journal of Clinical Psychiatry, 71*(10), 1313–1323.

46. Schottle, D., Schimmelmann, B. G., Karow, A., et al. (2014). Effectiveness of integrated care including therapeutic assertive community treatment in severe schizophrenia spectrum and bipolar I disorders: The 24-month follow-up ACCESS II study. *The Journal of Clinical Psychiatry, 75*(12), 1371–1379.

47. Bio, D. S., & Gattaz, W. F. (2011). Vocational rehabilitation improves cognition and negative symptoms in schizophrenia. *Schizophrenia Research, 126*(1–3), 265–269.

48. Kilian, R., Lauber, C., Kalkan, R., et al. (2012). The relationships between employment, clinical status, and psychiatric hospitalisation in patients with schizophrenia receiving either IPS or a conventional vocational rehabilitation programme. *Social Psychiatry and Psychiatric Epidemiology, 47*(9), 1381–1389.

49. Suresh Kumar, P. N. (2008). Impact of vocational rehabilitation on social functioning, cognitive functioning, and psychopathology in patients with chronic schizophrenia. *Indian Journal of Psychiatry, 50*(4), 257–261.

50. Glasner-Edwards, S., & Mooney, L. J. (2014). Methamphetamine psychosis: Epidemiology and management. *CNS Drugs, 28*(12), 1115–1126.

51. Roncero, C., Daigre, C., Gonzalvo, B., et al. (2013). Risk factors for cocaine-induced psychosis in cocaine-dependent patients. *European Psychiatry: The Journal of the Association of European Psychiatrists, 28*(3), 141–146.

52. In brief. (2011). Study strengthens evidence that early marijuana use increases risk of psychosis. *The Harvard Mental Health Letter, 27*(11), 7.

53. VanderKruik, R., et al. (2017). The global prevalence of postpartum psychosis: A systematic review. *BMC Psychiatry, 17*(1), 272.

54. Bergink, V., et al. (2016). Postpartum psychosis: Madness, mania, and melancholia in motherhood. *The American Journal of Psychiatry, 173*(12), 1179–1188.

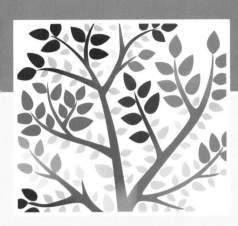

Addiction

Richard A. Pessagno

The financial cost of addiction is staggering. It is estimated that in United States the costs associated with substance abuse are estimated at over $740 billion annually[1]; this significant financial loss does not account for the stress, grief, and suffering endured by families and friends as a result of addiction. The purpose of this concept presentation is to develop a generalist nurse conceptual paradigm for the recognition and assessment of addiction on individual, family, and community levels. A conceptual understanding of addiction will enable nurses to analyze patient data for the planning and implementation of interventions necessary to ensure patient safety during emergency management and to motivate patients toward successful recovery from addiction during nonemergency management.

DEFINITION

Terminology related to the concept of addiction is controversial and subject to debate. For the purpose of this concept presentation, the term addiction is defined as "*a compulsive, abnormal dependence on a substance (such as alcohol, cocaine, opiates, or tobacco) or on a behavior (such as gambling, Internet, or pornography). The dependence typically has adverse psychological, physical, economic, social, or legal ramifications.*"[2] The American Psychiatric Association (APA) defines a wide range of mental disorders in the *Diagnostic and Statistical Manual of Mental Disorders (DSM)*; the terms *substance-induced disorders* and *substance use disorders* are used as diagnostic categories.[3] *Substance-induced disorders* involve the direct effects of the substance, and *substance use disorders* include cognitive, behavioral, and physiological symptoms associated with long-term use.[4] These distinctions are clarified further in the sections that follow. The term *intoxication* is used to describe behavioral and/or physical symptoms that result from substance use. *Craving* in the context of this concept is used to describe a desire to use a substance and is a symptom associated with substance use disorder. *Tolerance*, another symptom indicating substance use disorder, is defined as an increasing need for the substance to achieve its reward. A lack of reward from the same dose as previously taken would also be considered tolerance. *Withdrawal* refers to a syndrome of symptoms that occurs from a sudden cessation of taking the substance.[3]

SCOPE

This concept presentation examines addiction from the perspective of two broad categories—the substance maladictions and the behavioral addictions (Fig. 35.1). There is some controversy regarding whether

behavioral addictions exist, but as new developments occur in understanding brain neurochemistry, it is becoming more evident that substance addictions and behavioral addictions are the result of similar neurochemical processes.[4]

NORMAL PHYSIOLOGICAL PROCESS

Unlike most concepts presented in this book, the concept of addiction does not have a "normal" physiological process because addiction is never considered normal. However, there is an expected physiological process associated with addiction. Discussions of addiction physiology focus either on the exogenous signs and symptoms of substance abuse (shown later in Box 35.1) or on the endogenous neurochemistry underlying these signs and symptoms. The neurochemical relationship between addictive behaviors or substances and various neurotransmitters in the brain depends on complex models now being explored on the frontiers of addiction science.[5]

It is believed that neurochemical interactions related to addiction originate in the caudate nucleus, the nucleus accumbens, and the ventral tegmental areas of the brain—otherwise known as the reward centers. The reward centers are affected in different ways depending on which neurotransmitters and other brain areas are involved in various reward pathways. It is evident that the neurotransmitter dopamine plays a key role in many or all addictive processes, whether chemical addiction[5] or behavioral addictions.[4] Dopamine is directly associated with the euphoric reward known as being "high," and other neurotransmitters are associated with dopamine regulation. Examples of other neurotransmitters identified as involved in reward pathways include the endogenous opioids γ-aminobutyric acid, glutamate, acetylcholine, norepinephrine, and serotonin.

VARIATIONS AND CONTEXT

As mentioned previously, the scope of this concept is represented by two broad categories: substance addictions and behavioral addictions.

Substance Addictions

There are two major categories of problems stemming from substance addictions: substance-induced and substance use disorders.

Substance-Induced Disorders

Substance-induced disorders are temporary and reversible, caused by the immediate use of a substance (intoxication) and the immediate

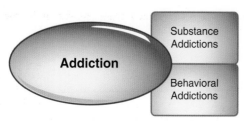

FIGURE 35.1 Scope of Addiction.

effect that occurs when the substance use is discontinued (withdrawal). The substance affects the central nervous system, causing physiological, psychological, and/or behavioral effects; the symptoms of intoxication or withdrawal are related to the specific substance or substances used. Thus these disorders can include not only the intoxication/withdrawal but also other conditions associated with intoxication and withdrawal, such as depression, anxiety, or psychosis.[5]

Substance Use Disorders

Substance use disorders result from continued, frequent use of a substance; the consequences occur over time as a cumulative effect as the addiction progresses. Substance use disorder combines abuse and dependence into a single diagnostic category with mild, moderate, and severe subclassifications. Although each substance is its own disorder (i.e., alcohol use disorder, heroin use disorder, opioid use disorder, etc.), the same overarching criteria for diagnostic purposes are used. According to the *DSM-5*, meeting 2 of 11 criteria within a 12-month period is indicative of substance use disorder. The severity is based on the number of criteria met (2 for mild, 4 for moderate, and 6 or more for severe).[3]

Behavioral Addictions

Although less clearly defined, there are many examples of behavioral addictions found in the literature. Like substance addictions, there are several behaviors that produce a reward response similar to the neurochemical processes previously described. An alternative perspective is that behavioral addictions actually represent impulse control disorders. This perspective has given rise to significant debate regarding the legitimacy of formally recognizing behavioral addictions. Although only one behavioral addiction (gambling disorder) was included in the *DSM-5* diagnostic criteria,[3] a less restrictive view is used for this concept presentation. Other behavioral addictions found in the literature (e.g., Internet addiction, gaming addiction, food addiction, and sex addiction) are included.

CONSEQUENCES

Depending on the individual and the particular addiction, the consequences of addiction are highly variable. However, an understanding of particular neurochemical processes known as *habituation* and *adaptation* forms a conceptual foundation for understanding all addictions. Habituation begins when neurons that receive a repetitive stimulus chemically inhibit their own receptors to restrict the stimulus. Habituation permits the organism to tolerate primal suffering such as hunger pain during a famine, but habituation also facilitates higher order functioning. For example, as a result of habituation, city dwellers are able to sleep in the presence of city sounds such as traffic noise or sirens.

If a repetitive stimulus persists, the neurons will permanently restrict a sufficient number of their own receptors to permit functioning of the organism in the presence of the stimulus; this is called *adaptation*. In evolutionary terms, adaptation began as a survival mechanism allowing the organism to establish a new equilibrium in the presence of an unceasing, long-term stimulus. Once adaptation to a repetitive stimulus

occurs, the stimulus must be increased to overcome the adaptation for there to be perception of the same stimulus. A user of cocaine who has adapted to a particular dose, for example, will no longer perceive a high on the same dose; therefore the dose of cocaine must be increased to get high. In turn, the brain neurochemically adapts to the increasing doses of cocaine in an addictive cycle known as *tolerance*. That is, habituation and adaptation cause tolerance.

Any behavioral reward, such as pleasure, is in fact a neurochemical process mediated by neurotransmitters; therefore, the brain will habituate and adapt neurochemically to repetitive behaviors such as gambling in the same way as it will adapt to ingested substances such as cocaine. Gamblers have to gamble more often for higher stakes to overcome the brain's adaptation to the gambling high. All the neurochemical consequences of substance use—whether alcohol, tobacco, cocaine, amphetamines, opiates, or others—apply to non-substance addictions such as money, power, relationships, sex, pornography, computer games, television, work, exercise, sports, and even addictive thought patterns such as worry or rumination.[4]

The processes of habituation, adaptation, tolerance, and withdrawal are well illustrated by an individual who is too anxious to sleep. The anxiety triggers the release of adrenaline as part of the fight-or-flight response, and insomnia results from the adrenaline. The brain recognizes the importance of sleep and will eventually block the anxiety stimulus so that sleep will occur. Some motor vehicle drivers have experienced this mechanism—the brain chemically overwhelms the alertness necessary to stay awake and accidents occur when drivers fall asleep at the wheel.

Tolerance and withdrawal enter the picture if a sedative is taken to artificially overwhelm the stimulus of anxiety to achieve sleep. In this case, instead of blocking the anxiety stimulus, the brain will block the sedative by signaling the release of more adrenaline. The need for increasing doses of the sedative to overcome the increasing level of adrenaline is tolerance. If the sedative is abruptly discontinued, the brain does not immediately stop signaling the release of adrenaline, and therefore the opposite effect of the sedative occurs in the form of restlessness and insomnia even if the original stimulus for anxiety is resolved. This restlessness and insomnia are called the rebound effects of withdrawing the sedative. After one or two nights, the neurons will readjust and these rebound effects will cease, but if the sedative is continued to artificially counter the rebound effects, then adaptation will take place and there will be addiction to the sedative.

RISK FACTORS

Examples of predisposing risk factors associated with addiction include family history of addiction, burnout, mood disorders, and stress.[5] Homelessness is also a significant risk factor for addiction.[6] Other risk factors identified by the National Institute on Drug Abuse (NIDA) include early aggressive behavior, lack of parental supervision, drug availability, and poverty.[7] Individuals with previous histories of dependence on opiates are at much higher risk for becoming addicted to opioid analgesics.[8] Use of illicit drugs, tobacco, and alcohol is much higher among adults with co-occurring severe psychological distress.[9] The unique challenges faced by those with co-occurring disorders are discussed in the Clinical Management section of this concept presentation.

Prevalence

The National Survey on Drug Use and Health (NSDU) provides a summary of substance use and mental health for individuals 12 and older in the United States. Alcohol and tobacco use are the most common substances used, while cannabis and misuse of prescription pain medication are the most prevalent illicit substances used in the United States.[10] Over 21 million Americans aged 12 and older have substance

BOX 35.1   Symptoms and Behaviors of Addiction

- Fatigue
- Insomnia
- Headaches
- Seizure disorder
- Changes in mood
- Anorexia, weight loss
- Vague physical complaints
- Overabundant use of mouthwash or toiletries
- Appearing older than stated age, unkempt appearance
- Leisure activities that involve alcohol and/or other drugs
- Sexual dysfunction, decreased libido, erectile dysfunction
- Trauma secondary to falls, auto accidents, fights, or burns
- Driving while intoxicated (more than one citation suggests dependence)
- Failure of standard doses of sedatives to have a therapeutic effect
- Financial problems, including those related to spending for substances
- Frequent reference to alcohol or alcohol use indicating preoccupation with and importance of alcohol in the person's life
- Problems in areas of life function (e.g., frequent job changes; marital conflict, separation, and/or divorce; work-related accidents, tardiness, absenteeism; legal problems, including arrest; social isolation; and estrangement from friends and/or family)

Modified from Lewis, S. L., Dirksen, S. R., Heitkemper, M. M. et al. (2014). *Medical-surgical nursing: Assessment and management of clinical problems* (9th ed.). St Louis: Mosby.

use disorders, yet only just over 11% receive treatment.[10] The misuse of prescription medication continues to rise and is most prevalent among those who misuse opioid prescription medication. Misuse of prescription medication is understood to be using medication other than has been directed by the prescribing provider, or the use of a prescription written for another individual.[10] In addressing the prevalence of behavioral addictions, there little research that articulates these data so the prevalence is not well-established. The more commonly recognized behavioral addictions are gambling, shopping, Internet use, video games, exercise, food addictions, and several subtypes of sex addiction.[4]

Substance Abuse Among Nurses

Substance use among healthcare professionals has been a long-standing concern for all health professions. The American Nurses Association (ANA) estimates that 10% to 15% of nurses are either recovering from substance use or have impaired practice.[11] States across the country are seeing a marked increase in substance abuse issues among nurses, leading to increasing numbers of nurses facing nursing board intervention.

Identifying risk factors for substance abuse among nurses is key if early intervention and prevention are to be achieved. Risk factors specific for nurses include job related stress and having access to controlled medication. Many nurses experience guilt and shame around their substance use; they often feel that have let patients and colleagues down or may be afraid of how colleagues will view them.[11]

ASSESSMENT

The first priority of nursing assessment for persons experiencing addictions is aimed at identifying those in need of emergency management so they can be referred immediately for stabilization. Nonemergency priorities of the assessment are aimed at identifying possible addictions by interview and screening so that treatment options for recovery can be explored. Screening tools are used during the history and examination;

these are discussed under Secondary Prevention in the Clinical Management section.

History

There are a number of general symptoms an individual with substance use or induced disorders may mention while taking a patient history (Box 35.1). The patient history also includes exploring the use of prescription and over-the-counter drugs, herbal and homeopathic products, caffeine, tobacco products, alcohol, and recreational drug use. However, the patient may consider the disclosure of addictions to be risky, so it is important to reassure the patient that the information is confidential. Even so, because of the presence of deception in addictive processes, patients are unlikely to disclose addictions accurately.[12] For this reason, it is recommended that the nurse build trust and rapport by using a therapeutic communication technique called motivational interviewing.

The use of motivational interviewing is discussed further (in the Clinical Management section) because it has been demonstrated to improve recovery significantly.[13] However, it is also recommended that the nurse use motivational interviewing methods during the assessment to identify the following defining characteristics for addiction: (1) tolerance and withdrawal, (2) deception of the self and others, and (3) relapse processes (loss of willpower). This interview technique allows the nurse to explore the defining characteristics as they arise without loss of rapport. The following discussion of the defining characteristics of addiction is provided to facilitate the assessment.

Tolerance and Withdrawal

Tolerance and withdrawal are the result of the neurochemical processes already discussed: habituation and adaptation. The nurse can identify tolerance when the patient acknowledges the need for increasingly more of the stimulus to achieve reward. Withdrawal symptoms occur when sufficient quantities are not obtained to achieve reward because of tolerance or because of reducing consumption. There are two categories of withdrawal symptoms: the stress reaction symptoms and the rebound symptoms. Stress reaction symptoms are mediated by the autonomic nervous system and result from the stress of stopping the addictive behavior. Stress reaction symptoms range from mild uneasiness and irritability to extreme agitation, rapid pulse rate, tremors, and panic.

Rebound symptoms occur when adaptive changes in the brain that counter the effects of the addiction continue despite cessation of the addictive substance or behavior. Therefore the effects of the rebound symptoms are the exact opposite of the effects of the addiction. If the addiction is stimulating, then rebound symptoms will be sedating and manifest as lethargy. If the addiction is sedating, then the rebound symptoms will manifest as agitation. This explains why stimulant addicts experience a "crashing" of mood and energy as a rebound symptom but also have anxiety as a stress reaction symptom. Agitation will be a rebound symptom to stopping the use of substances that are sedating, such as alcohol or benzodiazepines, and the agitation may be compounded as a reaction to the stress of stopping the substance.

Deception of the Self and Others (Denial)

Deception of the self and others may be loosely referred to as denial. Sometimes addicts deliberately deceive others to hide their addiction, but they may also deceive themselves. Individuals with substance use disorders may be dishonest, covert, engage in criminal activity, and/or turn away from family and friends in order to maintain their substance use. These individuals may find themselves engaging in activities (such as exchanging sex for drugs or robbery) that they would have never otherwise considered doing in order to maintain their substance use. Deception underlies tension, stress, and betrayal that is experienced among family and friends of individuals who have substance use disorders.

Relapse (Loss of Willpower)

Relapse processes are invariably linked to addiction, and they are addressed in the Clinical Management section because they are directly related to recovery.

Physical Examination

A routine physical exam may disclose evidence of addiction. Long-term use of toxic substances may harm the liver and result in symptoms of liver failure, such as jaundice, fatigue, abdominal discomfort, or ascites. Intravenous drug users may have damaged veins and be at risk for coronary complications that include endocarditis. Opiates and stimulants reduce appetite, so users of these substances tend to develop an undernourished, emaciated appearance. Physical signs typical of a withdrawal stress reaction should be noted, such as anxiety, palpitations, shakiness, increased heart rate, and diaphoresis. Other physical exam findings are listed in Box 35.1.

Diagnostic Tests

Diagnostic tests detect the presence of drug and alcohol metabolites in the blood and urine. Tests may also be ordered to detect addiction-related disorders, such as evidence of hepatitis, liver disease, and smoking-related disease.

CLINICAL MANAGEMENT

Primary Prevention

To prevent addiction, nurses need to understand the individual and social contexts in which addiction occurs. This section examines primary prevention from the community perspective and from the individual perspective.

Community Health

Successful models for the prevention of addiction promote healthy families in healthy communities.[14] Examples of large-scale community treatment programs shown to be effective in preventing addiction have been implemented in Australia[15] and Vancouver, British Columbia.[16] In the United States, the National Institute on Drug Abuse (NIDA) has established recommendations to support research-based community prevention.[7] NIDA suggests that a well-constructed community plan first identifies the specific drug problems in the community and then builds on existing resources to develop short-term goals and projects that include the assessment of outcomes.[7] Numerous examples of educational and community-based programs are offered on the NIDA website.[7]

Individual Positive Coping Strategies

Positive coping strategies are nonspecific and highly individualized to the individual, their past experiences and the specific situations. Ideally, positive coping strategies are used as opposed to turning to drugs or alcohol as a coping strategy. Coping strategies link to general strategies that optimize wellness, including maintaining good health, proper nutrition, and exercise. Additionally, maintaining positive personal relationships, positive social support networks, and maintaining positive self-esteem underlie positive coping strategies.

For nurses and other healthcare providers, personal coping strategies include developing a self-care philosophy that includes setting limits at work by saying "no" to unreasonable expectations; debriefing stress through supportive professional relationships; and developing rituals for coping with loss, grief, and death. It is recommended that all nurses reflect upon and further explore ideas for the positive management of

stress so that they can experience long and rewarding careers free from substance use.

Secondary Prevention (Screening)

The United States Preventative Services Task Force recommends screening all adults over age 18 for alcohol misuse.[17] Some evidence endorses the use of the National Institute on Alcohol Abuse and Alcoholism (NIAAA) Quantity and Frequency Questionnaire and the CAGE questionnaire by generalist nurses.[18] Box 35.2 presents these instruments with recommendations for their use to detect possible addictions by nurses. The CAGE questionnaire is easily adapted for screening of other substances and behaviors.[18] Initially developed by Ewing in 1984 to screen for alcohol addiction, the reliability and validity of the CAGE questionnaire have been established.[19] It does not distinguish between past and present problems, but it is an expedient and nonthreatening approach to assessing patients for the defining characteristics of any addiction.[18]

Collaborative Interventions

The clinical management of addictions and consequences of addictions by the generalist practice nurse consists of emergency management measures to stabilize life-threatening complications and nonemergency measures to facilitate the recovery from substance abuse.

Emergency Management

Generalist practice nurses are likely to encounter many different emergency scenarios related to adverse drug reactions and/or overdose. The primary goal of emergency management is to prevent life-threatening complications that occur as a result of substance consumption or that result as the substance clears the system.[20] Agency-specific protocols should be followed when indicated.

Presenting signs and symptoms depend on the doses of substance or substance combinations that may have been taken, and the nurse should institute basic life-support measures as needed until toxicology findings are confirmed and resuscitation efforts are directed by advanced

---

BOX 35.2 Alcohol Screening

NIAAA Quantity and Frequency Questions
1. On average, how many days per week do you drink alcohol?
2. On a typical day when you drink, how many drinks do you have?
3. What is the maximum number of drinks you had on any given occasion during the last month?

CAGE Questions
In the Last 12 Months:
1. Have you ever felt like you should **C**ut down on your drinking?
2. Have people **A**nnoyed you by criticizing your drinking?
3. Have you ever felt bad or **G**uilty about your drinking?
4. Have you ever had a drink first thing in the morning to "steady your nerves" or get rid of a hangover (**E**ye opener)?

Screen Positive if:
A positive response on one or more questions from CAGE and/or consumption:
Men >14 drinks/week or >4 drinks/occasion
Women >7 drinks/week or >3 drinks/occasion
Over 65 years old >7 drinks/week or >3 drinks/occasion

From National Institute on Alcohol Abuse and Alcoholism. Helping patients who drink too much: A clinician's guide. NIH Publication No. 07-3769. Retrieved from: http://pubs.niaaa.nih.gov/publications/practitioner/CliniciansGuide2005/guide.pdf

practice providers. Many agents impact the respiratory system, and respiratory management includes monitoring (rate, depth, and oxygen saturation) and support (oxygen administration, ventilation, and medication administration). Cardiovascular support includes monitoring (heart rate, blood pressure, and electrocardiograph) and support (intravenous fluids, medications, and/or resuscitation).

Opiate overdose. There is significant risk of death from respiratory arrest with opiate overdose. Naloxone is a rapid-acting drug that restores respiratory function almost immediately by blocking opiate receptors. Naloxone is used frequently used by paramedics, police officers and even family members as an emergency measure for opioid overdose in the community setting. Nurses and others who administer naloxone should be aware of the potential for injury to both the individual administering the drug and the individual receiving the medication due to the effects associated with this drug. The rapid reversal effect of the opiate is very uncomfortable and can cause fear and panic for the user when consciousness is restored.

Acute alcohol withdrawal syndrome. Acute alcohol withdrawal syndrome is a life-threatening condition that may occur unexpectedly whenever long-term, daily alcohol consumption is abruptly discontinued. This may occur in any setting—for example, on admission to the hospital for some other reason. Such patients may deny alcohol use for fear of legal implications or because of shame. Consequently, the nurse may be unprepared for the sudden onset of acute alcohol withdrawal syndrome (also known as delirium tremens).

When it occurs, the onset of alcohol withdrawal syndrome is highly variable, usually beginning within 6 to 9 hours of the last drink.[20] Signs that may lead the nurse to suspect the onset of alcohol withdrawal syndrome are alterations in mental status, tremors, seizures, tachycardia, and hypertension. Late signs such as bradycardia or hypotension are indicative of cardiovascular collapse and the impending need for resuscitation. Other signs of possible alcohol withdrawal syndrome are irritability, depressed mood, impaired concentration, dizziness, hyperreflexia, ataxia, pyrexia, anorexia, and insomnia.[20]

Wernicke encephalopathy and Korsakoff syndrome. Wernicke encephalopathy and Korsakoff syndrome are two stages of the same emergency problem: Heavy alcohol use leads to poor nutritional intake and also inhibits B vitamin absorption (especially vitamin B_1 [thiamine]). This leads to alcohol neuropathy from irreversible brain damage with manifestations of psychosis, ataxia, abnormal eye movements, and death. Therefore standard treatment for alcohol withdrawal for all patients should also include daily injections of B-complex vitamins.

Substance Abuse Recovery: The Nonemergency Management of Addictions

During substance abuse recovery, the individual struggles to achieve sufficient willpower to maintain long-term sobriety from addiction. The essence of this struggle is known as the relapse process, and an understanding of the relapse process is essential to understanding addiction. For some, addiction recovery may only involve attendance to group support meetings, whereas others may have much more complicated rehabilitation needs. Rehabilitation refers generally to a broad spectrum of treatment options that may be inpatient or outpatient and may include initial detoxification treatment, group therapy, individual therapy, mental health treatment, psychosocial rehabilitation, and others such as comprehensive community support services.[21]

The term *recovery* is used to depict an individual who is sober from an addiction and getting the help needed to maintain sobriety.[22] In successful recovery, craving is recognized as part of the relapse process, and therefore coping strategies are planned in advance to prevent use of the substance or behavior in response to craving. This process is an ongoing struggle as the individual moves through early sobriety from

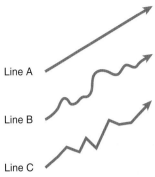

FIGURE 35.2 Recovery and the Relapse Process.

1 month to 1 year, sustained sobriety from 1 to 5 years, and stable sobriety that begins at approximately 5 years.[22]

It is a common misunderstanding among many patients and even some clinicians that recovery means simply the absence of addictive behavior, as depicted by line A in Fig. 35.2. Unfortunately, recovery is complicated by a distinct split between the will for freedom and the will of addiction. Consequently, the recovery from addiction is rarely or never a straight line to freedom, as depicted in line A of Fig. 35.2. Rather, as soon as anyone suffering from addiction begins to pursue freedom from it, the will of the addiction begins to draw him or her back into it. Therefore recovery is better demonstrated by lines B and C in Fig. 35.2 because these lines depict the two opposing forces of will that pull in one direction down toward addiction and in the other direction up toward freedom. It is important for the person in recovery to understand that this process is normal so that his or her self-esteem can withstand any feelings of failure that may result from the inevitable relapse into craving. The idea is that relapse is recognized on the emotional level as craving *before use reoccurs*, and therefore use can be prevented by implementing the positive coping strategies as planned. Success in doing this enhances self-esteem and strengthens recovery, whereas failure to understand this can damage self-esteem and undermine recovery.

Often, it is said that an individual who has been struggling with addiction "has entered rehab." What this means is that to a certain extent the individual has overcome his or her resistance to changing an addictive behavior and is now motivated to commit to a treatment recovery program. The overarching goal of any rehabilitation program is to establish and maintain sobriety by helping the patient manage the relapse challenges that will certainly arise. Rehabilitation may also include advanced practice care to manage any mood spectrum problems that emerge as addictive coping subsides. This specialized area of addiction care, which is known as the care for co-occurring disorders or dual diagnosis, is discussed in more detail later.

Motivational interviewing. It is well known that in modern health care, patient outcomes are greatly influenced by the patient's motivation to change lifestyle behaviors.[12] There are hundreds of randomized controlled trials of the motivational interviewing method in health care that endorse this simple truth: *Efforts to persuade patient to change increase their resistance to change.* Nurses can be more effective by building therapeutic relationship with the patient and then collaborating with the patient to identify what behavior can be improved or changed.[21]

It has been reliably demonstrated that whatever approach is selected in the treatment of addiction, the most significant factor is the motivation of the patient. Motivational interviewing is especially useful in the management of addictions.[23] Motivational interviewing does not involve convincing the patient to do something different. Motivational interviewing focuses on developing a collaborative relationship between the healthcare provider and honors the autonomy of the patient to make informed decisions about his or her behavior. In motivational interviewing, the nurse should listen more than talk. The patient will almost certainly have ambivalent feelings about his or her problem behaviors, and it is important to understand the ambivalence. In particular, the *benefits* of the addiction should be well understood for any plan of change to be effective.

A homeless woman addicted to amphetamines provides a poignant example of the benefits of addiction. In this example, the woman's addiction to amphetamines began when she was sleeping in parks and shelters, where her motivation to use the drugs emerged from a need to stay vigilant at night to avoid being raped, as had happened previously. In addition to the benefit of surviving the night, amphetamines were beneficial in providing her with a temporarily enhanced mood in an otherwise bleak and hopeless setting. Amphetamines provided her with temporary relief from symptoms of rape trauma syndrome. Once the individual's ambivalent situation is understood in this way, the patient and nurse can then collaborate to resolve the motivations underlying the addiction with a personal plan for recovery that anticipates relapse processes.

To enhance their abilities to do this, nurses are encouraged to participate in motivational interviewing workshops. As a brief overview, when patients are committed to change, the nurse is able help them to determine the best course of action, but most patients are not initially interested in change or they are ambivalent about changing. When the patient is not interested in changing, it is recommended that the nurse remain empathetic but raise doubt, provide information with permission, and let the patient know that he or she may return if an interest in change develops.[21]

When patients are ambivalent about changing addictive behaviors, the nurse should consider ways to tip the balance toward change without arguing. Arguing with an ambivalent person will put the person in a defensive position in which he or she is resistant to change. One way already discussed to tip the balance toward change is by analyzing the benefits of the addiction so that ideas for meeting the benefits by healthier means can be planned. Another technique is to develop a discrepancy between the patient's current behavior and important goals.

There are compassionate, respectful ways to point out discrepancies, and it is important that the nurse is authentic in his or her style of communication. In the example of the homeless woman who is addicted to amphetamines, lecturing her on the harm of amphetamines is likely only to alienate her and make her defensive. As an alternative, the nurse might ask this patient how she would like her life to be in 2 years. Chances are she would like to have a nice home and a job, providing the nurse with a point of leverage because there is a discrepancy between having a nice home and job while addicted to amphetamines.

The nurse should determine how motivated the woman is to achieve these goals and perhaps chat about how nice it would be to have her own apartment and a job. Patient motivation can be reported on a scale of 1 to 10. This opens the door to establish a discrepancy between amphetamine addiction and having a nice apartment and job. For example, the nurse might state, "Gosh, it would be really hard to hold down a job and pay rent while supporting an amphetamine addiction, wouldn't it?" Once the discrepancies are established, then resources for relapse prevention and support services can be arranged collaboratively.

Pharmacotherapy in substance abuse recovery. Relapse prevention is improved by reducing craving and withdrawal symptoms. This is the aim of pharmacotherapy in recovery.[21] A complete discussion of the full scope of pharmacotherapy in the routine treatment of addictions is beyond the scope of this concept presentation, and there are numerous text sources available for information on this subject.[21] The following is a brief overview to provide the nurse with a framework for deeper research:

- *Methadone*: Medications to treat opiate withdrawal either are substitutes for street opiates or are aimed at reducing the symptoms of withdrawal.[21] Methadone is a long-acting opiate that may be prescribed as a replacement; methadone can be gradually tapered once the withdrawal is stabilized.
- *Buprenorphine*: Buprenorphine may be prescribed rather than methadone; buprenorphine is a partial opioid agonist and, as such, higher doses can be administered with fewer side effects.[21]
- *Suboxone*: Buprenorphine may also be prescribed in a combined preparation with naloxone called Suboxone. Suboxone is taken sublingually, and the addition of the opiate antagonist naloxone in this preparation reduces the potential for abuse of buprenorphine alone by eliminating the opioid euphoria.
- *Clonidine*: The antihypertensive clonidine may also be prescribed for symptomatic relief of opiate withdrawal.
- *Nicotine*: Nicotine gum and nicotine patches may be prescribed to deliver nicotine into the body during withdrawal from tobacco products. These products are intended to alleviate withdrawal symptoms while tapering the dose of nicotine to zero. There are also nasal sprays and inhalers that serve the same purpose, but they are less popular.[21]
- *Bupropion*: Bupropion may also be prescribed for nicotine withdrawal; it is a non-nicotine replacement medication that reduces craving.
- *Naltrexone, nalmefene, and acamprosate*: Besides the emergency management for acute alcohol withdrawal, a number of pharmacologic approaches may be taken to facilitate the recovery from alcohol addiction. Naltrexone, nalmefene, and acamprosate are all used to reduce cravings for alcohol.
- *Disulfiram*: Disulfiram may be prescribed as aversion therapy for alcohol addiction meant to prevent impulsive drinking.[21] The intent of aversion therapy is to extinguish a negative behavior by pairing it with an unpleasant stimulus. Disulfiram works by disrupting the metabolism of alcohol so that toxic blood levels of alcohol metabolites occur in the bloodstream, causing severe headache, nausea, vomiting, palpitations, flushing, tachycardia, chest pain, and dizziness. Severe reactions that include convulsions and death may also occur, but these are rare. Taking disulfiram usually requires written consent to ensure that the patient is fully informed of the risks and aware that he or she must not consume anything containing alcohol. Therefore patient teaching is of critical importance. Such food items as vanilla extract and over-the-counter preparations of cough medicine and mouthwash often contain alcohol and are likely to induce the side effects of disulfiram and alcohol incompatibility. No form of alcohol should be consumed for at least 2 weeks after discontinuation of disulfiram.[21]

Co-Occurring Disorders

Also known as dual diagnosis, co-occurring disorders refer to the unique challenges faced by individuals who are chemically dependent and have serious psychological distress (SPD). There are two broad etiologies of co-occurring disorders. Persons with mental illness may turn to substance abuse to self-medicate the SPD, or the substance use may cause SPD. In either case, motivational interviewing is recommended as part of a comprehensive treatment approach to unravel the motivations that underlie the problem.[24]

Safe detoxification from the substances of abuse is usually the first step, but ongoing therapeutic communication skills such as active listening and affirmation will help establish trust so that the etiologies can be understood to avoid years of "revolving door" treatment for these individuals, sometimes labeled as "frequent flyers." By doing so, case management can be established to intervene in the underlying causes of the disorder. For example, there are likely to be logical benefits for the use of illicit drugs and alcohol for individuals with SPD.[24] Street drugs may alleviate symptoms of anxiety and psychosis. Intoxication may facilitate social interactions and mask psychosis as substance induced—among the users of street drugs, substance-induced psychosis is socially acceptable, whereas psychosis from "being mental" is not. An understanding of all the logical reasons *not* to stop taking street drugs will facilitate the development of treatment plans that are more likely to result in long-term remission by addressing these needs as logical within the patient's social ecology.

There are some contraindications for the use of motivational interviewing in dual diagnosis. The patient might be too psychotic to benefit from motivational interviewing.[24] If so, the psychosis will have to be stabilized before motivational interviewing can be of any significant value. These patients may also be too dangerous for motivational interviewing.[24] Dangerousness necessitates the removal of freedom, and this contradicts the principle of autonomy in motivational interviewing.

For patients who have a degree of orientation to reality despite their confusion or psychosis, the generalist nurse may modify the motivational interviewing method by frequently paraphrasing what the patient says to help maintain an organized dialogue. Nurses should try to keep motivational change talk very concrete and target compliance with medications and other treatments. To avoid escalating anxiety, nurses should avoid exploring despair and instead explore the patient's motivation for using street drugs. As in the ordinary motivational interviewing method, once the motivation is understood, then discrepancy can be established between the drug use and the patient's goals.[24]

INTERRELATED CONCEPTS

Addiction as a concept does not exist in isolation, and there are many other interrelated concepts, depending on the specific context of the patient situation. Three common interrelated concepts are **Stress and Coping**, **Family Dynamics**, and **Cognition**. When coping, family dynamics, or cognition become ineffective, the individuals within these systems are at risk for addiction. **Mood and Affect** also overlaps with a risk for addiction. Nurses will benefit by mentally applying the defining characteristics of addiction to these related concepts in their own analyses (Fig. 35.3).

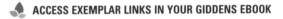

BOX 35.3 EXEMPLARS OF ADDICTION

Substance-Induced Disorders
- Alcohol-induced disorders
- Cocaine-induced disorders
- Heroin-induced disorders
- Inhalant-induced disorders
- Marijuana-induced disorders
- Methamphetamine-induced disorders
- Opioid-induced disorders
- Tobacco-induced disorders

Substance Use Disorders
- Alcohol use disorder
- Cocaine use disorder
- Heroin use disorder
- Inhalant use disorder
- Marijuana use disorder
- Methamphetamine use disorders
- Opioid use disorder
- Tobacco use disorder

Behavioral Addictions
- Food addiction
- Gambling addiction
- Gaming addiction
- Internet addiction
- Sex addiction
- Shopping addiction

ACCESS EXEMPLAR LINKS IN YOUR GIDDENS EBOOK

CLINICAL EXEMPLARS

There are numerous exemplars of addiction, representing both substance addictions and behavioral addictions; some of the most common are presented in Box 35.3. This list is brought to life by the story of a student in an addictions' concept class discussion who mentioned that her boyfriend was addicted to pornography. Inspired to change by the harm his addiction was causing their relationship, he drove to a distant city where he discarded his entire pornography collection in a dumpster. Evidently, it became clear to him that he was unable to defeat the will of his addiction without help when he found himself in that same dumpster at 3:00 AM rummaging for remnants of his precious pornography collection.

Stories such as this clearly illustrate tolerance, withdrawal, deception, loss of willpower, and relapse, but interrelated concepts are also clear. The boyfriend's will for freedom was motivated by the harm his addiction had on his family dynamics, mood, and cognition, but his coping abilities were not adequate to withstand the will of addiction. The nurse's role

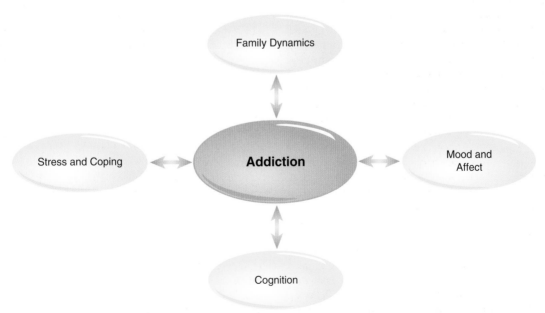

FIGURE 35.3 Addiction and Interrelated Concepts.

in this story is to recognize how these concepts interrelate so that the boyfriend's motivation to cope can be strengthened with a collaborative plan that will vary, depending on the local resources and the individual's sense of what will work for him.

Featured Exemplars

Tobacco Use Disorder and Tobacco Withdrawal

Tobacco use is the most common addictive disorder and the leading cause of preventable disease, disability, and death. Nicotine, a stimulant substance found in tobacco, increases arousal and alertness; increases heart rate, blood pressure, and cardiac output; and decreases appetite. Cigarette smoking is the most predominate form of tobacco use. It is estimated that 85% of smokers who try to quit on their own relapse within 1 week because of the withdrawal symptoms that include irritability, craving, depression, anxiety, cognitive and attention deficits, sleep disturbances, and increased appetite.[25]

Alcohol Intoxication

Alcohol intoxication is one of the most common substance-induced disorders. It occurs when alcohol is ingested faster than the liver can metabolize it. Physiological effects of alcohol intoxication are related to the dose. Euphoria, reduced social inhibitions, and flushed skin are associated with lower levels of alcohol intake. Drowsiness and progressive impairments in balance, coordination, judgment, and erratic or sometimes violent behavior occur with greater levels of alcohol intake. Sufficiently high levels of intake lead to nausea, vomiting, and potentially lethal depression of the central nervous system.

Alcohol Use Disorder

Alcohol use disorder (AUD) is one of the most prevalent of the substance use disorders. It is estimated that 15 million adults (older than age 18 years)[26] and more than 623,000 adolescents between ages 12 and 17 years had an AUD in 2015. AUD results from long-term excessive alcohol use and is characterized by the inability to cut down or stop drinking, craving, interference with family or job, alcohol tolerance, withdrawal, deception of the self and others, and relapse processes (loss of willpower).

Opioid Use Disorder

Opioid use disorder involves the misuse of a wide range of drugs from multiple sources, including prescription pain medications (e.g., codeine, morphine, and oxycodone), street drugs (e.g., heroin), and drugs to treat addictions (e.g., methadone). Opioids cause central nervous system depression, leading to analgesia, euphoria, drowsiness, relaxation, and detachment from the environment and impaired decision making. Over 2 million individuals ages 12 and older suffered from substance use disorder of prescription pain medication; 591,000 used heroin.[27]

Gambling Disorder

Compulsive gambling, a behavioral addiction, involves an uncontrollable urge to gamble despite social consequences. Gambling disorder is characterized by gaining a thrill from gambling risk; preoccupation with gambling; taking increasingly larger gambling risks; and using the behavior as a means to cope with problems, guilt, or depression. Gambling disorder closely resembles substance use disorders in the physiological response but also social consequences, including relationships, economic, and occupational. It is estimated that of the 80% of adults who have gambled, 2% or 3% have experienced a gambling problem—representing more than 1 million individuals with gambling disorders.[28]

CASE STUDY

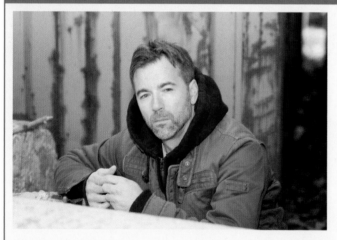

Case Presentation

Jim Wright is a 45-year-old male. He is married to Darla and has two children: 16-year-old Ryan and 9-year-old Jenny. The interview with Jim stemmed from a family therapy meeting to plan Jim's care in a substance treatment program. Jim is charming, funny, and talkative. His interview began with the CAGE questionnaire, and Jim affirmatively acknowledged all four CAGE questions. Jim further acknowledged more than two decades of heavy alcohol and substance use. He says he has tried Narcotics Anonymous and Alcoholics Anonymous meetings, "but they didn't help much." He says that after such meetings, he and other addicts would go out to drink and use drugs together.

Jim says tearfully that he has tried family therapy as well, "because of me our whole family is screwed up." As a youth, Jim was involved in gang activity; at age 16 years, he served time in the youth detention system for assault and battery and making threats with a deadly weapon. Jim has been arrested and incarcerated numerous times for reasons related to drug and alcohol use. While in jail, Jim would drink a fermented jailhouse concoction called "pruno" and use drugs with other inmates.

Jim has recently been released from jail and Darla has told him she does not want him around until he can stop drinking and using drugs. He plans ways to manipulate Darla into taking him back. His current plan is to be kind and generous with her at first, and he thinks he "might even have to get a job for a while." Knowing rules of confidentiality, Jim admitted that coming in for this interview was part of manipulating Darla.

"Alcoholism runs in the family," Jim says. Like others in his family, Jim has gone through alcohol withdrawal several times. "Withdrawal sucks," he says. "It can last a couple days or more. ... my skin feels like something is crawling on it, and my heart pounds. Last time I went through withdrawal I was in jail and almost died from a seizure. I needed some Valium for that, but since I was in jail they didn't care."

Case Analysis Questions

1. How does this case reflect relationship issues associated with substance use and addiction?
2. What risk factors are present in this case?

From NADOFOTOS/iStock/Thinkstock.

ACCESS EXEMPLAR LINKS IN YOUR GIDDENS EBOOK

REFERENCES

1. National Institute on Drug Abuse. (2017). *Trends and statistics.* Retrieved from: http://www.drugabuse.gov/related-topics/trends-statistics.
2. Venes, D. (Ed.), (2017). *Taber's cyclopedic medical dictionary.* Philadelphia: Davis.
3. American Psychiatric Association. (2013). *Diagnostic and statistical manual of mental disorders* (5th ed.). Arlington, VA: American Psychiatric Publishing.
4. Holden, C. (2010). Psychiatry: Behavioral addictions debut in proposed *DSM-V. Science, 327*(5968), 935.
5. National Institute on Drug Abuse. (2018). *Drugs, brains and behavior: The science of addiction.* Bethesda, MD: U.S. Department of Health and Human Services, National Institutes of Health. Retrieved from https://www.drugabuse.gov/publications/drugs-brains-behavior-science-addiction/preface.
6. National Coalition for the Homeless. (2017). *Addiction disorders and homelessness.* Retrieved from: http://nationalhomeless.org/wp-content/uploads/2017/06/Substance-Abuse-and-Homelessness.pdf.
7. National Institute on Drug Abuse. (2010). *Preventing drug abuse among children and adolescents.* Retrieved from: www.nida.nih.gov/prevention/risk.html.
8. Federation of State Medical Boards. (2013). *Model policy on the use of opioid analgesics in the treatment of chronic pain.* Washington, DC: Author. Retrieved from http://www.fsmb.org/Media/Default/PDF/FSMB/Advocacy/pain_policy_july2013.pdf.
9. Ruiz, M. A., Douglas, K. S., Edens, J. F., et al. (2012). Co-occurring mental health and substance use problems in offenders: Implications for risk assessment. *Psychological Assessment, 24*(1), 77–87.
10. U.S. Department of Health and Human Services. *Substance use and mental health estimates from the 2013 national survey on drug use and health: Overview of findings.* The NSDUH Report 2015. Retrieved from: https://www.samhsa.gov/data/sites/default/files/NSDUH-FFR1-2015/NSDUH-FFR1-2015/NSDUH-FFR1-2015.pdf.
11. Fearon, C., & Nicol, M. (2011). Strategies to assist prevention of burnout in nursing staff. *Nursing Standard, 26*(14), 35–39.
12. Boniface, S. (2013). How is alcohol consumption affected if we account for under-reporting? A hypothetical scenario. *European Journal of Public Health, 23*(6), 1101–1262.
13. Rollnick, S., Miller, W. R., & Butler, C. C. (2008). *Motivational interviewing in health care: Helping patients change behavior.* New York: Guilford.
14. Liddle, H. A. (2014). Adapting and implementing an evidence-based treatment with justice-involved adolescents: The example of multidimensional family therapy. *Family Process, 53*(3), 516–528.
15. Stafford, J., Allsop, S., & Daube, M. (2014). From evidence to action: Health promotion and alcohol. *Health Promotion Journal of Australia, 25*(1), 8–13.
16. Vancouver Coastal Health. (2011). *2011 Health watch.* Retrieved from: http://www.vch.ca/media/HealthWatchNOV2011.pdf.
17. United States Preventative Services Task Force. (2015). *Alcohol Misuse: Screening and Behavioral Counseling Interventions in Primary Care.* Retrieved from: https://www.uspreventiveservicestaskforce.org/Page/Document/RecommendationStatementFinal/alcohol-misuse-screening-and-behavioral-counseling-interventions-in-primary-care.
18. DiClemente. (2018). *Addiction and change: How addictions develop and addicted people recover* (2nd ed.). New York: Guilford.
19. Meneses-Gaya, C., Zuardi, A. W., Loureiro, S. R., et al. (2010). Is the full version of the AUDIT really necessary? Study of the validity and internal construct of its abbreviated versions. *Alcoholism, Clinical and Experimental Research, 34*(8), 1417–1424.
20. Mirjiellow, D., D'Angelo, C., Ferrulli, A., et al. (2015). Identification and management alcohol withdrawal syndrome. *Drugs, 75*(4), 352–365.
21. Espelin, J., & Halter, M. J. (2017). Substance related and addictive disorders. In M. J. Halter (Ed.), *Varcarolis' foundation of psychiatric mental health: A clinical approach* (8th ed.). Phildelphia: Elsevier.
22. Buddy, T. (2014). *What exactly is recovery? It's more than just being sober, panel says.* Retrieved from: http://alcoholism.about.com/od/faq/a/recovery.html.
23. Butler Center for Research. (2010). *Research update: Project MATCH: A study of alcoholism treatment approaches,* Hazelden Foundation. Retrieved from: www.hazelden.org/web/public/document/bcrup_0600.pdf.
24. Miller, W. R., & Arkowitz, H. (2015). Learning, applying, and extending. In H. Arkowitz, W. R. Miller, & S. Rollnick (Eds.), *Motivational interviewing in the treatment of psychological problems* (2nd ed., pp. 1–32.26). New York: Guilford.
25. National Institutes of Health, National Institute on Drug Abuse. (2012). *Tobacco/nicotine: Is nicotine addictive?* Retrieved from: http://www.drugabuse.gov/publications/researreports/tobacco/nicotine-addictive.
26. National Institute of Alcohol Abuse and Alcoholism. *Alcohol and your health 2017.* Retrieved from: https://www.niaaa.nih.gov/alcohol-health.
27. American Society of Addiction Medicine: *Opioid addiction 2016 facts and figures.* Retrieved from: https://www.asam.org/docs/default-source/advocacy/opioid-addiction-disease-facts-figures.pdf.
28. North America Foundation for Gambling Addiction Help. (n.d.). *Problem Gambling and Gambling Addiction.* Retrieved from: http://nafgah.org/.

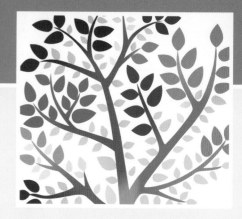

Interpersonal Violence

Paul Thomas Clements

Violence is pervasive and occurs across people of all ages, race, religion, geography, financial status, and gender identification. Ultimately, interpersonal violence (IPV) and intimate partner violence do not discriminate based on who the potential victims and offenders may be. The past several decades have demonstrated a significant increase in research and subsequent policy regarding IPV—specifically, enhanced assessment, targeted intervention, and utilization of referral. Yet there remains a pervasive lack of consistent clinical practice that includes targeted and sensitive assessment. Certainly, the challenges related to IPV are multifaceted. Perhaps violence itself is part of the human condition; however, it is, at the very least, destructive in nature. Although there are legal and moral rules, cultural traditions, political beliefs, and religious ramifications surrounding violence, it remains that such actions are always a potential manifestation of humanity. It would seem that the more society strives to understand IPV, the more complicated it seems to become. However, what is known is that IPV has been categorically established as a pervasive public health problem in the United States and globally.[1,2] The purpose of this concept presentation, regarding the role of the nurse relative to IPV, is to examine awareness, enhanced and targeted assessment, and identification of the foundations of intervention and referral.

DEFINITION

The World Health Organization's (WHO) Violence Prevention Alliance has defined *violence* as the intentional use of physical force or power, threatened or actual, against oneself, another person, or against a group or community that either results in or has a high likelihood of resulting in injury, death, psychologic harm, maldevelopment, or deprivation. Furthermore, it has categorized violence into three subtypes: self-directed violence, collective violence, and IPV.[3] When violence is defined as the use of power, then other concepts come into play including coercion and threats, intimidation, emotional abuse, isolation, economic abuse, and using any children as methods of control.[4] The WHO definition also encompasses the nature of IPV—for instance, physical, psychological, sexual, and neglect and/or deprivation. Intimate partner violence is recognized as a public health problem, but it is also a crime. Assault, battery, homicide, weapon use, kidnapping, and unlawful imprisonment are frequent crimes of domestic violence.[5] Since the majority of IPV occurs between two people who have some form of prior or existing relationship,[6] this concept does not pertain to abuse or violence by strangers, street crime, gang warfare, or military conflict.

SCOPE

IPV is a complex concept seen in many forms across the lifespan. In order to fully understand this concept, one must not restrict a view to that of only the *recipient* of the violence, but also necessarily consider the *offender* as well. For example, it is important to note that in one study, an estimated one in five men in the United States reported perpetration toward their intimate partner at least once in their lifetime.[7] When considering IPV, one must also consider the *nature* of the violence, the *environment* in which the violence occurs, and the *relationship* between the perpetrator and the recipient of the violence (Fig. 36.1).

Johnson[8] discusses a model of IPV that separates the violence into two types: *patriarchal terrorism* and *situational violence*. The first category includes cases in which the male partner attempts to dominate and assume control over his partner. The second category includes cases in which a situation produces an escalation of conflict and the partner initiates physical aggression based in the situational conflict. The first category is considered the most physically violent. Other studies have shown that as physical violence increases, danger of death also increases.[9,10] When considering the nature of the violence, there can be an overlap among the physical, sexual, and psychological components, and in children, direct acts of abuse and neglect often progress to become a regular part of the pattern of violence.

When considering IPV as a concept, the etiology of violence becomes an area of interest. Violence is closely related to criminality because most violence is criminal in nature. Throughout the 20th century, the dominant model for understanding violence and criminality had been a sociological model. Raine[11] proposed that violence and criminality may have a biological basis—a concept that continued to expand in the contemporary era of increased understanding of neurobiology and the expanding research on genetics.[12,13] Although the actual cause (or combination of contributing factors) remains unknown, what is known is that approaches for primary prevention continue to be minimally understood and the rate of IPV continues to be pervasive.

VARIATIONS AND CONTEXT

There are many categories of IPV that are seen across the lifespan. Many of these categories overlap and may, for example, include, child abuse/neglect, elderly abuse/neglect, youth violence, bullying, and sexual violence (Fig. 36.2).

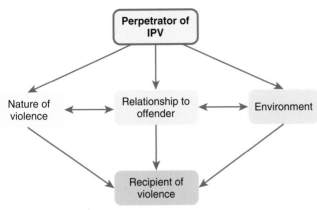

FIGURE 36.1 Scope of Interpersonal Violence *(IPV)*.

Child Abuse and Neglect

Child abuse and neglect encompass a wide variety of forms of child maltreatment, including physical abuse, sexual abuse, and neglect. The Federal Child Abuse Prevention and Treatment Act (CAPTA), which was amended by the Keeping Children and Families Safe Act of 2003, was again amended in a reauthorization act of 2010.[14] This document defines child abuse and neglect as occurring when there is any recent act or failure to act on the part of a parent or caretaker that results in death, serious physical or emotional harm, sexual abuse, or exploitation, or when there is any act or failure to act that presents an imminent risk of serious harm. According to the StopAbuse Campaign,[15] it is imperative for those working in health care to be aware of the pervasive myths and stereotypes that continue surrounding child abuse and neglect (Box 36.1).

Elder Abuse and Neglect

According to the National Council on Aging,[16] elder abuse includes physical abuse, emotional abuse, sexual abuse, exploitation, neglect, and abandonment. Offenders include youth, family members, and spouses—as well as staff at nursing homes, assisted living, and other facilities. National estimates indicate that 1 in 10 older adults experience elder abuse, and that women appear to be more likely to be abused.[16] Additional risk factors include individuals who have low social support, previous traumatic events (including IPV), functional impairment and poor physical health, living with a large number of household members other than the spouse, and lower income or poverty.[17] One of the most vulnerable populations are elders with disabilities, with an estimated 33% having ever experiencing IPV; however, prevalence estimates are influenced, and possibly underestimated, by the fact that many people with dementia or other intellectual, psychological, or emotional disability, are unable, frightened, or embarrassed to report abuse.[17] Ultimately,

elders can become prisoners to their caregivers, and death is often the end result of the abusive cycle.

Youth Violence

Youth violence is widespread in the United States. It is the third leading cause of death for young people between the ages of 15 and 24 and affects thousands of young people each day (and in turn, their families, schools, and communities).[18] Youth violence typically involves young people hurting other peers who are unrelated to them and who they may or may not know well. Youth violence can take different forms. Examples include fights, bullying, threats with weapons, and gang-related violence. A young person can be involved with youth violence as a victim, offender, or witness.[18] Patterns of behavior change over developmental stages; specifically, during teen and young adult years, violence seems to be most prevalent. In a 2013 survey, the Centers for Disease Control statistics regarding this public health issue were notable,[18] including the following:

- More than 599,000 young people aged 10 to 24 years had physical assault injuries treated in U.S. emergency departments—an average of 1642 each day.
- About 24.7% of high school students reported being in a physical fight in the 12 months before the survey.

BOX 36.1 Myths About Child Abuse

Myth: It's only abuse if it's violent.
Fact: Physical abuse is just one type of child abuse. Neglect and emotional abuse can be just as damaging, and since they are more subtle, others are less likely to intervene.

Myth: Only bad people abuse their children.
Fact: Not all abusers are intentionally harming their children. Many have been victims of abuse themselves, and don't know any other way to parent. Others may be struggling with mental health issues or a substance abuse problem.

Myth: Child abuse doesn't happen in "good" families.
Fact: Child abuse doesn't only happen in poor families or bad neighborhoods. It crosses all racial, economic, and cultural lines. Sometimes, families who seem to have it all from the outside are hiding a different story behind closed doors.

Myth: Most child abusers are strangers.
Fact: While abuse by strangers does happen, most abusers are family members or others close to the family.

Myth: Abused children always grow up to be abusers.
Fact: It is true that abused children are more likely to repeat the cycle as adults, unconsciously repeating what they experienced as children. On the other hand, many adult survivors of child abuse have a strong motivation to protect their children against what they went through and become excellent parents.

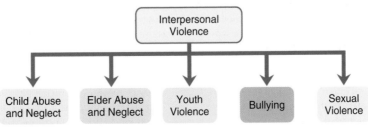

FIGURE 36.2 Categories of Interpersonal Violence Across the Lifespan.

- About 17.9% of high school students reported taking a weapon to school in the 30 days before the survey.
- 19.6% of high school students reported being bullied on school property, and 14.8% reported being bullied electronically.

Bullying

Bullying is now considered to be the most prevalent form of violence perpetrated globally by youth.[19] According to the U.S. Department of Health and Human Service's federal government website, StopBullying.gov,[20] bullying is unwanted, aggressive behavior among school-age children that involves a real or perceived power imbalance. The behavior is repeated, or has the potential to be repeated, over time. Both kids who are bullied and who bully others may have serious, lasting problems.

In order to be considered bullying, the behavior must be aggressive and include:

- *Imbalance of power*: This includes physical strength, access to embarrassing information, or popularity—to control or harm others. Power imbalances can change over time and in different situations, even if they involve the same people.
- *Repetition*: Bullying behaviors happen more than once or have the potential to happen more than once.[20]

Bullying includes actions such as making threats, spreading rumors, attacking someone physically or verbally, and excluding someone from a group on purpose. Bullying also consists of intimidation or domination toward an individual who is perceived as weak. Often, the perpetrator does this as a way to establish perceived superiority over another or to get something through coercion or force. Bullying tactics can be physical, verbal, or emotional—often through social and cyberbullying approaches. Subsequently, as a result of school shootings in the United States, professionals have turned their attention to school bullying.[21,22] Although most prevalent in school-age children and adolescents, adult bullying also exists and is reported in adults—most commonly in the workplace.[23]

Sexual Violence

The term *sexual violence* is an all-encompassing, non-legal term that refers to crimes like sexual assault, rape, and sexual abuse. Sexual assault can happen to anyone, regardless of age, gender identity, or sexual orientation. Men and boys who have been sexually assaulted or abused may have many of the same feelings and reactions as other survivors of sexual assault, but they may also face some additional challenges because of social attitudes and stereotypes about men and masculinity.[24]

The legal definition of *sex-related crimes* varies from state to state. There are often other crimes and forms of violence that arise jointly with sexual crimes.[25] Rape is a form of sexual assault, but not all sexual assault is rape. The term *rape* is often used as a legal definition to specifically include sexual penetration without consent. The definition of rape is: "The penetration, no matter how slight, of the vagina or anus with any body part or object, or oral penetration by a sex organ of another person, without the consent of the victim."[26] This definition includes any gender of victim or perpetrator, and includes instances in which the victim is incapable of giving consent because of temporary or permanent mental or physical incapacity, including due to the influence of drugs or alcohol or because of age. The ability of the victim to give consent must be determined in accordance with the state statute. Physical resistance from the victim is not required to demonstrate lack of consent.

Sexual violence can be committed by any person regardless of his or her relationship to the victim and in any setting, including, but not limited to, home and work. However, the majority of perpetrators are someone known to the victim. Approximately 7 out of 10 sexual assaults are committed by someone known to the victim, such as in the case of intimate partner sexual violence or acquaintance rape.[24] In other instances, the victim may not know the perpetrator at all. This type of sexual violence is sometimes referred to as *stranger rape*. Stranger rape can occur in several different ways:

- *Blitz sexual assault*: When a perpetrator quickly and brutally assaults the victim with no prior contact, usually at night in a public place.
- *Contact sexual assault*: When a perpetrator contacts the victim and tries to gain their trust by flirting, luring the victim to their car, or otherwise trying to coerce the victim into a situation where the sexual assault will occur.
- *Home invasion sexual assault*: When a stranger breaks into the victim's home to commit the assault.[25]

CONSEQUENCES

Physical Consequences

Physical consequences of IPV include the direct impact of physical traumatic injury and the accompanying pain, need for repair, and related recovery time. Certainly, the physiological symptoms can additionally be associated with stress and anxiety caused by IPV.[27] Common patterns of injury and related symptoms that have been identified in the literature range from sustaining minor injuries such as scratches, bruises, and swelling, to more severe injury if the abuse is frequent and harsh. Some of the most common injuries are bruises, lesions, and cuts, headaches, back pain, broken bones, gynecologic injuries, pregnancy complications, sexually transmitted diseases, gastrointestinal disorders, and heart or circulatory conditions.[27] In addition, in cases of attempted strangulation, there may be both significant physical and emotional sequelae.[28] It has been reported that the majority of fractures experienced by victims of assault involve the face, and typically these injuries involve the craniofacial region. Others have reported that the dominant cause of facial fractures in North America is IPV. The nature of fractures from IPV tends to be different in that the fracture is caused by a punch or kick to the face and prominent points are targeted, such as the cheek, the angle of the jaw, and the nose.[29] Other studies have found an increase in chronic health problems during midlife when previously exposed to IPV, which may be directly related to previous or ongoing physical injury.[30]

Sexual violence can occur in the context of child abuse and/or intimate partner violence, or it can occur as an isolated incident. In a multigenerational longitudinal study of females who had been sexually abused, it was noted that the health consequences depend on the age of the victim, the relationship between the victim and the perpetrator, the circumstances of the environment, and the severity and/or types of other violence accompanying the incident.[31] Unintended pregnancy and gynecologic complications—such as bleeding, infection, pain during intercourse, chronic pelvic pain, sexually transmitted diseases, HIV transmission, and urinary tract infections—are associated with sexual violence.[32] Violence that occurs during pregnancy can additionally have detrimental effects, not only on the mother but also on the fetus. Violence directed by an intimate partner toward the pregnant woman and her fetus, or during the first year after delivery, is often either not recognized by nurses or suspected but not addressed. Suspected intimate partner violence during pregnancy requires sensitive assessment and intervention by nurses and the interdisciplinary team, as numerous undesirable outcomes for both the mother and her fetus/baby have been identified—including, most significantly, an increased risk for homicide.[33] Educating nurses about intimate partner violence during pregnancy remains an ongoing challenge. Most nurses lack awareness of this significant public health problem, have limited knowledge and erroneous beliefs about battering during pregnancy, and are inexperienced in the assessment of at-risk women.[33,34]

Mental Health Consequences

Posttraumatic stress disorder (PTSD) is one of the most common mental health consequences of exposure to IPV.[35,36] The incidence of PTSD among those exposed to IPV varies based on the presence (or lack of) supportive factors; however, the nature, severity, and frequency of the of the violence is often predictive of the severity of the symptoms of PTSD. For instance, the use of a weapon during a violent assault or repeated episodes of sexual abuse may typically result in more severe symptoms than a one-time physical assault where the offender demonstrates sincere remorse.[36] Subsequently, repeated episodes of physical or sexual abuse may result in long-lasting physical and emotional effects. The characteristic symptoms of PTSD are threefold: *re-experiencing* the trauma, which includes intrusive and recurrent thoughts, images, and flashbacks of the violence; a biphasic response of *avoidance and numbing*; and *increased arousal*. These are manifest intrapsychically and interpersonally, including feelings of detachment and persistent avoidance of memories that relate to the violence while simultaneously experiencing increased arousal that can include insomnia, difficulty focusing, and hypervigilance.[37,38]

Depression is also a common reaction to IPV.[39] Depression inhibits the ability of abused individuals from formulating a plan to deal with the abuse. This inertia prevents the victim from taking proactive steps to leave the abusive situation or, if they do leave, the ability to place the violence into a perspective that allows them to reinvest in an enjoyable and productive lifestyle. Humphreys and Lee reported that the presence of social support mitigates the depressive effects of IPV.[40,41] When an individual experiences depression, there is an increased risk of suicide, and there are particularly increased suicide attempts in women experiencing IPV.[42,43]

Consequences of Bullying

Bullying is a serious problem for schools, parents, and public policy makers alike. A great deal of research has investigated the consequences of bullying; it has been shown that bullying behaviors in childhood and adolescence have ramifications in adulthood. There is strong evidence that childhood bullies are at risk of developing antisocial behaviors as adults.[44] In addition, adult childhood bullies are likely to have more criminal convictions and traffic violations than their less aggressive peers. The victims of bullying often view themselves as outcasts and failures. Victims often display signs of anxiety and depression in conjunction with isolationism, school absenteeism, loneliness, and suicidal ideation. Costello reported that bullying predicts poorer functioning up to 40 years from the bullying incident(s).[45] Poorer functioning includes psychological distress, depression, poor physical health, and poorer cognitive functioning.[44]

In an effort to understand the consequences of violence, it should be obvious that violence can be an initiating event that produces consequences on the offender as well as the victim. Being bullied is not a harmless rite of passage or an inevitable part of growing up, but throws a long shadow over affected children's lives. Victims, in particular chronic bullying victims, are at increased risk for adverse health and social functioning in adulthood. These problems are associated with great costs for the individual and society.[46]

Consequences of Interpersonal Violence Experienced by Infants and Children

It is a common misconception that infants and young children are minimally impacted by their limited life experiences and cognitive awareness of their environment. The issue of IPV and very young children is often ignored due to a set of erroneous beliefs:

1. that such young children are not affected by the violence due to their level of emotional and cognitive development;

2. that the needs of such young children cannot be adequately taken into consideration since they cannot express their own experiences; and

3. because the meaning of conflict to each individual child is considered highly subjective.[47,48]

As with adults, physical sequelae of childhood abuse are determined by the frequency and type of violence inflicted. Depending upon developmental factors, such as the level of verbal repertoire or understanding of social norms of "good and bad" or "right or wrong," the social and emotional consequences can be severe.

A history of childhood maltreatment often results in childhood delinquency and adult criminality.[46] Multiple studies have shown that children exposed to violence are more likely to become violent as adults.[46–48] Other common consequences of childhood sexual abuse are developmentally inappropriate sexual behavior, such as age-inappropriate knowledge, sexual preoccupation, and inappropriate displays of excessive masturbation.[38]

Neglected children often have learning problems, developmental delays, passivity, low self-esteem, and juvenile delinquency. Multiple emotional problems and social competency problems are associated with psychological maltreatment during childhood, such as anxiety, depression, low self-esteem, suicidal ideation, impulse control problems, substance abuse, eating disorders, isolating behavior, social phobia, aggression, and violent behavior.[49] Exposure to intrafamilial violence also often leads to behavioral problems such as anxiety, depression, and aggression.[49,50] Children experience many fears and worries that are otherwise developmentally inappropriate such as PTSD, which is often more detrimental than the violence itself.[38] Guilt is highly correlated with the severity of PTSD, and resolving guilt is difficult because of the child's inability to accept that the violence was beyond his or her control.[50]

Long-term health consequences of childhood abuse are often related to specific behavioral risk factors such as smoking, alcohol abuse, poor diet, and lack of exercise linking to many illnesses in adulthood, including ischemic heart disease, cancer, chronic lung disease, irritable bowel syndrome, and fibromyalgia.[49] The development of young children is strongly impacted by their caregiving environment. Exposure to IPV can have a detrimental impact on the cognitive and emotional development of infants and young children. Ultimately, "chronic childhood trauma interferes with the capacity to integrate sensory, emotional, and cognitive information into a cohesive whole and sets the stage for unfocused and irrelevant response to subsequent stress."[51, p.1]

RISK FACTORS

As mentioned previously, IPV spans all age groups, races, and ethnicities. It is not restricted to any one special interest group or any socioeconomic group and involves all genders (including those that vary along the LGBT continuum). Literally, all individuals have potential risk of experiencing IPV—as a recipient, perpetrator, or witness of violence. Violence has many complex linkages. Some factors are relative to one type of IPV, but in many cases, there are commonalities in that violence can share multiple and identical risk factors.

Populations at Risk
Infants and Children

Infants and children are at risk for abuse because of the power differential that exists with adolescents and adults. Due to their physical size and ongoing psychosocial development, they are typically unable to resist the abuse and unable or fearful to report it, relative to a pervasive expectation of actual retribution by the abuser. The most often ages for parents or caretakers to report child abuse were among infants from birth to 1 year of age, with the rate decreasing with increasing age.[52]

Although experts have considered toddlers to be at highest risk for abusive abdominal trauma (AAT), infants have higher rates of AAT hospitalization. Similar to other abusive injuries, young age, male gender, and poverty are risk factors for AAT.[52] Abusive head trauma (AHT), (more commonly known as shaken baby syndrome), resulting in head injury, is a leading cause of child abuse death in the United States. Nearly all victims of AHT suffer serious health consequences, and at least one of every four babies who are violently shaken dies from this form of child maltreatment.[53]

IPV has been documented to escalate in severity over time, with children and adolescents who are killed by their parents (also known as filicide) being battered to death (32.9%), physically assaulted (28%), drowned (4.3%), burned (2.3%), stabbed (2.1%), or shot (3.0%).[14] The peak age at which a child will most likely be killed by the mother or father is within the first few months of life. A child is 100 times more likely to be killed by a stepparent than by a genetically related parent. Compared to genetic parents, stepparents are six times more likely to abuse their genetically unrelated child younger than the age of 2 years.[14]

Older Adults

The elderly are often considered burdens and nonproductive members of society. This is reflective to the concept of ageism, which is the stigmatization of older people, and is likely an element of the etiology of elder abuse. Negative attitudes toward aging and the glorification of youth may contribute to elder abuse. They may be placed in nursing homes or other care centers, or be considered a significant burden for family members who must care for them. Elder abuse can occur in any of these situations and locations. Older adults, particularly those with impaired cognitive function and/or who lack independent functional ability, are at risk for abuse for similar reasons as infants and children; specifically, a power differential exists so that they may be physically unable to resist or lack the cognitive capacity to report. In addition, there may be a realistic fear for retaliation—physically, emotionally, or financially. Factors that place elders at risk for physical, sexual, emotional, and financial abuse include dependence on others (family members, caretakers, and agency staff), physical frailty, and cognitive limitations.[54,55] These dependency factors are barriers to detecting elder sexual abuse and can provide for increased risk of abuse with continued low rates of reporting and should be a focus for targeted assessment.[56,57]

Gender

For all age groups, rates of abuse are higher for males than females, and for children insured by Medicaid compared to those with private insurance. The overwhelming incidence of IPV is perpetrated by men to women; although men are victims but may under-report. In the United States, approximately one in three homicides of females is committed by an intimate partner, whereas approximately 5% of male homicide victims are killed by intimate partners.[8–10] Studies from developed countries have reported a higher incidence of elder abuse among males.[58] In consideration of child abuse, higher reports of maltreatment occurred for boys versus girls (51% vs. 48.3%, respectively), and 56% of the perpetrators were women.[59]

Individual Risk Factors
Substance Use

A common underlying factor associated with IPV involves the use/misuse of alcohol. Alcohol is legal for adults, and often easily, albeit illegally, obtained by youth, and has been reported to be a significant risk factor in IPV, child abuse, youth violence, and elder abuse.[60] Substance abuse has been found to co-occur in 40% to 60% of IPV incidents across various studies.[60] Several lines of evidence suggest that substance use and misuse plays a facilitative role in IPV by inhibiting impulse control, thereby increasing the risk for precipitating or exacerbating violence. The strong relationship between substance abuse and perpetration of IPV has been noted across healthcare settings, including primary health care, family practice clinics, prenatal clinics, and rural health clinics.[46,61] The incidence of IPV and relationship to substance abuse is also frequently observed and reported among individuals presenting at psychiatric and substance abuse treatment settings. For example, alcohol has been reported to be a risk factor in IPV, child abuse, youth violence, and elder abuse.[46,60,61]

Mental Health Conditions

Factors that have been identified as risk factors for a male abusing his intimate partner include young age, depression, personality disorders, and low academic achievement.[61,62] Studies have shown a link between those with mental health diagnoses and violence,[63] in that there is a high rate of lifetime victimization among psychiatric patients. However, evidence suggests that mental illness is exacerbated by exposure to violence, and it may also contribute to IPV. Diagnostically, aggressive behavior has been linked to schizophrenia, mania, alcohol abuse, organic brain syndrome, seizure disorder, and personality disorders. Further, among patients in acute psychiatric settings, young age, male sex, history of psychiatric illness, comorbid substance abuse, and positive symptoms (e.g., hallucinations, delusions, paranoia) have been shown as consistent predictors of violent behavior. Among these, the history of violence is often emphasized as the most significant predictor of future violence.[63]

Exposure to Violence in Childhood

Children can experience the harms associated with IPV through awareness of violence between caregivers, even if they have never directly observed any acts of violence."[64,p.1] In homes in which IPV occurs, children who are exposed to that violence often become additional recipients of that violence. Subsequently, exposure to intimate partner violence is increasingly being recognized as a form of child maltreatment; it is prevalent, and is associated with significant mental health impairment and other important consequences.[64] IPV of the adult partner (e.g., the mother) usually progresses to abuse of the child.[65] Individuals who were witness to and/or the victim of IPV during childhood are at greater risk of becoming perpetrators as adults; this is especially notable with intimate partner violence and child abuse.[66]

Sociocultural Factors

Cultural and social norms are highly influential in shaping individual behavior, including the use of violence. Norms can protect against violence, but they can also support and encourage the use of it. For instance, cultural acceptance of violence, either as a normal method of resolving conflict or as a usual part of rearing a child, is a risk factor for all types of IPV.[67] In North America, a sociocultural view of the etiology of IPV is rooted in the family and society in the form of a historical legacy of oppression and colonization. From the beginning of the colonization of the Americas, there has been a stratified caste system based on race, ethnicity, religion, and sexuality.[68] Europeans were privileged over non-Europeans and men over women. Therefore, the patriarchy was racialized. At an interpersonal and intrafamilial level, power leads to a culture that breeds violence. In particular, immigrant and refugee families are at risk for domestic violence because of their migration history and differences in cultural values and norms.[68] A high socioeconomic status has generally been considered to be protective against IPV, but not necessarily; generally, women living in poverty are disproportionately affected.[69]

"Cultural norms still exist that perpetuate the problem. For example, the tradition of not interfering in matters between family members that occur in private has led to reluctance for government, the criminal justice system, and other systems to respond to domestic violence, even after it became a crime. Music and the media continue to portray domestic violence as 'lover's quarrels' and domestic violence homicides-suicide as 'crimes of passion' by jilted men who think, 'If I can't have her, no one else will.' This 'romanticizing' of domestic violence allows it to be excused or explained away—something that is not done with any other type of assault and battery."[70,p.1]

ASSESSMENT

History

There are certain elements in the medical history that raise concern for physical abuse. Victims may provide a history of events that is incomplete or inconsistent with injuries seen. Many individuals who experience IPV are unable or afraid to provide an accurate account of events. Specific examples include a history of trauma that is inconsistent or implausible with the physical examination, a history of no trauma with evidence of injury, a history of self-inflicted trauma that is developmentally unlikely, and for children,[71] serious injuries blamed on siblings or playmates. This creates a serious situation in that direct questioning may not be the best way to determine incidence of abuse. Subsequently, targeted physical assessment (looking for bruises, injuries with inconsistent explanations) and a more overarching asking of questions can enhance determination of the need for additional investigation. For example, nurses often will ask an adult suspected victim directly "Have you ever been physically, sexually, or emotionally abused?" Since the patient has known the nurse for an extremely brief time, there may be an inherent lack of trust for revealing such information and a high level of uncertainty and anxiety regarding the consequences of doing so. Specifically, the patient may have been abused for years and never revealed this information—which may inhibit revealing the information to someone that they have just met. In addition, the patient may feel threatened by the abuser to maintain the secret. Subsequently, asking such sensitive questions in a more global manner can be much less anxiety producing by allowing the client to determine what information (if any) will be disclosed. For example, the nurse might matter-of-factly ask "Are there any times that you feel unsafe in your home? If so, we would be able to provide assistance to help with that situation" or "Have you ever been concerned for the safety of your children? If so, we could explore some approaches that could be helpful in making sure that they are safe." Another example could include "Sometimes people in a relationship make their partners feel afraid or scared. They might, for example, intimidate them, break or throw out their possessions, threaten to hurt them or someone they care about, hurt their pets, or physically attack them. Does anything like this happen in your relationship? If this has ever happened to you, could you share some information about that?"[72] If the patient chooses not to disclose, it is important to document any observations, both physical and emotional, and including direct quotes of relevant information, which can be significantly useful. The patient may return again as a result of subsequent abuse since the cycle of violence has been determined to escalate over time.[72]

Examination Findings

Examination findings for all IPV range from subtle to obvious. Some may manifest as old or new injuries that may seem mild to more significant (e.g., cuts, bruises, burns, or fractures) and may not raise concern. For this reason, it is critical to consider the history in relation to injuries seen. The nurse should also maintain a high degree of awareness for injuries that are not typically seen in the context of day-to-day living, such as unusual patterns of bruising or burn marks; inconsistent and/or implausible explanations are of significance. For example, a child who has a patterned injury of bruising behind the knee could not have

possibly received those from "falling off of a bicycle." Regardless of the explanation, all *suspected* child abuse must immediately be reported to the local or state Child Protective Agency because all nurses are mandated reporters.

In some cases, specific physical injuries are common. IPV often includes physical assault, which can include injuries to the head and attempted strangulation injuries. Both types of injuries can result in traumatic brain injury (TBI). The TBI sustained during IPV often occurs over time, which can increase the risk for health declines and post concussive syndrome (PCS). Abusive head trauma is also common in infants and young children. Abdominal injuries caused by punching or kicking, which lead to internal bleeding, are the second most common cause of death in child abuse. Burns are a common injury associated with abuse; in fact, it is believed that 10% of all physical abuse cases involve burns, usually with scalding water. Specifically, burns with a stocking pattern or circular burn marks always should raise suspicion.[73]

CLINICAL MANAGEMENT

Primary Prevention

The prevention of IPV is considered a key public health priority. The lead federal organization for violence prevention, established by the Centers for Disease Control and Prevention, is the National Center for Injury Prevention and Control (NCIPC). One of three divisions of the NCIPC is the Division of Violence Prevention (DVP). The strategic directions established by the DVP include reducing rates of various forms of violence (including child maltreatment, intimate partner violence, sexual violence, and youth violence) through individual, community, and societal change. A comprehensive discussion of the national strategic direction for DVP is beyond the scope of this concept analysis, but it is important for nurses to know these directions exist and are readily available on the CDC website.

What is of significant importance is that exposure and experience of violence is preventable in childhood and adolescence. The ultimate goal is to stop youth violence before it starts, as it often continues into adulthood.[18] According the U.S. Department of Justice (DOJ),[22] school engagement is a protective factor for victims and schools can mitigate the ill effects of bullying and related violence by changing school structure. The DOJ[22] highlighted what victims need from their schools. These include:

- A place of refuge where they can feel safe, appreciated, and challenged in a constructive way
- Responsible adults who can support and sustain them and provide them examples of appropriate behavior
- A sense of future possibility to persuade them that staying in school, despite the bullying, promises better things to come

These factors have demonstrated the capacity to facilitate bullied students and those who are victims of violence to overcome the potential for long-lasting effects of bullying.[22]

Secondary Prevention (Screening)

Evidence demonstrates that screening, during encounters in healthcare settings, increases the identification of women, children, and families-at-large experiencing IPV. The recommendation to include IPV screening in health care as routine practice is not new.[74] Research indicates that screening and counseling for IPV can identify survivors and, in some cases, increase safety, reduce abuse, and improve clinical and social outcomes.[75–77] Possible harms or unintended consequences of clinical assessment have been raised and considered in research trials, but thus far no evidence of such harm has emerged. Barriers for implementation of IPV screening and counseling are myriad, including clinician concerns about time; limited incentives for screening; either nonexistent or poorly implemented policies to guide clinicians and practices in conducting screening; and lack of knowledge and confidence about how to support a patient who discloses IPV,[78] which may reflect lack of awareness of reliable intervention services and cross-sector collaborations with victim service advocates. Addressing barriers and improving screening, counseling, and referral practices require attention to multiple levels within the healthcare delivery system to create a safe, trusting environment for patients.[77]

A large number of screening tools have been developed to screen for various types of IPV in a number of healthcare settings. Nurses should be aware of appropriate tools to use in various settings, such as emergency departments, school-based clinics, inpatient settings, or community-based clinics. A useful resource for screening tools is the *Intimate Partner Violence and Sexual Violence Victimization Assessment Instruments for Use in Healthcare Settings*, published by the Centers for Disease Control and Prevention.[79] This resource presents a variety of screening tools that have been tested and validated for multiple types of IPV and among various population groups (age and ethnic/cultural). It is beyond the scope of this concept presentation to describe each screening tool, but nurses are encouraged to become aware of the most appropriate screening tools used in their particular practice settings.

Collaborative Interventions

When IPV is suspected or identified, the priority intervention is to protect the infant, child, adult, or elder from further abuse. It is the legal and ethical duty of nurses and all health professionals to report suspected abuse. Each state has specific laws for mandatory reporting of child abuse and other forms of violence; as such, nurses must familiarize themselves with all related requirements. When the victim is a child or compromised elderly individual, referrals are made to the state agency child or human welfare departments for a formal investigation; based on these findings, the child or elderly person may be left in the home or removed and placed in another setting.

Emotional support and appropriate referrals are also needed for the patient and family. Survivors of both rape and other forms of intimate partner violence often blame themselves for behaving in a way that encouraged the perpetrator. It is important to remember, and immediately and repeatedly reinforce, that the victim is never to blame for the actions of a perpetrator. A focus on minimizing the physiological consequences is needed, particularly helping those who have consequently suffered emotionally, to experience and establish positive relationships.

BOX 36.2 Resources for Interpersonal Violence

The National Domestic Violence Hotline
1-800-799-7233 or TTY 1-800-787-3224
http://www.thehotline.org
National Child Abuse Hotline/Childhelp
1-800-4-A-CHILD (1-800-422-4453)
www.childhelp.org
Rape, Abuse and Incest National Network
1-800-656-HOPE (4673)
National Sexual Assault Hotline and Chat
https://www.rainn.org/
LGBTQI Domestic Violence
Adult Protective Services and Elder Abuse Hotline
1-800-222-8000
https://www.caregiver.org/adult-protective-services-and-elder-abuse-hotline-1

Education and referral for counseling are frequently needed to ensure adaptive coping strategies. Nurses can help patients and families gain access to appropriate community agencies and support groups as available. Common resources are presented in Box 36.2.

INTERRELATED CONCEPTS

Many of the sequelae of IPV result in other health and illness concepts. For instance, IPV could conceivably involve almost all health and illness concepts, depending on the physical and psychological effects of the violence. In fact, IPV sequelae are cumulative and long-lasting beyond the violence events.[1,12,30] Fig. 36.3 features important interrelationships to consider. Common psychological consequences of IPV include **Anxiety, Mood and Affect, Stress and Coping**. Individuals who experience IPV rely on coping strategies as part of the response to such events.[80] Interrelationships with several professional nursing concepts also are important to note. Nurses have a *legal* (**Health Care Law**) and *ethical* (**Ethics**) obligation to report abuses. Because of widespread prevalence, **Health Policy** initiatives have resulted in national strategies to address IPV.

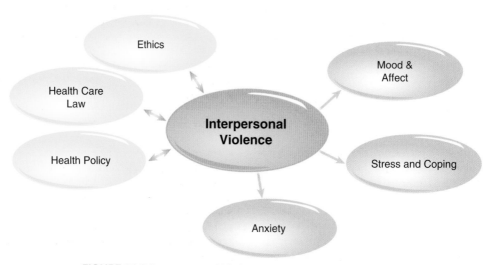

FIGURE 36.3 Interpersonal Violence and Interrelated Concepts.

BOX 36.3   EXEMPLARS OF INTERPERSONAL VIOLENCE

Child Abuse
- Physical abuse
- Sexual abuse
- Emotional abuse
- Neglect
- Bullying
- Youth violence

Intimate Partner Violence
- Physical violence
- Sexual violence
- Emotional abuse

Elder Abuse
- Physical abuse
- Sexual abuse
- Emotional abuse
- Neglect
- Abandonment
- Financial abuse

ACCESS EXEMPLAR LINKS IN YOUR GIDDENS EBOOK

CLINICAL EXEMPLARS

There are many examples of IPV, many of which have been described throughout this concept analysis. It is important to remember that this occurs across the lifespan and it can happen to any individual. Box 36.3 presents common exemplars of IPV.

Featured Exemplars
Child Abuse

It is difficult to know the actual figures of child maltreatment. Much of it is unreported. In 2008, the national rate of reports of child maltreatment was 10.3/1000 children.[81] In 2016, the U.S. Department of Health and Human Services reported the national estimate of children who received a child protective services investigation response or alternative response increased 9.5% from 2012 to 2016. Overall, for 2016, a nationally estimated 1750 children died of abuse and neglect, at a rate of 2.36/100,000 children in the national population.[14] An estimated rate of physical abuse of 49/1000 children was obtained when the following behaviors were included: hitting the child with an object, hitting the child somewhere other than the buttocks, kicking the child, beating the child, and threatening the child with a weapon.[14]

Neglect

It is difficult to differentiate neglect from abuse and neglect is often considered a form of abuse. Neglect is parental failure to meet a child's basic needs[82,83] or a caregiver's failure to meet a dependent adult's needs.[84] This can occur through commission of violence (i.e., active physical, emotional, sexual, or financial abuse), or through omission (i.e., neglect or purposeful withholding of necessary care and meeting of basic human needs).[83,84] Five subtypes of child neglect are physical neglect, psychological or emotional neglect, medical neglect, mental health neglect, and educational neglect.[81]

Bullying

Childhood bullying can have serious implications for bullies and their targets. Bullying involves a pattern of repeated aggression, a deliberate

intent to harm or disturb a victim despite the victim's apparent distress, and a real or perceived imbalance of power. Bullying can lead to serious academic, social, emotional, and legal problems. Research reveals a relationship between childhood bullying and adolescent suicide.[85,86] Most bullying occurs during childhood and adolescent years, with a peak among middle school children. In most cases, bullying occurs while at school, but this can also occur outside the school grounds, such as on the way to and from school or during extramural youth activities.[85] It is estimated that between 15% and 25% of students are bullied frequently, and nearly 20% reported bullying others often.

Youth Violence

Youth violence is a significant public health problem that affects thousands of young people each day, and in turn, their families, schools, and communities. Youth violence can take different forms, including fights, bullying, threats with weapons, and gang-related violence. A young person can be involved with youth violence as a victim, offender, or witness.[87] Worldwide, the highest rates of youth homicide are from Latin America (36.4/100,000 youths), and in the United States this rate is 11/100,000 youths.[88] According to the Centers for Disease Control and Prevention Youth Risk Behavior Survey (YRBS) in 2015,[89] nearly 8% of students had been in a physical fight on school property one or more times during the 12 months before the survey.

Intimate Partner Violence

Intimate partner violence occurs across all social, economic, educational, and professional settings. Physical or sexual abuse may be readily observed in some instances or well-hidden at other times; the emotional components of verbal, economic, and isolation abuse are often difficult to assess. According to 48 population-based studies from several countries, 10% to 69% of women reported being victims of intimate partner violence during their lifetime.[90] In the United States, the prevalence of intimate partner violence in minority women is higher than that in white women, with Hispanic women reporting a greater frequency of rapes and Native American women reporting more violent victimization.[91] It has been reported that intimate partner violence exposure causes more severe health consequences than other types of trauma.[92]

Sexual Violence

Sexual violence occurs across the lifespan. Men, women, and children are all affected by sexual violence. In 2018, one out of every six American women has been the victim of an attempted or completed rape in her lifetime, and approximately 3% of American men have experienced an attempted or completed rape in their lifetime.[93] Child Protective Services agencies substantiated, or found strong evidence to indicate that, 63,000 children a year were victims of sexual abuse. In addition, a majority of child victims are 12 to 17. Of victims under the age of 18, 34% of victims of sexual assault and rape are under age 12, and 66% of victims of sexual assault and rape are age 12 to 17. Older adults also are subjected to sexual abuse within their own homes, nursing homes, or community. Older adults are especially vulnerable to sexual violence, and elder sexual assault is one of the nation's most hidden crimes.

Elder Abuse

There are no national data on the prevalence or incidence of elder abuse, as lack of identification and the underreporting of elder abuse remains a significant challenge. In 2015, the rate of violent victimization against women age 65 and older was both higher than the rate for men in the same age group and 2.4 times greater than the previous year's rate.[94] Researchers estimate that elderly women experience maltreatment more frequently than men, and nearly 50% of individuals with dementia are abused or neglected by their caregivers.

CASE STUDY

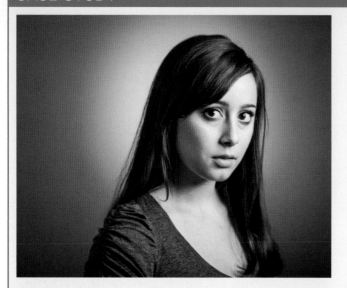

Case Presentation

Amanda Soto, a 22-year-old female, presents to an outpatient clinic with a chief complaint of headaches and problems sleeping. Yvonne Sanchez, the nurse at the clinic, remembers seeing Amanda in the clinic not long ago. She reviews Amanda's medical record before seeing her and notes that Amanda has been in the clinic four times in the past 5 months, each time with vague symptoms, and each time she was sent home with a nonspecific diagnosis. The nurse reviews her social history and sees that Amanda is married and has two children, ages 2 and 4 years, and works as a receptionist. Amanda has no medical conditions and takes no medications other than oral contraceptives.

When Yvonne enters the examination room, she observes Amanda sitting on the examination table with her knees held tightly against her torso and rocking

From Cameron Whitman/iStock/Thinkstock.

back and forth. Yvonne asks Amanda to describe the symptoms she has been experiencing. Amanda states her headaches have been occurring off and on for a while, and she describes them as "intense" and often keeping her awake at night. As she talks, Yvonne notes a flat affect in Amanda's communication pattern. She also notices bruising to her neck, just above the clavicle, and on her upper arms. When Yvonne asks Amanda the last time she experienced the headache, she tells Yvonne she cannot remember exactly, but perhaps 1 or 2 weeks ago.

Yvonne suspects Amanda may be experiencing violence. She pulls out the Partner Violence Screening tool, available at her office, and asks Amanda the following three questions:

1. Have you been hit, kicked, punched, or otherwise hurt by someone within the past year? If so, by whom?
2. Do you feel safe in your current relationship?
3. Is there a partner from a previous relationship who is making you feel unsafe now?

Amanda begins to cry and acknowledges she is in trouble. She states her husband has a drinking problem, and every couple of weeks, he gets drunk and becomes violent. He always feels badly after he becomes sober, but she has become frightened at what he will do to her or the children. She states that he has never hurt the children, but they see him regularly hit her. Amanda tells Yvonne she has contemplated leaving, but she does not think she can. She explains that her husband controls all of the money, and she has nowhere to go. She is sure she does not earn enough money to support herself and her children, and she is worried that he will track her down anyway. Amanda feels completely trapped and unable to remove herself from the situation.

Case Analysis Questions

1. What type of IPV does this case exemplify?
2. What were the clues that led Yvonne to suspect IPV?
3. What should Yvonne do as a next step?

🌿 **ACCESS EXEMPLAR LINKS IN YOUR GIDDENS EBOOK**

REFERENCES

1. Centers for Disease Control and Prevention: *Intimate partner violence*, 2018. Retrieved from: https://www.cdc.gov/violenceprevention/intimatepartnerviolence/index.html.
2. World Health Organization: *Violence against women: A 'global health problem of epidemic proportions*, 2018. Retrieved from: http://www.who.int/mediacentre/news/releases/2013/violence_against_women_20130620/en/.
3. World Health Organization: *Definition and typology of violence*, 2018. Retrieved from http://www.who.int/violenceprevention/approach/definition/en/.
4. National Center on Domestic and Sexual Violence. (n.d.). *Power and control wheel*. Retrieved from http://www.ncdsv.org/images/PowerControlwheelNOSHADING.pdf.
5. National Institute of Justice. (2017). *Intimate partner violence*. Retrieved from https://www.nij.gov/topics/crime/intimate-partner-violence/Pages/welcome.aspx.
6. The National Domestic Violence Hotline. (2018). *Get the facts and figures*. Retrieved from http://www.thehotline.org/resources/statistics/.
7. Singh, V., Tolman, R., Walton, M., et al. (2014). Characteristics of men who perpetrate intimate partner violence. *Journal of the American Board of Family Medicine*, 27(5), 661–668.
8. Johnson, M. P. (2008). *A typology of domestic violence: Intimate terrorism, violent resistance, and situational couple violence*. Boston: Northeastern University Press.
9. Summer, S. A., Macy, J. A., Dahlberg, L. L., et al. (2015). Violence in the United States: Status, challenges, and opportunities. *Journal of the American Medical Association [JAMA]*, 314(5), 478–488.
10. Sabri, B., Stockman, J. K., Campbell, J. C., et al. (2014). Factors associated with increased risk for lethal violence in intimate partner relationships among ethnically diverse black women. *Violence and Victims*, 29(5), 719–741.
11. Raine, A. (2013). *The anatomy of violence: The biological roots of crime*. New York: Random House Inc.
12. Pinto, L. A., Sullivan, E. L., Rosenbaum, A., et al. (2010). Biological correlates of intimate partner violence perpetration. *Aggression and Violent Behavior*, 12(5), 387–398.
13. Stuart, G. L., McGeary, J., Shorey, R. C., et al. (2014). Further investigation of genetics and intimate partner violence. *Violence Against Women*, 20(4), 420–426.
14. United States Department of Health and Human Services. (2016). *Child Maltreatment*. Retrieved from https://www.acf.hhs.gov/sites/default/files/cb/cm2016.pdf.
15. Stop Abuse Campaign. (2018). *Child abuse and neglect: How to spot the signs and make a difference*. Retrieved from http://stopabusecampaign.org/2018/02/12/child-abuse-and-neglect-how-to-spot-the-signs-and-make-a-difference/.

16. National Council on Aging. (2018). *Elder abuse facts.* Retrieved from https://www.ncoa.org/public-policy-action/elder-justice/elder-abuse-facts/.
17. National Center on Elder Abuse. (n.d.). *Research: Statistics and data.* Retrieved from https://ncea.acl.gov/whatwedo/research/statistics.html.
18. Centers for Disease Control and Prevention. (2017). *Youth violence.* Retrieved from https://www.cdc.gov/violenceprevention/youthviolence/index.html.
19. United Nations Educational, Scientific and Cultural Organization (UNESCO) (2017). *School violence and bullying: Global status report.* Retrieved from http://unesdoc.unesco.org/images/0024/002469/246970e.pdf.
20. Stopbulling.gov. (2018). *What is bullying.* Retrieved from https://www.stopbullying.gov/what-is-bullying/index.html.
21. Klein, J. (2012). *The bully society: School shootings and the crisis of bullying in America's schools.* New York: New York University Press.
22. United States Department of Justice. (2011). *Bullying in schools: An overview.* Retrieved from https://www.ojjdp.gov/pubs/234205.pdf.
23. Comaford, C. (2016). 75% of workers are affected by bullying: Here's what to do it about it. *Forbes.* Retrieved from https://www.forbes.com/sites/christinecomaford/2016/08/27/the-enormous-toll-workplace-bullying-takes-on-your-bottom-line/#14f7eeb55595.
24. Rape, Abuse and Incest National Network [RAINN]. (2018). *Sexual assault of men and boys.* Retrieved from https://www.rainn.org/articles/sexual-assault-men-and-boys.
25. Rape, Abuse and Incest National Network [RAINN]. (2018). *Sexual assault.* Retrieved from https://www.rainn.org/articles/sexual-assault.
26. Federal Bureaus of Investigation. (2012). *Attorney General Eric Holder announces revisions to the Uniform Crime Report's definition of rape: Data reported on rape will better reflect state criminal codes, victim experiences.* Retrieved from https://archives.fbi.gov/archives/news/pressrel/press-releases/attorney-general-eric-holder-announces-revisions-to-the-uniform-crime-reports-definition-of-rape.
27. LiveAbout. (2017). *The physical and emotions effects of domestic violence.* Retrieved from https://www.liveabout.com/the-physical-and-emotional-effects-of-domestic-violence-1102426.
28. The National Domestic Violence Hotline. (2016). *The dangers of strangulation.* Retrieved from http://www.thehotline.org/2016/03/15/the-dangers-of-strangulation/.
29. Arosarena, A. A., Travis, A. F., Yishung, H., et al. (2009). Maxillofacial injuries and violence against women. *Archives of Facial Plastic Surgery, 11*(1), 48–52.
30. Mathew, A., Smith, L. S., Marsh, B., et al. (2013). Relationship of intimate partner violence to health status, chronic disease, and screening behaviors. *Journal of Interpersonal Violence, 28*(12), 2581–2592.
31. Trickett, P. K., Noll, J. G., & Putnam, F. W. (2011). The impact of sexual abuse on female development: Lessons from a multigenerational, longitudinal research study. *Developmental Psychopathology, 23*(2), 453–476.
32. Adams Tufts, K. A., Clements, P. T., & Wessel, J. (2010). When intimate partner violence against women and HIV collide: Challenges for healthcare assessment and intervention. *Journal of Forensic Nursing, 6*(2), 66–73.
33. Clements, P. T., Holt, K., Hasson, C., et al. (2011). Enhancing assessment of maternal pregnancy homicide risk within nursing curricula. *Journal of Forensic Nursing, 7,* 195–202.
34. Shoffner, D. H. (2008). We don't like to think about it: Intimate partner violence during pregnancy and postpartum. *Journal of Perinatal and Neonatal Nursing, 22*(1), 39–48.
35. National Center for PTSD. (2015). *Intimate Partner Violence.* Retrieved from https://www.ptsd.va.gov/public/types/violence/domestic-violence.asp.
36. Babbel, S. (2018). Domestic violence: Power struggle with lasting consequences. *Psychology Today.* Retrieved from https://www.psychologytoday.com/us/blog/somatic-psychology/201105/domestic-violence-power-struggle-lasting-consequences.
37. van der Kolk, B. (1989). The compulsion to repeat the trauma: Re-enactment, revictimization, and masochism. *Psychiatric Clinics of North America, 12*(2), 239–411.
38. Burgess, A. W., Hartman, C. R., & Clements, P. T. (1995). The biology of memory in childhood trauma. *The Journal of Psychosocial Nursing and Mental Health Services, 33*(3), 16–26.
39. Flory, J. D., & Yehuda, R. (2015). Comorbidity between post-traumatic stress disorder and major depressive disorder: Alternative explanations and treatment considerations. *Dialogues in Clinical Neuroscience, 17*(2), 141–150.
40. Humphreys, J., & Lee, K. (2009). Interpersonal violence is associated with depression and chronic physical health problems in midlife women. *Issues in Mental Health Nursing, 30*(4), 206–213.
41. Varshney, M., Mahaptaar, A., Krshnan, V., et al. (2016). Violence and mental illness: What is the true story? *Journal of Epidemiology & Community Health, 70*(3), 223–225.
42. Humphreys, J., & Lee, K. (2009). Interpersonal violence is associated with depression and chronic physical health problems in midlife women. *Issues in Mental Health Nursing, 30*(4), 206–213.
43. American Association of Suicidology. (2014). *AAS Suicide and Sexual Assault/Interpersonal Violence Fact Sheet.* Retrieved from https://www.suicidology.org/resources/facts-statistics.
44. Wolke, D., & Lereya, S. T. (2015). Long-term effects of bullying. *Archives of Disease in Childhood, 100*(9), 879–885.
45. Costello, E. (2014). Adult outcomes of childhood bullying victimization. *American Journal of Psychiatry, 171,* 709.
46. Minh, A., Matheson, F. I., Daoud, N., et al. (2013). Linking childhood and adult criminality: Using a life course framework to examine childhood abuse and neglect, substance use and adult partner violence. *International Journal of Environmental Research and Public Health, 10*(11), 5470–5489.
47. Liu, J., Lewis, G., & Evans, L. (2013). Understanding aggressive behavior across the life span. *Journal of Psychiatric and Mental Health Nursing, 20*(2), 156–168.
48. Howell, K. H., Cater, Å. K., Miller-Graff, L. E., et al. (2013). The relationship between types of childhood victimisation and young adulthood. *The Journal of Criminal Behavior and Mental Health, 27*(4), 341–353.
49. Centers for Disease Control and Prevention. (2018). *Childhood abuse and Neglect: Consequences, 2018.* Retrieved from https://www.cdc.gov/violenceprevention/childabuseandneglect/consequences.html.
50. Street, A. E., Gibson, L. E., & Holohan, D. R. (2005). Impact of childhood traumatic events, trauma-related guilt, and avoidant coping strategies on PTSD symptoms in female survivors of domestic violence. *Journal of Traumatic Stress, 18*(3), 245–252.
51. Streeck-Fischer, A., & van der Kolk, B. A. (2000). Down will come baby, cradle and all: Diagnostic and therapeutic implications of chronic trauma on child development. *Australian and New Zealand Journal of Psychiatry, 34,* 903–918.
52. Gwirtman-Lane, W., Dubowitz, H., Langenberg, P., et al. (2012). Epidemiology of abusive abdominal trauma hospitalizations in United States children. *Child Abuse & Neglect, 36*(2), 142–148.
53. O'Malley, D. M., Kelly, P. J., & Cheng, A. L. (2013). Family violence assessment practices of pediatric ED nurses and physicians. *Journal of Emergency Nursing, 39*(3), 273–279.
54. National Institute on Aging. (n.d.). *Elder abuse.* Retrieved from https://www.nia.nih.gov/health/elder-abuse#types.
55. Wyandt, M. A. (2004). A review of elder abuse literature: An age old problem brought to light. *Californian Journal of Health Promotion, 2*(3), 40–52.
56. Marshall, C. E., Benton, D., & Brazier, J. M. (2000). Primary care—Elder abuse: Using clinical tools to identify clues of mistreatment. *Geriatrics, 55*(2), 42–44, 47–50.
57. Cohen, M., Levin, S., Gagin, R., et al. (2007). Elder abuse: Disparities between older people's disclosure of abuse, evident signs of abuse, and high risk of abuse. *Journal of the American Geriatrics Society, 55,* 1224.
58. Barkley-Burnett, L. (2017). Domestic violence clinical presentation. *Medscape.* Retrieved from https://emedicine.medscape.com/article/805546-clinical.

59. O'Doherty, L., Ramsay, J., Davison, L. L., et al. (2015). Screening women for intimate partner violence in healthcare settings. *The Cochrane Database of Systematic Reviews*, (7), CD007007.

60. Soper, R. G., & Fasam, D. (2014). Intimate partner violence and co-occurring substance abuse/addiction. *American Society of Addiction Medicine.* Retrieved from https://www.asam.org/resources/publications/magazine/read/article/2014/10/06/intimate-partner-violence-and-co-occurring-substance-abuse-addiction.

61. Xue, Y., Zimmerman, M., & Cunningham, R. (2009). Relationship between alcohol use and violent behavior among urban African American youths from adolescence to emerging adulthood: A longitudinal study. *American Journal of Public Health*, 99, 2041.

62. Miller, E., McCaw, B., Humphreys, B. L., et al. (2015). Integrating intimate partner violence assessment and intervention into healthcare in the United States: A systems approach. *Journal of Women's Health*, 24(1), 92–99.

63. Varshney, M., Mahaptaar, A., Krshnan, V., et al. (2016). Violence and mental illness: What is the true story? *Journal of Epidemiology & Community Health*, 70(3), 223–225.

64. Wathen, C. N., & MacMillan, H. L. (2013). Children's exposure to intimate partner violence: Impacts and interventions. *Pediatr Child Health*, 19(8), 419–422.

65. Amar, A., Bess, R., & Stockbridge, J. (2010). Lessons from families and communities about interpersonal violence, victimization, and seeking help. *Journal of Forensic Nursing*, 6, 110.

66. Howell, K. H., Barnes, S. E., Miller, L. E., et al. (2016). Developmental variations in the impact of intimate partner violence during childhood. *Journal of Injury & Violence Research*, 8(1), 43–57.

67. World Health Organization. (2009). *Changing cultural and social norms that support violence.* Retrieved from http://www.who.int/violence_injury_prevention/violence/norms.pdf.

68. Heise, L., & Garcia-Moreno, C. (2002). Violence by intimate partners. In E. Krug, L. Dahlberg, J. Mercy, et al. (Eds.), *World report on violence and health.* Geneva: World Health Organization.

69. Pan, A., Daley, S., Rivera, L. M., et al. (2006). Understanding the role of culture in domestic violence: The Ahisma Project for Safe Families. *Journal of Immigrant and Minority Health*, 8(1), 35–43.

70. Marshall University Women's Center. (2018). *Relationship violence and culture.* Retrieved from https://www.marshall.edu/wcenter/domestic-violence/relationship-violence-and-culture/.

71. Board on Children, Youth, and Families; Institute of Medicine; National Research Council. (2012). Recognizing and assessing child maltreatment. In *Child maltreatment research, policy, and practice for the next decade: Workshop summary.* Washington (DC): National Academies Press. Retrieved from https://www.ncbi.nlm.nih.gov/books/NBK201116/.

72. New York State Office of Children and Family Services. (n.d.). *Identifying domestic violence.* Retrieved from https://ocfs.ny.gov/main/dv/childWelfare/Identifying%20Domestic%20Violence%20FINAL.pdf.

73. Reece, R. (2011). Medical evaluation of physical abuse. In J. Myers (Ed.), *The APSAC handbook on child maltreatment.* Los Angeles: Sage.

74. Hamberger, L. K., Rhodes, K., & Brown, J. (2015). Screening and intervention for intimate partner violence in healthcare settings: Creating sustainable system-level programs. *Journal of Women's Health*, 24(1), 86–91.

75. Hamberger, L. K., & Phelan, M. B. (2004). *Domestic violence screening and intervention in medical and mental healthcare settings.* New York: Springer.

76. Ambuel, B., Hamberger, L. K., Guse, C. E., et al. (2013). Healthcare can change from within: Sustained improvement in the healthcare response to intimate partner violence. *Journal of Family Violence*, 28, 833–847.

77. Ambuel, B., Hamberger, L. K., Guse, C. E., et al. (2013). Healthcare can change from within: Sustained improvement in the healthcare response to intimate partner violence. *Journal of Family Violence*, 28, 833–847.

78. Morse, D. S., Lafleur, R., Fogarty, C. T., et al. (2012). "They told me to leave": How healthcare providers address intimate partner violence. *Journal of the American Board of Family Medicine: [JABFM]*, 25(3), 333–342.

79. Centers for Disease Control and Prevention. (2007). *Intimate partner violence and sexual violence victimization assessment instruments for use in healthcare settings.* Retrieved from https://www.cdc.gov/violenceprevention/pdf/ipv/ipvandsvscreening.pdf.

80. Campbell, J. C. (2002). Health consequences of intimate partner violence. *The Lancet*, 359, 1331–1336.

81. Hart, S., Brassard, M., Davidson, H., et al. (2011). Psychological maltreatment. In J. Myers (Ed.), *The APSAC handbook on child maltreatment.* Los Angeles: Sage.

82. U.S. Department of Health and Human Services. (2007). *Child maltreatment,.* Washington, DC: U.S. Government Printing Office.

83. Child Welfare Information Gateway. (2006). *Definitions of child abuse and neglect.* Retrieved from https://www.childwelfare.gov/pubPDFs/define.pdf.

84. National Adult Protective Services Association. (2018). *Get informed: What is abuse?.* Retrieved from http://www.napsa-now.org/get-informed/what-is-abuse/.

85. Jones, S. N., Waite, R., & Clements, P. T. (2012). An evolutionary concept analysis of school violence: From bullying to death. *Journal of Forensic Nursing*, 8(1), 4–12.

86. Cooper, G. D., Clements, P. T., & Holt, K. E. (2012). Examining childhood bullying and adolescent suicide: Implications for school nurses. *Journal of School Nursing*, 28(4), 275–283.

87. Centers for Disease Control and Prevention. (2018). *Youth violence.* Retrieved from https://www.cdc.gov/violenceprevention/youthviolence/index.html.

88. Flores-Ortiz, Y. (2004). Domestic violence in Chicana/o families. In R. Velasquez, L. Arellano, & B. McNeill (Eds.), *The handbook of Chicana/o psychology and mental health.* New York: Erlbaum.

89. Centers for Disease Control and Prevention. (2015). *School violence: Data and statistics.* Retrieved from https://www.cdc.gov/violenceprevention/youthviolence/schoolviolence/data_stats.html.

90. Hien, D., & Ruglass, L. (2009). Interpersonal partner violence and women in the United States: An overview of prevalence rates, psychiatric correlates and consequences and barriers to help seeking. *International Journal of Law and Psychiatry*, 32(1), 48–55.

91. Stockman, J. K., Hayashi, H., & Campbell, J. C. (2014). Intimate partner violence and its health impact on disproportionally affected populations, including minorities and impoverished groups. *Journal of Women's Health*, 24(1), 62–79.

92. Heise, L., & Garcia-Moreno, C. (2002). Violence by intimate partners. In E. Krug, L. Dahlberg, J. Mercy, et al. (Eds.), *World report on violence and health.* Geneva: World Health Organization.

93. Rape, Abuse, and Incest National Network (RAINN). (2018). *Scope of the problem: Statistics.* Retrieved from https://www.rainn.org/statistics/scope-problem.

94. National Center for Victims of Crime. (n.d.). *Elder victimization.* Retrieved from https://ovc.ncjrs.gov/ncvrw2017/images/en_artwork/Fact_Sheets/2017NCVRW_ElderVictimization_508.pdf.

Professional Nursing and Health Care Concepts

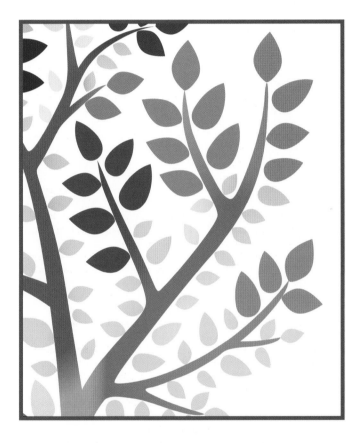

T he delivery of safe and effective health care is extremely complex. As the largest group of healthcare professionals, nurses play an especially important role within healthcare delivery. Healthcare delivery represents many critical elements that collectively describe the essence of professional nurse practice. The concepts within Unit III relate to these ideas and are closely associated with professional attributes and behaviors desired of all healthcare providers. As a group, the Professional Nursing and Health Care Concepts represent 21 concepts organized within four overarching themes. Unlike the Health and Illness Concepts, these are concepts associated with professional comportment—meaning the identity of nursing as a profession.

The first theme is *Nursing Attributes and Roles.* Concepts within this theme represent roles nurses play within healthcare delivery and the attributes or characteristics desired of professional nurses; these are the behaviors nurses incorporate into all patient care encounters. Specific concepts represented include *Professional Identity, Clinical Judgment, Leadership, Ethics, Patient Education,* and *Health Promotion.*

The second theme is ***Care Competencies.*** The term *competency* refers to being competent or well qualified to complete a skill or task. In the context of nursing and health care, competencies are identified knowledge, skills, and attitudes deemed important for safe and effective care. Specific concepts include *Communication, Collaboration, Safety, Technology and Informatics, Evidence,* and *Health Care Quality.* Although the concepts featured within this theme are not intended to be comprehensive of all competencies, some of the most common to all nurses, regardless of area of practice, are included.

The third theme is ***Health Care Delivery.*** These concepts represent the context of the application and care delivery situations or models. There are literally thousands of healthcare delivery concepts; those included are some of the most important to be aware of and include *Care Coordination, Caregiving, Palliative Care, Health Disparities,* and *Population Health.*

The final theme is ***Health Care Infrastructure.*** These concepts are foundational to healthcare delivery and the practice of nursing. *Health Care Organizations, Health Care Economics, Health Policy,* and *Health Care Law* represent specific concepts within this theme.

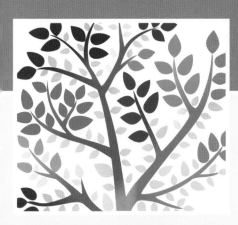

Professional Identity

Nelda Godfrey and Elizabeth Young

Professional identity is an attribute of a nurse professional that is initially acquired during one's nursing education. As a novice member of a professional group, the student nurse uses multiple experiences and reflections to embrace the characteristics, norms, and values of the nursing discipline and begins to think, act, and feel like a nurse.[1,2] The process of gaining this understanding is called professional identity formation, which together with professional identity encompasses what is sometimes referred to as professionalism. Professional identity is formed as a person transitions from layperson to a nurse professional during the educational process,[3] and it is fostered throughout the nurse's career as professional identity is challenged and matures through experiences within the profession.[4]

DEFINITION

Based on earlier work from medical colleagues,[1,2] professional identity in nursing is defined as *a sense of oneself, and in relation to others, that is influenced by characteristics, norms, and values of the nursing discipline, resulting in an individual thinking, acting, and feeling like a nurse.* Professional identity is part of the larger notion of identity, "an umbrella term used throughout the social sciences to describe an individual's comprehension of him- or herself as a discrete, separate entity."[5, p.119] Within the concept of identity one would find personal identity, with professional identity as a subset of personal identity (Fig. 37.1).[6]

SCOPE

Novice professionals in any discipline begin to form a sense of professional identity as their education and training begin. Professional identity is developed in many ways, although real and simulated experiences, reflection, and role modeling by professional colleagues seem to be the most meaningful strategies.[1,7–11] Nursing incorporates many, if not most, of these strategies in "clinicals," a highly valued[12,13] opportunity for experiential learning in clinical sites under the guidance of a preceptor or faculty member. In some schools, these experiences progress to apprenticeship opportunities[3] in which a student works the shift of a nurse in practice to better learn the knowledge, skills, and attitudes needed in that practice environment.

Today, *professional identity* and *professional identity formation* are replacing nursing terminology such as *professional role* and *professionalism*, largely because of important work from colleagues in academic medicine who determined that students needed to understand the nature of professionalism and internalize the value system of the medical profession.[1] Teaching and assessment efforts ensued, but faculty discovered that only part of what made up professionalism was addressed with these methods. Jarvis-Selinger et al. argue that focusing on role (a social construct) and competencies (behaviors), and assuming that the process of becoming a professional is a linear learning-related developmental process, is inadequate.[9] Instead, a broader focus should acknowledge the crisis nature of identity formation and that with every adoption of a new identity, an old identity has to be deconstructed that leads to discontinuity and crisis.

ATTRIBUTES AND CRITERIA

Professional identity is composed of five subcategories or attributes: doing, being, acting ethically, flourishing, and changing identities.

Doing

"Doing," or the consensus or sociological perspective, incorporates the societal and professional codes and standards that are part of the nursing discipline. It also includes a skill orientation, or a "doing" component.[14] Because of its sociological origins, *role*—how one functions as a part of a group—is central to understanding the "doing" part of professional identity, and it is seen in functionalistic approaches to accomplishing goals.[9,15] In the early stages of any new role, there is usually a strong focus on external expectations and tasks—the "doing."[9] An example is diploma nursing education of the 1950s, when each nurse or nursing student had a specific role or duty and needed to fulfill that role to be deemed successful. The "doing" orientation remains a part of professional identity formation in nursing today, but it does not entirely explain how laypersons become nurse professionals.[3,14,16]

Being

"Being," or the personal or psychological view of the nurse professional, explains what it means to do the right thing even when no one is looking.[14] Decisions and actions come from within, from a desire to do what is good. This attribute is about "being" a professional and about adopting attitudes and behaviors that reflect the value of how a professional thinks, feels, and acts. This perspective of a professional may incorporate rules and principles, but it is beyond the laws, codes, and standards within the discipline or society. In this case, it is more a personal sense of being a nurse and functioning within the norms and values that are characteristic of nursing as a discipline.[14] The

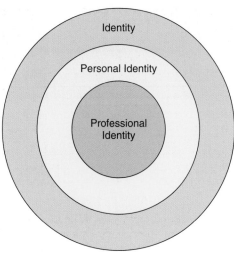

FIGURE 37.1 The Concept of Professional Identity as a Subset of Identity and Personal Identity.

BOX 37.1 Qualities Needed for a Sustainable Professional Life

- Deeply engage with the profession's public purposes.
- Develop a strong professional identity.
- See the world through the lens of the profession's moral purposes and standards.
- Use habits of response to patients, families, and colleagues that are aligned with the profession's standards and ideals.
- Plan to contribute to the ethical quality of the profession.

Adapted from Colby, A., & Sullivan, W. D. (2008). Formation of professionalism and purpose: Perspectives from the preparation for the professions program. *University of St. Thomas Law Journal*, 5(2), 415.

attitudes and behaviors associated with being a nurse professional can extend to other health professions. Fig. 37.2 shows the attributes of a healthcare provider using the terms of "healer" and "professional."[17] These attributes represent both the doing and being inherent in the professional identity of a nurse and other healthcare providers.[17]

Acting Ethically

Doing the right thing, or acting ethically, is a critical component of professional identity and professional identity formation. According to Socrates, "The really important thing is not to live, but to live well. And to live well [means] ... to live according to your principles." Living well means being attentive to what is considered right and good from both a societal and a professional perspective. For instance, it is not right to accept a date from a patient who is in your care in the hospital. Nor is it ethical to tell your family member details about a patient's condition. Society at large also recognizes acting ethically as a critical component

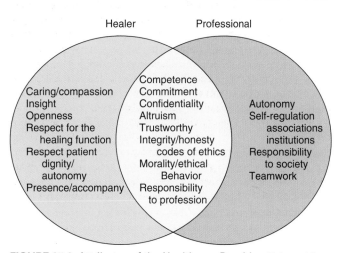

Attributes of a Healthcare Professional

Healer | Professional

Caring/compassion
Insight
Openness
Respect for the
  healing function
Respect patient
  dignity/
  autonomy
Presence/accompany

Competence
Commitment
Confidentiality
Altruism
Trustworthy
Integrity/honesty
  codes of ethics
Morality/ethical
  Behavior
Responsibility
  to profession

Autonomy
Self-regulation
  associations
  institutions
Responsibility
  to society
Teamwork

FIGURE 37.2 Attributes of the Healthcare Provider. (Adapted from Cruess, S. R., & Cruess, R. L. [2012]. Teaching professionalism—why, what, and how. *Facts, Views & Vision in ObGyn, 4*(4), 259–265.)

to the profession as nurses have been identified as the most honest and ethical profession in the Gallup Poll since 2002.[18]

Flourishing

Not only is it necessary to better understand the doing and being of the discipline of nursing, but also one must do so with a sense of positive and transformational growth. A transformational or human flourishing perspective is necessary for professional identity to move past the initial phases of formation. Not all professionals move to the expert stage of development; some opt to be experienced nonexperts who choose not to deepen their understanding of their profession.[19] Box 37.1 shows the five key qualities needed for sustainable, life-long growth as a professional. This perspective can also be found in Magnet Recognition Program materials, in which excellence and the effort to strive for excellence is a core value. These ideas are as old as the ancient Greeks, who believed that each person's life has a purpose and that the function of one's life is to attain that purpose. Flourishing is an important component of both forming and fostering professional identity.[14]

Changing Identities

From adolescence on, each time a new identity emerges, a reworking of the person's identity occurs in order to resolve this new developmental issue.[20] However, because each person has multiple identities (i.e., son, daughter, student, employee, grandchild, or parent) at any one time, identity formation for persons preparing for the professions looks more like disequilibrium and subsequent assimilation than a developmental transition.[1,9,20] Recognition of changing identities is the final attribute of professional identity and the process of professional identity formation.

THEORETICAL LINKS

The research base for professional identity formation is underdeveloped,[11] and no unified theoretical framework for understanding the process of professional identity formation exists.[8] However, a number of other theories strongly influence the current understanding of professional identity.

Marcia and Josselson note that identity issues first arise in late adolescence when society and adolescents expect beliefs and vision for future career goals will start to form.[20] For the adolescent and growing young adult, this occurs within an environment of exploration and commitment. It is manifested through four identity statuses: identity diffusion, foreclosure, moratorium, and identity achieved. *Identity diffusion* is characterized by a lack of interest in commitment, and even in exploration. The catchphrase for this would be "whatever seems good at the moment." The second identity status is *foreclosure*, in which

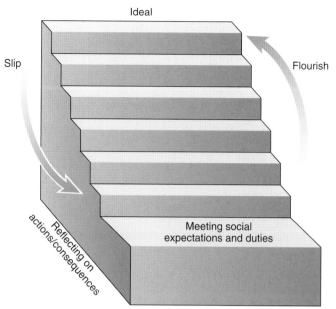

FIGURE 37.3 Stairstep Model of Professional Transformation. (Redrawn from Crigger, N., & Godfrey, N. [2011]. *The making of nurse professionals: a transformational, ethical approach.* Burlington, MA: Jones & Bartlett Learning, www.jblearning.com. Reprinted with permission.)

the person keeps talking about changing those around him or her and conspicuously not about making change him- or herself. *Moratorium*, the third identity status, is characterized by overwhelming anxiety that is "hard to sit through" with someone. The fourth status, *identity achieved*, means that the person is reasonably self-aware, has a sense of self, and can manage overwhelming anxiety should it occur.[20]

Crigger and Godfrey's work with a stairstep model of professional transformation for nursing (Fig. 37.3) visually represents dynamism in professional identity formation.[14] The main ethical traditions are represented in the model, along with the transformational nature of nursing with the reality of slips and progress (flourishing) that occur throughout the trajectory of one's career. Finally, the progress toward the ideal is a function of individual and group efforts, with influences from many experiences.[14]

From an intervention standpoint, Bandura's social learning theory, in which learning occurs through observations of others, and Mezirow's transformational learning theory, in which growth and development are outcomes of transformational learning when sufficient levels of cognitive functioning are present, form part of the theoretical basis for professional identity and professional identity formation interventions.[21,22]

CONTEXT TO NURSING AND HEALTH CARE

Three illustrations of the connection between professional identity with nursing and health care follow: (1) forming and fostering professional identity, (2) an interprofessional perspective on professional identity and professional identity formation, and (3) interventions to achieve professional identity formation.

Forming and Fostering Professional Identity

Forming a professional identity in beginning prelicensure nursing education is a challenge. First, the amount of empirical work in this area is limited, though growing. Second, it seems that a variety of terms have been used to describe the same phenomenon, making comparisons difficult. However, a small set of studies indicate that faculty incivility

can be a barrier to the development of professional identity[23]; observing the behaviors of registered nurses positively impacts students' development of their own sense of professional identity[10,24]; and, for students, the greatest barrier to growing a professional identity was the "unanticipated expectations" of the professional and academic nursing role. Students found that they needed to relinquish preconceptions and acclimate to their academic and professional climate in order to develop a sense of professional identity and to be successful.[25]

Even less is known about the impact of professional identity in nursing practice. Some data suggest that a robust professional identity can inoculate the nurse to bullying and incivility activity in the workplace. An example of one academic health center's professional identity statement for nurses is shown in Box 37.2.

An Interprofessional Perspective

Much of what is known about nursing and professional identity derives from interprofessional education and practice research. The term nurse is derived from the Latin word nutricia and from the Anglo Saxon nurice for "all things nourishing and good for the mind, body, and soul."[26, p.971] In contrast, the term physician is derived from the root of the Greek word physiology implying an individual who understands nature.[26]

The Core Competencies for Interprofessional Collaborative Practice have set a clear standard for interprofessional collaboration in education and practice settings in order for students to learn about, from, and with individuals from other professions to enable collaboration and improve health outcomes.[27] Early interprofessional education research findings indicate that novice learners may marginalize other professionals based on their group affiliation, and this may result from lack of knowledge and oversimplification.[28] Interprofessional education opportunities can address this issue in more focused ways and strategize about ways to diminish this behavior. Findings show that the stronger the perceived professional identity of the learner, the more confidence one has with interprofessional collaboration,[29] making the case for ensuring adequate professional identity formation efforts. Furthermore, medical students' early attachment with the nursing profession engenders more respect for it,[30] and nurses' greater levels of education (i.e., master's degree) yield higher scores on the Readiness for Interprofessional Learning Scale (RIPLS) and on the professional identity subscale,[31] indicating that higher levels of education may enhance interprofessional learning. Professional identity was greatest in students with cognitive flexibility (able to structure knowledge), previous work experience in these environments, better understanding of teamwork, and a greater knowledge of their own profession.[32]

Interventions to Achieve Professional Identity Formation

The following interventions will be helpful for students in building a professional identity:

- *Hear expectations clearly*: Most nursing education programs are highly complex and may seem difficult to understand. Listen carefully to expectations and advice for success.

- *Value debriefing and feedback from role models*: Studies have shown that role modeling is critically important in learning a profession. One study describes the most important component of the educational process as the "supportive yet challenging relationship" the learner has with the faculty member or mentor.[24] Recognize that these relationships are not only important in the future, but also a valuable part of the student's learning in the nursing program in the present.

- *Engage in reflection*: Reflection has been increasingly shown to positively influence student learning.[33] Sometimes the reflection will be guided, through assignments in and outside of class; other times, reflection will be expected to be spontaneous, such as in post conferences following clinical. Reflection is a time to internalize what is occurring with the patient and family and also what is happening and changing one's own perspective.

- *Actively adopt a professional identity*: There is increasing evidence that labeling what nurses do as part of nursing's standards and codes is an important step in building language within the discipline.[8,15,34] Adopting a clear sense of professional identity that includes growing understanding of how integrity, compassion, courage, humility, advocacy, and human flourishing fit within the identity of nursing will in turn clarify the nurse's purposes as he or she relates to patients, families, and healthcare colleagues.[35]

- *Understand your own responsibilities for learning and be accountable for them*: People's beliefs in their ability to influence events that affect their lives is known as self-efficacy.[36] Your ability to recognize your potential to grow and flourish will help propel you to greater personal and professional levels of self-efficacy.

- *Build relationships with those around you*: Building relationships is about understanding the importance of engaging in the learning environment and following through so that these relationships become stronger and more meaningful. Relationship building and engaging with others is an important part of identity formation. In their integrative review of professional identity formation in higher education, Trede et al. reported that students need authentic experiences on which to reflect, and active engagement that employs collaborative learning from practice environments.[11]

- *Develop personal self-care habits*: The American Nurses Association (ANA) Code of Ethics for Nurses[37] addresses the importance of nurses' self-care as part of nurses' ethical code. Caring for oneself is a key component of solidly developing a professional identity in any field.

- *Embrace any opportunity for experiences with patients*: Holden et al. report that both real and simulated unique experiences with patients are valuable in forming professional identity.[8] Early experiences with patients, or simulations, are also important in this component of professional identity development.

INTERRELATED CONCEPTS

The concept of professional identity is interrelated with four professional nursing and healthcare concepts (Fig. 37.4). **Clinical Judgment** depends on a deep and meaningful understanding of the professional identity of the nurse, incorporating health and illness concepts along with the norms and values that characterize the nurse as a designer, manager, and coordinator of care and as a member of a profession.[1,12] Principles of **Leadership** and **Ethics** govern the nurse's social contract with patients and families in his or her care, affirming that advocacy for the patient and family is a primary consideration for all decisions made within the healthcare environment.[19] **Communication** is fundamental to the nursing discipline and as such constitutes a substantial part of what actually happens in moment-to-moment nursing practice.

CLINICAL EXEMPLARS

There are many examples of professional identity in nursing practice. Box 37.3 presents some of the most common situations or examples seen in clinical practice, including language choice, attire (assurance), interaction, being "present," interacting in a professional way with the family, and acting as an agent for healing. It is beyond the scope of this text to provide details on all exemplars, but some are featured here.

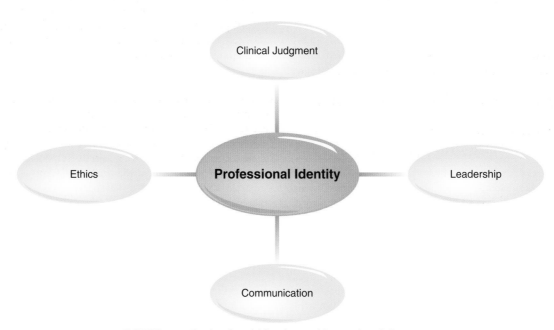

FIGURE 37.4 Professional Identity and Interrelated Concepts.

BOX 37.3 EXEMPLARS OF PROFESSIONAL IDENTITY

Integrity
- Following through with pain medication
- Calling the physician when the patient asks you to
- Checking the Code Cart by the prescribed time
- Giving medications within the 30-min window

Compassion
- Taking time to talk with a troubled family member
- Responding to a patient's call light with genuine interest
- Comforting a colleague who has just had a death in his or her family
- Using eye contact to apologize for a misstep with a colleague

Courage
- Speaking up when a colleague did not wash his or her hands before entering a patient room
- Conveying the details of the conversation a dying patient had with you to other members of the healthcare team
- Taking practice issues to the practice council to positively change practice on your nursing unit
- Speaking out about bullying occurring on the nursing unit

Humility
- Realistically viewing family members' ability to cope with a crisis
- Being nonjudgmental as staff deal with a unit-based crisis
- Clearly identifying your part in an error and not accepting more blame than is yours
- Seeing the larger picture when issues arise with patients, families, and coworkers

Advocacy
- Sharing with family members the details of a conversation you had with their loved one previously in the day
- Listening carefully to help family members carry out their wishes, and working with the hospital to do what you can to help that happen
- Communicating with the family about their loved one's surgery schedule, course of events, and expected finish time
- Working to get prescriptions filled before a homeless person leaves the hospital

Human Flourishing
- Encouraging patients in their difficult times
- Seeking additional resources for patients with limited discharge planning issues
- Encouraging coworkers to seek employee assistance options for difficulties they are having
- Creating a positive, encouraging environment for patients and families

ACCESS EXEMPLAR LINKS IN YOUR GIDDENS EBOOK

Featured Exemplars

Integrity
Considered a fundamental character trait, integrity is evident in nearly every nursing action. If one has integrity, she does what she says she will do and acts with consistency and purpose. Integrity is often the basis for trust—for families and patients and for coworkers. A breach of integrity can erode one's trust in another, making this exemplar a critical consideration when providing care to vulnerable patients and their families.[14]

Compassion
Not to be confused with sympathy or empathy, compassion is feeling what another is feeling and responding to it with the intent of doing something to help.[38] Compassion is akin to caring, although they are difficult to separate in concept analysis. Caring and the ethic of care are intricately intertwined with the notion of compassion, and together they constitute a sense of response and accompanying action with those in need.[14]

Courage
In the context of professional identity, courage has two meanings: (1) to affect change, and (2) "to stand in opposition for moral rightness."[14,p.125] Courage can also be categorized as physical or moral.[14] The nurse who put herself between the patient and falling debris from a tornado demonstrated physical courage. The nurse who escalated a patient care situation by consulting higher ranking members of the medical staff exhibited moral courage.

Humility
Sometimes misunderstood, humility is "like a buoy that rides the waves of disappointments and accomplishments."[14, p.121] When a person demonstrates humility, he or she views the world with equanimity, taking neither an overstated amount of credit nor blame for a particular situation.[14] Such an approach encourages a realistic view of circumstances, events, and the actions of others.

Advocacy
In situations in which nurse professionals employ advocacy, nurses and patients alike view this action as the "last line of defense" on behalf of the patient. This normative conception of the nurse as patient advocate is an example of a "signature image" of professional identity among nursing and other professions.[19]

Human Flourishing
The notion of human flourishing arises in conversation when virtues or normative views of a discipline are discussed. Grounded in the writings and beliefs of the ancient Greeks, the purpose of *being human* is to flourish. As nurses and fellow humans, we have a duty to do what is possible to foster outcomes that lead to human flourishing. Similar normative language is found in the ANA Code of Ethics for Nurses.[37]

CASE STUDY

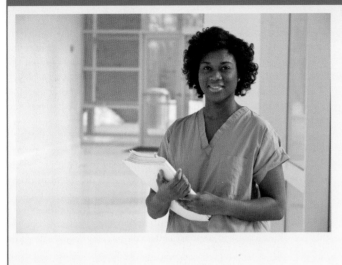

From Huntstock/Thinkstock

Case Presentation

Jane King is a 22-year-old female who has just begun her undergraduate nursing program. She is in her first clinical experience, and although she has been taught about giving bed baths, she is not sure that she is at all comfortable doing so. Her patient today is a 78-year-old male renal failure patient with limited mobility. Within her 8-hour assignment, Jane will need to complete all of her patient's personal care.

Jane has cared for young children in babysitting jobs since she was 11 years old, but has no experience caring for adults. She is particularly concerned about perineal care. Jane has had instruction—but what about the actual experience of doing perineal care? Because this is her first semester in her nursing program, she has not had much time to "feel, think, and act" like a nurse professional. However, this patient is in a difficult situation in which he needs her care. This is all new to Jane, and she does not know what to do.

Case Analysis Questions

1. Consider the attributes of professional identity. How do these apply to Jane's situation?
2. How could role modeling from the instructor or another nurse be helpful to Jane?

CASE STUDY

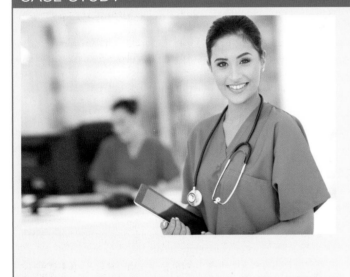

From michaeljung/iStock/Thinkstock

Case Presentation

Jackie Wilson is a junior nursing student who was assigned on Tuesday to her first day of operating room (OR) observation. The OR staff was excited that Jackie was able to see a liver transplant performed. Later that evening, Jackie shared with her family how interesting it was to see the transplant and to see the staff work so well together and function as a high-performing team. She also shared many details about the surgery and the patient, because, of course, the staff had been sharing these details with her.

Three days later, the academic health center released a press briefing to media outlets in the region reporting that the hospital had reached a milestone with a liver transplant performed on that Tuesday. That morning at work, Jackie's father told his colleagues that his daughter had been in the OR for that liver transplant, and he proceeded to communicate many of the details that Jackie had shared at the family dinner table.

Case Analysis Questions

1. What lapse in professional behavior occurred?
2. What strategies would be useful to help Jackie's understanding of professional identity?

CASE STUDY

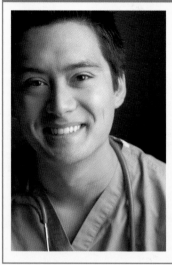

Case Presentation

John Roberts is a prelicensure nursing student who has been asked to be part of an interprofessional education activity at his school. His school has students going to many hospitals in the area for clinical experiences, and he also works in a local hospital as a nurse technician. He loves the clinical environment and is quite competent in his nurse technician role.

This interprofessional education activity includes students in occupational therapy, physical therapy, respiratory therapy, pharmacy, and nursing. In his work experience, John has worked (although minimally) with people who are in each of these fields, but he is sure that they do not have the "real picture" of what patients experience—particularly because he has often floated the hospital as he has worked his shift as a technician.

The small group portion of this interprofessional educational activity includes John, two occupational therapy students, and one physical therapy student. Going into the exercise, John is sure that he is the one who will have more knowledge and understanding than any of the other students.

Case Analysis Questions

1. How does John's attitude going into the learning activity link to the information shared in the interprofessional context of professional identity?
2. Ideally, what should John focus on doing to foster teamwork and collaboration with his fellow students?

From Photodisc/Thinkstock.

 ACCESS EXEMPLAR LINKS IN YOUR GIDDENS EBOOK

REFERENCES

1. Cruess, R. L., Cruess, S. R., Boudreau, J. D., et al. (2014). Reframing medical education to support professional identity formation. *Academic Medicine: Journal of the Association of American Medical Colleges, 89*(11), 1446–1451.
2. Merton, R. K. (1957). Some preliminaries to a sociology of medical education. In R. K. Merton, L. G. Reader, & P. L. Kendall (Eds.), *The student physician: Introductory studies in the sociology of medical education* (pp. 3–79). Cambridge, MA: Harvard University Press.
3. Benner, P., Sutphen, M., Leonard, V., et al. (2010). *Educating nurses: A call for radical transformation.* Stanford, CA: The Carnegie Foundation for the Advancement of Teaching.
4. Godfrey, N., & Crigger, N. (2012). Ethics and professional conduct: Striving for a professional ideal. *Journal of Nursing Regulation, 3*(1), 32–37.
5. Sharma, S., & Sharma, M. (2010). Self, social identity and psychological well-being. *Psychological Studies, 55*(2), 118–136.
6. Tsang, S. K. M., Hui, E. K., & Law, B. C. M. (2012). Positive identity as a positive youth development construct: A conceptual view. *Scientific World Journal, 2012,* Article ID 529691.
7. Baldwin, A., Mills, J., Birks, M., et al. (2014). Role modeling in undergraduate nursing education: An integrative literature review. *Nurse Education Today, 34,* e18–e26.
8. Holden, M., Buck, E., Clark, M., et al. (2012). Professional identity formation in medical education: The convergence of multiple domains. *HEC Forum: An Interdisciplinary Journal on Hospitals' Ethical and Legal Issues, 24,* 245–255.
9. Jarvis-Selinger, S., Pratt, D., & Regehr, G. (2012). Competency is not enough: Integrating identity formation into the medical education discourse. *Academic Medicine: Journal of the Association of American Medical Colleges, 87*(9), 1185–1190.
10. Keeling, J., & Templeman, J. (2013). An exploratory study: Student nurses' perceptions of professionalism. *Nurse Education in Practice, 13,* 18–22.
11. Trede, F., Macklin, R., & Bridges, D. (2012). Professional identity development: A review of higher education literature. *Studies in Higher Education, 37*(3), 365–384.
12. American Association of Colleges of Nursing. (2008). *Baccalaureate essentials for professional nursing practice.* Washington, DC: Author.
13. American Association of Colleges of Nursing. (2012). *Expectations for practice experiences in the RN to baccalaureate curriculum.* Washington, DC: Author.
14. Crigger, N., & Godfrey, N. (2011). *The making of nurse professionals: A transformational, ethical approach.* Sudbury, MA: Jones & Bartlett.
15. Khalili, H., Hall, J., & DeLuca, S. (2014). Historical analysis of professionalism in Western societies: Implications for interprofessional education and collaborative practice. *Journal of Interprofessional Care, 28*(2), 92–97.
16. Benner, P. (2011). Formation in professional education: An examination of the relationship between theories of meaning and theories of the self. *The Journal of Medicine and Philosophy, 36,* 342–353.
17. Cruess, S. R., & Cruess, R. L. (2012). Teaching professionalism-Why, what, and how. *Facts, Views, and Vision in OBgyn, 4*(4), 259–265.
18. Brenan, M.: *Nurses keep healthy lead as most honest, ethical profession.* Washington DC, 2017, December 26. Retrieved from http://news.gallup.com/poll/224639/nurses-keep-healthy-lead-honest-ethical-profession.aspx.
19. Colby, A., & Sullivan, W. D. (2008). Formation of professionalism and purpose: Perspectives from the preparation for the professions program. *University of St Thomas Law Journal, 5*(2), 404–426.
20. Marcia, J., & Josselson, R. (2013). Eriksonian personality research and its implications for psychotherapy. *Journal of Personality, 81*(6), 617–629.
21. Bandura, A. (1971). *Social learning theory.* New York: General Learning Press.
22. Merriam, S. B. (2004). The role of cognitive development in Mezirow's transformational learning theory. *Adult Education Quarterly, 55*(1), 60–68.
23. Del Prato, D. (2013). Student voices: The lived experience of faculty incivility as a barrier to professional formation in associate degree nursing education. *Nurse Education Today, 33*(3), 286–290.
24. Severinsson, E., & Sand, A. (2010). Evaluation of the clinical supervision and professional development of student nurses. *Journal of Nursing Management, 18,* 669–677.
25. Goodolf, D. (2013). Growing a professional identity: A grounded theory of the educational experience of baccalaureate nursing students, dissertation abstract. Chester, PA, Widener University.
26. Romano, C. A., & Pangaro, L. N. (2014). What is a doctor and what is a nurse? A perspective for future practice and education. *Academic Medicine: Journal of the Association of American Medical Colleges, 89*(7), 970–972.

27. Interprofessional Education Collaborative. (2016). *Core competencies for interprofessional collaborative practice: 2016 update.* Washington, DC: Interprofessional Education Collaborative.

28. Lingard, L., Resnick, R., & Espin, S. (2002). Forming professional identities on the health care team: Discursive constructions of the "other" in the operating room. *Medical Education, 36*(8), 728–734.

29. Jakobsen, F., Hanson, T. B., & Eika, B. (2011). Knowing more about the other professions clarified my own profession. *Journal of Interprofessional Care, 25*(6), 441–446.

30. Helmich, E., Derksen, E., Prevoo, M., et al. (2010). Medical students' professional identity development in an early nursing attachment. *Medical Education, 44*(7), 674–682.

31. Williams, C.: *Factors that relate to registered nurse readiness for interprofessional learning in the context of continuing professional development*, dissertation abstract. Berrien Springs, MI, 2014, Andrews University.

32. Adams, K., Hean, S., Sturgis, P., et al. (2006). Investigating the factors influencing professional identity of first year health and social care students. *Learning Health Social Care, 5*(2), 55–68.

33. Horton-Deutsch, S., & Sherwood, G. (2008). Reflection: An educational strategy to develop emotionally competent nurse leaders. *Journal of Nursing Management, 16*(8), 946–954.

34. Fitzpatrick, J. J. (2014). Educating our students regarding the standards of professional practice and professional performance. *Nursing Education Perspectives, 35*(3), 143.

35. Crigger, N., & Godfrey, N. (2014). From the inside out: A new approach to teaching professional identity formation and professional ethics. *Journal of Professional Nursing, 30*, 376–382.

36. Bandura, A. (2010). Self-efficacy. In *Corsini encyclopedia of psychology.* New York: Wiley.

37. American Nurses Association. (2015). *Code of ethics for nurses with interpretive statements.* Washington, DC: American Nurses Publishing.

38. Pellegrino, E. D., & Thomasma, D. C. (1993). *The virtues in medical practice.* New York: Oxford University Press US.

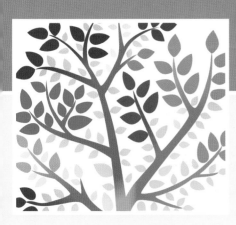

Clinical Judgment

Ann Nielsen and Kathie Lasater

The delivery of health care in general and the practice of nursing have become very complex. Larger numbers of patients with complicated medical conditions and healthcare financing and reimbursement have become major determinants of healthcare practices and policies; thus patients with interrelated comorbidities are now admitted to acute care settings for shorter periods of time, and sicker patients are cared for in community-based settings, such as home health and long-term care.[1] There is increasing evidence that acute deterioration in patients goes unrecognized by nurses, and therefore, nursing responses and/or referrals are delayed, putting patients' safety at risk.[2–4] More than simple knowledge acquisition is needed to support increased recognition and appropriate responses.[2]

The increased complexity requires nurses to provide care in situations in which patients' conditions may be changing rapidly. Ebright concluded that nurses in acute care medical–surgical settings must prioritize, or "restack," patient care tasks multiple times throughout a shift.[5] This restacking involves a myriad of unexpected events that necessitate reorganizing tasks, such as changes to patient schedules, changing patient conditions, multiple discharges and admissions, and patient care staffing issues. To restack tasks, nurses engage in a thinking process that results in crucial decisions or judgments about patient care, often with little time to think about or plan for the next steps. The foundation of safe and effective nursing practice is the ability to consistently make good clinical judgments. Clinical judgment as a concept is presented from a theoretical perspective to help the student gain an understanding of the complexities of this process.

DEFINITION

The concept of clinical judgment in general refers to interpretations and inferences that influence actions in clinical practice. The most recent nursing literature uses the term *clinical judgment* as an inference or interpretation made in a caregiving setting,[6–9] a process resulting in such an inference or interpretation,[8–10] or the capacity for making inferences or interpretations about patient care.[7,10] The definition of clinical judgment used for this concept presentation is "*an interpretation or conclusion about a patient's needs, concerns, or health problems, and/or the decision to take action (or not), use or modify standard approaches, or improvise new ones as deemed appropriate by the patient's response.*"[8, p.204]

Two other terms, clinical reasoning and critical thinking, are often used interchangeably in the literature with the term *clinical judgment*;

thus differentiation is needed.[11] *Clinical reasoning* is the thinking process by which a nurse reaches a clinical judgment.[9,12] It is defined as "an iterative process of noticing, interpreting, and responding—reasoning in transition with a fine attunement to the patient and how the patient responds to the nurse's actions."[10, p.230] Encompassed in clinical reasoning is the ability to perceive the relevance of scientific evidence and its fit with the specific patient situation.[10] *Critical thinking*, on the other hand, is a cognitive process used for analysis of an issue or problem, is knowledge based, and not dependent on a particular situation.[9,13] Critical thinking certainly can be valuable in nursing practice, but it should not be equated with clinical judgment as it is not situated or specific to a given patient, nurse, or care context.[9,10]

Herein lies the complexity of nursing: Clinical judgments require that the nurse recognize the unique situation of the patient using deep knowledge of a variety of interrelated physiologic and psychosocial concepts, which leads to a profound understanding of the clinical situation. In other words, clinical judgment requires the nurse to apply knowledge, both tacit and explicit, to the unique patient situation to make sense of it and respond appropriately in the specific context of care. Because of the diversity of patient care situations the nurse encounters, it should be noted there may be no one right clinical judgment or answer in a given situation.[10]

SCOPE

Standards-Based Approaches and Clinical Judgment

Early research on clinical judgment focused on trying to understand all the factors involved in clinical judgments about patient care, making them explicit. This resulted in a rules-based or standards-based approach that located the nurse and the individual needs of the patient outside the caregiving situation rather than situating the patient issue in a specific context of care. Decision making from this perspective involves selection from options of mutually exclusive possibilities, implying that there is one right decision. This approach often involves use of algorithms, decision trees, patient care guidelines, or standards of care. These tools provide clear-cut guidance or rules that standardize approaches to patient care within an institution, based on best practices for a typical patient population and focus on quality of care rather than the individual patient. Algorithms direct care in emergent situations, such as a cardiopulmonary arrest, that involve multiple personnel from several disciplines. These standardized tools are very useful to support safe patient care, especially for the beginning clinician who lacks knowledge and/or experience. However, their use may or may not result in the best possible care for a particular patient in a given situation. They also may limit options and creative solutions.

A principle that relates decision-making tools to clinical judgment is that if there is a rule or guideline that covers the situation, clinical judgment is not required. Furthermore, clinical judgment may be required in decision making whether or not a given standard is applicable or appropriate in a given patient care situation.[10] In fact, research has shown that although standards or guidelines may be useful beginning points, expert nurses rarely rely on them alone.[8,10] This is because the expert nurses nuance their understanding of the individual patient situation, coupled with practical experience and knowledge of standards to employ a much more interpretivist approach.[10]

Evidence-Based Practice and Clinical Judgment

All clinicians are expected to use the best evidence to inform practice. Use of evidence-based guidelines, informed by research, improves patient outcomes.[14] Evidence-based practice (EBP) is defined as a problem-solving approach to clinical decision-making that combines the best available scientific evidence with best available patient and practitioner experiential evidence toward optimal healthcare outcomes.[14] It is important to note that clinical judgment is an integral aspect of safe implementation of EBP.

Safe and effective nursing care requires scientific knowledge, as well as practical experience, to understand when particular research evidence is relevant.[2,10] The nurse must accurately assess the patient and care context and then apply EBPs that are most appropriate in a given situation. Clinical judgment also guides nurses to question current practices and consider when guidelines need to be updated based on current evidence.[10]

Interpretivist Perspective

Interpretivist approaches originate from the belief that life experiences are culturally bound, that individuals interpret these experiences on the basis of their encounters within a given culture,[15] and that one circumscribed approach is often not appropriate for everyone.[8] The nature of nursing care is not linear, and in fact, in numerous situations there are many unknowns; therefore approaches that consider multiple factors in clinical reasoning are frequently more appropriate.[8] Because there are often no clear-cut answers about nursing care or because of the influence of the individual patient circumstances and context of care, clinical judgments by nurses become very specific to a given patient care situation. Interpretivist approaches situate the nurse squarely in the context of care and account for what the nurse personally contributes to the caring encounter, including previous experiences, values, and emotions.[10] The creation or construction of understanding the patient and caregiving situation using empirical knowledge of the disease process and care approaches, knowledge of the patient, and knowledge of the clinical environment facilitates decisions about care, thereby setting the stage for what the nurse notices and how the nurse interprets and responds to what is noticed.[8,10]

Reasoning in interpretivist approaches may involve "rule of thumb" methods and be intuitive. It involves tacit or understood knowledge,[10,16] is often inductive in nature, and is referred to by some authors as engaged, practical reasoning that is reasoning based on experience.[8,10,17,18] In contrast, rules-based approaches tend to rely heavily on analytic reasoning that requires systematically dividing a situation into parts, examining alternatives, and weighing options.[8] One example of the analytic approach is diagnostic reasoning—considering the evidence that supports each diagnosis.[19]

Nursing Process and Clinical Judgment

Nursing process frames the overarching standards of practice of the nursing profession.[20] It involves assessment, nursing diagnosis, outcomes identification, planning, implementation, and evaluation and is a framework that is used to structure nursing care. Students will notice that nursing process is used in many textbooks to teach nursing care. Because the elements of both the nursing process and clinical judgment seem to be very similar on first look, it is important that students distinguish between the two. While nursing process is linear and can be useful in systematic problem solving problem-solving and planning care (often over time), considering care through the lens of clinical judgment allows nurses to examine more deeply the factors that go into clinical thinking and decision-making, often in "real time" as patient care is occurring.[8] The nursing process is more static in nature, whereas clinical judgment is a dynamic process that accounts for changes in the patient situation as they occur. The capacity for clinical judgment develops over time.[7,21]

ATTRIBUTES AND CRITERIA

Using the interpretivist perspective of clinical judgment and clinical reasoning from the nursing literature, clinical judgment has three significant defining attributes that are useful in understanding the concept:

- *Holistic view of the patient situation*: Clinical judgment is inherently complex and influenced by many factors related to the particular patient and caregiving situation, and it therefore requires a holistic view.[10,13,18,20] Making excellent clinical judgments requires a willingness to consider all factors involved in patient care, including certain characteristics of the nurse (theoretical and experiential knowledge, values, biases), the relationship with patient, as well as the context of care, and is much more than simply a combination of the individual aspects.[8,22]

- *Process orientation*: Clinical judgment is circular, interactive, and moves fluidly between and among all of the aspects of the process.[8,10,18] To make clinical judgments, the nurse employs a deep understanding of the individual patient situation and her own background, experience, and values. Patients and nurses are unique and bring different backgrounds to the caregiving situation. The nurse notices salient (or relevant) features of a unique situation based on these factors and intervenes. While the nurse observes the patient response, he or she determines what the next steps are going to be. These aspects do not have a linear relationship but, rather, continuously influence each other in complex ways. After the caregiving situation, the nurse connects the patient outcomes in a way that enhances further understanding of future patients' care, utilizing reflection.[8,10]

- *Reasoning and interpretation*: Clinical judgment involves reasoning and interpretation. As described previously, reasoning is the process that leads to clinical judgments. Nurses use at least three types of reasoning: analytic, intuitive, and narrative.[8] The type of reasoning used depends on the caregiving situation and the nurse's previous experience. When a situation is unfamiliar, the nurse (expert and novice alike) tends to rely on analytic reasoning processes, consider the possibilities, and deduce the solution. Based on broad and deep experience, the expert nurse may recognize a situation immediately and act intuitively and tacitly. Nurses may also process their reasoning in narrative form—that is, recognizing the significance of the situation at hand to the patient's experience with illness and engaging in interventions based on this understanding.[23,24]

- *Ethical comportment*: This attribute means that nurses come to a patient situation with an outlook of what is right or good for the patient that manifests in respect, responsiveness, and support toward that patient. This attribute arises from experience and practical learning from others,[10] as well as grounding in personal values.

THEORETICAL LINKS

Although there are a number of models describing clinical judgment in nursing, the Tanner Clinical Judgment Model (2006) will be used to explain the concept in this chapter. The Tanner Model is a comprehensive approach to clinical judgment that was developed based on three decades of clinical judgment research and through an extensive review of research done primarily with expert nurses in practice.[8] The model (Fig. 38.1) rests on assumptions about complexities in the environment of care and the interplay of multiple factors that affect nurses' clinical thinking. In the model, four aspects of clinical judgment are described. Influenced by background and contextual factors, the nurse *notices* various features of the caregiving situation, such as clinical assessment findings, lab work, data, patient demeanor, and family situation. Through clinical reasoning patterns, collecting additional clinical data as needed, and conferring with colleagues, the nurse develops an understanding of the particular clinical situation—a process called *interpreting*. Based on the interpretation of the situation, the nurse determines appropriate actions, which is termed *responding* in the model. The nurse observes the patient's reaction to the nursing action and decides if the action has addressed the primary concerns, if the action needs some refinement to adjust for the particular patient, or if a completely different response is required. This is referred to as *reflection-in-action*. Nursing reflection after-the-fact, *reflection-on-action*, helps the nurse to connect patient responses with outcomes in a way that contributes to the nurse's further understanding of patient care.[8] Despite the fact that these aspects are described in separate sections, they do not have a linear relationship but, rather, continuously influence each other in a complex manner. Thus the consideration of them as separate aspects may be artificial but is offered here as an in-depth means to better understand the concept.

Noticing

Noticing is most often the impetus for clinical reasoning and is critical to making an effective judgment to address a patient issue. Several important factors impact what the nurse notices. In fact, Tanner asserts that the factors behind the nurse's eyes are as important as what is in front.[8] These include the background of the nurse (including intrapersonal characteristics, ethical grounding for what is right, previous experiences, theoretical knowledge, biases, values), the nurse's relationship with the patient, and the context of care (for more detail about these precursors to noticing, see Box 38.1). Influenced by these factors,

BOX 38.1   Factors that Influence Noticing

Intrapersonal Characteristics of the Nurse
- Ethical grounding and personal sense of importance
- Trustworthiness—asking questions/seeking help when unsure
- Developmental maturity in thought and knowing processes; formulates opinions and values relative to the context of learning
- Skill in using various ways of knowing—empirical, experiential, and ethical

Theoretical and Experiential Knowledge of the Nurse
- Novice and less experienced nurses use deductive reasoning, rules, and comparisons of the patient with the textbook in a systematic analysis of the situation.
- Expert nurses look at the whole picture and use pattern recognition and intuition derived from their experiences to make judgments.

Knowing the Patient
- Knowing the range of patient's pattern of responses
- Knowing the patient as a person, including preferences and desires

Context or Environment of Care
- Setting in which the nurse interacts with the patient
- Unique aspects of nursing practice/patient care needs in a given setting

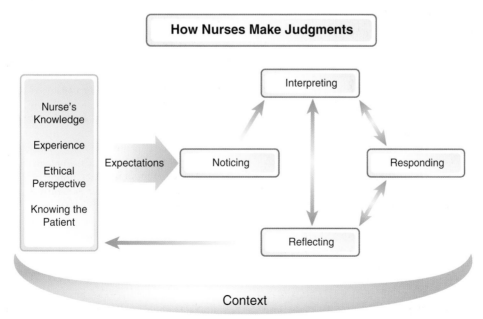

FIGURE 38.1 Tanner's Model of Clinical Judgment. (Adapted from Tanner, C. A. [2006]. Thinking like a nurse: A research-based model of clinical judgment. *Journal of Nursing Education, 45*[6], 204–211. Reprinted with permission from SLACK Incorporated.)

the nurse develops expectations about potential patient needs that set the stage for *noticing*. Expectations derived from the nurse's experiences with similar patients allow the nurse to anticipate the patient's appearance and needs, both currently and in the next hours and days. Without these experiences, the nurse uses theoretical, decontextualized knowledge, such as a list of general signs and symptoms for a medical diagnosis.

The nurse enters the care situation and collects pertinent information and patient data. Broad knowledge, based on experience and theoretical understanding as well as understanding a particular context, allows nurses to notice what factors are the most salient for a particular patient. Nurses select from a very broad set of data and patient assessment findings, searching for patterns that are consistent with previous experiences and using that information to guide care in the current situation. Less experienced nurses may have difficulty extracting the most important patient data and findings in a particular situation.[7,10,25]

Knowing the patient (whether it is knowing a given type of patient or knowing a specific patient) in a particular context influences what a nurse notices. For example, a home health nurse who has made visits to an older adult patient in his home over several months has a different level of "knowing the patient" than a nurse who sees a patient in an intensive care setting. Knowing the older adult allows the home health nurse to know the patient's baseline mental status and to notice subtle changes in cognition or affect. The nurse assuming care for this same patient in an intensive care setting might not realize that medication-related confusion demonstrated by the patient postoperatively is not typical for this patient and might assume that the patient has dementia or other cognitive impairment.

Based on what is noticed, the nurse may have an immediate grasp of the situation—recognition of a pattern or cluster of cues that signals a concern. On other occasions, the nurse, despite extensive experience, may have noticed that the situation is not as expected but does not quite have a clear grasp. Depending on this initial understanding, various reasoning patterns may be triggered. Once an issue is noticed, the nurse immediately gathers additional information and draws on her background, including theoretical knowledge, past experiences with similar patients, as well as her relationship and knowledge of this particular patient within the specific context of care, and ethical beliefs about what is right in this situation. Because each individual nurse and patient and the context of care are different, what happens next is also very unique; in many situations, there is no one correct way to provide patient care.

Interpreting

Using the particular patient data as well as germane theoretical and experiential knowledge, the nurse begins to assemble all the information, make sense of it, and establish priorities. For the expert nurse, certain data carry more weight than others with respect to the patient. For example, in the long-term care setting, a patient's age and kidney function may well impact the nurse's clinical judgment about using ibuprofen for pain relief even though the drug may be ordered. The nurse uses reasoning to make that determination.

According to Tanner, expert nurses draw on a variety of reasoning patterns (analytic, intuitive, and narrative) to interpret the meaning of what has been noticed.[8] The types of reasoning used seem to vary with the experience of the nurse.[10] For example, students and novice nurses, or more experienced nurses encountering unfamiliar situations, tend to rely on analytic reasoning based on theoretical knowledge. The nurse makes a hypothesis or best guess about the patient care situation and then tests the hypothesis. Sometimes this reasoning is not situation-specific but, rather, based on generalizations or rules. Expert nurses often use intuitive reasoning based on unstated but understood knowledge about the patient, the caregiving context, and

their previous experiences, sometimes very quickly.[10] A third type of reasoning, narrative reasoning, is a way of making sense of a situation through telling and interpreting stories.[8,23,24,26] Narrative reasoning supports deep understanding of caregiving situations.[8,10] Nurses hear patients' stories of their experiences with illness, how they understand their symptoms, what meaning they attribute to their illness, how they cope with it, and what resolution they hope for. This type of reasoning helps nurses understand the specific patient experience, setting the stage for individualizing care.[8] Nurses may also use narrative reasoning in their own reflections about patient care.

Responding

Once the patient data have been sorted and interpreted, the nurse uses his interpretation to respond to the particular patient issue through one or more nursing interventions. Depending on the level of expertise, the nurse may or may not be able to judge the effectiveness of the intervention before initiating it. For example, the nurse knows that the ordered pain medication is likely to help the newly admitted postoperative patient with a pain level of 8 out of 10. What the nurse may not know is what dose will be effective or the level to which it will reduce the patient's pain. The nurse's past experience with and knowledge about the effects of the pain medication will initially direct the dosage the nurse chooses. As the nurse comes to understand the unique patient's response to the medication and dosage required, the reasoning process moves from primarily analytic to more intuitive/narrative.

Reflecting

Many theorists have described reflective thinking and its usefulness. In fact, an early 20th-century educator made the bold statement that "reflective thinking alone is educative."[27,p.2] Other theorists consider that reflection and the ability to learn from one's actions are marks of a professional.[22,28] The clinical judgment model includes two types of reflection: reflection-*in*-action and reflection-*on*-action. Both have significant bearing on clinical judgment.

Reflection-in-Action

Reflection-in-action refers to the nurse's understanding of patient responses to nursing actions while care is occurring.[8] In observations and interactions with the patient, the nurse determines patient status and adjusts care accordingly. It is the thinking that happens in "real time" during patient care. Because of the ambiguous and complex nature of clinical judgments and the particular needs of each patient, reflecting is a critical step in evaluating the patient's reaction to the intervention. To continue the example of the postoperative patient, the nurse chooses a pain medication dose based on many factors; while administering the medication intravenously, the nurse is continually assessing and reflecting on the patient's response to medication, such as changes in facial expression, muscle relaxation, or verbal indications of relief. This is an example of reflecting-in-action. If the desired response is not achieved, the nurse may need to return to interpreting the data to respond with a different intervention.

Reflection-on-Action

Reflection-on-action is consideration of the situation after the patient care occurs. In reflection-on-action, the nurse contemplates a situation and considers what was successful and what was unsuccessful. Reflection-on-action is critical for development of knowledge and improvement in reasoning. It is how learning from practice is incorporated into personal experience for consideration in future patient care situations.[29] In the previous example, the nurse may take some time at the end of her shift to analyze why he or she intervened in a specific way for this particular patient and to consider whether the intervention was successful. Reflection-on-action is when significant learning from practice occurs and is critical to the development of increasing skillfulness as a nurse.[26,28,29] Often nurses spend more time reflecting on negative outcomes, but it is equally important to consider successful interventions to improve practice.

Nurses may use verbal narratives to engage in reflection-on-action, to make sense of their own experiences, and to process thinking. Listen to nurses in clinical settings when they talk; they often tell stories about their patients, especially if some aspect of care is perplexing. Telling stories is often a way of problem solving or learning from the experiences of others.

CONTEXT TO NURSING AND HEALTH CARE

All Nurses, All Settings

Clinical judgment is an integral aspect of nursing care of all patients and patient populations. Nurses in all specialty areas and practice settings—whether in public health nursing, community-based nursing, long-term care, or acute care—exercise clinical judgment; thus it is considered an essential skill of the professional nurse.[4] Clinical judgment, however, is not required for every patient care activity or intervention. Some nursing actions are obvious. For example, a postanesthesia recovery nurse knows that it is appropriate to take an immediate postoperative patient's vital signs quite frequently in the first few hours to recognize early signs of a problem. This is based on the nurse's knowledge that patients can sometimes have breathing or circulatory difficulties following administration of a general anesthetic and surgical interventions. The nurse also knows that the earlier such a sign or symptom is identified, the better the outcome for the patient. Recognition of an abnormal finding and actions taken subsequently are the result clinical judgments.

Environmental Context

As mentioned previously, the context or setting of care influences what a nurse notices. The specific environment of care also has a significant influence on care. Demanding environments of care can add increasing burden to making clinical judgments[4,5,8,9] and can actually interfere with competent clinical judgment.[30] On the other hand, context may also be a boon for easing the burden of clinical judgments. For example, consider the case of a patient experiencing a myocardial infarction in the emergency department, where a wide range of medications, including oxygen, are readily available. Monitoring devices are already on the patient and, in fact, may have signaled an impending life-threatening dysrhythmia. Nurses in this context are trained to respond quickly and confidently; because of the setting, they are anticipating emergent situations. By contrast, consider the nurse who encounters a person experiencing a myocardial infarction in a public setting, such as a park or a church. Very different actions must be employed, including deciding what to do first, who should call for help, who should be involved in the resuscitation process, and how long resuscitation should be continued.

Experience, Theoretical Knowledge, and Expertise

Clinical judgment, or thinking like a nurse, requires deep clinical knowledge and several types of thinking. Not surprisingly, deep clinical knowledge provides the nurse with the background needed to recognize patterns and therefore differences when they occur in patients, signaling the need for nursing care. As nurses become more experienced, clinical judgments become more intuitive, with nurses instantly recognizing patterns and grasping the meaning of situations they have previously encountered to immediately know what their response to the situation should be.[22] As such, it may appear that experienced nurses have not engaged in all aspects of clinical judgment, but, in fact, all aspects may occur almost simultaneously and subconsciously.[8]

Inexperienced nurses (novices) rely mostly on formal, theoretical knowledge and tend to treat all pieces of information with similar importance. They may have difficulty determining priorities in a given situation. Early in practice, it is more challenging to individualize and contextualize patient care. Expert nurses look at the whole picture and use pattern recognition and intuition derived from their experiences to make judgments, whereas those with less experience most often use deductive reasoning, rules, and comparisons of the patient with the textbook in a systematic analysis of the situation.[8,10,17,19] However inexperienced, students or novice nurses should pay attention to nagging or uncomfortable feelings when caring for patients and seek help for interpreting them.

Consider the experienced nurse in a clinic-based setting, such as an internal medicine clinic. Through honing his cardiopulmonary assessment skills over a number of years, the nurse has become familiar with the early signs of impending acute heart failure. A nurse new to that clinic may not as readily recognize the pattern of breathing correlated with patient color, including the slight blue tinge of oral mucous membranes, and complaints of increased fatigue with activities of daily living. The outcome of such experience may well be faster initiation of treatment for this patient, thereby preventing a hospitalization.

This concept has introduced the idea that students and novice nurses more often rely on theoretical knowledge or rules and analytic reasoning to make clinical judgments. That theoretical grounding is very important to student nurse practice and beyond. Understanding the principles of nursing care, communication, altered states of health, patient teaching, and other aspects of care is fundamental to becoming a nurse. As students and novice nurses acquire more experience, thinking, and clinical judgment, they use previous experiences, along with an understanding of this particular patient, the current context, and the best available, relevant evidence to ground their thinking about patient care. In fact, one study found that preceptors believed that new graduate nurses were ready for independent practice when they were able to integrate multiple sources of knowing and individualize care to the patient.[18] Evidence suggests that certain strategies promote development of clinical judgment.[6] With that in mind, the next section explores ways to facilitate clinical judgment development.

Developing Clinical Judgment

Developing clinical judgment is a process.[22,31,32] Novice nurses and nursing students often admire nurses who possess high-level clinical judgment skills. Taking advantage of a wide range of clinical learning opportunities and working closely with experienced nurses foster clinical judgment. Analyzing situations in which appropriate nursing actions are not obvious or clear-cut can enhance development of clinical judgment.[33] Nursing education combines theory with practice; learn to recognize how theory guides practice and how practice supports theories you have learned. Search for factors that impact the judgments that are made—including theoretical knowledge, nursing values, previous experiences, knowing the patient, and the patient care environment. Consider how these factors influence the situation. Seek insight and support from nurses with more experience to validate your thinking. Simulation is commonly used in nursing programs as an extension of learning in clinical situations. Learning through simulation scenarios can contribute to clinical judgment skills,[34–37] including skill in care of patients with acute deterioration.[3,38] The formation of clinical judgment is an essential skill for students to develop. In the future it will be incorporated in the nursing licensure examination (Box 38.2).

BOX 38.2   On the Horizon: NCLEX Testing for Clinical Judgment

From the discussion of clinical judgment presented in this chapter, one might surmise the difficulty involved in assessing levels of clinical judgment on a multiple choice question examination, such as a licensure exam. The National Council of State Boards of Nursing (NCSBN) that has responsibility for the RN licensing examination (NCLEX) in the United States has recognized a need to do this better. The Council has defined clinical judgment and created a model, primarily for assessment purposes, with hopes to improve testing in the future (Dickison, Haerling, & Lasater, 2019). The NCSBN states that "clinical judgment is defined by the skill of recognizing cues about a clinical situation, generating and weighing hypotheses, taking action and evaluating outcomes for the purpose of arriving at a satisfactory clinical outcome. Clinical judgment is the observed outcome of two unobserved underlying mental processes, critical thinking and decision making" (NCSBN, 2018, p. 3). At the present, the definition and a concomitant model are being tested (NCSBN).

Dickison, P., Haerling, K. A., & Lasater, K. (2019). The National Council of State Boards of Nursing Clinical Judgment Model. *Journal of Nursing Education, 58*(2), 72–78.
National Council of State Boards of Nursing (NCSBN). (2018). NCLEX RN® Examinations analysis and research. Next Generation NCLEX News. Retrieved from https://www.ncsbn.org/11998.htm.

Knowledge or Deep Understanding

Knowing how to respond to a patient issue requires deep knowledge of the complex interconnected factors that impact the issue.[39] This includes theoretical knowledge about the patient population, relevant physiology and pathophysiology, and potential nursing interventions.[10,40] For example, in maternal–newborn nursing, a deep understanding of the birthing process is essential. However, knowledge of interconnected concepts—such as the normal and problematic signs of impending delivery, the physiological transition of hormonal influences in the immediate postdelivery phase (both physical and psychological), and also the potential impact of a new member on the family's dynamics—will facilitate the nurse's clinical judgments in that context of care. In this example, the nurse will need specialty-specific knowledge about lab findings, subtle signs of depression, and community resources/supports that are available for new mothers. Deep knowledge provides a basis for focused assessments, including salient factors, and for interpreting findings that lead to appropriate clinical judgments specific to the patient's needs.

Learning to Recognize Patterns

Pattern recognition of specific conditions is a significant aspect of noticing and interpreting patient care needs and leads to a deeper understanding of patient issues.[41] To recognize patterns, the nurse relies on identification of specific cues (derived from patient data) that fit together to lead to better understanding of the patient situation. For example, a patient with septic shock will likely display a pattern of elevated heart rate, poor perfusion, decreased oxygen saturation, low blood pressure, and a left shift on the white blood cell count differential. Knowing this pattern alerts the student or nurse to note what signs or symptoms may be present or absent to determine an appropriate response. As students and nurses gain more practical experience, patterns related to nursing care become more apparent.

Applying Concepts to Nursing Practice

Search for opportunities to learn about patient care concepts; then compare and contrast how concepts present in various patients to see patterns.[41,42] For example, consider how a particular patient with sepsis matches the pattern of sepsis just described, as well as what signs or symptoms are different.[43] Then consider how the context (caregiving situation, your own values, knowing the patient and her specific personal qualities and needs, and your own past nursing and personal experiences with the concept) impacts the particular caregiving situation. This may help you to recognize how the specific situation influences the nursing response to the individual patient with sepsis.

Another opportunity to do this might occur on a pediatric rotation. On the unit, you may care for a child with respiratory problems that require oxygen, perhaps a child with asthma. Consider why your patient is receiving supplemental oxygen and other factors (physical, developmental, and pathophysiological) that impact oxygenation and oxygen administration to your patient. Then visit another student's patient who is also receiving oxygen, perhaps a child with pneumonia. Consider the same questions for your classmate's patient. Compare and contrast the two patients. What are the similarities? What are the differences? Why are they different? What learning will you apply to future situations?

Skillful Responding

An important aspect of responding involves setting priorities and modifying them as the situation changes. Pay attention to how nurses in the clinical setting prioritize patient care. Consider the factors they use to make decisions about planning and replanning their patient care. Discuss prioritization of care as a part of your daily routine in clinical. Identify the resources in the clinical setting that support skill-related decision making and performance, such as procedural references. Think about what you expect the patient response to the intervention might be, and then observe the actual response.[43,44]

Reflective Practice

Reflection is a learning activity included in many nursing programs and with good reason. Reflecting helps students to process and consolidate learning about caregiving situations.[4,26,28] Reflection on clinical experiences can support application of theoretical knowledge to clinical situations and improve prioritization of future nursing care.[29,45] As a student and as a practicing nurse, it is important to reflect on both successful and unsuccessful interventions during a caregiving experience. Nursing students are often acutely aware of their knowledge deficits as well as their shortcomings in performing a particular nursing skill. Although recognizing the need for improvement and analyzing how that will happen are critically significant parts of nursing practice, it is important to reinforce in one's mind those things that you did well.

Telling stories about practice is often a part of clinical postconference and journaling and is integral to reflective learning.[23,24,45] By being an active part of this important learning opportunity and considering carefully the patients described by classmates, students multiply their exposure to different patient issues and gain deeper understanding of nursing practice.[23,29,34,42,46,47] Questioning each other and expressing different possibilities can help students broaden their thinking about nursing care options.[42,47] Fostering personal habits of reflection during nursing school, whether individually in writing or in group discussions, provides a strong foundation for continued learning through reflection when one enters practice. Evidence shows that structured experiences in reflection and debriefing using a guide and/or a rubric may support development of clinical judgment.[4,37,47–49] Reflection-on-action is a type of self-evaluation. Evidence suggests that elements of clinical judgment can be measured.[7,21,32] Use of tools such as the Lasater Clinical Judgment Rubric[7] that provide clear description of levels of clinical judgment can help students and their teachers evaluate clinical judgment and identify goals for further growth.[32,47,50–52]

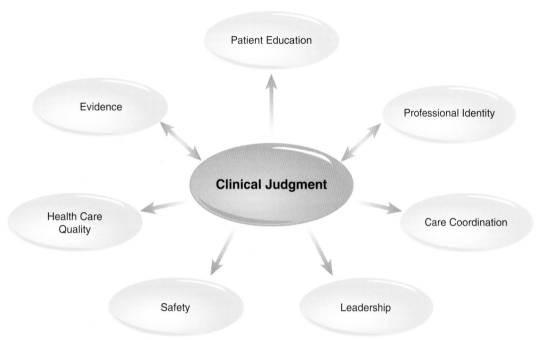

FIGURE 38.2 Clinical Judgment and Interrelated Concepts.

INTERRELATED CONCEPTS

Several concepts in this textbook are interrelated to the concept of clinical judgment—in fact, all concepts related to patient care activities have this link. Featured in Fig. 38.2 are seven concepts that are especially closely related to clinical judgment.

Clinical judgment is integral to the Safety of patients.[4] Consider the situation of an older adult getting up to walk postoperatively for the first time. The nurse may know that particular caution should be exercised because falls are very common in the hospital context, and there may be unit guidelines regarding fall prevention. From theoretical knowledge, the nurse knows that although falling is a danger when ambulating, there are significant dangers associated with immobility and staying in bed. In making the decision to get the patient up, the nurse considers factors, including the patient's level of consciousness, strength, pain control status, motivation, and environmental context. The nurse's previous experiences with ambulating older adult patients will significantly inform his decisions.

The nurse who is committed to high-quality patient care is alert to patterns that may indicate that there are concerns for Health Care Quality in a given hospital unit or agency. For example, if medications consistently arrive from pharmacy in mid-morning rather than early in the shift, some nurses become involved in other caregiving activities and then forget to administer the medications once they arrive on the unit. Based on theoretical knowledge, the nurse recognizes this as a systems problem. Experiential knowledge of unit culture and organization informs how the nurse takes action to communicate with the unit manager and the pharmacy to get medications to the unit on time.

Leadership choices are almost always fraught with multiple competing factors. For example, the charge nurse of an adult medical–surgical unit may have to consider the mix of nursing staff needed for a shift, given the acuity of the patients. What staffing combination will best serve the needs of the patients on the unit at any given moment? The charge nurse may need to respond by asking for help at a higher level if the staffing mix is inadequate. On the same unit, an individual nurse may delegate certain aspects of more stable patients' care to a certified nursing assistant, allowing greater focus on those more seriously ill. These kinds of leadership choices are dependent on knowing the patient(s) as well as the backgrounds of the nursing staff.

Determining when and how much Patient Education a patient and/or family needs frequently requires clinical judgment. A patient newly diagnosed with diabetes needs to know about diet, medication, exercise, and foot care, how to perform blood glucose monitoring, and medication administration. Because it is impossible for a patient to learn everything in one visit, the home health nurse must assess the patient's knowledge and prioritize which information is most important at a given time. Depending on the patient's ability and ease of learning, the nurse may need to use clinical judgment to refine her teaching to best address the patient's needs. Clinical judgment is exercised throughout the entire learning process—noticing how much the patient remembers from the last visit and assessing learning outcomes.

In making clinical judgments, nurses consider a variety of Evidence from research studies, clinical guidelines, and standards of care. The nurse may also use evidence from past experiences with "what works" for patient care within a particular unit culture, as well as practice experiences with a given patient ("knowing the patient") or understanding other contextual factors that impact a caregiving situation. The best available evidence may well impact how the nurse interprets a patient situation and responds to it, but other factors impact nursing actions as well. Using clinical judgment, values regarding individualizing patient care, and knowledge of the patient, the nurse identifies additional needs and resources and then advocates for the patient to meet the unique needs.

BOX 38.3   EXEMPLARS OF CLINICAL JUDGMENT

Clinical Skills
- Decisions about urinary or intravenous catheter placement, such as determination regarding size and type of urinary or intravenous catheter or whether placement is needed
- Decisions about timing and extent of bathing and personal care
- Assessment of a wound and determining next steps
- Selection of an appropriate dressing

Urgent/Emergent Situations
- Detection of subtle signs of sepsis
- Early treatment of patient hemorrhage
- Starting oxygen to respond to decreased saturation levels
- Early recognition of anaphylaxis

Communication
- Content and depth of patient teaching at discharge, pre- and postoperatively
- Advocacy for patient at care coordination conferences

- Communication with distraught or fearful patient or family
- Defusing potentially confrontational interactions

Medication Management
- Selection of dose when a range is ordered
- PRN decisions
- Holding a medication
- Early recognition of adverse reaction or side effect from medication

Management of Care and Nursing Leadership
- Delegation to ancillary nursing personnel
- Prioritization of care among patients
- Calling a physician
- Referral to another health professional (e.g., wound care specialist, dietitian)
- Decisions about patient assignments

ACCESS EXEMPLAR LINKS IN YOUR GIDDENS EBOOK

Clinical judgment is applied in situations in which the nurse relies on Professional Identity in interactions with patients and/or their families. Consider the patient who is newly diagnosed with late-stage lung cancer. The nurse caring for this patient should notice the patient's mood and level of interest to determine when the patient needs information about hospice care. The nurse may also have firsthand experience with a family member who had a similar diagnosis. Is there an appropriate opportunity for the nurse to relate to and encourage this patient's family, based on that experience, or is it better with this particular family to focus only on their experience? This situation requires careful noticing and interpretation.

Clinical judgment is used in Care Coordination situations to help the patient achieve optimal healthcare outcomes. When planning an older adult patient's discharge after a motor vehicle accident resulting in multiple fractures, the nurse may uncover information that is critical for coordinating the patient's care—information about a patient's home situation that will impact the older adult's recovery. Based on previous experiences with complicated patients, the nurse may request a case conference with members of the healthcare team, patient, and family to foster the transition for a quality outcome.

CLINICAL EXEMPLARS

Clinical judgment is applied in all areas of nursing practice; thus there are multiple examples. Box 38.3 presents five general areas in which nurses potentially apply clinical judgment within practice: application of clinical skills, recognizing and responding to urgent/emergent situations, communication, medication management, and management of care.

Featured Exemplars
Clinical Skills: Determining Type of Catheter

A nurse caring for an older adult postoperative patient with anesthesia-associated urinary retention needs to decide whether to catheterize the patient, and if so, if a straight catheterization procedure or placing a Foley (retention) catheter would be best. Nurses consider the evidence, unit standard for catheter placement, and their knowledge of the patient, including mobility, cognitive status, and preferences. From clinical experience, they estimate how long the typical older adult might experience anesthesia-related urinary retention. Contextual knowledge may include the time of day; for example, placement of a Foley catheter may allow the patient to rest through the night.

Management of Care: Patient Assignments

On a busy day in an adult surgical unit, the charge nurse must decide to whom a newly admitted patient should be assigned. She uses her background knowledge of general patient care on the unit and unit policy regarding nurse/patient ratios, and the current context of care involved in the patients on the unit. She also uses her knowledge of the nursing staff. Does someone have particularly strong organizational skills or knowledge about the anticipated care needs of the patient to be admitted? The experienced nurse leader realizes that safe patient assignment goes well beyond abiding by the unit guidelines for patient/nurse ratios.

Urgent/Emergent Situation: Child with Sepsis

The nurse caring for a 4-year-old being treated for leukemia notices a blood pressure (BP) of 70/40. To interpret this reading, the nurse uses background and theoretical knowledge (normal BP for 4-year-olds and knowledge of this patient's usual BP trends over time). The nurse considers contextual factors, including therapies the child is receiving that may lower BP. Prompted by theoretical knowledge of presenting signs of sepsis, his previous experiences with septic patients, and awareness of the patient's risk factors, additional data are collected to determine if the patient's symptoms resemble sepsis. With these additional data, the nurse contacts the physician to discuss the next steps in the care.

Clinical Skills: Community-Based Client

A volunteer nurse at a free clinic sees a client just released from jail and living in a single-room occupancy hotel. The client has an open wound on his left hip. The client lives alone and has no family or close friends nearby who can assist with wound care. The nurse must use her background knowledge to select an appropriate dressing from a wide range of available materials and her knowledge of the patient to help the patient change the dressing. Safe patient care includes ensuring that patients can manage their own care, sometimes in challenging circumstances.

CASE STUDY

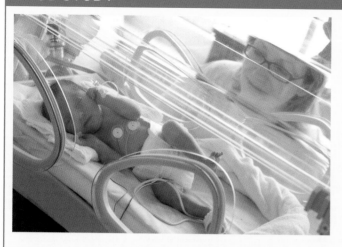

Case Presentation

Leon Rowen is a growing premature infant whose 32-year-old mother, Cassandra Rowen, is described by the nurses in the unit as "difficult." The baby is nearing discharge, but Cassandra is reported to be "resistant" to learning about how to feed and care for her infant. She has other children at home, but none of them was premature. A nursing care priority for the day is parental teaching about safe feeding of her premature baby.

Ruth, the nurse assigned to care for Leon, has worked in this unit for 10 years. She observes the entire caregiving situation and sees that Leon's condition is stable. Ruth meets Cassandra and notices she is quiet and sullen. Rather than beginning by explaining how to feed the baby, Ruth asks about Cassandra's other children and shares a little bit about the challenges of parenting her own children who are of similar ages as Cassandra's other children. Cassandra smiles and agrees. As time passes, Cassandra begins to talk about what a frightening experience having a premature baby has been. Ruth acknowledges those feelings. Cassandra smiles and begins to ask questions about how to care for Leon. Ruth answers those questions in a way that is tailored to what the mother has revealed about her family. Cassandra demonstrates feeding Leon in a developmentally appropriate way (side-lying position to prevent aspiration) based on Ruth's teaching. At the end of the shift, Ruth believes Cassandra has made significant progress toward competence in meeting her baby's unique needs. On her trip home, Ruth considers the experience. She realizes that prioritizing getting to know the mother and building a relationship by sharing a bit about herself as a parent helped to create emotional safety and trust so that Cassandra could talk about her apprehension as a first-time mother of a premature baby and then focus on learning infant care.

Case Analysis Questions

1. How does Ruth apply her knowledge and previous experience as a starting point for clinical judgment in this case?
2. In what way is there evidence that Ruth reflects on her experience to gain deeper understanding and further develop expertise?

From metin Kiyak/iStock/Thinkstock.

🌣 ACCESS EXEMPLAR LINKS IN YOUR GIDDENS EBOOK

REFERENCES

1. Institute of Medicine. (2010). *The future of nursing*. Washington, DC: Author.
2. Rattray, J. E., Lauder, W., Ludwick, R., et al. (2011). Indicators of acute deterioration in adult patients nursed in acute wards: A factorial survey. *Journal of Clinical Nursing, 20*(5–6), 723–732.
3. Lindsey, P. L., & Jenkins, S. (2013). Nursing students' clinical judgment regarding rapid response: The influence of a clinical simulation education intervention. *Nursing Forum, 8*(1), 61–70.
4. Razieh, S., Somayeh, G., & Haghani, F. (2018). Effects of reflection on clinical decision-making of intensive care unit nurses. *Nurse Education Today, 66*(2018), 10–14.
5. Ebright, P. R. (2010). The complex work of RNs: Implications for healthy work environments. *Online Journal of Issues in Nursing, 15*(1), Manuscript 4.
6. Capelletti, A., Engel, J., & Prentice, D. (2014). Systematic review of clinical judgment and reasoning in nursing. *The Journal of Nursing Education, 53*(8), 453–458.
7. Lasater, K. (2007). Clinical judgment development: Using simulation to create an assessment rubric. *The Journal of Nursing Education, 46*(11), 496–503.
8. Tanner, C. A. (2006). Thinking like a nurse: A research-based model of clinical judgment in nursing. *The Journal of Nursing Education, 45*(6), 204–211.
9. Victor-Chmil, J. (2013). Critical thinking versus clinical reasoning versus clinical judgment: Differential diagnosis. *Nurse Educator, 38*(1), 34–36.
10. Benner, P., Tanner, C., & Chesla, C. (2009). *Expertise in nursing practice: Caring, clinical judgment and ethics* (2nd ed.). New York: Springer.
11. Cazzell, M., & Anderson, M. (2016). The impact of critical thinking on clinical judgment during simulation with senior nursing students. *Nursing Education Perspectives, 37*(2), 83–90.
12. Simmons, B. (2010). Clinical reasoning: Concept analysis. *Journal of Advanced Nursing, 66*(5), 1151–1158.
13. Johansen, M., & O'Brien, J. (2016). Decision making in nursing practice: A concept analysis. *Nursing Forum, 51*(1), 40–48.
14. Dang, D., & Dearholt, S. (2018). *Johns Hopkins Nursing evidence-based practice: Models and guidelines* (3rd ed.). Indianapolis, IN: Sigma Theta Tau International.
15. Crotty, M. (1998). *The foundations of social research: Meaning and perspective in the research process*. London: Sage.
16. Braude, H. D. (2009). Clinical intuition versus statistics: Different modes of tacit knowledge in clinical epidemiology and evidence-based medicine. *Theoretical Medicine and Bioethics, 30*(3), 181–198.
17. Wolf, A. W. (2009). Comment: Can clinical judgment hold its own against scientific knowledge? *Psychotherapy, 46*(1), 11–14.
18. McNiesh, S. (2007). Demonstrating holistic clinical judgment: Preceptors perceptions of new graduate nurses. *Holistic Nursing Practice, 21*(2), 72–78.
19. Croskerry, P. (2009). A universal model of diagnostic reasoning. *Academic Medicine: Journal of the Association of American Medical Colleges, 84*(8), 1022–1028.
20. American Nurses Association (ANA). (2015). *Nursing: scope and standards of practice* (3rd ed.). Silver Spring, MD: ANA.
21. Lasater, K. (2011). Clinical judgment: The last frontier for evaluation. *Nurse Education in Practice, 11*(2), 86–92.
22. Boyer, L., Tardif, J., & Lefebvre, H. (2015). From a medical problem to a health experience: How nursing students think in clinical situations. *The Journal of Nursing Education, 54*(11), 625–632.
23. Wheeler, P., Butell, S., Epeneter, B., et al. (2016). Storytelling: A guided reflection activity. *The Journal of Nursing Education, 55*(3), 172–176.
24. Timbrell, J. (2017). Instructional storytelling: Application of the clinical judgment model in nursing. *The Journal of Nursing Education, 56*(5), 305–308.
25. Benner, P. (2001). *From novice to expert: Excellence and power in clinical nursing practice*. Upper Saddle River, NJ: Prentice Hall. [commemorative edition].

26. Bruner, J. (1996). *The culture of education.* Cambridge, MA: Harvard University Press.

27. Dewey, J. (1933). *How we think: A restatement of the relation of reflective thinking to the educative process.* Chicago.

28. Regnery Schön, D. (1983). *The reflective practitioner: How professionals think in action.* New York: Basic Books.

29. Glynn, D. (2012). Clinical judgment development using structured classroom reflective practice: A qualitative study. *The Journal of Nursing Education, 51*(3), 134–139.

30. Dillard, N., Sideras, S., Ryan, M., et al. (2009). A collaborative project to apply and evaluate the clinical judgment model through simulation. *Nursing Education Perspectives, 30*(2), 99–104.

31. Ashley, J., & Stamp, K. (2014). Learning to think like a nurse: The development of clinical judgment in nursing students. *The Journal of Nursing Education, 53*(9), 519–525.

32. Miraglia, R., & Asselin, M. (2015). The Lasater clinical judgment rubric as a framework to enhance clinical judgment in novice and experienced nurses. *Journal for Nurses in Professional Development, 31*(5), 284–291.

33. Foo, M., Tang, L., Vimala, R., et al. (2017). Educational intervention for clinical judgment skills. *Journal of Continuing Education in Nursing, 48*(8), 347–352.

34. Kelly, M., Hager, P., & Gallagher, R. (2014). What matters most? Students' rankings of simulation components that contribute to clinical judgment. *The Journal of Nursing Education, 53*(2), 97–101.

35. Lasater, K., Johnson, E., Ravert, P., et al. (2014). Role modeling clinical judgment for an unfolding older adult simulation. *The Journal of Nursing Education, 53*(5), 257–264.

36. Victor, J., Ruppert, W., & Ballasy, S. (2017). Examining the relationships between clinical judgment, simulation performance, and clinical performance. *Nurse Educator, 42*(5), 236–239.

37. AL Sabei, S., & Lasater, K. (2016). Simulation debriefing for clinical judgment development: A concept analysis. *Nurse Education Today, 45*(2016), 42–47.

38. Fisher, D., & King, L. (2013). An integrative literature review on preparing nursing students though simulation to recognize and respond to the deteriorating patient. *Journal of Advanced Nursing, 69*(11), 2375–2388.

39. Benner, P., Sutphen, M., Leonard, V., et al. (2010). *Educating nurses: A call for radical transformation.* San Francisco: Jossey–Bass.

40. Modic, M. B. (2013). Tanner's model of clinical judgment applied to preceptorship: Part 1. *Journal for Nurses in Professional Development, 29*(5), 274–275.

41. Modic, M. B. (2013). Tanner's model of clinical judgment applied to preceptorship: Part 2. *Journal for Nurses in Professional Development, 29*(6), 335–337.

42. Nielsen, A. (2016). Concept-based learning in clinical experiences: Bringing theory to clinical education for deep learning. *The Journal of Nursing Education, 55*(7), 365–371.

43. Modic, M. B. (2014). Developing skills in interpretation. *Journal for Nurses in Professional Development, 30*(1), 274–275.

44. Modic, M. B. (2014). Clinical judgment: Developing the skill of responding. *Journal for Nurses in Professional Development, 30*(2), 105–106.

45. Modic, M. B. (2014). Clinical judgment: Developing skills in reflection. *Journal for Nurses in Professional Development, 30*(3), 157–158.

46. Lavoie, P., Pepin, J., & Boyer, L. (2013). Reflective debriefing to promote novice nurses' clinical judgment after high-fidelity simulation: A pilot test. *Dynamics (Pembroke, Ont.), 24*(4), 36–41.

47. Nielsen, A., Lasater, K., & Stock, M. (2016). A framework to support preceptors' evaluation and development of new nurse's clinical judgment. *Nurse Education in Practice, 19*(2016), 84–90.

48. Lusk Monagle, J., Lasater, K., Stoyles, S., & Dieckmann, N. (2018). New graduate nurse experiences in clinical judgment: What academic and practice educators need to know. *Nursing Education Perspectives, 39*(4), 201–207.

49. Hines, C., & Wood, F. (2016). Clinical judgment scripts as a strategy to foster clinical judgments. *The Journal of Nursing Education, 55*(12), 691–695.

50. Bussard, M. (2018). Evaluation of clinical judgment in prelicensure nursing students. *Nurse Educator, 43*(2), 106–108.

51. Lancaster, R., Westphal, J., & Jambunathan, J. (2015). Using SBAR to promote clinical judgment in undergraduate nursing students. *The Journal of Nursing Education, 54*(3, Suppl.), S31–S34.

52. Lasater, K., Nielsen, A., Stock, M., & Ostrogorsky, T. (2015). Evaluating the clinical judgment of newly hired staff nurses. *Journal of Continuing Education in Nursing, 46*(12), 563–571.

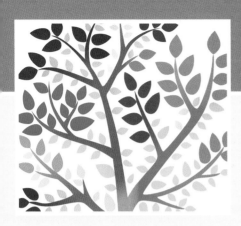

Leadership

Nancy Hoffart

Leadership is an old concept that applies to all aspects of life—from close to home, such as leading a family, to more distant situations, such as leading an international organization. Most people can name leaders in their experiences at school, work, and recreational and volunteer activities. Practical familiarity with the concept of leadership is gained through such experiences.

This concept presentation focuses on leadership as an essential aspect of the role of the registered nurse (RN). Nurses are called upon to be leaders as part of their daily work, and most RN competencies delineate leadership as an important capability for professional nurses. Nurses are expected to exhibit leadership when delivering patient care and when working with others to address issues that affect the practice of nursing.[1] Nurses have also been called on to play a leadership role in health policy and in shaping the healthcare system of the future.[2,3] This concept presentation introduces the general principles of leadership and their application in nursing and health care.

DEFINITION

Although there is a vast body of literature on leadership in work settings, a universally accepted definition of the term does not exist. For the purposes of this concept analysis, leadership is defined as *"an interactive process that provides needed guidance and direction."*[4,p820] Leadership involves three dynamic elements: a leader, a follower, and a situation. The leader provides guidance to followers, directing them toward a vision or goal and giving support to enable their success in the particular situation or setting.

SCOPE

The scope of leadership encompasses formal leadership and informal leadership (Fig. 39.1). Individuals who occupy designated administrative or management positions in an organization are considered to hold formal leadership positions. Chief executive officer, chief nurse executive, vice president for patient services, and nurse manager are common examples of formal leadership positions in health care. Depending on the location of the institution and type of setting, titles may vary. For example, in some settings, titles such as head nurse and nursing supervisor are still used. Other types of formal leadership positions are elected or appointed positions in professional nursing associations, such as president or committee chairperson and roles on boards, such as a community health center's board of directors.

Informal leadership by individuals who do not occupy a designated administrative or management position also occurs in organizations. Individuals are perceived as informal leaders by their supervisors and peers because of their capabilities and actions. An example is experienced staff nurses who are recognized as clinical leaders because of their expertise, their willingness to be spokespersons for other staff, or their involvement in important issues for patient care and nurses. Individuals who are perceived as informal leaders sometimes, but not always, move into formal leadership positions.

ATTRIBUTES AND CRITERIA

The following six attributes must be present for effective leadership to occur: followers, vision, communication, decision making, change, and social power. These attributes are presented in Fig. 39.2 and are described in the following sections.

Followers

There are no leaders without followers and no followers without leaders. In fact, most employees spend a large part of their work life as followers. Even leaders are followers in some settings, activities, and situations. Because followers and leaders are interdependent, each can influence the effectiveness of the other. Leaders, as discussed in the Featured Exemplars section, use different approaches to motivate, support, and reward their followers. How followers interact with leaders can be viewed on a continuum, with responses ranging from resistance to passivity to active participation in organizational activities. Consequently, success of an organization is closely tied to the interactions between leaders and followers.[5]

Fig. 39.2 uses a broken line to show a boundary between leaders and followers. The strength and permeability of the boundary between a leader and followers will depend on the leader's style. Autocratic leaders will maintain more distance from followers, interacting with them less than a leader who employs a democratic style. Transformational leaders also will have high interaction with followers.

Vision

A vision is a leader's ideological statement of a desired, long-term future for an organization. It is the future that a leader wants to create; thus, the vision is something to be worked toward over time. The aim of leadership, as indicated by its definition, is to guide and direct followers toward the organization's vision or toward goals instrumental

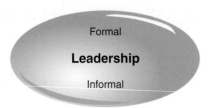

FIGURE 39.1 Scope of Leadership.

for attaining the vision. The importance leaders place on vision will depend on their leadership style. Articulating a clear vision is an essential component of transformational leadership, whereas in transactional leadership the leader is focused on performance goals for followers. To move followers toward a vision, a leader will use several processes. Three commonly used processes are communication, decision making, and change.

Communication

Communication is an essential function of effective leadership. In fact, leadership has been referred to as an ongoing conversation between a leader and followers. Leaders communicate with their followers, other leaders, the organization's clients, and people outside the organization to give and receive information. Fig. 39.2 depicts communication between the leader and followers as a process that spans the boundary between parties. The way in which a leader communicates with followers depends on the leader's style. Laissez-faire leaders have little communication with their followers. Authentic leaders use open communication and transparency to build trust with their followers.

Decision Making

All leaders make decisions that affect others and their organization's success. Good decisions are among the most critical features of good

leadership, but good decisions are also among leaders' most invisible actions. Like communication, decision making occurs at the boundary between a leader and followers (see Fig. 39.2) and varies depending on the leader's style. Democratic leaders use a participatory style of decision making. Autocratic leaders are more likely to make decisions without follower input. Laissez-faire leaders generally allow followers to make independent decisions except in a crisis.

Change

Change is the transition from an old state to a new state. Leaders guide the change process by working with their followers to move the organization or department toward the established vision and goals. A leader's change-management skills are vital in the change process. A leader influences change by using effective communication skills, understanding the organizational culture, considering alternate paths to achieve a goal, identifying and dealing with differences among followers, and creating leverage to motivate followers toward the vision.

Social Power

Social power is the potential influence of one individual over another. Leaders derive their social power from a variety of sources, as outlined by French and Raven's bases of power model (Table 39.1).[6] A leader's style influences how he or she will use power. For example, formal leaders' legitimate power is derived, in part, from the position they hold; transactional leaders use reward power, and authentic leaders use informational power.

THEORETICAL LINKS

Leadership theory has evolved in waves since the beginning of the 20th century. Each wave includes specific theories founded on common assumptions and incorporates different dimensions. As new waves of theory have emerged, they have not completely replaced previous waves

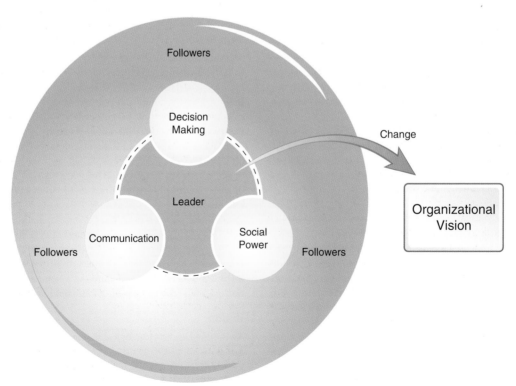

FIGURE 39.2 Attributes of Leadership.

TABLE 39.1 Bases of Social Power

Type of Power	Description
Coercive	Uses threat of punishment to get followers to respond. Followers expect to be punished by their leader if they fail to conform to leader's influence. Leader must monitor followers' work to allocate punishment. Followers who like their leader are more likely to respond to leader's threats than are followers who do not like their leader. Research has also shown that women are more responsive to coercive power than men.
Legitimate	Recognition that formal leaders have power over their followers because of the position they hold. A legitimate power relationship between two individuals can also be based on reciprocity (i.e., "You did 'X' for me, so I should do 'Y' for you"), equity (i.e., "I have done 'X' for you, so I have a right to ask you to do 'Y' for me"), and dependence (i.e., "I have an obligation to help others who cannot help themselves"). Internalized values dictate the extent to which individuals will respond to legitimate power.
Referent	Results when followers identify with or aspire to be like their leader. It does not require a direct relationship between leader and followers, or action on the part of the leader. Referent power is positive when followers voluntarily mold themselves to the leader. Referent power is negative when followers do not like or want to be like their leader.
Reward	Ability of one person to reward another for compliance with expectations. Leader must monitor the follower to give the reward. Like coercive power, reward power is stronger when followers like their leader, and women are more responsive to reward power than men.
Expert	Results when followers respond to their leader's directions because they perceive that the leader knows best. The range of expert power is limited to the leader's area of expertise. For example, one may have expert power as a registered nurse but not as an engineer. Like referent power, there is a negative variation on expert power. In this case, followers recognize the expertise of the leader but assume the leader will act in his or her own best interests rather than the followers' interests.
Informational	Based on the leader's ability to influence followers to act by using clear logic, rational argument, and information. Leader may present the information to followers directly or indirectly (e.g., through hints and suggestions). Use of indirect informational power is more effective than direct informational power when followers are trying to influence their leader.

Data from Raven, B. H. (1993). The bases of power: origins and recent developments. *Journal of Social Issues, 49*(4), 227–251.

but instead added to the understanding about this complex concept. As theory and research have advanced over time, the concept of leadership has changed. Leadership is no longer seen as a set of traits; it is now understood as a multifaceted, dynamic process. Today's leaders must know themselves, understand and relate effectively with their followers, and be responsive to varied situational dynamics and needs.

Great Man/Trait Theory

The oldest leadership theories illustrate the "great man" approach and are based on the assumption that leaders are born, not made. These theories hypothesize that when a situation demands leadership, a leader emerges to assume control; prior education or special preparation for leadership does not occur. Another key assumption of these theories is that traits can be used as criteria to select effective leaders. When the great man theory was first proposed, leaders were almost exclusively males from aristocratic backgrounds. Research based on the great man approach focuses on identifying traits of great leaders. Historically, this included physical characteristics (e.g., height) and demographic traits (e.g., male and aristocratic background). Now this research addresses personality (e.g., self-confidence and decisiveness), intellect (e.g., high IQ and reflection), and social attributes (e.g., friendliness and sense of humor). Gradually, the great man approach to leadership came to be termed "trait theory." Four attributes commonly identified by respondents throughout the world who were asked what qualities they look for and admire in leaders are (in rank order) honesty, forward looking, inspiring, and competent.[7] The many biographies of Florence Nightingale illustrate how trait theory has been used to describe her leadership characteristics (Box 39.1).[8] Recent nursing research shows that trait theory continues to be used to recommend qualities such as authenticity for today's nursing leaders.[9]

Behavioral Leadership

The second wave of leadership theory concentrates on leader behaviors. The core assumption of this wave is that effective leaders use different

BOX 39.1 An Example of the "Great Man" Theory in Nursing

Florence Nightingale is internationally recognized as the founder of modern nursing and is well known for her work in Scutari during the Crimean War, when she led an effort to provide better health care for British soldiers. Like many great man leaders, Miss Nightingale came from an aristocratic background, and although female, she and her only sibling, a sister, were educated and received encouragement from their father to read and study the texts that served as the educational core for men during the Victorian era.[8] Nightingale has been the subject of innumerable biographies, many of which attempt to identify the traits and attributes that made her the leader she became.

behaviors than ineffective leaders. Research using behavioral leadership theories has shown that effective leaders demonstrate high concern for employee needs, feelings, and morale (i.e., consideration) and address task accomplishment and organizational productivity (i.e., initiating structure). A contemporary behavioral leadership theory popular in nursing is emotional intelligence (EI).[10] EI is composed of five components: self-awareness, self-regulation, motivation, empathy, and social skill. The theory hypothesizes that to improve their effectiveness, leaders must develop their capabilities in all five components. EI has been used by nurse researchers to study the impact of nursing leadership styles on patient outcomes[11] and by nurse managers to encourage nursing staff to provide holistic patient care.[12] EI highlights the importance of knowing one's self, reflection, openness to feedback, and continuous learning in the leadership role.

Situational and Contingency Theory

The third wave of leadership theory, situational and contingency theory, aims to explain why some leadership approaches are effective in one situation and not in another. This wave takes into consideration the subtle and complex ways in which a leader's traits and behaviors, followers' needs and values, and situational parameters interact. It challenges the assumption that there is "one best way" to lead. For example, a leader is more likely to guide and monitor inexperienced nurses as they perform new responsibilities than he would when the nurses are experienced and performing routine responsibilities. Education and training to enhance leader effectiveness gained importance during this wave.

Charismatic and Transformational Leadership

The fourth wave of leadership theory is referred to as charismatic and transformational leadership. The underlying assumption is that leaders inspire, intellectually stimulate, and recognize the contributions of their followers. Charismatic leaders influence followers through their personality and charm; they develop an emotional relationship that motivates followers. Transformational leaders possess similar characteristics and, in addition, convey high expectations to their followers, challenging their perceptions about what can be attained and building their commitment to an organizational vision. Transformational nurse leaders encourage followers to grow professionally, which positively affects their job satisfaction and work performance.[13] Many, including the Magnet Recognition Program, have advocated for the use of transformational leadership in nursing.[14–16] Studies of charismatic and transformational nursing leadership have shown that they are associated with high nurse satisfaction, low nurse turnover, empowerment, and high productivity and effectiveness.[17]

Complexity Leadership

The complexity leadership approach is derived from complexity science, a way of thinking that reflects the dynamism and knowledge-based nature of the world in the 21st century. Using complexity science as a framework produces markedly different approaches to leadership than the theories presented previously. Complexity science assumes interconnectedness among the parts of a system and between the system and its external environment. Interaction among the interconnected parts can affect the entire system, often in substantial ways. Another assumption of complexity science is nonlinearity. Throughout the decades, organizational theory has been based on the assumption of predictability—that organizations are designed to work "like a well-oiled machine." Complexity science, however, recognizes that organizational processes are often nonlinear and unpredictable. Through the dynamic interplay of negative and positive feedback, an organization can make changes to keep abreast of the environmental context. Self-organization is another assumption of complexity science. Employees at the frontlines will self-organize to enable the organization to adapt to change, innovate, and create new capabilities.[18]

Leaders who apply complexity science will not direct or control the process of solving organizational problems. Instead, they recognize the interrelationship of workers and ideas, ensure communication and information flow to them, and foster innovative solutions to work challenges. The complexity leader brings workers together, helps them recognize their ability to find solutions to problems, and removes organizational barriers so the solution can emerge from the workers most affected by the problem.[18] Complexity science is beginning to appear in the nursing literature. In one report, the use of complexity science approaches helped newly licensed RNs manage patient care dilemmas that threatened the quality of patient care.[19] An investigation of care for nursing home residents showed that interaction strategies aligned with complexity science increased the staff's ability to deliver better care.[20]

CONTEXT TO NURSING AND HEALTH CARE

An expected role and competency of all nurses is leadership; it is a characteristic of nurses in all settings. The application of leadership begins in nursing school (with role formation) and continues throughout one's career. Three categories of nursing leadership are formal leadership, clinical leadership, and interprofessional leadership.

Formal Nursing Leadership

The increasing complexity and rapid change in healthcare demand effective leadership. The aims of nursing leadership are to ensure quality patient care and to create supportive practice environments for nurses. Nurses who hold executive-level leadership positions, such as chief nursing officer or vice president for patient care services, partner with other executives to establish the organizational vision, align the goals and operations of the nursing department with the organizational vision, and help formulate policies to advance the vision. Nurses in lower-level leadership positions, such as directors and nurse managers, report to the nurse executive. Their focus is to ensure that day-to-day patient care operations meet established standards, to empower staff to participate in improving patient care, and to create work environments that foster professional practice and nurse satisfaction.

The size and structure of the nursing leadership team depend on the size of the healthcare agency. For example, a small rural hospital may have only one formal nursing leader—a director who supervises all nursing staff. Home health and public health agencies that have offices in several communities may have designated nurse leaders for each site who report to an executive nurse leader at a central location. Urban quaternary medical centers and integrated healthcare systems may have four or five levels of nursing leadership, creating a hierarchy with considerable distance between the nurse executive and nurses who provide direct patient care.

Preparation for Formal Leadership

Jennings and colleagues reviewed 5 years of writing about leadership and management to identify the top categories of competencies recommended for nursing leaders.[21] These are presented in Box 39.2. Education and training are needed to cultivate these competencies. Academic education is the foundation for nurses who aspire to leadership positions. The position of the Council on Graduate Education for Administration in Nursing is that nurse managers should be minimally prepared at the bachelor's degree level but preferably at the master's in nursing level. Nurses seeking executive-level positions should hold a doctorate degree.[22]

Although some individuals have natural leadership tendencies, the most effective leaders are those who have participated in leadership training. Leadership development is essential for all levels of leadership. It is not a single event but, rather, an ongoing and interactive

---

BOX 39.2   Recommended Competencies for Nursing Leaders

- Personal qualities
- Interpersonal skills
- Thinking skills
- Setting the vision
- Communicating
- Initiating change
- Developing people
- Healthcare knowledge (clinical, technical, as a business)
- Management skills (e.g., planning, organizing)
- Business skills (e.g., finance, marketing)

Adapted from Jennings, B. M., Scalzi, C. C., Rodgers, J. D. III, et al. (2007). Differentiating nursing leadership and management competencies. *Nursing Outlook, 55*(4), 169–175.

process that enables the leader to learn, apply, and receive feedback that guides further learning. Studies have shown that nurses' participation in leadership development programs can bring significant and sustained improvements in leadership skills and competencies.[15,16,23]

Many leadership development options are available, including self-study, seminars, workshops, experiential learning, and mentorship from experienced leaders. Programs generally incorporate several components and extend over a period of time. Hospitals, community health agencies, and professional nursing associations offer leadership development workshops for new and aspiring leaders. Local programs such as that described by Schwarzkopf and colleagues have been designed to address the developmental needs of formal leaders at the unit level.[24] The program's aims were to enhance charge nurses' interpersonal and team management skills, give them tools to improve nurse–physician collaboration, and reduce charge nurse turnover. A 6-month statewide program in Kansas used a combination of in-person and online modules to prepare nurses in acute care, long-term care, public health, and school health for beginning leadership roles. Differences in competency ratings before and three months after program completion showed significant improvements in all three program-focus areas, managing the business of health care, leading people, and creating the leader within.[25] Several well-established national programs sponsored by universities, professional organizations, and health foundations enable executive nurses to broaden and deepen their leadership knowledge and competencies.[3]

The Impact of Formal Leadership on Outcomes

Several researchers have conducted studies to determine if there is a relationship between formal nursing leadership and RN outcomes. Investigations have shown that nursing leadership based on consideration for followers and leader visibility in the clinical setting is positively related to feelings of empowerment and autonomy, work commitment, staff nurse job satisfaction, and nurse retention.[17,26] Authentic leadership by nurse managers has also been shown to have a positive effect on RN job satisfaction and performance.[27] Nursing leadership based on emotional intelligence is positively associated with work environment characteristics that support professional nursing practice, such as more opportunities for staff development, good teamwork between nurses and physicians, positive work culture, and greater use of research in practice.[17,28]

The relationship between nurse leadership and patient outcomes has also been examined. An investigation of the impact of nurse leader tenure showed that when a nursing home's director of nursing had less than 1 year of experience at the facility, there were four times as many deficiencies in care compared to nursing homes whose director had 15 or more years of experience at the facility.[29] A systematic review of 20 studies showed that positive nurse leader practices were associated with fewer adverse patient events, particularly medication errors, decreased patient mortality, and higher patient satisfaction. The authors suggested that effective nurse leaders create practice environments that have sufficient nurse staffing, resources, and care delivery processes.[30]

Clinical Leadership

Clinical leadership has been defined as "the process by which staff nurses exert significant influence over other individuals in the healthcare team, and although no formal authority has been vested in them facilitate individual and collective efforts to accomplish shared clinical objectives."[31,p92] It is important to note that clinical leaders do not hold formal management positions; instead, they attain and maintain their status as leaders through clinical excellence, effective communication, and collaboration and coordination of care with other team members.[31]

The value of clinical leadership has risen in today's healthcare system because of the importance placed on the quality and safety of patient care and the need to ensure healthy work environments for professionals.

Clinical leaders are knowledgeable of the guidelines and clinical evidence that contribute to providing safe, high-quality care in their practice specialty. They use data about the outcomes of care and collaborate with others to continuously improve care processes. Their understanding of their own practice setting, cost drivers for nursing services, and factors that foster healthy work environments also contribute to their ability to be effective clinical leaders.[32]

Developing Clinical Leadership Skills

Every RN has the potential to be a clinical leader. A study of 32 nursing students and 21 RNs at different career stages was conducted to identify how students and nurses learn and practice clinical leadership.[33] A five-stage model emerged. The first stage is "I am aware of clinical leadership in nursing," described, primarily by students, as being able to discriminate between a positive and a negative nurse leader. Stage 2 is "integration of clinical leadership in my actions." In this stage, students and new nurses identified their personal strengths and weaknesses and identified a role model. Stage 3, described by senior students and new nurses, as "active leadership with patient/family, sometimes with colleagues." Patient/family successes inspired them to continue to develop, and they began identifying their own leadership style and competencies. Stage 4 is "active leadership with the team" and included mobilizing intra- and interprofessional teams, acting as a resource, and adapting leadership style to the context. Expert nurses described stage 5 as "embedded clinical leadership extended to organizational level and beyond." These clinical leaders take part in organizational decision making, propose changes that depart from the status quo, anticipate problems, manage conflicts, and act as mentors.[33]

Learning to be a clinical leader starts in the academic setting through coursework and guided experience.[34] After entering the practice setting, new nurses can participate in clinical leadership development opportunities offered by their employer, continuing education providers, and professional associations. Active and experiential learning are particularly important to enable aspiring clinical leaders to link theoretical knowledge with clinical practice. Mentorship from experienced clinical leaders, reflection on leadership actions, and feedback on leadership progress are important components of clinical leadership development programs.[35] Frequent and meaningful contact between leaders and the staff they lead also provides opportunities for aspiring leaders to observe and role model effective leadership behaviors and become more self-aware of their own style.[28] Clinical leaders are encouraged to develop their presentation and professional writing skills and to learn how to maintain a professional portfolio.[36]

Research on clinical nursing leadership is in its infancy, and to date it has focused on understanding the attributes and characteristics of clinical leaders, as reported previously in this concept presentation. A few studies have been conducted to assess the outcomes of clinical leadership development programs. For example, one comprehensive development program designed to prepare staff nurses for shared clinical leadership showed improvements in self-reported leadership behaviors such as accountability for clinical problem solving, confidence, negotiation skills, and interprofessional team skills. In turn, program participants reported that they were better able to meet patient needs, promote their recovery, and thereby positively influence patient satisfaction.[35]

Interprofessional Leadership

Today's healthcare system requires leadership that goes beyond a specific discipline or health profession. In many healthcare agencies and health sector businesses, nurses have interprofessional leadership responsibilities. For example, countless nurses in executive-level leadership positions in hospitals and home health agencies carry titles such as vice president for patient care services and, in addition to nursing, are responsible for other patient care departments, such as pharmacy, physical therapy, and chaplaincy. Nurses also move into formal leadership positions in areas such as clinical informatics and quality management. In these roles, nurses draw on their knowledge and experience as clinicians, their understanding of the healthcare system, and their leadership training to ensure safe and effective patient care.

Nurse leaders at all levels of the organization, formal and informal, are called on to become full partners in the interprofessional care environment.[3,37] Interprofessional collaboration reduces the use of redundant services and develops more creative solutions to complex patient care problems. In particular, patients with chronic conditions, patients who are critically ill, and the elderly population benefit from coordinated interprofessional care. Research has also shown that interprofessional collaboration can improve quality of care and patient outcomes.[38,39] Nurses are typically the healthcare providers who have the most frequent and sustained interaction with patients and their families. Thus, it is incumbent on nurse leaders to position the nursing staff to use their close relationships with patients and families as the vantage point for strengthening interprofessional collaboration and, in turn, the quality of healthcare services.

INTERRELATED CONCEPTS

Several concepts within this textbook are interrelated to the concept of leadership. These are presented in Fig. 39.3 and described here.

Health Care Organizations are the setting in which most nurse leaders work. Formal nurse leaders play an important role in the operations of healthcare organizations. Clinical nurse leaders usually emerge at the front lines of the organization where patient care is delivered.

Nursing is a practice discipline geared toward the delivery of health care, and the coordination of safe and effective patient care falls on the shoulders of leaders. As mentioned previously, there are multiple levels of leadership; thus, some leaders are further removed from direct patient care than others. Nonetheless, the efforts of nursing leaders ultimately link to the coordination of patient care. Care Coordination refers to the process of connecting healthcare services and resources to patients and is one of the distinctive contributions that clinical nurse leaders make in patient care.

Because Communication is an attribute of effective leaders (described previously), it is a key interrelated concept. Clear communication is central to effective leadership. Leaders who communicate unambiguous and consistent messages in a timely manner help followers understand the organization's direction, decision-making processes, and changes that may be underway. Listening is an essential aspect of communication. Only by listening to peers, followers, patients, and others will the leader understand all dimensions of a problem or opportunity. Effective leaders also provide mechanisms to foster clear communication throughout the organization.

Effective Collaboration within and among organizations, and within and across disciplines, is essential to efficient organizations. Skilled nurse leaders encourage and role model this behavior. Collaboration enhances communication and delivery of care.

Nurse leaders help ensure that the actions of the organization, unit, and individuals contribute to Health Care Quality. Formal and clinical nurse leaders are attuned to the standards and processes that an organization uses to provide high-quality care. They are involved in improvement initiatives and other change processes to meet the quality goals of their organization. Often, nurse leaders collaborate with others through professional organizations and regulatory bodies to establish the quality standards for nursing and health care.

Use of Evidence is important for effective leadership. Formal leaders use evidence about different leadership and management approaches to create organizational processes and work environments that contribute to satisfaction, productivity, and retention of nursing staff. Clinical leaders use research-based evidence and best practices to ensure healthcare quality and often guide other nurses in evidence-based practice.

Ethics is also important for effective leadership. Ethical integrity is a core element of all types of leadership. Formal leaders practice and role-model high ethical standards. Clinical and interprofessional leaders rely on their knowledge of ethical principles and decision-making models to protect and advocate for patients in all aspects of patient care.

Use of Technology and Informatics is important for all nurse leaders. They must have access to current data to inform decisions about patient care and the operations of the nursing organization. The widespread use of electronic medical records increases the availability of patient data to guide clinical leaders' care decisions and enable formal leaders to

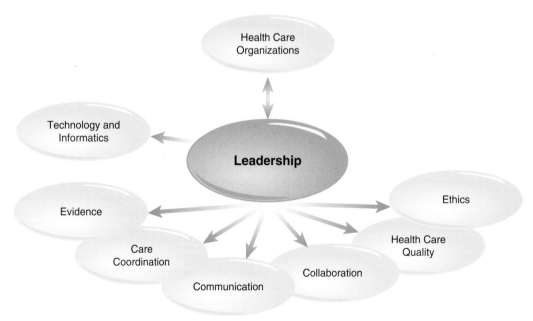

FIGURE 39.3 Leadership and Interrelated Concepts.

assess the effectiveness of the nursing care delivery system. Nurse leaders also use information technology to access and disseminate evidence and information that is critical for effective organizational operations.

CLINICAL EXEMPLARS

Every hospital, community health department, and long-term care facility is likely to have a variety of leadership positions. Box 39.3 presents common examples of formal, clinical, and interprofessional leaders.

Leaders are made, not born. Leadership in health care is not an act reserved only for designated administrators and managers. Clinical leaders are needed in every setting to ensure that quality patient care is delivered and that new evidence and research findings are adopted to improve patient care. It is incumbent on nurses who aspire to be leaders, and those who are leaders, to embrace opportunities to continue to develop their leadership skills. Research investigating the relationship between nursing leadership and nurse outcomes shows that people-oriented leadership approaches are positively associated with nurse satisfaction and retention and supportive work environments. An increasing number of studies also show that effective nurse leaders can positively influence patient satisfaction with care and other indicators of healthcare quality.

Featured Exemplars

Nurses experience situations in which different leadership styles are portrayed. The exemplars presented here are those most likely to be encountered.

> #### BOX 39.3 EXEMPLARS OF LEADERSHIP
>
> **Leadership Roles**
> *Formal Nurse Leader*
> - Chief nursing officer
> - Nursing director/assistant director
> - Nurse manager
> - Charge nurse/team leader
> - Dean
> - Associate dean
> - State board of nursing executive director
>
> *Clinical Nurse Leader*
> - Experienced staff nurse
> - Clinical nurse educator
> - Nurse navigator
>
> *Interprofessional Leader*
> - Director of clinical service line (e.g., primary care services)
> - Associate director of infection control department
> - Chairperson, quality improvement committee (e.g., ambulatory department)
> - Chairperson, reaccreditation steering committee
>
> **Leadership Styles**
> - Autocratic
> - Democratic
> - Laissez-faire
> - Transactional
> - Transformational
> - Authentic
> - Shared

ACCESS EXEMPLAR LINKS IN YOUR GIDDENS EBOOK

Autocratic Leaders

Autocratic leaders make all decisions and are generally most concerned with the tasks to be accomplished. They maintain distance from their followers, motivating them through the threat of punishment and offer of rewards as incentives. Traditionally, autocratic leadership was thought to be effective for leading new employees and large groups and for controlling work that needs to be coordinated among many departments. It is often used when a decision needs to be made quickly, such as in emergencies.

Democratic Leaders

Democratic leaders involve followers in the decision-making process by using a participatory leadership style. They show more concern about followers than do autocratic leaders. Democratic leadership is useful when the followers are experienced workers, particularly when they have professional education and socialization. It is effective when organizational success requires that followers are committed to the goal. Democratic leaders help followers develop technical and emotional maturity.

Laissez-Faire Leaders

Laissez-faire leaders do not interfere with employees and their work. They stand at a distance, giving followers freedom to make decisions and accomplish their work. They provide minimal information to followers and have little communication with them about their work. Typically, laissez-faire leaders wait until a crisis develops to make decisions. This leadership style works best when followers are highly experienced in their work, but it often results in employee apathy, inefficiency, and chaos.

Transactional Leaders

Transactional leaders focus on the daily operations of an organization and develop an exchange relationship with their followers. The transaction entails rewarding followers when they perform and correcting them when necessary. Transactional leaders focus on getting things done and satisfying their own and their followers' self-interests.

Transformational Leaders

Transformational leaders use approaches that change or transform individuals. They inspire and intellectually stimulate followers and recognize their contributions. Expectations are high and often challenge followers' assumptions about what can be attained. They communicate an organizational vision to their followers, moving them to accomplish more than expected. Their focus is long term and involves developing people and organizations.

Authentic Leaders

Authentic leaders are transparent and ethical in their dealings with followers. They are genuine, empathic, reliable, and believable. They are perceived by others to be open, optimistic, warm, and respectful. They focus on establishing relationships that embody trust and show commitment to the development of their followers.

Shared Leadership

A type of leadership associated with work teams is shared leadership, an approach in which employees are empowered to distribute leadership responsibilities broadly within a group. They lead one another to achieve a goal. Shared leadership is effective with professionals and with project-focused workgroups. It is highly interactive and enables employees to develop their skills and professionalism.

CASE STUDY

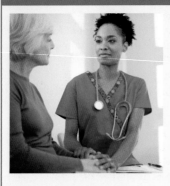

The case study is a clinical nurse leader who applied all three types of clinical leadership characteristics (clinical, follower/team, and personal qualities) to address a difficult patient/family situation.

Case Presentation

We had a very long-term patient in our medical/surgical intensive care unit (ICU) who was with us from early October until January 1 when he died. He had amyotrophic lateral sclerosis and a very aggressive, untreatable cancer, but he and his family were not willing to accept his diagnosis, thus kept him as a Full Code. His mind was intact until the last few days when he developed renal failure.

His wife was very difficult, constantly criticizing our care, constantly "checking him over," looking for a sheet crease or something to pin his deterioration on. She was so difficult, that most nurses gave up trying to even talk to her.

I spoke with my manager, who challenged me to understand her and to have her understand us and his prognosis. I remember telling my manager that I didn't need any more challenges, but I ended up taking it on! I spoke with all his doctors (even those who had "checked off" the case to understand their position[s]), used the Social Services and Case Management teams of nurses/social workers. I finally spoke with him alone to see what his end of life decision[s] were and then I spoke with her alone. He and she both wanted to maintain the Full Code status, so then we discussed his probable course. It took many conferences with her but she came to trust me and eventually called me "his favorite nurse." It taught me that patience is crucial and that was nothing I thought I had in my arsenal!

His room had a small window, but he hadn't been outside in many months other than his transfer from the ambulance from his rehab center to our hospital in October. The respiratory therapist and I decided to take him outside for some sun. We cleared it with the doctors, the charge nurse, and finally with the patient. He was terrified and I explained we'd bag him while he was outside and then he could see the life outside. He agreed. It was a major undertaking, but he smiled in the slightly overcast day. We bundled him in warm blankets and he was out there for about 15 minutes, with the wind blowing his hair and he beamed. His wife was thrilled and asked if we could do it again, so we repeated the adventure the following day with her. That day was sunny, so we stayed out longer. We had four to five trips outside over the next 2 weeks.

His deterioration was substantial after Christmas; his code status was changed to No Code and she asked for a priest to come to give him a final blessing. Eventually, she agreed, on January 1, to take him outside, off the ventilator, and allow him to go in peace in the sun where he had enjoyed some last pleasant days. It was a rainy day, but the sun came out for an hour and a half. He breathed for 45 minutes and had his family (real family and hospital family of RNs and "his" respiratory therapist, who had been with me on our first venture outside) around him when he finally passed away. It was one of the most beautiful experiences of my life and one I've learned a lot from!

Case Analysis Questions

1. What characteristics of clinical leadership did this RN show?
2. What interrelated concepts are illustrated through this example of clinical leadership?
3. What was the impact of this clinical leader's actions on the client and health-care team?

Reprinted with permission from National Council of State Boards of Nursing. (2009). *Report of findings from the post-entry competence study, research brief* (Vol. 38, p. 18). Chicago: Author.
From Fuse/Thinkstock.

🔷 **ACCESS EXEMPLAR LINKS IN YOUR GIDDENS EBOOK**

REFERENCES

1. American Association of Colleges of Nursing. (2008). *Essentials of baccalaureate education for professional nursing practice.* Retrieved from http://www.aacnnursing.org/Education-Resources/AACN-Essentials.
2. Holm, A. L., & Severinsson, E. (2010). The role of the mental health nursing leadership. *Journal of Nursing Management, 18,* 463.
3. Institute of Medicine. (2011). Transforming leadership. In *The future of nursing: Leading change, advancing health.* Washington, DC: National Academies Press.
4. Goethals, G. R., Sorenson, G. J., & Burn, J. M. (Eds.), (2004). *Encyclopedia of leadership.* Thousand Oaks, CA: Sage.
5. Kean, S., Haycock-Stuart, E., Baggaley, S., et al. (2011). Followers and the co-construction of leadership. *Journal of Nursing Management, 19,* 507.
6. Raven, B. H. (1993). The bases of power: Origins and recent developments. *Journal of Social Issues, 49,* 227.
7. Kouzes, J. M., & Posner, B. Z. (2007). *The leadership challenge* (4th ed.). San Francisco: Wiley.
8. Gill, G. (2004). Nightingales: *The extraordinary upbringing and curious life of Miss Florence Nightingale.* New York: Ballantine.
9. Waite, J., McKinney, N., Smith-Glasgow, M. E., et al. (2014). The embodiment of authentic leadership. *Journal of Professional Nursing, 30,* 282.
10. Akerjordet, K., & Severinsson, E. (2010). The state of the science of emotional intelligence related to nursing leadership: An integrative review. *Journal of Nursing Management, 18,* 363.
11. Cummings, G. G., Midodzi, W. K., Wong, C. A., et al. (2010). The contribution of hospital nursing leadership styles to 30-day patient mortality. *Nursing Research, 59,* 331.
12. Beydler, K. W. (2017). The role of emotional intelligence in perioperative nursing and leadership: Developing skills for improved care. *AORN Journal, 106,* 317.
13. Fischer, S. A. (2016). Transformational leadership in nursing: A concept analysis. *Journal of Advanced Nursing, 72,* 2644.
14. Clavelle, J. T., Drenkard, K., Tullai-McGuinness, S., et al. (2012). Transformational leadership practices of chief nursing officers in Magnet organizations. *The Journal of Nursing Administration, 42,* 195.
15. Martin, J. S., McCormack, B., Fitzsimons, D., et al. (2012). Evaluation of a clinical leadership programme for nurse leaders. *Journal of Nursing Management, 20,* 72.
16. Kelly, L. A., Wicker, T. L., & Gerkin, R. D. (2014). The relationship of training and education to leadership practices in frontline nurse leaders. *The Journal of Nursing Administration, 44,* 158.
17. Cummings, G. G., MacGregor, T., Davey, M., et al. (2010). Leadership styles and outcome patterns for the nursing workforce and work environment: A systematic review. *International Journal of Nursing Studies, 47,* 363.
18. Weberg, D. (2017). Innovation leadership behaviors: Starting the complexity journey. In S. Davidson, D. Weberg, T. Porter-O'Grady, & K. Malloch (Eds.), *Leadership for evidence-based innovation in nursing and health professions* (pp. 43–76). Burlington, MA: Jones & Bartlett Learning.
19. Kramer, M., Brewer, B. B., Halfer, D., et al. (2013). Changing our lens: Seeing the chaos of professional practice as complexity. *Journal of Nursing Management, 21,* 690.

20. Anderson, R. A., Toles, M. P., Corazzini, K., et al. (2014). Local interaction strategies and capacity for better care in nursing homes: A multiple case study. *BMC Health Services Research*, 14, 244.

21. Jennings, B. M., Scalzi, C. C., Rodgers, J. D., III, et al. (2007). Differentiating nursing leadership and management competencies. *Nursing Outlook*, 55, 169.

22. Council on Graduate Education for Administration in Nursing. (2012). Position statement on the educational preparation of nurse executives and nurse managers. *The Journal of Nursing Administration*, 42, 244.

23. Chappell, K. K., & Willis, L. (2013). The Cockcroft difference: An analysis of the impact of a nursing leadership development programme. *Journal of Nursing Management*, 21, 396.

24. Schwarzkopf, R., Sherman, R. O., & Kiger, A. J. (2012). Taking charge: Front-line nurse leadership development. *Journal of Continuing Education in Nursing*, 43, 154.

25. Shen, Q., Peltzer, J., Teel, C., & Pierce, J. (2018). Kansas nurse leader residency programme: Advancing leader knowledge and skill. *Journal of Nursing Management*, 26, 148.

26. Germain, P. B., & Cummings, G. G. (2010). The influence of nursing leadership on nurse performance: A systematic literature review. *Journal of Nursing Management*, 18, 425.

27. Wong, C. A., & Laschinger, H. K. S. (2012). Authentic leadership, performance, and job satisfaction: The mediating role of empowerment. *Journal of Advanced Nursing*, 69, 947.

28. Cummings, G. G., Olson, K., Hayduk, L., et al. (2008). The relationship between nursing leadership and nurses' job satisfaction in Canadian oncology work environments. *Journal of Nursing Management*, 16, 508.

29. Lerner, N. B., Trinkoff, A., Storr, C. L., et al. (2014). Nursing home leadership tenure and resident care outcomes. *Journal of Nursing Regulation*, 5, 48.

30. Wong, C. A., Cummings, G. G., & Ducharme, L. (2013). The relationship between nursing leadership and patient outcomes: A systematic review update. *Journal of Nursing Management*, 21, 709.

31. Chávez, E. C., & Yoder, L. H. (2015). Staff nurse clinical leadership: A concept analysis. *Nursing Forum*, 50, 90.

32. Grindel, C. G. (2016). Clinical leadership: A call to action. *Medsurg Nursing*, 25, 9.

33. Pepin, J., Dubois, S., Girard, R., et al. (2011). A cognitive learning model of clinical nursing leadership. *Nurse Education Today*, 31, 268.

34. Kling, V. G. (2010). Clinical leadership project. *The Journal of Nursing Education*, 49, 640.

35. George, V., Burke, L. J., Rodgers, B., et al. (2002). Developing staff nurse shared leadership behavior in professional nursing practice. *Nursing Administration Quarterly*, 26(3), 44.

36. Lannon, S. L. (2007). Leadership skills beyond the bedside: Professional development classes for the staff nurse. *Journal of Continuing Education in Nursing*, 38, 17.

37. Sorensen, R., Iedema, R., & Severinsson, E. (2008). Beyond profession: Nursing leadership in contemporary healthcare. *Journal of Nursing Management*, 16, 535.

38. Corcoran, J. R., Herbsman, J. M., Bushnik, T., et al. (2017). Early rehabilitation in the medical and surgical intensive care units for patients with and without mechanical ventilation: An interprofessional performance improvement project. *PM & R: the Journal of Injury, Function, and Rehabilitation*, 9, 113.

39. Wu, F. M., Rubenstein, L. V., & Yoon, J. (2018). Team functioning as a predictor of patient outcomes in early medical home implementation. *Health Care Management Review*, 43, 238.

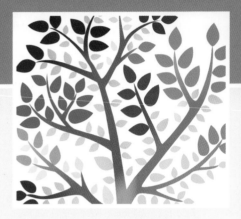

Ethics

Debra Bennett-Woods

Am I ever justified in withholding the truth from a patient? Should I respect the wishes of the family or the wishes of the patient? Is there a point at which the treatment I am providing causes more harm than good? What do I do when I suspect my best friend is caring for patients while under the influence of alcohol? When short-staffed, how do I divide my time among too many patients? Is there a limit to how many scarce resources I should provide to any one patient?

These are difficult questions, and not everyone will agree on the answers. On one level, these are practical problems and decisions that need to be made to do a job. However, on a deeper level, they are moral and ethical choices that speak to more than just our formal training and job description. They cannot be answered with simple logic or by referring to a policy or procedure manual. Rather, how you respond to such questions is a reflection of the core values, beliefs, and character that make you the person that you are and, ultimately, the professional that you become. The actions you take in response to ethically challenging situations often require great courage, compassion, or commitment. At the same time, failure to act or respond ethically can lead to serious and even dangerous errors, personal stress, and professional burnout.

Very few of us start our day wondering, "How can I harm someone today?" or "What unethical action should I take first?"[1] In fact, most of us would like to end the day feeling as though we made a positive difference in the world and satisfied that we did our best. We want the respect of our colleagues and patients. Most important, we want to feel at home in our own skin. We want a sense of personal and professional integrity—the feeling of wholeness we experience when our actions are consistent with our core beliefs and values. Technical proficiency in nursing is important but not enough, in and of itself, to guarantee this sense of integrity. To achieve the ideal of professional integrity, one also needs the skills and abilities of ethical practice, including moral sensitivity, ethical reflection, ethical analysis, and ethical decision making.

DEFINITION

Morality is a broad term without a single commonly recognized definition. Generally, the term *morality* is used to refer broadly to an accepted set of social standards or morals that guide behavior. *Ethics* and its various approaches deal more specifically with concepts of right and wrong. Although the terms ethics and morality, and the descriptors ethical and moral, are often used interchangeably, it is helpful to think of the various approaches to ethics as a foundation for morality and moral behavior. Thus, a simple working definition of ethics is *the study or examination of morality through a variety of different approaches.*[2] To understand morality, an understanding of underlying concepts, assumptions, and methods of the various approaches to ethics is needed.

Ethics is also a process involving critical thought and action. *Ethical sensitivity* helps us recognize when there is an ethical problem or dilemma, *ethical reflection and analysis* enable us to think critically to rank our ethical obligations and priorities, and *ethical decision making* is a method of ensuring that the action we take is well reasoned and can be justified. Finally, *moral courage* enables us to act on our decisions even under the most challenging circumstances.

Each individual has his or her own moral comfort zone, or personal morality, within which ethical reflection and analysis occur. This comfort zone is both influenced by societal concepts of morality and unique to the individual and his or her own ethical foundations. Most of us do not give much thought to our ethical comfort zone. We think of ourselves as being ethical without entirely understanding how we act ethically in practice or why we so often falter ethically when confronted with difficult choices. Knowing and understanding who you are as a moral being, how you think ethically, and why you make certain decisions are critical to ethical practice as a nurse.

The various approaches to ethics begin with *metaethics*, the branch of philosophy that considers fundamental questions about the nature, source, and meaning of concepts such as good and bad or right and wrong. Rather than making judgments about right and wrong, metaethics provides a foundation for how to think about right and wrong or good and bad, and it provides a common language to use when considering the ethical or moral dimensions of a situation.[1]

Normative ethics, on the other hand, deals with very specific judgments about right and wrong in everyday actions. Normative ethics uses the language of ethics, along with factual information, prior experience, commonly held values and beliefs, and acceptable standards of behavior, to make everyday judgments.[1]

Finally, when faced with a moral choice, *applied ethics* refers to the process of applying ethical theory and reasoning to daily life. Applied ethics is sometimes also referred to as *practical ethics*,[2] and it provides the justification for specific actions based on ethical reflection and reasoning.

SCOPE

The scope of ethics is broad, encompassing many different dimensions of our lives. For example, we all live and work within larger systems,

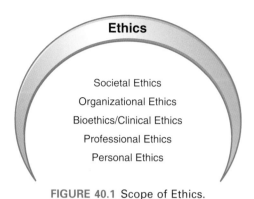

Ethics

Societal Ethics
Organizational Ethics
Bioethics/Clinical Ethics
Professional Ethics
Personal Ethics

FIGURE 40.1 Scope of Ethics.

each of which has its own moral and ethical dimensions. We are all members of a larger society, we work in organizational settings, and we function within the parameters of a particular profession. To fully understand the scope of ethics, one must consider how each of these dimensions interacts with us, as individuals, in shaping our ethical foundation and behavior (Fig. 40.1).

Societal Ethics

At the top, there are societal ethics that serve the larger community. Society provides a strong normative basis for ethical behavior through the legal and regulatory systems. Law is a minimum standard of behavior to which all members of society are held and that, generally, serves the interests of society as a whole. Laws prohibiting fraud and abuse or unauthorized release of medical information are examples of behaviors that society has deemed immoral and unethical. Legal standards such as the clinical standard of care, liability, negligence, and malpractice are based on legal and ethical obligations owed to patients. Other areas of our professional lives are guided by regulatory parameters such as the practice act that defines educational requirements and scope of practice as a nurse or the accreditation standards that determine how a healthcare facility must operate. Compliance with these minimum standards for practice is expected of all healthcare professionals and the organizations within which they practice.[3] Following the law is the most basic ethical standard required for the privilege of working as a licensed professional in health care. However, even as a minimum standard, law can create moral conflict for nurses, which is evident in issues such as abortion and provider-assisted dying, on which there remains broad disagreement within society.

Organizational Ethics

Organizational ethics involves a set of formal and informal principles and values that guide the behavior, decisions, and actions taken by members of an organization. These principles and values are expressed in the organizational systems, practices, policies, and procedures developed to ensure ethical operation. The billions of dollars spent annually as a result of healthcare fraud and abuse is an example of ethical failures at the level of the organization.[4] Ideally, organizational ethics directs all aspects of an organization and its culture, from its mission and values to how it treats customers and its employees, its financial practices, and how it responds to the needs of the larger community and the environment.[5]

Professional Ethics

Professional ethics refers to the ethical standards and expectations of a particular profession. Because professions have held a privileged role in society, their members are often held to a higher standard in terms of ethics. Therefore, ethics becomes a fundamental element of one's

professional identity and character as a nurse. As stated by Crigger and Godfrey, "The relationship between the patient and the nurse is, first and foremost, an ethical one."[6,p33] Ethical standards and expectations of practice are often expressed in a code of ethics or code of conduct that embodies the unique demands and philosophies of a particular profession. Unlike the minimum standard of the law, professional codes of ethics tend to offer general guidelines that are aimed at the highest ideals of practice. The Code of Ethics for Nurses of the American Nurses Association (ANA) establishes clear priorities in the ethical practice of nursing, such as compassion, respect, and primary commitment to the patient as well as advocacy for patient rights.[7] For example, the first provision in the ANA's Code of Ethics for Nurses states the following:

The nurse practices with compassion and respect for the inherent dignity, worth and unique attributes of every person.

Although this is an admirable ideal, how many of us can say that we live our lives or practice our professions in ways that *always* treat others with perfect compassion and respect, valuing every individual equally, and without any form of bias? Instead, it is the responsibility of the individual nurse to interpret this statement in terms of what it means in each unique situation and how well or poorly it is being demonstrated in his or her professional practice.

Bioethics and Clinical Ethics

Bioethics and its subcategory of clinical ethics are closely related to professional ethics. *Bioethics* deals broadly with ethical questions surrounding the biological sciences, emerging healthcare technologies, and health policy. *Clinical ethics* is involved primarily with decision-making at the bedside and other patient-specific issues. *Research ethics* is a specialized field within bioethics that examines the ethical conduct of research using human subjects and animals.

Personal Ethics

Finally, and perhaps most important, personal ethics describes an individual's own ethical foundations and practice. Our personal ethics continuously intersects with these other categories of ethics; however, they do not perfectly overlap, so there is much potential for conflict. In addition, the sources of our ethics change over time just as we continue to change with time.

ATTRIBUTES AND CRITERIA

The attributes of ethical nursing practice begin with the sources of ethics and involve skills and abilities needed to identify and distinguish ethical problems and dilemmas and then apply a disciplined approach to analysis and action.

Sources of Ethics

The beliefs, values, and methods that define ethical practice are influenced by a variety of sources. Natural intersections and places of agreement exist between the various sources; however, they can also conflict with each other, creating competing beliefs and inconsistency in the way we approach ethical issues (Fig. 40.2).

Family initially forms the most powerful influence on ethics, providing many of our earliest lessons about "right and wrong." A similar influence is the culture in which we are raised, including cultural practices related to our ethnicity, geographic area, socioeconomic status, and faith tradition. Peers become a source of ethical awareness and practice, especially as we move into adolescence, begin to look outside the family for direction, and are exposed to new experiences in the larger world. Education introduces new ways of thinking about difficult issues. Professional education, in particular, is charged with both your technical

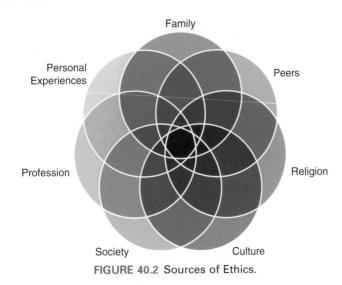

FIGURE 40.2 Sources of Ethics.

training and your awareness of the ethical practice of the profession. Once in the workplace, your colleagues and the organization where you work may further alter your views and your behaviors.

Ethical Problems and Dilemmas

An *ethical problem* is simply a problem with an ethical dimension. Most ethical problems have a reasonably clear solution, whereas others can be quite complex or involve competing ethical priorities. An *ethical dilemma* involves a problem for which in order to do something right you have to do something wrong. For example, to be loyal to one friend, you have to be disloyal to another. An example in patient care is determining whether aggressive treatment at the end of life will cause more harm than benefit. In other words, it is not possible to meet all of the ethical requirements in the situation. Instead, you must be sensitive to the ethical dimensions of the situation, able to use ethical concepts to analyze and reflect on the ethical conflicts within the dilemma, determine an ethically justifiable solution, and take action.

Ethical Analysis and Decision Making

When faced with an ethical problem or dilemma, it is helpful to apply a systematic approach of ethical analysis to the decision-making process. There are many different methods for ethical analysis.[8] A practical approach is to use some form of decision model, and there are a number of different decision models from which you might select.[9]

One popular model for clinical decision making is the four topics method of Jonsen et al.[10] The four topics are medical indications, patient preferences, quality of life, and contextual features. Within each topic, questions are posed that clarify factual aspects of the case with an emphasis on common ethical principles. Answering the various questions provides a framework within which different options for action can be considered.

Any approach to ethical analysis will depend heavily on one's ability to ask good questions. Asking the wrong question or failing to ask an important question will generally result in a wrong or incomplete answer. An *ethical question* is a question that challenges you to consider a particular ethical concept, principle, or perspective in your analysis. The following are examples of ethical questions:

- Do I have a duty to tell the truth?
- What is the greater harm?
- To whom is my primary loyalty?
- What are the best interests of my patient?

Framing good ethical questions is the key to strong ethical analysis, and the ability to use a variety of ethical concepts and theories naturally expands the range and quality of questions.

THEORETICAL LINKS

The study of ethics can be traced back to philosophers in the ancient world such as Aristotle in the West and Confucius in the East. In medicine, the Hippocratic Oath, although probably not written by Hippocrates himself, is dated to sometime near the fourth century BC.[11] The body of theory in ethics is vast, reflecting the diversity of human thought and action.

Think of each theory or principle as a camera lens. Different lenses have different magnifications and filters that allow us to view exactly the same scene but from a different angle or in a slightly different light. This body of ethical theory provides the "language of ethics" and allows us to explore situations from many different perspectives and points of view. The perspectives can be quite diverse; therefore, most of us feel more strongly about some principles and are drawn toward one or two theories at most. We may have a very difficult time even trying to think in the language of other theories. Ethical conflict occurs between parties when this language fails and each party simply cannot understand the other party's reasoning or point of view.

Ethical Principles

An ethical principle is a general guide, basic truth, or assumption that can be used with judgment to help determine a course of action.[12] Principles have long been used in bioethics and clinical ethics to describe the most common ethical concerns one must consider in most cases. Although all of the principles are important, they can conflict with each other in certain situations. The four principles most often cited are respect for persons, nonmaleficence, beneficence, and justice.[12] Less often mentioned, but equally important, is the principle of fidelity.

Respect for Persons

Respect for persons simply maintains that human beings have an unconditional moral worth that requires us to treat each individual person with great value, dignity, and respect.[13] The ethical principle of *autonomy* is an important extension of this principle and suggests that patients must be treated in a way that respects their self-determination by expressing their wishes and making informed choices about their treatment.[13] Another ethical principle closely related to autonomy is *veracity* or the principle of truth telling. A patient is not able to make an informed choice about treatment unless he or she has received the truth about his or her condition and the proposed treatment, and in a manner that is understandable to the patient.[13]

Nonmaleficence

Nonmaleficence directs us to act in ways that avoid harm to others, including even the risk of harm.[13] In health care, the primary focus is on harms such as pain, disability, or death; however, harm is difficult to define, and both patients and providers may be concerned about a wide range of perceived harms.[12] Another challenge in health care is that we are often required to inflict some harm and risk in order to benefit the patient and avoid a greater harm. However, these harms are not avoidable if we are to properly treat the patient, so we are required to carry out such treatments in ways that are unlikely to cause undue risk or needless harm.

Beneficence

Beneficence is an obligation to do good by acting in ways that promote the welfare and best interests of others.[12] Patients can reasonably expect that you, as a nurse, will promote their health and well-being. However, much like harm, the concept of good is difficult to define. A patient may define his or her best interests very differently than the nurse or other healthcare professional.[13]

Justice

The concept of *justice* is particularly complex, and there are no universally accepted definitions of what constitutes justice. However, at a minimum, the principle of justice is concerned with treating people equitably, fairly, and appropriately.[12] This means we owe our patients care and treatment that do not arbitrarily discriminate against them as an individual or as a member of a class of individuals. Returning to the ANA's *Code of Ethics for Nurses,* justice is the underlying principle that prohibits a nurse from treating patients differently based on their social or economic status, their personal attributes, or the nature of their health problems.[7] Each patient is entitled to the same level of care and consideration. Also of concern is the concept of distributive justice and the allocation of scarce healthcare resources. For example, should patients receive healthcare resources based on an equal share, what they need, or what they deserve based on contribution or effort? Related concepts include compensatory justice, such as occurs in a malpractice settlement, and procedural justice, which requires a system of fair treatment such as the system for allocating organs to people on the waiting list.[13]

Fidelity

Fidelity is the principle that requires us to act in ways that are loyal. In the role of a nurse, such action includes keeping your promises, doing what is expected of you, performing your duties, and being trustworthy.[13] Fidelity sounds easy enough, but it is probably the most frequent source of conflict for healthcare professionals because they owe loyalty to so many parties. In any particular situation, nurses may find themselves at odds between what they believe is right and what is in their own self-interest, what the patient or family wants, what other members of the healthcare team expect, what organizational policy dictates, or what the profession or the law requires.

Ethical Theories

There are many ethical theories, and we can only highlight a few major approaches in very simplified terms. Each theoretical approach offers a very different view of the same situation—views that may or may not lead to similar conclusions about an ethical problem or dilemma. For example, most of us have a preference for the consistency of rule-based approaches or the flexibility of consequence-based approaches. Likewise, some of us will be more comfortable with the highly contextual and emotionally engaged approach of relational ethics, whereas others are more comfortable with a highly rational and detached approach to ethical analysis.

Ethics of Duty

An ethics of duty is based on the ethical approach of deontology, in which moral duties are seen as self-evident, needing no further justification. Moral action is then based on acting according to a specific duty simply because it is the right thing to do.[13] Although the consequences of our actions are important, they are a secondary consideration to duty and our intention to do the right thing. The ethical question posed is, "What is my duty?" For example, if a nurse becomes aware that a friend and colleague has been diverting narcotics because she has developed an addiction, and the nurse reports her friend to her supervisor because that is what the organizational policy requires, she is complying with her ethical duty to report.

Ethics of Consequences

An ethic of consequences is based on a teleological view that moral actions are defined entirely on the basis of the outcomes or consequences of an action. Reaching a particular goal is what defines the ethical justification of an act regardless of your sense of duty or moral intent.[13] Consequence-based theories often weigh the advantages and disadvantages, or the harms and benefits, of different actions in the same situation. Utilitarianism, a common teleological theory, assumes that a moral action is one that results in the greatest good for the greatest number. The basic ethical question posed is, "What action will promote the greatest good with the least harm?" For example, if the nurse mentioned previously reports her friend because she is concerned that some patients are being harmed when their pain medications are diverted and all patients are at risk if her friend is practicing under the influence, then her actions are primarily based on a consideration of consequences. Her goal is to protect as many patients as possible rather than following a particular rule as a matter of duty. In fact, she might act outside of the policy if she believed reporting would not result in appropriate action by her supervisor.

Ethics of Character

Theories that emphasize character are classified under the general category of virtue ethics. Unlike the ethics of duty or consequences, which use external principles and rules to guide actions, virtue ethics relies on the character of the individual as the primary source of moral action.[13] Character develops over time based on life experiences and our willingness to reflect on our actions and motives. Virtues are character traits that predispose a person with good intentions to act with practical wisdom. Moral virtues include respect, honesty, sympathy, charity, kindness, loyalty, and fairness, whereas practical virtues include intelligence, patience, prudence, and shrewdness.[14] In general, a moral act must both promote good and intend good based on the moral predispositions of our character. The basic ethical question might be, "What is the wise action to take?"

Arguments are emerging for virtue theory to be the core of nursing ethics. Crigger and Godfrey argue for an emphasis on the virtues of compassion, integrity, humility, and courage.[6] In particular, the virtue of courage lies at the heart of ethical practice. It is one thing to know what one's intention should be and another to have the courage to act on that intention. The concept of virtue has been central to the definitions of professional, professionalism, and professional identity.[6] Common criticisms of virtue ethics are that character varies between individuals, leading to ethical inconsistency, and our choices may change over time with additional experience and character development. However, a strength of a virtue-based approach to nursing ethics is that it assumes character must be continually developed and refined in practice throughout a nurse's career. Ethics is a dynamic element of practice that cannot be reduced to simple habits of following rules or weighing outcomes. In the case of our nurse with the impaired colleague, a character-based approach would lead her to act based on a combination of her own good intentions to protect her friend, the patients, and the organization while also seeking the best possible outcome for all. She would be guided primarily by some combination of her own moral and practical virtues, and on the basis of her professional sense of identity, rather than by the externally dictated rules and consequences.

Ethics of Relationship

Ethical theories that emphasize relationship are focused on the nature and obligations inherent in human relationships and community. Examples of theories that are consistent with the history of nursing ethics include feminist ethics and social justice, both of which address vulnerability and issues of power affecting patients and communities.[15] The ethic of care approaches difficult ethical situations in a context-specific manner that searches for solutions in the particular details of the situation. Universal principles are used only to the extent they can be applied based on the unique circumstances of each situation. Primary attention is paid to preserving relationships, improving communication, enhancing cooperation, and minimizing harm to everyone involved while promoting an ideal of caring.[13] The basic ethical question in the ethic of care might be, "What is the caring response?"

Such an approach is very different from the highly abstract, rational, unemotional, and rule-oriented approach of most Western ethical traditions. Although duty-based, consequence-based, and, to a lesser extent, character-based approaches have dominated the fields of bioethics, clinical ethics, and medical ethics (physicians), nursing has long embraced an ethic of care and other relational approaches. Returning once more to our nurse with the impaired colleague, the ethic of care will direct her first toward gaining a full and empathetic understanding of the context of the situation, including the various relationships that must be protected and preserved if possible. She will seek open communication and a collaborative approach that emphasizes caring and minimizes harm to all parties. For example, she might first approach her friend and offer to accompany her to speak with the appropriate party in the organization to arrange for treatment and address the legal implications of her actions.

CONTEXT TO NURSING AND HEALTH CARE

Applied ethics addresses the process of ethical analysis and decision making in actual cases or with respect to specific topics. Although the range and complexity of ethical theory can be daunting, applied ethics is fairly straightforward insofar as you have a specific decision that needs to be made and you are free to incorporate any ethical concepts you consider relevant to making that decision.

Ethical Decision Making in Practice

There will be times when you must assess a situation and make a difficult ethical decision on your own. However, healthcare decisions are generally not made in a vacuum, and the nurse is often participating in ethical decision making as a member of an interprofessional patient care team or an administrative team. Although there is likely to be some conflict when people with different perspectives are involved, such conflict can be used to enhance the depth and breadth of the analysis by forcing everyone to consider the situation from various viewpoints. Therefore, group or team decision making can often result in a more refined solution.

When conflict within the team or between the team and the patient or patient's family cannot be resolved, an organizational ethics committee can be consulted to assist with mediating the conflict. Most acute care hospitals and some extended care facilities have an ethics committee onsite or they have access to one. An ethics committee does not make clinical decisions; however, the assigned consult team or the full committee can guide the discussion and act as mediator when there is conflict among the parties.

For organizational issues such as adherence to regulations, safety standards, quality of care, conflict of interest, or billing fraud and abuse, most organizations have a compliance committee or compliance officer, and they may even offer a compliance hotline for reporting of suspected violations. When the dilemma involves other professional issues, state and local chapters of professional associations may have similar ethics committees or experts with whom one can consult.

Ethical Issues in Nursing

A large study by Fry and Riley examined (1) the ethical issues encountered by registered nurses (RNs) in their practice, (2) the frequency that ethical issues occur in practice, (3) the degree to which RNs are concerned by these issues, (4) the way RNs handle ethical issues, and (5) the types of ethics education topics and resources that RNs perceive as helpful in practicing ethically.[16]

According to study findings, the following are the most frequent ethical issues experienced by RNs:

- Protecting patients' rights and human dignity
- Respecting/not respecting informed consent to treatment
- Providing care with possible risk to the nurse's health
- Using/not using physical or chemical restraints
- Working with staffing patterns that limit patient access to nursing care

Issues that RNs find most disturbing include the following:

- Coping with staffing patterns that limit patient access to nursing care
- Prolonging the living/dying process with inappropriate measures
- Not considering the quality of a patient's life
- Implementing managed care policies that threaten quality of care
- Working with unethical/impaired colleagues

More than 30% of the respondents reported encountering ethical issues in their practice one to four times per week or daily. In handling their most recently experienced ethical issue, more than 83% reported that they discussed the issue with nursing peers, whereas more than 66% discussed the issue with nursing leadership. On the other hand, more than 5% of the nurses reported that they did not deal with the ethical issue at all.[16]

Moral Distress

There has been much research on moral distress, with evidence of moral distress within all healthcare disciplines.[17–20] *Moral distress* occurs when you are unable to act upon what you believe is the morally appropriate action to take or when you otherwise act in a manner contrary to your personal and professional values due to perceived institutional, procedural, or social constraints.[7] In other words, you know what to do, but believe you cannot do it due to internal or external barriers. Self-doubt, lack of assertiveness, and the perception of powerlessness are examples of internal barriers. External barriers include inadequate staffing, lack of organizational support, poor relationships with colleagues, and policies that conflict with the care needs of patients.[17]

Situations that have been shown to cause moral distress are very similar to the common ethical issues noted previously. Many of them occur in end-of-life situations and involve what is perceived to be overly aggressive treatment and inappropriate use of resources. Working with other physicians and nurses who one considers incompetent is another common situation that has been shown to result in moral distress.[21]

The impact of moral distress occurs in two parts.[17] When the situation first occurs, moral distress can result in frustration, anger, guilt, anxiety, withdrawal, self-blame, and other stress-related symptoms. The second part of moral distress is referred to as *reactive distress* or *moral residue*, and it is characterized by lingering feelings that can accumulate over time with each subsequent experience of moral distress. At least three patterns of response to moral residue have been described. In the first pattern, a heightened response, leads healthcare professionals to engage in activities of conscientious objection, such as voicing opposition to a plan of care or refusing to follow orders. In the second pattern, they experience a desensitization with a tendency to be passive or to simply withdraw from situations in which they feel ethically challenged. The third pattern is characterized by strong, ongoing physical and

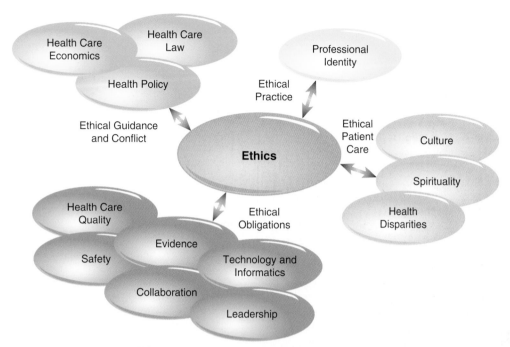

FIGURE 40.3 Ethics and Interrelated Concepts.

psychological stresses that often lead to burnout and leaving the profession.[17] In all cases, the healthcare professional's core values, integrity, and professional identity have been undermined.

Moral resilience is an emerging concept used to describe the ability of individuals to cope with ethical dilemmas and moral distress and restore integrity. Your ability to recognize ethical problems and apply ethical thinking and problem solving are two important strategies for avoiding moral distress.[22]

Because of the strong negative impact of unresolved moral distress on the job satisfaction and retention of nurses and other healthcare professionals, leaders in healthcare organizations are becoming aware of the need to create an organizational climate in which ethical issues can be openly discussed and resolved.[22–24] Interventions have included ethics debriefings, more support for ethics committees, and better access to ethics education and other resources.

INTERRELATED CONCEPTS

As evident in Fig. 40.3, ethics is closely intertwined with many other concepts related to nursing. Health Policy, Health Care Law, and Health Care Economics can all be the source of both ethical guidance and ethical conflict. For example, legal requirements may provide guidance in most situations but may create conflict in a specific situation that does not quite fit the context for which the legal requirement was intended. Professional Identity is contingent upon a conception of ethical practice.

The concepts Health Care Quality, Safety, Evidence, Collaboration, and Technology and Informatics are all grounded in ethical obligations such as preventing needless harm, acting in a patient's best interest, ensuring the best outcomes for the most patients, and serving as a good steward of scarce healthcare resources. The concept of Leadership has additional ethical obligations, such as balancing loyalties and the interests of patients, employees, the organization, and the community.

Patient care and the process of nursing are fraught with ethical problems and dilemmas. For example, the ethical practice of nursing requires that the nurse treat each patient with respect, recognizing and responding to each patient's unique experience of illness and injury; however, ethical challenges can arise at the intersections of patient care, Culture, and Spirituality, as well as in the face of Health Disparities.

CLINICAL EXEMPLARS

The scope of ethical issues in nursing can be generally examined across the broad categories of clinical, organizational, and health policy issues, with many issues falling into more than one category. Clinical issues can be further subdivided into those at the beginning of life, across the lifespan, and at the end of life. Box 40.1 provides an expanded list of examples of potential ethical issues faced in nursing practice. It is beyond the scope of this text to describe all of these exemplars; however, a few are featured here.

Featured Exemplars
Pain Management and Addiction
There is much focus on the "opioid crisis." For many complex reasons, the use and abuse of opioid pain medication has reached epidemic proportions, resulting in rapidly rising levels of addiction and overdose. A healthcare provider's basic obligation to relieve pain may well conflict with the best interests of a patient when pain management crosses the line into abuse or addiction. Health policy initiatives, regulatory interventions, and shifting or competing standards of care combine to render pain management unusually challenging for both individual providers and healthcare organizations.

Confidentiality
Confidentiality is an issue that can arise across the lifespan in many situations. A particularly complex dilemma involves mandatory reporting of potential domestic or elder abuse. The legal duty to report may be very much at odds with the patient's wishes and may result in unwanted intervention and disruption in the patient's life.

BOX 40.1 EXEMPLARS OF ETHICS

Clinical Ethics and Bioethics
Beginning of Life
- Abortion
- Assisted reproduction
- Child abuse
- Complications of pregnancy
- Emergency contraception
- Genetic enhancement
- Minor consent to or refusal of treatment
- Prenatal genetic selection
- Prenatal genetic testing
- Severely impaired newborns

Lifespan
- Confidentiality
- Cultural conflicts
- Decisional capacity
- Domestic and elder abuse
- Genetic testing
- Informed consent
- Pain management and addiction
- Patient noncompliance
- Patients as research subjects
- Protecting patient rights
- Provider bias

End of Life
- Advance directives
- Cardio pulmonary resuscitation orders
- Chronically critically ill
- Nonbeneficial treatment
- Organ allocation

- Organ procurement
- Proxy decision making
- Terminal sedation
- Withholding or withdrawal of life support

Organizational Ethics
- Allocation of scarce resources
- Conflict of interest
- Disclosure of medical errors
- Fraud and abuse
- Impaired providers
- Inadequate staffing levels
- Patient safety
- Provider conscience policies
- Uncompensated care
- Unrepresented patients
- Use of restraints

Health Policy Ethics
- Allocation of research funding
- Health care for the uninsured
- Health care for undocumented immigrants
- Health insurance reform
- High drug costs
- Medical marijuana
- Opioid abuse prevention, harm reduction, and treatment
- Privacy of health information
- Provider-assisted dying
- Reproductive rights
- Rural access to health care
- Drug shortages
- Tort reform (malpractice)

 ACCESS EXEMPLAR LINKS IN YOUR GIDDENS EBOOK

Advance Directives

Advance directives for health care pose many dilemmas at the end of life. A patient's autonomous wishes, or what we think the patient wanted based on the directive, may be strongly opposed by the family or the healthcare team. Even patients often change their minds when faced with the reality of their directive.

Uncompensated Care

Organizations face numerous ethical challenges. A common source of ethical conflict for healthcare organizations and their employees is ensuring high-quality and cost-effective operations while also maintaining safe levels of staffing, purchasing current technologies, and continuing to deliver necessary but unreimbursed care to uninsured or underinsured patients.

Conflict of Interest

Many ethical dilemmas at the bedside begin at the level of healthcare policy. For example, medical marijuana is now legal in nearly half of the United States; however, federal drug laws directly conflict with the ability of pharmacists and healthcare organizations to dispense it. In addition, there is a lack of strong evidence-based research for or against its use, particularly in children, posing ethical questions for both individual providers and organizations when treatment with the drug is requested by patients or parents.

CASE STUDY

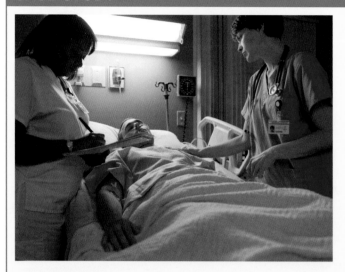

Case Presentation

Josh is a pleasant and intelligent 17-year-old male who was diagnosed with an aggressive bone cancer and underwent amputation of his left leg; however, his cancer has now metastasized to his chest, skull, and lungs. Josh and your son have been friends at school for years, and you knew him before his illness. Since then, you have been his nurse on occasion and he has talked to you about his disease. He has told you that talking about it upsets his parents and makes his friends uncomfortable, so it is nice to have someone with whom he can be honest. You have always been impressed with the maturity and insight he demonstrates.

Josh has been readmitted, his prognosis is grim, and he is experiencing a great deal of pain. Although you have not been assigned to care for him, you are aware that members of the clinical team have struggled with an ongoing request by Josh's parents that the healthcare personnel limit the information they share with him. Despite the many questions he asks, Josh has not been told the extent of the metastases or that he will likely die within a few weeks. Members of the care team have frequently omitted information and even lied to Josh at the insistence of his parents and with the reluctant agreement of his attending physician. Members of the care team have questioned the unit director several times; however, she continues to instruct them to respect the wishes of the parents to avoid any legal problems. Joshua's parents also insist that he continue to receive every possible intervention, and another clinical trial is being considered.

One evening, Josh notices you in the hall and calls you into his room. He confronts you and tells you he knows he is not being told everything. He says he believes he is dying and, although it frightens him, he is ready to die. He has not been able to attend school for several months, his friends no longer come to see him, he knows his younger brother and sister get very little attention because of him, and he is in nearly constant pain. He is tired of pretending to be "strong and brave." He has tried to talk to his parents, but they refuse to even listen to him. He says, "I trust you to tell me exactly what's happening and what I need to do to stop treatment, even if it is against my parents' wishes."

Case Analysis Questions

1. What is the primary ethical dilemma presented in this case?
2. Consider Fig. 40.1. Which of the elements of ethics presented in the Scope of Ethics apply to this case?
3. As a nurse, what ethical principles and concepts should be considered in your response and how should these be prioritized?

From Thomas Northcut/Digital Vision/Thinkstock.

 ACCESS EXEMPLAR LINKS IN YOUR GIDDENS EBOOK

REFERENCES

1. Bennett-Woods, D. (2008). Nanotechnology: *Ethics and society*. Boca Raton, FL: CRC Press.
2. Tubbs, J. B. (2009). *A handbook of bioethics terms*. Washington, DC: Georgetown University Press.
3. Darr, K. (2011). *Ethics in health services management* (4th ed.). Baltimore: Health Professions Press.
4. U.S. Department of Health and Human Services and U.S. Department of Justice. (April, 2018). *Health care fraud and abuse control program: Annual report for fiscal year 2017*. Retrieved from https://oig.hhs.gov/publications/docs/hcfac/FY2017-hcfac.pdf.
5. Morrison, E. E. (2016). *Ethics in health administration: A practical approach for decision makers*. Burlington, MA: Jones & Bartlett.
6. Crigger, N., & Godfrey, N. (2011). *The making of nurse professionals: A transformational approach*. Sudbury, MA: Jones & Bartlett.
7. American Nurses Association. (2015). *Code of ethics for nurses with interpretive statements*, Silver Spring, MD. Nursesbooks.org.
8. Sulmasy, D. P., & Sugarman, J. (2010). The many methods of medical ethics (or, thirteen ways of looking at a blackbird). In J. Sugarman & D. P. Sulmasy (Eds.), *Methods in medical ethics* (2nd ed.). Washington, DC: Georgetown University Press.
9. Johnson, C. (2015). *Meeting the ethical shadows of leadership* (5th ed.). Los Angeles: Sage.
10. Jonsen, A., Siegler, M., & Winslade, W. (2015). *A practical approach to ethical decisions in clinical medicine* (8th ed.). New York: McGraw-Hill.
11. Devettere, R. (2016). *Practical decision making in health care ethics* (4th ed.). Washington, DC: Georgetown University Press.
12. Beauchamp, T. L., & Childress, J. F. (2013). *Principles of biomedical ethics* (7th ed.). New York: Oxford University Press.
13. Bennett-Woods, D. (2005). *Ethics at a glance*, Denver, CO, Regis University, Center for Ethics and Leadership in the Health Professions. Retrieved from http://rhchp.regis.edu/HCE/EthicsAtAGlance/index.html.
14. Munson, R. (2016). Intervention and reflection: *Basic issues in medical ethics* (10th ed.). Belmont, CA: Wadsworth.
15. Grace, P. J. (2018). *Nursing ethics and professional responsibility* (3rd ed.). Burlington, MA: Jones & Bartlett.
16. Fry, S. T., & Riley, J. M. (2002). *Ethical issues in clinical practice: A multi-state study of practicing registered nurses*, Boston, Nursing Ethics Network. Retrieved from http://jmrileyrn.tripod.com/nen/research.html#anchor195458.
17. Epstein, E. G., & Hamric, A. B. (2009). Moral distress, moral residue and the crescendo effect. *The Journal of Clinical Ethics, 20*(4), 330–342.
18. Lamiani, G., Borghi, L., & Argentero, P. (2017). When health professionals cannot do the right thing: A systematic review of moral distress and its correlates. *Journal of Health Psychology, 22*(1), 51–67.
19. Oh, Y., & Gastmas, C. (2015). Moral distress experiences by nurses: A quantitative literature review. *Nursing Ethics, 22*(1), 15–31.
20. Whitehead, P. B., Herbertson, R. K., Hamric, A. B., et al. (2015). Moral distress among healthcare professionals: Report of an institution-wide survey. *Journal of Nursing Scholarship: An Official Publication of Sigma Theta Tau International Honor Society of Nursing / Sigma Theta Tau, 47*(2), 117–125.
21. Zuzelo, P. R. (2007). Exploring the moral distress of registered nurses. *Nursing Ethics, 14*(3), 344–359.
22. Lachman, V. D. (2016). Moral resilience: Managing and preventing moral distress and moral residue. *MEDSURG Nursing, 25*(2), 121–124.
23. Rushton, C. H., Schoonover-Shoffner, K., & Kennedy, M. S. (2017). A collaborative state of the science initiative: Transforming moral distress into moral resilience in nursing. *The American Journal of Nursing, 117*(2), S2–S6.
24. Stutzer, K., & Bylone, M. (2018). Building moral resilience. *Critical Care Nurse, 38*(1), 77–79.

CONCEPT

41

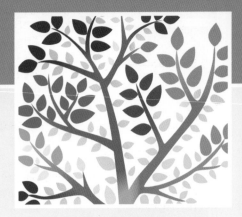

Patient Education

Barbara M. Carranti

Education empowers. Patient education is no exception. Effective patient education allows patients and their families the opportunity to control their own health, reduce risk for illness, improve longevity, and enhance overall wellness. Specifically, the goals of patient education are to learn and adapt by forming connections and associations that will facilitate changes in behavior, resulting in enhanced health and well-being or improved treatment of illness.[1] Thus, patient and family engagement and understanding knowledge of the problem is critical. In addition, understanding of past behaviors toward the problem and impact of the problem on function is also an essential element of nursing assessment for the education plan.[2] The importance of patient education is supported by *Healthy People 2030*. This science-based program, in existence for more than 40 years, has used evidence to establish objectives to improve the health of Americans. Patient education is the key to achievement of the overarching goals of *Healthy People*.[3]

DEFINITION

For the purposes of this concept presentation, the definition of patient education is "Anything that provides patients and families with information that enables them to make informed choices about their care, health, and wellbeing, and that helps them gain knowledge and skills to participate in care or healthy living processes."[4,p8] This is an intentional process whereby the patient is learning health-related information to support healthy lifestyle or behavior change. A similar term, *patient teaching*, is used interchangeably. The role of the nurse in patient education is to assist the patient in forming goals; assess patient need, motivation, and ability; plan educational interventions to achieve goals; and evaluate patient outcomes toward goal attainment. In short, nurses empower patients. This empowerment is accomplished by providing information to enhance wellness, reducing the risk for illness, and encouraging autonomy by enhancing self-care skills while maintaining a patient-centered approach.

SCOPE

As a concept, patient education can include provision of information in a wide range of formats and can be described from two perspectives: the delivery approach and educational domains. The process varies depending on multiple variables, including the intended outcome and the characteristics of the learner. For example, is the educational intervention intended to teach the patient a skill or impart knowledge related to a known health problem, increase the probability of successful treatment, prepare for discharge, or to promote a healthy lifestyle and enhance well-being? Thoughtful consideration of intended outcomes will enhance the patient's learning by matching an approach to intended goals. The nurse must ask, "What change in the patient is the desired outcome of this activity?" The type of education offered will require that the nurse match the approach, method, and evaluation to this desired outcome.[5]

Educational Approaches

Patient educational approaches can range from formal educational programming such as group lecture settings to informal, individualized one-on-one teaching and to self-directed learning by the patient that is facilitated by the nurse.[1] Formal patient education courses or classes are useful to address needs common to a group of patients or as individual teaching sessions. Formal courses are often taught using a curriculum/course plan with standardized content. In contrast, informal teaching often occurs in one-on-one sessions with the patient and/or family. Informal sessions may be planned or spontaneous, but they do not follow a specified formalized plan. An informal approach represents a large portion of patient education done by nurses. In fact, the majority of critical education occurs with each patient encounter when medications, diet, or treatment is explained or simply when answering questions about the patient's issues or concerns. Individual or self-directed education results when a patient or family obtains and/or completes an educational activity independent from the nurse or other healthcare providers. With the influence of consumerism and the availability of information, a great deal of education can occur through self-directed learning employing written material or media (e.g., Internet and video) designed to assist the patient with information about health topics, a particular disease, treatments, or a specific skill (Fig. 41.1).[1]

Because of the increasing dependence on technology in all aspects of life, the use of Internet resources for patient education cannot be ignored. A majority of adults in America use the Internet to find information on many aspects of life, including health, healthy lifestyles, and treatment options.[5] This use of technology expands the role of the nurse in patient education to include teaching on evaluation of Internet sources. Patients should be encouraged to search for information sources that list authors and their credentials and contact information. The source of information should also be listed, and any photographs, charts, graphs, or other graphics should contain helpful understandable information. Any links associated with the site should be functional, active links. It is also important that patients be taught to search for government (.gov),

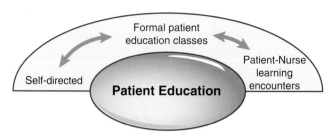

FIGURE 41.1 Scope of Patient Education Concept.

educational (.edu), and nonprofit (.org) sites because they are considered to be the most credible sources of information. Sites chosen for use in gathering information should be secure and should clearly identify how consumers can contact a site administrator.[6] Finally, appearance of a Health On the Net (HON) code can also help the provider and consumer to identify quality health information.[7]

For this discussion of approaches to patient education to be complete, the educated and motivated consumer should be considered. Many patients will be active consumers of health information and use self-directed approaches to education. Patients may present the nurse with articles, computer printouts, and other materials gathered in an attempt to learn about health promotion, symptoms, diagnoses, and treatments. These materials can be incorporated into the nurse's assessment of the patient and the educational plan. The tendency to pursue learning opportunities addresses motivation and presents the nurse with an opportunity to ask the patient to discuss what has been learned. This also gives the nurse the opportunity to teach the patient evaluative skills, looking at sources and content of the material for credibility and reliability.[6]

Learning Domains

Patient education can also be conceptualized from the perspective of learning domains—in other words, in terms of the type of learning a patient will need. The three main domains are cognitive, psychomotor, and affective (Fig. 41.2). Education intended to increase a patient's knowledge of a subject, for example, is cognitive in nature, and using methods such as written material, lecture, and discussion is appropriate. Skill teaching or psychomotor teaching requires that the patient have opportunities to touch and manipulate equipment and practice skills. A patient who must learn to change a dressing over a wound is an example. Education that is intended to change attitudes, such as viewing the lifestyle modifications associated with the treatment of coronary artery disease as a positive change rather than a burden, is known as the affective domain in education.[5]

To illustrate this, consider an example of a patient with a new diagnosis of a degenerative neurologic disorder that will require the patient to self-catheterize. The nurse will need to teach the patient the complex *psychomotor* skill of self-catheterization, and the teaching will be successful when the patient is able to competently demonstrate this skill.

Part of this teaching will include physiological information designed to enhance the patient's understanding of the necessity of this procedure (*cognitive* learning) as well as assistance with lifestyle alterations and coping to help the patient to adapt and continue to live fully (*affective domain*).[5]

ATTRIBUTES AND CRITERIA

For patient education to occur, there must be an identified need for learning. Although this need may be identified by the nurse, learning will not occur without readiness on the part of the learner. Ultimately, it is patient motivation that determines when, how, and if patient education will occur.[8] In addition to an identified need, the following are other major attributes of patient education:

1. Planning is involved.
2. The outcomes are goal oriented.
3. The patient is motivated to learn.

Like any other teaching-learning process, patient education requires that the teacher (nurse) know the intended audience and plan appropriately. This is a process that must be in place even in the most routine patient encounters. There must also be a goal, which is usually a change in behavior or attitude of some sort. The learners (patient and/or significant other) not only should be identified as the target of the teaching plan but also should be motivated by the outcome of the behavioral or attitudinal change. The nurse then develops the plan and evaluation to be consistent with the patient needs.

The nurse must determine the overall appropriateness of patient education. This requires asking, "Is the timing right, are the involved parties ready, and are the goals clear?" Only after these answers are determined can true education of the patient occur.

THEORETICAL LINKS

The goal of all patient education is to produce change. It is helpful to examine theories of behavior and learning in addition to nursing theory to understand patient need and motivation to change.

Theories of Health Behavior

The health belief model is used to help explain individual decisions to use health behaviors and screening opportunities. It has been adapted many times to explain compliance and behavior as they relate to health.[9] According to the health belief model, individual perceptions of susceptibility to and severity of disease are the primary motivators for making attempts to change health behavior. These motivators are modified by demographic, social, psychological, and structural variables that may heighten or dampen motivation. The primary motivation of patient perception then allows the patient to be open to cues to act, which of course leads to patient education opportunities.[10] For example, a patient who is aware that her risk for breast cancer is high because of genetics may be likely to participate in some form of education about risk for the disease. This education can enhance the patient's knowledge level to produce lifestyle changes that reduce risk. Put another way, the health belief model states that for an individual to change behavior related to health and wellness, there first must be a belief that illness can be avoided and that taking a particular action can reduce risk. Furthermore, the individual must believe that he or she is capable of making the needed change.

Nola Pender's health promotion model (HPM), developed in 1987 and revised in the late 1990s, is a model which "describes major components and variables that influence health promoting behaviors."[10,p237] The HPM is based on the health belief model that was expanded by Pender to include factors that can influence the patient's motivation to

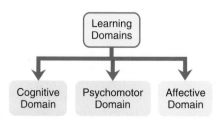

FIGURE 41.2 Learning Domains.

Learning Domains

Cognitive Domain | Psychomotor Domain | Affective Domain

change behavior, such as previous experience with behavior changes to address the problem, and the patient's perception of success in these attempts. This model also expands the view of patient motivation by including social supports and competing priorities as factors to consider.

Pender's model is focused on achieving optimum wellness rather than avoiding disease, which the original model stressed as the primary motivator for changing behaviors. Pender points out, for example, that consideration of the patient's prior experience with attempting to change health behaviors is a key factor for the nurse when planning strategy, including educational strategy. An obese patient with comorbidities of coronary artery disease and type 2 diabetes will likely be told to lose weight to avoid serious complications. The HPM dictates that part of the nursing assessment would be to ask the patient about prior attempts at weight reduction and perceived success of these efforts. The patient response to these inquiries will assist the nurse in development of educational interventions to address patient need. Pender also emphasizes that how the patient views the benefits and barriers to behavior change as well as the patient's own perception of ability to succeed will impact the nurse's plan for education.[11]

Nursing Theory

There are many theories that can be used as a basis for formulating patient education plans. Dorothea Orem's self-care deficit theory is based on optimizing the patient's ability to assume responsibility for his or her own care and that motivation is based on the anticipation of resuming this responsibility. Self-care is defined as "purposeful action performed in sequence with a pattern."[12,p110] Orem addresses the role of family and others in the patient's social support system as assuming the responsibility of the patient's care when the patient is unable, but also as a unit in need of nursing as the self-care needs of the family unit may be affected by the needs of one member. Utilization of Orem's theory can assist the nurse in determining the teaching needs of the patient/family and to use education as a method of patient/family support.[12]

CONTEXT TO NURSING AND HEALTH CARE

Education of patients is integral to professional nursing practice; this fact is illustrated in multiple documents, including the American Nurses Association's *Nursing: Scope and Standards of Practice*,[13] each state's Nurse Practice Act, the Institute of Medicine's *Future of Nursing* report,[14] and the *Quality and Safety Education in Nursing* competencies.[15] Nursing practice has been defined as "the protection, promotion, and optimization of health and abilities, prevention of illness and injury, alleviation of suffering through the diagnosis and treatment of human response, and advocacy in the care of patients, families, communities, and populations."[13,p1] These positive patient outcomes are often achieved through education.

Numerous agencies require that patients and families be provided with information required to make decisions about health care and treatment of illness.[16] Modifications in health care in terms of delivery style and financer expectations have also changed the role of the patient in participating in his or her own care. This new level of patient engagement in health care requires that patient education be a priority for the registered nurse in the provision of patient care.[4]

Consumerism has also made more individuals want to take control of their own health and wellness and is promoting more individuals to seek health education opportunities in many venues. Patient education, however, is a cornerstone of nursing practice and is one of the ways in which members of care teams collaborate to achieve quality patient care outcomes. Quality patient education requires appropriate assessment, planning, implementation, and evaluation of this often-complex process.

The educational process and the nursing process are essentially the same[16] and include learner assessment, planning, implementation, evaluation, and documentation. Each of these steps is discussed in detail.

Learner Assessment

Learner assessment begins with a comprehensive assessment of the patient's learning needs. This may include a formalized written assessment, may be incorporated as part of the health assessment interview, or certainly may be a stated need from the patient. The assessment should include patient resources (education level, literacy level, social support, and financial resources), educational resources, and nursing resources. Assessment data should be used to develop a teaching plan that is appropriate for the patient but also one that will meet the desired goal. To fully individualize the educational plan for a patient, the nurse will consider the age, stage of development, and motivation to change behavior.

Psychosocial Development

Educational interventions must attend to the patient's achievement of developmental tasks. Erikson's theory of development is based on an eight-stage process in which each stage requires the achievement of a particular task. Completion of each stage forms the foundation of the next stage.[17] An understanding of Erikson's theory of development assists the nurse in patient education by understanding approaches necessary to accomplish the goal. For example, the educational approach taken by the nurse in teaching a patient how to use a metered dose inhaler for delivery of steroids will be different for a school-age child than for a middle-aged adult. Using play-type activities to teach the procedure and identifying a celebrity or other role model who may need a similar treatment will appeal to the school-age patient. The middle-aged adult is more concerned with fitting this treatment into his or her normal life patterns. Finally, it is critical for the nurse to incorporate the patient's own culture to make the teaching process meaningful.

Pedagogy Versus Andragogy

An appropriate next step to follow when utilizing Erikson's theory of development is to ensure that the type of educational method used is appropriate to the individual stage of development. Pedagogy is the methodology used to assist children to learn, or the strategies of traditional teaching. Andragogy conversely describes adult learning.[18] This implies that the strategies used with great success for teaching children in classrooms may not translate to successful outcomes for the nurse teaching adults. The nurse should attend to the developmental level of the individual and tailor learning activities to account for these differences. In general, learning in the adult is focused on an immediate need to address a personal issue or to solve a problem. The nurse is viewed as one who can facilitate that goal rather than simply impart knowledge. All learning activity should be directed toward meeting the learning goals of the adult patient. It is also important to note that most adults enter any learning situation with a rich history of experiences that can be, and should be, drawn on by the nurse to enhance present learning.[1] Adults tend to learn best when there is a perceived need to learn the information (internal motivation) and the information perceived is pertinent to address an immediate problem or need, when learning is self-directed using learner-centered strategies with application, and when learning draws on the past experiences of the learner. The nurse further enhances learning in the role of a facilitator and by providing timely feedback.

Hierarchy of Needs

Maslow's hierarchy of needs theory is based on a simple premise that for higher level needs to be addressed, lower level needs must be met.

Maslow, a humanist, concluded that if environmental conditions are appropriate to meet basic needs, then individuals will be able to learn and self-actualize.[19] This is an important concept in all types of teaching and is clear in all levels of education. A school-age child has limited ability to concentrate if the child is hungry. A college student has limited ability to concentrate and learn after an all-night study session. Of course, this extends to patients as well. For example, inadequate oxygenation, safety deficits, and food, water, and elimination needs must be addressed before the patient can adequately learn. A patient who needs to learn a complex skill must have the needs of pain management and comfort met before he or she attempts to meet learning needs. The motivation for patient education may also be linked to survival, representing a much more basic level of need. For example, a patient learning to self-administer insulin for the first time may feel a great sense of accomplishment at mastering this complex task, but the ability to self-administer this drug is truly a matter of survival for the diabetic patient.

Generational Differences

Generational differences are also a consideration when approaching patient education. Much has been reported about differences in the learning styles between generations, relating not only to the age of the patient but also to the era in which the individual was raised, as well as the social and political experiences of a group.[20] Educational approaches may need to differ for those born before 1946; members of this age group usually are self-motivated and do not seek feedback for their performance. On the other hand, members of Generation Y are dependent on technology and desire immediate feedback.[20] This generational factor, perhaps more than any other, will dictate how the nurse approaches patient education.

Literacy Level

The ability to read and understand the written word is, of course, critical if the educational process is to include any written material. Based on the 2003 National Assessment of Adult Literacy, 43% of adults in the United States had literacy skills at the basic or below basic level.[21] It is also important to consider the patient's ability to understand and interpret health-related information and instructions—the individual's level of health literacy.[22] Although assessment of literacy levels can be very difficult in adult patients because of the stigma and shame often associated with limited reading ability, patients may give cues to limited literacy, such as avoiding reading materials provided (the patient may state "I forgot my glasses") or demonstrating repeated inability to follow written instructions. If there is a suspicion that the patient may not be able to read written material or that the information is written at a level that the patient cannot understand, the nurse must use alternate methods of instruction to ensure patient understanding. Although beyond the scope of this text, several methods exist for the nurse to quickly evaluate written material for readability for those with limited reading skills.

Barriers

There are a number of barriers to learning that must be considered as part of learner assessment. The lack of available social support systems, which may impair the patient's motivation to learn or ability to participate in classes or programs, is one common barrier. Lack of support may also limit the patient's ability to practice new skills. Additional patient-related barriers include cultural differences, lack of financial resources or time, and frequent interruptions. It may be within the patient's or the nurse's ability to control or remove these barriers to enhance patient learning and outcomes.

Barriers on the part of the nurse to participate in patient education include lack of time and multiple competing demands. The teaching role of the professional nurse is often not prioritized because of issues with staffing, payment, and perception of effectiveness of educational efforts. Furthermore, the nurse's professional motivation and confidence in education skills may pose a barrier to patient education. Again, assessing the nurse's attitudes can assist in identification of these professional barriers and development of interventions to overcome them.[1]

Planning

Planning is the determination of what methods will be used to meet the educational need. This includes deciding if the outcome is a cognitive (knowledge) change, a psychomotor (performance of a skill) change, or an affective (feeling or attitude) change. Determining the type of outcome dictates the approach as well as the goal. For example, a patient diagnosed with type 1 diabetes may need to learn about the overall pathophysiology of the disease so that he or she can appreciate the physical and lifestyle impact. However, the patient also needs to develop practical psychomotor skills (e.g., injection and testing) to cope with this disease. The nurse must plan not only to describe what diabetes is but also to demonstrate blood glucose testing and self-injection of insulin, allowing for practice and re-demonstration from the patient and perhaps significant others as well. The teaching methodology used should match the domain of learning.

Implementation of Educational Plan

Implementation or carrying out the plan is an area in which flexibility is key. The nurse will need to determine the length of educational sessions, content to be covered, and methodology for teaching. These plans may be influenced by numerous unpredictable factors, such as patient condition and competing priorities. The nurse must adjust the teaching session to accommodate the priorities of the patient.

Evaluation

Evaluation of learning outcomes should be consistent with the domain of learning as well. Psychomotor skills, for example, require that the patient be able to *do* something, such as perform a skill. Using a survey or other measurement tool to evaluate a skill will not adequately measure this outcome. Surveys and questionnaires can be used to measure affective behavior change as well as patient satisfaction with the teaching experience. Because the goal of patient education is behavior change, the evaluation of the process may need to be conducted over time and be dependent on multiple sources of data.

Returning to the example of teaching a patient diagnosed with type 1 diabetes, the nurse will likely include cognitive information about disease pathology to appropriately manage the condition. This patient will probably need to master the psychomotor skill of blood glucose monitoring and insulin injection. The nurse will also be concerned with the affective dimension of the diagnosis of chronic disease. Evaluation of all of these dimensions will require that the nurse observe the skills for level of mastery, discuss the "why" of diet and exercise with the patient on multiple occasions, evaluate the impact of the patient's daily decisions on disease management, and use repeated assessment of the patient's acceptance of the condition to fully evaluate behavior change.

No discussion of patient education would be complete without consideration of patient adherence. There are many factors that block patient adherence, such as lack of understanding, literacy, financial problems, lack of environmental or interpersonal support, previous experiences with treatment or self-management, and motivation.[3] These issues should be included in the assessment process and addressed in the educational plan for the patient in an attempt to enhance compliance.

Documentation

To ensure consistency in care, documentation of patient education is included in the patient record. This documentation should be comprehensive and include not only a description of the information that the patient was taught but also an assessment of the patient's motivation, ability to learn (any physical or cognitive issues that may inhibit the process), developmental level, and resources (personal and financial, if appropriate). A detailed plan should be included in the documentation so that other professionals can reinforce the process if education is to be continued across care settings. This should include goals and progress toward them. Finally, the patient response to the educational plan and adjustments to accommodate changes in patient condition or other factors should be included to ensure consistent, successful patient education outcomes.

INTERRELATED CONCEPTS

Patient education as a concept is central to the role of the nurse in the delivery of quality patient care (Fig. 41.3). The professional roles and attributes of Collaboration and Communication are essential in the development, planning, and delivery of patient education, whereas the nurse's role as an educator is central to his or her Professional Identity. The nurse works not only with the patient but also with teams of providers in determining care needs, and quality patient education is one of the results of this skilled collaborative effort. To accomplish this, the nurse's knowledge of Technology and Informatics along with the ability to teach patients and families the use of healthcare technology are critical when transitioning care from the acute care facility into the home. The result of current changes in health care requires the nurse to engage Leadership skills not only to assist patients and families but also to prepare the consumer for this evolution of health care.

The role of the nurse in Health Promotion, an area in which nurses generally take the lead, is also a critical professional dimension that is related to patient education. The nurse's knowledge and skill in recognizing opportunities to improve wellness, health, and function through lifestyle modification are used in all patient encounters and are a critical professional role in the education of patients.

Patient education incorporates the patient's attributes and resources. The nurse approaches each patient encounter as an opportunity to educate. This involves a determination of the patient's developmental level (Development) as well as an analysis of the dynamics of relationships (Family Dynamics) to assist in determination of supports and stressors. The patient's cultural background (Culture) and prior experiences with Adherence to prescribed regimens are also concepts that have a direct relationship to patient education and in fact form the foundation of the assessment and planning process.

CLINICAL EXEMPLARS

Examples of patient education exist in many formats for a broad range of topics, intended for use in a variety of ways. Box 41.1 represents some of the most common examples. Grouped by the primary focus as well as how the teaching/learning may be accomplished, Box 41.1 also highlights the numerous types, venues, and media types that can be considered in patient education.

Featured Exemplars

Although a discussion of all the exemplars presented in Box 41.1 is beyond the scope of this concept presentation, brief descriptions of a few of the most common and important exemplars are presented next. Refer to other resources for detailed information about these and any of the other exemplars.

Diabetes Education

Diabetes patient education is aimed at increasing the patient's ability to self-manage this endocrine disorder. Diabetes education programs

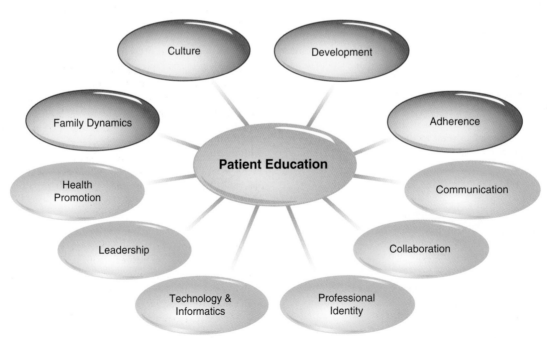

FIGURE 41.3 Patient Education and Interrelated Concepts. Professional nursing concepts are represented in blue; healthcare recipient concepts are represented in red.

BOX 41.1 EXEMPLARS OF PATIENT EDUCATION

Illness-Related
Formal Patient Education Programming
- Cancer support groups
- Cardiac education
- Coumadin classes
- Diabetes education
- Group preoperative teaching
- Ostomy support group

Informal Patient–Nurse Encounters
- Discharge teaching
- Disease-specific diet teaching
- High-tech home care teaching
- Medication teaching
- Symptom control
- Targeted written materials
- Wound care

Self-Directed Patient Education Activities
- Common literature (e.g., magazines, journals, newspapers)
- Instructional videos specific to condition or treatment
- Internet resources (e.g., American Cancer Society, American Heart Association)
- Self-help books (e.g., diet plans, herbal remedies, alternative and complementary treatment, coping with addiction)

Health Promotion
Formal Patient Education Programming
- Childbirth classes
- Complementary and alternative therapy
- Drug abuse avoidance
- Elder care classes
- Parenting classes
- Risk reduction activities
- Smoking cessation programs
- Strength/endurance building
- Weight reduction classes
- Wellness education programs

Informal Patient–Nurse Encounters
- Advanced care planning
- Age-specific screening needs
- Breast-feeding
- Counseling
- Genetic screening
- Health counseling
- Immunization teaching
- Preventing sexually transmitted diseases

Self-Directed Patient Education Activities
- Common literature (e.g., magazines, journals, newspapers)
- Exercise videos (e.g., aerobics, yoga, Pilates)
- Instructional videos specific to health-related topic
- Internet resources (e.g., WebMD, Real Age)
- Self-help books (e.g., diet plans, herbal remedies, alternative and complementary treatment, coping with addiction)
- Television (e.g., health-related programming, FIT TV)

ACCESS EXEMPLAR LINKS IN YOUR GIDDENS EBOOK

can take many forms, including group classes and one-to-one teaching. Typical topics included in diabetes education programs are the physiological alterations present in this disease, diet and medication management, monitoring of blood glucose, and risk reduction. Also critical to address in a comprehensive education plan is the psychosocial impact of this condition. If patients are unable to self-manage, family members and other support people can be educated to assist in the care.[23]

Genetic Screening (Testing) Education

Although nurses are an excellent source of general information regarding genetic testing and screening, it is important to advise patients to consult with a genetics counselor if they are considering genetic testing. This professional can provide the most accurate information about cost, confidentiality of results, and the risks and benefits of testing. General information that can be provided to patients involves the information that can be gleaned from genetic testing as it relates to risk of developing a particular disease and passing that risk on to offspring.[23]

Internet Resources

Many patients have the ability to actively research symptoms, diagnoses, and treatment options through use of the Internet. Although the Internet is often an excellent resource, the nurse remains an active partner in the education of the patient and family by answering questions, reviewing material and websites for accuracy, and assisting the patient and family to locate high-quality health information. It is also important to note that use of Internet resources requires access to a computer or mobile device and some comfort with technology.[23]

Complementary and Alternative Therapy

Inquiry into the use of complementary and alternative therapies should be part of a complete health assessment. This information is incorporated into a teaching plan for the patient. Teaching should include information about the specific type of complementary or alternative therapy (e.g., herbal supplements and meditation, acupuncture, or chiropractic intervention) and how these therapies may relate to more conventional treatments. For example, patients using herbal remedies should be instructed about the storage and use of these remedies and any potential medication or food interactions and also about potential complications of use in the perioperative period.[23]

Smoking Cessation Programs

Smoking cessation programs are designed to assist smokers to stop their use of cigarettes and other forms of tobacco. These programs provide education on the dangers and risks of tobacco use, but they are more focused on methods of stopping habitual use. Interventions may vary depending on the type or sponsor of the smoking cessation program, but they may include nicotine replacement, behavior modification, counseling, support, and relapse prevention. Education plans may also include non-nicotine drugs that may assist the patient to quit, such as some antidepressant medications.[23]

Cardiac Education

Information covered in cardiac education can include medication and treatment options as well as risk reduction. The following are all important topics to include in prevention programs as well as post-diagnosis education programs: alterations in lifestyle such as diet modification, weight loss, and control of diabetes; interpretation of common laboratory values (lipid profile); and sleep patterns and stress reduction. Concerns related to return to work, sexual activity, and exercise should be included in a comprehensive education plan. This information can be covered in group classes, which offer the benefit of support of others, or one-to-one teaching.[23]

CASE STUDY

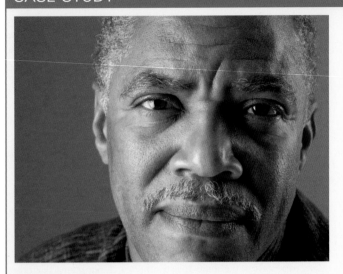

Case Presentation

Mr. Jacobs is a 55-year-old college-educated male recently diagnosed with colon cancer. He is scheduled for a colectomy with formation of a colostomy. Prior to meeting the patient, the nurse reviews the health record and notes that Mr. Jacobs is able to read English, has family support, and is currently not working. Mr. Jacobs' wife works in retail.

Mr. Jacobs is very health conscious, and his goals are to return to "normal" life. The nurse notes a comment made by Mr. Jacobs that "a colostomy is the one thing I said I would never live with." The nurse determines that these comments made by Mr. Jacobs require follow-up and asks for more information about what

Mr. Jacobs means by returning to a "normal" life. Mr. Jacobs and the nurse discuss that although his routines may need to be altered, he may find that he will be able to return to previous activities. Mr. Jacobs is hesitant to discuss sexual activity with the nurse, but reluctantly admits he is concerned about intimacy. Written information on sexual activity for those with colostomy and referral to a local support group will be included as part of the plan for Mr. Jacobs.

The nurse develops a teaching plan for Mr. Jacobs that includes the provision of written material about colon cancer, anatomy and physiology of the gastrointestinal tract, and alterations presented by having a stoma. Options for care of the stoma are also provided in writing. A second visit to demonstrate how the ostomy appliance is fitted, emptied, and changed is planned. A manikin abdomen will be used to demonstrate and practice stoma care with the patient. Mr. Jacobs is in the developmental stage of *generativity versus stagnation*.[21] When planning for his learning needs, the nurse uses multiple sources of information to teach Mr. Jacobs according to his level of education but also attends to the fact that psychomotor learning is required. To evaluate the outcome of the educational intervention conducted, the nurse follows up with Mr. Jacobs to determine his competency (both actual and perceived) in performing the necessary skills of care and Mr. Jacobs' emotional and attitudinal changes related to the ostomy and his illness. Plans are changed and adjusted according to Mr. Jacobs' progress toward his goals, incorporating family members while Mr. Jacobs becomes ready for this step.

Case Analysis Questions

1. Consider the attributes and criteria of this concept. How are these reflected in this case?
2. What learning domain needs are evident in this case?
3. What follow-up needs should the nurse anticipate in the post-operative period?

Source: Fuse/Thinkstock.

 ACCESS EXEMPLAR LINKS IN YOUR GIDDENS EBOOK

REFERENCES

1. Bastable, S. B., Gramet, P., Jacobs, K., et al. (2011). *Health professional as educator: Principles of teaching and learning*. Boston: Jones & Bartlett.
2. Marshall, L. C., Dall'Oglio, I., Davis, D., et al. (2016). Nurses as educators within health systems. *Reflections on Nursing Leadership*, *41*(4), 1–17.
3. U.S. Department of Health and Human Services: *Healthy People 2030 Framework*. Retrieved from https://www.healthypeople.gov/2020/About-Healthy-People/Development-Healthy-People-2030/Framework.
4. Marshall, L. C. (2016). *Mastering patient and family education: A healthcare handbook for success*. Indianapolis, IN: Sigma Theta Tau International.
5. Bastable, S. B. (2017). *Essentials of patient education* (2nd ed.). Boston: Jones & Bartlett.
6. Roberts, L. (2010). Health information and the internet: The 5 Cs website evaluation tool. *British Journal of Nursing*, *19*(5), 322–325.
7. *Health on the net foundation*, 2018. Retrieved from https://www.hon.ch/HONcode/Patients/Visitor/visitor.html.
8. Kitchie, S. (2019). Determinants of learning. In S. B. Bastable (Ed.), *The nurse as educator: Principles of teaching and learning for nursing practice* (5th ed.). Boston: Jones & Bartlett.
9. Heady, S. A. (2018). Health education. In C. L. Edelman & E. Kudzma (Eds.), *Health Promotion throughout the lifespan* (9th ed.). St. Louis, MO: Elsevier.
10. Wafer, M. A. (2019). Compliance, motivation and health behaviors of the learner. In S. B. Bastable (Ed.), *The nurse as educator: Principles of teaching and learning for nursing practice* (5th ed.). Boston: Jones & Bartlett.
11. Pender, N. J., Murdaugh, C. L., & Parsons, M. A. (2011). *Health promotion in nursing practice* (6th ed.). Upper Saddle River, NJ: Pearson Prentice Hall.
12. Hartweg, D. L. (2015). Orem's self-care deficit nursing theory. In M. C. Smith & M. E. Parker (Eds.), *Nursing theories and nursing practice* (4th ed.). Philadelphia, PA: Davis.
13. American Nurses Association. (2015). *Nursing: Scope and standards of practice* (3rd ed.). Silver Spring, MD: Author.
14. Institute of Medicine. (2010). *The future of nursing: Leading change, advancing health*. Washington, DC: National Academies Press.
15. QSEN Institute: *Quality and safety education in nursing*, nd. Retrieved from http://qsen.org/competencies/pre-licensure-ksas.
16. Bastable, S. B. (2019). *The nurse as educator: Principles of teaching and learning for nursing practice* (5th ed.). Boston: Jones & Bartlett.
17. Kudzma, E. C., Edelman, C. L., & Kudzma, E. C. (2018). *Health Promotion throughout the lifespan* (9th ed.). St. Louis: Elsevier.
18. Bastable, S. B., & Myers, G. M. (2019). Developmental stages of the learner. In S. B. Bastable (Ed.), *The nurse as educator: Principles of teaching and learning for nursing practice* (5th ed.). Boston: Jones & Bartlett.
19. Braungart, M., Braungart, R. G., & Gramet, R. (2019). Applying learning theories to health care practice. In S. B. Bastable (Ed.), *The nurse as educator: Principles of teaching and learning for nursing practice* (5th ed.). Boston: Jones & Bartlett.

20. Moreno-Walton, L., Brunett, P., Akhtar, S., et al. (2009). Teaching across the generation gap: Consensus from the Council of Emergency Medicine Residency Directors 2009 Academic Assembly. *Academic Emergency Medicine: Official Journal of the Society for Academic Emergency Medicine, 16*(12, Suppl. 2), S19–S24.

21. *The U.S. illiteracy rate hasn't changed in 10 years. Huffington Post*, 2013. Retrieved from https://www.huffingtonpost.com/2013/09/06/illiteracy-rate_n_3880355.html.

22. Bastable, S. B., Myers, G. M., & Poitevent, L. B. (2019). Literacy in the adult client. In S. B. Bastable (Ed.), *The nurse as educator: Principles of teaching and learning for nursing practice* (5th ed.). Boston: Jones & Bartlett.

23. Lewis, S. L., Dirksen, S. R., Heirkemper, M. M., et al. (2014). *Medical–surgical nursing: Assessment and management of clinical problems* (9th ed.). St Louis: Mosby.

CONCEPT
42

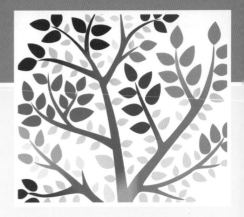

Health Promotion

Jean Giddens

During the past century, technological advancements have resulted in dramatic changes in nearly every aspect of our daily lives—particularly in the areas of transportation, communication, food production, and food acquisition. Technological advances have afforded humans with many conveniences incomprehensible 100 years ago. Along with these advances, there have been many consequences. Over time, the lifestyles of people worldwide have changed, resulting in a largely sedentary society with epidemic rates of obesity and many other related chronic diseases. According to the U.S. Department of Health and Human Services (USDHHS), unhealthy lifestyles and unhealthy environments are responsible for a large percentage of morbidity and mortality in the United States.[1]

Early technological advances in medicine fueled an initial interest in developing improved methods for the diagnosis and treatment of disease. As societal changes occurred, it became clear that a focus on health prevention was also necessary. Thus during the past several decades there has been a significant shift in national attention from the treatment of illness to the promotion of health.

Health promotion is a national health priority and foundational to the provision of care for people of all ages; it also influences health policy, economics, and distribution of resources. As the largest group of healthcare providers, nurses are central to meeting national health promotion goals through interactions with individuals, families, and communities. Not surprisingly, health promotion is included as part of the revised definition of nursing from the American Nurses Association (ANA), but is also specifically identified as a standard of professional nursing practice specifically identified by the ANA (Standard 5, Implementation; Health Teaching and Health Promotion).[2] The purpose of this concept presentation is to introduce health promotion and describe how this concept is applied within nursing practice.

DEFINITION

Initially, the concept of health promotion may seem simple—that is, a focus on improvement of health and prevention of disease. This concept, however, is actually very complex, involving multiple dimensions. For the purposes of this concept presentation, the World Health Organization's definition is proposed: *Health promotion is the process of enabling people to increase control over, and to improve, their health.*[3] Health promotion requires the adoption of healthy living practices and often necessitates a change in behavior. For this reason, long-term success of health promotion efforts is largely dependent on adaptation to change.

Disease prevention (also referred to as health protection) is considered a component of health promotion and refers to behaviors motivated by a desire to avoid illness, detect illness early, and manage illnesses when they occur.

To fully understand health promotion, one must have an understanding of various dimensions underlying this concept. Health promotion encompasses health, wellness, disease, and illness. First, what is meant by *health*? The World Health Organization defines *health* as "a state of complete physical, mental, and social well-being and not merely the absence of disease and infirmity."[4] Despite the fact that this definition is nearly 60 years old, it remains the most popular definition of health worldwide.[5] A similar term is *wellness*, but unlike health, there is no universally accepted definition. Wellness refers to a positive state of health of an individual, family, or community. It is multidimensional, encompassing several dimensions, including physical, mental, spiritual, social, occupational, environmental, intellectual, and financial. Wellness is seen as a continually changing state ranging from high-level to low-level wellness. *Disease* is a functional or structural disturbance that results when a person's adaptive mechanisms to counteract stimuli and stresses fail.[6] Although similar to disease, *illness* is seen as the physical manifestations and the subjective experience of the individual. Illness can be present in the absence of disease, and it is possible to have no illness when a disease is present. Likewise, many individuals experience wellness in the presence of an illness. For example, a person who has type 2 diabetes (a chronic illness) can experience high-level wellness. Low-level wellness is seen as an unfavorable state in which illness may result. Throughout the years, there has been ongoing debate about the relationship between health and illness—as paired entities at opposite ends of a single continuum or as separate entities.[7–9] The complex interrelationship of health, wellness, illness, and disease as components of health promotion would suggest the latter is a more realistic view. Fig. 42.1 shows a health-illness continuum with the variable of wellness added. From this perspective, one can see the interplay of having high or low-level wellness in a state of health or in a state of illness.

SCOPE

Health promotion is viewed broadly as behaviors that promote optimal health across the lifespan within an individual, family, community, population, and environment. The scope of health promotion (Fig. 42.2) is represented through levels of prevention, first defined by Leavell

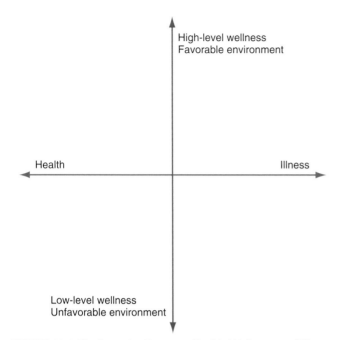

High-level wellness
Favorable environment

Health   Illness

Low-level wellness
Unfavorable environment

FIGURE 42.1 The Interplay Between Health, Wellness, and Illness. (From Endelman, C. L., & Kudzma, E. C. *Health promotion throughout the life span* [9th ed.]. St. Louis: Elsevier; 2018.)

and Clark: primary, secondary, and tertiary prevention.[10] Specific recommendations vary according to the level of prevention and the unique characteristics of an individual (e.g., age, gender or race, family history, or medical history), a community, or a population. Health promotion recommendations for population groups often are presented in the context of age groups, including infants, toddlers, school-age children, adolescents, adults, and older adults.

The terms community and population refer to collective groups of people identified by geography, common interests, concerns, characteristics, or values.[11] Thus, community may be a localized area or may involve groups of people without geographic boundaries. It is also important to recognize the entire world as a global community—meaning that events rarely occur in isolation of one country or region so a very broad perspective of potential impact must be considered.

Primary Prevention

Primary prevention refers to strategies aimed at optimizing health and disease prevention. The focus is on health education for optimal nutrition, exercise, immunizations, safe living and work environments, hygiene and sanitation, protection from environmental hazards, avoidance of harmful substances (e.g., allergens, toxins, and carcinogens), protection from accidents, and effective stress management. Specific

health promotion strategies are not linked to a single disease entity. For example, avoiding smoking helps to promote health and reduce the individual's risk for pulmonary, cardiovascular, and immunologic disease. Also, it is important to understand that a combination of strategies is usually advised for the prevention of specific conditions. For example, there are many known strategies that prevent or reduce one's risk for developing cardiovascular disease, including implementing a healthy diet, exercising regularly, and avoiding smoking; additional measures may be advised based on other personal risk factors.

Secondary Prevention (Screening)

The goal of secondary prevention is to identify individuals in an early state of a disease process so that prompt treatment can be initiated. Early treatment provides an opportunity to cure, limit disability, or delay consequences of advanced disease. Secondary prevention measures usually involve screening tests. Screenings are typically indicated and recommended if they are safe, cost-effective, and accurate and if the effort makes a substantial difference in the morbidity and/or mortality of conditions. Screenings are recommended for an individual, family, population, or community based on known risk factors.

To be considered accurate, a screening method must have a high degree of reliability and validity. A screening instrument, test, or method is considered reliable if the approach produces the same results when different individuals (with a similar skill set) perform the test. Validity reflects the ability of the test to accurately detect disease. Ideally, a screening measure will accurately differentiate individuals who have a condition from those who do not have a condition 100% of the time. *Sensitivity* is a measure related to the proportion of those with a condition who are correctly identified. A test with poor sensitivity fails to identify disease in people who actually have a condition—known as a false-negative result. *Specificity* refers to the ability to currently identify those who do not have a condition. If a screening measure has poor specificity, many people who are disease free will have a false-positive test result.

Tertiary Prevention

Tertiary prevention involves minimizing the effects of disease and disability; the focus of tertiary prevention is restorative through collaborative disease management. The aim is to optimize the management of a condition and minimize complications so that the individual can achieve the highest level of health possible. Specific strategies include rehabilitative efforts to increase adherence to medication, nutrition, physical activity, and other disease management strategies. Many strategies used as primary prevention strategies are also used for tertiary prevention. The difference is not the strategy itself but, rather, the intent, goal, and context of the strategy. For example, aerobic exercise is used as a primary prevention strategy to maintain health, but it may be a specific weight loss intervention for the obese patient or a rehabilitation strategy following an acute myocardial infarction.

Individual, Family, Community, Population, Environment

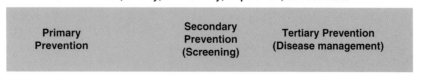

| Primary Prevention | Secondary Prevention (Screening) | Tertiary Prevention (Disease management) |

Lifespan Application

FIGURE 42.2 Scope of Health Promotion. Includes three levels (primary, secondary, and tertiary) applied across the lifespan with an individual, family, community, population, and environmental focus.

ATTRIBUTES AND CRITERIA

Attributes are qualities, characteristics, or elements that validate parameters of the concept. Health promotion is characterized by four elements:

- *Optimization of health*: The focus on optimizing health includes measures to maintain high-level wellness, measures to prevent illness, and strategies for early detection and management of disease when it occurs.
- *Evidence*: Health promotion guidelines are based on evidence; for this reason, recommendations are periodically updated to reflect new knowledge generated through research efforts. The recommendations are usually disseminated through practice guidelines for health professionals and via consumer-targeted media for the general public. In many cases, recommendations are presented as a matter of priority based on the level of evidence. For example, the U.S. Preventive Services Task Force (USPSTF) has five levels of evidence; each recommendation statement is accompanied by a recommendation grade that ranges from A to D or grade I (Box 42.1). As applied to two examples of cancer screening, USPSTF recommends biennial mammography screening for women aged 50 to 74 years (grade B recommendation)[12] and recommends selectively offering periodic prostate-specific antigen (PSA) for men 55 to 69 years old based on patient preferences (grade C recommendation) and is against routine PSA-based screening for prostate cancer in men 70 years and older (grade D recommendation).[13]
- *Patient/community centered*: Incorporation of health promotion measures must be valued and desired by the individuals impacted. On an individual level, personal motivation to incorporate the strategies is required. On a community level, leadership from individuals within the community is needed for successful implementation. It is critical that the wishes and desires of the targeted individual(s) are considered and understood. A patient/family/community assessment must be done in order to gain an understanding of the wishes and desires of the individual(s) impacted.[5]
- *Enculturation*: Designing and implementing health promotion require cultural competence and sensitivity to differences among cultures. Nurses must be willing to listen to and learn from patients and communities so that interventions are provided within appropriate languages and within the context of health belief practices.[6] Often, healthcare providers make recommendations for actions from their own perspective of what is appropriate and expected behavior—an ethnocentric perspective based on their own set of values and beliefs. Enculturation refers to the full internalization of values of a culture group. To be successful, health promotion plans incorporate the beliefs, attitudes, values, behaviors, and interpersonal dynamics into the planning, implementation, and evaluation of health promotion activities.

THEORETICAL LINKS

Numerous models and theories of health, health behavior, and health promotion have evolved during the past 30 years as the science and evidence of health promotion have expanded. Two areas of health promotion models include those focusing on the individual as a patient and those focusing on the community.

Individual-Focused Models

Models that focus on the individual typically share common themes, including cognition, decision-making, motivation, behavior, and environment. Although it is beyond the scope of this concept presentation to detail all the models and theories associated with health promotion, some of the most prominent, contemporary models are presented in Table 42.1.

Community-Focused Models

True community interventions focus on the community as a whole or the majority of the population within a community; this is in contrast to the application of interventions to individuals within a community. Community-focused models share common attributes, including (1) a focus on community values and norms, (2) legitimization of desirable behaviors and environmental changes, (3) participation of community leadership, and (4) a planned change in which community members have control.[14] A number of community-focused models exist for planning and dissemination of health promotion agendas; a few of these are presented in Table 42.2.

CONTEXT TO NURSING AND HEALTH CARE

Nurses have involvement in health promotion on a number of levels, including working with an individual or family to enhance health, working with communities and organizations to enhance health, and participating in the development and implementation of health policy. The most common roles of nurses include the assessment, planning, and implementation of interventions and the evaluation of health promotion strategies for individuals. In fact, nurses have a significant responsibility for enhancing the health of individuals across the lifespan; this occurs in the context of a therapeutic relationship and requires skillful communication by the nurse.

BOX 42.1   U.S. Preventive Services Task Force Grading

Grade A = Recommends
- There is high certainty that the net benefit is substantial.

Grade B = Recommends
- There is high certainty that the net benefit is moderate or there is moderate certainty that the net benefit is moderate to substantial.

Grade C = Selective Recommendation
- There is moderate certainty that the net benefit is small. There may be considerations that support providing the intervention for an individual patient depending on individual preferences and circumstances, but not for the general population.

Grade D = Recommends Against
- There is moderate or high certainty that the intervention has no net benefit or that the harms outweigh the benefits.

I Statement = Insufficient Evidence to Recommend For or Against
- The current evidence is insufficient to assess the balance of benefits and harms of the service. Evidence is lacking, of poor quality, or conflicting, and the balance of benefits and harms cannot be determined.

From U.S. Preventive Services Task Force: Grade Definitions, 2013. Retrieved from https://www.uspreventiveservicestaskforce.org/Page/Name/grade-definitions#grade-definitions-after-july-2012

TABLE 42.1   Models of Health Promotion Targeting the Individual

Model Name and Theorist	Brief Description
Health promotion model (Pender)	This model shows that healthy behaviors (behavioral outcomes) are influenced by integration of unique characteristics and experiences of an individual (prior behavior and personal factors) and by influences of behavior (perceived benefit and barriers to action, perceived self-efficacy, activity-related affect, and interpersonal and situational influences).
Transtheoretical model (Prochaska and DiClemente)	This model proposes that health-related behavior progresses through six stages of behavior change on a continuum from motivational readiness to change of a problem behavior. The six stages are precontemplation, contemplation, preparation for action, action, maintenance, and termination. These changes occur regardless of specific behavior change and have been observed both among individuals adopting healthy behaviors and among those stopping an unhealthy behavior (e.g., smoking).
Theory of reasoned action and planned behavior (Ajzen and Fishbein)	This theory is built on an understanding of attitudes and subjective norms and the influence these have on changes in behavior. According to the model, the intention to change is driven by the attitude toward the behavior and the subjective norm for the behavior.
Social cognitive theory (Bandura)	This is a social cognitive theory used to design individual behavioral change. Self-belief influences behavior; self-beliefs are formed through self-observation and self-reflection. The major concepts within this theory are self-direction, self-regulation, and self-efficacy.
Health belief model (Stretcher and Rosenstock)	This model explores behaviors of individuals who take actions to avoid illness and those who fail to take preventive actions and thus has been used to predict which individuals would or would not use preventive measures.

TABLE 42.2   Models of Health Promotion Targeting the Community

Model Name and Theorist	Brief Description
Social ecology models	These are models that emphasize social and cultural contexts of people within an environment—and recognition of multiple variables that influence health behaviors. Consideration for health promotion interventions includes an integration of environmental resources and lifestyles of individuals within that environment.
PRECEDE-PROCEED model (Green)	This is a nine-stage model designed to guide the planning to health programs by identifying the most appropriate intervention strategies. PRECEDE stands for predisposing, reinforcing, enabling constructs in ecosystem, diagnosis, and evaluation. PROCEED recognizes forces outside the control of individuals and stands for policy, regulation, organizational constructs in education, and environmental development.
Diffusion of innovations model (Rogers)	This is a model that emphasizes dissemination of health behavior interventions. Rogers' model identifies four steps of diffusion: (1) the innovation, (2) communication channels (spreading the word), (3) time, and (4) social systems. The underlying assumption of adoption is the perceived value placed on the new behavior or innovation.
Social marketing models	Social marketing models influence behavior change by influencing adoption of an idea by the general public. Foundational to social marketing models are product, price, place, and promotion. When applied to health promotion, the "product" is the desired application, the "price" is the cost (social and economic) to the community as a result of adoption, "place" refers to the location where the program(s) is available, and "promotion" refers to strategies used to entice individuals to accept the change through adoption.

National Healthcare Agenda and Healthcare Economics

Health promotion is a central focus of healthcare delivery that has been shown to add quality years of life and to decrease healthcare costs.[5] National goals and objectives for improving the health of Americans have been outlined in a series of reports beginning in 1979 with the publication of the first of the *Healthy People* series—*Healthy People: The Surgeon General's Report on Health Promotion and Disease Prevention*—and a companion document published in 1980—*Promoting Health/Preventing Disease: Objectives for the Nation*. Since that time, the USDHHS has published reports every 10 years outlining goals and objectives for the upcoming decade. The *Healthy People 2030* framework outlines five overarching goals for the nation to achieve by 2030; these goals are presented in Box 42.2. The five goals link to 41 topic areas, each with a set of objectives and target indicators to measure progress.[15]

The support for health promotion and illness prevention services is also demonstrated through the changes in coverage for such interventions by third-party payers. The impact of providing such services is continually evaluated; to maintain support, the cost of providing such

BOX 42.2   Overarching Goals for *Healthy People 2030*

1. Attain healthy, thriving lives and well-being, free of preventable disease, disability, injury, and premature death.
2. Eliminate health disparities, achieve health equity, and attain health literacy to improve the health and well-being of all.
3. Create social, physical, and economic environments that promote attaining full potential for health and well-being for all.
4. Promote healthy development, healthy behaviors, and well-being across all life stages.
5. Engage leadership, key constituents, and the public across multiple sectors to take action and design policies that improve the health and well-being of all.

From U.S. Department of Health and Human Services: *Healthy People 2030 Framework*. Accessed at https://www.healthypeople.gov/2020/About-Healthy-People/Development-Healthy-People-2030/Framework services (including to those who are uninsured or underinsured) must outweigh the consequences of the absence of such services, particularly in the face of rising healthcare expenditures. Such issues have been central to health policy debate.

Vulnerable Populations and Health Disparities

Vulnerable populations refer to groups of individuals who are at greatest risk for poor health outcomes. These people are more likely to develop health-related problems and experience significantly worse outcomes when they occur. Health disparities is a term (and a concept presented in this textbook) that refers to inequities in heath within vulnerable population groups. Vulnerable populations are often politically marginalized in society; they experience discrimination and intolerance and may not have basic human needs met. The most consistent predictor of life expectancy, morbidity, mortality, and nearly all indicators of health status is low socioeconomic status,[16,17] although race/ethnicity, education, and occupation are also powerful indicators. Thus, two of the most highly vulnerable populations are persons with low socioeconomic status and persons who are members of ethnic and racial minorities. Health policy to eliminate health disparities aims to increase accessible health services, requiring community involvement. Cultural competence is especially important to the elimination of health disparities because it facilitates integration of culturally appropriate interventions based on the values and beliefs of the targeted group. Thus, before working with vulnerable populations, nurses must be committed to developing skills in cultural competence.[18]

Assessment

Health assessment is the foundation for establishing a health promotion plan and the basis for application of health promotion into practice. Assessment can target an individual, family, or community.

Individual Assessment

The primary components of assessment for individuals include a comprehensive assessment of health status, health behaviors, and risk. Advances in genetic research have enhanced the ability to assess risk; thus, family history is a critical component of health assessment. In addition, assessment includes gaining an understanding of personal factors such as health preferences, values, and social relationships. The assessment of health is performed by nurses in nearly all settings and includes conducting a history and physical examination. Effective communication skills are essential to obtain necessary information for a successful health promotion process. The nurse–patient relationship is truly the context of care; the nurse must be sensitive to each person's goals and values.

Family Assessment

A family assessment is necessary to promote health within families. Family assessment includes gaining an understanding of health promotion and disease prevention activities within the family (including risk factors), family strengths, and the relationships among family members—how family members influence behaviors and decision-making of others. A genogram is a useful method to understand family members across multiple generations.[19]

Community Assessment

Community assessment is a necessary component of assessment when developing community-based health promotion strategies—usually in the context of community health nursing and public health nursing. Community assessment is conducted in participation with community representatives and through community data collection strategies including observation, interviews from community residents, and data collection using instruments that quantify data. Additional information about a community typically incorporated into an assessment includes the structure of a community; census; population/demographic statistics; morbidity rates; mortality rates; epidemiologic data; environmental data (e.g., pollution indices); and community resources such as healthcare services, government services (fire, police, and other emergency services), schools, and other local government agencies. These data can be collected from a variety of sources, including the Internet and city/government offices.

Health Promotion Interventions

Health promotion interventions are planned and initiated on the basis of data gained from assessment. Guidelines for health promotion interventions based on age or other risk factors are readily available for health professionals; nurses should know how to access and interpret the guidelines so these can be incorporated into patient care. The interventions described here are broadly applied to all levels of health promotion (primary, secondary, and tertiary) and can be applied to all targeted groups (individual, family, and community).

Education

Education is a cornerstone for health promotion; this is also one of the most important contributions of nursing. Education intersects with each area of health promotion—as a primary, secondary, and tertiary health promotion strategy. Education is applied to individuals (patient education), families, and communities. Nurses have an opportunity to assist individuals to optimize their health by educating individuals and families about healthy lifestyle choices and encouraging appropriate screening and management of disease when necessary. Teaching involves not only providing information but also helping to align resources and access so health services can be provided. This is especially important among individuals from vulnerable populations.

Vaccinations

Edward Jenner is credited with being the father of immunology because he was the first person to successfully develop a vaccination in 1798. Smallpox vaccination was a new and innovative way to prevent disease and provided the foundation for the science of immunology. Since that time, vaccinations have become one of the most effective primary prevention interventions; development and research efforts for new immunizations are ongoing. Nurses are commonly involved in this area of health promotion by providing patient education regarding immunizations, allaying fears of immunization, identifying those who are in need of immunization, and administering vaccines. Vaccinations are recommended for individuals across the entire lifespan from infancy through geriatric populations. Although it is beyond the scope of this concept presentation to describe all vaccinations, nurses should know where to find and interpret current immunization guidelines. The Centers for Disease Control and Prevention (CDC) provides regular updates to recommended immunization guidelines for all age groups and is readily found on the website (http://www.cdc.gov).[20]

Screening

Screening is a secondary prevention strategy; the goal is for disease detection in the early stages of the disease process. Screening usually involves testing that has high reliability and validity—and screens for important conditions in which early detection is paramount. The benefits must outweigh the consequences and must be feasible from an economic and resource perspective. Specific routine screening guidelines have been developed for individuals across the lifespan. The USPSTF offers reliable screening recommendations, as do many other government agencies and organizations such as the CDC, the American Cancer Society, the American Heart Association, and the American Academy of Pediatrics. Screening is also done based on an individual's risk. Genetic screening, for example, is not routinely performed on all individuals, but it is indicated in cases in which the history supports the need.

Nutritional Health

It is estimated that more than 60% of all deaths are associated with chronic diseases such as cardiovascular disease, cancer, lower respiratory disease, and diabetes;[21] a large percentage of these diseases are caused or exacerbated by poor or unhealthy nutritional behaviors. According to the National Center for Health Statistics,[22] 20.6% of children between ages 12 and 19 years, 18.4% of children between ages 6 and 11 years, and 13.9% of children between ages 2 and 3 years are overweight. Children who are overweight or obese are at significant risk for many health-related problems as adults. For these reasons, one of the most important health promotion interventions is nutrition counseling.

The *Dietary Guidelines for Americans 2015–2020* provides the basis for dietary recommendations and guides state and federal policies related to nutrition.[23] New guidelines for 2020–2025 were being developed at the time this book was published. A consumer-friendly translation of the *Dietary Guidelines*, known as *ChooseMyPlate*, serves as a useful tool for dietary teaching and planning and can be found at the following website: http://www.choosemyplate.gov.

The promotion of an adequate diet is included in nearly all health promotion plans—either as a primary or as a tertiary prevention focus. For example, a healthy individual whose weight is within normal range may set a goal to increase the servings of fruits and vegetables consumed each day to meet the dietary recommendations found in *MyPlate*. Another individual who is obese and has cardiovascular disease may reduce saturated fats and calorie consumption as a treatment measure with a goal to reduce weight and decrease levels of serum lipids. In addition to improving dietary intake, other topics related to nutrition include dietary supplements, food safety, and nutritional screening.[6]

Physical Activity

The human body was designed to move; therefore, it should be no surprise that regular physical activity is an essential component of maintaining optimal physical and psychological health. Physical activity encompasses any bodily movement involving skeletal muscles and energy expenditure. Physical activity occurs as part of routine daily activities, occupational activities, and recreational activities. Exercise training (purposeful bodily movement with the intention to improve physical fitness) is recommended for individuals across the lifespan and also is an important component to maintaining a healthy weight.

The benefits of physical activity are well documented for individuals across the lifespan. According to the USDHHS, there is strong evidence that regular physical activity among children and adolescents results in improved bone health, improved cardiorespiratory and muscular fitness, improved cardiovascular and metabolic health biomarkers, and increased favorable body composition.[24] For adults and older adults, there is strong evidence that regular physical activity lowers the risk for multiple conditions, including coronary heart disease, stroke, hypertension, elevated lipids, type 2 diabetes, metabolic syndrome, breast and colon cancers, weight gain, and depression.[24] There is also a reduced risk for falls and improved cognitive function. In addition to being a primary prevention strategy, physical activity and exercise are also common tertiary health promotion interventions. Examples include physical activity as part of cardiac rehabilitation or following a stroke and physical therapy following joint replacement surgery.

Pharmacologic Agents

In addition to immunizations, many pharmacologic agents are useful for health promotion efforts. Details of drugs are primarily discussed in specific concept chapters, but two common examples are provided here.

Drugs used for smoking cessation. Several U.S. Food and Drug Administration (FDA)-approved medications are available to assist smoking cessation. Most of these drugs are nicotine replacement therapy for short-term use to reduce nicotine craving and provide relief of symptoms from nicotine withdrawal. These are available in the form of patches, gums, or lozenges.[25]

Drugs used for weight loss. There are several FDA-approved medications for weight loss. Most drugs are used to reduce appetite by making the patient feel full and several (phentermine, benzphetamine, diethylpropion, and phendimetrazine) are only for short-term use (up to 12 weeks) as appetite suppressors. However, one approved drug (orlistat) is a lipase inhibitor that blocks the ability of the body to absorb fat. This is recommended for long-term use (up to 1 year) for adults and children older than age 12 years.[26]

INTERRELATED CONCEPTS

Several important concepts interrelated to health promotion are presented in Fig. 42.3. Health promotion actually is linked to every health and illness concept within this book as a matter of prevention, screening, or tertiary care. Interrelationships with the health and illness concepts Nutrition and Mobility are especially important based on the health promotion interventions discussed in the previous section. Healthcare recipient concepts Development, Culture, Adherence, and Self-Management are interrelated and form a concept cluster; these impact the type of health promotion interventions and approaches offered, as well as factors that influence the success of behavior change. Self-management and adherence are particularly important in the area of disease management.

Patient Education, a professional nursing concept, is based on patient attributes and significantly influences the success of health promotion interventions. Recommended health promotion guidelines are based on Evidence, and the effectiveness of health promotion recommendations is evaluated. Because of evidence, health promotion guidelines are implemented through Health Policy. A significant amount of evidence exists showing the connection between Health Disparities among vulnerable populations, thus underscoring the need for measures to enhance health promotion access and practices. These concepts form a natural concept cluster (Fig. 42.3). Health promotion is also interrelated to Health Care Economics. The delivery of health promotion interventions must be financed, and these interventions should be cost-effective.

CLINICAL EXEMPLARS

Considering the recommendations across the lifespan, there are literally thousands of exemplars for health promotion. Box 42.3 presents some of the most common exemplars of health promotion for individuals. Major exemplars for the promotion of health for individuals are often considered in terms of primary prevention, secondary prevention, and tertiary prevention. Box 42.3 is not comprehensive and does not include community or environmental health promotion strategies. Specific details for all exemplars presented can be found in multiple textbooks and on many websites devoted to health promotion.

Featured Exemplars
Vaccination

Vaccination represents standard health promotion measures for individuals of all ages. Vaccines provide immunity, or the ability to resist infection from many dangerous communicable diseases. The specific vaccines given to an individual are dependent on age, previous

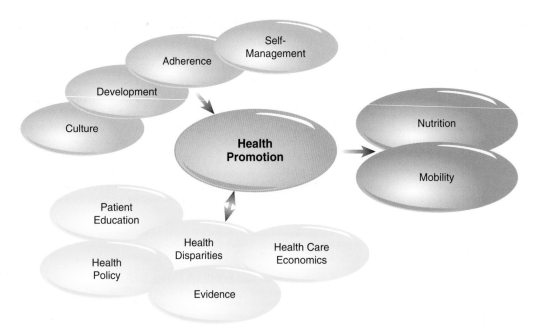

FIGURE 42.3 Health Promotion and Interrelated Concepts. Interrelationships among healthcare recipient concepts (in *blue*), health and illness concepts (in *purple*), and professional nursing concepts (in *yellow*).

BOX 42.3   EXEMPLARS OF HEALTH PROMOTION

Primary Prevention
Prenatal
- General prenatal care
- Folic acid supplementation
- Vaccinations (e.g., rubella, hepatitis B)
- Abstinence from smoking, alcohol, and other drugs
- Nutrition counseling
- Genetic counseling

Infants/Children/Adolescents
- Injury prevention (e.g., car seats, seat belts, helmets, life jackets)
- Environmental exposures (toxins/poisoning)
- Vaccinations (health protection)
- Physical activity
- Nutrition counseling
- Avoidance of smoking and other substance use
- Dental/oral care

Adults/Older Adults
- Injury prevention (e.g., safety belts, fall prevention measures)
- Physical activity
- Nutrition counseling
- Vaccinations

Secondary Prevention (Screening)
Prenatal
- Ultrasound screening
- Rh factor and antibody screening
- Sexually transmitted infection screening

Infants/Children/Adolescents
- Developmental screening
- Hearing screening
- Vision screening

- Body mass index screening
- Blood pressure screening
- Depression screening
- Substance abuse screening

Adults/Older Adults
- Hearing screening
- Vision screening
- Body mass index screening
- Blood pressure screening
- Depression screening
- Substance abuse screening
- Blood lipid screening
- Cognitive function screening
- Functional assessment screening
- Cancer screenings (e.g., breast, colon, prostate, skin, oral)

Tertiary Prevention
Prenatal
- Diabetes management
- Hypertension management
- Substance use/abuse management

Infants/Children/Adolescents
- Chronic disease management
- Obesity management
- Nutrition counseling
- Physical activity

Adults/Older Adults
- Chronic disease management
- Obesity management
- Nutrition counseling
- Physical activity

 ACCESS EXEMPLAR LINKS IN YOUR GIDDENS EBOOK

vaccinations, health status, medical history, lifestyle, type of employment, and travel history. Immunization schedules are available from the Centers for Disease Control for various age groups, including infants and children, adolescents, and adults.[20]

Oral Hygiene

Oral hygiene is an important health promotion measure for people of all ages and includes brushing teeth, flossing, drinking fluoridated water, dental sealants, and regular visits to a dental care professional. Oral hygiene prevents dental caries (considered the most common chronic condition in childhood) and periodontal disease (which affects an estimated 47% of adults older than age 30 years).[27] Periodontal disease is considered a risk factor in several systemic diseases such as cardiovascular disease and diabetes.[28]

Nutrition Counseling

Patient education regarding optimal dietary intake is one of the most common forms of health promotion and includes both primary prevention and tertiary prevention (disease management). Although most individuals as early as childhood are aware of the importance of eating a healthy diet, many children, adolescents, adults, and older adults have diets that are not optimal for a variety of reasons, including access to healthy foods; poor food choices; or conditions interfering with appetite, intake, digestion, or elimination.

Physical Activity

Physical activity is a fundamental health promotion measure for all individuals. Physical activity helps to control weight and improves cardiovascular health, musculoskeletal strength and agility, sleep, and mental health. Common activities include walking, running, cycling, swimming, and weight training. School-based, community-based, and employer-based programs to increase physical activity are examples of the greater awareness of physical activity as an important health promotion activity.

Blood Pressure Screening

Screening for hypertension involves regular blood pressure assessment. This is one of the most common health screenings because of its relative ease and cost-effectiveness. The USPSTF recommends blood pressure screening every 2 years after age 20 years.[29] Although it is not clear the optimal age to begin routine blood pressure screening in children, that American Academy of Pediatrics recommends annual blood pressure screening in the ambulatory setting starting at age 3; for children under three, blood pressure measurements should be taken at well-child visits if they are at increased risk for hypertension.[30]

Breast Cancer Screening

Screening measures to detect breast cancer depend on an individual's age and risk factors. A clinical breast exam, conducted by a healthcare professional, involves palpation of the breasts and axilla for the presence of lumps. A mammography is a radiographic test that detects tumors in the breast tissue that are too small to feel. Magnetic resonance imaging is used among women with high-risk factors for breast cancer. The USPSTF recommends screening mammography every other year for women aged 50 to 74 years.[12]

Colorectal Cancer Screening

Colorectal cancer screening efforts focus on detecting and removing precancerous polyps in the colon and early detection of colorectal cancer. Screening measures include high-sensitivity fecal occult blood testing, sigmoidoscopy, or colonoscopy. Routine screening is recommended for all adults beginning at age 50 years and continuing through age 75 years.[31]

CASE STUDY

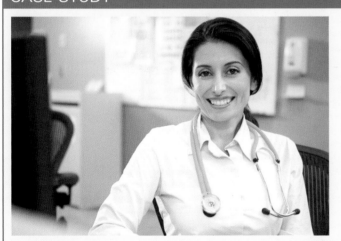

Case Presentation

Natalie Jemez, DNP, a pediatric nurse practitioner, works for a community-based health center. After hearing about the death of a 12-year-old boy who suffered head trauma at the local skateboard park, Natalie and her colleagues at the community center decided to initiate an injury reduction program targeting local youth and their families. Specifically, they were interested in raising awareness regarding traumatic brain injury and providing a mechanism to increase helmet use among children skateboarding, riding scooters, and riding bicycles at the city park. Natalie wrote a grant in partnership with the local school district to secure state funds for a 3-year project that would achieve the following four goals: (1) development of informational brochures to be mailed to the families of children attending the local schools, (2) development of an age-appropriate information video "Helmet Heads" to be shown to children within the school system, (3) providing a mechanism for parents to purchase helmets at a significant discount from a local retailer, and (4) purchasing a large number of helmets for free use (by checking the helmets out at the local park service center) while children and their families are at the park.

Natalie was awarded grant funding for a 3-year project. As the program was implemented, other community stakeholders (including the local hospital, the orthopedic physician group, and the neurosurgeon physician group) became interested and provided additional funds to purchase additional protective equipment and to track data regarding use of equipment and number and types of reported injuries.

Case Analysis Questions

1. Considering the scope of health promotion in Fig. 42.2 (primary, secondary and tertiary), what does this health promotion project represent?
2. What are the primary health promotion interventions represented in this case?

ACCESS EXEMPLAR LINKS IN YOUR GIDDENS EBOOK

REFERENCES

1. U.S. Department of Health and Human Services. (2010). *Healthy People2020*. Washington, DC: U.S. Government Printing Office.
2. American Nurses Association. (2015). *Nursing: Scope and standards of practice* (3rd ed.). Silver Spring, MD: Author.
3. World Health Organization. (1986). *Ottawa charter for health promotion*. Geneva: Author.
4. World Health Organization. (2006). *Constitution of the World Health Organization*. Retrieved from http://www.who.int/governance/eb/who_constitution_en.pdf.
5. Pender, N. J., Murdoaugh, C. L., & Parsons, M. A. (2015). *Health promotion in nursing practice* (7th ed.). Upper Saddle River, NJ: Pearson.
6. Endelman, C. L., & Mandle, C. L. (2018). *Health promotion throughout the lifespan* (9th ed.). St. Louis: Elsevier.
7. Oelbaum, C. H. (1623). Hallmarks of adult wellness. *The American Journal of Nursing, 74*, 1974.
8. Sullivan, M. (2003). The new subjective medicine: Taking the patient's point of view on health care and health. *Social Science and Medicine, 56*(7), 1595–1604.
9. Dunn, H. L. (1980). *High level wellness*. Thorofare, NJ: Charles B. Slack.
10. Leavell, H., & Clark, E. (1953). *Textbook of preventative medicine*. New York: McGraw-Hill.
11. World Health Organization. (1974). *Community health nursing: Report of a WHO expert committee*, report No. 559, Geneva, Author.
12. U.S. Preventive Services Task Force. (2016). *Final update summary: Breast cancer: Screening*. Retrieved from https://www.uspreventiveservicestaskforce.org/Page/Document/UpdateSummaryFinal/breast-cancer-screening1?ds=1&s=breast%20cancer%20screening.
13. U.S. Preventive Services Task Force. (2018). *Final update summary: Prostate cancer: Screening*. Retrieved from https://www.uspreventiveservicestaskforce.org/Page/Document/UpdateSummaryFinal/prostate-cancer-screening1?ds=1&s=prostate%20cancer.
14. Minkler, M., Wallerstein, N., & Wilson, S. (2008). Improving health through community organization and community building. In K. Glanz, B. K. Rimer, & F. M. Lewis (Eds.), *Health behavior and health education theory, research, and practice* (4th ed., pp. 287–312). San Francisco: Jossey–Bass.
15. U.S. Department of Health and Human Services. (2019). *Healthy people 2030 framework*. Washington, DC: Author. Retrieved from https://www.healthypeople.gov/2020/About-Healthy-People/Development-Healthy-People-2030/Framework.
16. Braverman, P. A., Cubbin, C., Egerter, S., et al. (2010). Socioeconomic disparities in health in the United States: What the patterns tell us. *American Journal of Public Health, 100*, S186–S196.
17. Braverman, P. A., Egerter, S. A., & Mockenahaupt, R. E. (2011). Broadening the focus: The need to address the social determinants of health. *American Journal of Preventive Medicine, 40*(Supp 1), S4–S18.
18. Liu, J. J., Davidson, E., Bhopal, R., et al. (2016). Adapting health promotion interventions for minority groups: A qualitative study. *Health Promotion International, 31*(2), 325–5334.
19. Wilson, S., & Giddens, J. (2017). *Health assessment for nursing practice* (6th ed.). St Louis: Elsevier.
20. Centers for Disease Control and Prevention. (2018). *Immunization schedules*. Retrieved from https://www.cdc.gov/vaccines/schedules/.
21. Centers for Disease and Control Prevention. (2018). *Leading causes of death of males and females in the United States*. Retrieved from https://www.cdc.gov/healthequity/lcod/.
22. Hales, C. M., Carroll, M. D., Fryar, C. D., et al. *Prevalence of obesity among adults and youth United States, 2015-2016*. Retrieved from https://www.cdc.gov/nchs/data/databriefs/db288.pdf.
23. U.S. Department of Agriculture and U.S. Department of Health and Human Services. *2015-2020 dietary guidelines for Americans, 8th edition*. Retrieved from https://health.gov/dietaryguidelines/2015/resources/2015-2020_Dietary_Guidelines.pdf.
24. U.S. Department of Health and Human Services. (2008). *Physical activity guidelines for Americans*. Retrieved from http://www.health.gov/paguidelines.
25. U.S. Department of Health and Human Services. (2017). *Want to quit smoking? FDA-approved products can help*. Retrieved from http://www.fda.gov/forconsumers/consumerupdates/ucm198176.htm.
26. National Institutes of Health. (2016). *Prescription medications to treat overweight and obesity*. Retrieved from https://www.niddk.nih.gov/health-information/weight-management/prescription-medications-treat-overweight-obesity.
27. Eke, P., Dye, B., Wei, L., et al. (2012). Prevalence of periodontitis in adults in the United States: 2009–2010. *Journal of Dental Research, 91*(10), 914–920.
28. Nazir, M. A. (2017). Prevalence of periodontal disease, its association with systemic diseases, and prevention. *International Journal of Health Sciences, 11*(2), 72–80.
29. U.S. Preventive Services Task Force. (2017). *Final recommendation statement: High blood pressure in adults: Screening*. Retrieved from https://www.uspreventiveservicestaskforce.org/Page/Document/RecommendationStatementFinal/high-blood-pressure-in-adults-screening.
30. Flynn, J. T., Kaelber, D. C., Baker-Smith, C. M., et al. (2017). Clinical practice guideline for screening and management of high blood pressure in children and adolescents. *Pediatrics, 140*(3), pii: e20171904.
31. U.S. Preventive Services Task Force. (2016). *Final update summary: Colorectal cancer: Screening*. Retrieved from https://www.uspreventiveservicestaskforce.org/Page/Document/UpdateSummaryFinal/colorectal-cancer-screening2?ds=1&s=colorectal%20cancer.

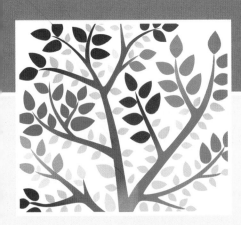

Communication

Lorraine P. Buchanan and Nelda Godfrey

Communication is an essential form of human behavior—so fundamental to human social systems that our world would be barely recognizable without it. As a fundamental behavior, communication is so pervasive that the profound impact on our ability to engage with our world cannot be underestimated. Communication is unavoidable within the context of social life.[1] Human social interaction is accomplished through the relationships that develop between people, and these relationships are mediated by communication. These relationships vary from the intimacy of family to the more distant or more formal relationships between members of a community or nation. However, all of these relationships are dependent on communication for the creation and coordination of social interaction through the exchange of messages between participants. This exchange of information allows for the creation and coordination of social action, the integration of disparate individuals into social groups, and the subsequent formation of social relationships. Therefore, communication is the essential process that ties people together, whether the ties create a family, an organization, a culture, or a nation.

DEFINITION

There are many definitions of communication in the literature, and these really only vary slightly. A synthesized definition would need to include the use of symbols to convey meaning through an interactive process. Because there is no way to directly communicate mind-to-mind with others, people must communicate through the use of symbols.[2] These symbols are used to create a message that is transmitted to others, usually through spoken or written language but also through gestures, facial expressions, or body movements.[3] Symbolic interaction between people becomes an expression of mind states and a means to transmit ideas. Thus, for the purposes of this concept presentation, communication is defined as *a process of interaction between people in which symbols are used to create, exchange, and interpret messages about ideas, emotions, and mind states.*

SCOPE

Communication encompasses all means by which people exchange messages with each other. The scope of the communication concept ranges from effective communication to no communication. Ineffective communication lies within this continuum. Forms of communications include verbal, nonverbal, symbolic, and metacommunication (Fig. 43.1).

Verbal language includes spoken and written word, conveying meaning through a collection of words. Vocabulary and intonation are examples that impact verbal communication. Nonverbal communication includes all communication that is not spoken or written. This form of communication is powerful and often complex, and can include influences such as eye contact, personal space, and facial expressions. Symbolic communication adds to what is understood by incorporating art and music to enhance meaning.[4] Metacommunication consists of the factors that comprise the context of the message. Because the ultimate goal of communication is to create meaning, the particular context or situation in which the communication act is occurring will have an effect on the meaning derived from the message.[4] Metacommunication factors that affect how messages are received and interpreted include internal personal states (e.g., disturbances in mood), environmental stimuli related to the setting of the communication, and contextual variables (e.g., the relationship between the people in the communication episode).

ATTRIBUTES AND CRITERIA

As defined, communication simply describes the transmission of ideas between people. However, the concept of communication becomes very complex when studied in-depth and is therefore a major field of study for academics and professionals in specialized fields such as speech therapy and linguistics. There are three attributes of communication that form the basis of study in the nursing sciences: a process of complementary exchange, context, and learned skill.[4]

Process of Complementary Exchange

The process of complementary exchange occurs between people. In the exchange, each participant is, in turn, either a sender or a receiver. In the act of communication, the reception and transmission of messages between participants is dynamic, cyclic, reciprocal, and interactive, where dialogue serves to support the creation of shared meaning. The sender encodes a message using symbols (both verbal and nonverbal) and transmits the created message to the receiver. As each transmission is completed, the receiver perceives the message, interprets the symbols, and then responds with another act of encoding and transmission of a response to the sender. The implication is that the meaning created for participants during the communication act is negotiated during the exchange while messages are perceived, decoded, and interpreted.[5] Because meaning results from negotiation, effective communication depends on mutual engagement and on the authenticity of each

415

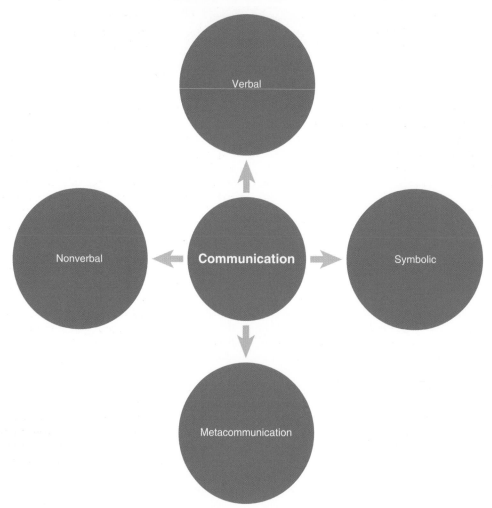

FIGURE 43.1 Forms of Communication.

participant's contributions during an exchange. The interpretation of meaning explains why communication by nurses to patients is subject to distortion or misinterpretation when the patient is ill, anxious, or distracted by pain. Communication messages and responses between nurses and patients can be misread or negatively perceived.[6]

Context

The metacommunication aspect, or context of communication, is important to the quality of meaning derived by participants during the process of complementary exchange. Contextual factors are those characteristics of the environment in which the communication occurs that affect perception and subsequent interpretation of messages by participants. Context can include factors such as the relationship between participants, internal mood states, mental and physical condition, experience and education, and external noise emitted from the environment.

Communication between people is both subject to and a reflection of relationships. The relationship could be relatively distant, or more intimate. Relational roles can affect the communication process. Symmetrical roles can yield equal relationships, while complementary relationships when one person is in a higher position than another can involve status and power and thus affect communication between the participants. For example, children might fear upsetting their parents

with some kinds of information because of the consequences of parental responses.[3,4]

Learned Skill

Communication is a learned skill that develops over time and through interactions with others. It is a complex interaction between a person's genetics and culture.[2] Becoming an expert communicator requires knowledge of the communication process and reflection of ones' communication experiences.[3] Gaining awareness of all the factors that influence communication help people better understand the message being communicated. Cognitive, behavioral, and cultural factors all influence communication. For nursing students, it is important to learn medical terminology to communicate with other healthcare professionals. A nurse should also be aware of intrapersonal communication, often called self-talk, because of the impact it could have on the nurse's way of thinking about the nursing care provided.[4,5]

THEORETICAL LINKS

The most basic theory of communication is a linear process model that describes a *sender* transmitting a *message* to a *receiver* (Fig. 43.2).[1] The process starts with a sender encoding a message, either verbally or

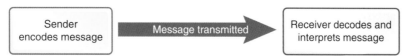

FIGURE 43.2 Basic Communication Theory.

nonverbally, and sending it to the receiver through some medium, such as voice or print. Upon perceiving the message, the receiver decodes and interprets the message, creating meaning from the symbols.

This simplistic representation fails to convey the true richness of the communication exchange as a means to create shared meaning among participants. As noted previously, there are a great many factors that affect the perception and interpretation of messages. A simple model such as this does not reflect the iterative complexity of communication acts in which messages are passing back and forth between participants in the exchange.[3] Actual communication episodes involve multiple acts of perception and interpretation, in addition to the creation of a mutually negotiated meaning. A more accurate representation is shown in the complex model of communication (Fig. 43.3), in which the interactive process depicts the influence of multiple factors on the meaning created during the interaction between participants.

To be effective, communication needs to be an active, two-way process with an exchange of clear, concise, accurate, timely, usable information between patients and healthcare professionals. Effective communication is correct when it is concrete, courteous, and complete. The negotiation of shared meaning in the communication encounter is impaired if the purpose of the communication is unclear or the symbols used for expression of the message are inappropriate.[7] A poorly worded memo can create much confusion among members of a workgroup because the true meaning of the message is questionable. Course syllabi that fail to provide clear direction because of incomplete information or errors will result in uncertainty for students. For nonnative speakers, the colloquialisms common to any foreign language can be inexplicable and the source of error and embarrassment. In all these situations, clarity and the goals of the message transmitted can be lost, and the ultimate meaning of the message distorted.

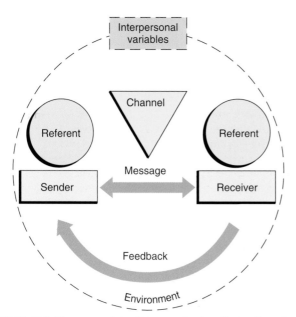

FIGURE 43.3 **Elements of the Communication Cycle.** (From Potter, P. A., Perry, A. G., Stockert, P., & Hall, A. [2019]. *Essentials for nursing practice* [9th ed.]. St. Louis: Elsevier.)

CONTEXT TO NURSING AND HEALTH CARE

Health care is a major social activity established for the purpose of helping people with their health concerns. It encompasses a variety of social structures that reflect the myriad of specialized relationships necessary for supporting the delivery of healthcare services. Nurses can expect to engage in multiple acts of communication daily in their work environments, perhaps even more so than in their personal lives. For nurses, effective communication is critically important. The professional role requires that nurses develop and practice a variety of communication skills that will ensure successful role function as well as the delivery of quality patient care. Because health care is relationship based, communication competence is highly valued for nurses, whether that communication is with patients or with other members of the healthcare services environment. Patient safety and health care quality, the electronic health record, and advocacy are also key elements of communication in today's healthcare environment.[5]

Communication Competence

Communication competence in nursing means that communication is both *effective* and *appropriate*. Effectiveness is achieved when the goals of the communication are met. Appropriate means the communication has been adapted to the people and situation involved in the act of communication.[1] Because communication is a learned skill, instruction begins early in nursing education related to a variety of behaviors and attitudes that produce the framework for communication competence in the nurse. Communication competence among nurses continues to evolve with experience and professional development throughout a nursing career. Professional nurses can expect to be tasked with the need to communicate as a caregiver and as a member of a healthcare profession, both of which require skill in interpersonal communication. As a caregiver, nurses are expected to effectively and appropriately communicate with patients and families and with members of the healthcare team. As members of the profession, nurses are expected to competently voice the concerns of patients, families, and communities to others both within the profession and in the larger health services' sector. Achieving communication competence in nursing is important for optimizing safety and quality in health care and for creating the voice and authority needed to advocate for better systems and safer workplaces.

Patient Safety and Health Care Quality

The Institute of Medicine (IOM) captured national attention in 2001 with the report, *To Err Is Human: Building a Safer Health Care System.*[8] In this report, the IOM noted that an estimated 98,000 medical errors each year were leading to unnecessary injury and even death for patients in the U.S. healthcare system. IOM reports since then have critically evaluated the safety and quality problems inherent to our healthcare systems, especially how these problems are related to the actions of healthcare professionals, including nurses.[9,10] Communication is frequently cited as a cause of errors in the delivery of health care, including being the leading cause of *sentinel events*, defined as unusually serious, unexpected events that occur during episodes of care. Sentinel events—such as wrong-site surgery, adverse drug events, or patient falls—not only result in harm to the patient but also lead to increased health care costs. Consequently, communication competence has become a critical skill that promotes quality of care and patient safety.[11]

One recommendation by the IOM is to educate health professionals to use practices and tools that support effective communication. A tool that supports consistent and accurate communication between professionals is the SBAR communication technique (Table 43.1). SBAR—which stands for Situation, Background, Assessment, and Recommendation—provides a framework for communication between members of the healthcare team. This easy-to-remember, concrete cue can be helpful in any communication, but especially when the patient situation is critical and requires immediate attention and action. By using this method, all healthcare professionals can better develop a culture of teamwork and patient safety.[12]

Electronic Health Record

Another fundamental communication skill for nurses is accurate and timely documentation in the patient record. Now that most inpatient settings are using an electronic health record (EHR), the potential for improving communication among healthcare providers in a variety of settings is enhanced. A digital record of a person's health history can facilitate timely transmission of complete and accurate information between providers. For example, the EHR provides a means for emergency personnel to access prior history and medical condition for patients who are too ill or too injured to provide a complete medical history. However, the speed of digital transmission and the potential for widespread dissemination of electronic records also create increased concerns related to accuracy and confidentiality. Documentation errors or omissions in the EHR can jeopardize patient safety and the quality of care

provided because multiple providers access these records and then make healthcare decisions based on inaccurate or faulty information. Nurses working with an EHR need to be cognizant of these potential threats to the quality of care and patient safety.

Advocacy

Communication competence is a necessary component for nurses to effectively function in the role of advocate. Advocacy is the act of speaking for others to assist them to meet needs, and it is an expectation for all who assume the role of professional nurse. The advocacy might be in the form of interceding with members of the healthcare team on behalf of patients or families, advocacy on behalf of these same members of the healthcare team, or even advocacy on behalf of the profession. The ability to speak out assertively, credibly, and authoritatively is a highly valued communication skill critical to effective advocacy. Principles of assertive communication are routinely taught in basic nursing education courses with continued refinement of the skill through professional development and graduate education.[4,5]

INTERRELATED CONCEPTS

Communication is the exchange of information between participants that leads to a negotiated, mutual understanding of a situation or phenomenon. As such, there are related concepts that are closely associated with communication (Fig. 43.4).

Communication is the structure that supports social interaction. Social interaction is the primary means for both Collaboration and Care Coordination. Nurses collaborate with patients and families in the development of a plan of care. Nurses also collaborate with members of the healthcare team, often functioning as the link between the patient and the rest of the team. As the link, nurses routinely coordinate care to ensure that the care is appropriately and safely delivered and that it is beneficial to patients. The importance of effective collaboration and care coordination to quality care and patient safety cannot be overemphasized. It is crucial that communication between the patient and the healthcare team as well as communication between the members of the healthcare team be clear, accurate, and timely. Errors, omissions, and gaps in communication can lead to dangerous and costly errors in care.[4]

TABLE 43.1	**SBAR Communication Tool**
Element	**Description**
Situation	What is happening at the current time?
Background	What are the circumstances leading up to this situation?
Assessment	What does the nurse think the problem is?
Recommendation	What should we do to correct the problem?

SBAR, Situation, background, assessment, and recommendation.
From Institute for Healthcare Improvement: *SBAR Toolkit*, 2014.
Retrieved from www.ihi.org/knowledge/pages/tools/sbartoolkit.aspx.

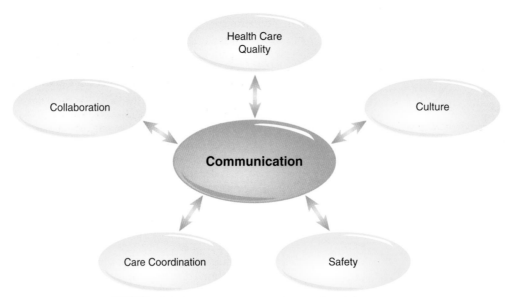

FIGURE 43.4 Communication and Interrelated Concepts.

Culture and communication exist in a symbiotic relationship. Cultures develop on the basis of an infrastructure of communications. Communications, especially the symbols used in language, dress, and patterns of behavior, are expressions of culture. Behavioral expectations and norms, values and traditions, the way relationships are built and maintained, the definition of personal space as dictated by cultural norms, and even the significance of words and gestures are possible because people are able to transmit ideas, values, emotions, and needs through communication acts. The relationship between culture and communication has important implications for nurses. As a profession that interacts with people from all cultures, nurses will frequently encounter different, culturally based communication practices. Nurses need a fundamental appreciation of cultural differences and the potential effect of these differences on care. By recognizing these differences, nurses are able to proactively address potential misperceptions and misunderstandings that might arise during the implementation and evaluation of care. Communications in organizations are affected by the prevailing culture and also serve to help mold the organizational culture. This is particularly important in health care because of the links between communication, organizational culture, Safety, and Health Care Quality. Communications and systems for communications must allow for clear, timely, and accurate communications between professionals working together in order to deliver quality patient care, unimpeded by contextual factors such as power and status. Effective communication is fundamental to safe systems, leading to the adoption of improved communication strategies by healthcare organizations to ensure quality care.[4]

CLINICAL EXEMPLARS

Communication for nurses encompasses a wide range of practices, most of which support effective interactions with others. Exemplars of communication represent situations within the context of professional nursing practice. A list of exemplars is presented in Box 43.1. Some of these exemplars are featured next.

Featured Exemplars

Assertive Communication

Assertive communication refers to a process in which positive and negative ideas and feeling are expressed in an open and direct way. Intentionally using assertive communication helps the nurse to advocate for the patient with other healthcare professionals. Many personal factors can play a role in a nurse's communication with others. Some of the influencing factors on communication are culture, gender, personality type, and level of self-confidence. Assertive communication respects the rights of all involved while allowing the sender to stand up for his or her beliefs.[4,5]

Therapeutic Communication

Therapeutic communication is a dynamic and interactive process in which words and actions are used by clinicians and patients to

BOX 43.1 EXEMPLARS OF COMMUNICATION

- Assertive communication
- Therapeutic communication
- Intrapersonal communication (self-talk)
- Interpersonal communication
- Interprofessional communication
- Electronic health record documentation
- Handoff/Reporting

ACCESS EXEMPLAR LINKS IN YOUR GIDDENS EBOOK

collaboratively achieve identified healthcare outcomes. Therapeutic communication becomes an important part of the healing process for patients and families. This type of communication promotes understanding and builds relationships that lead to positive patient outcomes.[13]

Interpersonal Communication

Embedded in relationships, interpersonal communication is the verbal and nonverbal interaction that occurs among human beings. This interaction can be one-to-one or occur within groups. Interpersonal communication and the resulting relationships begin at birth with the infant and parent, and they continue throughout the lifespan, satisfying the human need for connection with others. Many types of interpersonal relationships exist, including friendships, family, romantic, and, in nursing practice, nurse–patient relationships.

Electronic Health Record Documentation

Skill in using the EHR is a requirement in today's healthcare environment. Not only does the nurse need to adequately and thoroughly document patient care and patient condition, he or she must also be attentive to the need for accuracy and the overall need of the healthcare system to be able to retrieve a complete record of nursing care and patient condition. Most documentation systems incorporate a series of conventions and rules for use, and nurses must be fully aware of the expectations for documentation.

Handoff/Reporting

Nurses communicate with one another via end-of-shift or end-of-day report—often called the handoff. This is the process of nurse-to-nurse communication in which patient data are shared between shifts and at other points of transition, with the primary intent of ensuring accuracy and continuity of care. A common process for handoff reporting is the SBAR, described previously. Handoff and reporting are key components to effective communication and are directly related to safety, health care quality, and patient outcomes.[5,12]

CASE STUDY

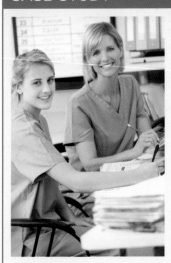

Case Presentation

Jenna Wright is a new graduate nurse eagerly anticipating her first day of work. She has been hired as a nurse in the surgical intensive care unit (ICU) of a large hospital and was selected for a 6-month residency program for new nurses offered by the hospital.

Jenna reports to her new nursing unit early on her first day. She waits at the nurses' station for her assigned preceptor, Diane Miller, who has 20 years of nursing practice experience. Diane was chosen by the unit manager to be Jenna's preceptor because of her communication skills and effective mentorship. Diane is familiar with the "first-day jitters" common with new nurses, so she also arrives slightly early and meets Jenna at the nurses' station. Diane walks directly to Jenna, smiles,

and greets her: "Hi, you must be Jenna. I'm Diane and I will be your preceptor during your residency. I have worked on this unit for the last 5 years and find I really enjoy the challenge of the surgical ICU." Jenna smiles shyly and nods her head, "I am so excited to be here…. It's great to finally be starting out, no longer a student." Diane laughs and nods her head, "Oh yes, I know. Students are fun to have on the unit but I also know there are limits on what they can do. Getting to spread your wings and learn this new role can be very exciting and we want you to be excited. We want you here and we are going to work really hard to get you oriented to the unit and help you get your 'feet on the ground.' We have a great team of nurses on this unit and we expect a lot of each other. We want you to be a part of that team and to learn and grow in the position. After all, that helps all of us, right? So let's find a place for your things and then we will go to report. You know, I think there is another new nurse working in the medical ICU. Let's see if we can arrange to have lunch with her and her preceptor."

Case Analysis Questions

1. What are three attributes of effective communication noted in the case?
2. What is one verbal and one nonverbal communication example in the case?
3. What is the impact of culture in this case?

Source: monkeybusinessimages/iStock/Thinkstock.

 ACCESS EXEMPLAR LINKS IN YOUR GIDDENS EBOOK

REFERENCES

1. Wood, J. (2016). *Interpersonal communication: Everyday encounters* (7th ed.). Boston: Wadsworth.
2. Samovar, L., Porter, R., & McDaniel, E. (2013). *Communication between cultures.* Boston: Wadsworth.
3. Arnold, E. (2016). Theory-based perspectives and contemporary dynamics. In E. Arnold & K. Boggs (Eds.), *Interpersonal relationships: Professional communication skills for nurses* (pp. 1–22). St Louis: Elsevier.
4. Finkelman, A. (2019). *Leadership and management in nursing.* Upper Saddle River, NJ: Prentice-Hall.
5. Crowe, C. (2017). Communication. In P. Potter, A. Perry, P. A. Stockert, & A. M. Hall (Eds.), *Fundamentals of Nursing, 9e.* St. Louis: Elsevier.
6. Boggs, K. (2016). Bridges and barriers in therapeutic relationships. In E. Arnold & K. Boggs (Eds.), *Interpersonal relationships: Professional communication skills for nurses* (pp. 202–216). St Louis: Elsevier.
7. Boggs, K. (2016). Professional guides for nursing communication. In E. Arnold & K. Boggs (Eds.), *Interpersonal relationships: Professional communication skills for nurses* (pp. 22–39). St Louis: Elsevier.
8. Institute of Medicine. (2000). *To err is human: Building a safer health care system.* Washington, DC: National Academies Press.
9. Institute of Medicine. (2001). *Crossing the quality chasm: A new health care system for the 21st century.* Washington, DC: National Academies Press.
10. Institute of Medicine. (2004). *Keeping patients safe: Transforming the work environment of nurses.* Washington, DC: National Academies Press.
11. Joint Commission Center for Transforming Health Care. (2017). *Hand-off communications.* Retrieved from http://www.centerfortransforminghealthcare.org/news/press/handoff.aspx.
12. Institute for Healthcare Improvement. *SBAR: situation-background-assessment-recommendation.* Retrieved from http://www.ihi.org/sites/search/pages/results.aspx?k=sbar.
13. Arnold, E. (2016). Developing communication skills. In E. Arnold & K. Boggs (Eds.), *Interpersonal relationships: Professional communication skills for nurses* (pp. 75–97). St Louis: Elsevier.

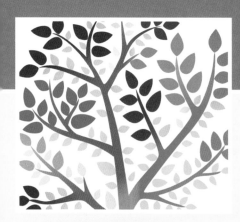

Collaboration

Judy Liesveld

When thinking about the profession and practice of nursing, the words "collaboration" and "nursing" seem inseparable. Nurses work with patients, families, communities, and other professionals in a multitude of settings from state-of-the-art hospitals to remote rural home settings and clinics. Collaboration involves building models of health care using the best ideas of our patients and our partners in the healthcare setting. Understanding collaboration is perhaps the key component for reducing errors in patient care. Collaboration remains an unclear concept with varying meanings and perspectives among health professionals. Exploration of the concept of collaboration will help to crystallize its meaning and its potential for advancing the nursing profession and for improving the health outcomes of our patients.

DEFINITION

The word *collaborate* is derived from the Latin word *collaborare*, meaning "to labor together." Collaboration usually has the connotation of working with others in an intellectual endeavor. Nurses labor with patients, families, and healthcare workers such as physicians, pharmacists, social workers, physical therapists, medical assistants, and other lay health workers using knowledge, reasoning, and critical thinking skills to promote or restore health. For the purposes of this concept presentation, collaboration in nursing is the *development of partnerships to achieve best possible outcomes that reflect the particular needs of the patient, family, or community, requiring an understanding of what others have to offer.* Collaboration also involves a joint responsibility for patient outcomes.[1]

SCOPE

The scope of collaboration spans four overarching categories, each based on collaboration with the nurse: nurse–patient, nurse–nurse, interprofessional, and interorganizational collaboration (Fig. 44.1).

Nurse–Patient Collaboration

Nurses are inherent collaborators. The American Nurses Association (ANA) identifies six standards for nursing practice known as the nursing process: assessment, diagnosis, outcomes identification, planning, implementation, and evaluation.[2] Opportunity for nurse–patient collaboration exists at each level of the process. Nurses particularly collaborate with patients as fully functional members of the healthcare team in making healthcare decisions.[3] For example, nurses collaborate with patients regarding health promotion and disease prevention behaviors, treatment strategies and options, lifestyle changes, and end-of-life decision making.

The historical context for nurse–patient collaboration is rich and extensive. Florence Nightingale encouraged collaboration with the patient, assessing what is needed or wanted.[4] In an early use of nurse–patient collaboration, Hildegard Peplau described a component of the working phase of her nursing theory as the patient participating with and being interdependent with the nurse.[5] Also, in her human-to-human relationship model of nursing, Joyce Travelbee defined nursing as an interpersonal process whereby the nurse assists an individual, family, or community to prevent or cope with the experience of illness and suffering and, if needed, to find meaning in these experiences.[6] Throughout the years, many other nurse theorists have examined and defined the nurse–patient relationship with elements of nurse–patient collaboration existing in many of the theories.

Nurse–Nurse Collaboration

Nurse–nurse collaboration, or intraprofessional collaboration, is also important to consider. How do nurses collaborate together? Nurses develop nursing teams on hospital units, in clinics, and in community settings that provide collaboration and support in patient caregiving. Nurses from various specialty areas also collaborate: nurse managers, nurse researchers, nurse educators, advanced practice nurses, as well as novice nurses with expert nurses.[7]

Mentoring

Mentoring is a special type of collaboration, or creative partnership, typically between a novice nurse and an expert nurse, that has been recognized as beneficial to the development of professional nurses.[8] Mentoring is described as purposeful activities that facilitate the career development, personal growth, caring, empowerment, and nurturance that are important to nursing practice and leadership.[9] The purpose of mentoring is to enable a smooth transition from novice nurse to a knowledgeable practitioner who is self-reflective and self-confident and who is able to negotiate both professional and patient relationships.[9] Despite the valuable benefits of mentoring, challenges to successful and constructive mentorships exist. Ketola stated that mentoring needs to go beyond the acquisition of knowledge and skills and include the socialization of a nurse transmitting the values, norms, and accepted modes of behavior for the professional nurse.[10] Jakubik also encouraged mentoring to progress from the traditional approach of fostering support, competency, and job retention to a more modern approach of

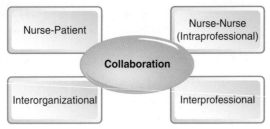

FIGURE 44.1 Scope of Collaboration.

promoting career development and advancement, similar to mentoring in the business world.[11]

Shared Governance

Shared governance, another type of collaboration found in nursing, is a model that fosters a decentralized style of management that creates an environment of empowerment.[12] Shared governance is seen as an important component of professional practice and pursuit of Magnet designation from the American Nurses Credentialing Center.[13] The goal of shared governance is to transition from a traditional hierarchical management style to one in which nursing staff are more involved in decision-making processes and managers are facilitative, rather than controlling.[14] Nurses practicing in a shared governance environment truly labor together and collectively develop collaborative relationships. Collaborating in the shared governance model, nurses can help improve quality of care and clinical effectiveness, facilitate the development of knowledge and skills, and increase professionalism and accountability.[15] Shared decision making, the cornerstone of shared governance, is an essential element to improve the healthcare system of the future.[14]

Interprofessional Collaboration

The true essence of collaboration involves working across professional roles. With interprofessional collaboration (IPC), individual areas of expertise are represented along with diverse perspectives influenced by professional orientation, experience, age, gender, education, and socioeconomic status.[16] The goal of IPC is to form a partnership between a team of health providers and a patient in a participatory, collaborative, and coordinated approach to share in decision-making of health and social issues.[17] The scope of IPC is vast and could include professionals from nursing, medicine, pharmacy, occupational therapy, physical therapy, dentistry, social work, education, law, or many others interacting with the patient and family. IPC can encounter challenges such as imbalance of power and authority, confusion of roles and responsibilities, and tension with boundaries when delivering patient care.[18]

Globally, health policy makers have recommended IPC as a primary approach to improve quality and safety in patient care. Anecdotally, nurses and other health professionals know that IPC improves patient outcomes as well as professional job satisfaction. A recent Cochrane Review of IPC,[18] however, found minimal impact of IPC strategies in improving patient care delivery. Following a rigorous literature search, nine studies with 5540 participants were reviewed. IPC strategies were found to slightly improve patient functional status, particularly in stroke patients, health professionals' adherence to best practices, and shared use of healthcare resources. Uncertainty of IPC improving patient assessed quality of care, continuity of care, or collaborative working relationships was found due to lack of clear evidence. Further rigorous research involving mixed methods studies, with longer periods of adjustment to new IPC strategies prior to undertaking research, was recommended.[18]

A growing trend in professional healthcare curricula is to offer interprofessional courses as a means of facilitating mutual respect,

understanding, and commitment to common goals; joint problem solving; mutual give and take; shared accountability; and collegial communication.[17] Many accrediting organizations, including the Commission on Collegiate Nursing Education, are incorporating interprofessional education (IPE) as a requirement for baccalaureate and graduate nursing programs.[19] Best practices to deliver IPE are being researched and developed. General opinion in IPE is that students benefit from learning to collaborate in an academic setting before they are expected to practice together in a care delivery setting. Studies have shown positive changes in medical students' attitudes toward their nurse colleagues when introduced to the diverse roles on interprofessional teams. Pfaff and colleagues found that new graduate nurses were more confident in IPC if their unit educator and manager had close proximity and were easily accessible, if different healthcare disciplines were worked with daily, and if satisfaction with the team existed.[20]

Many undergraduate nursing programs are combining interprofessional learning with simulation.[21] A recent integrative review of the literature of nine studies showed that the combination of interprofessional learning and simulation successfully increased collaboration and understanding of roles, improved communication and enhanced learning in practice between nursing students and other health professionals.[21]

Interorganizational Collaboration

Consideration of interorganizational collaboration is important in today's healthcare environment. Pooling of resources and information between organizations can benefit patients and communities at regional, national, or international levels. Interorganizational collaboration often takes place in the form of coalitions or consortiums. For example, nurses have been involved in coalitions addressing healthcare disparities, diabetes prevention, teen pregnancy, immunization rates, and health care for the homeless. Healthcare consortiums often exist in communities or regions to ensure integrated care delivery, information, and networking among healthcare deliverers. Academic, practice, and industry settings are recently collaborating to share big data sets that can be used in research to improve precision in measuring quality, patient outcomes, and cost of nursing care.[22]

ATTRIBUTES AND CRITERIA

The Interprofessional Education Collaborative Expert Panel, a panel representing 15 different professional entities (including the nursing, social work, pharmacy, medical, osteopathic, public health, and dental professions), identified four competencies or attributes necessary for effective IPC.[1] These attributes are transferable to intraprofessional collaboration, and they represent the ingredients (attributes) needed for successful collaboration. They are (1) values/ethics, (2) roles/responsibilities, (3) communication, and (4) teamwork/team-based practice. These are further described with several specific competencies mentioned for each attribute.

Values/Ethics

Values and ethics, undergirded with mutual respect and trust, are an important component in creating a professional and interprofessional identity. These values and ethics are embedded in patient-centeredness and strive for safer, more efficient, and more effective systems of care. Demonstration of interprofessional values would be evidenced by professionals working together and applying principles of altruism, excellence, caring, ethics, respect, communication, and accountability to achieve high-level health and wellness in individuals and communities.[1] The ethical principles considering health care as a right and balance in the distribution of resources are also important. Respect for diversity that is found in the individual expertise each profession contributes to care delivery is also considered. Ten competencies were identified for the attribute of values/ethics. The following four are highly pertinent for collaborative practice:

- Embrace the cultural diversity and individual differences that characterize patients, populations, and the healthcare team.
- Respect the unique cultures, values, roles/responsibilities, and expertise of other health professions.
- Work in cooperation with those who receive care, those who provide care, and others who contribute to or support the delivery of disease prevention and health services.
- Demonstrate high standards of ethical conduct and quality of care in one's contributions to team-based care.

Roles/Responsibilities

Collaboration requires an understanding of how professional roles and responsibilities support patient-centered care. Clearly articulating one's professional role and responsibilities to other professions and conversely understanding other professions' roles is a key element for effective collaboration. Recognizing legal boundaries and limits of professional expertise is also needed. Understanding that roles and responsibilities might change based on a specific care situation is important. The following three competencies are representative of roles and responsibilities in collaboration:

- Engage diverse healthcare professionals who complement one's own professional expertise, as well as associated resources, to develop strategies to meet specific patient care needs.
- Use the full scope of knowledge, skills, and abilities of available health professionals and healthcare workers to provide care that is safe, timely, efficient, effective, and equitable.
- Communicate with team members to clarify each member's responsibility in executing components of a treatment plan or public health intervention.

Communication

Communication has been defined as a core aspect of collaborative practice. A common language for team communication that avoids professional jargon is considered a key to safe and effective communication. Dismantling professional hierarchies created by demographic and professional differences is also valued in interprofessional communication. All professions and team members are equally empowered to speak up in firm, respectful ways regarding patient care issues. Finally, consideration of health literacy and effective use of communication technologies are viewed as important components of interprofessional communication. The following three competencies are shared as examples of collaborative communication:

- Organize and communicate information with patients, families, and healthcare team members in a form that is understandable, avoiding discipline-specific terminology when possible.
- Listen actively, and encourage ideas and opinions of other team members.
- Recognize how one's own uniqueness, including experience level, expertise, culture, power, and hierarchy within the healthcare team, contributes to effective communication, conflict resolution, and positive interprofessional working relationships.

Teams and Teamwork

Learning to be a good team player is an important component of collaboration. Teamwork behaviors involve collaboration in the patient-centered delivery of care and also in coordinating care with other health professionals so that gaps, redundancies, and errors are avoided. Teamwork also involves shared accountability, shared problem solving, and shared decision-making. The process of teamwork can occur in microsystems such as hospital units or with increasing complexity between organizations and communities. The following three competencies are representative for collaborative teamwork:

- Describe the process of team development and the roles and practices of effective teams.
- Engage other health professionals—appropriate to the specific care situation—in shared patient-centered problem solving.
- Apply leadership practices that support collaborative practice and team effectiveness.

THEORETICAL LINKS

Theory of Collaborative Decision Making in Nursing Practice

Kim's theory of collaborative decision making in nursing practice offers a solid framework for the concept of collaboration.[23,24] Kim developed her theory in the early 1980s, following society's renewed interest in human rights and demand for informed consent. Kim recognized that many different types of nursing care decisions are made for patients that influence their health in various ways and that patients have the resources required to be active participants in making healthcare decisions affecting the outcomes of nursing care.[23] Collaboration was defined as a process in which two or more individuals work together for the attainment of a goal—a process by which a joint influence on an action is produced. Kim's theoretical framework included the initial context of participant, both the patient and the nurse and their accompanying role expectations and attitudes, knowledge, personal traits, and definition of the situation. This initial context then influenced the context of the situation, including organizational components of decision making and the nursing care decision type, such as immediate- or long-term effects. Next, the primary outcomes of the decision-making process, the level of collaboration, and the nature of the decision were assessed. Kim stated that collaborative decision making could be assessed on a continuum in which the lowest level of collaboration is expressed as complete domination of decision making by the nurse and the highest level of collaboration is expressed as an equally influencing joint decision making.[23] Finally, the patient outcomes, the result of the primary outcomes, were determined: goal attainment, feelings of autonomy and control, satisfaction, health status, and recovery.

Kim's model specifically addresses collaboration between the patient and the nurse but could extend to collaboration with other family members or health professionals at the context of participant level, such as patient, caregiver, and nurse. Kim proposed several research questions to develop a knowledge base for the theory of collaboration in nursing.[23] These questions continue to hold relevancy for collaboration with patients, nurses, and other health professionals. The following is a list of some of these questions:

- Are there opportunities for patients to collaborate in making nursing care decisions?
- Do nurses believe in the value of patients' collaboration in making nursing care decisions?
- What are the relationships between the patients' collaboration in making nursing care decisions and patient outcomes?
- What are the consequences to nurses of patients' collaborations in making nursing care decisions?

Interprofessional Education Collaborative Model

The Interprofessional Education Collaborative developed a model that incorporates the four attributes of collaboration as previously described.[1] The model was derived from social theories of learning and complexity theory.[25] These theories recognize the social and experiential nature of interprofessional collaboration and the complex healthcare environment

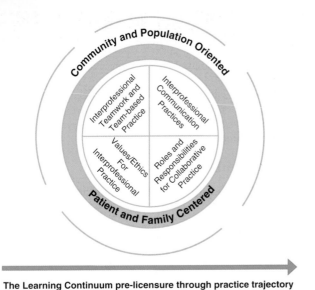

The Learning Continuum pre-licensure through practice trajectory

FIGURE 44.2 Interprofessional Collaborative Practice Domains. (From Interprofessional Education Collaborative Expert Panel. [2011]. *Core competencies for interprofessional collaborative practice: Report of an expert panel.* Washington, DC: Interprofessional Education Collaborative.)

in which it occurs. The attributes of communication, roles and responsibilities, values/ethics, and teamwork and team-based practice are equally distributed in a fluid circle surrounded by patient- and family-centered care (Fig. 44.2). A final outer layer including the importance of community- and population-oriented care is included. A straight arrow representing the learning continuum from prelicensure through practice trajectory is situated at the bottom of the circle in Fig. 44.2.

CONTEXT TO NURSING AND HEALTH CARE

The implications for collaboration and the nursing profession are expansive. The ANA's *Code of Ethics for Nurses* specifically addresses the importance of collaboration.[26] The code addresses the complexity of healthcare delivery systems, requiring a multidisciplinary approach

with the strong support and active participation of all health professions. The code states that within the context of collaboration, nursing's unique contribution, scope of practice, and relationship with other health professions needs to be clearly articulated, represented, and preserved. Nurses are encouraged to work together to ensure all relevant parties have a voice in informed decision making and patient care issues. Nurses are also encouraged to promote collaborative planning to ensure the availability and accessibility of quality health services. The code also addresses the importance of intraprofessional collaboration—that is, collaboration of practice nurses with educators, researchers, and administrators—because effective care is accomplished through the interdependence of nurses in differing roles.

The Quality and Safety Education for Nurses (QSEN) initiative anticipates that collaboration will have a major impact on positive patient outcomes and improve quality of care.[27] To date, conclusive results from research have been difficult to determine because of various definitions of collaboration, difficulty in measuring levels of collaboration, and small sample sizes.

Despite the difficulties of defining and measuring collaboration, there are hundreds of published narratives and reports involving interprofessional collaboration. Nursing is embracing the values and ethics of interprofessional collaboration by recognizing the roles of other team members and other disciplines. Effective communication with patients and families and other health professionals, and nurturing relationships to develop safe care, contributes to the health of individuals and communities.[28]

Collaboration also has potential to benefit health care at the organizational level. Achieving a sense of belonging and team identify is however more difficult at the organizational level because differences can exist between corporate cultures, geographical distances can be challenging, and formal paths of communication can be difficult to navigate. Research of collaboration between nurses and healthcare professionals from other organizations is encouraged as nurses have much to contribute to interorganizational collaboration.[29]

INTERRELATED CONCEPTS

Because there are many closely related concepts, collaboration is at times a fluid concept. Fig. 44.3 presents these interrelationships. **Professional Identity** involves use of nursing's full scope of knowledge,

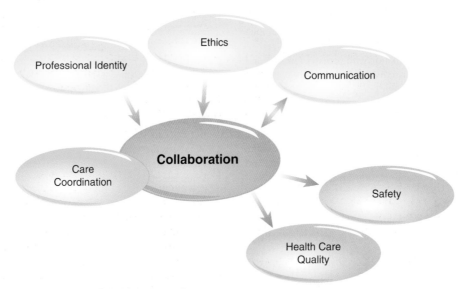

FIGURE 44.3 Collaboration and Interrelated Concepts.

skills, and abilities while clearly articulating the role of nursing in collaboration and respecting the boundaries of diverse professions. Ethics involves nurses' ethical comportment when working in cooperation with various professions, patients, and families. Altruism, excellence, caring, respect, and accountability are important considerations. Communication is also an important ingredient of collaboration because individuals from diverse backgrounds and professions need openness and clear communication skills and strategies for collaboration to occur.

The concept of Care Coordination is closely aligned and intertwined with collaboration; it is not possible to achieve highly efficient coordination of care without clearly effective collaboration among healthcare professionals and resources. Care coordination involves ensuring appropriate delivery of services and information, as well as coordination of resources to ensure optimal health and care across settings and time. These efforts occur while nurses, patients, and interprofessional teams collaborate to resolve a specific caregiving situation.

The outcomes of collaboration include healthcare quality and safety. Health Care Quality is a desired outcome when collaboration occurs. Serious quality problems continue to plague the healthcare industry despite highly trained and technically skilled professionals. Error prevention, specifically reducing sentinel events and near-miss events, requires a whole systems' approach that seeks to understand the parts and their interactions, as well as the broader context in which they are embedded. Questions involving the expectations, assumptions, habits, behaviors, history, and tradition that influenced an adverse situation must be asked. A better understanding of the whole is needed for intelligent leadership and quality results in today's healthcare organizations. Collaboration with diverse professionals and patient-centeredness can make this happen. Safety is also a concept that is influenced by collaboration. Multiple threats to patient safety and errors occur at all levels of healthcare delivery. The Institute of Medicine (IOM), along with the QSEN initiative, has changed from an emphasis on errors to widespread system change to ensure safety. A culture of safety is being promoted. The IOM encourages training programs for effective communication and collaboration including transitions and handoffs. Collaboration is at the heart of resolving safety issues and creating a culture of safety in nursing and health care.

CLINICAL EXEMPLARS

The concept of collaboration with patients, nurses, and other professionals clearly has the potential to improve the safety and quality of healthcare delivery. Nurses must continue to find ways to clearly articulate the nursing component of health care in collaborative arenas. Involvement of nurses in the development of models of collaboration and development of collaborative interventions is needed. These collaborative strategies will continue to benefit patients, nursing, other professions, and healthcare organizations. There are many examples of collaboration within nursing and health care. These are presented as exemplars in Box 44.1, using the categories previously discussed.

Featured Exemplars
Patient Care Handoffs

Handoffs using communication tools such as SBAR (Situation, Background, Assessment, and Recommendation) offer opportunity for collaboration in many situations. Collaborative handoffs can occur between nurses during shift change, between nurses when transferring patients to different units or facilities, between nurses and providers when receiving orders on patients, or between nurses and other healthcare workers when communicating critical information about patients. Many entities, such as the Joint Commission, the Institute for Health Improvement,

BOX 44.1 EXEMPLARS OF COLLABORATION

Nurse–Patient Collaboration
- Collaboration on plan of care
- Collaboration from time of assessment to discharge plan
- Home care models
- Community partnerships
- Community-based participatory research

Nurse–Nurse Collaboration
- Quality improvement project
- Mentoring programs
- Dedicated information exchange: meetings, memos, e-mail
- Shared governance
- Patient care handoff
- Student nurse collaborative learning

Interprofessional Collaboration
- Rapid response teams
- Ethics committees
- Specialty care teams
- Patient rounding
- Team meetings for information exchange
- Quality improvement committee to discuss near-miss or sentinel events
- Patient care handoff
- Disaster preparedness teams
- Interprofessional education
- Interprofessional practice

Interorganizational Collaboration
- Regional, national, or international coalitions
- Healthcare consortiums

ACCESS EXEMPLAR LINKS IN YOUR GIDDENS EBOOK

and nursing's QSEN initiative, recognize collaborative handoffs as an important strategy for the safety of patients.

Interprofessional Education

Participation in interprofessional education (IPE) events in educating nurses, medical students, pharmacy students, and many other healthcare professions is an outcome goal in almost every healthcare college or university. Students are exposed to many different disciplines and their role in caring for patients. Students collaborate with each other on a variety of interprofessional projects, including quality and safety initiatives, community health projects, disaster preparedness, collaborative care in clinical settings, and many other interprofessional opportunities. IPE is recognized as an important educational component as students enter the workforce and collaborate for the best outcomes for patients, families, and communities.

Community Partnerships

Healthcare professionals from many disciplines come together to work on a common initiative important to their community, such as a collaborative initiative on child abuse and neglect. In such an example, the collaborative collectively works on goals and strategies to ameliorate this identified community problem. Other examples of community collaboratives include homelessness, access to health care, nutrition in schools, and care of the elderly. The potential for positive healthcare outcomes for local, national, and international communities is endless with individuals and communities working toward a common goal.

Patient Rounding

Patient rounding refers to the process of purposeful rounds to see each patient in each room or area on a regular basis. Patient rounding is often done by interprofessional teams to monitor progress and clearly communicate goals and a plan for each patient. Patient rounds are frequently mentioned as a means for collaboration, but reviews are mixed with regard to whether this is an effective strategy for collaboration.[18] Patient rounding may also be done by a nursing staff with the goal to check on patients on a predetermined basis (e.g., hourly) to determine if they have any needs, such as addressing pain level and assisting them with basic needs.

Specialty Care Team

A specialty care team is an interprofessional team of healthcare professionals who work together around a specific type of patient or population need. Specialty team members represent various disciplines (medicine, nursing, pharmacology, physical therapy, occupational therapy, nutrition, social work, etc.) and contribute to the team by sharing their area of expertise, thus providing the best collective thinking for patient care. Examples of specialty care teams include pediatric, geriatric, pain, wound care, pulmonology, oncology, cardiac, and palliative care teams.

CASE STUDY

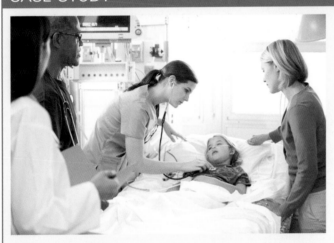

Case Presentation

Melanie is a 4-year-old girl with cystic fibrosis and developmental delays. She is from a small rural community. Melanie is currently hospitalized at a large tertiary care center for a "tune-up" consisting of vigorous chest physiotherapy and antibiotics. Kayla is an experienced registered nurse mentoring Janelle, a new graduate nurse who has not worked with patients with cystic fibrosis. Together they are working with Melanie's parents on a nursing plan of care

during the hospitalization. The Child Life program has also been included in Melanie's plan of care to ensure developmental appropriateness for Melanie's hospital experience.

The pediatric pulmonary team (consisting of the pulmonologist, social worker, nutritionist, nurse practitioner, and nurse educator) meets with Melanie's parents and the pediatric unit nursing staff to discuss the need for a gastrostomy tube because of Melanie's poor weight gain and past aspiration episodes. Via telehealth modalities, Melanie's primary care provider, a pediatric nurse practitioner from Melanie's hometown, joins the team conference. Kayla has also linked Melanie's family with a parent advocacy group and has invited a representative to be present at the meeting to ensure understanding of the presented information. Melanie's parents ask many questions regarding the gastrostomy tube placement. The questions are met with open, honest answers using evidence-based information as appropriate. Joint decision making occurs with agreement to have the surgery scheduled. At the end of their shift, Kayla and Janelle handoff information to the oncoming nurse at Melanie's bedside. The parents are present to hear and contribute to the report and plans for Melanie's care. Kayla and Janelle leave work feeling a sense of joy and accomplishment.

Case Analysis Questions

1. Reflecting on the scope of the concept, what type of opportunities for collaboration are evident in this case?
2. Which attributes of collaboration are apparent in this case?

Source: monkeybusinessimages/iStock/Thinkstock.

 ACCESS EXEMPLAR LINKS IN YOUR GIDDENS EBOOK

REFERENCES

1. Interprofessional Education Collaborative Expert Panel. (2016). *Core competencies for interprofessional collaborative practice: 2016 Update.* Washington, DC: Interprofessional Education Collaborative.
2. American Nurses Association. (2015). *Nursing: Scope and standards of practice* (3rd ed.). Washington, DC: Author.
3. Agency for Healthcare Research & Quality. (2017). *Guide to patient and family engagement in hospital quality and safety.* Rockville, MD: Author.
4. Nightingale, F. N. (1992). *Notes on nursing: What it is and what it is not* (Com ed.). Philadelphia: Lippincott. (original work published 1859).
5. Peplau, H. E. (1988). *Interpersonal relations in nursing.* New York: Springer. (original work published 1952, New York, Putnam's Sons).
6. Travelbee, J. (1971). *Interpersonal aspects of nursing* (2nd ed.). Philadelphia: Davis.
7. Benner, P. (1984). *From novice to expert: Excellence and power in clinical nursing practice.* Menlo Park, CA: Addison-Wesley.
8. Cervera-Gasch, A., Macia-Soler, L., Torres-Manrique, B., et al. (2017). Questionnaire to Measure the Participation of Nursing Professionals in Mentoring Students. *Investigación y educación en enfermería, 35*(2), 182–190.
9. Hale, R. (2018). Conceptualizing the mentoring relationship: An appraisal of evidence. *Nursing Forum, 53,* 333–358.
10. Ketola, J. (2009). An analysis of a mentoring program for baccalaureate nursing students: Does the past still influence the present? *Nursing Forum, 44*(4), 245–255.
11. Jakubik, L., Weese, M., Eliades, A., & Huth, J. (2017). Mentoring in the career continuum of a nurse: Clarifying purpose and timing. *Pediatric Nursing, 43*(3), 149–152.
12. Weaver, S., Hess, R., Williams, B., et al. (2018). Measuring shared governance: One healthcare system's experience. *Nursing Management, 49*(10), 11–14.
13. American Nurses Credentialing Center. (2019). *2019 Magnet application manual.* Silver Spring, MD: American Nurses Credentialing Center.
14. Dechairo-Marino, A., Raggi, M., & Mendelson, S. (2018). Enhancing and advancing shared governance through a targeted decision-making redesign. *The Journal of Nursing Administration, 48*(9), 445–451.

15. Disch, J. (2010). Teamwork and collaboration competency resource paper. *Quality and Safety Education for Nurses.*

16. Canadian Interprofessional Health Collaborative. (2010). *A national interprofessional competency framework.* Vancouver, British Columbia, Canada: Author.

17. Sterchi, L. (2007). Perceptions that affect physician–nurse collaboration in the perioperative setting. *AORN Journal, 86*(1), 45–57.

18. Reeves, S., Pelone, F., Harrison, R., et al. (2017). Interprofessional collaboration to improve professional practice and healthcare outcomes. *The Cochrane Database of Systematic Reviews,* (6), CD000072.

19. *Commission on Collegiate Nursing Education: Accreditation,* 2018. Retrieved from https://www.aacnnursing.org/CCNE-Accreditation.

20. Pfaff, K., Baxter, P., Jack, S., et al. (2014). Exploring new graduate nurse confidence in interprofessional collaboration: A mixed methods study. *International Journal of Nursing Studies, 51,* 1142–1152.

21. Granheim, B., Shaw, J., & Mansah, M. (2018). The use of interprofessional learning and simulation in undergraduate nursing programs to address interprofessional communication and collaboration: An integrative review of the literature. *Nurse Education Today, 62,* 118–127.

22. Jenkins, P., Garcia, A., Farm-Franks, D., et al. (2018). Academic/practice/industry collaboration to develop nursing value research data warehouse governance. *Nursing Economic, 36*(5), 207–212.

23. Kim, H. (1983). Collaborative decision-making in nursing practice: A theoretical framework. In P. Chinn (Ed.), *Advances in nursing theory development* (pp. 271–283). Rockville, MD: Aspen.

24. Kim, H. (1987). Collaborative decision-making with clients. In K. J. Hannah (Ed.), *Clinical judgment and decision-making: The future with nursing diagnosis* (pp. 58–62). New York: Wiley.

25. Sargeant, J. (2009). Theories to aid understanding and implementation of interprofessional education. *The Journal of Continuing Education in the Health Professions, 29*(3), 178–184.

26. American Nurses Association. (2015). *Code of ethics for nurses with interpretive statements.* Washington, DC: Author.

27. Cronenwett, L., Sherwood, G., Barnsteiner, J., et al. (2007). Quality and safety education for nurses. *Nursing Outlook, 55,* 122–131.

28. Jakubowski, T., & Perron, T. (2018). Interprofessional collaboration improves healthcare. *Reflections on Nursing Leadership.* Retrieved from https://www.reflectionsonnursingleadership.org/features/more-features/interprofessional-collaboration-improves-healthcare.

29. Karam, M., Brault, I., VanDurme, T., & Macq, J. (2018). Comparing interprofessional and interorganizational collaboration in healthcare: A systematic review of the qualitative research. *International Journal of Nursing Studies, 79,* 70–83.

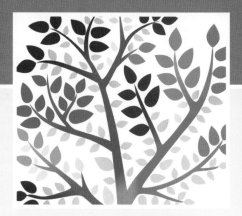

CONCEPT

45

Safety

Gail Elizabeth Armstrong and Gwen Sherwood

Patient safety has always been fundamental to the delivery of responsible health care, but over the past two decades new knowledge, skills, and attitudes have enhanced how it is understood and operationalized. New theories and frameworks inform current applications of safety science that describe the impact of complex systems as a context of health care, how errors and near misses are recognized and reported, ways to manage the myriad of human factors that impact safe care delivery, and competencies required for health professionals to work in cultures of safety. These concepts undergird the new safety science for health care adapted from the approach to safety first developed in other high-performance industries and are now being adapted to healthcare systems. Important shifts in these advances focus not only on considering personal responsibility and accountability in the delivery of safe care but also on how to direct efforts to system improvements to mitigate the possibility of errors. Nursing has historically focused on maintaining patient safety and integrating new concepts of keeping patients safe. Safety science require all healthcare professionals to adopt the new knowledge, skills, and attitudes to achieve practice changes identified in national reports from the Institute of Medicine (IOM). The new focus extends personal responsibility and accountability to incorporate safety from a systems perspective so that analysis of events includes system changes to prevent future occurrences.

DEFINITION

Many of the safety concepts used to improve today's healthcare system originate from the IOM's groundbreaking work in patient safety. Beginning with the 2000 publication *To Err Is Human*, the IOM alerted the healthcare industry and the public to the problem of deaths from preventable errors. In this report, the IOM offers a definition of safety as "freedom from accidental injury."[1] An expanded definition of patient safety is offered in this report's appendix: "Freedom from accidental injury; ensuring patient safety involves the establishment of operational systems and processes that minimize the likelihood of errors and maximizes the likelihood of intercepting them when they occur."[1,p11] In *Crossing the Quality Chasm* (2001), the IOM defines safe care as "avoiding injuries to patients from the care that is intended to help them."[2,p5] An important emphasis in this IOM report is the expectation of consistent safety in our healthcare systems:

The health care environment should be safe for all patients, in all of its processes, all of the time. This standard of safety implies that

organizations should not have different, lower standards of care on nights and weekends or during time of organizational change.[2,p45]

In a third report in this series, *Keeping Patients Safe* (2004), the IOM defines safe care as care that maintains a focus on using evidence in clinical decisions to maximize the health outcomes while also reducing the potential for harm. In its exploration of safe care, this IOM report addresses errors of commission (did not provide correct care) as well as errors of omission (did not provide care).[3]

The National Patient Safety Foundation (NPSF), formerly an independent, not-for-profit organization with a mission to improve the safety of care for all patients, merged with the Institute for Healthcare Improvement. NPSF defines patient safety as the "prevention of health care errors, and the elimination or mitigation of patient injury caused by healthcare errors."[4] To further clarify this definition, NPSF defines healthcare errors as unintended healthcare outcomes caused by a defect in the delivery of care to a patient. Healthcare errors may be errors of commission (doing the wrong thing), omission (not doing the right thing), or execution (doing the right thing incorrectly). Errors may be made by any member of the healthcare team in any healthcare setting.[4] A recent concept analysis of the concept of patient safety includes prevention of medical errors and avoidable adverse events, collaborative efforts by individual healthcare providers and a strong, well-integrated healthcare system.[5]

The NPSF report, *Safety Is Personal: Partnering With Patients and Families for the Safest Care*, emphasizes how collaboration with patients and families through ongoing engagement can transform safety outcomes. Specific action items are clearly identified to enable health leaders, clinicians, and policymakers to accentuate the overlap of engagement and patient safety as interrelated phenomena. A key component is how providers, especially nurses, work with the patient and family as a safety ally; they can be invited to observe and report gaps or omissions in care to help avoid errors and near misses.[6]

The work of defining safety and safe care by the IOM is relevant for all healthcare professionals and emphasizes safety from the patient's perspective. In nursing, a Robert Wood Johnson Foundation-funded national initiative, Quality and Safety Education for Nurses (QSEN), builds on IOM's work and defines safety as "minimizing risk of harm to patients and providers through both system effectiveness and individual performance."[7] This competency definition is further explicated by the necessary knowledge, skill, and attitude elements to demonstrate safety in one's practice and can be found on QSEN's website

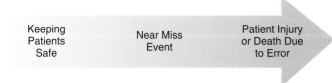

FIGURE 45.1 Scope of Safety.

3. Preventive errors occur when there are failures to provide prophylactic treatment and inadequate monitoring or follow-up of treatment.
4. Communication failure (meaning a lack of communication or a lack of clarity in communication) can lead to many types of errors.

By employing a standardized system for classifying different types of errors, best practices can be developed to address safety compromises in healthcare systems.

Placement of Errors

Along with types of error, the placement of errors may be described as active or latent. This distinction is important in further understanding the etiology of healthcare errors and appropriate improvements. In health care, active errors are made by those providers (e.g., nurses, physicians, and technicians) who are providing patient care, responding to patient needs at the "sharp end," which is at the point of care (Fig. 45.2).[11,12] Latent conditions are the potential contributing factors that are hidden and lie inactive in the healthcare delivery system, originating at more remote aspects of the healthcare system, far removed from the active end.[13] Latent errors—more organizational, contextual, and diffuse in nature or design-related—are called errors occurring at the "blunt end."[11] A latent failure is a flaw in a system that does not immediately lead to an accident but establishes a situation in which a triggering event may lead to an error.[14] Identifying errors as either active or latent in origin allows more accurate identification and correction of the exact system that needs improvement. Most bedside nurse clinicians operate at the sharp end of health care and are involved with active errors or inherit latent errors that can manifest as active errors. For example, a nurse who administers the incorrect medication because of a failure to check the medication order is involved in an active error. However, a medication error can occur in which a latent error leads to an active error. For example, a latent error can lead to an active error if a Pyxis (or other medication administration system) is incorrectly stocked with a look-alike, sound-alike medication that a nurse mistakenly administers based on what should have been stocked in a certain Pyxis compartment. As nurses learn about differences between active and latent errors, they can more accurately identify and contribute to processes or systems for improvement.

Improving safety is a continual balance of individual competence and awareness of safety with the need for system improvements—for example, safety is a partnership between individuals and the systems in which they work. Recent models for improving safety across the complex systems in health care emphasize addressing system safety because of increased awareness of latent errors. A 2017 Institute for

(http://qsen.org). Definitions regarding the levels of errors are also important to understand and include:
- **Adverse event**: An event that results in unintended harm to the patient by an act of commission or omission rather than by the underlying disease or condition of the patient.[8]
- **Near miss**: An error of commission (did not provide care correctly) or omission (did not provide care) that could have harmed the patient, but serious harm did not occur as a result of chance (e.g., the patient received a contraindicated drug but did not experience an adverse drug reaction), prevention (e.g., a potentially lethal overdose was prescribed, but a nurse identified the error before administering the medication), or mitigation (e.g., a lethal dose was administered but discovered early and countered with an antidote).[8]
- **Sentinel event**: A sentinel event is an unexpected occurrence involving death or serious physical or psychological injury, or the risk thereof. Serious injury specifically includes loss of limb or function. The phrase "or the risk thereof" includes any process variation for which a recurrence would carry a significant chance of a serious adverse outcome. Such events are called "sentinel" because they signal the need for immediate investigation and response.[8]

Ongoing focus on patient safety has resulted in a decrease in adverse events in hospital care. For example, according to a 2015 National Healthcare Quality and Disparities Report, the overall rate of hospital-acquired conditions (including catheter associated urinary tract infections, pressure ulcers and adverse drug events) decreased by an estimated 17% between 2010 and 2014.[9]

SCOPE

The concept of safety is broad and encompasses the ideal of keeping all patients safe to the unfortunate reality that errors can lead to injury or death (Fig. 45.1). Several key elements associated with this perspective include gaining an understanding of the types of errors, placement of errors, and ways of building a culture of safety.

Types of Errors

In nursing, safety has focused on the safe execution of specific procedures and tasks. However, recent safety work has emphasized the variety of errors that compromise patient safety and the range of variables that impact the occurrence of errors in health care. Understanding types of errors in health care is a vital element in addressing individual practice and improving healthcare systems. In its early report, the IOM cites a pioneer in the field of patient safety, Lucian Leape, who identified four types of errors:[10]
1. Diagnostic errors are the result of a delay in diagnosis, failure to employ indicated tests, use of outmoded tests, or failure to act on results of monitoring or testing.
2. Treatment errors occur in the performance of an operation, procedure, or test; in administering a treatment; in the dose or method of administering a drug; or in avoidable delay in treatment or in responding to an abnormal test.

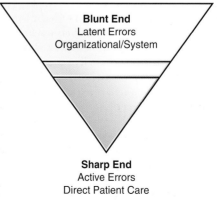

FIGURE 45.2 Active and Latent Errors.

Healthcare Improvement (IHI) white paper, *A Framework for Safe, Reliable and Effective Care*, focuses on two foundational domains for preventing errors: healthcare culture and the learning system.[15] The report emphasizes that in addition to teaching individuals and teams, advances are needed for designing safer healthcare systems to address the many kinds of errors that occur.

Culture of Safety

A common focal point in the advancements in safety over the past decade is a clearer focus on patient outcomes for healthcare clinicians and facilities. Historically, a culture of blame has been pervasive in health care. When an error occurred, the focus was often on identifying the clinician at fault and meting out discipline.[16] With greater focus on the role of safety in patient outcomes, healthcare teams now investigate what went wrong rather than just blaming the individual clinician who executed the error. Balancing the historical emphasis on blame within the broader context of a culture of safety is vital to effectively addressing error occurrence. A commonly cited definition of safety culture derives from the Health and Safety Commission of Great Britain and is utilized by the Agency for Healthcare Research and Quality (AHRQ): "The safety culture of an organization is the product of individual and group values, attitudes, perceptions, competencies, and patterns of behavior that determine the commitment to, and the style and proficiency of, an organization's health and safety management."[17] Research into the impact of the development of a culture of safety within a hospital indicates that higher levels of patient safety culture are associated with higher safety performance, and hospitals where employees reported more fear and shame had a significantly higher risk of safety problems.[18]

From an organizational context, a culture of safety acknowledges the influence of complex systems and human factors that influence safety. In a culture of safety, the focus is on teamwork to accomplish the goal of safe, high-quality care. When errors or near misses occur, the focus is on what went wrong rather than on who committed the error. The focus shifts from identifying fault to establish blame and determine discipline to acknowledging and reporting errors and near misses to improve the system. Accountability is a critical aspect of a culture of safety; recognizing and acknowledging one's actions is a trademark of professional behavior.

Safety culture literature identifies seven aspects that define the concept and thus contribute to a culture of safety in a healthcare organization: Leadership, teamwork, an evidence base, communication, learning, a just culture, and patient-centered care.[19] Safety culture is complex and is built through support from the organization leadership, policy, and the bedside clinician.[19] Empowering staff to participate in an error-reporting system without fear of punitive action is an essential aspect of creating a culture of safety. In surveying nurses and physicians, a barrier to reporting medication errors and near-miss events is the fear of professional or personal punishment.[20-22] As the largest segment of the healthcare workforce, nurses are central to creating and maintaining a culture of safety in any healthcare setting. From the bedside to the administrative suite, nurses can contribute to all aspects of a culture of safety.

ATTRIBUTES AND CRITERIA

What knowledge, skills, and attitudes are required for nurses to effectively contribute to safety in health care? The QSEN project has been the national leader in defining the competency for safety by specifying the knowledge, skill, and attitude objectives for prelicensure students. A national expert panel of thought leaders in each competency used an iterative process to reach consensus on the essential knowledge, skill,

and attitude objectives that all nurses need to contribute to developing systems of safety in health care.

Knowledge

Historically, the emphasis in nursing has been on the safe execution of discrete skills. However, contemporary nurses need to be knowledgeable in examining human factors and other basic safety design principles as well as make the distinction with commonly used unsafe practices (e.g., workarounds and dangerous abbreviations). Nurses need to be able to describe the benefits and limitations of selected safety-enhancing technologies (e.g., barcodes, computerized provider order entry, medication pumps, and automatic alerts/alarms). Educating nurses in effective strategies to reduce reliance on memory (e.g., checklists) encourages nurses to understand safety as an individual as well as a systems phenomenon. As nurses become more knowledgeable about safety at the systems level, they can delineate general categories of errors and hazards in care (e.g., active vs. latent and diagnostic, treatment, and preventive errors). Nurses need to be able to describe factors that create a culture of safety (e.g., open communication strategies and organizational error-reporting systems). Nurses must understand the processes used in understanding the cause of error and allocation of responsibility and accountability through such processes as root cause analysis (RCA) and failure mode effects analysis (FMEA). An important facet of nurses' knowledge is their appreciation of the potential and actual impact of national patient safety resources, initiatives, and regulations to effectively use and contribute to these important facets of standardized safe practices.

Skills

Nurses need skills to utilize tools that contribute to safer systems. For example, nurses must develop skills in the effective use of technology and standardized practices that support safety and quality as well as effectively use strategies to reduce risk of harm to self or others. Communication failures are the leading cause of inadvertent patient harm.[23] It is vital for nurses to develop skills to communicate observations or concerns related to hazards and errors to patients, families, and the healthcare team. Nurses' ability to engage patient participation in safety measures is an essential element of effective patient participation and improves outcomes.[24] Nurses have the responsibility to use organizational error-reporting systems for near miss and error reporting and to participate in analyzing errors and designing system improvements (e.g., RCAs). Nurses are responsible for their own individual practices while also contributing to the development of safer systems. Applying the national patient safety resources to his or her professional development will also enhance the capacity to focus attention on safety in care settings.

Attitudes

Nurses' personal and professional attitudes are instrumental in shaping their nursing practice and recognizing the cognitive and physical limits of human performance. Safety systems utilize principles of standardization and reliability—doing things in the same evidence-based way to get the same result every time—as part of error prevention strategies. Professionals value their own role in preventing errors and realize the difference that one person can make in prevention, even for one patient and family. Developing an attitude of collaboration across the healthcare team to ensure safe coordination of care contributes to safe care. It is the collective and shared environmental scanning and vigilance by all team members (e.g., patients, families, and all disciplines and staff) that prevents errors. As nurse clinicians perceive their own local practices as components of the broader national safety initiatives, patient outcomes can be incrementally improved at the local and national levels.

THEORETICAL LINKS

Theoretical links that further explicate safety include human factors, crew resource management, and high reliability organizations.

Human Factors

Principles of human factors have been adapted from engineering and expanded to address processes in health care by studying the interrelationship between people, technology, and the environment in which they work.[25] Human factors consider the ability or inability to perform exacting tasks while attending to multiple things at once. Human factors offer a systematic approach to studying process and outcome effectiveness for greater error prevention and greater efficiency. Within human factors healthcare research, attention is paid to all levels of care provision: external environment, management, physical environment, human–system interfaces, organizational/social environments, the nature of the work being done, and individual characteristics and aspects of performance.[13] Recent human factors research in patient safety has focused on the ability of systems to anticipate the potential for failure through focusing on usability of technology, human error, and clinician performance and resilience.[26]

In employing a human factors framework to health care, the emphasis is on both supporting healthcare professionals' performance and eliminating hazards. Human factors is another example of the interdependence between individuals and systems. Supporting healthcare professionals' performance in systems design includes physical performance, cognitive performance, and social/behavioral performance.[27] Simultaneously, consideration should be given to designing systems that avoid hazards. A hazard is anything that increases the probability of errors or patient/employee injury.[27] The dual consideration of supporting healthcare professionals and eliminating hazards is a qualitative shift to the development of systems that do not respond reactively to error occurrence but instead work proactively to avoid errors in an anticipatory way through the purposeful design of safer systems. A culture of safety requires organizational leadership that gives attention to human factors such as managing workload fluctuations, seeking strategies to minimize interruptions in work, and attending to communication and coordination across disciplines including power gradients and excessive professional courtesy.

Applying a human factors framework to guide research in appreciating and quantifying processes that lead to error will increase our understanding of the complexity of nurses' work in the acute care environment. Ebright and colleagues identify eight patterns that represent to the intersection of human factors and the complexity of nursing work in the acute care environment:[14]

- Disjointed supply sources
- Missing or nonfunctioning supplies and equipment
- Repetitive travel
- Interruptions
- Waiting for systems/processes
- Difficulty in accessing resources to continue care
- Breakdown in communication
- Communication media

Using a human factors paradigm to guide research highlights how work complexity can threaten patient care continuity and contribute to medical error.[14] Nurses confront challenging human factors situations every day that impact safety, such as multitasking, distractions, complacent attitudes, fatigue, task fixation that limits environmental scanning, and failure to follow up or follow protocol. Helping nurses understand human factors can inform their understanding of safety and further facilitate nursing's contributions toward the development of safer healthcare delivery systems.

Crew Resource Management

Crew resource management (CRM) training was developed in the aviation industry to standardize procedures, standardize communication, decrease errors, and increase efficiency. Within aviation, crew resource management has been defined as a set of instructional strategies designed to improve teamwork by applying well-tested training tools (e.g., performance measures, exercises, and feedback mechanisms) and appropriate training methods (e.g., simulators, lectures, and videos) targeted at specific content (i.e., teamwork knowledge, skills, and attitudes).[28] CRM emphasizes the role of human factors in high-stress, high-risk work environments. The work environments of health care and aviation share the characteristics of high stress, complexity, the need for highly functioning teams, the importance of accurate and precise communication, and the high cost of system failures.[29]

CRM has been used to improve team functioning in operating rooms, emergency departments, labor and delivery, and perioperative areas. CRM programs are tailored to an individual organization to consider specific human factors that contribute to errors and near misses in that particular environment.[30] Critical reviews of CRM training programs in health care indicate the need for further study to validate effectiveness[28] to determine the transfer of the learned behavior to provision of care.

Application of CRM principles to guide improvement work in healthcare settings is becoming more common. A 2013 unit-based project applied sterile cockpit principles to protect nurses from distractions during medication administration through the use of "Do Not Disturb" signs and donning of orange vests by nurses administering medications.[31] In tracking the type and frequency of distractions, there was a decrease in the number of distractions over time as well as a decrease in medication error rates. The generalizability and sustainability of CRM interventions is a common question because unit culture and staff buy-in can vary dramatically between agencies.

High Reliability Organizations

High reliability organizations (HROs) manage work that involves hazardous environments (e.g., nuclear power plants and air traffic control agencies) in which the consequence of errors is high but the occurrence of error is low.[32,33] AHRQ offers resources for hospitals or other organizations to adapt and apply the principles and characteristics of HROs.[34] Five characteristics describe the mindset of HROs:

- HROs exhibit sensitivity to operations. Beyond policies and manuals, there is a "situational awareness" among HROs in which process anomalies and outliers are quickly identified. Sensitivity to operations both reduces the number of errors and facilitates prompt recognition to avoid larger consequences from errors.
- HROs are preoccupied with failure and focused on predicting and eliminating errors rather than being in the position of reacting to errors. HROs view near misses as opportunities to improve current systems by examining strengths and weaknesses and addressing gaps.
- HROs have a reluctance to simplify. These high-functioning organizations accept the complexity inherent in their work and do not accept simplistic solutions for challenges intrinsic to complex systems. In complex work environments, different team members may have information at different times.
- Effective HROs exhibit deference to expertise and cultivate a culture in which team members and organizational leaders defer to the person with the most knowledge of the current issue or concern. The team member with the most information may not be the individual with the highest rank, deemphasizing hierarchy.
- HROs exhibit a commitment to reliance. HROs pay close attention to their ability to quickly contain errors and return to functioning despite setbacks.[32,34]

HROs share power and standardized communication. Especially in the acute care setting, nurses are often the most informed bedside clinicians to a potential error and have an obligation to speak up to share critical information. HROs have an explicit value of safety at the organizational level. Organizational leadership aligns safety goals with mission and vision so that safety is explicitly valued throughout all areas and levels of the organization. A hospital is a system, a set of interdependent components that interact to achieve a common goal. Hospitals are composed of interdependent components such as service lines, nursing care units, ancillary care departments, and outpatient care clinics that interact to achieve a common goal of care delivery. The way in which these separate but united system components interact and work together is a significant factor in delivering high-quality safe care, and the more that clinicians understand the interrelationships, the more effectively they can coordinate care. HROs have a multilevel focus on safety; it is pervasive in the culture, and all employees demonstrate a mindful approach to their work so that they catch where the next error may occur and implement prevention strategies.

CONTEXT TO NURSING AND HEALTH CARE

Just Culture

Data about errors have not always been accessible to healthcare professionals or to healthcare consumers. To create a culture of safety, adverse events must be reported so they can be analyzed for lessons learned and new procedures drafted to improve the system. "Just culture" refers to a system's explicit value of reporting errors without punishment, and therefore, as noted above, is a signature component of a safety culture. A just culture is one in which people can report mistakes or errors without reprisal or personal risk.[34] Just culture does not mean individuals are not accountable for their actions or practice, but it does mean that people are not punished for flawed systems. A just culture promotes sharing and disclosure among stakeholders, including the patient and family.[34]

A just culture seeks to balance the need to learn from mistakes and the need to implement corrective or disciplinary action.[3] The IOM recommends that in most cases front-line workers should be protected from disciplinary action when they report injuries, errors, and near misses, even if they were personally involved, to encourage transparency in the system. These recommendations are based on literature review of other high-risk industries such as aviation safety, nuclear power, and high-reliability military operations. Without such protections, injury-reporting rates may drop and thus impede the ability to prevent future injuries. The IOM provides exceptions to such protection, however, if an error involves criminal behavior, active malfeasance, or cases in which an injury is not reported in a timely manner.[3]

Consequences for errors in a just culture are commonly addressed by a model proposed by David Marx. Marx differentiates *human error* from *at-risk* behavior and *reckless* behavior. Human error is inadvertent action: a slip or lapse. At-risk behavior is behavioral choice that increases risk when risk is not recognized or is mistakenly believed to be justified. Reckless behavior is a behavior choice to consciously disregard a substantial risk. Each level of error involves differing responses from leadership. Human error is best remedied by training, redesigning the system, and improving procedures. At-risk behavior is best mitigated by creating incentives for healthy behaviors, increasing situational awareness, and providing education. Marx suggests remedial or punitive action in instances of reckless behavior.[35]

Transparency in Health Care

Transparency in healthcare is increasingly considered an ethical responsibility, because it leads to improved outcomes, fewer errors,

more satisfied patients, and lower costs.[36] Transparently sharing information with patients allows them to make informed decisions about where and from whom to receive their care. This information should include information on a system's performance on safety, evidence-based practice, and patient satisfaction. The Hospital Compare website, operated by the U.S. Department of Health and Human Services (http://www.hospitalcompare.hhs.gov), makes Health Care Quality Information from the Consumer Perspective (HCAHPS) available to consumers.

More than just making quality information available to consumers, transparency is also defined as open communication and information sharing with patients and their families about their care, including adverse and sentinel events. Timely, open, honest communication with patients and families about adverse events helps restore trust. Professionals trained in the principles and practice of transparency, usually risk management staff, communicate with the patient and family as soon as an adverse event is recognized and the patient is ready physically and psychologically to receive this information, usually within 24 hours. There are specific recommendations to help healthcare professionals understand how transparency can be operationalized in a healthcare system and fit within the framework of just culture. Patients should be told what happened, and those involved should take responsibility, apologize, and explain how the organization will respond and what will be done to prevent future events.[37]

Transparency and disclosure are interrelated experiences. Rick Boothman and colleagues have developed a standardized model around transparency and disclosure (often referred to as the *Michigan model*) that focuses on compensating patients quickly and fairly when inappropriate care causes injury, supporting clinical staff when the care was reasonable, and reducing patient injuries by learning from patients' experiences. This transparent disclosure model has demonstrated a decrease in rate of new claims, a decline in lawsuits, and decreased overall compensation costs.[38]

INTERRELATED CONCEPTS

Safety is a multidimensional term as applied in health care with several interrelated concepts. The concepts featured in this text that are most closely interrelated with safety are shown in Fig. 45.3.

Health Care Quality is very closely interrelated to safety—so much so that they really overlap. Health Care Quality is defined as identifying the gap that occurs between ideal care and actual care delivered. Quality improvement is an approach to practice that measures the variance in ideal and actual care and implements strategies to close the gap. Quality measures include benchmarks from other areas of the same institution or from peer institutions across the healthcare industry.

How well healthcare professionals work together accounts for as much as 70% of healthcare errors.[1] For this reason, Communication, Collaboration, and Care Coordination are closely related to safety. Standardized communication can ensure safe handoffs between providers or between settings, provide clear direction in seeking and sharing information between providers, and instill collaborative behaviors for speaking up to prevent errors from occurring. Ineffective communication, hierarchy, and disruptive behavior are challenges to patient safety. Care coordination requires cross-disciplinary communication, knowing scope of responsibility, and organizational support for speaking up when safety is compromised.[18] Collaboration begins with self-development based on emotional intelligence to monitor appropriate reactions and responses to team members. Nurses need skills in problem solving, conflict resolution, and negotiation to be able to coordinate safe care across interprofessional teams. Sharing team leadership based on the provider most expert in the situation is consistent with HROs.

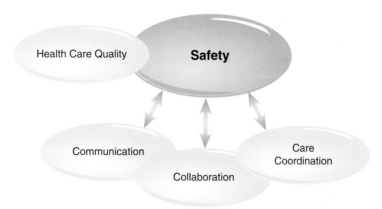

FIGURE 45.3 Safety and Interrelated Concepts.

BOX 45.1 EXEMPLARS OF SAFETY

Point of Care
- Prevention of decubitus ulcers
- Medication administration
- Fall prevention
- Invasive procedures
- Diagnostic workup
- Recognition of/action on adverse effects
- Communication with patients/families
- Communication with other healthcare providers

Systems Level
- Care coordination
- Documentation/electronic records
- Team systems
- Work processes
- Communication process
- Environmental systems
- Error reporting/analysis
- Regulatory systems
- National quality benchmarks

ACCESS EXEMPLAR LINKS IN YOUR GIDDENS EBOOK

CLINICAL EXEMPLARS

Because multiple exemplars exist for safety and injury prevention within health care, it is not possible to list them all. Box 45.1 presents the most common safety issues at the point of care and the systems level. A few of the most important exemplars are briefly described here.

Featured Exemplars
Fall Prevention

Prevention of falls is a safety concern in all living environments, especially for older adults. The American Geriatrics Society (http://www.americangeriatrics.org) offers evidence-based clinical practice guidelines for older adults living independently, in assisted living, in long-term care facilities, and for those being cared for in the acute care environment. These guidelines address recommended screening, elements of a focused history, physical examination, and functional assessment. In addition, the guidelines synthesize common fall prevention interventions and tailor them for various living situations: adaptation of the environment; minimization of psychoactive medications; attention to postural hypotension; management of foot problems and footwear; and exercises that emphasize balance, strength, and gait training.

Medication Administration

Medication administration is an essential aspect of nurses' work, especially in the acute care setting. Medication errors are the most common errors in the hospital setting, and they usually involve the frontline nurse clinician. From 26% to 32% of medication errors occur at the administration stage and involve nurses.[39] Interventions to decrease medication administration errors often focus on technology such as bar code medication administration or computer physician order entry, standardization of medication administration practices, or alterations to the nurses' environment to decrease distractions or interruptions. Recent research indicates that medication administration errors are reduced by both system improvement as well as clinician-focused interventions.[40]

Care Coordination

Poorly coordinated care systems contribute to safety compromises in the delivery of care. Integrated care systems are an effective method to address such system gaps. The development of care coordination models has grown out of the need to address fragmented service delivery, cost inefficiencies, and poor health outcomes. Care coordination can be defined as a set of activities purposefully organized by a team of personnel that includes the patient to facilitate the appropriate delivery of the necessary services and information to support optimal health care across settings and over time.

Team Systems

Healthcare professionals provide care in teams. Safety outcomes are often closely tied to effective team functioning. Understanding team systems in health care is complex because of the high degree of variability in settings, microsystem culture, care delivery, and members of the care team. Effective team systems in health care contribute to safe, patient-centered outcomes. Evidence suggests that high-functioning teams in health care are related to clear role definition, timely information about a patient's changing health status, mutual respect among team members, consistent feedback, and participation of patient or family on the team, when desired.[41]

Error Reporting

Adverse outcomes in health care can only be addressed when reported; thus error reporting is essential to error prevention. A reluctance to report errors may be attributed to a perceived lack of impact of the error on the patient or a patient outcome, a fear of a punitive response by leadership or a system, or a personal sense of embarrassment about the error.[42] There is also wide variation in how errors are defined, which information should be reported, and the best approaches to mitigating the effects of errors.[42] Addressing reluctance to error reporting at the unit culture level through implementation of just culture concepts is one evidence-based approach to this complex issue.[43]

CASE STUDY

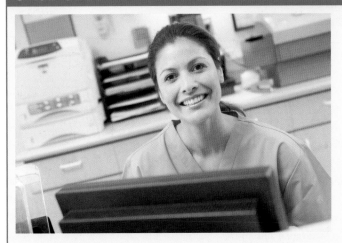

Case Presentation

Gloria considers herself an expert nurse on her medical/surgical unit. She has been a registered nurse (RN) on this unit for 12 years and has seen some important changes in how care is provided. Keeping up with these changes is an important part of Gloria's practice, and many RNs look to Gloria for guidance in understanding the latest evidence.

Lately, Gloria has been concerned about the occurrence of decubitus ulcers on her unit. She knows that there are several strategies that must be employed to effectively address this deleterious patient outcome. When caring for Mr. Brown, a postoperative spinal stenosis patient, Gloria knows that at the individual practice level it is important that she establish a schedule of turning this patient every 2 h. Gloria is aware this nursing intervention at the individual clinician level is effective in preventing decubitus ulcers.

As Gloria goes off shift after caring for Mr. Brown, she thinks about the importance of clear communication with the rest of the healthcare team about decubitus ulcer prevention for Mr. Brown. Therefore, to address safety at the healthcare team level, Gloria posts a reminder above his bed listing the turning schedule so that all healthcare team members follow the same protocol to turn Mr. Brown every 2 h.

While Gloria cares for Mr. Brown for consecutive shifts, she thinks about the variety of ways that nurses can work with other members of the healthcare team to prevent decubitus ulcers. On his second postoperative day, Mr. Brown's surgeon mentions to Gloria that because he has been prescribed steroids, he is at especially high risk for developing decubitus ulcers. Gloria decides to address this safety concern for Mr. Brown at the unit level, and she seeks input on his care from the physical therapist to learn about skin protection products and from the dietitian to address nutritional strategies to help prevent decubitus ulcers in Mr. Brown.

When speaking with the physical therapist and dietitian about decubitus ulcer prevention for Mr. Brown, both colleagues mention the increase in occurrence of decubitus ulcers on this medical/surgical unit. Gloria works with her manager and the quality improvement department to track the decubitus ulcer rate on her medical/surgical unit for the previous 6 months, and plans to compare this rate with state and national quality benchmarks for decubitus ulcer prevention. She is also aware that many studies have been published by the Institute for Healthcare Improvement on best practices for decubitus ulcer prevention. Once Gloria has retrieved the data from her own unit to compare to other benchmarks, she will collaborate with her manager and RN colleagues to identify some systematic strategies that can be adopted on her unit. Gloria demonstrates that she understands how to address safety needs at the individual clinician level as well as at the systems level that improves patient outcomes.

Case Analysis Questions

1. In what ways does Gloria exemplify the incorporation of safety into her clinical practice?
2. Review Fig. 45.3. Which interrelated concepts are evident in this case? Are there other concepts representing in this book that also apply to this specific situation?

From monkeybusinessimages/iStock/Thinkstock.

 ACCESS EXEMPLAR LINKS IN YOUR GIDDENS EBOOK

REFERENCES

1. Institute of Medicine. (2000). *To err is human: Building a safer health system*. Washington, DC: National Academies Press.
2. Institute of Medicine. (2001). *Crossing the quality chasm*. Washington, DC: National Academies Press.
3. Institute of Medicine. (2004). *Keeping patients safe: Transforming the work environment of nurses*. Washington, DC: National Academies Press.
4. National Patient Safety Foundation. (n.d). *Our definitions*. Retrieved from http://s197607105.onlinehome.us/au/mission_definitions.php.
5. Kim, L., Lyder, C. H., McNeese-Smith, D., et al. (2015). Defining attributes of patient safety through concept analysis. *Journal of Advanced Nursing, 71*(11), 2490–2503.
6. National Patient Safety Foundation's Lucian Leape Institute. (2014). *Safety is personal: Partnering with patients and families for the safest care*. Retrieved from http://www.npsf.org/?page=safetyispersonal.
7. Cronenwett, L., Sherwood, G., Barnsteiner, J., et al. (2007). Quality and safety education for nurses. *Nursing Outlook, 55*(3), 122–131.
8. The Joint Commission. (2011). *Sentinel events*. Retrieved from http://www.jointcommission.org/assets/1/6/2011_CAMBHC_SE.pdf.
9. Agency for Healthcare Research and Quality. (2016). *National healthcare quality and disparities report and 5th anniversary update on the national quality strategy*. Rockville, MD: Author.
10. Leape, L., Lawther, A. G., Brennan, T. A., et al. (1993). Preventing medical injury. *Quality Review Bulletin, 19*(5), 144–149.
11. Cook, R., & Woods, D. (1994). Operating at the sharp end: The complexity of human error. In M. Bogner (Ed.), *Human error in medicine* (pp. 255–310). Hillsdale, NJ: Erlbaum.
12. Reason, J. (1997). *Managing the risks of organizational accidents*. Burlington, VT: Ashgate.
13. Henrickson, K., Dayton, E., Keyes, M. A., et al. (2008). Understanding adverse events: A human factors framework. In R. G. Hughes (Ed.), *Patient safety and quality: An evidence-based handbook for nurses*. Publication No. 08-0043. (pp. 1-67–1-85). Rockville, MD: Agency for Healthcare Research and Quality.
14. Ebright, P. R., Patterson, E. S., Chalko, B. A., et al. (2003). Understanding the complexity of registered nurse work in acute care settings. *The Journal of Nursing Administration, 33*(12), 630–638.
15. Frankel, A., Haraden, C., Federico, F., et al. (2017). *A framework for safe, reliable and effective care*. White paper. Cambridge, MA: Institute for Healthcare Improvement and Safe & Reliable Healthcare.
16. Barnsteiner, J. H. (2010). *Safety competency resource paper*. Washington, DC: American Association of Colleges of Nursing QSEN Education Center.
17. Health and Safety Commission Advisory Committee on the Safety of Nuclear Installations. (1993). *Organizing for safety: Third report of the ACSNI study group on human factors*. Sudbury, UK: HSE Books.
18. Singer, A., Lin, S., Falwell, A., et al. (2009). Relationship of safety climate and safety performance in hospitals. *Health Services Research, 44*(2), 399–421.

19. Sammer, C., Lynken, K., Singh, K., et al. (2010). What is patient safety culture? A review of the literature. *Journal of Nursing Scholarship, 42,* 156–165.

20. Cohoon, B. D. (2003). Learning from near misses through reflection: A new risk management strategy. *Journal of Healthcare Risk Management, 23*(2), 19–25.

21. Schmidt, C. E., & Bottoni, T. (2003). Improving medication safety and patient care in the emergency department. *Journal of Emergency Nursing, 29*(1), 12–16.

22. Bullock, L. M. (2011). Transform into a culture of safety. *Risk Management, 42*(7), 14–15.

23. Leonard, M., Graham, S., & Bonacum, D. (2004). The human factor: The critical importance of effective teamwork and communication in providing safe care. *Quality and Safety in Health Care, 13,* i85–i90.

24. Vaismoradi, M., Jordan, S., & Kangasniemi, M. (2014). Patient participation in patient safety and nursing input — A systematic review. *Journal of Clinical Nursing, 24,* 627–639.

25. Karsh, B. T., Holden, R. J., Alper, S. J., et al. (2006). A human factors engineering paradigm for patient safety: Designing to support the performance of the healthcare professional. *Quality and Safety in Health Care, 15*(Suppl. 1), i59–i65.

26. Carayon, P., Xie, A., & Kianfar, S. (2014). Human factors and ergonomics as a patient safety practice. *BMJ Quality & Safety, 23,* 196–205.

27. Salas, E., Prince, C., Bowers, C., et al. (1999). A methodology for enhancing crew resource management training. *Human Factors, 41,* 161–172.

28. Rivers, R. M., Swain, D., & Nixon, W. R. (2003). Using aviation safety measures to enhance patient outcomes. *Association of Operating Room Nurses Journal, 77*(1), 158–162.

29. Oriol, M. D. (2006). Crew resource management. *The Journal of Nursing Administration, 36*(9), 402–406.

30. Salas, E., Wilson, K. A., Burke, C. S., et al. (2006). Does crew resource management training work? An update, an extension and some critical needs. *Human Factors, 48*(2), 392–412.

31. Fore, A. M., Sculli, G. L., Albee, D., et al. (2013). Improving patient safety using the sterile cockpit principle during medication administration: A collaborative, unit-based project. *Journal of Nursing Management, 21,* 106–111.

32. Baker, D. P., Day, R., & Salas, E. (2006). Teamwork as an essential component of high-reliability organizations. *Health Services Research, 41*(4), 1576–1598.

33. Oster, C. A., & Braaten, J. S. (2016). *High reliability organizations: A healthcare handbook for patient safety & quality.* Indianapolis, IN: Sigma Theta Tau Press.

34. Agency for Healthcare Research and Quality. (2008). *Becoming a high reliability organization: Operational advice for hospital leaders.* Rockville, MD: U.S. Department of Health and Human Services. Retrieved from http://archive.ahrq.gov/professionals/quality-patient-safety/ quality-resources/tools/hroadvice/hroadvice.pdf.

35. Marx, D. (2001). *Patient safety and the "just culture": A primer for health care executives.* New York: Columbia University.

36. National patient safety foundation's Lucian Leape institute. (2015). *Shining a light: Safer healthcare through transparency.* Boston, MA: National Patient Safety Foundation.

37. Harvard Hospitals. (2006). *When things go wrong: Responding to adverse events.* Burlington, MA: Massachusetts Coalition for the Prevention of Medical Errors.

38. Boothman, R. C., Imhoff, S. J., & Campbell, D. A. (2012). Nursing a culture of patient safety and achieving lower malpractice risk through disclosure: Lessons learned and future directions. *Front Health Services Manage, 28*(3), 13–28.

39. Hughes, R. G. (2008). Nurses at the "sharp end" of patient care. In R. G. Hughes (Ed.), *Patient safety and quality: An evidence-based handbook for nurses.* Publication No. 08-0043. Rockville, MD: Agency for Healthcare Research and Quality. Retrieved from http://www.ncbi.nlm.nih.gov/ books/NBK2672.

40. Keers, R. N., Williams, S. D., Cooke, J., & Ashcroft, D. M. (2013). Causes of medication administration errors in hospitals: A systematic review of quantitative and qualitative evidence. *Drug Safety, 36*(11), 1045–1067.

41. Sevin, C., Moore, G., Shepherd, J., et al. (2009). Transforming care teams to provide the best possible patient-centered, collaborative care. *The Journal of Ambulatory Care Management, 32*(1), 24–31.

42. Wolf, Z. R., & Hughes, R. (2008). Error reporting and disclosure. In R. G. Hughes (Ed.), *Patient safety and quality: An evidence-based handbook for nurses.* Publication No. 08-0043. (pp. 2-333–2-379). Rockville, MD: Agency for Healthcare Research and Quality.

43. Boysen, P. G. (2013). Just culture: A foundation for balanced accountability for patient safety. *The Ochsner Journal, 13,* 400–406.

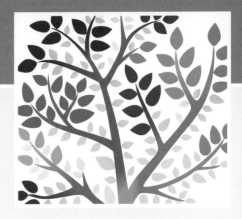

Technology and Informatics

Jennie De Gagne

Healthcare providers have always gathered patient data and information to provide the best care possible. What has changed over time is the use of technology to gather, process, and manage data and information. With the advent of new technologies in health care, information technology (IT) has become essential to providing safe, effective, efficient, and quality care, and with it, a new discipline of informatics has emerged. Health professionals with expertise and experience in computer and information science became focused on furthering and broadening their specialty area of practice with informatics. The field of health IT and informatics is rapidly advancing and must include a workforce prepared to meaningfully use these evolving technologies. There is a growing requirement for practicing nurses, nurse educators, nurse researchers, and nurse administrators to ensure that expected competencies in informatics are met. Despite widespread use of the term informatics, few seem to understand exactly what it means.

DEFINITION

Technology describes the knowledge and use of tools, machines, materials, and processes to help solve human problems. It can be applied to a specific discipline such as educational technologies, medical technologies, or health technologies. Technology is the product of creative human action, and it is sustained by human action.[1] For the purpose of this concept presentation, the focus is on *health information technology (health IT)* as the essential antecedents for health informatics. Currently, health informatics cannot exist without health IT.

Health IT provides the umbrella framework to describe the comprehensive management of health information and its secure exchange between consumers, providers, government and quality entities, and insurers. Health IT is generally viewed as the most promising tool for improving the overall quality, safety, and efficiency of the health delivery system.[2-4] The efficacy and effectiveness of health IT tools are also being examined in terms of their engagement of patients, the families, and caregivers in their healthcare decisions.

Informatics, like technology, also is a broad term and is derived from the French word *informatique*—it is the science that encompasses information science and computer science to study the process, management, and retrieval of information.[5] Currently the term informatics as it relates to health care is ubiquitous and ambiguous because of the many health professions and related disciplines that use health data. In this concept presentation, the focus is on health informatics.

Health informatics is a discipline in which health data are stored, analyzed, and disseminated through the application of information and communication technology (Box 46.1). It involves the use of technology and information systems to support the healthcare industry. Health informatics encompasses the interprofessional study of the design, development, adoption, and application of IT-based innovations in healthcare services delivery, management, and planning.[6] Informatics communities, such as the American Medical Informatics Association (AMIA), use the term health informatics to refer to applied research and practice of informatics across the clinical and public health domains.[7] As a broad term, health informatics includes the discipline of informatics as applied to biomedical research, clinical care, and public health.[7]

SCOPE

The scope of this concept is represented by the idea that health IT and health informatics intersect with the science of health to provide powerful tools and processes for advancing health practices and serve as an infrastructure to support and promote a continuously learning healthcare system (Fig. 46.1).[8]

Health IT and informatics tools are used by various groups and serve as part of the infrastructure of a healthcare delivery system. These groups include consumers, patients and their families, caregivers, healthcare professionals, administrators, and any personnel supporting the delivery of health care. One such tool is the electronic health record (EHR), which is a central component of the health IT infrastructure. An EHR is an individual's official, digital health record and is shared among multiple facilities and agencies. Other tools include the electronic medical record (EMR), which is an individual's health record within a Healthcare provider's facility, and decision support tools to guide practice and decision making. Tools for patients, their families, and caregivers, as well as consumers, consist of mobile health tools such as wellness monitoring devices (e.g., physical activity monitors such as Fitbit), personal health records, patient portals, and physiologic monitoring (e.g., pulse oximetry, digital stethoscope, and glucose monitors) and sensors. In addition, there are infrastructure health information technologies such as health information exchanges (HIEs) that support the sharing of health data across healthcare institutions, data warehouses that are repositories of stored data, and communication networks. The plethora of health IT and informatics tools provide the opportunity for engaging consumers in health care and creating a connected health system.

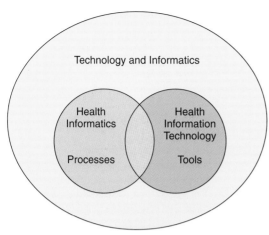

FIGURE 46.1 Scope of Technology and Informatics.

BOX 46.1 Informatics Definitions

- *Technology* is the knowledge and use of tools, machines, materials, and processes to help solve human problems.
- *Health information technology (health IT)* is the application of information processing involving both computer hardware and computer software that deals with the storage, retrieval, sharing, and use of healthcare data, information, and knowledge for communication and decision making.
- *Informatics* is derived from the French word *informatique*. Simply stated, informatics is the science that encompasses information science and computer science to study the process, management, and retrieval of information.
- *Health informatics* is a discipline in which health data are stored, analyzed, and disseminated through the application of information and communication technology.
- *Informatician* is a person who works in the field of informatics, sometimes called an informaticist.
- *Information science* is an interprofessional science primarily concerned with the analysis, collection, classification, manipulation, storage, retrieval, and dissemination of information.
- *Computer science* is a branch of engineering that studies computation and computer technology, hardware, and software, as well as the theoretical foundations of information and computation techniques.

ATTRIBUTES AND CRITERIA

Health IT is a precursor or antecedent to health informatics and is summarized in Table 46.1. The defining characteristics and consequences of health IT are reflected in the analysis of health informatics. The results of the health IT and informatics concept analysis suggest the following attributes: hardware and software, data standards and terminology, policies and procedures, privacy and security, informatics workforce, and organizational skills.

Hardware and Software

Health IT is the application of information processing involving computer hardware, computer software, communications, and networking technologies that enables the storage, retrieval, sharing, and use of healthcare data, information, knowledge, and wisdom for communication and decision making.[9] Certified *clinical information systems (CISs)* offer the best set of tools for achieving quality outcomes and are at the heart of health IT and informatics. CISs consist of information technology that is applied at the point of clinical care. They include EHRs, clinical data repositories, decision support programs, handheld and mobile devices for collecting data and viewing reference material, and imaging modalities, as well as collaborative communication between patients and providers such as electronic messaging systems and patient portals. Increasingly, care is provided in multiple settings, thus creating a need for clinicians to share data with providers at other locations. Advances in computer networking, broadband, and wireless communication technologies have now made it possible for clinicians to access these data via any device at any time from any location—whether in the office, the hospital, at home, or even when traveling out of town.

An increasing number of digital tools are being used as part of health information technologies and used by patients and their families, caregivers, and consumers. These digital tools include patient portals including secure messaging that are available on numerous devices (e.g., tablets, smartphones, and desktop or laptop computers) and mobile applications software that collects and shares patient-generated health data (PGHD) (e.g., daily glucose readings, food consumptions, and physical activities measures) with other consumers or their healthcare providers. The mobile applications can also be used to connect patients or consumers with social network groups. The use of these digital tools in the connected health world helps patients and families, caregivers, and consumers to manage their health, wellness, and health conditions,

---

TABLE 46.1 Health Information Technology Summary

Antecedent	Defining Characteristics	Outcomes
• Need for a tool, machine, materials, and/or processes to improve health care • Information science • Computer science • Health discipline science (e.g., nursing, medicine) • Information technology specialist • Informed patients, families, and caregivers	• Technology (hardware and software) that supports discipline of health informatics (e.g., electronic health record) • Clinical point-of-care tools • Interoperable and connected • Evolutionary and updated to provide new functionality • Interoperable systems and tools • Technology-competent and engaged patients, families, and caregivers	• Improves health provider's workflow • Improves healthcare quality • Prevents medical errors • Reduces healthcare costs • Increases administrative efficiencies • Decreases paperwork • Improves disease tracking • Creates cultural, social, organizational, and intellectual change • May be used in unintended ways • Serves as an infrastructure for a learning health system • Promotes and supports patient and family engagement in health decisions • Connected health

especially chronic illnesses such as heart disease, stroke, and diabetes. Digital tools that collect PGHD may be used for personal management and may or may not be shared with providers. Healthcare providers also may use remote monitoring tools and sensor technologies to monitor patients in their homes.

Standardized Information Systems and Terminology

The proliferation of clinical information systems has created a pressing need for standardization of patient information systems and terminology. Standardized terminology within the EHR is critical for communicating care to the interprofessional team and exchanging health information. The universal requirement for quality patient care, efficiency, and cost containment makes it imperative to express data, information, and knowledge in a meaningful way that can be shared across disciplines and care settings.[10] EHRs must use consistent, codified terminology to eliminate ambiguity and to ensure greater interoperability. The many different ways of organizing data, information, and knowledge are built on taxonomies and nomenclature developed over decades using a clear coding scheme. The terminologies recognized by the American Nurses Association (ANA) are listed in Table 46.2.

Policies

Responsibility for developing an overall policy infrastructure that supports health IT and health information exchanges primarily lies with the Office of the National Coordinator for Health IT (ONC). ONC has worked closely with the Centers for Medicare and Medicaid Services (CMS) to assist in establishing policies related to Medicare and Medicaid payment for "meaningful use" of EHRs. ONC rules specify the standards, implementation specifications, and other criteria for EHR systems and technologies to be certified, whereas CMS rules specify how hospitals, physicians, and other eligible professionals must demonstrate their meaningful use of these technologies to receive Medicare and Medicaid payment incentives. These EHR incentive programs have been renamed as the Promoting Interoperability (PI) programs to better reflect patients' access to health information.[11]

In addition to meaningful use criteria and certification standards, the ONC health IT policy committee has issued recommendations regarding health information extension centers, workforce training, and privacy and security. Once the policies are established at the federal level, states, professional organizations, and institutions adopt and adapt these fundamental practices at the local level to reduce barriers to health information exchange.

Privacy and Security

A major concern with healthcare information, as with other highly sensitive personal data, involves privacy and security. The privacy and security rules issued under the Health Insurance Portability and Accountability Act (HIPAA) of 1996 along with multiple state laws create a complex network of laws and regulations that address patient privacy and consent for the use of identifiable personal health information. In 2013, HIPAA rules were modified to reflect new technologies and to enhance personalization and the quality of health care.[12] Building and maintaining the public's trust in health IT requires comprehensive privacy and security protections that establish clear rules on how patient data can be accessed, used, and disclosed.

Informatics Workforce

An informatics workforce with the right skill set is critical to the advancement of health IT and informatics. During the past decade, a great deal of work has been done in nursing and other disciplines to define informatics competencies; however, currently there is no single consolidated list of competencies. Several professional organizations are working toward identifying informatics competencies, such as the American Medical Informatics Association (AMIA) and the Health Information Management Systems Society (HIMSS). In nursing, the ANA has defined the scope and standards for an informatics nurse and an informatics nurse specialist.[13] In 2006, the Technology and Informatics Guiding Education Reform (TIGER) initiative advocated that all nurses need informatics knowledge and skills to practice in a technology-intensive healthcare environment. In addition, the Quality and Safety Education

TABLE 46.2   ANA-Recognized Terminologies

Terminology	Terminology URL	Nursing Process Within Terminology	Date Recognized by ANA
CCC: Clinical Care Classification	http://www.sabacare.com	Diagnoses, interventions, and outcomes	1992
ICNP: International Classification of Nursing Practice	https://www.icn.ch/what-we-do/projectsprogrammes/ehealth	Diagnoses, interventions, and outcomes	2000
NANDA: NANDA International	http://www.nanda.org	Nursing diagnoses	1992
NIC: Nursing Interventions Classification	https://nursing.uiowa.edu/cncce/nursing-interventions-classification-overview	Interventions	1992
NOC: Nursing Outcomes Classification	https://nursing.uiowa.edu/cncce/nursing-outcomes-classification-overview	Outcome indicators	1997
Omaha System	http://www.omahasystem.org	Problem classification scheme Intervention scheme Problem rating scale for outcomes	1992
PNDS: Perioperative Nursing Data Set	https://www.aorn.org/education/individuals/continuing-education/online-courses/introduction-to-pnds	Diagnoses, interventions, and outcomes	1999
SNOMED CT: Systematic Nomenclature of Medicine Clinical Terms	https://www.snomed.org/snomed-ct	Assessment concepts, diagnoses, interventions, and outcomes	1999

for Nurses (QSEN) initiative and American Association of Colleges of Nursing's documents have determined informatics competencies for nurses being prepared at the prelicensure and graduate levels. In 2016 a European Union–United States collaboration on eHealth (i.e., EU*US eHealth Work Project) began to map the current structure and gaps in health IT skills and training needs globally.[14] As a result of the various initiatives, informatics competencies have been developed for all levels of nursing as well as competencies for specialization as an informatics nurse and an informatics nurse specialist.

Informaticians are informatics specialists with advanced education and training who collaborate with other healthcare professionals and IT specialists to enhance and support patient-centered quality health care. Informaticians use their knowledge of patient care (e.g., nursing and medicine) combined with their understanding of informatics concepts, methods, and tools to analyze, design, implement, and evaluate information and communication systems that enhance individual and population health as well as provide efficient administrative services.[15] The hallmark of nursing informatics practice is its cross-disciplinary nature, with nurse informaticians often leading the team to create practical informatics solutions for use by many disciplines.[13] For physicians, clinical informatics was recognized in 2011 in the United States as a board-certified medical subspecialty.[16] Nurses can become certified in nursing informatics through the American Nurses Credentialing Center (ANCC).

Peopleware and Organizational Skills

Informatics is not limited to the hardware and software; it includes people and organizational skills. When talking about widespread use of health IT and informatics, technical skills alone are not sufficient for implementation success. Peopleware, a key component of successful implementation, is a term used to refer to anything that has to do with the role of people in the development and use of computer hardware and software systems. Peopleware involves the sociologic side of informatics implementations and includes issues such as productivity, teamwork, group dynamics, project management, organizational factors, human interface design, and human-machine interaction. When introducing new technologies into an organization, the peopleware issues become as important and at times more important than the technological issues. Learning to manage people is crucial to managing technological change.[17] Table 46.3 summarizes the concept analysis of health informatics and its impact on nursing practice and on consumer and patient health.

TABLE 46.3 Health Informatics Summary[a]			
Antecedents	**Defining Characteristics**	**Nurse Outcomes**	**Patient Outcomes**
Certified health IT hardware and software (clinical information system and computer applications)	Interoperable electronic health record and tools that allow for formal representation of data/information/ knowledge/wisdom	Clinical decision support tools at point of care	Consumers adopt personal health record
		Reduces duplication of services	Decreased cost of health care
		Evidence-based practice	Patient-centered, personalized health care and user-generated data
		Opportunity for shared learning environment	
Standard terminology for data collection and electronic exchange of health information	Data structure that allows for uniform input and retrieval of health data	Mechanism to determine costs of nursing and other healthcare services	Better understanding of healthcare benefits and services
	Algorithms that support evidence-based clinical decision making and provide safety checks	Accurate, timely, and up-to-date information at point of care	Improved quality of health care and reduced medical errors
Policies for data transmission and use	Policy framework for development and adoption of health IT infrastructure and health information exchange	Ensures security and privacy of health information and exchange	Confidentiality of health data
Broadband capacity for widespread electronic data transmission and download	Sufficient bandwidth requirement to achieve full functionality of health IT applications	Ability to transfer health data among providers and across healthcare systems	Health data available at point of care
Persons with specialized education in informatics	Informatics specialist as team member	Maximize use of clinical information system	
Persons with technical knowledge and skill	Health information management and health IT professionals as team members		
End users with basic informatics competencies and discipline-specific knowledge and wisdom	Clinicians (nurses) with knowledge of phenomena of nursing in their area of practice as a team member	Broad-based team approach to patient care to support clinical judgment and meaningful use	
Patient, families, and caregivers informed about health and healthcare decisions	Patient, families, and caregivers central to the healthcare team		Improved patient engagement
Organizational culture that supports a learning healthcare system	Dynamic interprofessional team-oriented digital culture focused on peopleware and organizational skills	Use of data to inform clinical care and support research and knowledge development	Improved patient education, self-management, and health literacy

[a]*Health informatics* is a discipline that sorts, enhances, processes, operates on, organizes, makes usable, and retrieves information related to human health and illness through the application of technology for the purpose of sharing data, information, knowledge, and wisdom among health providers, among consumers, and across organizations.
IT, Information technology.

THEORETICAL LINKS

Classic theories that underpin the concept of informatics are from information science and computer science. Other sciences that play a role in the implementation of informatics are cognitive science and organizational science. Discipline-specific science, such as nursing science or medical science, is what differentiates informatics in the specialty areas of practice or domains of informatics and provides the fundamental building blocks for knowledge and wisdom.[13,18]

Information Science

Information science is a branch of applied mathematics and electrical engineering that involves the quantification of information. It is a collection of mathematical theories, based on statistics, concerned with methods of coding, transmitting, storing, retrieving, and decoding information. Its application includes the design of systems, such as clinical information systems, that are involved with data transmission, encryption, compression, and other information processing techniques. Recent advances in health ITs and health information exchanges have resulted in an enormous increase in healthcare data requiring large storage capacities, powerful computing resources, and accurate data analysis algorithms. Every clinical decision is based on this availability of the information that is transmitted. If the exchange of information works well, clinical care is solidly based on best evidence, whereas poor transmission of clinical data can lead to poorly informed decisions.[18]

Computer Science

Computer science is the study of the theoretical foundations of information and computation as these techniques relate to implementation and application of computer systems. It is frequently described as the systematic study of algorithmic processes that create, describe, and transform information. Computer science is a broad field of study that focuses on computation, algorithms and data structures, programming methodology and languages, and computer elements (hardware, software, and networks) and architecture. It also includes fields such as software engineering, artificial intelligence, computer networking and communications, database systems, and human-computer interaction.[19]

Cognitive Science

Cognitive science is the interprofessional study of mind, intelligence, and behavior from an information processing perspective. It encompasses how people think, understand, remember, synthesize, access, and respond to stored information and knowledge. Cognitive science provides the scaffolding for the analysis and modeling of complex human performance in technology-mediated settings. Theories from cognitive science inform and shape design, development, implementation, and assessment of health information systems. The mind is frequently compared to a computer, and experts in cognitive science try to model human thinking using the artificial networks of the computer.[18]

Organizational Science

Organizational science is an emerging field that focuses on behavior of organizations and includes a wide variety of topics, such as individual, group, and organizational decision making; the management of human resources; and the design of organizations and interorganizational networks. Understanding an organization and particularly understanding how culture, behavior, and social change impact an organization are essential requirements for successful implementation of health IT and health informatics within and among organizations.[20] Health care has been determined to be a complex adaptive system and as such involves patients, providers, and policymakers alike to ensure that every healthcare decision is guided by timely, accurate, and comprehensive health information to guarantee patient-centered care in a timely, efficient, and equitable manner. Informatics specialists with knowledge and skills in analyzing organizational culture, planning change within the organization, building and working in interprofessional teams, and leading information system development and implementation are key resources for the organization. For healthcare professionals and healthcare systems to embrace and meaningfully use informatics and other emerging technologies, a change in culture is critical.[21]

CONTEXT TO NURSING AND HEALTH CARE

Nurses are involved in informatics in terms of their own professional roles and responsibilities and with their interprofessional roles and responsibilities with other healthcare professionals within a healthcare institution. To best understand this, it is important to examine the evolution of health informatics and the domains of informatics and specific application in nursing.

Historical Perspective: The Evolution of Technology and Informatics in Health Care

One could argue that early ideas related to informatics date back more than 150 years (Fig. 46.2). Various health ITs have been available since the 1970s; the support for widespread use of information and communication technologies is a more recent occurrence. During the past decade, a convergence of driving forces has served as a major catalyst to move the healthcare informatics agenda forward and ensure that all healthcare professionals have the necessary "21st century knowledge and skills for practice in a complex, emerging technologically sophisticated, consumer-centric, global environment."[22,p58] Since 2000 the Institute of Medicine has consistently highlighted the use of health ITs as one solution for ensuring safe and quality health care. Starting with *To Err Is Human: Building a Better Health System*,[23] using appropriate technologies has been one recommended solution to reduce errors and ensure patient safety. In *Crossing the Quality Chasm*,[24] there was general consensus that the current healthcare system was in need of reform. It is stated throughout the report that to achieve this reform, the healthcare system must make

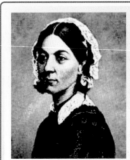

"In attempting to arrive at the truth, I have applied everywhere for information, but in scarcely an instance have I been able to obtain hospital records fit for any purposes of comparison. If they could be obtained they would enable us to decide many other questions besides the ones alluded to. They would show the subscribers how their money was being spent, what amount of good was really being done with it, or whether the money was not doing mischief rather than good."
Florence Nightingale (1863).

Longman, Green, Longman, Roberts and Green: Notes on Hospitals, 1863, London, p. 176

FIGURE 46.2 The First Nurse Informatician.

"effective use of information technologies to automate clinical information and make it readily accessible to patients and all members of the care team. An improved information infrastructure is needed to establish effective and timely communication among clinicians and between patients and clinicians."[24,p12]

This points not only to the need for the meaningful use of the EHR but also to the need to examine the use of communication tools and patient portals to foster communication between patients and clinicians, as well as the need to transform health professional education. The Institute of Medicine report entitled *Best Care at Lower Cost: The Path to Continuously Learning Health Care in America*[8] continues to support an informatics infrastructure to ensure

"the development of a learning healthcare system which generates and applies the best evidence for the collaborative healthcare choices of each patient and provider; drives the process of discovery as a natural outgrowth of patient care; and ensures innovation, quality, safety, and value in health care."[25,p39]

In 2009 the American Recovery and Reinvestment Act authorized the CMS to provide a reimbursement incentive for physician and hospital providers in becoming "meaningful users" of an EHR.[11] As part of this act, the adoption of EHRs and other initiatives, such as meaningful use, was of paramount importance and served as the current catalyst for all hospitals, clinics, and providers to use EHRs.

According to the current draft of the Federal Health Information Technology Strategic Plan 2015–2020, the overall vision is that "health information is accessible when and where it is needed to improve and protect people's health and well-being."[26,p3] The mission is to "improve health, health care, and reduce costs through the use of information and technology."[26,p3]

The increased use of digital technology in society also is driving the integration of technology in health care. The Pew Research Center has noted three technology revolutions that have occurred since 2002: (1) greater access to broadband, which has increased access to the Internet and promoted its use in various facets of people's lives; (2) mobile connectivity and the concept of any time–anywhere access; and (3) the presence of social media and social networks in daily life.[27] These three revolutions have impacted patients and their families, caregivers, and healthcare providers as increasingly more adults are using digital tools to not only access health information but also to manage their own health data and be an active participant in their health care.

Domains of Informatics

Health informatics is evolving as a discipline, and its definition and standards are a work in progress. Although there is currently no universally accepted taxonomy for the major domains of informatics, for the purposes of this concept presentation, AMIA's five domains of informatics are used: translational bioinformatics, clinical research informatics, clinical informatics, consumer health informatics, and public health informatics.[7]

The domains overlap in various ways and are not exclusive to one another.[7] All domains integrate computer science and information science to manage and communicate data, information, and knowledge; however, they differ in the integration of the discipline-specific science and discipline-specific practice. The field of informatics has recently grown to reflect the substantive contribution of the various health disciplines to the generation and use of healthcare data and related information, which has helped to differentiate the often-confusing terminology. In the following discussion, each domain is defined and the major subtypes, if applicable, are described.

Translational Bioinformatics

AMIA refers to translational bioinformatics as the development of storage, analytic, and interpretive methods to optimize the transformation of increasingly voluminous biomedical and genomic data into proactive, predictive, preventive, and participatory health.[7] Translational bioinformatics is evolving with the support of the National Institutes of Health road map for medical research. The end product of translational bioinformatics is newly found knowledge from integrative efforts that can be disseminated to a variety of stakeholders, including biomedical scientists, clinicians, and patients.

Clinical Research Informatics

Clinical research informatics relates to informatics whose objective is to advance the biomedical/health sciences through the humane and ethical use of informatics. Included are issues relating to the use of information and knowledge, as well as the sound and socially appropriate collection and maintenance of person-specific and/or deidentified patient data. EHRs will enhance the availability of clinical data for research and quality improvement initiatives.

Clinical Informatics

Clinical informatics is the application of information and communication technologies to the delivery of healthcare services. It is also referred to as applied clinical informatics and operational informatics. Despite some variations, informatics, when used in healthcare delivery, is essentially the same regardless of the health professional group involved, whether dentists, pharmacists, physicians, nurses, or other health professionals. Clinical informatics is concerned with information use in health care by clinicians, which includes topics ranging from clinical decision support to digital images commonly used in radiology, pathology, dermatology, and ophthalmology; from clinical documentation to computerized provider order entry (CPOE) systems; and from system design to system implementation and adoption issues.

Consumer Health Informatics

Consumer health informatics (CHI) is a form of health IT geared toward delivering better healthcare decisions based on the consumer's perspective.[7] It is well recognized that consumer informatics stands at the crossroads of other disciplines, such as nursing informatics (NI), public health, health promotion, health education, library science, and communication science, and is perhaps the most challenging and rapidly expanding field in health informatics. NI is the specialty that integrates nursing science with multiple information and analytical sciences to identify, define, manage, and communicate data, information, knowledge, and wisdom in nursing practice.[13] NI supports consumers, patients, nurses, and other providers in their decision making in all roles and settings. The support is accomplished through the use of "information structures, information processes, and information technology."[13,p7] CHI is paving the way for health care in the age of connected health by the inclusion of technologies that focus on patients as the primary users of health information.[28]

Public Health Informatics

Public health informatics and its corollary population informatics are the application of information, computer science, and technology to public health science to improve the health of populations. Application of the principles and practices of public health informatics leads to the development of new tools and methodologies that enable the development and use of interoperable information systems for public health functions such as biosurveillance, outbreak response, and electronic laboratory reporting.

Informatics in Nursing Practice

Nurses use various health IT tools to support their clinical practice. EHRs are the most common tool and are more inclusive of the clinical data and information collected on a patient by numerous healthcare professionals to facilitate clinical decision making. Within EHRs, nurses also use nursing documentation systems to record the process and outcomes of their care. To facilitate the provision of care, evidence-based practice guidelines and alerts are incorporated to help nurses conduct their assessments, diagnose, and determine the nursing interventions to achieve optimal patient outcomes.

With the introduction of meaningful use criteria, EHRs are also becoming accessible to patients and their families, as well as to caregivers and consumers. Patients, families, caregivers, and consumers are part of the interprofessional team and engage in healthcare decision making. The engagement of patients is not a new concept, but in recent years, health ITs have made health information and patient records more accessible, thus giving patients the tools they need. Accessing social media sites, patient portals, and mobile health devices are all ways that engaged patients can participate in their health care.

The use of health ITs across professionals, patients/consumers, and healthcare institutions is creating a connected healthcare delivery system. Connected health maximizes the use of technology-enabled tools to provide healthcare delivery beyond the walls of any one health institution.[29] The concept of connected health is integral to the notion of providing accessible health information for patients and families.

The transformation of health care is enabled by the future of health IT and informatics. Widespread and meaningful use of fully functional EHR systems combined with a robust infrastructure for broad-based health information exchange has the potential to improve the quality, safety, and efficiency of health care for all Americans. As more organizations adopt EHRs, health professionals will have greater access to patient information, allowing faster and more accurate diagnoses and treatment. Patients will also have access to their own information and will have the choice to share it with family members securely over the Internet.

This will allow better coordination of care for themselves and their loved ones. EHRs are becoming increasingly widespread across the healthcare system because of their efficiency in disseminating knowledge and promoting safe patient care. Health ITs, network connectivity, and an informatics infrastructure provide the necessary strategies to transition to a continuously learning health system, one that aligns science and informatics, patient-clinician partnerships, incentives, and a culture of continuous improvement to produce the best care at lower cost.[8]

INTERRELATED CONCEPTS

Many interrelated concepts bear some relationship to health IT and health informatics but do not necessarily share the same set of attributes. Related concepts identified here include data, information, knowledge, wisdom, trust, health, health care, meaningful use, bandwidth, and interoperability.

Interrelated concepts that are found in this book include Clinical Judgment, Leadership, Communication, Collaboration, Safety, Evidence, Care Coordination, Health Care Quality, Ethics, Health Policy, and Health Care Law (Fig. 46.3). It is also important to note that the health and illness concepts in Section 2 of this book are interrelated concepts in that they provide the substance for the data, information, knowledge, and wisdom components that form the framework for meaningful use of health informatics.

CLINICAL EXEMPLARS

Box 46.2 displays some common exemplars of health IT and informatics that may be encountered in clinical practice. This list is not complete and is ever changing and expanding as new technology and new interfaces are developed and implemented in health care. Emerging new models of healthcare delivery will require informatics tools for improving quality and efficiency. Additional information for all exemplars presented can be found in multiple textbooks and websites related to health IT and informatics.

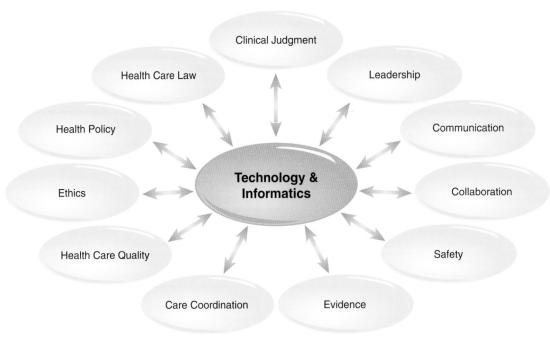

FIGURE 46.3 Technology and Informatics and Interrelated Concepts.

BOX 46.2 EXEMPLARS OF TECHNOLOGY AND INFORMATICS

Clinical Informatics
- Bar code medication administration
- Clinical decision support systems
- Computerized acuity systems
- Computerized nursing documentation
- Computerized provider order entry systems
- Disease/patient registries
- Electronic health record systems
- Electronic prescribing
- Health information exchange
- Telehealth tools
- Population health management tools

Consumer Health Informatics
- Personal health records
- Patient portals
- Patient-generated health data tools (i.e., PatientsLikeMe)
- Social media tools for online support

- Health and wellness apps
- Chronic disease management apps
- Home and self-care monitoring devices
- Smart devices and sensors
- Public health informatics

Biosurveillance Tools
- Geographical information system tools
- Predictive modeling tools
- Disaster preparedness tools
- Immunization registries

Bioinformatics Tools
- Homology and similarity tools
- Protein function analysis tools
- Structural analysis tools
- Sequence analysis tools
- Data mining and data analytics tools

 ACCESS EXEMPLAR LINKS IN YOUR GIDDENS EBOOK

Featured Exemplars

Computerized Nursing Documentation

Computerized nursing documentation technology enables nurses to document all activities associated with the nursing process and serves as a repository for stored nursing data and information that can facilitate clinical decision making and interprofessional communication. Nurses can use an electronic documentation system to capture and store assessment data and to transform these data into clinical information associated with diagnoses, nursing activities, and a plan of care to enable patients to reach desired outcomes. Electronic documentation systems facilitate effective, efficient, safe, and quality care to patients.

Bar Code Medication Administration

Bar code medication administration (BCMA) technology allows nurses to effectively and safely administer medications to patients. BCMA ensures that the right provider is giving the right patient the right medication in the right dose and right route at the right time for the right reason and documents the result of that administration. The BCMA system reduces errors and adverse drug effects.

Clinical Decision Support Systems

Clinical decision support systems (CDSSs) provide electronic tools that can provide the information and knowledge to assist the nurse in clinical decision making. CDSSs can include such tools as computerized alerts, reminders, clinical guideline protocols, condition-specific order sets, and diagnostic tools. CDSSs can significantly impact improvements in quality, safety, efficiency, and effectiveness of health care. Health ITs designed to improve clinical decision making are particularly attractive for their ability to provide a platform for integrating evidence-based knowledge into care delivery.[30]

Electronic Health Record Systems

EHR systems are real-time, patient-centered records that make information available instantly and securely to authorized users. EHR is more than a digital version of a patient's paper chart because its system is built to go beyond standard clinical data collected in a provider's office while it can be inclusive of a broader view of a patient's care. EHR systems can decrease the fragmentation of care by improving care coordination. EHRs have the potential to integrate and organize patient health information and facilitate its instant distribution among all authorized providers involved in a patient's care.[31]

CASE STUDY

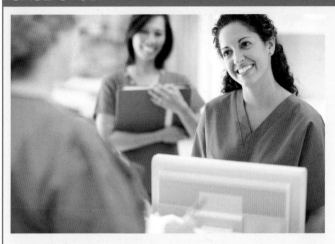

Case Presentation

The University Medical Center uses an electronic health record certified by the Office of the National Coordinator of Health Information Technology. To demonstrate nursing's contribution to patient care, the chief nursing officer supports the Council for Nursing Informatics and provides trained informatics nurses to help the Council achieve the goals of safe patient care and quality nursing data. University Medical Center is a Magnet hospital and is actively engaged in a patient safety program, including the National Database for Nursing Quality Indicators (NDNQI) quality metrics.

Cassandra Mendoza, MSN, RN, is one of the informatics nurse specialists. Her current informatics project is to design and implement a falls risk management protocol in the EHR that also collects data to submit to NDNQI. She first meets with the nursing staff to determine the evidence supporting falls risk management. Based on this evidence, they select a falls risk assessment tool and other data that need to be collected to document and manage the falls risk. They determine the levels of risk are none, moderate, and high risk, and they define order sets for each risk level. Next, Cassandra interviews and observes the staff to determine the workflow surrounding the assessment, documentation, and management of a falls risk.

With this information, she begins to design the screens for the assessment and order sets to facilitate accurate data entry and present the information in a way that all clinicians can understand and can use to make accurate clinical judgments about the care of the patient at the point of care. As she evaluates the evidence, she determines the data elements and their values (assessment questions and possible patient observation) and the appropriate data types (e.g., numeric, free text, and coded response list). For each question and coded response list, she matches each concept to a standardized language. Next, she ensures that the design reveals the nursing process and maps each component to the Reference Information Model of Health Level Seven. She adds a decision support rule that states, "When the falls risk assessment score indicates a risk, Falls Risk is added to the patient problem list and an order set for the indicated risk level is presented to the nurse for approval." Finally, she determines the staff members who may view and interact with the protocol to ensure confidentiality.

After Cassandra completes the implementation of the protocol, she meets with the nursing staff again to evaluate whether the protocol meets their needs and represents the evidence for falls risk management. After the final approvals for the protocol, she builds the screens in the EHR and implements a training program for the staff. Three months after implementation, Cassandra evaluates the protocol and its use by the staff. The number of falls had been reduced by 15%, all of the NDNQI falls metrics were collected electronically (saving money on data collection from charts), nurses were very satisfied with the decision support that saved them time by automatically adding the risk to the problem list and entering orders, and patient satisfaction increased by 10% based on free text comments about the staff's thoughtfulness in keeping patients safe.

Case Analysis Questions

1. Referring to Fig. 46.1, in what way does Cassandra incorporate the processes and tools into this project?
2. What would be barriers in implementing the new fall protocol in the EHR? Which evidence and strategies might help to minimize these challenges?

Source: Fuse/Thinkstock.

 ACCESS EXEMPLAR LINKS IN YOUR GIDDENS EBOOK

REFERENCES

1. Merriam–Webster. (n.d.). *Technology.* Retrieved from https://www.merriam-webster.com/dictionary/technology.
2. Buntin, M. B., Burke, M. F., Hoaglin, M. C., et al. (2011). The benefits of health information technology: A review of the recent literature shows predominantly positive results. *Health Affairs (Project Hope), 30,* 464–471.
3. Chaudhry, B., Wang, J., Wu, S., et al. (2006). Systematic review: Impact of health information technology on quality, efficiency, and costs of medical care. *Annals of Internal Medicine, 144,* 744.
4. Shekelle, P. G., Jones, S. S., Rudin, R. S., et al. the Southern California Evidence-Based Practice Center. (2014). *Health information technology: An updated systematic review with a focus on meaningful use functionalities.* Washington, DC: U.S. Department of Health and Human Services. Retrieved from http://www.healthit.gov/sites/default/files/systematic_review_final_report_508_compliant.pdf.
5. Saba, V. K. (2001). Nursing informatics: Yesterday, today, and tomorrow. *International Nursing Review, 48,* 177.
6. Proctor, R. (2009). *Definition of health informatics. Personal communication to Virginia Van Horne, Content Manager, HSR Information Central, Bethesda MD.* Retrieved from https://hsric.nlm.nih.gov/hsric_public/display_links/717.
7. American Medical Informatics Association. *The science of informatics.* Retrieved from https://www.amia.org/about-amia/science-informatics.
8. Institute of Medicine. (2013). *Best care at lower cost: The path to continuously learning health care in America.* Washington, DC: National Academies Press.
9. Thompson, T. G., & Brailer, D. J. (2004). *The decade of health information technology: Delivering consumer-centric and information-rich health care—Framework for strategic action.* Washington, DC: U.S. Department of Health and Human Services.
10. Lundberg, C. B., Warren, J. J., Brokel, J., et al. (2008). Selecting a standardized terminology for the electronic health record that reveals the impact of nursing practice on patient care. *Online Journal of Nursing Informatics, 12*(2).
11. Center for Medicare and Medicaid Services. (2018). *Promoting Interoperability (PI).* Retrieved from https://www.cms.gov/Regulations-and-Guidance/Legislation/EHRIncentivePrograms/index.html.
12. U.S. Department of Health and Human Services. (2013). *HIPAA regulations.* Retrieved from https://www.federalregister.gov/articles/2013/01/25/2013-01073/modifications-to-the-hipaa-privacy-security-enforcement-and-breach-notification-rules-under-the.
13. American Nurses Association. (2015). *Scope and standards of nursing informatics practice* (2nd ed.). Silver Spring, MD: Nursebooks.org.
14. O'Connor, S., Hübner, U., Shaw, T., et al. (2017). Time for TIGER to ROAR! Technology informatics guiding education reform. *Nurse Education Today, 58,* 78–81.

15. Gardner, R. M., Overhage, M., Steen, L. B., et al. (2009). Core content for subspecialty of clinical informatics. *Journal of the American Medical Informatics Association, 16,* 153.

16. Gundlapalli, A. V., Gundlapalli, A. V., Greaves, W. W., et al. (2015). Clinical informatics board specialty certification for physicians: A global view. *Studies in Health Technology and Informatics, 216,* 501–505.

17. Lorenzi, N., & Riley, R. (2000). Managing change: An overview. *J ournal of the American Medical Informatics Association, 7*(2), 116–124.

18. McGonigle, D., & Mastrian, K. (2018). *Nursing informatics and the foundation of knowledge* (4th ed.). Boston: Jones & Bartlett.

19. Shortliffe, E. H., & Blois, M. S. (2014). Biomedical informatics: The science and the pragmatics. In E. H. Shortliffe & J. J. Cimino (Eds.), *Biomedical informatics: Computer applications in health care and biomedicine* (4th ed.). New York: Springer.

20. McCarthy, M., & Eastman, D. (2010). *Change management strategies for an effective EMR implementation.* Chicago: Healthcare Information Management Systems Society.

21. Walker, P. H. (2011). Strategies for culture change. In M. Ball, J. V. Douglas, & P. H. Walker (Eds.), *Nursing informatics: Where caring and technology meet* (4th ed.). New York: Springer.

22. Warren, J., & Connors, H. (2007). Health information technology can and will transform nursing education. *Nursing Outlook, 55*(1), 58–60.

23. Institute of Medicine. (2000). *To err is human: Building a safer health system.* Washington, DC: National Academies Press.

24. Institute of Medicine. (2001). *Crossing the quality chasm: A new health system for the 21st century.* Washington, DC: National Academies Press.

25. The Learning Health Care System in America. (2012). *Institute of Medicine activity description.* Retrieved from http://www.nationalacademies.org/hmd/Activities/Quality/LearningHealthCare.aspx.

26. Office of the National Coordinator for Health Information Technology (ONC), Office of the Secretary, U.S. Department of Health and Human Services. (2015). *Federal health IT strategic plan 2015–2020.* Retrieved from http://www.healthit.gov/sites/default/files/federal-healthIT-strategic-plan-2014.pdf.

27. Pew Research Center. (2014). *Three technology revolutions.* Retrieved from http://www.pewinternet.org/three-technology-revolutions.

28. Brennan, P. F., & Greenes, R. A. (2014). Consumer health informatics. In E. H. Shortliffe & J. J. Cimino (Eds.), *Biomedical informatics: Computer applications in health care and biomedicine* (4th ed.). New York: Springer.

29. Partners Healthcare. (2018). *Connected health.* Retrieved from http://connectedhealth.partners.org.

30. HealthIT.gov. (2018). *Clinical decision support.* Retrieved from https://www.healthit.gov/topic/safety/clinical-decision-support.

31. HealthIT.gov. (2017). *Benefits of EHRs.* Retrieved from https://www.healthit.gov/topic/health-it-basics/benefits-ehrs.

CONCEPT

47

Evidence

Ingrid Hendrix

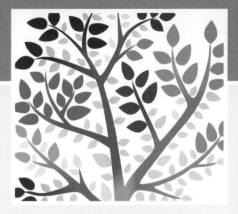

Evidence has become a ubiquitous term in health care and society as a whole. Public fascination with forensics and police and legal proceedings has proliferated in the media. Evidence uncovered at crime scenes or in autopsy rooms is vital to solving cases. Evidence can describe the course of events leading to a crime or a death and can solve the riddle of who committed the offense. An emphasis on evidence also permeates every aspect of health care. Evidence serves a similar function in health care as it does in the legal system. It provides confirmation or substantiation of the usefulness of an intervention, the projected course of a disease, or the link between environmental insults and illness.

The phrase "evidence-based" is applied to every health discipline: evidence-based medicine, evidence-based nursing, evidence-based dentistry, and the more inclusive evidence-based practice or evidence-based health care. But what is evidence? This concept presentation examines evidence broadly and includes how the term is defined, describing the various forms of evidence and the way it is used in health care. Understanding approaches to recognize and classify evidence in clinical or educational situations aids in incorporating evidence in useful and meaningful ways.

DEFINITION

The concept of evidence is probably most closely associated with law and the sciences. In the legal system, evidence is used to establish guilt or innocence. In the sciences, evidence establishes expected benefit or harm. Evidence is defined as a testimony of facts tending to confirm or disprove any conclusions, or something that furnishes verification. When used as a verb, evidence means to attest or prove. These definitions describe most aptly why evidence-based practice (EBP) is so fundamental to health care. Evidence supports or disputes the efficacy of a treatment, the use of a diagnostic tool, the transmission of a disease, or any number of scenarios relevant to health care. Similarly, in the legal arena, evidence is a highly regarded and essential element in judging a situation. Evidence is "Information (in the form of personal or documented testimony or the production of material objects), tending or used to establish facts in a legal investigation."[1] Distilling this definition into its key elements, evidence is information given to establish fact. Synonyms for evidence include affirmation, attestation, confirmation, corroboration, data, documentation, information, substantiation, and testimony. However, evidence is more than just data or documents. Aikenhead states that evidence, as opposed to data, is scrutinized by comparing it with other information and thus is more credible than raw data.[2] Examples of this definition of evidence in forensic and legal arenas can be witness testimony, phone records, toxicology reports, or DNA samples. In clinical practice and health research, evidence is usually exemplified by research studies. Clinical experience and expert opinion can be considered as evidence, but these forms of evidence are usually given less merit because of their subjective nature.

Evidence-based nursing has been defined as "the conscientious, explicit, and judicious use of theory-derived, research-based information in making decisions about care delivery to individuals or groups of patients and in consideration of individual needs and preferences."[3,p152] Scott defines evidence-based nursing as "an ongoing process by which evidence, nursing theory, and the practitioners' clinical expertise are critically evaluated and considered, in conjunction with patient involvement, to provide delivery of optimum nursing care for the individual."[4,p1089] A commonality among these definitions is the use of evidence to guide practice while incorporating key elements of patient involvement and the expertise of nurses.

SCOPE

Consider the scope of evidence as a range from the discovery and generation of evidence on one end of the spectrum, to the delivery of care at the bedside on the other end (Fig. 47.1). Discovery of evidence is often referred to as "bench" research when discovery is on a molecular or cellular level. Moving bench evidence to studying its application in clinical practice is known as translational research. This is a bidirectional process because the focus of bench research is based on clinical problems observed, and advances in clinical practice are dependent on bench research. In health care, research can be done by an individual, but recently greater emphasis and value have been placed on collaborative and interprofessional research, particularly with translational research efforts.

ATTRIBUTES AND CRITERIA

An attribute is a quality or characteristic that is associated with the concept that helps to clarify or confirm the concept. Several attributes of evidence exist (Box 47.1). Major attributes of evidence include replicability, reliability, and validity:

- *Replicability*: Evidence is built on research findings. Findings can only be verified if they can be repeated. If other researchers are

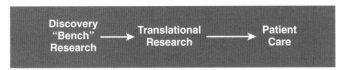

FIGURE 47.1 **Scope of Evidence.** Scope extends from the discovery of evidence to the application of evidence into patient care through patient care standards.

unable to achieve the same results using the same methodology as the original study, the evidence presented by that study is called into question.

- *Reliability*: Evidence must also be consistently and accurately measured.[2] Even clinical experience, as a form of evidence, must demonstrate that the same treatment applied to similar patients over time leads to similar outcomes.
- *Validity*: For evidence to be valid, it must successfully measure what the study set out to measure. For example, a test designed to measure intelligence may actually be measuring the subjects' ability to remember a fact, and so is not a valid measure of intellect.

Minor attributes of evidence include that it is publicly available, understandable, and usable.

THEORETICAL LINKS

Various models of evidence-based practice have been developed to help nurses understand how to incorporate evidence into nursing practice on a routine basis. Some models address EBP from the standpoint of an individual, whereas others address it from an organizational viewpoint. Six of the most commonly cited models are the ACE Star Model of Knowledge Transformation, The Stetler Model, The Advancing Research and Clinical Practice Through Close Collaboration (ARCC) Model, the Promoting Action on Research Implementation in the Health Services Framework (PARIHS) Framework, the Johns Hopkins Nursing Evidence-Based Practice Model and Guidelines, and the Iowa Model of EBP. Two of these models are presented here.

The Johns Hopkins Nursing Evidence-Based Practice Model and Guidelines

This model provides a systematic method for applying evidence in the clinical, research, and educational settings.[5] Developed in collaboration with clinical and academic nurses, the Johns Hopkins model uses a mentored, stepwise approach called the PET Process, standing for the three phases of the model: The *Practice Question*, *Evidence*, and *Translation*. The model addresses three common barriers to implementing EBP in nursing—lack of knowledge, overwhelming amounts of information, and time constraints. The 2017 revision incorporates new evidence and reflects its use in clinical settings as well as providing staff nurses with a robust set of tools to facilitate gathering and evaluating

evidence. The key elements of this model are individual mentoring and support from nursing leadership.

The Iowa Model of Evidence-Based Practice

The Iowa model takes a broader and more institutional approach to implementing EBP.[6] The flowchart of the model begins with either of two types of triggers—problem focused or knowledge focused. These triggers are initiated by events such as clinical problems, accrediting agency requirements, organization or national initiatives, or new evidence from the literature. Nurses can easily follow the steps of the flowchart to identify if there is a sufficient evidence base to guide a change in practice, to determine steps to take if there is insufficient evidence, and to establish outcomes to monitor after initiating a change. Another unique element of this model is consideration of the relevance of the question to the organization, which in turn guides the level of support that can be expected when piloting, adopting, and instituting the projected change and evaluating outcome data. The 2015 revision of the model provides even more feedback loops and detailed instructions for incorporating EBP as well as inclusion of patient preferences.

CONTEXT TO NURSING AND HEALTH CARE

To provide safe, quality care, nurses must base their practice decisions on evidence. The context of evidence in nursing is nurses using the available evidence and producing new research evidence.

Origins of Evidence

Examining the origins and definitions of the phrase "evidence-based" is useful in determining the meaning of evidence within the context of health care. Although there has been a recent emphasis placed on the use of evidence in clinical practice, this is not a new phenomenon. Examples of evidence-based medicine and evidence-based nursing can be found throughout history. One historical example is illustrated by the discovery of the link between an absence of hand washing and the transmission of infection. In the 1800s, Ignaz Semmelweis, a physician, was alarmed by the high rate of childbed (i.e., puerperal) fever in women delivered by physicians compared to those attended by midwives.[7] Semmelweis questioned the cause of this disparity, an essential element in uncovering the evidence to prove or disprove his theory. He observed the women dying of this fever were attended by physicians and students who had previously been in the dissection lab. These physicians and medical students did not wash their hands after working on cadavers and were spreading contaminants from the cadavers to the laboring women. The mothers who had a lower rate of puerperal fever were attended by midwives who did not attend the cadaver lab. Semmelweis did not purposely randomize the women but, rather, discovered the difference between the two groups through observation. Upon instituting mandatory handwashing with soap and lime, the puerperal fever rates dropped precipitously. Unfortunately, his discovery was not enthusiastically adopted, perhaps due to professional jealousy.[7] Semmelweis was forced to move to another city, where he implemented hand-washing techniques and reduced the prevalence of puerperal fever significantly.[8] He questioned existing and entrenched practices, examined the variables involved, and then changed his practice based on the evidence he uncovered.

Florence Nightingale is well-known for her work in establishing the nursing profession and being instrumental in hospital reform. Her work and writings provide a classic example of evidence-based nursing. She used observations and statistics as evidence to support her demand for improved hospital conditions to reduce infections and mortality.[9] Nightingale began evidence-based reporting during her work in the Crimean

War, but she continued throughout her career to incorporate evidence in lobbying for hospital design reform, patient record systems, nursing care, and patient outcomes.[10]

The more recent emphasis on using evidence to guide practice came from Dr. Archie Cochrane, a British epidemiologist who called on the medical profession to incorporate more evidence, in the form of randomized controlled trials, into the care of patients. He was concerned that many healthcare professionals were not implementing evidence from research that could improve patient care and instead turned to colleagues for information or relied on historical methods of treatment. His advocacy led to the creation of the database which bears his name, the *Cochrane Database of Systematic Reviews*.[11]

Types of Evidence

An expectation of the professional nurse is to incorporate evidence into his or her practice. Evidence can present in many ways; it is important to recognize and understand the various types. Evidence created from research studies presents in two major ways: through primary and secondary literature.

Primary Literature

Primary literature constitutes original research studies on which the secondary literature is created. Two broad types of primary literature represent research studies that are the building blocks of evidence: quantitative research and qualitative research.

Quantitative research. Quantitative research has been defined as being "focused on the testing of a hypothesis through objective observation and validation."[12,p17] Some examples of the types of studies that make up this category include randomized controlled studies, cohort studies, longitudinal studies, case–control studies, and case reports (Fig. 47.2).

Randomized controlled double-blind studies are considered the "gold standard" for quantitative research. The reason is that the methods used to conduct these types of studies introduce the least amount of bias. Patients are randomly assigned to the experimental or control group, and both researchers and subjects are "blind" to the intervention. Minimal bias in research studies allows the user of this information to have more confidence in the evidence created by that research. As Gugiu explains, "by 'credible evidence' we mean results for which the study design, conduct, and analysis has minimized or avoided biases

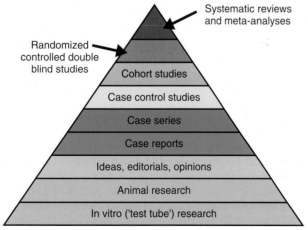

FIGURE 47.2 Evidence Pyramid. (From SUNY Downstate Medical Centre: *Guide to research methods.* Retrieved from http://library. downstate.edu/EBM2/2100.htm.)

that would otherwise raise doubt in their veracity beyond a reasonable doubt."[13,p234] Other study designs introduce more variables and thus the potential for increased bias. For example, case reports study only a few subjects, making it difficult to draw meaningful conclusions to other patients.

Qualitative research. Qualitative research answers questions that cannot be answered using a quantitative study design. Qualitative research focuses on a person's experience and uses analysis of textual, or non-numeric, data, such as interviews, surveys, or questionnaires. As Astin points out, the evidence provided by qualitative studies is not "less than" that produced by quantitative studies, rather it provides the important perspective of the patient experience which should be used in addition to quantitative research.[14] Examples of qualitative study methods are ethnography, phenomenology, grounded theory, and case study.

Mixed methods research. Increasingly, mixed methods studies are being conducted that feature both quantitative and qualitative approaches. These types of studies can corroborate and confirm the findings between the two methods. It is an important design for gaining a deeper understanding of the issue being studied.[15] As an example, quantitative data could supply the evidence as to how often a service is used, and the qualitative data enhances these results by providing the experiences of patients using that service.

Secondary Literature

Busy professionals tasked with providing evidence-based care face an enormous body of literature to guide their practice. This information explosion in the health sciences has led to the development of several types of secondary literature designed to summarize findings from individual or multiple studies. Three categories of secondary literature are evidence summaries, systematic reviews and meta-analyses, and practice guidelines.

Evidence summaries. Evidence summaries are classified as secondary literature because they summarize original research studies. Summary publications have emerged in recent years to address the explosion of information and timely incorporation of evidence into practice. Publications such as *Evidence-Based Nursing, WORLDviews on Evidence-Based Nursing*, and *ACP Journal Club* review individual studies and summarize the results for their readers.

Systematic reviews and meta-analyses. Systematic reviews and meta-analyses provide a synthesis of the quantitative evidence.[16] Systematic reviews include the available evidence on a topic in the form of randomized controlled trials that are summarized using a systematic methodology. Rather than conducting one very large study, the results of many studies are evaluated and a conclusion is drawn about the effectiveness of a particular treatment. The number of systematic reviews is expanding with initiatives such as the Cochrane Collaboration, the Campbell Collaboration, and the Joanna Briggs Institute. Topics found in a systematic review tend to focus on areas of research that would be of the most interest to the greatest number of practitioners. Meta-analyses, similar to systematic reviews, summarize evidence from multiple studies. What differentiates a meta-analysis from a systematic review is that it focuses on combining the statistical results of numerous studies and analyzes that evidence.

Practice guidelines. Practice guidelines are another type of summary publication. They are designed to summarize findings of the research and advise practitioners on the current standard of care. Ideally, guidelines result in a faster integration of new evidence into practice and address issues of cost and variation in practice. Guidelines are often developed by government agencies or societies, such as the U.S. Preventive Services Task Force, the American College of Obstetricians and Gynecologists, or the National Association of Pediatric Nurse Practitioners. These organizations create guidelines by using evidence from the literature in the form of research studies and expert opinion to craft the publications. Practice guidelines are considered the standard of practice for a particular treatment. Unlike systematic reviews or meta-analyses, practice guidelines are less structured in their design. Databases, such as PubMed, have the option to limit a search to practice guidelines or associations post guidelines on their websites.

Levels of Evidence

Unfortunately, not all evidence produced is of equal quality. Conclusions drawn from research are not necessarily valid just because they originate from a study. For this reason, levels of evidence have been created to help the busy practitioner determine the quality of a study. Hierarchies, based on how much trust can be placed in the results of a study design, have been developed. Unfortunately, there has been no standardization, and therefore different organizations have created their own versions. Initiatives such as GRADE (Grading of Recommendations, Assessment, Development, and Evaluation) are attempting to consistently measure the quality of research studies.[17] This system classifies studies as strong or weak based on the methodology of the study—such as sample size and blinding of the researchers and/or study subjects. Designed as a tool for developers of systematic reviews and guidelines, the system is useful for anyone trying to appraise the evidence presented in individual studies. For quantitative studies, numerous websites show detailed tables of what has become known as levels of evidence.[18,19] Levels of evidence provide an evidence hierarchy, with items at the top showing study designs that promote the least amount of bias, to the ones at the bottom being most subjective in the evidence they provide. The design of qualitative studies makes them less well suited for categorization into these levels of evidence, but articles and free online checklists are available to help guide readers in evaluating these types of studies.[20,21]

Another level of evidence is applied to secondary literature, particularly practice guidelines. In this context, a grade or level is assigned to a recommendation to help a healthcare professional understand how well the recommendation is supported by the collective research. For example, the U.S. Preventive Services Task force has a grading of evidence A, B, C, D, and I (Box 47.2).

Evidence on the Internet

Levels of evidence are designed to be applied to original research studies—the primary literature. With the exponential growth of published research studies, many healthcare professionals look to search engines such as Google to find the information that they need. This can be a risky practice. Anyone can post information on the Internet and create very authoritative-appearing websites, even if the information provided is false or misleading. Checklists, such as the CRAAP (Currency, Relevance, Authority, Accuracy, Purpose) Test, help individuals evaluate the credibility of online health information.[22] First, check the date the website was last updated, usually found at the bottom of the page. Currency is an important element of information found on the Web, especially in regard to health information. Determine the author and sponsor of the information. This is not always easy to discern. Looking at the *About Us* or *Contact Us* page of a website can provide clues. As with research studies, information found online should limit bias as much as possible. For example, if the information about a particular drug is provided by the pharmaceutical company selling that product, it would be prudent to evaluate that information with such a bias in mind. Looking at a website's domain can help determine the source of the information—for example, *.edu* for educational institutions or *.gov* for government websites. Determine who is providing the content of the website. Is it a healthcare professional, a concerned individual, or a government agency and are they providing facts or opinions? Content on a website should be validated with evidence, such as

---

BOX 47.2 U.S. Preventive Services Task Force Grading of Evidence

Grade A = Recommends
- There is high certainty that the net benefit is substantial.

Grade B = Recommends
- There is high certainty that the net benefit is moderate or there is moderate certainty that the net benefit is moderate to substantial.

Grade C = Selective Recommendation
- There is moderate certainty that the net benefit is small. There may be considerations that support providing the intervention for an individual patient depending on individual preferences and circumstances, but not for the general population.

Grade D = Recommends Against
- There is moderate or high certainty that the intervention has no net benefit or that the harms outweigh the benefits.

I Statement = Insufficient Evidence to Recommend for or Against
- The current evidence is insufficient to assess the balance of benefits and harms of the service. Evidence is lacking, of poor quality, or conflicting, and the balance of benefits and harms cannot be determined.

From U.S. Preventive Services Task Force: Grade Definitions, 2013. Retrieved from https://www.uspreventiveservicestaskforce.org/Page/Name/grade-definitions#grade-definitions-after-july-2012

---

references to research studies. Otherwise, the information should be considered opinion. Organizations such as the Health on the Net Foundation (https://www.hon.ch/en/) provide a seal of approval to websites adhering to their standards of quality. Adding their toolbar to a web browser provides a quick visual that the information on the site has met certain quality criteria.

Nurses as Researchers: Evidence Discovery

Many nurses are involved in research. Involvement may include leading a research study as a principal investigator, being a collaborating investigator on a study, or contributing to a study through data collection. Leading research studies requires a specific skill set acquired by completing graduate education at the doctoral level and following research protocols outlined by an institutional oversight committee, such as an institutional review board. Most researchers are affiliated with an academic health sciences center, private organizations and foundations with dedicated research departments, or government agencies dedicated to research.

Quality improvement projects differ from research studies in a number of ways. The aim of quality improvement projects is to improve patient care at the local level (i.e., hospital units) and the improvement is based on current knowledge rather than creating new knowledge. A familiar model for QI projects is the PDSA (Plan, Do, Study, Act). There is seldom outside funding involved and the methodology is iterative rather than following a rigid protocol. Institutional Review Board approval is not always required of quality improvement projects, but that varies with the project and the institution.

Nurses as Consumers of Evidence

All nurses must be skilled as consumers of evidence. Understanding research designs and learning to incorporate high-quality evidence into practice can make creating nursing research a less daunting endeavor. For nurses, being a consumer of the evidence generally assumes two forms: (1) practice policies and procedures and (2) finding solutions to practice problems.

Policies and Procedures

Policy and procedure manuals in healthcare agencies outline the practice standards for various care activities; nurses are expected to follow policies and procedures for the agency in which they practice. Policies and procedures should be regularly updated to reflect the current evidence and standards of practice and approved by a committee charged with this oversight. Nurses have a role in developing and maintaining policy and procedure guidelines by serving on such committees or volunteering to participate in updates. In this context, nurses must be skilled research consumers in order to make accurate and efficient recommendations for policy updates.

Finding Solutions to Practice Questions or Problems

There are many occasions when practicing nurses identify practice-related problems that require solutions. Nurses should use available evidence to systematically approach a question of patient care. The steps are outlined as follows:

1. Develop an answerable question.
2. Search the literature to uncover evidence to answer the question.
3. Evaluate the evidence found.
4. Apply the evidence to the practice situation.
5. Evaluate the outcome.

Step 1: Develop an answerable question. The first step in finding evidence is determining a question to ask. This may seem straightforward and obvious, but this step is an obstacle for many people. Most people start searching for information, or evidence, with only a vague idea of what they are seeking. It would be similar to searching for someone's house and knowing only that the person is located in the southeast part of town. One could spend days trying to find the exact location with such vague directions—and one would probably quit the search without success. To find the most direct route, one must start with a good map. A good map begins with the question, "Where do you want to go?" The best way to find evidence is to be clear about what information is needed. The question needs to be specific or answerable without being too vague or so specific that the probability of finding information about the topic would be unlikely. Entering a search query such as "breast cancer" or "diabetes" would lead to an overwhelming abundance of information. What particular aspect of breast cancer or diabetes is of interest: treatment, supportive services, or prevention strategies? Before searching for the evidence, define the question to be answered and map a strategy to get there.

There are two types of questions to consider, background and foreground questions. Background questions are those that provide foundational knowledge. An example of a background question is "What is scleroderma?" These types of questions can most easily be answered by a textbook, review article, or a reputable website. Foreground questions address issues of a more specific nature, such as "Is drug *x* more effective than drug *y* in treating scleroderma?" These questions are best answered by searching the primary literature, which is found in databases indexing research studies, such as PubMed or the Cumulative Index to Nursing and Allied Health Literature (CINAHL).

A strategy that can be helpful in designing an answerable foreground question is using the PICO formula. The acronym stands for *p*opulation, *i*ntervention, *c*omparison, and *o*utcome. Defining these elements clarifies the question. The following is an example of a PICO question: "For inpatients (P), is turning every 2 hours (I) more effective than air mattresses (C) for preventing pressure ulcers

(O)?" Another formula used to develop an answerable question is the PICOT formula. The difference here is the addition of the T, which represents time. This represents the time frame in which the patient or population of interest is observed to determine if the outcome of interest is achieved. The following question is an illustration of the PICOT formula: In new mothers (P), do home visits by a nurse practitioner (I) versus no home visits (C) decrease the incidence of child abuse (O) in the first year postpartum (T)? For qualitative studies, the SPIDER formula was created. SPIDER stands for *S*ample, *P*henomenon of *I*nterest, *D*esign, *E*valuation, *R*esearch type. These elements more accurately reflect the design of a qualitative study than does the PICO formula that was created to help create quantitative research search strategies.

Step 2: Search the literature. Once a question is developed, the next step is searching the literature. With a question mapped out, it is easier to determine which key words to use in the search. Including synonyms for terms will help expand a search, combine them using the OR Boolean operator, i.e., ambulatory OR outpatient. Use the Boolean operator AND between key words to narrow a search, i.e., nurses AND advocacy. Quotes around phrases search for those words next to each other, such as "kangaroo care." Healthcare professionals use many acronyms; spelling out abbreviations can avoid unrelated articles. For example, a search on the topic "AIDS" will result in articles discussing hearing aids or walking aids, for example, in addition to articles on the disease. Searching the phrase *acquired immunodeficiency syndrome* will retrieve articles focused on the disease. If retrieval is too limited, remove a key word of less importance to the question. A large retrieval can benefit from limits such as language, age groups, or dates of publication.

It is virtually impossible to keep current with new findings and different approaches to patient care. On the topic of evidence-based nursing alone, the number of articles in the PubMed database has expanded from 1 in 1996 to 5828 in 2018. Bibliographic databases are designed to help access and catalog the rapidly expanding body of literature. However, it is an imperfect system. There are many databases with different focus areas, and each has a different search engine, or interface, to learn. As a result, many clinicians resort to Google or Wikipedia because of the fast, user-friendly interfaces. However, there are drawbacks to using search engines such as Google. The amount of information retrieved is usually quite large. Using Google Scholar, a subset of Google, reduces somewhat the volume of information retrieved, but results are still sizeable. This can be beneficial for an initial search to discover how much is available on a topic. But databases such as PubMed provide multiple options for fine tuning results, such as age groups or study design. Mastrangelo et al. reported that Google Scholar has a higher recall than PubMed but that PubMed's retrieval is more precise.[23]

Using databases specifically focused on healthcare research is more efficient, but it requires some training. Most searchers use only key words, but using the subject heading search feature of a database can significantly narrow a search and yield more targeted results. Consulting with a medical librarian or using tutorials provided by the database producer saves valuable time in locating evidence to guide practice. Searching the literature is more an art than a science, and it requires creativity and perseverance. As with any skill, practice will increase satisfaction with the outcome.

Step 3: Evaluate the evidence found. Once information has been located as evidence for a change in practice, that information should be evaluated for its quality and applicability to a particular patient situation. The following questions are commonly used to evaluate studies: Are the results of the study or systematic review valid? What are the results, and are they meaningful and reliable? Are the results clinically relevant to my patients? *American Journal of Nursing* has created a website compiling articles from their journal to help nurses assess the quality of the information found in research studies.[24] The American Medical Association has also published the book *Users' Guides to the Medical Literature*, which is a compilation of articles from *Journal of the American Medical Association* covering topics on how to read and understand the information found in published studies. As stated previously, not all evidence is created equal, and nurses need to be critical consumers of the information they uncover. By reading these sources, nurses can improve their skills in critically evaluating the literature.

Step 4: Apply the evidence found. If sufficient evidence is found to guide a change in practice, the next step of EBP is to apply that evidence to a particular patient situation. Although evidence provides proof of the validity of a course of action, it is not the sole reason for treatment decisions. A key element in any practice situation is the incorporation of patients' preferences for their health processes and outcomes: "Nurses play a pivotal role in empowering patients, engaging them in their care, and ensuring that they are fully activated to be personally accountable for their own health."[25,p110] An individual should be provided with the evidence and advice of a well-informed healthcare professional to support his or her decision to move forward with the care he or she desires. It is the responsibility of the healthcare professional to use the most appropriate and current evidence to guide practice and optimize care.

Step 5: Evaluate the evidence. To complete the process, the nurse evaluates the outcome. Evaluation includes appraisal of the degree of success of the intervention and the patient's satisfaction with the outcome in addition to assessment by the nurse of the efficacy of the evidence. Outcomes, both successful and unsuccessful, provide a source of new evidence for others to use. Repeatedly following the steps of EBN will facilitate its use.

INTERRELATED CONCEPTS

Many concepts relate to and work in synergy with evidence; in fact, nearly everything in health care is shaped by evidence. In addition to

guiding individual practice, evidence also impacts health care on a more global scale. Four concepts featured in this textbook have especially important interrelationships: Safety, Health Policy, Technology and Informatics, and Health Care Economics. Fig. 47.3 illustrates the multidirectionality of evidence. The arrow pointing outward illustrates how evidence provides the foundation and evolution for these concepts. The arrow pointing toward evidence indicates that these concepts provide evidence to their efficacy; thus, their connection to the evidence is not static. Outcomes inform future research to update previous evidence and thus a constant flow of evidence is maintained.

In 2003, the Institute of Medicine (IOM) released the report, *Keeping Patients Safe: Transforming the Work Environment of Nurses.*[26] The IOM used evidence from a variety of industries, other IOM reports, and expert testimony to develop policy recommendations related to nurse/patient ratios, work hours, and overtime—all factors that influence the delivery of safe patient care (Safety). The Agency for Healthcare Research and Quality point out on their Patient Safety Network how important nurses are to patient safety since they spend the most time with patients and are therefore the best at alerting the rest of the healthcare team to a patients' deteriorating status. They also summarize numerous articles identifying nurse staffing ratios as an essential element in patient safety.[27] Patient safety initiatives and the pursuit of quality health care are all built on the foundation of evidence.

Evidence provides a foundation for the creation of Health Policy. Benefits of new treatments and diagnostic tests are evaluated by examining the evidence proving their efficacy for policymakers to approve their use. Policies developed to guide practice are based on evidence found in the literature. Policymakers should incorporate all types of evidence appropriate to the topic, but also balance the evidence with practical constraints such as values of the community, costs, and ethics.[28] Federal agencies and numerous global agencies, such as the World Health Organization, have developed initiatives to improve the uptake of scientific evidence into the development of health policy.[29,30]

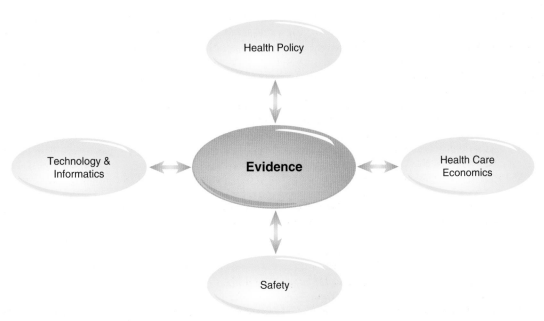

FIGURE 47.3 Evidence and Interrelated Concepts.

Technology and Informatics is another concept related to evidence. Technology in the context of evidence allows for increased access to the literature through online databases, web content, electronic books, and online journal articles. Sophisticated search engines provide end users with increasingly intuitive interfaces that are faster and use increasingly sophisticated algorithms to locate information. Handheld devices allow information to be accessed from anywhere the user is located. Ideally, evidence informs the use and adoption of technology, with new technology incorporated into practice once it is tested for its validity and utility. The specialty of nursing informatics "integrates nursing science with multiple information management and analytical sciences to identify, define, manage, and communicate data, information, knowledge, and wisdom in nursing practice."[31] Informatics has been the driving force behind such innovations as the development of the electronic medical record (EMR), wearable monitors, and patient portals. Data from these systems and others, often referred to as "big data" for its size, speed of creation, and variety, is a rich source of information to guide local, national, and international efforts at studying and improving patient care. But while such data exists, system silos and platform heterogeneity challenge researchers to combine these gold mines of disparate data into a cohesive and useable database.

Evidence plays a vital role in Health Care Economics through cost containment. Policymakers, governments, institutions, and the public are all demanding evidence to support healthcare resource decisions. One example of the relationship between economics and evidence is research showing that care provided by nurse practitioners, practicing to the full extent of their license, is more economical than care provided by primary care physicians, a significant issue in an era of healthcare reform.[32,33]

CLINICAL EXEMPLARS

An exemplar is a specific example of a concept, and there are literally thousands of evidence exemplars. Although research studies, practice guidelines, and expert opinions are general categories of evidence exemplars, the studies or practice guidelines themselves are the exemplars. For example, in the category of practice guidelines alone, PubMed indexes 24,000 guidelines. Box 47.3 presents common exemplars linked to this concept.

Featured Exemplars
Randomized Controlled Trial
Double-blinded randomized controlled trials are considered the gold standard for evidence related to therapies because these types of studies represent the least amount of design bias. Study subjects are randomly placed (randomized) into either a treatment or a control group of the study, so neither the subjects nor the researchers decide the subject placement, thus reducing the influence of preconceived ideas about the likely outcomes. Double-blinded studies are designed so that neither the researcher nor the subject knows which treatment is being given; thus they are both "blinded." By removing these sources of design bias, more confidence can be placed in the results of the study.

Longitudinal Study
Studies of a group of people over a specified period of time can be used to detect long-term health changes, such as the effects of exposure to particular environmental factors or lifestyle choices. Groups of people who are exposed and who are not exposed may be observed over time to determine if their health outcomes differ. The time frame can be as long as decades, as in the case of the Framingham Heart Study, started in 1948, or the Nurses' Health Study, started in 1976.

BOX 47.3   EXEMPLARS OF EVIDENCE

Quantitative Research Studies
- Randomized controlled trial
- Cohort study
- Case–control study
- Case study
- Longitudinal study

Qualitative Research Studies
- Ethnography
- Phenomenology
- Grounded theory
- Case study

Practice Guidelines
- Standards of medical care in diabetes (American Diabetic Association)
- Lipid screening and cardiovascular health in childhood (American Academy of Pediatrics)
- Guideline for human papillomavirus (HPV) vaccine use to prevent cervical cancer (American Cancer Association)

Expert Opinion/Commentaries
Healthcare Policies
- Healthy People 2030

ACCESS EXEMPLAR LINKS IN YOUR GIDDENS EBOOK

Ethnography

Ethnographic studies are a type of qualitative research methodology. This type of study has historically been used by anthropologists to study cultural groups, such as indigenous peoples. In health care, the cultural groups can be patients in a particular unit or groups of nurses. A key element of ethnography research is that the researcher studies the group in question over a long period of time and usually will join the group to become a participant observer. Nursing examples of ethnography research include observing interruptions in the work environment of nurses and the use of various knowledge sources by newly graduated nurses' in decision-making.[34,35]

Practice Guidelines

Practice guidelines are recommendations for clinicians on the current best practices for treatment. Guidelines, using the latest evidence available on a particular topic, are usually created by the consensus of experts. They can be developed by government agencies, nonprofit agencies, hospitals, or professional societies. Often, they are sponsored by government agencies to standardize the best treatment available and disseminate research findings as quickly as possible.

Expert Opinion

Opinion is at the opposite end of the spectrum of reliability from double-blind randomized controlled trials, due to the inherent bias. Individuals who are considered experts in their field by their peers produce evidence based on their experience. Although experience is an important and valid form of evidence, it needs to be considered in light of how it is produced. Examples of expert opinions are book chapters, review articles, and guidelines.

CASE STUDY

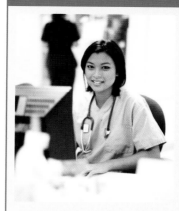

Case Presentation

Mika Kimura, a registered nurse working in the neurosurgical intensive care unit (NSICU), observes that many of the patients under her care need to be transferred from their beds to wheelchairs. However, most of these patients have very little motor control and are unable to assist the nurses with transfers. As a result, she observes more absences among her coworkers attributable to back injuries. Mika realizes there is a need for change and is curious about how other similar units address this issue. She asks her coworkers who have worked in other units if they have seen a solution to this problem. No one reports a satisfactory solution.

Mika turns to the evidence from the published literature to determine if anyone has conducted a study to address this problem. The question she develops is, "In intensive care units, specifically neurosurgical ICUs, is there a method of transferring patients that does not cause injury to the nurse?" She starts her search in the PubMed database and types in the key words "neurosurgical icu," "patient transfers," and "nurses." This yields a few hits but nothing very useful. Thus she decides to broaden her search to include any ICU, and this time spells out "intensive care unit" and tries the key word of "lift*." By using an asterisk, Mika retrieves articles that use the word *lift* or *lifts* or *lifting* or *lifted*. She omits the word "nurse" because she can still use the information if the article refers to other healthcare employees. She finds a few articles that she wants to examine in more depth, so she links to the full text of those articles and prints them. Later that evening, when it is quieter on the unit, she reads the articles. Mika learns that many hospitals have developed "no lift" policies and have also purchased moveable lift devices. One article discusses the cost-effectiveness of using a lift versus dealing with staff absences attributable to back injuries and workers' compensation claims. Mika then determines how many employees in her unit in the past year have missed work because of injuries caused by transfers. Armed with this information, she approaches the unit manager to request that the hospital purchase a lift that can be rolled from room to room. Based on the evidence that she provided to prove her point—both from the literature and from hospital injury reports—Mika's request is approved and a lift is purchased. Not only has she won the thanks of her coworkers but also she has saved the hospital substantial money in lost time from occupational injuries.

Case Analysis Questions

1. Mika exemplifies the idea of nurses as consumers of evidence. Consider the steps in a systematic approach outlined early in this concept presentation. In what way is this consistent with what Mika did?
2. The last step in a systematic approach is evaluating outcomes. How should it be determined if the acquisition of a lift has made a difference?

From Ablestock.com/Thinkstock.

ACCESS EXEMPLAR LINKS IN YOUR GIDDENS EBOOK

REFERENCES

1. OED Online. (2018). *Evidence*. Retrieved from http://www.oed.com. libproxy.unm.edu/view/Entry/65368?rskey=ynYW5q&result=1&isAdvanced=false#eid.
2. Aikenhead, G. S. (2005). Science-based occupations and the science curriculum: Concepts of evidence. *Science Education, 89*, 242–275.
3. Ingersoll, G. (2000). Evidence-based nursing: What it is and what it isn't. *Nursing Outlook, 48*, 151–152.
4. Scott, K., & McSherry, R. (2009). Evidence-based nursing: Clarifying the concepts for nurses in practice. *Journal of Clinical Nursing, 18*, 1085–1095.
5. Dang, D., & Dearholt, S. (2017). *Johns Hopkins nursing evidence-based practice: Model and guidelines* (3rd ed.). Indianapolis, IN: Sigma Theta Tau International.
6. Iowa Model Collaborative, Buckwalter, K. C., Cullen, L., et al. Authored on behalf of the Iowa Model Collaborative. (2017). Iowa model of evidence-based practice: Revisions and validation. *Worldviews on Evidence-based Nursing, 14*(3), 175–182. https://doi.org/10.1111/wvn.12223.
7. Manor, J., Blum, N., & Lurie, Y. (2016). "No good deed goes unpunished": Ignaz Semmelweis and the story of puerperal fever. *Infection Control and Hospital Epidemiology, 37*, 881–887.
8. Loudin, I. (2013). Ignaz Philip Semmelweis' studies of death in childbirth. *Journal of the Royal Society of Medicine, 106*, 461–463.
9. Aravind, M., & Hung, K. C. (2010). Evidence-based medicine and hospital reform: Tracing origins back to Florence Nightingale. *Plastic and Reconstructive Surgery, 125*, 403–409.
10. McDonald, L. (2001). Florence Nightingale and the early origins of evidence-based nursing. *Evidence-Based Nursing, 4*, 68–69.
11. Shah, H. M., & Chung, K. C. (2009). Archie Cochrane and his vision for evidence-based medicine. *Plastic and Reconstructive Surgery, 124*, 982–988.
12. Hamer, S., & Collinson, G. (2005). *Achieving evidence-based practice: A handbook for practitioners* (2nd ed.). Edinburgh, UK: Baillìere Tindall Elsevier.
13. Gugiu, P. C., & Gugiu, M. R. (2010). A critical appraisal of standard guidelines for grading levels of evidence. *Evaluation and the Health Professions, 33*, 233–255.
14. Astin, F., & Long, A. (2014). Characteristics of qualitative research and its application. *British Journal of Cardiac Nursing, 9*, 93–98.
15. Halcomb, E., & Hickman, L. (2015). Mixed methods research. *Nursing Standard, 29*, 41–47.
16. Askie, L., & Offringa, M. (2015). Systematic reviews and meta-analysis. *Seminars in Fetal and Neonatal Medicine, 20*, 403–409.
17. Goldet, G., & Howick, J. (2013). Understanding GRADE: An introduction. *Journal of Evidence-Based Medicine, 6*, 50–54.
18. Association of perioperative Registered Nurses. (2015). *Evidence Rating*. Retrieved from https://www.aorn.org/guidelines/about-aorn-guidelines/evidence-rating.
19. Phillips, B., Ball, C., Sackett, D., et al. (2009). *Oxford Centre for Evidence-Based Medicine—Levels of evidence*. Retrieved from http://www.cebm.net/oxford-centre-evidence-based-medicine-levels-evidence-march-2009.
20. Moon, M., Wolf, L., Zavotsky, K., et al. (2013). Evaluating qualitative research studies for use in the clinical setting. *Journal of Emergency Nursing, 39*, 508–510.
21. Critical Appraisal Skills Program. (2018). *CASP Qualitative Checklist*. [online] Retrieved from https://casp-uk.net/wp-content/uploads/2018/03/CASP-Qualitative-Checklist-Download.pdf.
22. Lewis State College. *Ron E. Lewis Library*. Thinking critically about web information—Applying the CRAAP test. (n.d.). Retrieved from http://library.lsco.edu/help/web-page-rubric.pdf.

23. Mastrangelo, G., Fadda, E., Rossi, A., et al. (2010). Literature search on risk factors for sarcoma: Pubmed and Google Scholar may be complementary sources. *BMC Research Notes, 3,* 131–134.

24. American Journal of Nursing (Ed.). *Evidence Based Practice: Step by Step.* Retrieved from https://www.nursingcenter.com/evidencebasedpracticenetwork/home/tools-resources/collections/ajn-ebp-series.aspx.

25. Pelletier, L., & Stichler, J. (2014). Ensuring patient and family engagement. *Journal of Nursing Care Quality, 29,* 110–114.

26. Page, A. (Ed.), (2004). *Keeping patients safe: Transforming the work environment of nurses.* Washington, DC: National Academies Press.

27. Agency for Healthcare Research and Quality. (2017). *PSNet (Patient Safety Network): Nursing and patient safety.* Retrieved from https://psnet.ahrq.gov/primers/primer/22/nursing-and-patient-safety.

28. Bedard, P. O., & Ouimet, M. (2016). Persistent misunderstandings about evidence-based (sorry:informed!) policy-making. *Archives of Public Health, 74,* 31–37.

29. World Health Organization. (2018). *Evidence-informed policy networks (EVIPNet).* Retrieved from http://www.who.int/evidence/en/.

30. Agency for Healthcare Research and Quality. (2018). *EPC Evidence-based reports.* Retrieved from http://www.ahrq.gov/research/findings/evidence-based-reports/index.html.

31. American Nurses Association. (2015). *Nursing informatics: Scope and standards of practice* (2nd ed.). Silver Spring, MD: American Nurses Association.

32. Timmons, E. J. (2017). The effects of expanded nurse practitioner and physician assistant scope of practice on the cost of Medicaid patient care. *Health Policy, 121,* 189–196.

33. Perloff, J., Desoches, C. M., & Buerhaus, P. (2016). Comparing the cost of care provided to Medicare beneficiaries assigned to primary care nurse practitioners and physicians. *Health Services Research, 51,* 1407–1423.

34. Hopkinson, S. G., & Wiegand, D. L. (2017). The culture contributing to interruptions in the nursing work environment: An ethnography. *Journal of Clinical Nursing, 26,* 5093–5102.

35. Voldbjerg, S. L. (2016). Newly graduated nurses' use of knowledge sources: A metaethnography. *Journal of Advanced Nursing, 72,* 1751–1765.

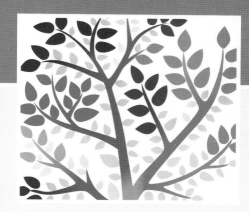

Health Care Quality

Rebecca S. Miltner

Quality is one of the most important issues in health care today. Healthcare organizations and services have a duty to the communities they serve to provide high-quality care to all residents at the lowest cost. The quality of health care is intertwined with patient preferences, access to services, and the cost of care. In other words, the delivery of quality care is irrelevant if the patient cannot access care, the cost is prohibitive (either through insurance or self-pay), or the patient does not want it. Thus both the medical provider and the nurse who want to do the best for the patient may be at odds with the patient, society norms, and best practices.

Countries and healthcare systems struggle with the issues of cost, access, and quality. In 2016, in the United States, healthcare expenditures were estimated at 17.8% of its gross domestic product, or $9403 per person.[1] Although the United States spends more per person than any other industrialized country, 10% of people under the age of 65 years are without any form of health insurance to pay for care.[1] Even worse, healthcare error may be the third leading cause of death with 210,000 to 400,000 deaths per year estimated to be linked to poor quality of care.[2]

Numerous government laws and regulations, accreditation standards, and professional standards are in place to monitor quality and protect the public from harm. Hospitals and other healthcare organizations must establish structures and processes to show evidence that standards for quality are in place and upheld. Nurses are a crucial link in meeting the needs of patients and ensuring patient safety, patient-centered care, and communication as part of the healthcare team. The purpose of this concept presentation is to help students gain a general understanding of healthcare quality.

DEFINITION

The importance of healthcare quality dates back to Florence Nightingale. During the Crimean War in the mid-1800s, most soldiers died of infections, not battle injuries. Nightingale insisted on meticulous sanitation and attention to the patients' needs. In a short period of time, deaths among the wounded at Scutari were reduced from 33% of the wounded to 2%.[3] Nightingale documented this improvement with meticulously kept records. These accomplishments were initially not well received by the medical establishment, but Nightingale is now recognized not only for modern nursing practice, but also infection control, epidemiology, and hospice care.[3]

Defining quality is challenging because the meaning of "quality" can vary based on the context of care, personal expectations, and regulatory requirements. Patients, clinicians, and managers may define healthcare quality in different ways. The patient may value how much time providers spend with them or how they speak to them. Physicians may value providing the cutting-edge medical interventions to optimize patient outcomes. The nurse at the bedside might view quality as the delivery of safe, caring, and competent care. The nurse manager might see quality as a ratio of volume of care in relation to the available resources or the score on a patient experience survey. One definition of healthcare quality is limiting to these many different perspectives. However, the most widely accepted definition of healthcare quality is from the Institute of Medicine (IOM) which states that quality is *the degree to which health services for individuals and populations increase the likelihood of desired health outcomes and are consistent with current professional knowledge.*[4] This definition remains appropriate because it infers that health services must be examined at the individual and larger population levels, suggests that desired health outcomes will vary based on individual preferences and current care options, and points out that all healthcare professionals should be lifelong learners to keep up with the current evidence for their practice.

SCOPE

The patient and their family expect that every encounter with the healthcare system will be safe and of high quality. As noted above, this is not the case. Health care is one of the most complex systems because of the individual patients' needs and preferences, the number and type of healthcare professionals involved, and the organizations' missions and resources. Therefore, the scope of healthcare quality is broad and encompasses most healthcare activities from direct patient care to health policy at the state, national, and international levels. As depicted in Fig. 48.1, healthcare quality begins with the individual patient and family. The patient is the focus of healthcare services, and their direct interaction is with professionals in clinics or nursing units. The patient's health is affected by their socioeconomic status and educational and work opportunities as well as environmental factors. The

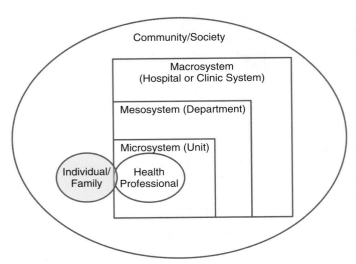

FIGURE 48.1 Scope of Healthcare Quality from a Systems Perspective.

patient's behavior and cultural preferences also impact their health and well-being. The patient comes to the healthcare system with these environmental, socioeconomic, and behavioral attributes that impact the care needed.

The first part of the system that the patient interacts with is usually a primary care clinic or hospital unit. These clinics or nursing units are sometimes called microsystems which are a small group of professionals who work together on a regular basis to provide care to discrete populations of patients.[5] These microsystems are responsible for monitoring their processes and outcomes of care and taking steps to improve things that are not working well. These microsystems are embedded in departments or mesosystems and larger organizations known as macrosystems. The meso- and macrosystems provide administrative support functions such as personnel services, product and supply acquisition, and other managerial functions. The leaders at these higher levels are accountable to regulatory agencies, stakeholders, and the community for the quality of care at their organizations. Leaders should role model the importance of everyone's attention to quality and safety as well as ensure that clinical staff have resources needed to provide high-quality care. Within the larger society, healthcare quality is impacted by policies and legislation that facilitates access and quality and finds appropriate mechanisms to pay for care. People at all levels of the healthcare system must be engaged in ongoing efforts to improve quality.

ATTRIBUTES AND CRITERIA

In *Crossing the Quality Chasm*, the IOM (now known as the National Academy of Medicine) identified six characteristics or attributes for quality health care that are widely used as the basis for quality assessment and measurement: safe, timely, effective, efficient, equitable, and patient-centered. This is often referred to as the STEEEP healthcare principles or aims (Box 48.1).[4]

Safe

All patients should expect care to be delivered without error and free of injury.[4] Unfortunately, thousands of errors occur every day in the U.S. health system from seemingly minor incidents such as not completing ambulation orders to administering the wrong medication that leads to patient death.[2] Safe healthcare delivery requires competent clinicians who demonstrate appropriate knowledge of the health/illness status of the patients they are treating and practice within the appropriate scope of practice based on their licensure or certification. More importantly and challenging, safe healthcare delivery requires interprofessional teamwork and collaboration at all levels of the organization.

Timely

Timeliness of care refers to reducing wait time for healthcare delivery services. This principle is particularly important to avoid harmful delays that can occur with certain medical conditions. There are many delays in the healthcare system. Patients wait for parking, they wait in the clinic to get registered, they wait to be put in a room, and they wait to be seen by the healthcare provider. If they need diagnostic testing, to fill a prescription, or to see a physical therapist, they will probably wait again. Professionals may also have to wait. For example, they may wait for lab test results to make decisions for the plan of care. When health care is delivered in a timely manner, wait times and harmful delays for both the patient and the provider of care are reduced and care is offered before unnecessary complications occur.[4]

Effective

Effective health care is care based on offering evidence-based services that address the most important healthcare concerns to individuals and the most vulnerable population groups. Effective care involves integration of curative and preventative services and refraining from providing services to those who are not likely to benefit. In other words, effective care avoids underuse and overuse of healthcare services.[4]

Efficient

Efficiency in healthcare delivery refers to avoiding waste of resources for care delivery, such as time, cost, supplies, and even treatment. Using a standard process and products for securing IV catheters instead of letting every nurse pick their own products can save money and time. On a larger scale, care coordination for patients with chronic conditions can reduce redundancy in diagnostic tests, prevent unnecessary hospitalizations, and improve the patient's quality of life. Efficiency reduces waste and improves value in the healthcare system.[4]

Equitable

Equitable care is providing care that does not vary in quality because of gender, ethnicity, geographic location, and socioeconomic status.[4] Equitable care serves people with limited resources with the same essential treatment options that people with more personal resources have available to them.

Patient-Centered Care

Patient-centered care is responsive to individual patient preferences, needs, and values. These considerations guide all clinical decisions. It also means treating patients with respect and dignity. Patient-centered care requires partnering with the patient and his or her family in every aspect of care.[4]

BOX 48.1	**Attributes of Healthcare Quality**	
• Safe		• Efficient
• Timely		• Equitable
• Effective		• Patient-Centered

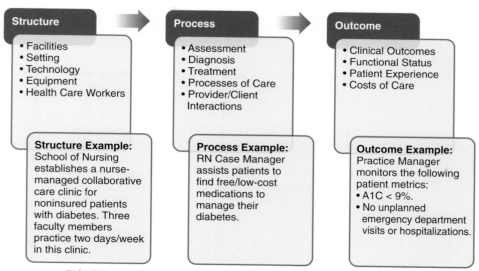

FIGURE 48.2 Donabedian Model of Structure-Process-Outcome.

THEORETICAL LINKS

Avedis Donabedian's quality assessment model has been the predominant theoretical framework for healthcare quality research and improvement for over 50 years. Evaluation of the quality of care requires looking at the structures of care, the processes of care, and the outcomes of care.[6] According to Donabedian, *structure* is the characteristics of the settings in which the care is delivered. *Process* is the health care provided and includes both the technical aspects of care and the interpersonal aspects of care, and a health *outcome* is the effect of care on the health status of individuals or populations.[7] The Structure-Process-Outcome model identifies ways to define, categorize, and measure quality which is increasingly important with the focus on the value of healthcare services. The model is depicted in Fig. 48.2 with an example of how it might be used to assess the quality of a nurse-managed collaborative care clinic.

Structure

Structure is defined as the characteristics of settings in which care is delivered. These include the facility characteristics such as size, governance and management structure, equipment, supplies, staff, provider knowledge and attitudes, and other contextual characteristics. Structure affects both processes and outcomes of care. For example, if a school of nursing decides to open a nurse-managed clinic for uninsured patients with diabetes, resources such clinic space, administrative support, equipment, and supplies must be identified as well as determining how the clinic will be staffed. Without these basic resources, the clinic cannot operate.

Process

Process is the health care provided as well as support functions and includes the services offered, the technical quality of the services (i.e., the staff and providers perform the technical aspects of the task or job), the quality of interpersonal interactions, and the adequacy of patient education, access, safety, and promotion of continuity of care (i.e., appropriate referral and follow-up). Donabedian suggested that the processes of care should be the primary focus of quality assessment.[8] In our example of a nurse-managed clinic, there are many interdependent processes including, but not limited to, registration, triage, and the episode of care with the provider. Developing a new process to help

uninsured patients obtain free or low-cost diabetes medications and supplies can directly impact patient outcomes.

Outcomes

Outcomes are the end result of an encounter with the healthcare system and are impacted by both the processes of care and structures of care. For example, if no primary care providers, clinics, or hospitals are located in a rural area, the people who live in the area may have undiagnosed and treated hypertension, diabetes, and other chronic conditions. The most commonly tracked outcomes are mortality, morbidity, functional status, disease, patient experience, and costs. In our example of a nurse-managed clinic, the outcomes of interest may be hemoglobin A1C values less than 9% or unplanned emergency room visits or hospitalizations related to diabetes. These outcomes are important for the health and well-being of the patients, but they also help the clinicians evaluate the effectiveness of the care they are providing.

CONTEXT TO NURSING AND HEALTH CARE

Quality is a component of almost every aspect of healthcare services. In the United States, healthcare services are provided in a variety of for-profit or not-for-profit private entities and public systems. Reimbursement for services also varies based on the patient's insurance status. This patchwork of services and reimbursement makes it difficult to systematically improve the quality of care, despite concentrated efforts over the last two decades to improve quality.[9] As part of the Patient Protection and Affordable Care Act (ACA) 2010, a National Quality Strategy was developed to improve the delivery of healthcare services, patient outcomes, and population health.[10] More than 300 organizations had input into the first plan that laid out three aims commonly known as the Triple Aim.[10]

- Better care: Improve the overall quality by making health care more patient-centered, reliable, accessible, and safe.
- Healthy People/Healthy Communities: Improve the health of the U.S. population by supporting proven interventions to address behavioral, social, and environmental determinants of health in addition to delivering higher-quality care.
- Affordable Care: Reduce the cost of quality healthcare for individuals, families, employers, and government.

There are many laws and regulations that govern how healthcare organizations operate, and many are directly related to ensuring the quality of care provided in the organization. System leaders are responsible for providing the resources and creating the work environment that allows healthcare workers to deliver high-quality care. All healthcare providers are responsible for delivering safe, effective, efficient, patient-centered care. Nurses are the front-line defense against actual and potential risks to patients. This requires an understanding of, and willingness to participate in, activities that promote and ensure high-quality patient care. Individual nurses have to go beyond just providing care based on the organization's policies and procedures. Nurses need to identify unsafe practices and respond appropriately to ensure a safe outcome for patients, oneself, and others. Nurses also need to understand the outcomes of care on their unit. For example, a nurse may ask, Does my medical unit have a higher number of falls than other medical units? If so, what does the evidence suggest we can do to reduce the number of falls on our unit? Finally, all nurses must be lifelong learners to keep up with current available knowledge related to the patient population they work with.

Regulatory Agencies

Multiple oversight bodies and regulatory agencies exist to ensure the safety of the public. These regulatory agencies license healthcare facilities for operation (e.g., specific state licensing regulations) and can fine organizations or restrict services and suspend operations if there is a failure to meet expected standards. For example, hospitals can lose accreditation status and Medicare or Medicaid reimbursement can be withheld if the delivery of patient care does not meet national quality standards.

The Centers for Medicare & Medicaid Services (CMS), part of the Department of Health and Human Services, is a key government entity with a large impact on healthcare quality.[11] Over one-third of the U.S. population get their health insurance through Medicare, Medicaid, or other public insurance.[12] Because of the size of the population covered as well as the need for fiscal responsibility with tax dollars, CMS has been leading efforts to link reimbursement to improved quality. One initiative is value-based purchasing (VBP), which links incentive payments to hospital quality.[13] Hospital quality is assessed through measures of mortality outcomes for specific diseases (e.g., heart failure and pneumonia), selected clinical process of care measures (e.g., catheter-associated urinary tract infection), and patient experience scores (e.g., HCAHPS Communication with Nurses).[13] The quality of nursing care directly impacts most of the measures used by the VBP program and whether or not the hospital loses reimbursement dollars for low performance or gains financial incentives for exemplary performance.

Other public agencies that regulate care provided in hospitals and in community-based settings include the Occupational Safety and Health Administration (OSHA), the Centers for Disease Control and Prevention (CDC), the U.S. Food and Drug Administration (FDA), the U.S. Department of Justice (DOJ), and the U.S. Drug Enforcement Administration (DEA). Many state and local public agencies also regulate care as well as health professions. Nurses are directly overseen by the Board of Nursing; nurses must maintain current license and practice by the standards set within the state.

Advisory Bodies

Advisory bodies have an important role in influencing standards for the delivery of quality health care. Although the focus of various advisory bodies varies, contributions to quality health care include efforts such as studies and recommendations regarding best practices for the improvement of health care, establishment of healthcare performance measures, provision of data on care and outcomes, and collaborative learning efforts.

One of the most influential advisory bodies is the National Academy of Medicine (NAM), formerly known as the IOM. The NAM is an independent, nonprofit organization that conducts studies and provides unbiased and authoritative advice to improve the nation's health.[14] Many of the studies that NAM undertakes begin as specific mandates from Congress, whereas others are requested by federal agencies and independent organizations. Examples of landmark studies that have directly influenced healthcare quality include *To Err Is Human: Building a Safer Health System*,[15] *Crossing the Quality Chasm: A New Health System for the 21st Century*,[4] and *Keeping Patients Safe: Transforming the Work Environment of Nurses*.[16] Other advisory groups include the American Nurses Association (ANA), the Institute for Healthcare Improvement (IHI), and the National Quality Forum (NQF).

Science of Improvement

There is wide variation in the healthcare services provided and the cost of care across the United States.[17] This variation includes situations in which evidence-based interventions are not consistently provided, may be used at a variable rate related to differences in professional opinion, or may be overused because of excessive supply and demand.[17] Reducing unnecessary variation is at the core of improvement work. Quality improvement (QI) is a data-driven, formal approach to the analysis of performance and the systematic efforts to improve outcomes and processes.[18] Quality improvement methods and tools originated in the Western Electric Company in the 1920s by Walter Shewhart, and were advanced and spread by W. Edwards Deming after World War II in postwar Japan. In the 1980s, American industries recognized the value of continuous QI techniques, and Deming's ideas began to take hold in the U.S. Healthcare systems soon began looking at these ideas to improve their own processes. While there was initial skepticism about the relevance of using manufacturing tools in the complex healthcare environment, there is a growing body of knowledge about improvement science.[19] Today health professions' education accreditation standards expect schools to expose students to improvement methods, and many federal funding programs also expect improvement methods are used to support the work proposed by those seeking funding.

There are four key principles of successful quality improvement: understand the systems and processes, focus on the customers (patients), build the teams, and use data to drive decision-making.[20] Data are critical in QI activities and can be quantitative or qualitative or both. Data are used to describe how well current systems are working (baseline performance), what happens when changes are applied (did the change lead to improvement), and to document successful performance and allow comparison across sites.[20]

QI programs and methods vary across healthcare organizations, and include Continuous Quality Improvement (CQI), Six Sigma (DMAIC), Lean (The Toyota Production System), and the Model for Improvement. The Model for Improvement is the most common framework for organizational QI because of its relative simplicity. In this model, the QI team must address three questions:

1. *"What are we trying to accomplish?"* (Create an aim statement or goal for the educational improvement effort.)
2. *"How will we know a change is an improvement?"* (Identify measures that determine whether the change led to improvement.)
3. *"What change can we make that will result in improvement?"* (Identify and test changes in the current process that may lead to improvement.)

Once an aim, measure(s), and tests of change have been identified, the QI team engages in a series of learning cycles known as Plan-Do-Study-Act (PDSA) cycles (Fig. 48.3). PDSA cycles examine whether or

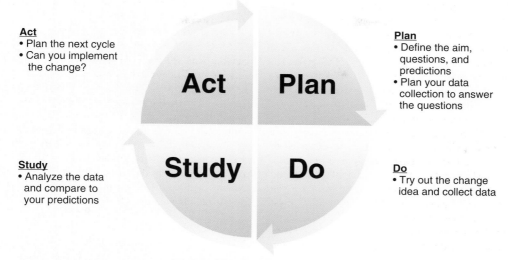

Act
- Plan the next cycle
- Can you implement the change?

Plan
- Define the aim, questions, and predictions
- Plan your data collection to answer the questions

Study
- Analyze the data and compare to your predictions

Do
- Try out the change idea and collect data

FIGURE 48.3 Plan-Do-Study-Act.

not a proposed test of change actually results in the desired outcome. PDSA cycles are ideally implemented on a small scale, often in rapid succession, and over a short period of time.[20,21] These types of QI activities are common in practice settings, and each professional is expected to participate on improvement teams at all levels of high-performing healthcare organizations.

INTERRELATED CONCEPTS

Health Care Quality has close relationships with many other concepts featured in this textbook, including most in Section 3: Professional Nursing and Health Care Concepts. At the national level, Health Policy is used to provide overarching goals and set priorities for the allocation of valuable health resources. Health Care Economics is concerned with issues related to the scarcity of resources in the allocation of health and health care. Health Care Law covers multiple legal issues related to health care including health insurance, patient protections, financing, and much more. One of the key aims of healthcare quality is to reduce Health Disparities. Health Care Organizations and delivery systems provide the framework for the delivery of health care. Technology and Informatics provides tools to help deliver quality health care. Leadership at all levels of the practice setting is key to ensuring high quality of care; leaders set the standards of care, provide resources such as staff and supplies, and role model the attitudes and behaviors that should exemplify a focus on high-quality care. Using current Evidence to provide the most appropriate interventions is fundamental to healthcare quality. Population Health is concerned with the health outcomes and well-being of groups of people. Care Coordination facilitates efficient use of healthcare services. Clinical Judgment, Communication, and Collaboration are essential competencies for every professional to ensure quality within the healthcare setting. Safety is one of the key attributes of healthcare quality and focuses on preventing patient harm. These interrelationships are depicted in Fig. 48.4.

CLINICAL EXEMPLARS

In the United States, nurses can expect to encounter healthcare quality in any setting and whenever they interact with a patient. Nurses will encounter regulations and standards that their healthcare organization must meet along with nurse-sensitive indicators for which they are personally responsible. A sample of exemplars, based on categories previously described, is listed in Box 48.2. It is beyond the scope of this text to describe all these in detail, but several are briefly presented next.

Featured Exemplars
The Joint Commission
The Joint Commission (TJC) is an independent, not-for-profit organization that develops standards for quality and safety and evaluates organizations based on these standards.[22] After CMS, this organization has the second greatest influence on healthcare quality in the United States. Healthcare organizations that want to participate in and receive payment from the Medicare or Medicaid programs must be certified as complying with the Conditions of Participation (CoPs), or standards, set forth in federal regulations. TJC is an approved accreditor for CMS Medicare certification. The TJC survey process includes an onsite survey focused on patient safety and quality and evaluates actual care processes and technology for the purpose of evaluating the organization's compliance with standards. The surveyors also provide guidance to help staff improve the organization's performance.[22] TJC accreditation and certification is recognized nationwide as a symbol of quality that reflects an organization's commitment to meeting certain performance standards.

Agency for Healthcare Research and Quality
The Agency for Healthcare Research and Quality (AHRQ) is the lead Federal agency charged with improving the safety and quality of the healthcare system.[23] AHRQ is the primary funder of health services research to understand how to make care safer and improve quality. One example is the Re-Engineered Discharge (RED) project to help hospitals improve their discharge processes to reduce unnecessary readmissions.[24] AHRQ also creates materials and training programs to help professionals put research into practice. AHRQ worked with the Department of Defense to create the TeamSTEPPS program designed to improve teamwork skills and communication among healthcare professionals.[25] AHRQ also generates data used by providers and policymakers to improve care. An example of this work is the Hospital Consumer Assessment

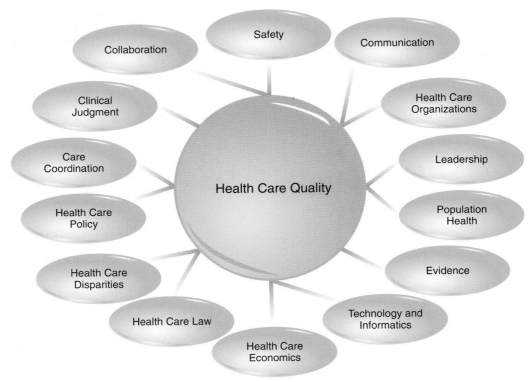

FIGURE 48.4 Health Care Quality and Interrelated Concepts.

BOX 48.2 EXEMPLARS OF HEALTH CARE QUALITY

Regulatory Agencies
- Centers for Medicare and Medicaid Services (CMS)
- The Joint Commission (TJC)
- U.S. Food and Drug Administration (FDA)
- Centers for Disease Control and Prevention (CDC)
- Occupational Safety and Health Administration (OSHA)
- National Committee for Quality Assurance (NCQA)
- State Boards of Nursing and other state level professional boards

Advisory Bodies
- American Nurses Association (ANA)
- Agency for Healthcare Research and Quality (AHRQ)
- National Academy of Medicine (NAM)
- Institute for Healthcare Improvement (IHI)
- The Quality and Safety Education for Nurses Institute (QSEN)
- National Quality Forum (NQF)

Quality Frameworks and Methods
- Baldrige
- ANCC Magnet designation
- Quality Improvement
- Plan-do-study-act (PDSA)
- Model for Improvement
- Lean Six Sigma

Point of Care
- CMS Value-Based Purchasing
- Patient Experience (CAHPS surveys)
- Hospital Acquired Conditions (HAC)
  - Pressure Ulcers stage III and IV
  - Falls with Injury
  - Catheter Associated Urinary Tract Infection (CAUTI)
  - Central Line Associated Blood Stream Infection (CLABSI)

 ACCESS EXEMPLAR LINKS IN YOUR GIDDENS EBOOK

---

of Healthcare Providers and Systems (HCAHPS) which is the primary survey used to assess the patients' experience of care in the hospital.[26]

The Institute for Healthcare Improvement

The IHI was founded in 1991 as a not-for-profit organization focused on redesigning healthcare organizations to reduce errors and wasted resources, and decrease costs.[27] IHI first focused on spreading best practices through building improvement communities. IHI initiatives include the 5 Million Lives campaign aimed at reducing 5 million unnecessary deaths related to poor quality and safety. IHI also aims to build improvement capability by providing educational and consultative support to health professional schools and healthcare organizations. The IHI Open School offers 30 web-based training courses on patient safety, QI, person-centered care, and other topics which are free to most students. Over 500,000 students and professionals have taken IHI Open School courses.[28]

The Quality and Safety Education for Nurses Institute

The Quality and Safety Education for Nurses (QSEN) project began in 2005. The overall goal is to prepare nursing students with the knowledge, skills, and attitudes (KSAs) necessary to continuously improve the quality and safety of the healthcare systems.[29] Quality and safety competencies for pre-licensure and graduate nursing have been established (Box 48.3) and are embedded in nursing program accreditation standards as well as part of the NCLEX test plan. The QSEN Institute continues this work today as a collaborative focused on education, practice, and scholarship with the aim to improve quality and safety of healthcare systems. The website is a central repository of information on the core QSEN competencies, KSAs, teaching strategies, practice innovations, and faculty development resources designed to best support this aim.[30]

The National Quality Forum

The NQF is a not-for-profit membership-based organization focused on meaningful quality measurement.[31] As an advisory body, NQF has been instrumental in advancing efforts to improve quality through performance measurement and public reporting. There are over 430 member organizations including government agencies, professional organizations, healthcare systems, insurance companies, and other healthcare services entities. NQF has become the central repository for healthcare measures that are considered scientifically sound, have been standardized for use across facilities/settings, and are relevant to improving quality of care. Currently NQF has endorsed more than 500 measures.[31] Some of these measures are associated with the quality of nursing care including falls, falls with injury, pressure ulcer/injury, central line associated blood stream infection, and catheter-associated urinary tract infection.

BOX 48.3 QSEN Competencies

- **Patient-Centered Care**: Recognize the patient or designee as the source of control and full partner in providing compassionate and coordinated care based on respect for patient's preferences, values, and needs.
- **Teamwork and Collaboration**: Function effectively within nursing and interprofessional teams, fostering open communication, mutual respect, and shared decision making to achieve quality patient care.
- **Evidence Based Practice**: Integrate best current evidence with clinical expertise, patient/family preferences, and values for delivery of optimal health care.
- **Quality Improvement**: Use data to monitor the outcomes of care processes and use improvement methods to design and test changes to continuously improve the quality and safety of healthcare systems.
- **Safety**: Minimizes risk of harm to patients and providers through both system effectiveness and individual performance.
- **Informatics**: Use information and technology to communicate, manage knowledge, mitigate error, and support decision making.

CASE STUDY

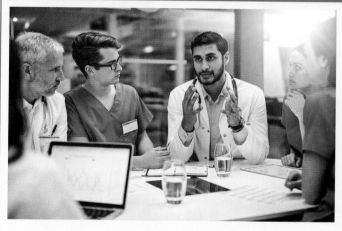

Case Presentation

An interprofessional team including staff nurses, nurse managers; physicians; a Wound, Ostomy, Continence Nurse (WOCN); a pharmacist; a dietician; a supply technician; and a quality management specialist were assigned to work on reducing hospital-acquired pressure injuries in their facility. They decided to review 50 random charts for pressure injury prevention interventions and 50 wound care consults. The data suggested that nurses were consulting WOCN frequently for incontinence-associated dermatitis (IAD) mistaking it for stage 1 pressure ulcers. The team decided to look more carefully at this problem in one medical intensive care unit. They used QI methods including observing the process and interviewing the staff and patients involved. They also collected data about the number of patients who had incontinence and who had redness in their perineal area; they found that 50% of patients with incontinence had redness in the perineal area. The team further investigated the current care processes for incontinence and found no standardized process for cleaning up an incontinent patient and no consistent product use to prevent dermatitis. The team searched the literature for the best evidence for skin care for incontinent patients. The evidence suggested that use of a cleanser, moisturizer, and skin barrier would reduce IAD.

For the first PDSA cycle, the team implemented a protocol based on the three products (cleanser, moisturizer, and skin barrier) available at the hospital. While the nurses were willing to try this protocol, it was soon clear that the new process was cumbersome and time consuming for nurses to use because the products came in multi-use bottles stored in the medication room and took too many steps to complete.

For the second PDSA cycle, the team implemented a protocol based on one product that incorporated all three elements in a single disposable wipe. The bulk of any solid waste was removed, and the nurse used one to three wipes to finish the cleansing process. The ongoing assessment during this cycle showed that nurses were satisfied with the product, and most patients did not develop IAD. Further time and motion studies showed that the new product saved money too. The use of the single disposable wipe was $0.95 cheaper than the use of the three multi-use bottles. Nursing time for cleaning up an incontinent patient with the wipes was also reduced by 4.5 min compared to the three products. Using a run chart with data plotted over time, team leaders presented the data from this improvement activity to the hospital administration, and the single product was approved for use across all adult nursing units in the hospital (Fig. 48.5).

Case Analysis Questions

1. What steps did this team take to understand the current process of caring for patients with incontinence?
2. What was the test of change in the first PDSA cycle? What did the team learn?
3. What change did the team test in the second PDSA cycle? Did it work?

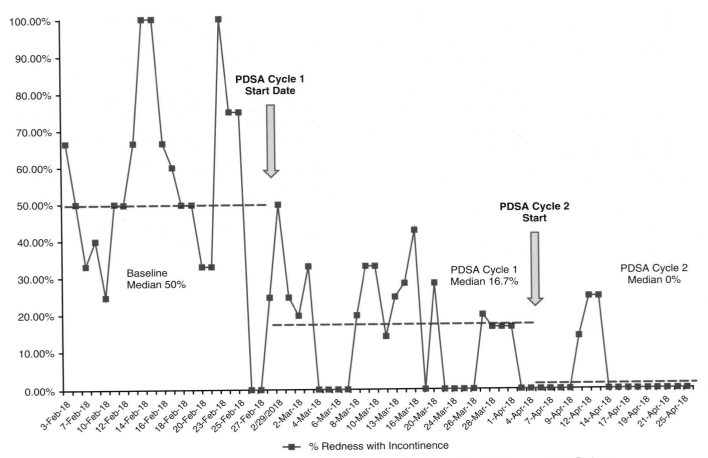

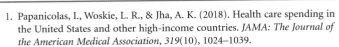

FIGURE 48.5 Medical Intensive Care Unit Incontinence Associate Dermatitis (IAD) Improvement Project: % of patients with IAD. *PDSA*, Plan-Do-Study-Act.

🌿 **ACCESS EXEMPLAR LINKS IN YOUR GIDDENS EBOOK**

REFERENCES

1. Papanicolas, I., Woskie, L. R., & Jha, A. K. (2018). Health care spending in the United States and other high-income countries. *JAMA: The Journal of the American Medical Association, 319*(10), 1024–1039.
2. James, J. (2013). A new evidence based estimate of patient harms associate with hospital care. *Journal of Patient Safety, 9*(3), 122–128.
3. Gill, C. J., & Gill, G. C. (2005). Nightingale in Scutari: Her legacy reexamined. *Clinical Infectious Diseases: an Official Publication of the Infectious Diseases Society of America, 40*(12), 1799–1805.
4. Institute of Medicine, Committee on Quality of Health Care in America. (2001). *Crossing the quality chasm: A new health system for the 21st century.* Washington, DC: National Academies Press.
5. Nelson, E. C., Batalden, P. B., Godfrey, M. M., & Lazar, J. S. (2011). *Value by design: Developing clinical microsystems to achieve organizational excellence.* San Francisco, CA: Jossey-Bass.
6. Donabedian, A. (1966). Evaluating the quality of medical care. *The Milbank Quarterly, 44*(3 Suppl.), 166–203.
7. Donabedian, A. (1988). The quality of care: How can it be assessed? *JAMA: The Journal of the American Medical Association, 260*(12), 1743–1748.
8. Donabedian, A. (1980). *Explorations in Quality Assessment and Monitoring: The Definition of Quality and Approaches to its Assessment.* Ann Arbor, MI: Health Administration Press.
9. Chassin, M. R. (2013). Improving the quality of health care: What's taking so long? *Health Affairs, 32*(10), 1761–1765.
10. Agency for Healthcare Research and Quality. (2018). *National Quality Strategy.* Retrieved from https://www.ahrq.gov/workingforquality/about/nqs-fact-sheets/fact-sheet.html.
11. Centers for Medicare & Medicaid Services (2018). *CMS program history.* Retrieved from https://www.cms.gov/About-CMS/Agency-Information/History/index.html.
12. Kaiser Family Foundation (2016). *Health Insurance Coverage of the Total Population.* Retrieved from https://www.kff.org/other/state-indicator/total-population.
13. Centers for Medicare & Medicaid Services. (2017). *Hospital Value Based Purchasing.* Retrieved from https://www.cms.gov/Outreach-and-Education/Medicare-Learning-Network-MLN/MLNProducts/downloads/Hospital_VBPurchasing_Fact_Sheet_ICN907664.pdf.
14. National Academy of Medicine (2018). *About the National Academy of Medicine.* Retrieved from https://nam.edu/about-the-nam/.
15. Institute of Medicine, Committee on Quality of Health Care in America. (2000). *To err is human: Building a safer health system.* Washington, DC: National Academies Press.
16. Institute of Medicine, Committee on Quality of Health Care in America. (2004). *Keeping patients safe: Transforming the work environment of nurses.* Washington, DC: National Academies Press.
17. Wennberg, J. E. (2010). *Tracking medicine: A Researcher's quest to understand healthcare.* New York, NY: Oxford University Press.
18. Devers, K. J. (2011). *The state of quality improvement science in health: What do we know about how to provide better care?* Robert Wood Johnson

Foundation & Urban Institute. Retrieved from https://www.rwjf.org/content/dam/farm/reports/issue_briefs/2011/rwjf71781.

19. Perla, R. J., Provost, L. P., & Parry, G. J. (2013). Seven propositions of the science of improvement: Exploring foundations. *Quality Management in Health Care*, *22*(3), 170–186.

20. U.S. Department of Health and Human Services Health Resources and Services Administration (2011). *Quality Improvement*. Retrieved from https://www.hrsa.gov/sites/default/files/quality/toolbox/508pdfs/qualityimprovement.pdf.

21. Taylor, M. J., McNicholas, C., Nicolay, C., et al. (2014). Systematic review of the application of the plan–do–study–act method to improve quality in healthcare. *BMJ Quality & Safety*, *23*(4), 290–298.

22. The Joint Commission (2018). *About the Joint Commission*. Retrieved from https://www.jointcommission.org/about_us/about_the_joint_commission_main.aspx.

23. Agency for Healthcare Research and Quality (2018). *About AHRQ*. Retrieved from https://www.ahrq.gov/cpi/about/index.html.

24. Jack, B., Paasche-Orlow, M., Mitchelle, S., et al. (2013). *An overview of the Re-Engineered Discharge (RED) Toolkit*. Rockville, MD: Agency for Healthcare Research and Quality; March AHRQ Publication No.

12(13)-0084. Retrieved from https://www.ahrq.gov/sites/default/files/publications/files/redtoolkit.pdf.

25. King, H. B., Battles, J., Baker, D. P., et al. (2015). *TeamSTEPPS™: Team strategies and tools to enhance performance and patient safety*. Agency for Healthcare Research and Quality. Retrieved from http://www.ahrq.gov/teamstepps/instructor/fundamentals/index.html.

26. Agency for Healthcare Research and Quality (2018). *CAHPS: Surveys and Tools to Advance Patient-Centered Care*. Retrieved from https://www.ahrq.gov/cahps/index.html.

27. The Institute for Healthcare Improvement (2018). *About IHI*. Retrieved from http://www.ihi.org/about/Pages/default.aspx.

28. The Institute for Healthcare Improvement (2018). *IHI Open School*. Retrieved from http://www.ihi.org/education/ihiopenschool/Pages/default.aspx.

29. Cronenwett, L., Sherwood, G., Barnesteiner, J., et al. (2007). Quality and safety education for nurses. *Nursing Outlook*, *55*(3), 122–131.

30. The QSEN Institute (2018). Retrieved from http://qsen.org/.

31. National Quality Forum (2018). Retrieved from http://www.qualityforum.org/Home.aspx.

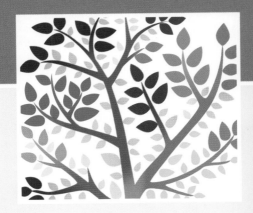

Care Coordination

Kimberly D. Davis and Pamela Parsons

Care coordination is recognized as a professional standard and essential competency of the registered nurse.[1-3] Current healthcare reform has driven the need to improve quality of care delivery while reducing inappropriate use of healthcare services. Care coordination is recognized as essential for organizing care and information around patients' needs and preferences.[4] Additionally, care coordination is one of the six priorities identified by the National Quality Strategy (NQS) as needed to provide more affordable care, improved health for people and communities, and better patient-centered care.[5] The Institute of Medicine has estimated that care coordination initiatives have the potential savings opportunity of $240 billion.[6] The Patient Protection and Affordable Care Act (ACA) identifies care coordination as fundamental in helping the healthcare industry shift away from a fee-for-service mindset and toward value-based care delivery models.[7] Without the adoption of care coordination models, fragmented service delivery, cost inefficiencies, and poor health outcomes will continue. This concept presentation explores the defining characteristics, attributes, and theory supporting care coordination, highlighting clinical exemplars and other related concepts.

DEFINITION

There are many names and descriptions for care coordination and its definition continues to evolve, particularly as stakeholders become interested in healthcare improvement strategies. Examination of professional organizations which have endorsed definitions to guide practice and measurement of care coordination show evidence of its complexity and the need to adopt a multidimensional approach to coordinating care. Following a systematic review which identified over 40 definitions of care coordination, the Agency for Healthcare Research and Quality (AHRQ) Care Coordination Measures Atlas cites the definition for care coordination broadly as: "...the deliberate organization of patient care activities between two or more participants (including the patient) involved in a patient's care to facilitate the appropriate delivery of healthcare services. Organizing care involves the marshalling of personnel and other resources needed to carry out all required patient care activities and is often managed by the exchange of information among participants responsible for different aspects of care".[8,p6] The authors emphasize that in order to meet patient needs and deliver high-quality, high-value health care, consideration must be given to the patient and family's perspective, the healthcare professional's perspective, as well as the system representative's perspective.

For the purposes of clarifying direct measurement of care coordination, the National Quality Forum (NQF) issued a report that addressed performance measurement gaps in care coordination. The definition of care coordination endorsed in this report is "the deliberate synchronization of activities and information to improve health outcomes by ensuring that care recipients' and families' needs and preferences for healthcare and community services are met over time".[9,p2] Recommendations include a need to focus efforts to better provide comprehensive assessment, monitoring of care plans, linkages to services, measurement of progression toward goals, and a shared accountability which requires skillful interprofessional communication. In addition, in an effort to address the diversity of patient needs, care coordination must appropriately link communities and healthcare systems while staying true to the patient's goals.[9]

Nursing, with its holistic and comprehensive approach to person-centered care, is positioned to assume an integral role in the development and implementation of care coordination models. In 2018 the American Nurses Association published *Care coordination: A blueprint for action* in which the authors synthesized AHRQ and NQF definitions, analyzed the current landscape, and produced six actionable steps for nurses to consider in the advancement of care coordination initiatives. These issues consider the importance of "patient, family, and caregiver engagement"; "competency and readiness" of the registered nurse; "teams and teamwork"; "documentation and health information technology (HIT)"; "quality and performance measurement"; and "payment." Further, this blueprint acknowledges the importance of expanding and supporting the role of the registered nurse in care coordination strategies.[10]

SCOPE

The scope of care coordination is dependent on the needs and complexity of the individual (Fig. 49.1). An individual with minimal healthcare needs may be mostly self-sufficient and require consultation with perhaps one member of the interprofessional team. Alternatively, individuals with complex healthcare needs and multimorbidity often require multiple members of the healthcare team to best coordinate an extensive list of services and resources. The goal for any healthcare system is to coordinate care well, especially during transitions between health settings. Although the need for efficient coordination of care exists for all patients, it is especially important for the management of individuals with complex chronic conditions with consideration of barriers associated not just with physical conditions, but mental illness and the impact of social determinants of health.

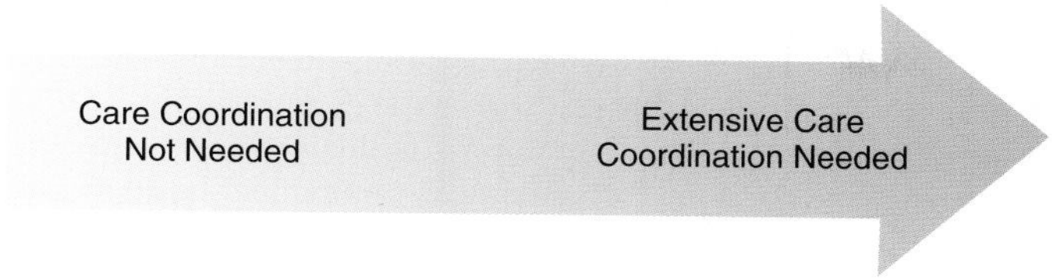

FIGURE 49.1 Scope of Care Coordination.

BOX 49.1 **Key Attributes of Care Coordination**

- Patient-centered/individualized plan of care
- Evidence-based care
- Efficiency
- Improved health outcomes
- Value-based care delivery
- Interprofessional team-based care

ATTRIBUTES AND CRITERIA

An attribute is a characteristic associated with a concept that clarifies the concept. Several common attributes are in nearly all care coordination models (Box 49.1).

Optimal care coordination features patient-centered, evidence-based care highlighted by efficiency which results in the achievement of the NQS goals for improved quality of health care; better health of individuals, communities, and populations; and delivery of health care that is affordable.[5] Additionally, care coordination efforts will demonstrate movement toward value-based care delivery and away from fee-for-service as a response to the goals of the ACA.[7] Efficiency is conceptualized broadly to include efficiency in communication among providers, consumption of medical treatment and associated costs, and a consideration of time as a resource.

THEORETICAL LINKS

Transitions between health settings and transitions in health status are recognized areas of high need for care coordination in order to ensure the individual's clinical stability and to address potential gaps in services. The AHRQ's Care Coordination Measures Atlas supports the idea that care coordination must be considered in the context of care transitions and identifies that transitional care may occur across or within settings, among those involved in the patient's care, and may be longitudinal with transitions occurring between episodes of care.[8] It is therefore useful to consider a theoretical framework for care coordination that provides analysis in the context of transitional care, such as is provided by Radwin and colleagues.[11] The two fundamental domains described within this theoretical framework include continuity of care and activities of the clinician, both of which must simultaneously occur across care transitions. Continuity of patient care requires connected health care and should provide consistency for the patient and healthcare team. For example, treatment plans should be communicated between settings and among the healthcare team so that it is clear that patient information has been adequately shared. Relationships should be maintained between patient and clinician to promote consistency. Activities of the clinician must include skilled interprofessional communication, covering provision of care during transitions, clearly delineating who on the team is accountable for aspects of the patient care, and connecting the patient to resources.[11] Most importantly, utilizing a reliable theoretical framework provides a means to link activities related to

patient care delivery to measurable outcomes, strengthening the evidence related to care coordination and quality care.

Within the context of these two central domains, efforts to achieve patient-centered care and assess patient outcomes must be considered both before and after transitional care. Additionally, consideration of patient and healthcare system characteristics must be applied in order to inform patient-centered care and patient outcomes. Organizational support is integral to successful implementation of care coordination activities. Optimally, when care is organized within this theoretical framework, communication among the interprofessional team is enhanced resulting in improved quality of the patient care experience as individual needs are met.

CONTEXT TO NURSING AND HEALTH CARE

Target of Care Coordination Efforts

Care coordination is important for everyone. During the life course, every person will have at least a temporary need for improved coordination and communication between providers, settings, or periods of time during an illness. Thus we are all at risk for, at a minimum, an episodic illness with at least temporary needs for care coordination. However, the structure of health care in the United States today and the workforce supporting it does not allow for everyone to be supported by a fully integrated care coordination program or model of service delivery.

Individuals particularly vulnerable to fragmented, uncoordinated care on a chronic basis are often at highest risk of negative health outcomes. Care coordination services and case management are cost-intensive, necessitating risk stratification strategies to target services for those with demonstrated high need. Currently, as evidence mounts and the translation, adoption, adaptation, and implementation of care coordination models is accepted throughout the country, the priority population will need to be those most vulnerable and frail. This may include a targeted focus on serving children with special healthcare needs, the frail elderly population, those in crisis situations or catastrophic events, and people at the end of life before other high-risk populations. People in the second tier of risk and need for care coordination are individuals with complex conditions or life situations elevating the likelihood of negative outcomes, including people with cognitive impairments, complex medical or mental health conditions, disabilities, low incomes, or unstable health insurance coverage. Unfortunately, it is only a matter of time before the latter high-risk group will also become vulnerable and in greater need, and the risk increases for people in the general population.

The paradigm shift in healthcare financing and delivery of holistic patient-centered, family-focused care is slowly evolving; there is a noticeable shift occurring as healthcare teams consider how to implement value-based care and how to best improve healthcare quality outcomes. Recent evidence supports that over 70% of poor outcomes are related to issues outside of clinical care delivery that impact daily living, known as the social determinants of health. Factors related to environment and health behaviors include poverty, housing stability, access to healthy foods, and transportation, all of which impact overall health.[12] To be successful, these factors must be included in assessment with appropriate connection to resources as needs are identified. Registered nurses are in key roles to complete these assessments and connect individuals to services and resources. It will take time and continued research to fully implement care coordination for everyone, at all levels of need and in all healthcare settings. Holistic care coordination is targeted toward those most likely to benefit, which includes those who are most vulnerable: low-income, facing health disparities related to social determinants of health, those with chronic illness and multimorbidity, children, and frail older adults.

Care Coordination Models

Effective care coordination models will demonstrate quality healthcare delivery by documenting improved patient outcomes and promoting cost effectiveness. However, care coordination models are complex due to constraints of healthcare financing, inherent difficulty working in interprofessional teams, and lack of interoperability of health information systems. Review of the literature reveals many effective models of care coordination that have achieved documented improved patient outcomes and cost effectiveness; however, many challenges still exist with implementation of these models, and the role of the registered nurse in care coordination models is still evolving. The American Academy of Nursing cites multiple examples of nurse-led care coordination models that have had significant positive impact on patient outcomes.[13]

To understand and evaluate the different care coordination models, it is important to recognize that people—patients and consumers—live and have needs beyond the healthcare system. Healthcare services are just one component in our society of services supporting health. Care coordination for some people may require the knowledge and organization of social services such as those in sectors of education, employment, and the community from housing to utilities, transportation, or insurance of all types. For others, care coordination requires knowledge and organization of medical needs such as prescriptions, medical equipment, and chronic disease self-management. When coordinating care for a person's needs that may fall within these different arenas, care coordination models for consideration should ideally include integrated models which include social, behavioral, and medical services (Fig. 49.2). Fig. 49.3 illustrates the balance in an ideally functioning integrated model that is proactive, focuses on patient wellness using evidence-based methods, employs effective communication, and appoints appropriate use of resources.[14]

Community-Based Models

Leadership and organizing responsibility for community-based models of care coordination can be at the local or state level. For example, Area Agencies on Aging are often designated as coordinators and administrators of care coordination programs that can then be standardized at some level across a state. County social service agencies also assume care coordination responsibilities and are often able to serve as a single entity for multiple funding sources, such as waiver services, block grants, state-funded services, and Medicaid. Having a single entity coordinate all relevant social services can reduce the likelihood of redundancy and duplication of efforts. Advances in technology and electronic social networking interfaces will continue to facilitate opportunities for partnership and referral to social services. Community-based models of care coordination are an important part of promoting health and independence in the community.

The Transitional Care Model (TCM) led by Dr. Mary Naylor is an example of a nurse-led model of care coordination which aims to facilitate older adult patients who are transitioning from a hospital admission back to home by providing relationship-based care by an advanced practice registered nurse (APRN) in the patient's home. Although results have shown significant cost savings by decreasing hospital readmissions, barriers to implementation include reimbursement for such services.[15,16]

Integrated Models

Models committed to the integration of health care, social support, and community clinical and nonclinical services are still evolving. They offer significant promise for supporting holistic, patient-centered, family-focused care, but building bridges between services and settings is fraught with barriers. In the United States, most challenges stem from having different service types financed from different sources. Coordination is further complicated by the scope of authority for managing the different services and the level of involvement of each agency or organization. An example is the need to coordinate services across community programs supported philanthropically, social services supported with government financing, and medical services supported by a health system. It can also be difficult to determine the setting in which the coordination should reside and ultimately the relationship or nature of the partnership that should exist between agencies and service organizations. Fully integrated models need to be able to coordinate a full range of services across settings and over time; they should also be funded and financed by different entities and inclusive of service providers (both clinicians and nonclinical community leaders), patients, and their caregivers.

An evolving example of an integrated model that has gained national support is the Patient-Centered Medical Home (PCMH) which notably incorporates five specific functions: comprehensive care from an interprofessional healthcare team; patient-centered care that appreciates each

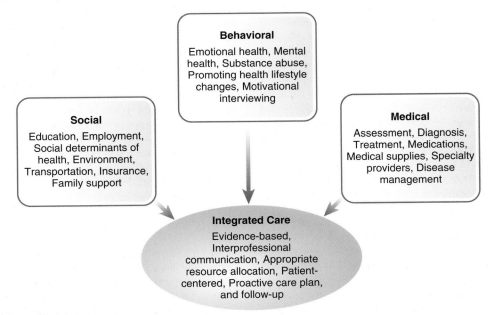

FIGURE 49.2 An Ideally Functioning Integrated Care Coordination Model.

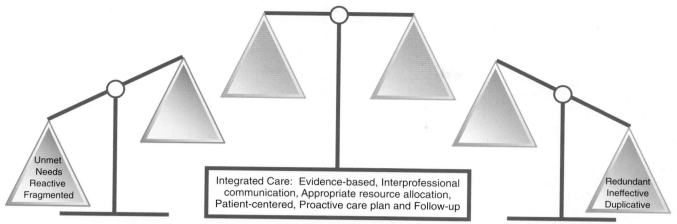

FIGURE 49.3 Balance and Imbalance of Care Coordination Attributes.

patient's unique needs and supports self-management goals; coordinated care that assists patients with access to the healthcare system and community services; accessible services which allow patients timely access to the healthcare team; and a commitment to quality and safety improvement initiatives through the use of evidence-based care and performance measurement.[17,18] A well-documented example is the Program of All-Inclusive Care for the Elderly (PACE). The PACE program is provider based and integrates both acute and long-term healthcare and social services. Working in contract with Medicare and Medicaid, the program is designed to support people age 55 years or older who qualify for admission to a nursing home but prefer to continue residing in the community.[19]

Additionally, Accountable Care Organizations (ACOs) have received national support as a means to provide integrated high-quality care coordination services by "assign(ing) responsibility for a population of patients to healthcare providers, with payments depending on the cost and quality outcomes for that population."[20,p40] The population of patients served by the ACO will determine the types of healthcare partnerships needed to best meet the clinical needs, and so ACOs will vary in composition. Potential healthcare settings which may become part of the ACO include preventive care, behavioral health, primary care, acute care, and post-acute care.[20] It is important to note that the need for primary healthcare settings to provide integrated mental health care, behavioral health, and substance abuse has been well documented and the PCMH and ACO models are in position to address this integration.[21]

Role of Nurse in Care Coordination

The nurse's role in effective care coordination must include use of evidence-based guidelines with consideration of best practices, particularly during transitional care. Additionally, the nurse must utilize skills in comprehensive assessment to inform creation of the patient care plan and to assist in goal setting. Patients must be taught how to self-manage their chronic conditions with a special emphasis on medication management. When care coordination programs are implemented, the nurse must be able to guide structure of the intervention and implementation, followed by program evaluation to show both improved quality of patient care and assessment of healthcare utilization with associated costs. The nurse will utilize information technology to enhance communication among the interprofessional healthcare team members as well as between the patient and healthcare team. Effective care coordination will be obvious when improved patient outcomes are achieved. Necessary skills of the care coordinator include effective management of populations, skill in a variety of communication styles in order to

effectively lead and work with interprofessional healthcare teams, and the ability to provide patients and caregivers with coaching and education regarding self-management all while linking patients and families to community resources. Additionally, care coordinators must have a working knowledge of health insurance and various methods of payment. The care coordinator should also possess basic skills in research and evaluation so as to be able to justify the role as well as contribute to the body of science by disseminating findings of program outcomes. Above all the nurse must document care coordination activities so as to show justification for the role.[8,10,14,22]

INTERRELATED CONCEPTS

Care coordination is a generic term that is sometimes used interchangeably both with specific types, such as case or disease management, and with related concepts that share a subset of defining attributes. The most closely related concepts and the ways they distinctly differ from care coordination are discussed here and illustrated in Fig. 49.4.

At the center of the care coordination is the patient. Patient factors affecting care coordination are shown at the top in Fig. 49.4. These concepts influence care coordination at the individual level and are affected by both personal and interpersonal situations; they include Functional Ability, Development, ability for Self-Management, Adherence to treatment plan, Family Dynamics, and the influences of Culture. Concepts shown at the bottom of Fig. 49.4 are those related to care coordination at a community and systems level. Delivery of care is influenced and associated with Health Care Quality, Evidence-based practice, Technology and Informatics, Communication, and Collaboration. Access to care is determined in part by Health Policy, Health Care Law, Health Disparities, and Health Care Organizations. Additional concepts at the systems level include Health Promotion, Patient Education, and Safety. Each concept is associated with care coordination at either the individual or the systems level and guides implementation and outcomes.

CLINICAL EXEMPLARS

The need for care coordination can be seen across the lifespan, ranging from simple plans involving just the patient and primary care provider to complex plans involving a team of specialized healthcare services in multiple locations. Box 49.2 presents a variety of exemplars associated with care coordination. The following featured exemplars provide insight on clinical conditions and situations associated with care coordination.

Patient Factors

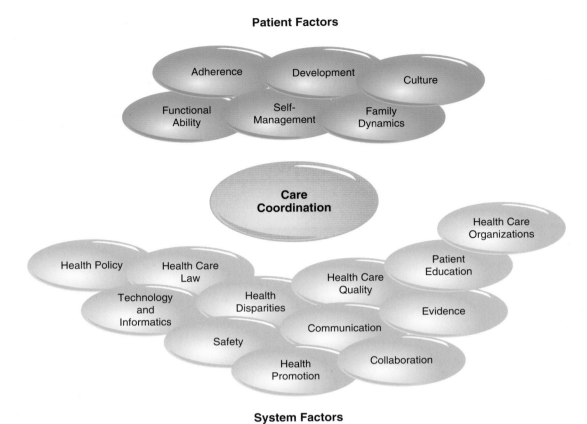

System Factors

FIGURE 49.4 Care Coordination and Interrelated Concepts.

Featured Exemplars

High-Risk Pregnancy

Pregnant women who have a high-risk pregnancy require more monitoring to promote the best possible outcome. Care coordination may include patient education, dietician or nutritionist referral, and coordination of specialty testing. A social work consult may be necessary for Women, Infants, and Children (WIC) and Medicaid program initiation.

Preterm Infants

Preterm infants typically have a myriad of needs. Depending on gestational age, preterm infants may be born with problems associated with breathing, feeding, temperature regulation, heart, brain, blood, and immunity. Care coordination may include specialty care, home health nursing or private duty nursing, family teaching, and social support.

Special Needs Children

Children with special needs "require interfacing among multiple care systems and individuals, including the following: medical, social, and behavioral professionals; the educational system; payers; medical equipment providers; home care agencies; advocacy groups; needed supportive therapies/services; and families."[23,pe1451] Common conditions include autism, cerebral palsy, cystic fibrosis, Down syndrome, epilepsy, learning disabilities, intellectual disabilities, hearing loss, speech disabilities, and visual disabilities.

Frail and Elderly

The frail and elderly spend the most healthcare dollars per capita. According to the National Council on Aging, 80% of Medicare beneficiaries have at least one chronic disease, and 70% have two or more. Additionally,

caring for chronic diseases accounts for 66% of healthcare-associated costs.[24] The frail and the elderly are vulnerable to negative outcomes following falls and serious illness, making this population ideal for care coordination to prevent such events and to assist with aging in place so as to avoid unnecessary institutionalization.

Transitional Care

Preventing hospital readmissions through incentivized transitional care coordination is a targeted area for improvement across government initiatives and strategies, including the ACA, the U.S. Department of Health and Human Services, and the CMS.[25] The Hospital Readmissions Reduction Program (HRRP) provides financial incentives to hospitals to reduce 30-day hospital readmissions in the following priority areas: acute myocardial infarction, chronic obstructive pulmonary disease, heart failure, pneumonia, coronary bypass graft surgery, and total hip or knee arthroplasty.[26] Kaiser Permanente Southern California recommends a standardized discharge summary, medication reconciliation, post discharge hotline, post discharge phone call within 72 hours, and timely primary care or specialist follow-up less than 7 days after discharge to reduce readmission rates.[27]

Mental Illness

According to the Substance Abuse and Mental Health Services Administration, patients with mental illness are at increased risk of early death from treatable chronic diseases and substance use conditions, however, integrated care is lacking in the primary care setting.[21,28] Care coordination is beneficial for integrating mental health and substance abuse care with primary medical care through screening, referral, and follow-up.

End-of-Life Care

End-of-life care espouses many aspects of care, including physical, psychosocial, spiritual, and cultural needs of both the patient and the family. It can be extremely costly, particularly if patient needs are not communicated or coordinated well. Hospice and palliative care can take place in all healthcare settings, as well as in the home. Clinical guidelines of care established by the National Consensus Project for quality palliative care recommend a multidimensional and interprofessional approach to care coordination during end of life to improve quality and decrease healthcare costs.[29]

BOX 49.2 EXEMPLARS OF CARE COORDINATION

Approaches to Care Coordination
- Case management
- Care management
- Discharge planning
- Integrated care
- Managed care
- Medical home
- Transitional care

Population Groups Most in Need of Care Coordination
- Children with special needs
- Disabled people
- Frail elderly
- High-risk pregnancy
- Preterm infant

Common Situations Requiring Care Coordination
- Catastrophic event
- Cancer care
- Cerebral vascular accident
- Chronic obstructive pulmonary disease
- Diabetes mellitus
- End-of-life care (hospice, palliative care)
- Heart failure
- Mental illness
- Myocardial infarction
- Substance use
- Traumatic brain injury

ACCESS EXEMPLAR LINKS IN YOUR GIDDENS EBOOK

CASE STUDY

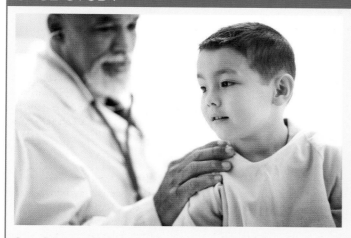

Case Presentation

Shane is a 5-year-old boy who is having difficulty ascending the stairs to his family's second-story apartment. After diagnostic testing, Shane's family is informed that he has Duchene muscular dystrophy. Shane receives care from a medical home, and his team consists of a pediatrician, pediatric nurse practitioner, nurse, neurologist, physiologist, physical and occupational therapists, social worker, care coordinator, Shane, and Shane's family. The primary provider, in this case an advanced practice registered nurse (APRN), oversees the team, and the care coordinator facilitates organization. Mutually agreed upon goals include optimizing independence and attending school with his peers. The team communicates recommendations and changes in care through a patient care portal available to the medical home, inpatient, and outpatient services. This program also monitors prescriptions and provides prompts for the APRN when vaccinations and wellness activities are due.

During his initial evaluation, physical therapy makes recommendations for bracing. The social worker discusses when and how to file for social services programs such as Medicaid and disability. The social worker also contacts the local elementary school to make arrangements for bus transportation and accommodations so Shane can begin kindergarten in the fall. The care coordinator contacts the local chapter of the Muscular Dystrophy Association (MDA) for assistance with family and school support. The MDA also has supporters who assist the family's church to make the children's area accessible and help the family search for wheelchair-accessible housing within its school district. In addition, the care coordinator assists the APRN with compiling the documentation necessary for insurance approval of medications, durable medical equipment, and a physical and occupational therapy visit at the patient's home for family teaching. The care coordinator schedules a follow-up appointment in 3 months and will call Shane's mother in 3 weeks to determine if the current plan is meeting the needs of Shane and his family.

Summer camp and sports are important activities of childhood that can be facilitated through national and community programs for children with special needs. The MDA, Special Olympics, and other charitable organizations coordinate with the family and medical team to ensure safe and appropriate activities while complying with current medical treatment. When Shane enters high school, his care coordinator will work with the medical team, family, school counselor, and support group to help Shane develop a vocational plan for transitioning from school to higher education or the workforce, as well as a plan for independent living. Shane will also start transitioning from pediatric to adult care during this time; because both practices are located in his medical home, the same framework for care and electronic medical records are utilized, easing the transition and decreasing errors.

Case Analysis Questions

1. Consider the attributes of Care Coordination presented earlier in this chapter. Describe which attributes are evident in this case.
2. What type of care coordination model is represented by this case? What elements lead you to this assessment?

From Fuse/Thinkstock.

ACCESS EXEMPLAR LINKS IN YOUR GIDDENS EBOOK

REFERENCES

1. American Association of Colleges of Nursing. (2008). *The essentials of baccalaureate education for professional nursing practice.* Retrieved from http://www.aacnnursing.org/Portals/42/Publications/BaccEssentials08.pdf.
2. American Nurses Association. (2012). *Position statement: Care coordination and nurses' essential role.* Retrieved from https://www.nursingworld.org/~4afbf2/globalassets/practiceandpolicy/health-policy/cnpe-care-coord-position-statement-final–draft-6-12-2012.pdf.
3. American Nurses Association. (2015). *Scope and Standards of Practice* (3rd ed.). Silver Spring, MD: American Nurses Association.
4. Camicia, M., Chamberlain, R., Finnie, M., et al. (2013). The value of care coordination: A white paper of the American Nurses Association. *Nursing Outlook, 61*(6), 490–501.
5. About the National Quality Strategy. Content last reviewed March 2017. Agency for Healthcare Research and Quality, Rockville, MD. Retrieved from http://www.ahrq.gov/workingforquality/about/index.html.
6. National Quality Forum. (2014). *NQF-Endorsed measures for care coordination*: Phase 3, 2014- Technical report. (Funded by the Department of Health and Human Services under contract HHSM-500-2012-00009I, Task Order HHSM-500-T0008.).
7. Patient and Protection and Affordable Care Act. (2010). Pub. Law No. 111-148.
8. McDonald, K. M., Schultz, E., Albin, L., et al. (2014). *Care coordination measures atlas, version 4* (Prepared by Stanford University under subcontract to American Institutes for Research on Contract No. HHSA_290-2010-00005I). AHRQ Publication No. 14-003-EF. Rockville, MD, Agency for Healthcare Research and Quality.
9. National Quality Forum. (2014). Priority setting for healthcare performance measurement: Addressing performance measure gaps in care coordination. (Funded by the Department of Health and Human Services under contract HHSM-500-2012-00009I, Task 5.).
10. Lamb, G., & Newhouse, R. (2018). *Care coordination: A blueprint for action for RNs.* Silver Spring, MD: American Nurses Association.
11. Radwin, L. E., Castonguay, D., Keenan, C. B., & Hermann, C. (2016). An expanded theoretical framework of care coordination across transitions in care settings. *Journal of Nursing Care Quality, 31*(3), 269–274.
12. County Health Rankings Model. (2018). A Robert Wood Johnson Foundation program. Retrieved from http://www.countyhealthrankings.org/explore-health-rankings/what-and-why-we-rank.
13. American Academy of Nursing. (2015). *Care coordination- Raise the voice: Edge runners.* Retrieved from www.aannet.org/initiatives/edge-runners/carecoordination.
14. Kurtzman, E., Dailey, M., Baxter, A., et al. (2013). *Framework for measuring contributions to care coordination.* Silver Spring, MD: American Nurses Association.
15. Naylor, M. D., Brooten, D. A., Campbell, R. L., et al. (2004). Schwartaz JS: Transitional care of older adults hospitalized with heart failure: a randomized, controlled trial. *Journal of the American Geriatrics Society, 52*(5), 675–684.
16. Naylor, M. D., Hirschman, K. B., Hanlon, A., et al. (2014). Comparison of evidence-based interventions on outcomes of hospitalized, cognitively impaired older adults. *Journal of Comparative Effectiveness Research, 3*(3), 245–257.
17. Agency for Healthcare Research and Quality (AHRQ). (n.d.). *Defining the PCMH.* Retrieved from https://pcmh.ahrq.gov/page/defining-pcmh.
18. PCMH Roadmap. (2016). Patient-centered Medical Homes and the Care of Older Adults: vision of the John A. Hartford Foundation Patient-Centered Medical Home Change AGEnts Network. Co-chairs Dorr, D. & Schreiber, R. Retrieved from https://changeagents365.org/resources/patient-centered-medical-home-network/Roadmap_PCMH_Change%20AGEnts.pdf.
19. Center for Medicare and Medicaid (CMS). (n.d.). PACE (Program of All-Inclusive Care for the Elderly). Retrieved from https://www.medicare.gov/your-medicare-costs/help-paying-costs/pace/pace.html.
20. Muhlestein, D., De Lisle, K., & Merrill, T. (2018). Assessing provider partnerships for Accountable Care Organizations. *Managed Care, 27*(3), 40–49.
21. Crowley, R. A., & Kirschner, N. (2015). The integration of care for mental health, substance abuse, and other behavioral health conditions into primary care: Executive summary of an American College of Physicians position paper. *Annals of Internal Medicine, 163*(4), 298–299.
22. Lamb, G. (2015). *Care coordination: The game changer—How nursing is revolutionizing quality care.* Silver Spring, MD: American Nurses Association.
23. American Academy of Pediatrics. (2014). Patient- and family-centered care coordination: A framework for integrating care for children and youth across multiple systems. *Pediatrics, 133*(5), e1451–e1460.
24. National Council on Aging (NCOA). (2018). *Healthy aging fact sheet.* Retrieved from https://www.ncoa.org/wp-content/uploads/Healthy-Aging-Fact-Sheet-final-2018.pdf.
25. Kocher, R. P., & Adahi, E. Y. (2011). Hospital readmission and the Affordable Care Act: Paying for coordinated quality care. *JAMA: The Journal of the American Medical Association, 306*(16), 1794–1795.
26. Centers for Medicare and Medicaid (CMS). (2018). *The Hospital Readmissions Reduction Program (HRRP).* Retrieved from https://www.cms.gov/Medicare/Quality-Initiatives-Patient-Assessment-Instruments/Value-Based-Programs/HRRP/Hospital-Readmission-Reduction-Program.html.
27. Tuso, P., Huynh, D. N., Garofalo, L., et al. (2013). The readmission reduction program of Kaiser Permanente Southern California—Knowledge transfer and performance improvement. *The Permanente Journal, 17*(3), 58–63.
28. Substance Abuse and Mental Health Services Administration. (2018). *Can We Live Longer? Integrated Healthcare's Promise.* Retrieved from https://www.integration.samhsa.gov/Integration_Infographic_8_5x30_final.pdf.
29. National Consensus Project. (2013). *Clinical practice guidelines for quality palliative care* (3rd ed.). Pittsburgh, PA: National Consensus Project for Quality Palliative Care.

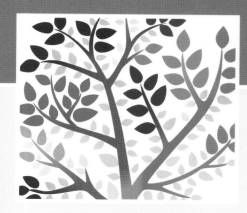

Caregiving

Ishan C. Williams, Fayron Epps, Mijung Lee

An estimated 43.5 million Americans provide unpaid care for an adult or child with functional and/or cognitive limitations. These dedicated caregivers provide care as an extension of and partner with long-term services and supports (LTSS) systems. Approximately 60% of caregivers are women, and 40% are men. The average age of the caregiver is 49.2 years, but spousal caregivers are older (average age of 62.3 years).[1]

The need for family caregivers will escalate dramatically in the coming years because of the increase in our aging population and an overwhelmed formal healthcare system. People with chronic, debilitating diseases are being treated more effectively and they are living with rather than dying from these diseases. It is important for nurses to be aware of the role that caregivers play in healthcare delivery, the impact of this role on caregivers' lives, and supportive interventions that are needed to care for caregivers.

DEFINITION

Dentrea describes caregiving as providing unpaid support and assistance to family members or acquaintances who have physical, psychological, or developmental needs. Dentrea differentiates caregiving for a disabled child across his or her lifespan as different from routine child care, which is considered parenting.[2] Similarly, the National Alliance for Caregiving defines caregivers as "those who provide unpaid care to a relative or friend to help them take care of themselves."[1,p3] The definition of caregiving offered by Hermanns and Mastel-Smith is "a multidimensional concept that encompasses the action or process of helping those who are suffering."[3,p2] Furthermore, they explain that "caregiving is made up of actions one does on behalf of another individual who is unable to do those actions for himself or herself."[3,p5]

SCOPE

The scope of caregiving ranges from a temporary/limited caregiving role for an individual with an acute illness or condition to a long-term or permanent caregiving role (Fig. 50.1). Examples of acute limiting conditions/illnesses include acute myocardial infarction, burns, influenza, pneumonia, and traumatic injuries. Chronic conditions/illnesses often requiring caregiving support include dementia, Parkinson disease, cancer, diabetes mellitus, and stroke. Family caregiving is central to long-term care in the United States and the main source of assistance for the elderly and disabled. Family caregivers make enormous sacrifices to

assist their loved ones and to care for them at home. Caregiving is known as the universal occupation that most of us take part in at some point in our lives.[4] It is estimated that 14% of family caregivers provide care for children with special needs younger than age 18 years, whereas 50% provide care for one's parent(s).[3]

Types of Caregivers

The caregiving role may be shared among family members so that it may be episodic. Caregivers are often categorized by their relationship to the person receiving care (care recipient). Although some caregivers may not have a familial relationship to the patient, the most common types of caregivers are spousal caregivers, adult children caregivers, grandparent caregivers, and parent caregivers.

Spousal Caregivers

Spousal caregivers are commonly caring for their spouse with significant physical and/or cognitive disorders yet have their own significant health issues. Typically, spousal caregivers are older, have lower educational levels and income, and are less employed than nonspousal caregivers. Despite those vulnerabilities, about 65% of the spousal caregivers provide medical/nursing tasks such as wound care and complex medication management.[5] Spousal caregivers frequently have their own lifestyle interrupted and are emotionally affected themselves while serving as the primary caregiver for their spouse. With the increase in military war casualties, there is a new population of very seriously wounded service members who require extensive care and rehabilitation. Young spouses are now becoming caregivers for their husbands or wives with multiple physical injuries, including traumatic brain injuries. In addition to the physical injuries, the emotional wounds inflicted by war, combat stress, and the effects of the injuries are challenging for these young families. Spousal caregivers often have to face the reality that they have lost the husband or wife that they once knew.

Adult Children Caregivers

Adult children are often caregivers for their elderly parents. The increase in this phenomenon is due, in part, to medical and technological advances that have extended life expectancy. In the United States, a large proportion of the "baby boomer" generation is now 65 years or older, and thus, the population over the age of 65 is expected to increase to 74 million by 2030.[6]

The impact of the caregiving role can be overwhelming for adult children caregivers who have to assume multiple roles and responsibilities

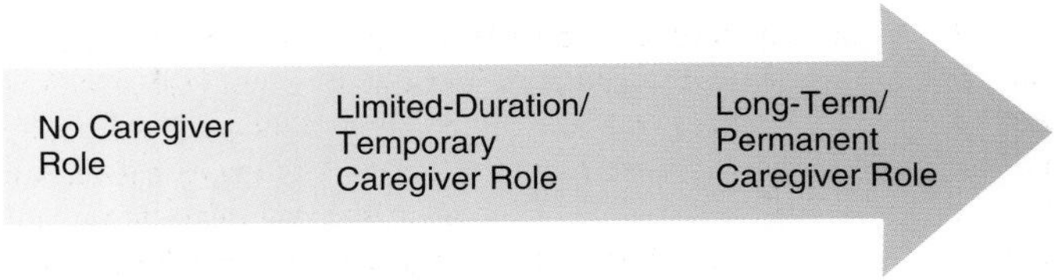

FIGURE 50.1 Scope of Caregiving Role.

while juggling employment and family responsibilities. They have to change their lives to meet the needs of their parent(s). Most adult children caregivers are in the "sandwich generation"—they must care for their children as well as their parents, either in their own home or in the home of their parents. Adult children caregivers also may experience forms of loss, including the following:

- Loss of their parent(s) as they knew him or her before the illness
- Loss of their jobs (or needing to cope with job changes)
- Change in their social networks

Adult children caregivers may be at higher risk of impaired health behaviors because their role as caregivers hinders the amount of time available for engaging in personal and preventative health behaviors.[7]

Grandparent Caregivers

Today, many grandparents are raising their grandchildren and providing care in a variety of ways. Approximately 5.8 million grandparents live with a grandchild. More than 6.5 million children throughout the United States live in households maintained by grandparents or other relatives. In approximately one-third of these homes, no parents are present.[8]

The most common reasons why grandparents become the primary caregivers are that their own children have died, have abandoned the grandchildren, have a mental illness or substance abuse problem, or are in prison. Other factors leading to grandparent-led households include child abuse and neglect. There has also been an increase in the number of pregnant teenagers unprepared for parenthood and an increase in unemployment and poverty, contributing to growing numbers of parents unable to care for their own children.[9] Grandparents are often overwhelmed in the role of caring for their grandchildren. This feeling of being overwhelmed may occur because they are

- raising their grandchildren on a fixed income and facing financial hardships;
- experiencing the effects associated with normal aging and/or the health problems that make caring for their grandchildren difficult;
- worrying about who will be the caregivers when they die or are physically unable to provide care; or
- raising children who may have mental, behavioral/emotional, or physical problems.[9]

In addition, a more subtle stressor occurs when grandparents become primary caregivers of children in that they lose the special relationship and unique role of being the grandparent. Grandparents may also be challenged with needing legal assistance and guardianship rights for their grandchildren in order to register them in school, apply for affordable housing, qualify for special community resources, and obtain medical care.

However, not all the demands of being a grandparent caregiver are negatives. Despite the challenging and stressful role grandparents endure to raise their grandchildren, aging caregivers frequently perceive caregiving as a rewarding experience.[9]

Parental Caregivers

Approximately 3.7 million Americans take care of a child because of a medical, behavioral, or other disability.[1] A primary role of parents is the provision of care for their children. However, parents become "caregivers" for their children when the children are at an age at which they would normally be expected to care for themselves. This can be due to a disability such as severe physical or cognitive limitations. It can also happen later in life from an accident (e.g., a spinal cord injury), a debilitating illness, or severe physical or emotional trauma experienced in military combat.

Stressors of parent caregivers of children will be unique to their situations. For parent caregivers of children with lifelong disabilities, stressors may include the fear of what will happen to their children when they outlive the parents. Parents of adult children who have experienced severe trauma or illness may suddenly be thrust into the parenting role again. Then these parents must decide how and when to relaunch their children into independence under a new context. Parental caregivers are in need of greater support at a community level, which can only be generated if healthcare practitioners and service providers have a better understanding of caregivers' experiences and perspectives.[10]

ATTRIBUTES AND CRITERIA

Concept attributes are identified characteristics that enhance a shared understanding and meaning to those discussing, observing, or experiencing the concept. In other words, attributes are the structural elements of a concept that are consistently described or observable. Antecedents describe experiences that lead to the concept, whereas consequences describe the human experience subsequent to the concept.[11]

The need for love, affection, empathy, compassion, and holistic care are identified as requisite emotions or antecedents to the concept of caregiving.[3] The attributes of the caregiver are specific to the person and are contextually based dependent on the caregiver/care recipient relationship and other relationships in the family. Caregivers have the following attributes or characteristics:

- Having the ability to care
- Adapting to a situation
- Being a good listener
- Showing affection
- Being responsible for someone other than self
- Being strong, protective, organized, patient, and understanding
- Serving as an advocate
- Assisting with activities of daily living
- Providing emotional and social support
- Managing and coordinating healthcare services[12]

THEORETICAL LINKS

Several classical theoretical frameworks have been suggested to assess the psychological burden or rewards, as well as other factors related to family caregiving. The stress process model is one that identifies the positive and negative aspects of caregiving.[13] Caregiver stress is seen as the outcome of a multifactorial process that comprises caregiver resources, socioeconomic characteristics, and primary and secondary stressors to which a caregiver is exposed. Primary stressors are described as challenges directly related to the caregiving process, whereas secondary stressors are divided into two categories—the additional burden of roles and responsibilities external to caregiving and the psychological stress involving the depreciation of self-concept.[13]

Lazarus and Folkman proposed another theoretical model highlighting the concepts of stress, appraisal, and coping.[14] Stress is defined as a stimulus that can serve as a positive drive or a negative event. Stressors can be acute (sudden onset or time limited) or chronic. Prolonged caregiving is a chronic stressor. Psychological stress is a particular relationship between the person and the environment that is appraised by the person as taxing or exceeding his or her resources and endangering his or her well-being.[14] See Concept 30, Stress and Coping for additional information regarding stressors and coping responses.

The theory of caregiving dynamics describes the positive forces that make possible the change and growth of the caregiving relationship.[15] The model represents the relationship of caregiver and care recipient in the past, present, and future. The major concepts of the theoretical framework include commitment, expectation management, and role negotiation supported by the related concepts of self-care, new insight, and role support that maintains a caregiving relationship along the trajectory of an illness. Commitment refers to the caregiver intrinsic motivation to adapt and make changes to prioritize the care recipient's needs. Expectation management encompasses five dimensions: envisioning tomorrow, getting back to normal, taking one day at a time, gauging behavior, and reconciling treatment twists and turns. Role negotiation is defined as actions taken by the caregiver leading to patient recovery and independence.[15] The concepts presented in this theory serve as communication points with family caregivers, with the opportunity to explore their associated feelings and to discuss ways of promoting the caregiving experience.

CONTEXT TO NURSING AND HEALTH CARE

Caregiving involves daily demands that collectively become the experiences of the caregiver. Nurses can play an important role by maintaining an awareness of those experiences as well as connecting the caregiver with resources and providing supportive interventions for the caregiver.

Caregivers' Experience

As caregivers assume responsibilities for another person, they experience a tremendous amount of change in their lives. Caregiving involves unique experiences that may not be what most people expected during their lifetime. The realities of caregiving can be very rewarding with opportunities for positive change, or it can produce a negative effect on the caregivers' physical and emotional health.

Caregivers' Perception and Coping

How caregivers deal with the experiences and realities of caregiving depends on their perception of the experience and their coping abilities. *Perception* is the mental process of viewing and interpreting a person's environment.[12] Caregiver experiences (potential stressors) are not stressful unless the individual *perceives* them as stressful. What is stressful for one person may not be stressful for another. Important factors that may influence how caregivers perceive and react to the challenges of caregiving include their level of knowledge; their level of anticipatory loss and grief; and the availability of material, practical, and spiritual resources needed for self-care.[16]

Another factor that influences their perceptions and experience is their coping style and abilities. Coping can be either positive or negative. Positive coping includes activities such as exercising and spending time with friends and family. Negative coping may include substance abuse and denial.

Uncertainties and Inadequate Understanding

Caregivers often face uncertainties about the present and future along with an inadequate understanding of the disease. Caregivers simply do not know what is going to happen. For example, in the case of patients with dementia, patients' behaviors often change daily. There can be many fluctuations in the disease, especially early in its course. Sometimes the person can seem quite cognitively intact with no noticeable indication that anything is wrong. Then there may be other days when the person is combative and barely able to function. Many caregivers are unprepared to deal with variations in changes in cognitive status, and they become confused and hurt by the strange and/or difficult behaviors of the patient. Caregivers who do not understand a given diagnosis often can refuse to accept that certain symptoms are the result of a disease process.[10] This can result in caregivers feeling guilty, and they often express the idea that if they loved the person more and were more patient with him or her, then the individual would be less irritable or combative. Receiving a clear diagnosis and understanding the implications of a given disease process can provide caregivers with a sense of validation regarding their experience.[10]

Caregivers' Financial and Social Distress

Caregivers often experience negative financial consequences. The majority of family caregivers work full- or part-time. Nearly 50% of those caring for an adult older than age 50 years are working, with the majority working full-time.[17] They report being late for work or needing to leave early, needing to take time off because of their caregiving responsibilities (e.g., to take their loved one to healthcare provider appointments), reducing their hours or taking a less demanding job, declining a promotion, altering work-related travel, quitting their job entirely, or taking an early retirement. Grandparents find their retirement funds dwindle rapidly to cover the unexpected costs of raising their children's children. Many older adults do not have long-term care insurance, so the financial responsibilities of their care need to be paid for by the family. The caregiver may need to sell the family home to pay for health care or long-term care for the person with the disease, with their life savings quickly depleted.[18]

When caregiving responsibilities increase, caregivers may also become isolated as they sacrifice time with family and friends and give up their vacations, hobbies, social life, and sense of self. Giving up a professional career or work in general can have different consequences depending on the caregiver and his or her social support network. Evidence indicates that giving up work can in some cases increase the perceived burden and psychosocial and monetary distress.[10]

Changing Family Roles, Relationships, and Dynamics

When a person becomes very ill, his or her original roles and responsibilities in the family cannot be maintained and therefore need to be restructured. The family patriarch may no longer be able to fulfill that role; the family may struggle to find a new leader and existing roles are forced to change. For example, a woman who has never managed finances may now need to balance the checkbook. She may also need to learn how to do home and car repairs. Men, if in traditional roles, may have to learn how to cook and clean. Grandparents may also be unfamiliar with the roles of children being raised in today's world, which may be quite different from their past childrearing experiences. In addition, they may experience difficulty resolving legal issues and obtaining medical care for their grandchildren.

Many different situations exist with regard to how care is provided within a family. Some families share the responsibilities. Often, the primary care will fall to (or be designated to) one person with or without helpful (or often unhelpful) input from other family members.[12] These other family members may not be willing to be involved in the care, but their comments can be very stressful to the person who has become the primary caregiver. A common situation with spousal caregivers is that they find that their children do not help with the caregiving of their father or mother. Children may distance themselves because they cannot emotionally handle seeing their parent in a "sick" role. Parents may believe that their children are very busy with their own lives (career and children) and they cannot expect them to do anything. Spousal caregivers may believe it is their responsibility and they do not want to seem overbearing or demanding of their children.

Family members frequently do not communicate with each other about the needs of the patient or other important issues, such as the delegation of responsibilities and emotions related to the issues. This results in tension, which results in stress for the caregiver.[12] Ideally, one or several family members assume the central role of caregiver (usually a spouse or one of the care recipient's children) with the support and cooperation of the remaining members of the family. They share the burden of caregiving by providing emotional, financial, and spiritual support. They also relieve the primary caregiver for short periods of time in order to provide for respite and a recovering opportunity needed to focus and/or renew the primary caregiver's physical and emotional strength.[19]

The journey to achieve equilibrium after a drastic change that alters the family dynamics is a difficult one. Kim and Rose conceptualize this progression as family homeostasis. It involves processes and mechanisms that are based on knowledge of family dynamics, with an appraisal of those involved in the caregiving and receiving process, and the families' desire for stability or equilibrium.[19]

The burden of caregiving changes over time, requiring a constant adjustment of the family dynamics and also the relationship between the caregiver and healthcare providers.[20] An important issue among adult children is who will care for the mother or father. Even with the best of intentions, families can struggle. Preexisting patterns in the family, such as a history of disagreements or unresolved issues, influence how a family responds after a person is diagnosed with a disease and requires caregiving. If problems such as poor or bad relationships existed before the disease, they are probably going to worsen after the diagnosis of the disease.[21] Preexisting disagreements that are resolved during this process can help a family adjust to the new living situation and arrangements while improving communication and overall satisfaction.[21]

Influence of Culture on the Caregiving Experience

Culture permeates every aspect of the caregiving experience, from the initial demands placed on the caregiver to the final perception of the overall experience and the outcomes for the caregiver.[22] The culture in which the caregiver was socialized as a young person determines how caregiving duties are assumed, managed, and perceived. People from a culture that values individualism, competition, and independence may view the role of being a caregiver differently from people who come from collectivistic cultures in which interdependence and family take precedence over individual achievement. Although becoming a caregiver is an expectation in some cultures, caregivers in other cultures may feel captive in their role and perceive only the negative aspects of caregiving.[22]

A value shared in some cultures (e.g., Asian and Hispanic/Latino culture) is *familism* or *filial responsibility*. This value refers to the central role of family in an individual's life and the individual's reliance on family as a priority. The Asian and Hispanic/Latino caregivers rely more heavily on unofficial sources of support, which include children, family members, and spouses, which is consistent with larger familial and kin networks among caregivers of color than non-Hispanic white caregivers.[23]

In addition, the support and resources that caregivers seek are largely determined by cultural values. The stressors in the caregiving experience are common to the vast majority of caregivers regardless of racial or ethnic background. However, how the caregiver perceives the situation and whether and when resources are mobilized to cope with the demands of caregiving are influenced by the cultural meaning given to the situation. The sense of duty and responsibility toward family members, especially parents, may determine whether a caregiver believes caregiving

is an honor, a duty, an obligation, or a burden. The meaning attached to the caregiving experience is greatly influenced by cultural values.[24]

Outcomes of Caregiving

Caregiving can have both positive and negative consequences or outcomes. How caregivers perceive their caregiving experience may influence their abilities to focus on the positive aspects of caregiving, such as a sense of peace that they care for their family member. The caregiving experience has benefits and possible gains, but these outcomes have received little attention. The positive aspects associated with the caregiving experience may act as a buffer against overwhelming burden and traumatic grief.[25] Caregivers who have a positive approach to life are better able to cope with caregiving demands and are motivated to maintain their caregiving role.[26] A comprehensive review of quantitative studies reported posttraumatic growth of bereaved caregivers and a sense of existential meaning associated with the caregiver role, including a sense of pride, esteem, mastery, and accomplishment.[27] Using the stress process model, Haley and colleagues examined spousal caregiver depression and life satisfaction in the hospice setting and reported that caregivers found meaning and benefits of caregiving.[28] Concentrating on the positive aspects can "reframe" their role and help it seem more manageable and meaningful. It strengthens the bonds between caregiver and care recipient and elicits feelings of fulfillment at a personal level and satisfaction derived from the act of assisting others.[29]

In contrast, caregivers may become physically, emotionally, and financially overwhelmed with the responsibilities and demands of caring for a family member. Risk for negative, as well as positive, health events related to caregiving responsibilities is not homogeneous, and it varies depending on the activities involved and the coping abilities and resources available to caregivers.[29] Signs of caregiver stress include irritability, inability to concentrate, fatigue, and sleeplessness. Stress can progress to burnout and result in negligence and abuse of the family member by the caregiver. The combined action of multiple stressors, including monitoring and managing the patient's signs and symptoms, as well as emotional and spiritual needs can exhaust the caregiver's coping system and provoke a crisis for caregivers.[30] An understanding of the antecedents, attributes, and consequences of family caregiving are helpful when conducting a family caregiver assessment.

Nursing and Caregiver Support

Nursing care is framed within a holistic approach that includes the nurse, the patient, the caregiver, and the family as a whole.[31] When the nurse assesses a patient, he or she should include an assessment of the caregiver.

The nurse should listen attentively to the caregivers' stories. These stories provide clues as to what their lives are like and provide them the opportunity to share their perceptions, experiences, and coping as caregivers. Box 50.1 presents questions one may include when assessing a caregiver. The creation of a plan of care is developed in collaboration with members of the interprofessional team. The team includes, but is not limited to, the nurse; the medical doctor; physical, speech, and occupational therapists; the social worker; and a spiritual advisor or clergy. The plan of care attempts to identify the obvious and hidden needs or concerns of the caregiver and allows for the formulation of interventions that can reduce the impact of the caregiving process on the caregiver or family.[12]

Initially, caregivers may not identify with the term "caregiver." They may view themselves only as carrying out expected family responsibilities rather than as a caregiver. How does a nurse know when caregivers need help? The Alzheimer's Association has developed 10 signs of caregiver stress (Table 50.1). These are indicators that if the caregiver is not helped, he or she may develop serious health problems. Caregivers are

BOX 50.1 Assessment of Family Caregivers

- What is your experience with being a caregiver?
- What are you doing to cope and how well are you coping?
- How well do you maintain your own nutrition, rest, and exercise?
- What is your level of social interaction versus social isolation?
- How much support do you get from outside sources (e.g., other family members, friends, church members)?
- How well are you taking care of your own healthcare needs (especially those with chronic illnesses of their own)?
- Are you aware of and do you use community and/or Internet resources?
- Do you know about resources available for respite (someone caring for your loved one while you have time to yourself)?
- What kind of help or services do you think you need now and in the near future?

Adapted from Lewis, S. L., Bucher, L., Heitkemper, M. M., et al. (2017). *Medical-surgical nursing: assessment and management of clinical problems* (10th ed.). St Louis: Mosby.

TABLE 50.1 Signs of Caregiver Stress

Sign	Description	What the Caregiver May Say
Denial	About the disease and its effect	"I know that Mom is going to get better."
Anger	At the person with the disease or others	"If he asks me that question one more time, I will scream."
Social withdrawal	From friends and family that once brought pleasure	"I don't care about getting together with the neighbors anymore."
Anxiety	About facing another day and what the future holds	"What happens when he needs more care than I can provide? What happens if I'm not here to provide his care?"
Depression	Begins to break the spirit and affects the ability to cope	"I don't care anymore."
Exhaustion	Makes it nearly impossible to complete necessary daily tasks	"I'm too tired to do anything."
Irritability	Leads to moodiness and triggers negative responses and reactions	"Leave me alone!!"
Sleeplessness	Caused by a never-ending list of concerns	"What if she wanders out of the house, falls, and hurts herself?"
Lack of concentration	Makes it difficult to perform familiar tasks	"I was so busy, I forgot we had an appointment."
Health problems	Begin to take their toll both mentally and physically	"I can't remember the last time that I felt good."

Adapted from the Alzheimer's Association. Staying strong: Stress relief for a caregiver. Available at http://www.alz.org/national/documents/aa_brochure_stressrelief.pdf.

frequently unaware that they have reached a breaking point. The first step in helping family caregivers is to identify persons as caregivers—either by healthcare professionals or by the caregiver him- or herself. Caregivers have been referred to as "hidden patients" because a common characteristic of caregivers is primarily having concern for their family member and often ignoring their own needs or being ignored by healthcare professionals.[32,33]

Identifying and Accessing Resources

Caregivers often need outside assistance and have difficulty asking for help because they do not want to be a burden on others; are afraid of being rejected if they ask for help; may be embarrassed or feel guilty for having a sick person in the family, especially when the disease has cognitive, memory, or behavior components; believe it is their duty to be the single provider of care; or do not have the financial resources to pay for assistance.

Many caregivers suffer in silence because they may not know *how* to ask for help or *where* to look for help, or they do not know that help is available for them. Nurses should encourage caregivers to seek and accept the support of family, friends, and community resources when needed. It is important for caregivers to understand that exhaustion and burnout are common consequences if they attempt to do everything themselves. Nurses can and should act as facilitators who can access and provide information about local, regional, and national sources of help and resources for caregivers and care receivers.[19]

In many cases of end-of-life caregiving, palliative care and hospice are options that are not mentioned or offered to the caregiver. The nurse can be in a unique position to provide information and support that can help reduce the burden of care and enhance the rewards of caregiving through the development of an individualized plan of care.[34]

Caring for the Caregiver

Another way nurses can assist caregivers is to help them to understand and cope with the stressors of caregiving. Nurses can communicate a sense of empathy to the caregiver by allowing discussion about the burdens and rewards of caregiving. There is not enough research focused on how caregiving affects the health and well-being of the caregiver. The authors state that there is need for research on posttraumatic stress disorder, differences between short- and long-term periods of caregiving burden, how caregivers react when they become receivers of care from healthcare professionals, and the effect of repeated episodes of caregiving responsibility.[35]

Nurses must monitor the caregiver for indications of declining health and emotional distress. A strategy to reduce stress is to help caregivers acknowledge feelings of stress and plan self-care activities.[36] Support groups provide self-help by sharing experiences and information, offering understanding and acceptance, and suggesting solutions to common problems and concerns. Encourage the caregiver to seek help from the formal social support system regarding matters such as respite care, housing, healthcare coverage, and finances. Respite care, which is planned temporary care for the patient, can allow the caregiver to regain a sense of equilibrium. Respite care includes adult day care, in-home care, and assisted living services. In addition, caregivers need to be encouraged to take care of themselves in all aspects of life.

Caregivers' quality of life is the cornerstone of effective caregiving interventions. Improved mental and physical health is essential in order for caregivers to continue to provide care. It is essential for healthcare providers to teach caregivers techniques to manage stressors and day-to-day challenges.[36] The care that nurses offer to family caregivers occurs on several levels:

- *Caring for the caregiver physically*: Nurses should reinforce the importance of eating a healthy diet at regular times, exercising to help relieve stress, and obtaining adequate sleep as essential. Lack of activity has been identified as one of the factors affecting caregivers' mood and propensity to depression.

- *Caring for the caregiver emotionally*: Nurses can speak to caregivers about keeping a journal, which can help caregivers express feelings that may be difficult to express verbally. Humor is important, and its occasional use in some situations can provide distraction and relieve stress-filled situations. Humor can motivate caregivers and keep them focused on the importance of keeping a positive attitude.[37] Nurses should encourage caregivers to continue their social activities, interests, and hobbies to maintain a sense of balance in their own lives.
- *Caring for the caregiver socially*: Nurses can promote social support of caregivers. Physical contact with others provides emotional support and acknowledgment of the caregiver's own need for comfort and assurance. The main support sources for caregivers include friends, family, and healthcare professionals.[38]
- *Caring for the caregiver cognitively*: Nurses can encourage the caregiver to appraise his or her perception of situations and try to maintain a positive perspective. Caregivers adapt to circumstances through a conscious procedure while dynamically making sense of the caregiving situation.[39]
- *Caring for the caregiver spiritually*: Nurses can nourish the spirits of family caregivers, help them to maintain a sense of awe about life, connect with the transcendent, and participate in spiritual or religious experiences that are important to the caregivers. Spiritual support from communities of faith can be a valuable resource for caregivers.

INTERRELATED CONCEPTS

Many concepts presented in this textbook are related to the concept of caregiving and are presented in Fig. 50.2. Three concepts that are closely linked to caregiving are Family Dynamics, Culture, and Spirituality. Caregiving can trigger many changes in family structure and family roles. Culture influences a person's definition of family, the relationships among family members, and the perception of the caregiver's responsibilities or identity. Some caregivers report positive feelings such as a sense of purpose when cultural values and religiosity support positive family dynamics.

Caregivers can be motivated to provide care for different reasons. Some caregivers report that their strong desire to provide care is due to a positive pre-illness/disability relationship with the care recipient and vice versa, and for others, caregiving is their main reason for living. Some may experience feelings of emptiness and lack of purpose the moment they do not have someone to care for.[40] Other reasons for Adherence to the caregiver role include feeling that their designated role is unavoidable, the need to keep a promise, or the lack of alternatives. These motives usually create a tense environment in which the caregiver may provide a minimum level of care, or there is a chance of neglect.[40] The caregiver may also feel unable to keep up with their own disease Self-Management.

The Stress and Coping concept is closely interrelated because of the actual or perceived threat to the caregiver's mental, emotional, and spiritual well-being and can result in a series of physiological responses, including Fatigue. The emotional and physical strain is caused by a person's response to pressure (stressors) in the environment. It leads

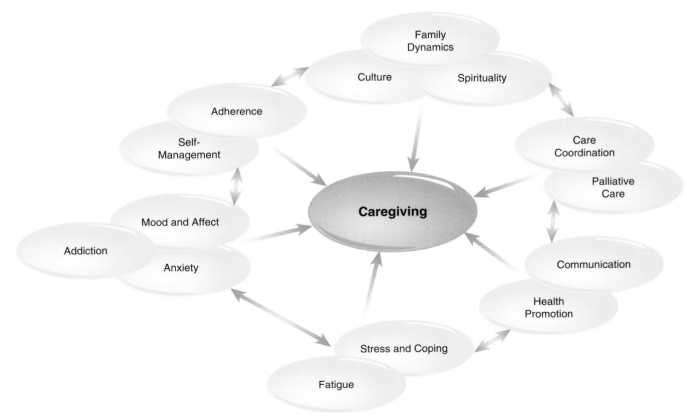

FIGURE 50.2 Caregiving and Interrelated Concepts.

to rapid changes throughout the body affecting almost every body system. Coping is the process through which a person manages the demands placed on the person–environment relationship and the emotions generated by a given situation and is influenced by a person's cognitive appraisal of an event. One's cognitive appraisal subsequently influences emotional arousal.[14]

Caregivers' **Mood and Affect** is influenced by their ability to cope with the experience. Mood swings can be expressive emotional responses to heightened tension and stress-related defensive mechanisms. Caregivers may become overwhelmed and experience great **Anxiety**, which may result in **Addictions** of different kinds and may be a reflection of caregiver burnout, low self-esteem, or a history of psychosocial problems exacerbated by the act of caregiving.

Establishing effective **Communication** between the caregiver, the care receiver, and the healthcare provider is essential in order to support the positive aspects of caregiving and minimize negative aspects. Through an effective communication channel, all involved parties can be educated so that they can be aware of all of the complex intricacies of the caregiving process and understand the responsibilities associated with caregiving. **Health Promotion** is the expected result of an effective communication process and education.

Deciding which is the right moment to request a **Palliative Care** consult in the case of patients with declining health status can make a major difference in the healthcare and treatment decisions going forward. Vigilant exploration of worrisome signs and symptoms and the analysis of functional and physical limitations can signal the need for the involvement of a palliative care specialist to coordinate the care that is appropriate on a case-by-case basis. **Care Coordination** can be achieved when the needs of the patient and his or her family caregivers are discussed with other members of the interprofessional team. The results are positive outcomes for patients and their caregivers and efficient use of healthcare resources.

CLINICAL EXEMPLARS

A wide variety of conditions and situations contribute to the need for an individual to require caregiving, and the variability in the level of care needed is influenced by multiple variables, including age and underlying health status. Although it is not possible to list all conditions or illnesses that require caregiving, Box 50.2 presents very common exemplars. It is beyond the scope of this textbook to describe all exemplars listed, but some of the most important are featured here.

Featured Exemplars
Impaired Physical Mobility
Many diseases and rehabilitative states involve some degree of immobility. Examples include strokes, traumatic injuries, multiple sclerosis, Parkinson disease, Huntington disease, amyotrophic lateral sclerosis, and cerebral palsy. With impaired mobility, individuals experience a decrease in muscle mass, strength, and function; their joints become stiffer and contracted; and their gait changes. The restrictions on movement affect the performance of activities of daily living (ADLs), and in some medical conditions or advanced medical conditions care recipients are totally dependent on caregivers.

Impaired Cognitive Status
Changes in cognition can be highly stressful for caregivers. Individuals with moderate to severe changes in their level of cognition often require special care, which includes 24-hour-a-day supervision, special communication techniques, and management of their difficult behaviors. They can become aggressive and unpredictable, and they will become totally dependent on their caregivers for assistance of ADLs, which

---

BOX 50.2   CAREGIVING EXEMPLARS

Short-Term Caregiving Needs
- Acute myocardial infarction
- Burn injury
- Influenza
- Pneumonia
- Recovery from surgery
- Sepsis
- Traumatic injury (nondisabling)

Long-Term Caregiving Needs
General Chronic Conditions
- Blindness
- Cancers
- Chronic kidney disease
- Chronic obstructive pulmonary disease
- Diabetes
- Heart failure

Impaired Cognitive Status
- Alzheimer disease
- Dementia
- Huntington disease
- Traumatic brain injury
- Stroke

Impaired Physical Mobility
- Amputation
- Amyotrophic lateral sclerosis
- Cerebral palsy
- Multiple sclerosis
- Parkinson disease
- Stroke
- Spinal cord injury
- Traumatic brain injury

Mental Health Conditions
- Depression (severe)
- Post-traumatic stress disorder
- Schizophrenia
- Substance abuse

 ACCESS EXEMPLAR LINKS IN YOUR GIDDENS EBOOK

---

include bathing, eating, transferring from bed to a chair or wheelchair, toileting, and other personal care. Examples include traumatic brain injury, dementia, Alzheimer disease, Parkinson disease, and stroke.

Post-Traumatic Stress Disorder
Post-traumatic stress disorder (PTSD) occurs when individuals are exposed to traumatic events that engender extreme levels of fear for the safety of self and others. Although PTSD is treatable, it can become a chronic and disabling condition. In severe cases, PTSD leads to disability, and individuals may experience symptoms such as nightmares, hyperarousal, re-experience reminders of the trauma, flashbacks of the event, and increased startle reflexes. After a traumatic injury or experience, individuals must cope with psychological and physical factors, prolonged hospital stays, delayed recovery time, and treatment-related stressors. Frequently, the combination of physical and psychological

factors can be disabling for the affected individual, and he or she becomes the responsibility of a caregiver.

Impaired Respiratory Function

Impaired respiratory function can be the result of several diseases and conditions. Examples include chronic obstructive pulmonary disease, pneumonia, asthma, and cystic fibrosis. Respiratory failure can be acute or chronic. In severe cases of lung disease, long-term care may be needed to provide continuous breathing support through mechanical ventilation. In the majority of these cases, individuals who require mechanical ventilation or continuous oxygen support to sustain their lives require the assistance of formal and informal caregivers.

Substance Abuse

Substance abuse refers to the damaging and harmful use of psychoactive substances, including alcohol and illicit drugs. The negative consequences of drug abuse are not only limited to the abuser; rather, they influence the families of the abuser particularly. Family members have an increased prevalence of experiencing domestic violence, stress, family cohesion problems, and, in the case of children, behavioral problems. In addition, close family members of drug-addicted individuals sometimes become the sole caregivers of abusers due to financial, legal, and physical restraints.[41]

CASE STUDY

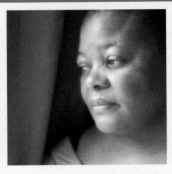

Case Presentation

Maria, age 44 years, recently immigrated from the Caribbean to south Florida to live with her parents, grandmother, aunt, sister, and two teenage sons. Maria is a single mother and is struggling to find employment due to her language barrier. The family's main source of income is the Social Security benefits obtained from her parents, grandmother, and aunt. The Social Security pensions that the family receives are currently the minimum amount assigned by the federal government due to the limited employment histories of the retirees. Maria's father, Joseph, age 74 years, had stomach cancer 5 years ago and requires weekly injections of vitamin B12 and a specialized diet to maintain his nutritional health. Maria's 72-year-old mother, Luisa, suffers from depression and does not help around the house. Maria's grandmother recently turned 100 years old and requires moderate assistance with her activities of daily living. Approximately 1 month ago, Maria's 83-year-old Aunt Elsa (who has advanced Alzheimer disease) suffered a subdural hematoma as a result of a fall. After 1 month in the trauma unit and the inpatient rehabilitation center, Aunt Elsa's Medicare benefits expired and she had to be relocated home because the family could not afford her care in a skilled inpatient facility.

Elsa's health condition has deteriorated significantly since her accident. She now has a tracheotomy tube, requires permanent oxygen, tube feedings, and needs 24-hour care due to her bedbound status. Maria's sister Laura is 52 years old, unemployed, and undergoing chemotherapy for breast cancer. Laura has a 15-year-old daughter, whose father lives in another country and does not provide any financial support.

Three months after Maria arrived in the United States, her sister Laura passed away from breast cancer, leaving Maria in charge of the entire household, which now consists of three teenagers currently attending high school and three elderly individuals.

Six months after Maria's arrival from the Caribbean, she has become the sole caregiver of her entire family and has gained 30 pounds. She is always stressed, and she constantly complains to her sons and niece that she has no help and that she has become a slave as a punishment by God. Sometimes, she spends the entire day without speaking to anyone, and whenever she has a chance, she locks herself in her room to eat and watch TV.

Case Analysis Questions

1. Maria's situation represents multiple types of caregiver roles. What caregiving roles are represented?
2. Referring back to the scope of the concept, presented in this chapter, where on the continuum does Maria fit?
3. What caregiver support options would most benefit Maria?

From ands456/iStock/Thinkstock

 ACCESS EXEMPLAR LINKS IN YOUR GIDDENS EBOOK

REFERENCES

1. National Alliance for Caregiving. (2015). Executive summary: *Caregiving in the U.S.*. Retrieved from http://www.caregiving.org/wp-content/uploads/2015/05/2015_CaregivingintheUS_Final-Report-June-4_WEB.pdf.
2. Dentrea, P. (2007). Caregiving. In G. Ritzer (Ed.), *Blackwell encyclopedia of sociology*. Malden, MA: Blackwell Publishers.
3. Hermanns, M., & Mastel-Smith, B. (2012). Caregiving: A qualitative concept analysis. *The Qualitative Report, 17*(75), 1–18.
4. Family Caregiver Alliance. (2009). *Caregiving*. Retrieved from https://caregiver.org/caregiving.
5. Reinhard, S. C., Levine, S., & Samis, S. (2014). *Family caregivers providing complex chronic care to their spouses*. Washington, DC: AARP Public Policy Institute. Retrieved from https://www.aarp.org/content/dam/aarp/research/public_policy_institute/health/2014/family-caregivers-providing-complex-chronic-care-spouses-AARP-ppi-health.pdf.
6. Alzheimer's Association. *2018 Alzheimer's disease facts and figures*. Retrieved from https://alz.org/media/HomeOffice/Facts%20and%20Figures/facts-and-figures.pdf.
7. Do, E. K., Cohen, S. A., & Brown, M. (2014). Socioeconomic and demographic factors modify the association between informal caregiving and health in the sandwich generation. *BMC Public Health, 14*, 362.
8. Generations United. (2011). *Grandfacts: Data, interpretation, and implications for caregivers*. Retrieved from http://www2.gu.org/OURWORK/Grandfamilies.aspx.
9. Scommegna, P., & Nadwa, M. (2011). The health and well-being of grandparents caring for grandchildren. *Today's Research on Aging, 23*.
10. Williams, K. L., Morrison, V., & Robinson, C. A. (2014). Exploring caregiving experiences: Caregiver coping and making sense of illness. *Aging & Mental Health, 18*(5), 600–609.
11. Bonis, S. A. (2013). Concept analysis: Method to enhance interdisciplinary conceptual understanding. *ANS. Advances in Nursing Science, 36*(2), 80–93.
12. Sherman, D. W., & Cheon, J. (2014). Family caregivers. In M. Matzo & D. W. Sherman (Eds.), *Palliative care nursing: Quality care to the end of life* (4th ed., pp. 147–167). New York: Springer.

13. Pearlin, L. I., Mullan, J. T., Semple, S. J., et al. (1990). Caregiving and the stress process: An overview of concepts and their measures. *The Gerontologist, 30,* 583–594.

14. Lazarus, S., & Folkman, S. (1988). The relationship between coping and emotion: Implications for theory and research. *Social Science & Medicine, 26*(3), 309–317.

15. Williams, L. A. (2007). Whatever it takes: Informal caregiving dynamics in blood and marrow transplantation. *Oncology Nursing Forum, 34,* 379–387.

16. Epiphaniou, E., Hamilton, D., Bridger, S., et al. (2012). Adjusting to the caregiving role: The importance of coping and support. *International Journal of Palliative Nursing, 18*(11), 541–545.

17. Feinberg, L., & Rita, C. (2012). *Understanding the impact of family caregiving on work.* AARP Public Policy Institute. Retrieved from https://www.aarp.org/content/dam/aarp/research/public_policy_institute/ltc/2012/understanding-impact-family-caregiving-work-AARP-ppi-ltc.pdf.

18. Kapp, M. B. (2013). For love, legacy, or pay: Legal and pecuniary aspects of family caregiving. *Care Management Journals, 14*(3), 205–208.

19. Kim, H., & Rose, K. M. (2014). Concept analysis of family homeostasis. *Journal of Advanced Nursing, 70*(11), 2450–2468.

20. Rosser, M., & Walsh, H. (2014). *Fundamentals of palliative care for student nurses.* Hoboken, NJ: Wiley-Blackwell.

21. Moore, H., & Gillespie, A. (2014). The caregiving bind: Concealing the demands of informal care can undermine the caregiving identity. *Social Science & Medicine, 116,* 102–109.

22. U.S. Department of Health and Human Services, Office of Minority Health. (2015). *What is cultural competency?* Retrieved from http://minorityhealth.hhs.gov/omh/browse.aspx?lvl=1&lvlid=6.

23. Miyawaki, C. E. (2016). Caregiving practice patterns of Asian, Hispanic, and non-Hispanic white American family caregivers of older adults across generations. *Journal of Cross-cultural Gerontology, 31*(1), 35–55.

24. Pharr, J. R., Dodge Francis, C., Terry, C., & Clark, M. C. (2014). Culture, caregiving, and health: Exploring the influence of culture on family caregiver experiences. *ISRN Public Health, 2014.*

25. Roth, D. L., Dilworth-Anderson, P., Huang, J., et al. (2015). Positive aspects of family caregiving for dementia: Differential item functioning by race. *The Journals of Gerontology. Series B, Psychological Sciences and Social Sciences, 70*(6), 813–819.

26. Lloyd, J., Patterson, T., & Muers, J. (2016). The positive aspects of caregiving in dementia: A critical review of the qualitative literature. *Dementia (Basel, Switzerland), 15*(6), 1534–1561.

27. Stajduhar, K. I., Martin, W. L., Barwich, D., et al. (2008). Factors influencing family caregivers' ability to cope with providing end-of-life cancer care at home. *Cancer Nursing, 31*(1), 77–85.

28. Haley, W. E., LaMonde, L. A., Han, B., et al. (2003). Predictors of depression and life satisfaction among spousal caregivers in hospice: Application of a stress process model. *Journal of Palliative Medicine, 6*(2), 215–224.

29. Buyck, J., Bonnaud, S., Boumendil, A., et al. (2011). Informal caregiving and self-reported mental and physical health: Results from the Gazel Cohort Study. *American Journal of Public Health, 101*(10), 1971–1979.

30. Li, Q., Mak, Y., & Loke, A. (2013). Spouses' experience of caregiving for cancer patients: A literature review. *International Nursing Review, 60*(2), 178–187.

31. Gulanick, M., & Myers, J. (2017). *Nursing diagnosis care plans: Diagnoses, interventions, and outcomes* (9th ed.). St Louis, MO: Mosby.

32. Saban, K., Sherwood, P., DeVon, H., et al. (2010). Measures of psychological stress and physical health in family caregivers of stroke survivors: A literature review. *The Journal of Neuroscience Nursing: Journal of the American Association of Neuroscience Nurses, 42*(3), 128–138.

33. Van Vliet, D., de Vugt, M. E., Bakker, C., et al. (2010). Impact of early onset dementia on caregivers: A review. *International Journal of Geriatric Psychiatry, 25*(11), 1091–1100.

34. McGuire, D., Grant, M., & Park, J. (2012). Palliative care and end of life: The caregiver. *Nursing Outlook, 60*(6), 351–356.

35. Baker, P. R., Francis, D. P., Hairi, N. N. M., et al. (2017). Interventions for preventing elder abuse: Applying findings of a new Cochrane review. *Age and Ageing, 46*(3), 346–348.

36. Lowder, J., Buzney, S., & Buzo, A. (2005). The caregiver balancing act: Giving too much or not enough. *Care Management Journals, 6*(3), 159–165.

37. Liptak, A., Tate, J., Flatt, J., et al. (2014). Humor and laughter in persons with cognitive impairment and their caregivers. *Journal of Holistic Nursing, 32*(1), 25–34.

38. Kemp, C. L., Ball, M. M., Morgan, J. C., et al. (2018). Maneuvering together, apart, and at odds: Residents' care convoys in assisted living. *The Journals of Gerontology. Series B, Psychological Sciences and Social Sciences,* gbx184.

39. Yu, D. S. F., et al. (2018). Unravelling positive aspects of caregiving in dementia: An integrative review of research literature. *International Journal of Nursing Studies, 79,* 1–26.

40. Czekanski, K. (2017). The Experience of Transitioning to a Caregiving Role for a Family Member with Alzheimer's Disease or Related Dementia. *The American Journal of Nursing, 117*(9), 24–32.

41. American Psychological Association. (2018). *Family members of adults with substance abuse problems.* Retrieved from http://www.apa.org/pi/about/publications/caregivers/practice-settings/intervention/substance-abuse.aspx.

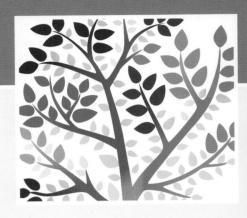

Palliative Care

Constance Dahlin and Patrick Coyne

Palliative care is an integrated approach to address the physical, psychological, emotional, social, cultural, and spiritual needs of patients and families experiencing serious, life-threatening, progressive or chronic illness.[1] Palliative care is offered to patients and families across the lifespan, and across the illness trajectory beginning at the diagnosis of serious disease into the bereavement period for families.[1] The issues affecting the care of patients with serious, life-threatening, and chronic illness are expected to intensify during the next several decades, particularly given the aging population. It is predicted that by 2030, for the first time in history, people aged 65 years or older will outnumber the young.[2] Unlike a century ago, when most people died of infections, accidents, or other rapidly lethal diseases, the leading causes of death in the United States are now cardiovascular disease, cancer, cerebrovascular diseases, chronic obstructive lung disease, unintentional injuries, and dementia.[3]

From a global perspective, it is estimated that 40 million people worldwide will need palliative care as a result of chronic, noninfectious diseases.[4] In the United States, palliative care has permeated across acute care in the United States with 67% of hospitals with over 50 beds having palliative care teams, leaving about 30% without palliative care teams.[5] Strides are being made for palliative care development in the community. Palliative care models have developed in the home, the clinic, the skilled facility as well as other settings.

DEFINITION

Palliative care is a holistic approach to care that focuses on the physical, emotional, social, cultural, and spiritual needs of both the patient and his or her family members across the illness trajectory.[6] The Center for Medicare and Medicaid offers the following definition of palliative care:

> *Palliative care means **patient and family-centered care** that optimizes quality of life by anticipating, preventing, and treating suffering. Palliative care throughout the continuum of illness involves addressing physical, intellectual, emotional, social, and spiritual needs **and to facilitate patient autonomy, access to information, and choice.**[6,7]*

The definition of palliative care recognizes the multidimensionality of the illness experience. Moreover, palliative care is appropriate for end-stage organ diseases such as end-stage heart, lung, liver, or kidney disease, as well as neurodegenerative diseases or life-threatening infections such as HIV/AIDS.[1] Like hospice, palliative care was originally associated with end-of-life care or when curative treatments were no longer beneficial, effective, or desirable. However, in its current conceptualization, palliative care promotes quality of life in a person with a serious illness through exquisite pain and symptom management, optimization of functional status, and support for patients and families.

SCOPE

The changing demographics of populations, changing illness trajectories, advances in health care, and longer life expectancies have created a need for palliative care offered across the lifespan, from neonates to the frail elderly. Palliative care is offered from the time of diagnosis with a life-threatening illness until death and into the bereavement period for families.[1] Moreover, palliative care is accessed across many health settings and the continuum of care from the clinic, home, long-term care, rehabilitation setting to the hospital, including adult and pediatric day care. With palliative care as the umbrella term for care of patients' serious illness, hospice is recognized as last stage of palliative care for patients with a terminal diagnosis at the end of life.

In the past, there were many diseases or conditions for which there was no cure. Therefore, when there were no further treatments to offer a cure, the prevalent medical thought was that there was nothing more to do. Many of these patients participated in goals of care to decide next steps to make the awful decision of forgoing treatment. The patient was offered "comfort care," "supportive care," "end-of-life" or hospice care, in which there was still much to offer. Hospice care, as the gold standard of terminal care, meant these patients received expert pain and symptom management, psychosocial support for him or herself and the family, spiritual support, and home support to prevent admission to the hospital or long-term care setting. However, it seemed unethical that only patients who were dying received such comprehensive care.

In the 1990s, hospice care moved from the home to the academic setting. This new care was called palliative care with the goal to offer this type of comprehensive care to all patients, not just terminally ill patients. The term *palliate* means to moderate or ease symptoms. *Palliative care* means to "cloak," "soothe," or "alleviate" the pain and suffering associated with serious, progressive, life-threatening or chronic illness.[8] Through the National Consensus Project for Quality Palliative Care (NCP) *Clinical Practice Guidelines for Quality Palliative Care*, first released in 2004, it was recognized that palliative and hospice care were part of a continuum of care, with palliative care beginning "upstream" at diagnosis. Palliative care is present in hospitals, rehabilitation settings, skilled nursing facilities, offices, and clinics and is now moving into the community in patients' homes, group homes, and adult and pediatric day programs, to name a few. Palliative care can work with patients under the care of hospice programs and home health agencies. However, it is recognized that some people will decline hospice or home health services, but still receive palliative care.

ATTRIBUTES AND CRITERIA

Palliative care is a comprehensive, holistic interdisciplinary approach to care of patients and families across the lifespan who have serious, life-threatening, progressive, or chronic illness or conditions.[1] Palliative care is a team approach to care and this approach is unique as the family is a part of the care delivered. Palliative care can transform the current disease-focused approach to a patient-centered philosophy, in which the needs of the patient and patient and family goals form the basis of the patient's care plan.[9] Patient-centeredness broadens the focus of care and requires well-defined coordination across specialties and disciplines as well as access to specialty palliative care clinicians such as nurses, physicians, social workers, and chaplains.[1] To promote, maintain, and even restore the patient's and family's quality of life, an interdisciplinary model to care is essential. Optimal functioning of a team requires outstanding training, communication, and the role delineation of each team member.[6] Palliative care encompasses the following attributes: (1) state of the art treatment tailored to the individual; (2) support for the family and/or caregivers; and (3) interdisciplinary team approach.[5] Further attributes of palliative care include the following:

- Optimal assessment and management of physical and psychological symptoms (i.e., pain, dyspnea, nausea/vomiting, constipation, anxiety, agitation, and depression)
- Eliciting and advocating for the wishes and preferences of patients and developing a comprehensive and individualized plan of care
- Assisting patients in advance care planning including the delegation of a surrogate decision-maker, clarifying values, preferences, and beliefs in advanced directives, and out of hospital orders for life-sustaining treatment with the completion of appropriate documents specific to each state
- Promoting effective communication among patient, families, and members of the interdisciplinary team
- Promoting continuity of care and care coordination across transitions of care[1,4]

THEORETICAL LINKS

The National Consensus Project for Quality Palliative Care has played a major role in moving palliative care upstream. The *Clinical Practice Guidelines*, a theoretical framework for palliative care clinical practice, education, and research, was established for palliative care across the lifespan and healthcare settings. There have been four editions of the Guidelines, in which each revision reflects the maturity and evolution of the field. Now there are Guidelines specific to the community being developed. The guidelines promote high-quality care; reduce variation in new and existing programs; encourage continuity of care across settings; and facilitate collaborative partnerships among palliative care programs, community hospices, and a wide range of other healthcare delivery settings.[1] Another goal of the guidelines has been to promote recognition, stable reimbursement structures, and accreditation initiatives through projects such as the National Quality Forum (NQF).[10] In 2006, the NQF created the Framework for Hospice and Palliative Care using the NCP *Clinical Practice Guidelines* as a foundation. However, at this point, these are outdated as they no longer reflect the growth and maturity of the field over the last decade. The Joint Commission

uses the NCP *Clinical Practice Guidelines* as the basis of Advanced Certification in Palliative Care for hospitals and in the community for home health and hospices.[11,12] The Hospice and Palliative Nurses Association (HPNA), which is the professional organization for all nursing levels of specialty hospice and palliative care, uses the *Clinical Practice Guidelines* as an education framework. In particular, there is an registered nurse and advanced-practice registered nurse pathway for development into specialty palliative nursing practice, from novice to expert, in their competencies and education products. Other organizations have implemented *The Clinical Guidelines* into practice and operationalized the domains to provide optimal palliative care, including the basis of education and nursing competencies.[13]

CONTEXT TO NURSING AND HEALTH CARE

In 2014, more than 20.4 million people needed palliative care, 69% of whom were older than 60 years of age and 6% of whom were children.[4] Millions of Americans are living with one or more chronic debilitating diseases, and 7 out of 10 Americans can expect to live with their diseases several years before dying.[2] When coupled with the advancing age of the 8 million baby boomers, who now qualify for Medicare, this will create a huge demand on healthcare resources and community-based services. These demands will force changes in patterns of care for patients living for several years with chronic illness and their complications before dying.[2] The early referral to palliative services can make a difference in the treatment approach, resulting in positive healthcare outcomes even in the face of serious illness or impending death. Nurses are often the first clinicians that patients meet and therefore have an essential role in providing education to patients and families to facilitate their engagement in early palliative care when appropriate. It is essential that nurses have primary palliative care education to assure access to quality care across all settings.[14]

Palliative Care as a Team-Based Approach

To promote quality of life, the comprehensive needs of patients and families are addressed by an interdisciplinary palliative characterized by a collaborative process that includes information exchange and coordinated care planning to achieve patient- and family-centered care. Services commonly offered by the palliative care team are presented in Box 51.1. The central focus of the team is to engage and partner with patients and families to provide effective and efficient care coordination.[15,16] This is facilitated by effective communication and attention to the linguistic, health, and educational literacy of the patient and family.[17-19] The interdisciplinary team must have an appropriate number of dedicated and palliative care specialty educated staff available.[1] Education must include cultural awareness and competence in order to deliver culturally sensitive care.[1,20,21]

Core Services

The palliative care team often represents a variety of disciplines in which the four core services include chaplaincy, social work, nursing, and medicine.

- *Chaplaincy*: Clergy and spiritual care providers are members of the clergy, chaplains, and other spiritual advisors providing spiritual counseling and support for the patient and his or her family, as well as other members of the interdisciplinary team when they experience moral or ethical distress. Spiritual issues often are intertwined with other patient symptoms and can be masked by both physical and psychoemotional responses. Spiritual care goes beyond identification of the patient's or family's faith background to an understanding of the meaning and purpose in life, sense of hope, faith, love, trust, and forgiveness.[1] All healthcare providers can offer

BOX 51.1   Common Palliative Care Services

- Advance care planning—surrogate decision maker, advance directives, out of hospital orders for life sustaining treatment (POLST/MOLST forms)
- Physical assessment and management of symptoms with focus on proactive planning (pharmacological, nonpharmacological)
- Psychological assessment and management of symptoms with focus on proactive planning (pharmacological, nonpharmacological)
- Care coordination
- Resource access (community and health system)
- Counseling (patient and/or family)
- Rehabilitation services (physical therapy, occupational therapy, speech and language pathology, nutrition)
- Important conversations (goals of care, advanced illness, disagreement in care)
- Patient/family education
- Medication management (reconciliation, safe prescribing or deprescribing, safe disposal)
- Respite services
- Volunteer services

compassionate care that touches the human spirit of patients and families, whereas spiritual care providers have a deep understanding of human emotional and spiritual needs and issues.

- *Nursing*: Registered nurses and advanced practice registered nurses assess and evaluate the ongoing needs of the patient and family, including physical, emotional, social, cultural, and spiritual well-being; advocate for the patient and family; and provide referrals to other health professionals when needed.[9,22,23]
- *Social services*: Social workers provide psychological care for the patient and family, helping to identify areas of need, such as communication, behavioral issues, educational, financial, guardianship, and other legal issues, including assistance with housing and access to community support and resources. In the event of death, social workers also provide support with the grief and bereavement process.[24]
- *Medicine*: Doctors of medicine and doctors of osteopathy offer diagnosis, care planning, and oversight of care for patients and families including education, trajectory of illness, and prognosis.[25]

Expanded Services

With each patient there may be a larger circle of care providers. This team expands and contracts depending on the situation. All members of the interdisciplinary team contribute their expertise and knowledge in assisting patients and family members to establish goals of care and identify treatment wishes and preferences that facilitate patient/family choice and autonomy.[1] This includes:

- *Psychological support*—psychologists or psychiatrists who provide support to enable coping for the patient and family;
- *Care coordination and case management*—manage care across transitions;
- *Rehabilitation services*—physical, speech, and occupational therapists;
- *Expressive therapies*—child life, art, and music therapists; pharmacists; and
- *Volunteers*—bereavement counselors; family support specialists; and volunteers.[26,27]

Levels of Palliative Care

Two levels of palliative care include primary palliative care and specialty palliative care.[14,28,29]

- *Primary palliative care providers*: These are healthcare professionals who may be advanced practice registered nurses, registered nurses, physicians, physician assistants, social workers, or chaplains with a working knowledge of issues surrounding patients with serious illness. They may assess, diagnose, manage, or treat conditions or problems of issues such as advance directives, common pain syndromes, and symptoms. Depending on their location, they may work closely with nursing and other members of the interdisciplinary team with a working knowledge of palliative care.[14,28,29]
- *Specialty palliative care providers*: These are providers who may also be any member of the team from diverse specialty services or who are specialists in palliative care. They have expert knowledge in the physical, spiritual, emotional, psychological, and cultural aspects of palliative care. They provide consultation to others such as the primary care team, disease specialty teams, and home teams in the complex management of pain, symptoms management, advanced illness, and communication related to the serious illness trajectory.[14,28,29]

Strategic Directions for Palliative Care

The Institute of Medicine's 2014 report regarding the care of patients with serious and advanced illness recommended that the provision of palliative care should be covered by every health insurer.[30] Furthermore, standards of care should be evidence-based and continuously updated based on emergent research findings, and healthcare providers must achieve competence in palliative care. Thus, at least generalist or primary palliative care competencies should be achieved by all nurses and other healthcare providers across all healthcare settings.[30] Since nursing and palliative care are intertwined, there has been national work and collaboration to consider the education of nurses.

In 2017, the American Nurse Association and Hospice and Palliative Care Nurses Association released *A Call for Action: Nurses Leading and Transforming Palliative Care*. The document emphasizes an interdisciplinary model of clinical practice in which palliative care practitioners collaborate to provide evidence-based care to create a plan of care that reflects patients' wishes and preferences.[14] In addition, it describes the current state of palliative care and the mandate for all nurses to have primary palliative care skills. It recognizes that nurses at all levels must receive palliative care education in their preparation education in order to deliver primary palliative care and some may choose to practice specialty palliative care.[14] One recommendation of the American Nurses Association and the Hospice and Palliative Nurses Association is that all nurses pursue End-of-Life Nursing Education Consortium (ELNEC) training, which is available for critical care nurses, geriatric nurses, pediatric nurses, general nursing practice, and advanced practice nursing.[14]

Changing Models of Care

Historically, the hospice care model was initially based on the cancer disease trajectory, when treatment options were limited, cure was illusive, and death was inevitable. Now cancer care has changed with emerging new treatment modalities, and cancer is considered a chronic illness. In fact, cancer patients now have a more unpredictable prognosis trajectory and are similar to patients with other chronic diseases such as chronic obstructive pulmonary disease (COPD) and heart failure. These patient populations often experience disease exacerbations and recovery or partial recovery over a long trajectory. Patients may live for many years with their chronic disease and have varying fluctuations in their functional status. Each time these patients encounter an exacerbation of their disease and enter into the acute care setting, their disease may become less responsive to curative or disease-specific measures.

Changes in care models will require attention to the cost-effective management of chronic diseases and their associated symptoms.[31] When palliative care is consulted at the time of diagnosis of a serious or life-limiting illness, research has demonstrated higher satisfaction and decreased symptoms burdens.[32–35] Furthermore, the needs of family caregivers are often not assessed or supported. In these situations, palliative care offers expert pain and symptom management while improving quality of life for patients and supporting their families across the illness trajectory.[36,37]

Ongoing education about the role of palliative needs will foster early referral to palliative care. This promotes better continuity of care and partnership between clinical and community services. For individuals receiving palliative care across the lifespan, continuous evaluation of the care plan by members of the interdisciplinary team is essential to ensure that it reflects "best practices" and "evidence-based" interventions while recognizing and addressing the individual needs of patients and families facing serious illness across the illness–dying trajectory.

INTERRELATED CONCEPTS

Palliative care is a concept that is related to the eight domains to palliative care with the National Consensus Project for Quality Palliative Care (Box 51.2). The interrelated concepts associated with Palliative Care are organized around these domains. Domains are shown as boxes; the concepts presented within this book (shown as ovals) are linked to these eight themes (Fig. 51.1).

Domain One, Structure and Processes of Care focuses on interdisciplinary team engagement and collaboration with patients and family members. Concepts such as Health Care Quality, Caregiving, and Care Coordination are included in this domain.

Domain Two, Physical Aspects of Care and Domain Three, Psychological and Psychiatric Aspects of Care focus on the physical, psychological, and psychiatric assessments and treatment of the whole person. These domains integrate a variety of concepts, such as Fatigue, Sleep, Nutrition, Elimination, Pain, Mood and Affect, Anxiety, and Stress and Coping. These concepts present common symptoms and difficulties for patients in palliative care and require the best thinking of palliative care practitioners. The use of evidence supports high-quality interventions in palliative care, resulting in improved quality of life.

Domain Four, Social Aspects of Care focuses on the family as the unit of care and developmental needs. Nurses identify, support, and capitalize on family strengths in collaboration with social work. Interrelated concepts include Family Dynamics and Development.

Domain Five, Spiritual Aspects of Care focuses on meaning and purpose of life and its expression in terms of religion, Spirituality, and humanity with a focus of spiritual care, sometimes in collaboration with spiritual providers.

Domain Six, Cultural Aspects of Care focuses on the far-reaching aspects of Culture. It includes age, gender identification, sexual orientation, political affiliation, ethnicity, and the various dimensions of literacy—health, financial, and cognitive.

Domain Seven, Care of the Patient Nearing the End of Life focuses on pre-death, peri-death, and post-death. This is an area of nursing focus and important presence from living with life-limiting illness to actively dying to death for patients, families, and colleagues. Associated concepts are Culture and Spirituality.

Domain Eight, Ethical and Legal Aspects of Care focuses on goals of preferences of patients in terms of their care and the role of the nurse to promote communication on these difficult topics. In addition, there is discussion of the complex ethics that accompany palliative care such as withholding or withdrawing life-sustaining treatments. Finally, there is the acknowledgment of providing care within both the legal and ethical aspects of palliative care. Concepts include Ethics, Health Policy, Health Care Law, and Health Disparities.

BOX 51.2 Eight Domains of Palliative Care

1. Structure and processes of care
   Program structure, palliative process, education and training of team members, comprehensive care delivery
2. Physical aspects of care
   Assessing and managing pain, dyspnea, constipation, etc., through established tools
3. Psychological and psychiatric aspects of care
   Assessing and managing anxiety, depression, and other common psychological symptoms or normal psychological reactions of patients/families to serious illness, through established tools and including the establishment of organized grief and bereavement tools
4. Social aspects of care
   Assessing patient and family with a family assessment, to ensure social determinants of care support the care needs of the patient and family
5. Spiritual, religious, and existential aspects of care
   Understanding and assessing the multidimensionality of spirituality and religion and the needs of patients and families, religious practices or rituals, appropriate assessment, and the provision of spiritual and existential support
6. Cultural aspects of care
   Understanding and assessing the multidimensionality of culture, appropriate assessment, to assure decision making and preferences of patient or family regarding the disclosure of information and truth-telling, language, and rituals
7. Care of the Patient Nearing the End of Life
   Recognizing advanced illness to ensure communication and respect in planning use of time consistent with the patient's wishes. Proactive planning for end of life in terms of site, social, cultural, and spiritual detail. Ensuring attention to social, cultural, spiritual, physical, and psychological needs at the end of life; and providing bereavement support to caregivers
8. Ethical and legal aspects of care
   Determining and documenting patient/surrogate preferences for goals of care, treatment options, and setting of care; promoting advanced care planning; and signing of appropriate documents.
   Understanding the ethical and legal aspects of palliative and organizational resources

Data from National Consensus Project for Quality Palliative Care. (2018). *Clinical practice guidelines for quality palliative care* (4th ed.). Richmond, VA: National Coalition of Hospice and Palliative Care.

CLINICAL EXEMPLARS

Since palliative care is practiced in the acute setting, clinic setting, home setting, and long-term settings, examples of palliative care delivery in locations with diverse conditions are offered. Box 51.3 identifies some of the most common diagnoses associated with palliative care.

Featured Exemplars
Stroke

Stroke, otherwise known as a cerebral vascular accident (CVA), results in ischemia to the brain. Patients may experience varying degrees of paralysis or weakness and depending on the affected area of the brain, may also experience subsequent physical, emotional, behavioral, and motor sensory effects. CVAs often occur in conjunction with other comorbidities and without warning necessitating critical care. Moreover, patients and their families are faced with life-altering and catastrophic changes. In these situations, palliative care provides holistic care of the patient and family to help them cope with the residual effects of the

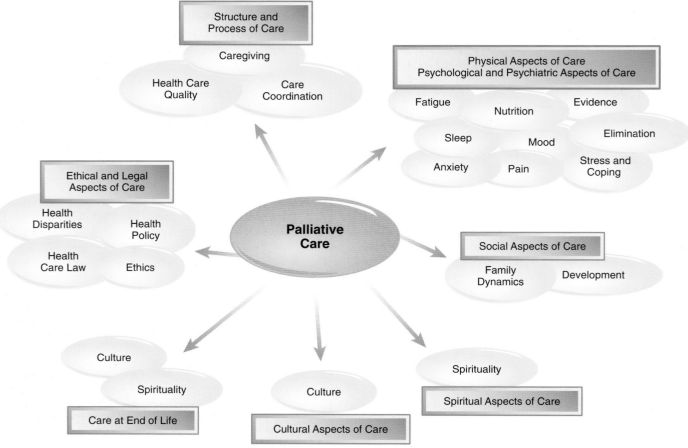

FIGURE 51.1 Palliative Care and Interrelated Concepts.

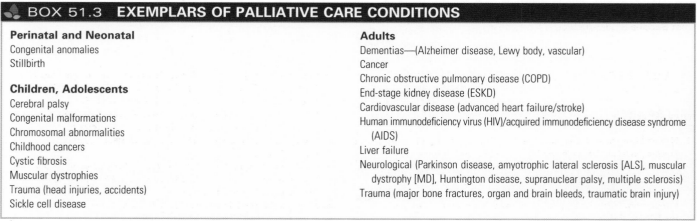

BOX 51.3   EXEMPLARS OF PALLIATIVE CARE CONDITIONS

Perinatal and Neonatal
Congenital anomalies
Stillbirth

Children, Adolescents
Cerebral palsy
Congenital malformations
Chromosomal abnormalities
Childhood cancers
Cystic fibrosis
Muscular dystrophies
Trauma (head injuries, accidents)
Sickle cell disease

Adults
Dementias—(Alzheimer disease, Lewy body, vascular)
Cancer
Chronic obstructive pulmonary disease (COPD)
End-stage kidney disease (ESKD)
Cardiovascular disease (advanced heart failure/stroke)
Human immunodeficiency virus (HIV)/acquired immunodeficiency disease syndrome (AIDS)
Liver failure
Neurological (Parkinson disease, amyotrophic lateral sclerosis [ALS], muscular dystrophy [MD], Huntington disease, supranuclear palsy, multiple sclerosis)
Trauma (major bone fractures, organ and brain bleeds, traumatic brain injury)

 ACCESS EXEMPLAR LINKS IN YOUR GIDDENS EBOOK

CVA. In addition, it focuses on discussions of goals of care and expectations while determining the plan of care.[38]

Heart Failure

Heart disease is one of the leading causes of morality, yet just a small percentage enter hospice. Physical symptoms include shortness of breath, chest pain, fatigue, depression, and edema. Most symptoms can be managed by cardiac protocols. Moreover, acute events often result in various procedures such as automatic implantable cardioverter-defibrillator (AICD), pacemaker, and ventricular assist device. Often there had been no discussion of their long-term benefits and burdens. Palliative care can promote advance care planning and discussions on goals of care to help with promoting quality of life.[38,39]

Pulmonary Disease

Pulmonary disease includes obstructive and restrictive diseases which result in lung damage, making it difficult to efficiently breathe. Physical symptoms associated with pulmonary disease include shortness of breath, low oxygen in the blood, cough, pain, weight loss, and infections. Patients may also experience psychological symptoms of depression, anxiety, insomnia, and social isolation. Palliative care aims to improve quality of life through pharmacologic and nonpharmacologic management. Interdisciplinary team members are essential to help with energy conservation, dietary modifications, counseling, and emotional/spiritual distress.[40,41]

Dementia

There are many types of dementia—Alzheimer, Lewy body, and vascular are very common. Dementia is primarily diagnosed in older adults who experience progressive cognitive impairment, memory loss, and decreased level of functioning. Palliative care promotes optimal functioning, structure, and promotion of a safe environment. Advance care planning becomes paramount with ongoing discussions of goals of care. Patients and families can benefit from palliative care symptom management, family support, and proactive management of future care needs. In addition, since the trajectory of dementia is attenuated, families need assistance to secure resources and respite.[42]

CASE STUDY

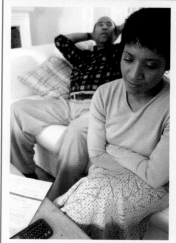

Case Presentation

Alfred Kennedy is a 46-year-old male school principal who is married and has young children. Over the past year, Mr. Kennedy began to experience swallowing difficulties, hand weakness, and falls. After a workup over several months, the diagnosis of amyotrophic lateral sclerosis (ALS) was made.

With the diagnosis, Mr. Kennedy developed situational depression which was managed with antidepressants. He had discussions with the ALS team about advance care planning, in particular about a tracheostomy and a gastrostomy tube. He met with physical therapy to work on strength training and a nutritionist to discuss strategies to manage dietary needs.

Following an appointment with a nurse practitioner, a comprehensive assessment indicates that Mr. Kennedy continues to have depressive symptoms. He has forgone his prescribed medications, he spends more time in bed, and has less energy. He is worried about his family, his employment, and his long-term and short-term disability insurance. He has many questions about the cause of his disease and the burden he is placing on his family. A referral is made to social work and chaplaincy. Social work offers resources to Mrs. Kennedy including durable medical equipment, assistive devices, and information on disability. The chaplain performs a life review with Mr. Kennedy.

With the help of the palliative care team, Mr. Kennedy has less anxiety and depression. Mrs. Kennedy is less overwhelmed. They are relieved by the provision of physical, psychosocial, spiritual, and emotional support. They also find the patient-centered and family-focused care plan alleviates their worry about constantly renegotiating goals of care.

Case Analysis Questions

1. What attributes of palliative care are evident in this case?
2. Review Fig. 51.1. How do the domains and interrelated concepts (shown in the illustration) apply in this case?

From Buccina Studios/Photodisc/Thinkstock.

 ACCESS EXEMPLAR LINKS IN YOUR GIDDENS EBOOK

REFERENCES

1. National Consensus Project for Quality Palliative Care. (2018). *Clinical practice guidelines for quality palliative care* (4th ed.). Richmond, VA: National Coalition of Hospice and Palliative Care.
2. Ortman, J., Velkoff, J., & Hogan, H. (2014). An Aging Nation: The older population in the United States—population estimates and projections. *Current Population Reports*; Retrieved from: https://www.census.gov/prod/2014pubs/p25-1140.pdf.
3. U.S. Department of Health and Human Services, Center for Disease Control and Prevention. National Center for Health Statistics. (2017). *Health, United States, 2016: With Chartbook on Long-term Trends in Health*. Retrieved from: https://www.cdc.gov/nchs/data/hus/hus16.pdf#019.
4. Worldwide Palliative Care Alliance and World Health Organization. (2014). *Global Atlas of Palliative Care at the End of Life*. In: London, England: Worldwide Palliative Care Alliance. Retrieved from: http://www.who.int/cancer/publications/palliative-care-atlas/en/.
5. Center to Advance Palliative Care. (2015). *America's Care of Serious Illness: State-by-State Report Care on Access to Palliative Care in Our Nation's Hospitals*. Retrieved from: https://reportcard.capc.org.
6. Department of Health and Human Services, Center for Medicare and Medicaid Services. (2012). *CMS Manuel System, Pub-100-07 State Operations, Provider Certification*. Center for Clinical Standards Quality / Survey and Certification Group. Retrieved from: https://www.cms.gov/Medicare/Provider-Enrollment-and-Certification/SurveyCertificationGenInfo/Downloads/Survey-and-Cert-Letter-12-48.pdf.
7. Center for Medicare & Medicaid Services. (2019). *Medicare & You*. Retrieved from: https://www.medicare.gov/sites/default/files/2019-05/10050-Medicare-and-You.pdf.
8. Merriam-Webster Dictionary. (2019). *Palliate*. Retrieved from: https://www.merriam-webster.com/dictionary/palliate.
9. American Nurses Association, Hospice and Palliative Nurses Association. (2014). *Palliative nursing: Scope and standards of practice—An essential resource for hospice and palliative nurses* (5th ed.). Silver Spring, MD: American Nurses Association and Hospice and Palliative Nurses Association.
10. National Quality Forum. (2006). *A National Framework and Preferred Practices for Palliative and Hospice Care Quality: A Consensus Report*. Washington, DC: NQF.
11. The Joint Commission. (2012). *Palliative care certification manual*. Oakbrook Terrace, IL: The Joint Commission.
12. The Joint Commission. (2018). *Community-Based Palliative Care Certification Option for Home Health & Hospice. Standards Available Now!*

Retrieved from: https://www.jointcommission.org/community-based_palliative_care_certification_option_july_1_2016/.

13. Dahlin, C. (2019). National consensus project for quality palliative care: Assuring Quality Palliative Care through *Clinical Practice Guidelines*. In B. & J. Paice (Eds.), *Oxford textbook of palliative nursing* (5th ed., pp. 3–12). New York, NY: Oxford University Press.

14. American Nurses Association, Hospice and Palliative Nurse Association. (2017). *A Call for Action—Nurses Lead and Transform Palliative Care*. https://www.nursingworld.org/~497158/globalassets/practiceandpolicy/health-policy/palliativecareprofessionalissuespanelcallforaction.pdf.

15. Zachariah, F., Gallo, M., Loscalzo, M., & Crocitto, L. E. (2014). Embedding palliative care into care coordination. *J Clinic Oncol, 32*(31_suppl), 62.

16. Mazanec, P., Lamb, G., Haas, S., et al. (2018). Palliative nursing summit: Nurses leading change and transforming care the nurse's role in coordination of care and transition management. *J Hosp Palliat Nurs, 20*(1), 15–22.

17. Chou, S. W., & Gaysynsky, A. (2016). Health literacy and communication in palliative care. In E. Wittenberg, J. Goldsmith, et al. (Eds.), *Textbook of palliative care communication*. New York, NY: Oxford University Press. CHECK.

18. du Pré, A., & Foster, E. (2016). Transactional communication. In E. Wittenberg, J. Goldsmith, et al. (Eds.), *Textbook of palliative care communication* (pp. 14–21). New York, NY: Oxford University Press.

19. Fage-Butler, M. A., & Jense, N. M. (2016). Patient- and family-centered written communication in the palliative care setting. In E. Wittenberg, J. Goldsmith, et al. (Eds.), *Textbook of palliative care communication* (pp. 102–110). New York, NY: Oxford University Press.

20. Palos, G. (2016). Cultural considerations in palliative care and serious illness. In E. Wittenberg, B. Ferrell, J. Goldsmith, et al. (Eds.), *Textbook of palliative care communication* (pp. 153–160). New York, NY: Oxford University Press.

21. Nuebauer, K., Dixon, W., & Coronoa, R. (2016). Boudurtha: Cultural humility. In E. Wittenberg, B. Ferrell, J. Goldsmith, et al. (Eds.), *Textbook of palliative care communication* (pp. 79–89). New York, NY: Oxford University Press.

22. Dahlin, C., & Lentz, J. (2013). National guidelines and APRN practice. In C. Dahlin & M. Lynch (Eds.), *Core curriculum for the advanced hospice and palliative registered nurse* (2nd ed., pp. 639–660). Pittsburgh, PA: Hospice and Palliative Nurses Association.

23. Dahlin, C., & Lentz, J. (2015). National guidelines and RN practice. In P. Berry & H. M (Eds.), *The core curriculum for the hospice and palliative registered nurse* (4th ed., pp. 359–380). Pittsburgh, PA: Hospice and Palliative Nurses Association.

24. Stewart, D. (2017). Bereavement, grief and loss. In P. J. Coyne, B. Bobb, & K. Plakovic (Eds.), *Conversations in palliative care* (4th ed., pp. 229–234). Pittsburgh, PA: Hospice and Palliative Nurses Associaton.

25. Marie Oliver, D., Tatum, P., Kapp, J., & Wallace, A. (2010). Interdisciplinary collaboration: The voices of hospice medical directors. *The American Journal of Hospice and Palliative Care, 27*(8), 537–544.

26. Bullington, J., & Yoder, C. (2017). The role of volunteers in palliative care. In P. J. Coyne, B. Bobb, & K. Plakovic (Eds.), *Conversations in palliative care* (4th ed., pp. 295–305). Pittsburgh, PA: Hospice and Palliative Nurses Association.

27. Coyne, E. (2017). How volunteer services can improve and advance palliative care programs. *J Hosp Palliat Nurs, 19*(2), 166–169.

28. Quill, T., & Abernathy, A. P. (2013). Generalist plus specialist palliative care—Creating a more sustainable model. *NEJM, 368*(13), 1173–1175.

29. Dahlin, C. (2015). Palliative Care—Delivering comprehensive oncology nursing care. *Sem in Onc Nursing, 31*(4), 327–337.

30. Institute of Medicine. (2014). *Dying in America—Improving quality and honoring individual preferences near end of life*. Washington, DC: The National Academies Press. http://www.nationalacademies.org/hmd/Reports/2014/Dying-In-America-Improving-Quality-and-Honoring-Individual-Preferences-Near-the-End-of-Life.aspx.

31. Dahlin, C. (2016). Palliative care models. In M. Boltz, D. Zwicker, & T. Fulmer (Eds.), *Evidence-based geriatric nursing protocols for best practice* (5th ed.). New York: Springer Publishing Company.

32. Bakitas, M., Lyons, K. D., Hegel, M. T., et al. (2009). Effects of a palliative care intervention on clinical outcomes in patients with advanced cancer: The Project ENABLE II randomized controlled trial. *JAMA: The Journal of the American Medical Association, 302*(7), 741–749.

33. Delgado-Guay, M. O., Parsons, H. A., Li, Z., et al. (2009). Symptom distress, interventions, and outcomes of intensive care unit cancer patients referred to a palliative care consult team. *Cancer, 115*(2), 437–445.

34. Temel, J., Greer, J., Muzikansky, A., et al. (2010). Early palliative care for patients with metastatic non-small cell lung cancer. *New Engl J Med, 363*(8), 733–742.

35. Morrison, R. S., Dietrich, J., Ladwig, S., et al. (2011). Palliative care consultation teams cut hospital costs for Medicaid beneficiaries. *Health Affairs, 30*(3), 454–463.

36. Gelfman, L. P., Meier, D. E., & Morrison, R. S. (2008). Does palliative care improve quality? A survey of bereaved family members. *J Pain Sympt Manag, 36*(1), 22–28.

37. Higginson, I. J., Finlay, I. G., Goodwin, D. M., et al. (2003). Is there evidence that palliative care teams alter end-of-life experiences of patients and their caregivers? *J Pain Sympt Manage, 25*(2), 150–168.

38. McClung, J. A. (2012). End of life care in the treatment of advanced heart failure in the elderly. *Card Rev*, Journal Article.

39. Fahlberg, B. (2016). Palliative care in the cardiac specialty care unit. In C. Dahlin, P. Coyne, & B. Ferrell (Eds.), *Advanced practice palliative nursing* (pp. 90–100). New York, NY: Oxford University Press.

40. Whitehead, P. (2016). Palliative care in the medical, surgical, and geriatric care unit. In C. Dahlin, P. Coyne, & B. Ferrell (Eds.), *Advanced practice palliative nursing* (pp. 74–82). New York, NY: Oxford Univerisity Press.

41. Rocker, G., Simpson, C., & Horton, R. (2015). Palliative care in advanced lung disease. *Chest, 148*(3), 801–809.

42. Brody, A. (2016). Cognitive impairment. In C. Dahlin, P. Coyne, & B. Ferrell (Eds.), *Advanced practice palliative nursing* (pp. 506–515). New York, MY: Oxford Univerisity Press.

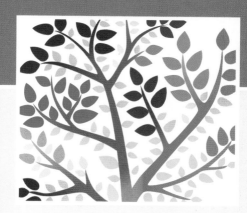

Health Disparities

Eun-Ok Im and Sangmi Kim

ealth disparities refer to gaps in the quality of health and health care among population groups that often parallel differences in socioeconomic status, racial/ethnic background, and education level. Health disparities are prevalent throughout the world between countries and within countries. For example, when comparing the countries Malawi and Japan, there is a 36-year gap in life expectancy (47 years in Malawi compared to 83 years in Japan).[1] Within countries, health disparities occur by social status, family income, race/ethnicity, gender, disability, or sexual orientation.[1] Significant health disparities in the morbidity and mortality of the U.S. population also exist. The Centers for Disease Control and Prevention reports health disparities and inequalities in various diseases; risk factors; environmental factors; social and behavioral determinants; and healthcare access by sex, race/ethnicity, income, education, disability status, and other social characteristics.[2] For example, premature death (before age 75 years) from stroke and coronary heart disease is higher in non-Hispanic African Americans compared to non-Hispanic whites.[2] As another example, the incidence of diabetes is highest among men, those aged older than 65 years, non-Hispanic African Americans, those of mixed race/ethnicity, and the disabled.[2]

Health disparities have long been a focus of nursing care; in fact, a number of nursing studies on health disparities in various populations have been conducted.[3,4] However, health disparities have rarely been explored as a major concept in nursing. When PubMed was searched with key words of "health disparity," "nursing," and "concept analysis," only nine articles were retrieved, and only one of these was a concept analysis of health disparities.[5] Even when the search was expanded with the key words of "health disparity," "nursing," and "concept," only 26 articles were retrieved, and only two articles pertained to the concept of health disparity.[5,6] Here, the concept of health disparities is examined in the context of nursing.

DEFINITION

Various definitions of health disparities exist in the literature. The Institute of Medicine defined health disparities as "racial or ethnic differences in the quality of health care that are not due to access-related factors or clinical needs, preferences, and appropriateness of intervention."[7] In *Healthy People*, health disparities are defined as "differences that occur by gender, race or ethnicity, education or income, disability, living in rural localities, or sexual orientation."[8] Common to these definitions is the notion of differences in health status between one or more

population groups compared to a more advantaged group, and most mention social justice and equity as components.

Since the mid-1990s when the term health disparities first came into use, it has generally been assumed to refer to health or healthcare differences between racial/ethnic groups, including differential access to screening and/or treatment options, or unequal availability of culturally or linguistically knowledgeable and sensitive health personnel.[9,10] However, equating health with health care draws attention primarily to diseases and healthcare services to alleviate the existing health inequality in the United States and could overlook the contribution of social determinants of health (e.g., race/ethnicity, socioeconomic status, or gender) to health disparities. Because the delivery of health care is a major source of health disparities, the term *healthcare disparities* is often used. That is why the National Library of Medicine and the National Institutes of Health (NIH) recently provided two separate definitions related to health disparities as *healthcare disparities* and *health status disparities*. Healthcare disparities are defined as "differences in access to or availability of facilities and services."[6] Health status disparities are defined as "the variation in rates of disease occurrence and disabilities between socioeconomic and/or geographically defined population groups."[6]

Interestingly, the Health Resources and Services Administration (HRSA) recently replaced their definition of health disparities with that of health equity on their website. As an opposite concept of health disparities, health equity was defined as *"the absence of disparities or avoidable differences among socioeconomic and demographic groups or geographical areas in health status and health outcomes such as disease, disability, or mortality."*[11] All these terms and their distinctions are necessary to an understanding of the impact of health disparities in nursing practice.

SCOPE

From the broadest and most simplistic perspective, the scope of health disparities is represented by unavoidable and avoidable disparities (Fig. 52.1). This categorization can be easily applied to most cases. For example, disparity in health outcomes by age may be unavoidable because aging as the biological process is not subject to intervention. Disparity in health outcomes due to unsafe living environments could be an avoidable cause of inequality. An avoidable disparity raises ethical questions of needless harm and injustice. Indeed, many health disparities are avoidable, and continuous efforts are necessary to identify existing health disparities that are preventable.

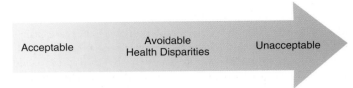

FIGURE 52.1 Scope of Health Disparities.

ATTRIBUTES AND CRITERIA

Carter-Porkras and Baquet asserted that health disparity should be viewed by "a difference in environment, access to, utilization of, and quality of care, health status, or a particular health outcome that deserves scrutiny."[12,p427] These criteria could be used to identify health disparity. That is, if differences are observed in "environment, access to, utilization of, and quality of care, health status, or a particular health outcome,"[12] then we could say that a health disparity might exist.

Before determining existence of a health disparity, however, it is critical to examine if the identified difference is inequality or inequity. As briefly stated above, some health inequalities are unavoidable since their underlying causes are biological variations or free choice, which may make changing the health determinants impossible or ethically or ideologically unacceptable. On the other hand, other health inequalities are not only unnecessary and avoidable, but also unjust and unfair. Their driving forces are external environmental factors/conditions that are outside the control of the individuals concerned.[13,14] Thus, White-head's seven determinants of health disparities are useful as attributes for health disparity:[13]

1. Natural, biological variation
2. Health-damaging behavior that is freely chosen
3. The transient health advantage of one group over another when one group is first to adopt a health-promotion behavior
4. Health-damaging behavior in which the degree of choice of lifestyles is severely restricted
5. Exposure to unhealthy, stressful living and working conditions
6. Inadequate access to essential health services and other basic services
7. Natural selection, or health-related social mobility, involving the tendency for sick people to move down the social scale

The determinants of health disparity by Health Canada are also useful attributes to determine existing health disparity (although some overlap with Whitehead's determinants exists).[13,15] These include income and social status; social support networks; education; employment and working conditions; social environments; physical environments; personal health practices and coping skills; healthy child development; biology and genetic endowment; health services; gender; and culture.

THEORETICAL LINKS

There are several different theories associated with health disparities that are used in nursing, and each theory has strengths and limitations in explaining health disparities.[16] Three prominent theories used in nursing to explain health disparities are presented here.

The Social–Ecological Model

The social–ecological model aims to explain dynamic interrelations among various personal and environmental factors. This model basically evolved from the ecological systems theory of child development by Bronfenbrenner, who proposed five socially organized subsystems

related to human development: microsystem, mesosystem, exosystem, macrosystem, and chronosystem.[17,18] Each of these five systems interacts within the context of the person's life and provides diverse options and sources of growth. The interactions within and between systems are bidirectional and have impact from and toward the person. The meso-system is beyond the dyad or two-party relation and links over two systems that a person lives.[17,18] Also, mesosystems link the structures of the person's microsystem. The macrosystem consists of cultural values, customs, and laws, and includes the overall patterns of ideology and organization that distinguish an individual society or social group. The chronosystem includes time as a dimension as it relates to environmental contexts.[17,18] The chronosystem could be either external or internal. For instance, the timing of a family member's death could be an external chronosystem, and physiological changes due to aging could be an internal chronosystem.

The social–ecological model has been widely used in nursing research and practice related to health disparities because it provides an understanding of interrelationships of individuals and systems, and it can provide a perspective to identify health disparities at each system level and directions for interventions at each system level. For example, the social–ecological model allows nurses to identify cultural barriers in access to health care at the level of macrosystem and to develop an intervention to tackle the cultural barriers to reduce subsequent health disparities.

The Structural–Constructivist Model

The structural–constructivist model is based on an assumption of dual nature of human existence.[16] The model adopts a constructivist perspective that the reality of life is based on a mental representation constructed by combinations of socially shared understandings within a society. Simultaneously, the model adopts a structural perspective that people are constrained by the external structures in which they are embedded (e.g., social relations created by the shared and distributed expectations of others). Health disparities literature featuring this model asserts that the concept of race/ethnicity is socially or culturally constructed with the underlying logic that when we can control the ways in which race/ethnic groups differ, racial/ethnic disparities will disappear. This perspective/model strongly supports the idea of social and cultural construction of race/ethnicity that frequently results in health disparities observed in healthcare systems,[19,20] and it gives direction for nursing research and practice in understanding health disparities in both clinical and community settings.

The Cultural Competence Model

The cultural competence movement grew out of early efforts to bridge the divide between the largely biomedical, white, middle-class American culture perspectives of clinicians and the perspectives of patients (mainly immigrants) whose experience and language put them at a substantial cultural distance from American health care.[21] Cultural competence expanded in the late 1980s through the 1990s in three ways. First, the populations of interest expanded from primarily immigrants to essentially all racial/ethnic minority groups. Second, the conceptual boundary expanded beyond culture per se to such issues as prejudice, stereotyping, and the social determinants of health. Third, the scope expanded beyond the interpersonal domain (between patients and healthcare providers) to health systems and communities. Cultural competence in health care entails (1) understanding the importance of sociocultural influences on patients' health beliefs and behaviors, (2) considering how these factors interact at multiple levels of the healthcare delivery systems (organizational, structural, and clinical), and (3) devising interventions that take these issues into account to ensure the delivery of high-quality health care to diverse patient populations.[22]

BOX 52.1   Key Elements of Cultural Competence for Interpersonal Interactions and Organizations

Interpersonal Interactions

- Explore and respect patient beliefs, values, meaning of illness, preferences, and needs
- Build rapport and trust
- Find common ground
- Awareness of one's own biases/assumptions
- Knowledgeable about different cultures
- Awareness of health disparities and discrimination affecting minority groups
- Use of interpreter services when needed

Organizations

- Diverse workforce reflecting the diversity of patient populations
- Healthcare facilities convenient and attentive to communities
- Language assistance available for patients with limited English proficiency
- Ongoing staff training regarding the delivery of culturally and linguistically appropriate services

From Saha, S., Beach, M. C., & Cooper, L. A. (2008). Patient centeredness, cultural competence and healthcare quality. *Journal of National Medical Association, 100*(11), 1275–1285.

Despite the existence of several different models of cultural competence, several key elements are shared at interpersonal and organizational levels (Box 52.1).[21] Interpersonal interactions focus on the ability of a provider to bridge cultural differences to build an effective relationship with a patient. Healthcare organizations focus on meeting the needs of diverse groups of patients. Nevertheless, the cultural competence model has been criticized due to its exclusive emphasis on healthcare providers to improve health disparities.[23]

CONTEXT TO NURSING AND HEALTH CARE

Health disparities witnessed in the context of nursing and health care mainly represent healthcare disparities. These occur in various nursing settings and/or situations and are roughly categorized into the following four cases: unavoidable and acceptable, unavoidable and unacceptable (unjust), avoidable and acceptable, and avoidable and unacceptable.

Unavoidable and Acceptable

The health disparities that are unavoidable and acceptable should not be a concern for nurses. For example, in an emergency room, nurses could observe health disparities in emergency visits by age; in general, older people make more emergency visits compared with younger people. In this situation, age becomes a determinant of the disparity, and aging is unavoidable and acceptable.

Unavoidable and Unacceptable

Health disparities that are unavoidable and unacceptable can also happen in healthcare settings and should be a concern for nurses. For example, the high prevalence of diabetes among Hispanic populations might be partially due to genetic factors so that such a disparity in the prevalence of diabetes could be unavoidable. However, a persistently higher risk of diabetes in these populations due to inappropriate diabetes management (e.g., lack of accessibility and affordability of health care and wholesome foods in the neighborhoods) is unacceptable, which raises a red flag for nurses.

Avoidable and Acceptable

Most health disparities that are avoidable are not viewed as acceptable. Only in unique or unusual circumstances can avoidable health disparities be considered acceptable. For example, a health disparity could exist among people involved and those not involved in a natural disaster. When a natural disaster occurs, unequal health outcomes among residents in the affected area may be acceptable even though the disaster and resultant health disparity could be avoidable if a proper contingency plan were in place at the local, state, or national level.

Avoidable and Unacceptable

Health disparities that are avoidable and unacceptable unfortunately occur in healthcare settings, and these are the targets of interventions. For example, a disparity in cancer pain management exists between Asians and whites. This difference is attributable to Asian cultural values and attitudes related to cancer pain and pain medication distinguished from the cultural values of whites. The disparity is avoidable if Asian cancer patients are adequately educated and instructed on cancer pain management strategies, including pain medication and complementary and alternative medicine. Also, this disparity is unacceptable because this gives an unnecessary burden of pain to Asian cancer patients that could be easily managed by using existing strategies. Several avoidable and unacceptable disparities are worth further exploration from the perspective of healthcare disparities because they are frequently seen and experienced by nurses.

Lack of Health Insurance and High Healthcare Costs

Health insurance is the most significant contributing factor to poor quality of care. Uninsured people are less likely to get adequate care for disease prevention (e.g., cancer screening, dental care, counseling about diet and exercise, and flu vaccination) and/or for disease management (e.g., diabetes care management), and they are more likely to visit the emergency department and be admitted to the hospital for ambulatory care-sensitive conditions.[24,25] Many racial/ethnic, low socioeconomic status, and other minority groups lack adequate health insurance compared with their counterparts. For example, Hispanics and non-Hispanic African Americans have substantially higher uninsured rates compared to Asian/Pacific Islanders and non-Hispanic whites.[2] Also, minorities are disproportionately enrolled in lower-cost health plans that place greater per-patient limits on healthcare expenditures and available services.[7]

Even with health insurance, the financial burden of health care is high and continuously increasing. High premiums and out-of-pocket payments can be a significant barrier to accessing needed medical treatment and preventive care.[24] From 2006 to 2011, the percentage of people younger than age 65 years whose family's health insurance premium and out-of-pocket expenses were more than 10% of total family income was more than 3.5 times as high for poor individuals and low-income individuals and more than twice as high for middle-income individuals compared to that of high-income individuals.[24]

Lack of Transportation to Healthcare Providers

The lack of access to affordable transportation could physically isolate people of color, households in rural areas, and people with disabilities from healthcare facilities. It also forces families to spend a large percentage of their budget on cars and other expensive options rather than actual healthcare costs. An increasing number of people are unable to reach healthcare providers and healthcare services because they reside in non-walkable areas with limited public transportation. Individuals of low socioeconomic status, households in rural areas, and people with disabilities could face significant hurdles because many cannot drive and/or because public transportation is often unavailable, inaccessible, or unreliable.[26]

The poorest one-fifth of U.S. families spend approximately 42% of their income on transportation. This massive expenditure on transportation can wipe out their already limited budget for out-of-pocket medical expenses, nutritious foods, and healthy recreational activities. Because affordable housing is increasingly located far from main transportation lines and jobs, low-income people and people of color are more likely to have long commutes, which reduces their time for exercise, shopping for healthy foods, and additional earning opportunities.[26]

Ineffective Provider-Patient Communication

Sociocultural differences between healthcare providers and patients often influence patient and provider communication. People from different backgrounds frequently have differences in their recognition of symptoms, thresholds for seeking care, comprehension of management strategies, expectations of care (e.g., preferences for or against diagnostic and therapeutic procedures), and adherence to preventive measures and medications.[27] Furthermore, patients with different sociocultural backgrounds from those of healthcare providers may not feel comfortable asking questions or disclosing personal health information. Due to the pressures of a fast-paced clinical setting, healthcare providers frequently experience difficulty determining what the patient does not understand and addressing this knowledge gap adequately. The printed health information materials that are frequently used in an effort to bridge the knowledge gap may be too complex or scientific for patients to understand.[28,29] Thus, when sociocultural differences between healthcare providers and patients are not appreciated or communicated effectively in clinical encounters, patient dissatisfaction, poor adherence, poorer health outcomes, and racial/ethnic disparities in health care easily happen.[27]

Language Barriers

Patients who face language and cultural barriers are less likely than others to have a usual source of medical care. They receive preventive services at reduced rates and have an increased risk of nonadherence to medication. Among patients with psychiatric conditions, those who encounter language barriers are more likely than others to receive a diagnosis of severe psychopathology.[30] Ad hoc interpreters, including family members, friends, untrained members of the support staff, and strangers found in waiting rooms or on the street, are commonly used in clinical encounters. However, the use of such unqualified interpreters results in increased medical errors, less effective patient–clinical provider communication, and poorer follow-up and adherence to clinical instructions, as well as possible conflicts with patient privacy rights.[30,31]

Biased Clinical Decision Making

Clinical decisions are shaped by the attributes of patients (e.g., age, sex, socioeconomic status, race/ethnicity, language proficiency, religion, nationality, and insurance status), healthcare providers (e.g., specialty, level of training, clinical experience, age, sex, and race/ethnicity), and practice settings (e.g., location, organization of practice, form of compensation, performance expectations, and incentives).[27,32] Thus, health disparities, especially healthcare disparities, often result from healthcare providers' bias or prejudice against minorities, greater clinical uncertainty when interacting with minority patients, and beliefs or stereotypes about the health or health behaviors of minority patients. If a healthcare provider has difficulty accurately understanding his or her patient's symptom(s) or is less sure of his or her patient's signal, then the provider is likely to place greater weight on his or her prior beliefs, which may differ by the provider's age, gender, socioeconomic status, and race/ethnicity, than on information gathered in a clinical encounter. This reliance on prior beliefs may result in discordance between health services and patient needs.[7]

Stereotyping often leads to biased clinical decision-making. Stereotyping refers to the process by which people use social categories (e.g., gender or race/ethnicity) in acquiring, processing, and recalling information about others. Both implicit and explicit negative attitudes and stereotypes of healthcare providers significantly shape interactions with patients, influence how information is recalled, and guide expectations and inferences in systematic ways.[7] Stereotyping often occurs subconsciously, unlike prejudice or discrimination. If it is left unchecked, stereotyping has a detrimental clinical effect on certain groups deemed as less worthy of diagnostic or therapeutic procedures or resources.[27]

Biased clinical decision-making also derives from the bias in health care, operationalized as discrimination on the basis of patient attributes. Patients with certain sociodemographic features have a propensity to be assessed, diagnosed, referred, and treated not only differently but also at a lower level of quality or to a lesser degree of adherence to established standards of care than different groups of people with comparable health problems.[32]

Prejudice, which refers to unjustified negative attitudes based on a person's group membership, is another source of biased clinical decision making. An example of prejudice related to race/ethnicity is the belief that African American patients are less intelligent, less educated, more likely to abuse drugs and alcohol, more likely to fail to comply with medical advice, and more likely to lack social support than white patients, regardless of an individual patient's actual income, education, and personality.[7]

Patient's Mistrust and Refusal

In response to historical factors of discrimination, segregation, and medical experimentation or to real/perceived mistreatment by healthcare providers, African American patients may convey mistrust, refuse treatment, or comply poorly with treatment. As a result, healthcare providers may become less engaged in the treatment process such that patients are less likely to be provided with more vigorous treatments and services.[7]

INTERRELATED CONCEPTS

Many concepts discussed in this book are interrelated to the concept of health disparities. Some of the most closely interrelated are presented in Fig. 52.2 and described further. Health disparities are closely linked to **Culture**. Nursing scholars have suggested that marginalization due to cultural differences could decrease the opportunities to receive equitable health care, which subsequently leads to health disparities.[22,33] They also claim that marginalization due to cultural differences and subsequent disadvantages including financial, environmental, and linguistic barriers result in health disparities.[33–35] Furthermore, cultural differences frequently give rise to issues with **Communication** between healthcare providers and patients, and the miscommunication could cause health disparities.[36] Stereotypes, bias, or prejudice of healthcare providers can be activated or increased by miscommunication with patients, which can then lead to diminished **Health Care Quality** provided to the patients.[34]

The lack of **Health Promotion** in disadvantaged populations (e.g., physical inactivity of African American adolescents in poor urban areas) also results in health disparities. The poor health outcomes or increased morbidity and mortality among ethnic minorities are frequently due to lack of health promotion activities and/or risky health behaviors in these populations.[2] **Health Policy** and **Health Care Law** powerfully influence healthcare utilization, particularly for vulnerable populations

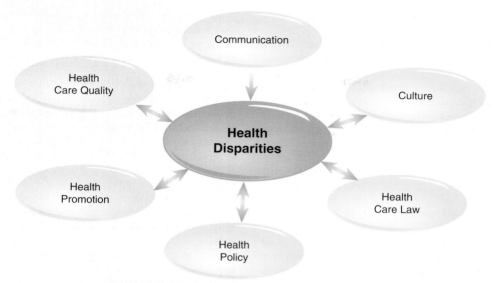

FIGURE 52.2 Health Disparities and Interrelated Concepts.

including minorities, people with low SES, and people with disabilities. The Affordable Care Act exemplifies the critical role of health policies and healthcare laws in addressing health disparities. The Affordable Care Act was expected to extend health insurance coverage to an additional 25 million people by 2019.[37] However, with recent changes in the Affordable Care Act as well as other related policy and governmental budget changes, this figure could change in the near future.

CLINICAL EXEMPLARS

Despite numerous types of health disparities, only the avoidable and unacceptable health disparities are presented in Box 52.2 because these are the ones that healthcare providers, including nurses, frequently encounter in clinical and community settings. Furthermore, these are the health disparities that healthcare providers need to target to intervene. A detailed discussion of each exemplar of health disparities is beyond the scope of this textbook; however, some of the most important exemplars across the age span are briefly described here.

Featured Exemplars
Unequal Receipt of Early and Adequate Prenatal Care
Early and adequate prenatal care is defined as the prenatal care initiated by week 28 of pregnancy and in which a woman has at least 80% of the expected number of prenatal visits.[24] Early and adequate prenatal care helps to promote healthy pregnancies through screening and management of risk factors and conditions and through education and counseling on healthy behaviors during and after pregnancy. Common barriers to getting prenatal care as early as desired (or at all) are limited resources, transportation issues, and not knowing that one is pregnant.[38]

Unequal Receipt of Recommended Immunizations
Immunization protects recipients from illness and protects others in the community who are not vaccinated. Beginning in 2007, the recommended vaccines that should be completed by the age of 19 to 35 months include diphtheria–tetanus–pertussis vaccine (DTaP), polio vaccine, measles–mumps–rubella (MMR) vaccine, *Haemophilus influenza* type B (Hib) vaccine, hepatitis B vaccine, varicella vaccine, and pneumococcal conjugate vaccine (PCV).[24] However, according to the Centers

---

BOX 52.2 EXEMPLARS OF HEALTH DISPARITIES

- Breast cancer mortality
- Breast cancer screening
- Cardiovascular disease
- Diabetes
- Early and adequate prenatal care
- Healthcare access
- Health insurance coverage
- Immunizations
- Infant, fetal, and perinatal mortality
- Intimate partner violence
- Invasive cervical cancer
- Mental health services
- Obesity
- Pain management
- Pap smear screening
- Pregnancy-related mortality rate
- Preterm birth rates
- Preventive care
- Prostate cancer mortality
- Quality of palliative care
- Safe neighborhood
- Smoking
- Social support system

 ACCESS EXEMPLAR LINKS IN YOUR GIDDENS EBOOK

for Disease Control and Prevention (CDC), children living below the federal poverty level had a lower coverage of nearly all vaccines compared with those at or above the poverty level in 2014. For instance, the coverage of vaccines (with ≥4 doses of DTaP, ≥3 doses of polio vaccine, ≥1 dose of MMR, the primary and full series of Hib, ≥4 doses of PCV, ≥2 doses of Hepatitis A, the rotavirus series, and the combined seven-vaccine series) was lower among children below the poverty level.[39]

Unequal Pain Management

Judgments about pain are frequently influenced by the characteristics of patients (e.g., race/ethnicity), situations (e.g., medical evidence), and healthcare providers (e.g., experience).[40] In the face of such uncertainties, latent/implicit stereotypes may be activated, advantaging patients who fit positive stereotypes (e.g., pro-white) and disadvantaging patients who do not (e.g., African Americans).[40] For example, African Americans and Hispanics are seen as more likely to require scrutiny for potential drug abuse. Consequently, primary care providers are more likely to underestimate pain intensity in African Americans and Hispanics than in other sociodemographic groups, leading to less and passive pain management in the former.[40,41]

Unequal Breast Cancer Screening

Women without health insurance are much less likely to get a mammogram than women with health insurance. In the United States, breast cancer is the most common cancer in Asian American women, but these women have relatively lower rates of breast cancer screening than African American and white women.[42,43] Furthermore, disparities in breast cancer screening reportedly result from low income, lack of a local mammography center, lack of transportation to a mammography center, lack of a usual healthcare provider, lack of a recommendation from a healthcare provider to get mammography screening, lack of awareness of breast cancer risks and screening methods, and cultural and language differences.[43]

Unequal Quality of Palliative Care

Racial/ethnic minorities tend to receive lower-quality palliative care across multiple domains, including satisfaction, communication, and pain management. Compared to whites, African Americans report less satisfaction with the quality of communication, including the extent to which healthcare providers listen and share information, with greater disparities in racially discordant patient–provider relationships. Moreover, racial/ethnic minorities are disadvantaged in terms of the access to hospice care. Minority patients have lower rates of hospice use than their white counterparts across diagnoses, geographic areas, and settings of care.[44] For instance, African American women with breast cancer were less likely to enter hospice; however, they were more likely to undergo an intensive care unit admission, more than one emergency visit or hospitalization in the last 30 days of life, and die in the hospital.[45] Racial/ethnic differences in knowledge, cultural beliefs, and treatment preferences are regarded as barriers to the use of palliative care.[44]

CASE STUDY

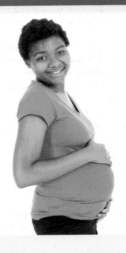

Case Presentation

Jones Antoinette, a 21-year-old pregnant African American woman, visited an obstetric clinic for prenatal care for the first time at 30 weeks of gestation. Her baseline vital signs were normal. She was assigned to a white nurse midwife for her prenatal care throughout the remaining pregnancy until her delivery.

The nurse midwife interviewed and assessed Jones' sociodemographic characteristics, past medical history, health behaviors, and psychological health status. Jones had a medical history of abnormal glucose tolerance and asthma, but she has not seen a healthcare provider to treat the asthma because she lacks health insurance. Prior to her pregnancy, she smoked five cigarettes a day, but she stopped smoking when she learned she was pregnant. She also said that she drank often during the weekends but has cut back. She complained of depressive feelings and sleep disturbances due to several life crises. She is at risk of losing her part-time job and has not had steady income for months. She has a car, but she often gets rides because she cannot afford gas. She wants to move from her current apartment because there is high crime activity in her apartment complex—even drug use in the hallways. Her asthma has become worse due to poor housing conditions. Furthermore, her boyfriend was recently arrested and has been asking her for money for legal help. Under these circumstances, she was not sure if it was right to carry this baby.

After the interview, the nurse midwife ordered a regular diabetes check, which should have been conducted at week 28 of gestation. The patient's history of abnormal glucose tolerance has a potential to put Jones and her fetus at high risk. The nurse midwife informed Jones of cystic fibrosis screening as well. This genetic test is not mandatory, but it is encouraged. Jones listened to the nurse midwife carefully and asked if it would be good for her baby. After getting information on the test, Jones wanted to be tested. The nurse midwife provided the test consent form and printed information on the screening test. Jones signed the consent form without reading the printed information. Before leaving, the nurse midwife asked if Jones had any questions or concerns, and Jones said "no." After meeting with the nurse midwife, Jones met a nurse coordinator who was responsible for scheduling of the next appointment and additional tests, case management, and patient education. When the nurse coordinator double-checked whether Jones really wanted cystic fibrosis screening, Jones said that she did not hear about the test from the nurse midwife.

Case Analysis Questions

1. What risk factors for health disparities associated with prenatal care exist for Jones?
2. How can the change in Jones' response regarding the prenatal testing for cystic fibrosis be explained?
3. What interventions would be helpful to Jones now and throughout her prenatal care?

From michaeljung/iStock/Thinkstock

 ACCESS EXEMPLAR LINKS IN YOUR GIDDENS EBOOK

REFERENCES

1. World Health Organization. (n.d.). *Fact file on health inequities.* Retrieved from http://www.who.int/sdhconference/background/news/facts/en.

2. Centers for Disease Control and Prevention. (2013). *CDC health disparities and inequalities report—United States 2013.* Retrieved from http://www.cdc.gov/mmwr/pdf/other/su6203.pdf.

3. Ancheta, I. B., Carlson, J. M., Battie, C. A., et al. (2015). One size does not fit all: Cardiovascular health disparities as a function of ethnicity in Asian-American women. *Applied Nursing Research, 28*(2), 99–105.

4. Cameron, B. L., Carmargo Plazas, M. D. P., Salas, A. S., et al. (2014). Understanding inequalities in access to health care services for aboriginal people: A call for nursing action. *Adv Nurs Sci, 37*(3), E1–E16.

5. Fink, A. M. (2009). Toward a new definition of health disparity: A concept analysis. *Journal of Transcultural Nursing, 20*(4), 349–357.

6. National Library of Medicine, National Institutes of Health. *Health Disparities*. Retrieved from https://www.nlm.nih.gov/hsrinfo/disparities.html.

7. Institute of Medicine. (2002). *Unequal treatment: Confronting racial and ethnic disparities in health care*. Washington, DC: National Academies Press.

8. U.S. Department of Health and Human Services. (2000). *Healthy People 2010: Understanding and improving health* (2nd ed.). Washington, DC: Author.

9. Adler, N. E., & Stewart, J. (2010). Health disparities across the lifespan: Meaning, methods, and mechanisms. *Annals of the New York Academy of Sciences, 1186*, 5–23.

10. Braveman, P. (2006). Health disparities and health equity: Concepts and measurement. *Annual Review of Public Health, 27*, 167–194.

11. U.S. Health Resources and Services Administration. *Office of Health Equity, Definitions*. Retrieved from https://www.hrsa.gov/about/organization/bureaus/ohe/index.html.

12. Carter-Pokras, O., & Baquet, C. (2002). What is a "health disparity"? *Public Health Reports, 117*(5), 426–434.

13. Whitehead, M. (1991). The concepts and principles of equity and health. *Health Promotion International, 6*(3), 217–228.

14. World Health Organization. (n.d.). *Health Impact Assessment (HIA) Glossary of terms used*. Retrieved from http://www.who.int/hia/about/glos/en/index1.html.

15. Canadian Institute for Health Information. *Improving the health of Canadians*. Retrieved from http://publications.gc.ca/Collection/H118-14-2004-1E.pdf.

16. Dressler, W. W., Oths, K. S., & Gravlee, C. C. (2005). Race and ethnicity in public health research: Models to explain health disparities. *Annual Review of Anthropology, 34*, 231–252.

17. Swick, K. (2004). *Empowering parents, families, schools and communities during the early childhood years*. Champaign, IL: Stipes.

18. Roberts, M. C., & Steele, R. G. (2009). *Handbook of pediatric psychology* (4th ed.). New York: Guilford.

19. Gravlee, C. C. (2005). Emic ethnic classification in southeastern Puerto Rico: Cultural consensus and semantic structure. *Social Forces; a Scientific Medium of Social Study and Interpretation, 83*, 949–970.

20. Gravlee, C. C., & Dressler, W. W. (2005). Skin pigmentation, self-perceived color, and arterial blood pressure in Puerto Rico. *American Journal of Human Biology : the Official Journal of the Human Biology Council, 17*, 195–206.

21. Saha, S., Beach, M. C., & Cooper, L. A. (2008). Patient centeredness, cultural competence and healthcare quality. *Journal of the National Medical Association, 100*(11), 1275–1285.

22. Betancourt, J. R., Green, A. R., Carrillo, J. E., et al. (2003). Defining cultural competence: A practical framework for addressing racial/ethnic disparities in health and health care. *Public Health Reports, 118*(4), 293–302.

23. Meade, M. A., Mahmoudi, E., & Lee, S.-Y. (2015). The intersection of disability and healthcare disparities: A conceptual framework. *Disability and Rehabilitation, 37*(7), 632–641.

24. Agency for Healthcare Research and Quality. (2016). *National healthcare disparities report*. Retrieved from https://www.ahrq.gov/research/findings/nhqrdr/nhqdr16/index.html.

25. Kaiser Family Foundation. (2017). *Key facts about the uninsured population*. Retrieved from https://www.kff.org/uninsured/fact-sheet/key-facts-about-the-uninsured-population/.

26. The Leadership Conference Education Fund. (2011). *The road to health care parity: Transportation policy and access to health care*. Retrieved from http://civilrightsdocs.info/pdf/docs/transportation/The-Road-to-Health-Care-Parity.pdf.

27. Betancourt, J. R., & Renfrew, M. R. (2011). Unequal treatment in the US: Lessons and recommendations for cancer care internationally. *Journal of Pediatric Hematology, 33*(Suppl. 2), 149–153.

28. Egbert, N., & Nanna, K. M. (2009). Health literacy: Challenges and strategies. *Online Journal of Issues in Nursing, 14*(3), 1–10.

29. Eiser, A. R., & Ellis, G. (2007). Cultural competence and the African American experience with health care: The case for specific content in cross-cultural education. *Academic Medicine: Journal of the Association of American Medical Colleges, 82*(2), 176–183.

30. Flores, G. (2006). Language barriers to health care in the United States. *The New England Journal of Medicine, 355*(3), 229–231.

31. Steinberg, E. M., Valenzuela-Araujo, D., Zickafoose, J. S., et al. (2016). The 'Battle' of managing language barriers in health care. *Clinical Pediatrics, 55*(14), 1318–1327.

32. Alspach, J. G. (2012). Is there gender bias in critical care? *Critical Care Nurse, 32*(6), 8–14.

33. Meleis, A. I. (1996). Culturally competent scholarship: Substance and rigor. *Adv Nurs Sci, 19*(2), 1–16.

34. Hall, J. M. (1999). Marginalization revisited: Critical, postmodern, and liberation perspectives. *Adv Nurs Sci, 22*(2), 88–102.

35. Hall, J. M., Stevens, P. E., & Meleis, A. I. (1994). Marginalization: A guiding concept for valuing diversity in nursing knowledge development. *ANS. Advances in Nursing Science, 16*(4), 23–41.

36. Sharby, N., Martire, K., & Iversen, M. D. (2015). Decreasing health disparities for people with disabilities through improved communication strategies and awareness. *International Journal of Environmental Research and Public Health, 12*(3), 3301–3316.

37. National Bureau of Economic Research. *Impacts of the Affordable Care Act on Health Insurance Coverage in Medicaid Expansion and Non-Expansion States*. Retrieved from http://www.nber.org/papers/w22182.pdf.

38. U.S. Department of Health and Human Services, Health Resources and Services Administration, Maternal and Child Health Bureau. (2014). *Child health USA*. Retrieved from https://mchb.hrsa.gov/chusa14/.

39. Hill, H. A., Elam-Evans, L. D., Yankey, D., et al. (2016). Vaccination coverage among children aged 19–35 months—United States, 2015. *MMWR. Morbidity and Mortality Weekly Report, 65*, 1065–1071.

40. Tait, R. C., & Chibnall, J. T. (2014). Racial/ethnic disparities in the assessment and treatment of pain: Psychosocial perspectives. *The American Psychologist, 69*(2), 131–141.

41. Mack, D. S., Hunnicutt, J. N., Jesdale, B. M., & Lapane, K. L. (2018). Non-Hispanic Black-White disparities in pain and pain management among newly admitted nursing home residents with cancer. *Journal of Pain Research, 11*, 753–761.

42. American Cancer Society. (2017). *Breast cancer facts & figures*. Retrieved from https://www.cancer.org/research/cancer-facts-statistics/breast-cancer-facts-figures.html.

43. Komen Susan, G. *Comparing breast cancer screening rates among different groups*. Retrieved from https://ww5.komen.org/BreastCancer/DisparitiesInBreastCancerScreening.html.

44. Johnson, K. S. (2013). Racial and ethnic disparities in palliative care. *Journal of Palliative Medicine, 16*(11), 1329–1334.

45. Check, D. K., Samuel, C. A., Rosenstein, D. L., & Dusetzina, S. B. (2016). Investigation of racial disparities in early supportive medication use and end-of-life care among medicare beneficiaries with stage IV breast cancer. *Journal of Clinical Oncology, 34*(19), 2265–2270.

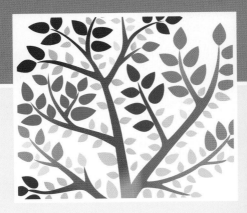

Population Health

Elizabeth Reifsnider

Population health is a concept that is emerging as significant to the future of nursing's adaptation to new ways to assess, diagnose, plan interventions, and evaluate; in other words, conducting the nursing process. Although nurses are well equipped to use the nursing process for individuals, population health will require the same ability to perform assessments of populations, diagnose population-level problems, plan and complete interventions for a specified population, and then evaluate the success of the intervention and revise accordingly. To be effective practitioners at the population level, nurses must understand many other concepts presented in this text. Health disparities and social determinants of health occur among populations but are expressed as individual health outcomes. Healthcare organizations must attend to the health of the populations they serve or they will not succeed in delivering care that is high-quality, patient-centered, cost-effective, and evidence-based. Health policy should strive to improve the health of the population or at least address the health needs of the population. Improving population health is not a simple task. The complex causes of robust or ill health require many different interventions and approaches. These interventions and approaches can vary from funding policy and legislation at the national level to health behavior of individuals and local healthcare agencies.[1]

Nursing care is increasingly moving from acute care institutions (tertiary care medical centers) toward the community. Many patients that would have been hospitalized previously for an extended period are being treated for the most acute problems and then discharged to home and community care. Other health problems are addressed through outpatient surgery or at smaller, emergency health centers. As the need for nursing care moves into the community, nurses will need to understand how to address the health needs of the population and plan for care delivery. Population health aims to improve the health of the entire population and reduce health inequities among population groups. To reach these objectives, it looks at and acts upon the broad range of factors and conditions that have a strong influence on our health.

DEFINITION

Health means many different things to many people and the same is true for the term population. If you consider how people think about health, their conceptions of health can vary from health as being free of illness to the ability to do daily work and having total well-being.[2] When one thinks of population health, it needs to be viewed as not only being free from disease, but the ability to adapt, respond to, and control health challenges.[3] The World Health Organization (WHO) in its 1946 charter defined health as "a state of complete physical, mental, and social well-being and not merely the absence of disease or infirmity."[4] The same confusion about meaning can occur with "population." Population is commonly used to mean the number of people living in a certain geographic area (e.g., the population of this town is 34,562), but when considering population health, it often means individuals having characteristics in common, such as individuals with type 2 diabetes who all live in a specified area.[5] Population health considers the health outcomes of a group of people,[1] and nurses who are concerned about improving the health of the group need to understand how to address health care and health outcomes at a population level.

The definition of population health was first coined in 2003 by Kindig and Stoddard as the means to consider the health outcomes of a group of people and to understand how health outcomes (illnesses or less-than-desired health) are distributed among the group.[6] Although it may be convenient to think of health as a steady state, a population health approach views health as a capacity or resource, which allows someone to acquire skills and pursue one's goals. When health is seen in this manner, then population health can be seen as the range of social, economic, and physical environmental factors that benefit and contribute to health.[3]

It may be helpful to consider the definition of population health as the health of groups of people, composed of the physical, social, and economic environments that surround them and influence their health outcomes. In Canada, population health is defined by the health of a population, measured by health status indicators and influenced by environments that surround the population as well as individual health practices, genetics and biology, early childhood development, and access to and delivery of health services.[7] In the United States, the Centers for Disease Control and Prevention (CDC) defines population health as an interdisciplinary approach that allows health departments to align practice to policy to influence health locally.[8] The goal of the alignment is to connect partnerships among healthcare providers, academia, business, and local government to achieve positive health outcomes. Focusing on population health allows significant health concerns to be recognized and addressed to overcome issues that create poor health conditions among the population.[9]

As the concept of population health is relatively new, its definition varies and people may mean different things when they discuss population health. For this chapter population health is defined as "...*health outcomes of a defined group of people along with the distribution of health*

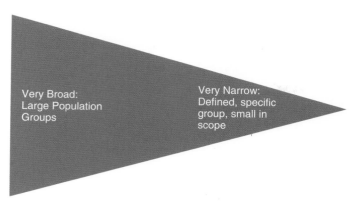

FIGURE 53.1 Scope of Population Health.

outcomes within the group."[1] Health equity, the realization that all people may achieve the same health outcomes if provided with equal opportunities, is essential for understanding population health. According to the WHO, health equity infers that everyone should have a fair chance to attain their full health potential and that no one should be disadvantaged from achieving this potential.[1]

SCOPE

As indicated by the concept of a population, which conveys the meaning of people in a defined group (e.g., population of a city, county, state, nation, etc.), the scope of population health can be very broad (i.e., the health of the population of the United States) or very narrow (i.e., the health of the population in a defined census tract or in a specific hospital unit) (Fig. 53.1). The scope is malleable and can refer to whatever grouping of people is chosen by the lens of an organization that is interested in the population's health under its purview. In addition to the number of people within a defined population grouping, the scope of population health also refers to the health issue that is being examined. If a healthcare organization wants to study the health of the population for which it is responsible, it may want to know, for example, the prevalence of chronic diseases among the population or the incidence of preventable communicable diseases. Many different organizational units study population health at distinct levels or particular sub-units of a population (e.g., all adults ages 65+) to determine the status of the population's health as well as establish goals for health improvement. For all of these examples, the scope will vary. It is essential that nurses understand the scope of the population being considered to know the appropriate metrics for measurement and potential treatment approaches.

ATTRIBUTES AND CRITERIA

The concept of population health is centered on its emphasis to maintain and improve the health status of the population. In addition to maintenance and improvement, population health also seeks to reduce health disparities and create health equity. According to the Canadian Ministry of Health, whose approach to population health is more robust and developed as compared with the United States' approach, the major attributes of population health are as follows[10]:

1. Deciding on the key indicators of health to use for population health evaluation
2. Addressing determinants of health to link health concerns to their determinants
3. Using the best evidence on which to base population health management

4. Investing in disease prevention, health protection, and health promotion to lessen the development of preventable and chronic diseases
5. Collaborating across sectors (such as government agencies, local healthcare organizations, individual healthcare practitioners) to build alliances for health
6. Applying multiple strategies to address health disparities and guide interventions focused at a population level
7. Increasing health literacy and involving the public in creating strategies to address population health improvement
8. Evaluating health outcomes and reporting results and health statistics

The major criterion for population health is that it is comprehensive; it not only evaluates health status of a population but it also addresses how to improve the population's health in collaboration with the population involved. Although it includes acute as well as chronic illnesses in its evaluation, disease prevention and health protection and promotion remain its key emphasis. Population health strives to ensure the highest level of wellness among the population.

THEORETICAL LINKS

The theories that are most closely linked to population health are the Social Ecological Model of Health (also known as the socioecological model) and the Social Determinants of Health conceptual framework. These two theories are closely related to each other and mirror many of the same concepts.

Socioecological Model

The socioecological model is based on the Ecology of Human Development, a conceptual model that was advanced by Bronfenbrenner.[11] This framework strives to explain how children develop through interactions with parents and family and the interactions that parents have with environments where the child is not present. However, these environments influence the child's development through their influence on the parents. In this theory, human development is examined by focusing on three aspects: (1) an individual's perspective of the environment; (2) the environment surrounding that individual; and (3) the dynamic interaction between the individual and the environment.[12] Thus, development is defined as an ongoing change in the way a person perceives and deals with or adapts to the environment.

The Ecology of Human Development was adapted by multiple researchers into a Social-Ecological Model (SEM) that is broader than one focused on child development, but retains the emphasis on the dynamic interaction between an individual and the environment surrounding the individual. In broad strokes, the SEM can be conceptualized as nested circles with the individual and his/her unique characteristics as the innermost circle. In ascending order, as the circles enlarge surrounding the center, are the levels of family/close peers, neighborhood, organizations/work, larger community of residence, physical environment of residence, and the environment of all the descending circles such as the government and culture (see Fig. 53.2).[12,13]

Social Determinants of Health Conceptual Framework

The conceptual framework of determinants of health is also closely related to population health. According to the CDC[14] and *Healthy People*,[15] the determinants of health consist of biological, socioeconomic, psychosocial, behavioral, and social in nature. They are displayed as follows:

- *Biology and genetics:* examples include sex and age
- *Individual behavior:* examples include alcohol use, injection drug use (needles), unprotected sex, and smoking

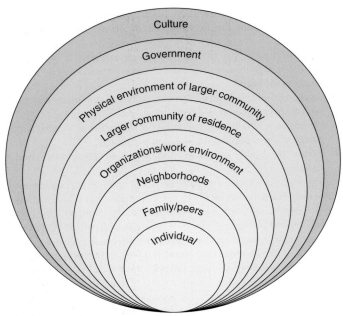

FIGURE 53.2 Socioeconomic Model.

TABLE 53.1 **Population Health and Related Practice Areas**

Focus Area	Definition
Population Health	The health outcomes of a defined group of people and how the outcomes are distributed throughout the group.
Public Health	An emphasis on disease prevention, health protection, and health promotion using evidence to benefit society, usually supported by government agencies.
Community Health	A collaborative enterprise that is comprised of multiple sectors in the community as well as an interdisciplinary approach that uses public health sciences and evidence to work with communities to benefit the health of all members of the community.[17]
Global Health	Evidence-based disease prevention, health protection, and health promotion on a global scale, accomplished through collaborative efforts of sovereign countries.
Population Health Management	Efforts by healthcare organizations, accountable care organizations, and insurers to keep individuals as healthy as possible for as long as possible.

- *Social environment:* examples include discrimination, income, and gender
- *Physical environment:* examples include where a person lives and crowding conditions
- *Health services:* examples include access to quality health care and having or not having health insurance

The WHO's Commission on Social Determinants of Health[16] portrayed its conceptual model as linked boxes leading to the distribution of health and well-being among a population. The socioeconomic and political context (governance, health policy, and social/cultural norms and values) influences the individual level of social position, education, occupation, income, gender, and race/ethnicity, which are affected by the next level of material circumstances, biological factors, and behaviors, all of which, through the healthcare system, lead to the distribution of health and well-being. An imbalance in any of these factors can have a detrimental effect on health and well-being. If someone lives in a social environment that does not support health promotion or disease prevention, has a low income and poor health literacy, develops a chronic illness through genetic predispositions allied with poor health behavioral choices, their health and well-being will suffer. Population health draws its theoretical foundation from these understandings—that an individual's health is influenced by the multiple social and environmental factors that surround the individual. Factors are not equally distributed, and their lack of equitable distribution leads to poor health for some, and access to health services is an important element in assuring health and well-being on a population level.

CONTEXT TO NURSING AND HEALTH CARE

Population health in the context of nursing and health care is apparent in multiple areas. It varies depending on a nurse's scope of responsibility and general area of practice. A nurse working in acute care with a defined population (such as neurological intensive care) may not realize that he/she is practicing population health when the nurse wonders why more elderly neurological patients are referred to the unit than younger patients. The nurse may think of how neurological patients

need different rehabilitation services than will patients with other conditions, and they become the population of focus. Population health should not be viewed as a concept that applies only in the abstract or at a national/global level, but also in daily practice. Populations exist at all levels of a socioecological model, and at each level, nursing care is needed. Nurses assess the health of a defined population and strive to improve the health of that population. Nurses use population health concepts in all aspects of their practice, from wondering if a patient has symptoms of a communicable disease to conducting population-wide evaluation of the prevalence of communicable diseases. Nurses apply population health when they work at all levels of health care, from a unit and hospital level of population up to national level or global level (Table 53.1).

Community/Public Health

A particular context in which nurses practice population health is in public health nursing and community health nursing. The Quad Council Coalition (QCC) of Public Health Nursing Organizations is composed of four organizations that set a national policy agenda for public health nursing. The organizations that comprise the QCC are the Association of Public Health Nurses (APHN), the Public Health Nursing Section of the American Public Health Association (PHN Section), the Alliance of Nurses for Healthy Environments (ANHE), and the Association of Community Health Nursing Educators (ACHNE). The QCC published competencies for nurses who work as community or public health nurses,[18] and the competencies describe daily functions in community organizations and state and/or local public health agencies. The functions include home visiting for acute, chronic, or follow-up care; population-based services such as immunization clinics for schoolchildren; or holding community-wide immunization clinics for influenza prevention. Community/public health nurses work directly with at-risk populations carrying out disease prevention, health protection, and health promotion efforts at all levels of prevention (primary, secondary, and tertiary). They also conduct basic data collection and contact follow-up on communicable incidence and prevalence; field-work such as planning, implementing, and/or evaluating health education programs for diverse groups; program planning, implementation, and evaluation; outreach activities to ensure that populations at risk receive referrals to needed service; and assessment of population needs. The emphasis in the practice of community/public health nursing is on assessment of population health needs, assurance that these health needs are met, and policy development to reduce health risks to populations.

Public Health Nurses

Although the competencies are the same, there are differences between community health and public health. Public health is a part of a recognized public unit (state, county, city, etc.) and is legally responsible for ensuring the public's health. Public health workers conduct many different functions but commonly emphasize infectious disease prevention and eradication, monitoring environmental factors like water quality and air pollution from a health perspective, or working with policymakers to address a wide range of wellness issues. Nurses in public health work to assure conditions that will allow for optimal health such as *disease prevention*: prevention of the spread of disease through immunizations, contact follow-up, and treatment for those who have been exposed to infectious diseases such as syphilis or tuberculosis; *health protection*: providing education to public groups on the importance of health protective practices such as avoiding injuries, skin cancer prevention and screening, or tobacco cessation and avoidance; or *health promotion*: health education programs on the importance of healthy diets for children along with types of and places for physical activity that will improve overall health. Effective public health nurses emphasize disease prevention and health promotion for the whole community, as defined by the political unit. Public health nurses aim to create better conditions for health aimed at the environment, human behavior and lifestyle, and access to health care.

Public health is the traditional home for nurses who enjoy working with a focus on population health. As illustrated earlier in this chapter, public health is concerned with the health of the population and strives to prevent disease, protect health, and promote health in an entire population as well as in specific subpopulations that are at risk for poor health based on social determinants of health. On a routine basis, public health nurses conduct home visits and provide many ambulatory clinic services (immunizations, well baby, sexually transmitted infections, and prenatal care) as well as respond during infectious disease outbreaks through contact follow-up, screening, treatment, and communicating with community groups. Public health nurses work at city, county, state, and national levels, and at each level they assess the health of the population, provide assurance that the population receives the needed services, and promote health policy adoption among communities.

Community Health Nurses

Community health nurses (CHNs), although adhering to the same competencies as public health nurses, often have a broader area of responsibility. Community health nurses may take responsibility for addressing health equity and social determinants of health through working for community or faith-based agencies that are not affiliated with any government or political unit. Community health nurses may center their practice on increasing a population's access to healthy food and after-school activities as well as working to create common spaces that promote community well-being.

Collaboration is essential in community health nursing, and the CHNs need to be knowledgeable about coalition-building and community efforts that build community agency to solve problems. They may work with community organizations, school systems, faith-based

organizations, local governments, healthcare providers, etc., to accomplish these goals. One thing that public health nurses and CHNs have in common is a great need for cultural awareness and cultural humility, as they work with all members of a community and respond to requests for services, from home visits to policy work, in response to community needs. Both CHNs and public health nurses use evidence to meet the interests and needs of a community.

In the United States, nurses fill many roles in population health, and many more nurses understand how the term "population health" applies to all patients, families, communities, and organizations. Indeed, it is difficult to envision a healthcare system that does not consider population health in its mission and vision. The use of the socioecological model as a framework allows a perspective on the clinical applications of population health.

Hospitals and Ambulatory Clinics

Hospital and clinic management must understand the population metrics and health dynamics of the patients they serve to maintain viability. The type of patient mix, level of skilled nursing care needed for patients, specialty services, ancillary services, and even the ebb and flow of emergency department admissions and discharges depend on the population who use hospital and associated clinical services. With changes in reimbursements tied to inpatient days, patient satisfaction, and readmissions, improving the health of the patient population within the hospital as well as its surrounding community becomes crucial for its economic survival. As more procedures shift from inpatient to outpatient, nurses employed in ambulatory care facilities need to understand how presenting patients may echo common health concerns within a specific subpopulation and be alert for issues that may be associated with subpopulations. Individual nurses employed by hospitals and clinics can improve the health of the population they serve by not only providing skilled nursing care but also reflecting on how their patients mirror the health of the population they represent.[19]

Home Settings

Although home health care (HHC), visiting nurse services (VNS), and hospice all conduct nursing care in the home setting, the population health applications may be different. HHC is often used for patients who need additional nursing care and are expected to return to wellness or learn from nursing instruction how to care for themselves but are no longer ill enough for hospitalization. The health of this population, with temporary illness concerns, can be expected to return to a level of wellness that will enable them to become independent in their own health care. Community patients who receive home visiting services, such as Nurse-Family Partnership,[20] often represent an underserved and vulnerable population, such as low-income, first-time mothers. It is essential for nurses who practice home visiting services to understand the health and social risks faced by their population of focus and know how to apply health promotion and disease prevention practices to improve health outcomes for mothers, children, and families. Patients admitted to hospice typically are not expected to live more than six months. Patients facing terminal illnesses require a population focus on how to maintain social, spiritual, and family-focused attention to health. When nurses understand how health encompasses all levels of wellness, more than physical, population health for hospice patients can be achieved.

School Health

A focus on a population of children is necessary for optimum school health.[21] For many children, the school nurse becomes their only healthcare provider. School health nurses not only meet the children's need for immunizations, health screenings, minor illness, and trauma, the nurse must also be alert for signs of disease outbreaks and constantly monitor for disease prevention as well as teach health promotion. Health protection and injury prevention are important areas of practice as well. If the school nurse does not understand the population of children in the school and know the health issues of the community's population surrounding the school, the nurse will be ill-prepared to protect and promote the children's health. In addition, the nurse needs to attend to the children's education and learning and determine if health issues are undermining children's educational pursuits.

Case Managers/Care Coordinators

Managing the health outcomes of a panel of patients is the role of case managers and care coordinators. Nurses in these roles understand the healthcare needs of their panel and work to maintain the highest level of health for their patients. Population health in this context implies that the nurse knows the health issues experienced by a subpopulation very thoroughly and is able to promote their health to the most optimal level.

Population Health Management

Another context of population health for nurses is population health management. Population health management and population health care are sometimes used interchangeably with population health. These terms refer to a narrower meaning of population health than the concept covers. These terms tend to more heavily focus on health and medical care and particular groups of patients.[1]

Population health management is the act of identifying and addressing the health of individuals within defined populations, but this can be done in many different ways.[22] Healthcare organizations (hospitals, clinics and ambulatory care agencies, nursing homes, and hospice agencies), accountable care organizations, and insurers are vitally interested in providing the most effective and cost-efficient care for the populations they serve. Nurses participate in population health management by using data to stratify patients by risk, developing insights into obstacles faced by some portion of the community, and targeting interventions to certain subpopulations to produce the best results for the population of interest.[22]

A population health management effort involves developing realistic, scalable population health programs for segments of the population that the agency serves, such as diabetes management programs for diabetics. In addition to health programs, individualized treatment plans that recognize determinants of health (social, cultural, environmental, and behavioral) may be needed when health education and support are insufficient to improve health. Patient-centered care plans, although sharing a population health focus, acknowledge barriers that may be present with some segments of the population that hinder them from accomplishing disease prevention, health protection, and health promotion efforts.[23] Successful population health programs can be accomplished when patients are engaged and have the resources needed to adhere to treatment plans.

Community collaborations and creating links across all sectors of health care are essential for population health management. Gaps in care can exacerbate any underlying health problems or lead to a worsening of a previously stable health issue. Collaboration and linkages can allow a healthcare organization to continue to address health problems even when an individual is no longer receiving care from the organization. As insurers see the benefit of keeping people healthy and supporting their care in a community setting, more focus is given to population health management outside of tertiary care centers. Often nurses function as care coordinators or case managers to address healthcare needs of specialized populations. These nurses are practicing population health management while they address the healthcare needs of the patients on their caseload to meet the goal of keeping them as healthy as possible and to maintain their outpatient status as long as it is feasible. Collective action with community social networks can leverage individual nurses practicing population health management by linking those who need social support with others. This has been associated with improvements in people's mental health and emotional well-being and reductions in social isolation.[1]

INTERRELATED CONCEPTS

Several concepts presented in this text are related to population health. The most closely related concepts are illustrated in Fig. 53.3, and their

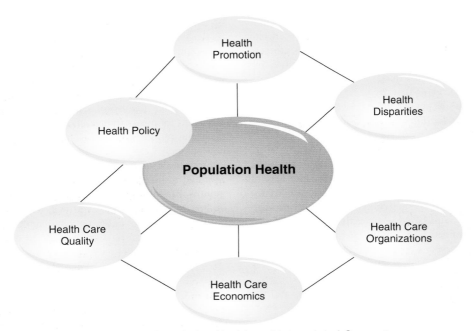

FIGURE 53.3 Population Health and Interrelated Concepts.

relationship is described in more detail. Health Promotion, along with health protection (e.g., seat belt use, food and water safety, and pollution reduction) and disease prevention (e.g., vaccinations and recall of tainted foods) contributes to improving health among a population of individuals. Illnesses can spread quickly among populations, and protection and prevention are essential to prevent mortality and reduce morbidity. Health promotion is geared to help populations achieve and maintain their highest level of wellness, so they can be resilient in the face of illness. Health Disparities threaten the health of populations as they cause unequal distributions of illness based on where people live, work, and spend free time. When health disparities are present, some populations are less resistant to disease and more likely to suffer preventable illnesses or succumb to earlier morbidity and mortality. Health Care Organizations can contribute to improving population health through their attention to health disparities among the populations they serve. When healthcare organizations focus on common causes of illness among their patients to reduce the prevalence of the illnesses, they must examine the commonalities among the population they serve. This in turn leads to improved Health Care Quality, wherein better quality of care can improve the health of specific populations or a segment of a certain population. Health Care Economics support the existence of healthcare organizations and drive the quality of health care. Prevention is cheaper than cure, but the prevention must be spread throughout a population and have a population focus for it to be effective. Health Policy underpins all these concepts because policy sets the direction for action. If health policy emphasizes health promotion for all the population and creates goals and metrics to reduce health disparities, then health for all can be achieved.

CLINICAL EXEMPLARS

Considering that population health represents health outcomes of groups of people, there are countless potential exemplars represented by this concept. Some of the most common exemplars of population health are presented in Box 53.1, but this in no way represents a comprehensive list. In the section that follows, a few of these exemplars are briefly presented.

Featured Exemplars
Prevention of Communicable Diseases

In the past few decades, new infectious diseases such as HIV/AIDS have emerged and rapidly spread among the population, originally among select sub-populations but then among anyone at risk of contact with contaminated bodily fluids. Other diseases that have a long history with humans, such as tuberculosis, have adapted and are still causing millions of deaths each year.[24] Only a population health focus, where everyone is considered "at risk" and in need of health protection and disease prevention, can prevent the rising morbidity and mortality. Maintaining constant surveillance with a population health mindset is the initial line of defense against the emergence of potentially deadly infections.

Immunization

Immunization is the most effective means to prevent communicable disease because immunization protects an individual from becoming infected with the disease-causing agent. The most effective way to become immunized, other than contracting the disease and surviving it, is to become vaccinated against the disease. Bacteria and virus do not respect geographical, political, economic, social, or any other types of artificial boundaries enacted by humans. But for immunization to be effective on a population health level, 90–95% of the population needs to be immunized to prevent the spread of an infectious agent. This is known as "herd immunity."[25]

Prevention of Non-Communicable Diseases

Of the top ten leading causes of death in the United States, five are from non-communicable diseases that can be addressed through health promotion, which is an essential component of a population health approach. Heart disease (#1), chronic lower respiratory disease (#4), stroke (#5), diabetes (#6), and end stage renal disease (#9) can be addressed through maintaining healthy weight, being physically active for 150 minutes weekly, avoiding tobacco, and little or no alcohol intake.[26] The most effective ways to reduce these diseases are through wide-spread publicly available health education, community approaches to creating healthy lifestyles, and policies that advocate smoke-free environments.

Substance Abuse/Misuse

Community programs and local policies have reduced rates of substance abuse initiation and harm. Prevention programs that are coordinated by community agencies such as schools, healthcare systems, faith organizations, and social service organizations can deliver comprehensive and unified prevention programs than can be sustained over time. When a community unites to address the problem at a population level, which acknowledges that all individuals may be at risk, then programs can be established that reach more people than individually focused treatment efforts.[27] Prevention programs and interventions can have a strong impact and be cost-effective, but only if evidence-based components are used and if those components are delivered in a coordinated and consistent fashion throughout the at-risk period.

Accidents and Suicide

Accidents and suicide (unintentional and intentional harm) are the third and tenth leading causes of death in the United States.[26] Both are closely related to substance abuse when alcohol abuse is also considered as a substance abuse. Safer roads and automotive vehicles, along with more severe penalties for driving under the influence of alcohol, have reduced vehicle accidents. Although most suicide attempts are through intentional drug overdoses, when firearms are used, they are the most lethal, with 85% of suicides succeeding when firearms are used.[28] Prevention strategies for suicide prevention are directed to building community capacity to create supportive, protective environments and strengthen economic supports among other strategies.[29]

BOX 53.1 EXEMPLARS OF POPULATION HEALTH

- Prevention of accidents and suicide
- Communicable disease prevention
- Food and restaurant inspections
- Health data collection and statistics
- Health planning and administration
- Immunizations
- Infection control in hospital settings
- Non-communicable disease prevention
- Public health laws (e.g., seat belts and car seats)
- School-wide screenings and vaccine administrations
- Substance abuse education and prevention

 ACCESS EXEMPLAR LINKS IN YOUR GIDDENS EBOOK

CASE STUDY

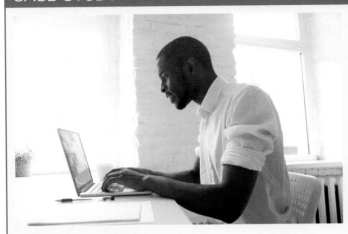

Case Presentation

Kris is a public health nurse in a small county health department and is responsible for all public health nursing functions in the county. Kris is notified by a local healthcare provider that a patient being treated for nausea, vomiting, and jaundice has just tested positive for Hepatitis A (HepA), caused by the hepatitis A virus (HAV), and a communicable disease that is required to be reported to the county and state health departments and to the CDC. Kris also knows that it is highly contagious and needs immediate follow up. Kris contacts the healthcare provider that provides the patient's name and contact information. Kris visits the patient and discovers that the patient is a fast food handler and had diarrhea while preparing food. With a thorough history taken of the time before the patient became ill, the onset of illness, and the patient's continued work during illness, Kris realizes that there is a high risk of HAV spreading among the population of the county and creating a high level of illness.[30] Kris knows that people who consumed food prepared by the patient need immediate intervention with Immunoglobulin G (IgG) to prevent illness, and others who may have come in contact with the patient need to be immunized with the HepA vaccine if they are not immune through previous administration of the vaccine or have had Hepatitis A, which confers lifelong immunity.

Kris knows that communicating the news to the public without panic, setting up IG clinics and additional immunization clinics, and additional contact follow up are more than one public health nurse can do. Kris calls upon the resources of the state health department to assist with communication, contact follow up, and establishment of additional clinics because the state health department is responsible for disease prevention and health protection by addressing all communicable diseases in the state. With Kris' prompt action and population health focus, a wide-spread epidemic of HepA was prevented and many previously un-immunized persons obtained not only HepA vaccination but also other needed immunizations.

Case Analysis Questions

1. What levels of population health (as illustrated in the socioecological model) did Kris address and how would all levels apply to this case?
2. How did Kris practice assessment, assurance, and health policy implementation?
3. With what subpopulations did Kris interact, and how was their health protected and promoted?

🌿 **ACCESS EXEMPLAR LINKS IN YOUR GIDDENS EBOOK**

REFERENCES

1. The King's Fund. (2017). *What does improving population health really mean?* Retrieved from https://www.kingsfund.org.uk/publications/what-does-improving-population-health-mean.
2. Laffrey, S. C. (1986). Development of a health conception scale. *Research in Nursing and Health, 9*(2), 107–113.
3. Frankish, J., Green, L., Ratner, P., et al. (1996). *Health impact assessment as a tool for population health promotion and public policy.* Vancouver: Institute of Health Promotion Research, University of British Columbia.
4. Grad, F. P. (2002). The preamble of the constitution of the World Health Organization. *Bulletin of the World Health Organization, 80*(12), 981–984.
5. *Merriam-Webster Dictionary.* (2018). Britannica Online Academic ed: Encyclopædia Britannica, Inc.
6. Kindig, D., & Stoddart, G. (2003). What is population health? *American Journal of Public Health, 93*(3), 380–383.
7. Public Health Agency of Canada. (2013). *What is the population health approach?* Retrieved from https://www.canada.ca/en/public-health/services/health-promotion/population-health/population-health-approach/what-population-health-approach.html.
8. Centers for Disease Control and Prevention, National Center for HIV/AIDS VH, STD, and TB Prevention. (2008). *NCHHSTP Social Determinants of Health.* Retrieved from https://www.cdc.gov/nchhstp/socialdeterminants/definitions.html.
9. Friedman, D. J., & Parrish, R. G. (2010). The population health record: Concepts, definition, design, and implementation. *Journal of the American Medical Informatics Association, 17*(4), 359–366.
10. Health Canada. (2018). *Social determinants of health and health inequalities.* Retrieved from https://www.canada.ca/en/health-canada.html.
11. Bronfenbrenner, U. (1979). *The ecology of human development: Experiments by nature and design.* Cambridge, MA: Harvard University Press.
12. Reifsnider, E., Gallagher, M., & Forgione, B. (2005). Using ecological models in research on health disparities. *Journal of Professional Nursing, 21*(4), 216–222.
13. Sallis, J. F., Cervero, R. B., Ascher, W., et al. (2006). An ecological approach to creating active living communities. *Annual Review of Public Health, 27*, 297–322.
14. Koo, D., O'Carroll, P. W., Harris, A., et al. (2016). An environmental scan of recent initiatives incorporating social determinants in public health. *Preventing Chronic Disease, 13*, E86.
15. Centers for Disease Control and Prevention, National Center for Health Statistics. (2018). *Healthy People 2020*, Social Determinants of Health. Retrieved from https://www.healthypeople.gov/2020/topics-objectives/topic/social-determinants-of-health.
16. Commission on Social Determinants of Health. (2008). *Closing the gap in a generation: Health equity through action on the social determinants of health. Final Report of the Commission on Social Determinants of Health.* Geneva: World Health Organization.
17. Goodman, R. A., Bunnell, R., & Posner, S. F. (2014). What is "community health"? Examining the meaning of an evolving field in public health. *Preventive Medicine, 67*(Suppl. 1), S58–S61.
18. Quad Council Coalition Competency Review Task Force. (2018). *Community/Public Health Nursing Competencies.* Retrieved from http://www.quadcouncilphn.org/documents-3/2018-qcc-competencies/.
19. Reifsnider, E., & Garcia, A. A. (2015). What's in a name? Does population health have the same meaning for all stakeholders? *Public Health Nursing, 32*(3), 189–190.
20. Miller, T. R., & Hendrie, D. (2015). Nurse family partnership: Comparing costs per family in randomized trials versus scale-up. *The Journal of Primary Prevention, 36*(6), 419–425.
21. Magalnick, H., & Mazyck, D. (2008). Role of the school nurse in providing school health services. *Pediatrics, 121*(5), 1052–1056.

22. Bresnick, J. (2017). *How Do Population Health, Public Health, Community Health Differ?* Retrieved from https://healthitanalytics.com/news/how-do-population-health-public-health-community-health-differ.

23. Taylor, M. E., Gomez, A. M., & Bengtson, R. J. (2017). *Identify Sociodemographic Challenges to Manage Patient Risk: Understanding Sources of Risk to Deliver Better Care.* Retrieved from https://www.connance.com/wp-content/uploads/2017/10/con-wp-IDIngSocioChallenges-EM171013.pdf.

24. Centers for Disease Control and Prevention. (2018). *Division of Tuberculosis Elimination. Data and Statistics.* Retrieved from https://www.cdc.gov/tb/statistics/default.htm.

25. Hu, Y., Lu, P., Deng, X., et al. (2018). The declining antibody level of measles virus in China population, 2009-2015. *BMC Public Health, 18*(1), 906.

26. Heron, M. (2018). Deaths: Leading causes for 2016. *National Vital Statistics Reports: From the Centers for Disease Control and Prevention, National Center for Health Statistics, National Vital Statistics System, 67*(6), 1–77.

27. U.S. Department of Health and Human Services (HHS), Office of the Surgeon General. (2016). Vision for the future: A public health approach. In *Facing Addiction in America: The Surgeon General's Report on alcohol, drugs, and health.* Washington, DC: US Department of Health and Human Services. Chapter 7.

28. Drexler, M. (2018). Guns & suicide: The hidden toll. *Harvard Public Health.* Retrieved from https://www.hsph.harvard.edu/magazine/magazine_article/guns-suicide/.

29. Centers for Disease Control and Prevention. (2018). *Suicide: Prevention Strategies.* Retrieved from https://www.cdc.gov/violenceprevention/suicide/prevention.html.

30. Delaware Health and Social Services, Division of Public Health. (2011). *Immune Globulin (IG) Frequently Asked Questions.* Retrieved from https://www.dhss.delaware.gov/dph/files/immunegifaq.pdf.

Health Care Organizations

Teresa Keller

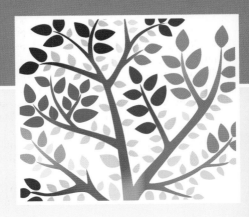

Healthcare organizations (HCOs) are complex and dynamic, a product of the interactions of mission and values, internal and external environments, and the motivations and actions of those who work in these organizations. The delivery of healthcare services in the United States is driven by the need to provide a broad spectrum of care in a variety of settings to diverse consumers. The delivery of these services requires a highly specialized, professional workforce financed by a mix of private and public funding and subject to oversight and regulation by many different public and private authorities. Whether they are rural clinics catering to migrant laborers, large urban teaching hospitals, or multisite integrated health systems providing a spectrum of services, HCOs face challenges that require them to adapt and innovate or face extinction.

The results are new service delivery arrangements, new kinds of healthcare workplaces, new types of service providers, and new treatments and services hardly imagined in prior times, all of which represent some innovation meant to serve a market, a population, or a social need. HCOs are social systems created by people and managed by people; therefore, the HCO is a socially created entity with no meaning outside of the collective actions and aspirations of the people involved. The significance of this perspective of the organization is that all people involved with an HCO, as members of a dynamic social system, are able to make meaningful contributions to the success of the HCO. As members of the largest professional workforce, nurses can have a strong and positive influence on the HCO as it evolves and innovates.

DEFINITION

Organizations can be defined as a group of people who come together for a purpose[1] or as a collection of people brought together for a predetermined purpose in a defined environment.[2] Common to both of these definitions is that organizations are composed of people and have a purpose. Organizations could be further defined as having a socially determined structure provided by formal properties, such as rules, policies, and procedures, and by informal properties, such as customs, norms, and values.[1] A more robust definition for organizations is that they are structured social arrangements that use systematic strategies to combine and coordinate a mix of resources (people and capital) to provide specific products or services. For the purposes of this concept presentation,

the definition of HCO is *a purposefully designed, structured social system developed for the delivery of healthcare services by specialized workforces to defined communities, populations, or markets.*

SCOPE

There are so many different ways to organize an HCO that the result is a large variety of distinctive organizations in the U.S. healthcare services sector, purposely designed to meet the need for healthcare services in a community or population or market.[1] There are HCOs specifically designed to deliver healthcare services, such as hospitals and clinics, and those that are designed for a health-related purpose but not to deliver services, such as pharmaceutical companies or manufacturers of medical equipment.

Obviously, a discussion of the concept of the HCO can be quickly complicated by all the different possible purposes and forms of organization. The variety of distinctive organizations with specific purposes defies simple classification. To establish a scope for this complex topic, only organizations that provide a range of healthcare services for health promotion, illness, and wellness care are considered. This encompasses a variety of organizations, including (but not limited to) hospitals, home health agencies, clinics or ambulatory care centers, nursing homes, and organizations that serve a particular market or population.

ATTRIBUTES AND CRITERIA

All organizations have defining attributes. Each has a purpose, a structure, and members who do the work of the organization. HCOs are no different from other kinds of organizations in this regard. As social systems, HCOs operate in environments from which resources are obtained and from which challenges are presented that require an organizational response. In daily operations, HCOs must be able to acquire resources, produce services, and change as necessary to sustain their existence within the challenging U.S. healthcare services sector.

Major Attributes

HCOs are distinguished from other types of organizations by their unique purpose, by their specialized workforce, and by a level of public trust that separates HCOs from other types of organizations.

Purpose

The purpose of HCOs is to help others by providing healthcare services. This distinguishes the HCO from other types of organizations involved in the business of health care. The primary purpose of companies that sell health insurance is to sell an insurance product. Schools for health professions have a primary educational purpose. The purpose of accreditation and public regulatory agencies is to support the work of the HCO, but they do not directly deliver healthcare services. An HCO provides healthcare services to manage illness or promote health, whether those services are childhood immunizations, surgical interventions, diabetes education, family planning advice, or any of a wide variety of other healthcare services offered to individuals, families, and communities. This purpose remains the same—to provide healthcare services—regardless of profit status or ownership arrangements.

Specialized Healthcare Workforce

HCOs are notable for the highly specialized workforce needed to deliver healthcare services. The work produced in an HCO is complex, variable, and, at times, urgent in nature.[1] The margin for error is narrow with little tolerance for mistakes that can lead to life-threatening and costly consequences. Health professionals who work in HCOs undergo extensive education and experiential learning. The knowledge and skills that these specialized workers bring to the HCO are necessary for the effective delivery of services in an ambiguous, challenging work environment. The compelling need for this specialized workforce increases the costs for HCOs, but it also benefits the organization in terms of maintaining standards and ensuring quality services.[3] An additional benefit is that the strong professional ideals of these workers promote and strengthen the service values that support the purpose of the HCO.

Furthermore, the work of managing the health of humans is not easily divided as people present with health problems that affect the whole person, their families, and perhaps the entire community. The need to treat a person, rather than a disease or problem, is central to the work of healthcare professionals. This creates an interdependence among these workers that is another notable characteristic of HCOs.[1] Although labor might be divided among numerous specialized personnel, the need to address the person or patient as a whole means that each of these professionals is dependent on the knowledge and skills of others. An interprofessional approach to the treatment of human health problems not only is a distinguishing feature of the HCO but also serves to increase the complexity of the organization.

Although the HCO is uniquely defined by its specialized workforce of healthcare professionals, a discussion of the healthcare workforce is not complete without reference to the numerous other personnel essential to the effective functioning of the HCO. For example, the human resource department of any large HCO provides critical services necessary for the daily operations of the HCO because most healthcare professionals expect to receive a salary and benefits. Dietary and housekeeping personnel provide important services within the HCO that support the work of healthcare professionals as do the administrators responsible for ensuring adequate supplies and equipment. Because the HCO is a specialized organization with unique functions, all of these workers could be considered a part of the specialized healthcare workforce.

Public Trust

The historical development of HCOs demonstrates a long record of service to others. Early organizations were created by religious orders or by social service groups to provide services to society's most vulnerable members—the ill and infirm. The work of these early organizations gained the confidence of the public that their altruistic purpose was to serve others by providing care and comfort, regardless of personal circumstances. These laudable efforts helped to establish a social contract between the public and HCOs, from which HCOs have benefitted in both financial terms and public regard.

Currently, the level of public trust in HCOs has eroded with the growth of managed care, national corporate chains of for-profit HCOs, and allegations of fraud and abuse by healthcare providers.[4] However, people still turn to their physicians and nurses for help and advice, and they still seek services offered by HCOs for health concerns. This indicates that the social contract is still intact, if a little worn. As such, HCOs are still distinguished by their relatively positive image of institutions designed to provide valuable and needed services to others. As mentioned previously, all organizations must generate income to remain viable, so the for-profit/not-for-profit status of the HCO is less important than managing the tensions created by financial issues versus the need to preserve altruistic values. HCOs that provide quality healthcare services and are good corporate citizens will be able to maintain their positive image and their part of the social contract, regardless of their profit status.

Minor Attributes

The minor attributes of HCOs differ from major attributes in terms of HCOs' relationship to other kinds of organizations. The major attributes of HCOs discussed in the preceding section are identified with health care and the healthcare services sector. The minor attributes of HCOs are those that define them as forms of purposeful organizations and are features they share in common with other types of organizations.

Structure

Structure is the collective of formal rules and policies that govern organizational practices and that promote the effective management of materials and resources. Structure also creates various roles and associated responsibilities that are required for organizational function. Different organizational roles carry varying levels of authority for decision making relative to the assigned responsibilities of those roles. Organizational rules, policies, and authority are necessary for the integration of diverse functions and activities across the organization into a coordinated system capable of supporting the purpose of the organization. However, too much structure can be stifling, causing the HCO to be so encumbered by rules and regulations that hamper meaningful action.[5] An organization needs sufficient structure to support important processes and operations; otherwise, it will disintegrate into anarchy. A balance needs to be maintained that provides the structure necessary for sustaining the HCO while not producing unnecessary constraints.

The requirement for supportive structures that minimize constraints is especially important for HCOs because of the type of personnel working within these organizations. As noted previously, the workforce of HCOs is composed of a large number of healthcare professionals. These professionals possess valuable knowledge and skills that are critical to the delivery of healthcare services. These professionals also have a strong allegiance to a set of professional values. Most healthcare professionals possess a state-licensed authority to manage their own practice and are responsible for the outcomes of their work.

For an HCO, this means management authority and control is relatively weak in relation to professional authority because decision making related to practice is not subject to control by those outside the profession.[3] This requires additional lines of authority to be established within the HCO; for example, nurses are accountable to nursing officers, and physicians are accountable to medical executives. This is true for most of the institutional arrangements that create authority within an HCO. Professional control of licensed practice is the basis for the interdependency between health professionals in the HCO, but it can also fuel the typical conflicts and "turf wars" seen in an HCO.[1]

The result of these divided lines of authority is that management control by those outside of the profession is limited to those work activities that lie outside the professional's scope of practice. For example, nurses can expect that their professional practice will be directed and evaluated by other nurses and that they will be accountable for maintaining the standards of the profession. However, they can also expect that they will need to meet the requirements established by non-nursing administrators for other expected work behaviors, such as the use of vacation time or maintaining appropriate licensure.

Organizational Environments

Organizations possess an internal environment, but they also interact with an external environment. The internal environment of the HCO consists of an integrated web of factors such as organizational culture (where *culture* is defined as a set of values, beliefs, and practices), systems such as information systems or the human resources management system, and structural elements such as role responsibilities, rules, and practices. All of these factors affect the decisions and responses of the HCO to demands and challenges encountered during daily operations.[6]

The external organizational environment consists of those external forces, conditions, or events that affect the organization, such as economic trends or new laws and government regulations. Examples of external environmental forces are a widespread economic recession and government funding changes that affect HCOs. These kinds of forces in the external environment provide resources and/or feedback as inputs to the organization and are major factors that drive organizational change.

There is an ongoing interplay between the internal and external environments of the HCO, where organizational decisions and operations are affected by perceived forces from the external environment.[6] Organizations integrated into their environments will also change those environments in some ways, adding to the complexity of the relationship. For example, a national economic recession can prompt workers to expand their work hours, either by increasing the hours they work or by seeking additional employment. This holds true for nurses. If experienced professional nurses are working more hours or seeking additional employment, the effect on the HCO could be human resources changes, that results in fewer new and inexperienced nurses being hired. The decline in demand for new nurses has the potential to affect the admission decisions of nursing schools or the funding decisions made by government organizations that support nursing education. As these resources are curtailed, there are fewer new nurses prepared and, subsequently, fewer new nurses for the HCO to hire to replace nurses who leave or retire.

Before the 20th century and the rise of organized healthcare delivery, the healthcare industry was unregulated, healthcare workers were less knowledgeable, and healthcare markets were small and relatively simple.[5] Currently, multiple interacting forces in the healthcare environment have profound effects on HCOs, especially because they increase uncertainty and create instability. While HCOs evolve to meet the challenges presented by their environments, they are still expected to maintain the service orientation that is fundamental to their purpose. An example of the internal pressures created by external environmental demands is tying government reimbursements to HCOs for meeting evidence-based standards of quality care and ensuring optimal patient safety. Meeting quality and safety standards is highly desirable, but it is also costly in terms of training personnel, providing additional staffing, and building work processes that support quality care and patient safety. This creates tensions within the HCO while workers seek to meet expectations for safe and effective care with limited additional resources.[7]

HCO policies created to meet environmental challenges might conflict with professional values or with legal guidelines, requiring actions to negotiate and resolve the conflict. New technologies might need to be adopted that require a shift of resources from one part of the organization to another. The need to change (rapidly in some cases) in response to environmental effects means that HCOs are complex and their work environments are notably ambiguous.

THEORETICAL LINKS

The industrial revolution led to the development of large organizations. As these organizations grew, they became the vehicle through which many different kinds of human activities are organized and coordinated. This prompted social scientists to study the phenomenon of purposive, organized systems and create theories to explain these systems. A complete description of the organizational theories of the past 100 years is beyond the scope of this concept presentation. Instead, an overview of the major directions in theory development related to organizations is useful in understanding the HCO concept.

Bureaucracy

Early conceptualizations of organizations were that they were closed systems and were a rational, machine-like collection of components to be coordinated and controlled through authoritative management.[2] Max Weber, German sociologist and economist, developed the first theoretical model of bureaucracy in the early 20th century. Weber described the principles of organization that created efficiency in work design and were thought to be the most effective way to organize work. He also described the distribution of authority in bureaucracies, noting that authority grounded in position and divided into hierarchies was preferable to authority derived from personal characteristics. Weber viewed the bureaucracy as the organizational design most likely to create the stability needed to sustain an organization.[2] Bureaucratic design was common to large organizations that developed during the industrial revolution because the manufacturing and distribution of goods required a rational system of centralized control to effectively acquire resources and efficiently convert them to a finished product.[2,8] Bureaucratic organizations were made of functional parts or divisions, all welded together through management control made possible by hierarchical authority. These organizations were believed to be capable of achieving a high degree of coordinated precision in production, leading to the common metaphor of a "well-oiled machine."

The drawback to this model of rational efficiency is that it takes little account of the organization as a social system within an environment. Bureaucratic theory mainly focuses on authority and control to achieve efficient production within a closed system. The human dimension of the organization is not well-defined outside of the role of management. Other organizational theorists of that time attempted to describe and explain the social dynamics of organizations, but the main theoretical approach taken was mechanical and emphasized the role of management in attaining maximal productivity from workers through planning and control.[8] The effects of environmental factors on the production and efficiency of an organization were also not considered by these early theorists. The bureaucratic organization was a self-contained, closed system.

Systems Theory

The view of organizations as social systems had an early beginning with the human relations school of organizational theorists. This group focused their study on the needs and desires of people who work in the organization. From this field of study grew an understanding that the organization has social components that interact and that these components are affected by factors from the outside environment.[8] These social components (people, relationships, and roles) interact with environment, technology, and organizational structure in an integrated manner to create a unified, dynamic system.[1,5] An open system's perspective paved the way for interesting new theories that not only intrigue organizational theorists but also provide new ways to organize and empower the people who work in these systems (Fig. 54.1).[6]

Complex Adaptive Systems

Current organizational theory describes the organization as having biological characteristics that allow the organization to react and change when stimulated. This understanding defines a new way of viewing organizations as organic and lifelike entities that are open to the environment and capable of transforming themselves in light of perceived opportunities and threats. Organizations can "read" and interpret the environment, and they can adjust and adapt through the coordinated action of their interdependent parts.[1] The changes that occur within an organization in response to environmental stimuli are necessary for sustaining the organization just as metabolic processes within the human body change to allow the body to adapt to environmental challenges. In the case of the HCO, the need for change and adaptation requires that all organizational members be engaged and motivated to meet the organization's goals. Viewing the organization as a living social system recognizes the creative energy of the people who innovate to produce desirable products and services in uncertain, changing environments. Understanding the HCO as a complex, adaptive system is probably the most realistic of the organizational theories developed to date because it can account for the complexity created by interrelated and interdependent social systems responding to internal and external stimuli.

CONTEXT TO NURSING AND HEALTH CARE

In the context of health care, HCOs can be broadly classified by their mission, financial structure, and ownership.

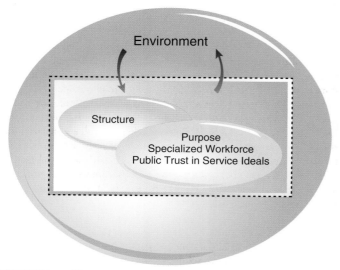

FIGURE 54.1 Health Care Organizations: Open Systems Model.

Mission

The purpose of an HCO is determined by the organization's mission, vision, and values.[9] Mission statements issued by HCOs describe each organization's purpose based on a vision of what the HCO is meant to achieve. Mission statements also describe the values that drive the work of the organization, such as quality and excellence. Even if the HCO is a for-profit, privately owned corporation that pays dividends to shareholders, the mission statement will reflect values commonly associated with helping others, such as service and professionalism. Because mission statements reflect strategic vision, they focus and drive the work of the HCO toward organizational goals. Mission statements that reflect values and primarily benefit shareholders, such as seeking higher profits, would drive the work of the HCO in a direction that may conflict with the goal of helping others with their healthcare needs. Mission statements that prominently feature service ideals and values and promote assistance and support to others serve to sustain the primary purpose of the HCO.

Financial Structure

Another way to classify HCOs is by their financial purpose as either for-profit or not-for-profit entities. The difference between the not-for-profit and the for-profit HCO is not the profits generated but, rather, how the profits are distributed. For-profit HCOs are designed to generate profits for shareholders while also providing healthcare services. Not-for-profit HCOs also generate profits, but these are used for organizational purposes, such as building additional facilities, providing improved services, or acquiring new equipment.

In reality, this distinction between for-profit and not-for-profit HCOs is less clear because all HCOs must pay attention to financial viability. The need to generate revenues to meet expenses is important to all organizations, whether for-profit or not-for-profit, because the failure to cover expenses creates risks to the continued existence of HCOs. Unprofitable HCOs that collect less revenue than what is required to meet expenses—even if they are publicly supported—will eventually have to close or be reorganized.

Ownership

In addition to their mission and financing, HCOs can also be classified as publicly or privately owned. Publicly owned HCOs are organizations that are supported by government funding. The typical example of this type of ownership is the tax-supported county or state hospital that provides generalized healthcare services or specific health services, such as behavioral and mental health. State and local public health departments could also be considered publicly owned HCOs. Investor-owned corporations are considered privately owned, but private ownership could also include HCOs owned by religious or social organizations. Privately owned HCOs are not generally supported by public funding.

The defining characteristics of mission, finance, and ownership noted previously can be combined to create a myriad of HCOs designed to meet the challenges of the healthcare environment. The variety seen in HCOs can be illustrated using hospice as an example. Hospice services provide specialty care to a specific population—the terminally ill and their families. As an HCO, the hospice might be for-profit and privately owned (by investors) and any profits generated by services are returned to the investors in the form of dividends, or the hospice might be nonprofit and privately owned by a religious organization and any profits realized are returned to the HCO to improve the quality of services and infrastructure or to sustain other services offered by the organization. Both of these types of hospice provide the same unique service and play a distinct role in the healthcare community, although they vary by ownership and profit status. Furthermore, a hospice could be a part of an integrated, national network of HCOs delivering a full spectrum of coordinated healthcare services. Regardless of the structure and institutional arrangement, as an HCO, the hospice must be ready to manage costs and maintain services while evolving as the health services environment changes.

Regardless of the mission, financing, or ownership, nurses can be found in almost any kind of HCO, where they are responsible for ensuring the safe and effective delivery of care. The nursing profession in the United States is the largest health professional group. Nurses are working throughout the health services sector and in all HCOs because their knowledge and skills are integral to the delivery of healthcare services.[10]

However, nursing contributions to successful HCOs go beyond providing bedside, patient-focused care to include active management and administration of patient care and patient units, conducting research, and collaborating with other professionals to coordinate and deliver safe and effective patient care. Nurses work as case managers, infection control specialists, managers of information technology, human resources specialists, and quality/risk managers. Nurses are also directors and executives, advanced practice providers, and administrative specialists in HCOs and HCO networks. Furthermore, professional nurses affect the environments of HCOs by creating partnerships with other institutions, educating future nurses in universities and community colleges, and working with public policy decision makers to create policies that enhance health services environments. It is likely that professional nurses will be associated in some way with HCOs for most, if not all, of their professional nursing careers.

INTERRELATED CONCEPTS

Other organizational concepts featured in this textbook are important to understand the HCO as a dynamic social system (Fig. 54.2).

Contemporary Leadership is required for HCOs—a leadership that creates inspiration, is able to sustain motivation to achieve results, and values the contributions of all members. Leaders have to be able to

"read" the environment and interpret the trends or changes for others. They must be able to lead others through turbulent and uncertain environments and must be able to adapt to change as readily as their followers.[11]

Timely, current, and accurate Communication is an essential component of safe and effective care delivery. Delayed, diminished, or compromised communication not only hampers the organization's activities and productivity but also can lead to serious deficiencies in patient care. Ineffective communication is linked to many instances of catastrophic errors in patient care, such as wrong-site surgery or unexpected patient death.[11]

Collaboration can be defined as partnerships developed for the purpose of achieving optimal patient care outcomes.[12] It is essential that nurses be able to collaborate with other members of the HCO, the patient, and the patient's family to deliver quality health care that is safe and effective. The ability to collaborate also creates the conditions necessary for effective mentoring of new nurses and for professional control of practice.

Technology and Informatics is essential to the HCO for ensuring the delivery of safe patient care, and the collection and meaningful use of patient care information provides the basis for much of the evidence used in healthcare decision making. The era of the electronic health record has arrived and is proving to be a disruptive innovation that will fundamentally change how health care is delivered. Clinical informatics provides data and statistics about healthcare services and the outcomes of these services.[13] Coupled with new government payment systems, these outcomes will drive the products and services provided by HCOs.

In 2001, the Institute of Medicine issued a clarion call for an increased focus on Health Care Quality. Since then, many HCOs and healthcare leaders (including nurses) have worked to identify gaps in care that lead to patient care errors and to propose solutions to address the conditions that lead to these errors. Many of these proposals are aimed at correcting the problems in organizational design and function that promote an error-prone environment in HCOs. For instance, the strategies developed for improving communications in

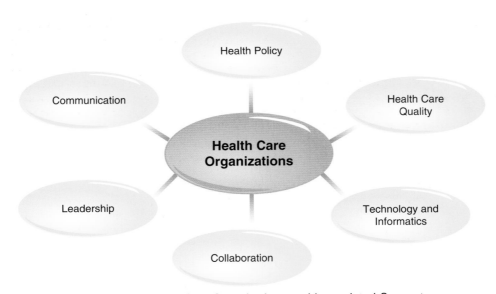

FIGURE 54.2 Health Care Organizations and Interrelated Concepts.

handoffs are meant to promote greater patient safety during transfers between units.[7]

Health Policy is a major force driving change in HCOs. Obvious pressures are changes to HCO revenue related to the increased focus on reimbursements for quality outcomes or on changes to health insurance markets that result in greater access to health care. Less obvious are the pressures that arise from other policy decisions. To illustrate, consider the impact of decisions by a state board of nursing on the nursing workforce. Suppose a board of nursing moves to require a bachelor's degree as a condition of professional licensure. A decision such as this will greatly affect the staffing patterns and pay scales of nurses hired by an HCO.

CLINICAL EXEMPLARS

Examples of HCOs are numerous. As defined previously, an HCO can be any type of organization developed for the delivery of healthcare services and employing a workforce of health professionals to achieve this mission. These include hospitals, clinics and ambulatory care centers, nursing homes, public/community health agencies, hospice, and HCOs developed to meet the needs of a unique market or population (Box 54.1). These are the more familiar types of HCOs in which nurses are likely to be employed. These facilities can be classified by ownership, financial purpose, and services delivered, but when combined with their organizational mission and purpose, the variety to be found among HCOs expands greatly.

Featured Exemplars
Hospitals

Hospitals have traditionally been viewed as tertiary care centers for the treatment of acute illness and disability. Hospitals can be large or small and urban or rural, but they are all driven by a particular mission. For example, research and teaching hospitals are large HCOs usually associated with academic health centers whose mission includes the education of health professionals as well as the delivery of healthcare services. Community hospitals offer general medical and surgical services to a surrounding community, but most will not have a research or teaching mission. Hospitals can also specialize in the care of a particular health condition, a market, or a population.

Clinics and Ambulatory Care Centers

Clinics and ambulatory care centers are generally viewed as HCOs with a mission to deliver services in an outpatient setting. For example, federally qualified health centers offer primary care services such as well-child examinations, immunizations, and the diagnosis and management of chronic conditions such as diabetes. Another example of a clinic is a nurse-managed center offering a range of primary care services for adults, children, and families. Clinic facilities and ambulatory care centers are not usually equipped to provide prolonged acute care, so

patients requiring these types of services are referred to a hospital for treatment.

Nursing Homes

Nursing homes and assisted living facilities offer long-term, skilled nursing services most often to the frail and ill elderly population. However, adults with conditions requiring prolonged periods of skilled nursing care may also be admitted to nursing homes.

Hospice

Hospice is a type of HCO with a specific mission—to provide end-of-life services to patients and their families. The intent is to provide palliative care to patients with terminal illnesses and to provide support for their families.

Specialty Healthcare Organizations

Other HCOs with highly specialized purposes include the U.S. Department of Defense HCOs that provide healthcare services to military members and their families and Indian Health Services HCOs that provide healthcare services for Native American populations. These HCOs most often confine service delivery to the specified population and are designed with the unique needs of these populations in mind. For example, the HCOs that make up the network of the U.S. Department of Veteran Affairs facilities offer services only to military veterans.

BOX 54.1 EXEMPLARS OF HEALTH CARE ORGANIZATIONS

Hospitals
- Teaching/academic medical centers
- Community hospitals (rural and urban)
- Specialized care (rehabilitation)

Nursing Homes
Clinics and Ambulatory Care Facilities
- Federally qualified health centers
- Nurse-managed centers
- Retail walk-in clinics (urgent care)
- Same-day surgery centers

Hospice
Specialty Health Care Organizations
- U.S. Department of Defense military Health Care Organization (HCO)
- U.S. Department of Veterans Affairs
- Indian Health Services

 ACCESS EXEMPLAR LINKS IN YOUR GIDDENS EBOOK

CASE STUDY

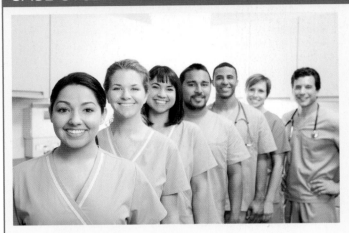

Case Presentation

A form of HCO that offers nurses the opportunity to fully realize their professional role is the Magnet organization. Magnet organizations are those HCOs, primarily hospitals, that have adopted organizational practices that promote excellence in nursing practice. The HCO that adopts Magnet principles is committing to an organizational design and structure that empowers nursing staff to achieve higher levels of performance through engagement and participation. The Magnet designation is only obtained after a process of learning and self-evaluation followed by changes to the organization's structure.[14] These design changes provide a decentralized authority structure created to support participative management and professional autonomy for nurses. Nurses working in Magnet facilities are expected to be active participants in organizational processes, to govern themselves, collaborate with other professional colleagues, and be both responsible and accountable for the outcomes of nursing care.

Magnet designation is an empowerment model that captures the main features of the complex adaptive system. Adopting Magnet principles meant to attract and retain excellent nurses is, fundamentally, the recognition that professional nursing is a valuable and scarce resource essential to the effective function of the HCO.[14] Nurses are not simply workers in the system but are instead a critical component of the organization that makes substantial contributions to the success of the HCO. To achieve this recognition, an HCO must be able to demonstrate the full integration of professional nursing into its operations through authority structures that move decision making, power, and control of practice to nurses throughout the organization. This is usually accomplished through the creation of governance councils in which all nursing staff are able to voice their concerns with care issues and then make decisions that will affect how care is delivered in that facility. Professional decision making is no longer the exclusive domain of the nursing executive and directors. Instead, there is a flattening of hierarchical relationships related to authority and control over practice, with more of the responsibilities for care outcomes being assumed by nursing staff.

The HCO must also demonstrate that appropriate processes are in place that allow for the development of innovative care strategies and that nurses can implement and review the results of their innovation efforts. Quality management in Magnet organizations is robust, and nurses are fully involved in creative activities that encourage continuous quality improvement and the achievement of excellence in nursing care. These facilities promote the continuing professional development of their nurses by supporting education and career-ladder programs.[13]

Case Analysis Questions

1. Which major and minor attributes of healthcare organizations are represented in this case study?
2. Consider the interrelated concepts shown in Fig. 54.2. Which concepts are represented in this case? What additional interrelated concepts apply?

From Steve Hix/Fuse/Thinkstock.

🍃 **ACCESS EXEMPLAR LINKS IN YOUR GIDDENS EBOOK**

REFERENCES

1. Charns, M., & Young, G. (2012). Organizational design and coordination. In L. Burns, E. Bradley, & B. Weiner (Eds.), *Health care management: Organization design and behavior* (6th ed., pp. 64–90). Clifton Park, NY: Delmar.
2. Olden, P., & Diana, M. (2019). Classical theories of organization. In J. Johnson & C. Rossow (Eds.), *Health organizations: Theory, behavior and development* (pp. 23–34). Sudbury, MA: Jones & Bartlett.
3. Spetz, J., & Chapman, S. (2015). The health care workforce. In J. Knickman & A. Kovner (Eds.), *Jonas and Kovner's health care delivery in the United States* (11th ed., pp. 213–223). New York: Springer Publishing.
4. Hutchinson, M. (2018). The crisis of public trust in governance and institutions: Implications for nursing leadership. *Journal of Nursing Management, 26,* 83–85.
5. Johnson, J. (2019). Complexity and Postmodern Theories of Organization. In J. Johnson & C. Rossow (Eds.), *Health organizations: Theory, behavior and development* (pp. 47–58). Sudbury, MA: Jones & Bartlett.
6. LaMarche, P., & Maillet, L. (2016). The performance of primary health care organizations depends on interdependencies with the local environment. *Journal of Health Organization and Management, 30*(6), 836–854.
7. Havily, C., Anderson, A., & Currier, A. (2014). Overview of patient safety and quality of care. In P. Kelly, B. Vottero, & C. Christie-McAuliffe (Eds.), *Introduction to quality and safety education for nurses: Core competencies* (pp. 1–37). New York: Springer.
8. Diana, M., & Olden, P. (2019). Modern theories of organization. In J. Johnson & C. Rossow (Eds.), *Health organizations: Theory, behavior and development* (pp. 35–46). Sudbury, MA: Jones & Bartlett.
9. Kopaneva, I., & Sias, P. (2015). Lost in translation: Employee and organizational constructions of mission and vision. *Management Communication Quarterly, 229*(3), 358–384.
10. Institute of Medicine. (2010). *The future of nursing: Leading change, advancing health.* Washington, DC: National Academies Press.
11. Altmiller, G. (2014). Interprofessional teamwork and collaboration. In P. Kelly, B. Vottero, & C. Christie-McAuliffe (Eds.), *Introduction to quality and safety education for nurses: Core competencies* (pp. 131–160). New York: Springer.
12. Liesveld, J. (2016). Collaboration. In J. Giddens (Ed.), *Concepts for nursing practice* (2nd ed., pp. 438–444). St Louis: Elsevier.
13. Skiba, D., & Connors, H. (2016). Technology and informatics. In J. Giddens (Ed.), *Concepts for nursing practice* (2nd ed., pp. 453–462). St Louis: Elsevier.
14. American Nurses Credentialing Center. (2018). *Magnet Recognition Program.* Retrieved from https://www.nursingworld.org/organizational-programs/magnet/.

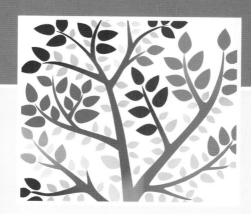

Health Care Economics

Teresa Keller

Economics is a social science that studies how valuable and scarce resources are managed in human social systems. In the United States, demand for health care exceeds the available supply, meaning those goods and services are considered to be both valuable and scarce. Healthcare finance involves strategies and methods used to pay for these scarce and valuable resources. Both of these entities exist in a symbiotic relationship where they affect each other in meaningful ways.

Most people in the United States finance their health care through some form of insurance, either provided by their employers, government and military programs, or by out-of-pocket payment. The healthcare market is complicated and involves insurance companies, employers, a variety of levels of government, and institutional stakeholders. The result is an untidy system of health insurance coverage that profoundly affects access, equity, and quality of care within the health services sector. Even with the major overhaul of the healthcare insurance market by the Patient Protection and Affordable Care Act of 2010 (Public Law 11-148), commonly known as the ACA, gaps in coverage still exist and there are still issues with access to quality, affordable care for all.[1,2] Determination of those who qualify for access to healthcare markets, the amount of care received, and how to pay for it are moral and practical challenges to financing health care for all.

Economics, as a discipline, provides insight into the issues of the distribution of health care because the fundamental problem of resource scarcity requires making choices in the healthcare market. Healthcare resources are limited, creating a situation in which scarcity propels the prices and costs associated with financing health care. Healthcare economics is concerned with both efficiency (getting the most out of a fixed amount of resources) and distribution (determining who receives resources and who will be denied).[3]

DEFINITION

Healthcare economics focuses on how people deal with scarcity and finite resources. For the purpose of this concept presentation, healthcare economics is defined as *the study of supply and demand of resources and its effect on the allocation of healthcare resources in an economic system*.[3,4] The term *healthcare finance* refers to the arrangements made to pay for these goods and services.

SCOPE

The scope of healthcare economics includes the availability (or scarcity) of healthcare resources, access to the resources, and the financing or payment mechanisms, to pay for these resources (Fig. 55.1). Whether or not there is payment influences utilization of resources, regardless of the availability and distribution of health care. Therefore healthcare economics and finance are twin sides of the same coin and are appropriately considered together. The delivery and financing of healthcare resources is highly influenced by the actions of government, as well as public and private organizations, because they define and control payment for healthcare services. Individual responses to price/cost and supply/demand signals in a healthcare market (behavioral economics) are also within the scope of this concept.[4]

ATTRIBUTES AND CRITERIA

The attributes commonly associated with the concept of healthcare economics are markets, price and cost, supply and demand, and efficiency versus equity in the production and distribution of healthcare goods and services. In a healthcare market, financing is driven by these attributes and their effect on the behavior of market participants. Each will be considered separately for the purpose of identifying and understanding each attribute. However, each of these pairs of attributes has effects on the others resulting in complex interactions (Box 55.1 and Fig. 55.2).

Markets

In traditional economic theory, the exchange of goods and services is thought to take place in a competitive *market*. In this market, buyers and sellers have full knowledge of the goods and services offered, prices are determined by the perception of value by both sides, and every participant can enter or exit at will.[3,4] Prices stabilize when neither participant in the exchange will receive additional benefits from changes to the price. The basic assumption of this model is that it operates free from outside influence and without producing undue burden for participants.[4] This assumption does not hold true for healthcare markets.

Many factors distort the processes that drive healthcare markets. Entry into the market is often limited to those individuals who are insured or able to pay the price for goods and services.[3] Knowledge of conditions in the market is often limited to producers, governments, insurers, and professional healthcare providers, whereas buyers and consumers often have less knowledge of the conditions that influence the prices they pay.[4] Insurance coverage shields healthcare consumers from the true cost of health care; therefore their decision to buy is distorted. Government intervention in healthcare markets always distorts the relationship between price and costs, further complicating individual

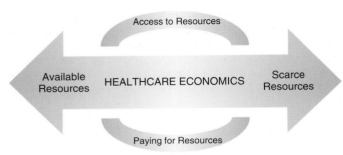

FIGURE 55.1 Scope of Health Care Economics.

decision making and affecting producer costs and the price paid by buyers.[3]

Price and Cost

The price of a good or service is a combination of the seller's production costs plus an additional increment that represents the seller's profit. In a market, price settles at the level of acceptance by both the seller and the buyer, an equilibrium point where neither side will benefit from a price change.[3,4] In healthcare markets, price is highly influenced by factors unrelated to the basic exchange between participants.

For example, consider the cost and price of a cough syrup. Most healthcare consumers know little about pharmaceuticals, increasing the risk that a consumer could experience harm from taking too much of a given medication. In an effort to protect healthcare consumers, a government regulatory agency determines that the particular formulation of cough syrup must only be sold with a provider prescription. Limited access created by government decree means the supply of cough syrup is available only for those purchasers who obtain a prescription. As the supply of cough syrup is limited and assuming demand does not change, the price of the medication increases and the producer's profit is enhanced. Requiring a prescription for cough syrup creates additional costs for the consumer because they now must visit a provider for an exam and prescription, perhaps taking time from their work schedule or adding to their childcare costs. The consumer ends up paying for

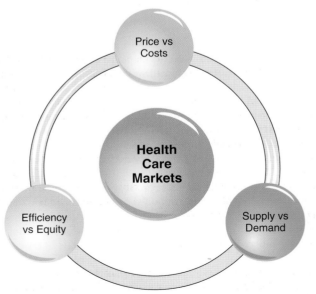

FIGURE 55.2 Relationship Among Attributes of Health Care Economics.

the producer's costs and profit margin plus additional costs related to limited access.[3]

Supply and Demand

In a competitive market, the unit price for a particular good or service will vary until it settles at a point where quantity demanded by consumers will equal the quantity supplied by producers. This results in an economic equilibrium between quantity desired and quantity supplied.[3,4] Two important relationships will determine the price of goods and services at equilibrium. Increasing demand will result in driving up the price of a good because the supply does not meet the demand for that product. The production of that item will increase as producers seek to maximize their profits by selling to meet rises in demand. The price point will stabilize where supply meets demand.[4]

In healthcare markets, the relationship between supply and demand is often distorted and price equilibrium is not easily achieved.[3,4] In the cough syrup example, limiting access to cough syrup will reduce demand because the buyer must also assume additional costs to obtain a prescription for cough syrup. Adding a pharmacy to the transaction as a middleman also increases the costs for consumers and may lead to a decrease in demand, not because of the relationship between demand and supply, but because the middleman adds their costs to the price of a product. Some buyers will be priced out of the market by the additional costs. Some producers may decide to exit the marketplace, thereby limiting choice for the consumer and affecting the supply of cough syrup even more.

Efficiency and Equity

Efficiency in the production and distribution of healthcare resources can be thought of as avoiding waste (including waste of equipment, supplies, and people) or as using healthcare resources to get the best value for the money. Equity is assuring that everyone will have access to the healthcare resources they need and that these goods and services do not vary in quantity or quality among different individuals.[3,4]

Efficiency and equity are another pair of intertwined concepts as the economic question is how to balance both. Efficient production assumes a trade-off between quality and costs that could lead to very expensive or low-quality products. Efficient distribution could result in limited access or the provision of less than optimal amounts of a resource.[3,4] Suppose the makers of cough syrup find that the price for a key ingredient in their medication has increased. To maintain their profits, they could decide to substitute a cheaper ingredient of lower quality. When this new formulation is sold, the cheaper ingredient leads to respiratory distress for a subset of buyers. In this case, maintaining efficiency in the production process results in additional healthcare resources needed to treat the buyers for a medication effect that likely would not happen if the ingredients of the cough syrup had not changed. Additional costs and wastage might also accrue to the producers if they must refund the money spent by consumers on their product and recall unsold quantities of the cough syrup.

Inequities in the cough syrup market may result when pursuing efficient distribution of a product.[5] The producers of cough syrup determine that their best profits are derived when their medication is

BOX 55.1	**Attributes of Health Care Economics**

- Markets
- Price and cost
- Supply and demand
- Efficiency and equity

sold in medium to large cities and that their costs increase when delivering their product to rural areas. To maintain their profits and continue production, the makers of cough syrup may elect to forgo delivery of their product to clinics and drugstores in towns with less than 25,000 people. The end result is unequal access to cough syrup for people who live in small towns and rural areas.

THEORETICAL LINKS

An important theoretical link to the concepts of healthcare economics is *risk*. Risk is the uncertainty and unpredictability of a loss (e.g., the loss of a home due to fire). Typical healthcare risks are generally related to the debilitating effects of serious health conditions and their effect on an individual's or family's quality of life. For example, if the health of one of the income earners in a household deteriorates, there is likely to be a loss of income to sustain the family. Health insurance mediates this risk by providing the financing necessary to pay for needed healthcare resources.[3–5]

CONTEXT TO NURSING AND HEALTH CARE

Healthcare economics and finance affect all areas where nurses practice as well as the individual nurse and his or her family. Nurses delivering patient care in an organization may be unaware of the many issues of economics and finance that they encounter on a daily basis. Nurses will often learn of the economic and finance issues that directly affect their patients at discharge, such as insufficient resources to pay out-of-pocket costs or to purchase medications. Nurses will experience almost daily a constant concern for achieving efficiencies in practice, reducing unnecessary waste, and working together to reduce the costs of care. In addition, as healthcare consumers themselves, nurses will have to make choices and trade-offs about the resources they use to keep themselves and their families healthy.

Patient Protection and Affordable Care Act of 2010 (Public Law 11-148)

The ACA has been a profound influence on healthcare economics and finance as well as the nursing practice environment in the United States. The goal of the ACA was to reform health insurance markets in the United States. Changes from reform included provisions to expand access to health care for most of the U.S. population, abolish some insurance practices that limit enrollment in insurance plans, and address the need for promoting quality, cost-effective care in the U.S. health services sector.[3]

Access

The ACA expanded access by subsidizing state Medicaid expansions, requiring mandatory purchase of health insurance by individuals, and by creating state level exchanges where individuals and small firms could purchase health insurance.[3,6]

Insurance Reforms

The ACA eliminated two insurance industry practices that are meant to limit industry costs but also resulted in limiting access for the chronically ill. The first, *cherry-picking,* is the selection of the healthiest individuals for enrollment in a health insurance program. The second, *limitations or even denial of coverage for preexisting conditions*, is meant to exclude high-cost individuals from a given pool of insured individuals.

These practices have been used for many years prior to the ACA to control the risk of higher healthcare costs for insurance companies.[5] After the implementation of the ACA, there was an initial uptick in expenditures from enrollment growth as more previously uninsured

individuals obtained and used health insurance.[1,2] The duration of time that people with preexisting conditions were uninsured dropped,[2] while the provisions of the ACA that included mandates for employer and individual purchases of insurance helped eight million more Americans obtain health insurance in just the first year of state exchange operations. As of 2016, the growth of healthcare expenditures has slowed, and the percent of gross domestic product (GDP) devoted to health care has dropped from an estimated 19% in 2010 to 17.9% in 2016.[7] The percentage of people with health insurance amounted to approximately 91% of the eligible U.S. population.[8]

Quality, Cost-effective Care

Current health policy initiatives to reduce market distortions are directed at both supply and demand. *Value-based purchasing* or *pay for performance* is a financial strategy meant to encourage the efficient delivery of high-quality goods and services.[9] It is designed to enhance efficiency through better coordination of care among patients, providers, and clinicians, including nurses. Incentives are offered in the form of additional reimbursement to clinicians and hospitals for the provision of appropriate and high-quality healthcare services.[10,11]

Nurses contribute directly to the organization's performance that results in high-value, high-quality care and allows for optimized reimbursements from government and private payers. Many of the measures of quality tied to reimbursement are considered to *be nurse-sensitive indicators*. Currently, Medicare will not cover the cost of preventable hospital-acquired conditions, mistakes, and infections that can occur during a patient's hospitalization.

For example, if a patient admitted to a hospital develops a pressure ulcer during his or her hospital stay, Medicare will not pay for the costs associated with treating the pressure ulcer. Other nurse-sensitive indicators included in Medicare quality measures are falls from bed, catheter-associated urinary tract infections, blood incompatibility mistakes, and vascular catheter-associated infections. This is placing an additional financial burden on hospitals because nurses need the time to assess all of these indicators on an ongoing basis and hospitals must code for infections and other conditions as "present on admission" so they are not liable for a reduction in their payment. Therefore staff nurses have a profound effect on an organization's efforts to achieve pay-for-performance standards, including education, documentation, team collaboration, and patterns of care.

INTERRELATED CONCEPTS

Several concepts featured in this textbook have a relationship with the concepts of healthcare economics and finance. Health Policy is used to provide overarching goals and to set priorities and values for the allocation of health resources. Health Care Quality is concerned with issues related to ensuring standards of care, and outcomes are achieved in the delivery of health care. Health Care Organizations provide the framework for the delivery of health care. Care Coordination involves the marshaling of personnel and other resources needed to carry out all required patient care activities. Health Care Law affects healthcare economics because it governs the insurance industry and is illustrated in the application of healthcare funding and reform. These interrelationships are depicted in Fig. 55.3.

CLINICAL EXEMPLARS

The ability to deliver patient care is affected by a wide variety of factors related to healthcare economics and finance. These include financial strategies that distort healthcare markets, such as government regulations and public and private insurers. In addition, healthcare financing,

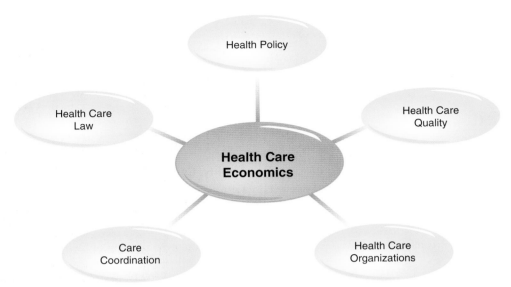

FIGURE 55.3 Health Care Economics and Interrelated Concepts.

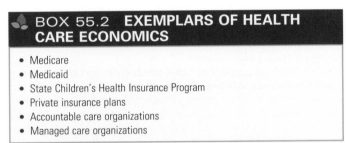

which includes government-sponsored care, managed care, and private insurance, is the driving force behind healthcare economics. Payment mechanisms dictate the use of care, and this influences the availability and scarcity of resources. These exemplars are shown in Box 55.2 and further described next.

Featured Exemplars

Medicaid

Medicaid is the nation's major public health insurance program for low-income Americans. Enacted in 1965, Medicaid has improved access to health care for low-income individuals, financed innovations in healthcare delivery, and functioned as the nation's primary source of long-term care financing. Medicaid is funded by state and federal government resources. The expansion of Medicaid by the ACA resulted in increased access to healthcare resources for those individuals and families whose income did not meet the Medicaid threshold for enrollment.[1]

State Children's Health Insurance Program

The State Children's Health Insurance Program (SCHIP) was enacted in 1997 to provide coverage to uninsured low-income children who did not qualify for Medicaid. Like Medicaid, SCHIP is jointly funded by state and federal governments and eligibility is determined by income and need.

Medicare

Medicare provides healthcare coverage for all people ages 65 years or older, people who are permanently disabled, and individuals with

end-stage renal disease. It is a federal health insurance program that individuals or their spouses have paid into through employment or self-employment taxes.[9] Medicare includes hospital insurance (Part A), supplemental medical insurance (Part B), Medicare Advantage plans (Part C), and outpatient prescription drug coverage (Part D). Part A includes hospital coverage, and Part B includes outpatient coverage and is optional—the recipient must contribute a premium each month to preserve coverage. Patients with Part A may opt to add Part B, which covers 80% of the fees for outpatient services.[9]

Accountable Care Organizations

Accountable care organizations (ACOs) are organizations of healthcare providers that are accountable for the quality, cost, and overall care of Medicare patients, for whom they provide the bulk of primary care services.[9] ACOs must have defined processes for promoting evidence-based medicine and reporting data to evaluate the quality, cost, and coordination of care. ACOs that meet specified quality standards will receive a share of the savings if Medicare's cost for the care of their assigned patients is below a certain benchmark.[9-11]

Managed Care Organizations

In managed care, healthcare providers and insurance companies share the financial responsibility for health care. Patients pay a monthly premium for healthcare insurance and are able to choose from several different plans under the managed care system, including preferred provider organizations (PPOs) and health maintenance organizations (HMOs). Patients receive health care from a list of providers who participate in the PPO or HMO.[4] The price for healthcare goods and services are set beforehand by the insurance company. Providers may suffer losses if their costs for providing care exceed the payment received.[4,9]

Private or Indemnity Health Insurance

Private health insurance may be purchased on a group basis (e.g., by a firm to cover its employees) or purchased by individual consumers. Most Americans with private health insurance receive it through an employer-sponsored program.[9] The ACA has expanded access to Medicaid and private insurance markets for individuals and families who were previously unable to obtain insurance benefits from their employer.[12]

CASE STUDY

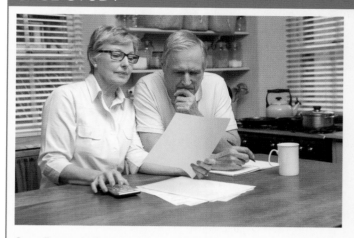

Case Presentation

Raymond Wiley operates a small business in a rural area. In his community, there is a 10-bed hospital that has a two-bed intensive care unit (ICU). A large hospital with comprehensive services is located in a nearby city 100 miles away.

Mr. Wiley became ill with fever and cough. Because his regular physician was out of town, he went to the local hospital, where he was diagnosed with pneumonia and admitted. Mr. Wiley received supportive care, but after three full days with no apparent improvement, the admitting physician transferred him to the city hospital for a referral with a pulmonologist.

Mr. and Mrs. Wiley wanted to drive to the city hospital in their private vehicle, as opposed to having Mr. Wiley transported by ambulance. Their rationale was

based on the fact that Mrs. Wiley could drive, Mr. Wiley was stable, and their insurance did not cover ambulance transport unless it was a medical emergency. Up to this point, Mr. Wiley had only received supportive care; his intravenous line had been capped, and he was taking oral antibiotics. The Wileys' request to drive themselves was refused, and Mr. Wiley was transported by ambulance; they were charged $1300 for the transport.

Once Mr. Wiley arrived at the city hospital, it took 2 days for the pulmonologist to see him because the admitting unit mixed up his name with another patient. A computed tomography scan was completed, which revealed he had a large mass and pleural effusion. Mr. Wiley was then seen by a thoracic surgeon, who scheduled him for a thoracotomy the next day—a Sunday. This required assembling an on-call surgical team at the higher weekend rate. Following surgery, Mr. Wiley was in the ICU. He experienced several postoperative complications precipitated by the initial delay in correct diagnosis and treatment. On postoperative day 11, an order was written to transfer Mr. Wiley out of the ICU to the medical unit, but because of a shortage of nursing staff on the medical unit, he remained in the ICU for two additional days before being transferred to a medical unit and discharged home later that day.

Case Analysis Questions

1. Recall the attributes of healthcare economics and finance. How are these attributes reflected in this case study?
2. Two hospitals are the settings for this story. Describe the efficiency versus equity issues of each.
3. How did inefficiencies and gaps in coverage affect the costs of care for Mr. and Mrs. Wiley and also the costs of care for each hospital?

From 4774344sean/iStock/Thinkstock.

 ACCESS EXEMPLAR LINKS IN YOUR GIDDENS EBOOK

REFERENCES

1. Mazurenko, O., Balio, C., Agarwal, R., et al. (2018). The effects of Medicaid expansion under the ACA: A systematic review. *Health Affairs*, *37*(6), 931–937.
2. Vistnes, J., & Cohen, J. (2018). Duration of uninsured spells for nonelderly adults declined after 2014. *Health Affairs*, *37*(6), 951–956.
3. Feldstein, P. (2015). *Health policy issues: An economic perspective* (6th ed.). Chicago: Health Administration Press.
4. Rice, T., & Unruh, L. (2016). *The economics of health reconsidered* (4th ed.). Chicago: Health Administration Press.
5. Jacobs, P., Cohen, M., & Keenan, P. (2017). Risk adjustment, reinsurance improved financial outcomes for individual market insurers with the highest claims. *Health Affairs*, *36*(4), 755–763.
6. Sparer, M., & Thompson, F. (2015). Government and health insurance: The policy process. In J. Knickman & A. Kovner (Eds.), *Jonas & Kovner's health care delivery in the United States* (11th ed., pp. 29–51). New York: Springer Publishing.
7. Centers for Medicare and Medicaid Services. *National health expenditures: 2016 highlights*. Retrieved from: https://www.cms.gov/research-statistics-data-and-systems/statistics-trends-and-reports/nationalhealthexpenddata/.
8. U.S. Census Bureau. *Health Insurance Coverage in The United States: 2016*. Report # P60-260. Retrieved from: https://www.census.gov/library/publications/2017/demo/p60-260.html.
9. Knickman, J. (2015). Health care financing. In J. Knickman & A. Kovner (Eds.), *Jonas & Kovner's health care delivery in the United States* (11th ed., pp. 231–251). New York: Springer Publishing.
10. Clancy, C., & Fraser, I. (2015). High quality health care. In J. Knickman & A. Kovner (Eds.), *Jonas & Kovner's health care delivery in the United States* (11th ed., pp. 273–295). New York: Springer Publishing.
11. Anderson, A., O'Rourke, E., Chin, M., et al. (2018). Promoting health equity and eliminating disparities through performance measurement and payment. *Health Affairs*, *37*(3), 371–377.
12. Hartman, M., Martin, A., Espinosa, N., et al. (2018). National health care spending in 2016: Spending and enrollment growth slow after initial coverage expansions. *Health Affairs*, *37*(1), 150–160.

Health Policy

Teresa Keller and Nancy Ridenour

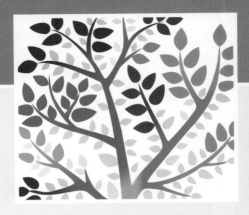

Health policies are the result of a government's interest in promoting optimal health in populations. Poor health can disrupt an individual's ability to participate in personal and civic activities and can also have a major impact on family members and communities. Widespread ill health threatens entire communities and even larger social systems, potentially disrupting the delicate web of social obligations and activities that are the supporting infrastructure of modern life.[1] The creation of public policies that address health concerns has become an accepted responsibility for governments and a means for ensuring some level of security from the personal and public consequences of ill health.

In the United States, decisions about health policy are made at various government levels and by a variety of political institutions.[2] Health policy is determined through laws, regulatory actions, judicial decisions, and administrative actions of government agencies.[3] Health policy decision-making in the United States is also affected by numerous cultural and social trends that arise from technological change, shifting demographics, economic pressures, and consumer demands.[4] The results are health policies that support a decentralized health services sector in which there is no single source of decision-making power. The healthcare policies created within this dynamic environment are meant to address policy goals through a political process of negotiation and compromise, subjected to public review and comment and, ultimately, acceptable to the widest possible majority of interested parties. However, the outcome of widespread, decentralized health policy decision making can also be that the policies are fragmented, complex, contradictory, and even unconstitutional.

This slow and sometimes cumbersome process reflects the realities of the healthcare environment in the United States. A mix of private and public systems, the healthcare environment is constantly changing and constantly creating new opportunities for innovations that are both a part of and in response to the political and cultural values of Americans. It is also this type of health policy environment that provides opportunities for nurses to intervene in the interests of their patients, families, and vulnerable populations as well as for the interests of the nursing profession. To effectively participate and advocate in the health policy decision-making process, nurses should have a clear understanding of the concept of health policy, including its definition, major characteristics, and ways it is differentiated from related concepts.

DEFINITION

A clear definition of health policy needs to account for the variety of ways that health policy is determined and controlled in the public sector. Health policy can be generally defined as a form of public policy, differentiating it from other kinds of decision-making. A classic and basic definition of public policy is what governments decide to do or not to do.[5] Public policy can also be defined as the choices made by a society or social entities that relate to public goals and priorities, as well as the choices made for allocating resources to those goals and priorities.[6] Health policy would, therefore, be the result of choices and resource allocation decisions made to support health-related goals and priorities. Longest and Darr define health policy as public policies pertaining to health that are the result of an authoritative, public decision-making process.[7] A realistic definition of the concept health policy is *goal-directed decision-making about health that is the result of an authorized, public decision-making process.* Health policy is further defined as *those actions, nonactions, directions, and/or guidance related to health that are decided by governments or other authorized entities.*

Examples of this definition of health policy include decisions related to federal subsidies for the education of health professionals, state regulations that cover insurance benefits, and court decisions that overturn these same state regulations based on constitutional arguments. This definition also includes a variety of other health policies related to Medicare reimbursements to nurse practitioners, state-mandated immunizations for schoolchildren, and the decisions of a state or federal court that establish the rights of families to make healthcare decisions for their children or elderly parents. This definition also provides for government *inaction,* as is the case when a legislative committee defers a decision on a health-related matter or when a proposed health program is not adopted by a government agency because of resource restraints. All of these examples demonstrate the public, goal-oriented, and authoritative nature of health policy decision-making. They are also examples of the divided nature of health policy decision-making in the United States.

SCOPE

Health policy as a concept can first be considered within the realm of public decision-making by political authority, including executive order, legislation, and judicial process or regulatory rule-making agencies. Health policy determined through a presidential executive order or by legislation is easily recognizable as the legitimate responsibility of elected leadership. Health policy that is the result of regulatory actions or results from the administrative decisions of government agencies is not as visible. However, the decisions made in other policy arenas may have significant impact on the distribution and quality of healthcare services.

The scope of health policy is wide and as varied as numerous entities responsible for decisions, funding, enactment, and oversight as well as the many populations and individuals who are affected by these decisions. Health policy decisions can have both macro-level (Medicare program funding) and micro-level effects (copayments for episodes of care) and can be made on the basis of economics, social justice, political trends, and/or changing social values. Health policy can also be the source of much political conflict because it has the potential to affect a large number of people, depending on the health policy goal.

Because health policy is the result of authoritative, public decision-making, a simple way to categorize it is to use the major types of political institutions established in the United States for making policy decisions. These major government institutions decide, implement, and regulate policies, including health policy, and are legally authorized to do so by constitutional arrangements. Each of these authorities uses a public process for decision-making. The major public authorities operating at the federal, state, and local levels are (1) state and national legislatures, (2) state and national as well as local courts and judiciary, (3) the executive branches of federal and state governments, and (4) regulatory agencies.[3]

Legislatures

The U.S. Congress and state legislatures are deliberative bodies that establish laws to serve some policy goal. Along with the authority to create laws, legislatures are also tasked with determining the appropriate funding for a legislative act and providing oversight for policies that are administered by government agencies. Health policy that results from law is legally binding as long as it is consistent with the authorizing constitutional framework.[3] The multiple perspectives embodied by the independently elected legislative representatives ensure the consideration of a diversity of different values in the political process.[2]

Courts and Judiciary

Health policy is the result of the political integration of values and interests. The enactment of new health laws can result in the establishment of new rights related to health programs or benefits. At the same time, it might be necessary to ensure preservation of previously established rights. Court systems play an important role in the development of health policy because federal and state courts are often the staging ground for determining rights in health policy disputes. Judiciary review can be addressed to widely varying concerns, including challenging unreasonable government action, supporting the establishment of newly created rights through legislation, and ensuring protections provided by healthcare law.[8]

Executive Branch

The executive branch of federal and state governments is responsible for the execution of laws passed by legislatures. Government executives, such as state governors and the U.S. president, oversee a vast apparatus of agencies and personnel tasked with the implementation of laws. The chief executive plays a major leadership role in health policy because of the legitimate powers of the office. Chief executives develop and implement institutional budgets, control the vast resources of the executive branch, and are usually able to use veto authority to influence policy changes. The office is also a clearly identified leadership position that provides the chief executive with a stage from which to influence the direction of health policy goals and decision-making.

Regulatory Agencies

Regulatory agencies either can be a part of the executive branch or may be independent or semi-independent organizations. These agencies are established by legislatures to implement and enforce laws through a rule-making process.[3] The rules developed by these agencies are made through public administrative processes and have the force of law. Health care is a highly regulated industry, so many health policies are established through administrative rule making by regulatory agencies. Decisions related to nursing licensure by state boards of nursing are an example of administrative rule making.

ATTRIBUTES AND CRITERIA

Health policies relate to a health concern or issue and are meant to address a public policy goal. Health policies result from a public decision-making process that directs the action or inaction of governments. The following are the *major attributes* of health policy:

1. Decisions are made by authorized government institutions such as legislatures or courts or by government-authorized entities (i.e., state boards of nursing).
2. The decision-making process is subject to public review and public input.
3. Health policies address a public policy goal.
   Minor attributes of health policy include the following:
1. Health policies are subject to ongoing review by governing institutions and by the public.
2. Health policy goals change according to changes in political and social values, trends, and attitudes.

THEORETICAL LINKS

The attributes described previously provide one means for understanding the concept of health policy. The concept can be further understood by developing an understanding of the process by which health policy is made. Anderson provides a simple framework for understanding how health policy is created through sequential stages of activities.[9] In the first step or stage, *agenda setting*, a health-related issue is identified, usually as a problem. Nurses can be especially effective in this stage by helping to frame the issue. Framing the issue means creating a particular perspective for the issue; for example, that assisted suicide is ethically justified because patients have a right to make their own healthcare decisions. In this case, a controversial issue is framed as an ethical concern.

Once defined and framed, an issue is refined through a political process that involves negotiation and debate as well as the mobilization of support from interested politicians and interest groups. The next stage is *policy formulation*, in which different policy interventions are proposed and considered. *Policy adoption* is the next stage; during this stage, a proposed intervention is selected. Selection is followed by *policy implementation* (carrying out the proposed intervention), and the process ends with *policy evaluation* or determining if the policy achieved the desired policy goals (Fig. 56.1).

This simple process model does not fully describe the complexities of health policy, but it does provide a structure for clarifying the concept. As defined previously, health policies result from political processes. A basic understanding of health policy is impossible without the consideration of key political concepts that affect policy development and implementation in the United States. These concepts are basic to the operations of constitutionally grounded governments in the United States and are necessary for ensuring health policies that account for the myriad of perspectives present in a multicultural, democratic society.

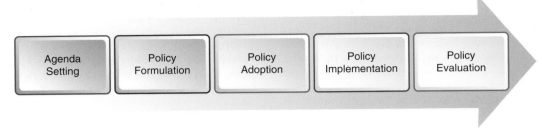

FIGURE 56.1 The Policy Process.

These include the dynamics of intergovernmental relationships, social expectations created by a system of participative governance, and effect of dominant cultural values on political processes.

Intergovernmental Relationships

The United States consists of 50 sovereign states and a federal government, united by a mutually agreed upon constitution. The U.S. Constitution provides for a division of power between the federal government and the states that seek to balance one against the other. The result is divided and limited government powers that create the need for political collaboration through systems of intergovernmental relations. The concept of *federalism* explains the dynamics of these intergovernmental relationships. Since 1965, federal funding for health policy initiatives has increased significantly. Policy initiatives requiring collaborative federal-state relations may result in state governments ceding some of their decision-making authorities in return for federal funding. The reverse can also be true: The federal government may delegate more decision-making responsibilities regarding health policies to state governments.

This results in a complex mix of collaborative strategies supported by a web of shared responsibilities between state and federal governments.[10] The effect on health policy can be profound, leading to ongoing policy changes as authority and discretionary power shift. For example, the Patient Protection and Affordable Care Act of 2010 made significant changes to health insurance markets that are traditionally regulated by state governments as part of constitutional divisions of authority.[11]

Participative Governance

State and federal constitutions also help governments operate through *consent of the governed.* Government power, especially in the United States, is limited to that allowed by the governed U.S. citizens. Representatives of the governed are elected through a public voting process to conduct the business of government and to be accountable to voters for their decisions. Citizens are also expected to attend to the actions of government and participate in the political process. Paying attention and participating include a range of activities, from the simple act of voting in elections to more active political participation such as lobbying or running for office. Participative governance is fundamental to American democratic institutions because government powers are limited and subject to the will of the governed. It is a necessary check on government power that promotes the interests and values of the citizenry rather than a few elected officials. Health policies created by governments, that do not gain support from the governed, do not enjoy much prolonged success.

Values

The dynamic relationship between the levels of government and sustained participative governance provides for the negotiation of diverse values through the political process. All health policy in the United States should be viewed as a product of negotiated values. Fairness and efficiency are the two competing values that are at the heart of most public policy decisions.[12] These values are decision drivers, and the source of much health policy conflict because decision makers must be accountable for the prudent use of public funding while also considering the needs of different constituencies. The values of fairness and efficiency are subject to interpretation and highly influenced by time, social trends, cultural expectations, economic priorities, and political situations. To ensure fairness in health policy might mean that legal rights are preserved, whether an individual right or communal rights established by law. Fairness might be interpreted as equitable distribution of health resources or as improved access to those resources. Establishing a fair policy might mean a trade-off with efficiency. Less efficient health policies may be more impartial, but they are also more costly. The additional costs must be balanced against the benefits to be derived from the policy. American democratic institutions are uniquely crafted to provide the forums necessary to manage diverse interests in open, clearly identified political processes.

Dynamic Tension

Federalism, participative governance, and the need to negotiate values produce a dynamic tension between competing health policy interests at the intersection of access, cost, and quality (Fig. 56.2). For example, providing access to care for uninsured Americans will require increased government expenditures and increases the need for tax revenue. Depending on state and national policy goals, increasing access to health care for the uninsured would bring into play the forces of federalism, politics, and economic interests from both public and private sectors. Current national concerns with the quality of health care are another major focus of U.S. health policy since the publication of two Institute of Medicine (IOM) reports that emphasized the morbidity and mortality caused by medical errors.[13,14] In an effort to address the issues of quality care while also managing costs, the federal government has issued new

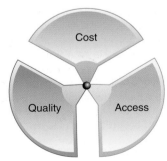

FIGURE 56.2 The Dynamic Tension among Cost, Quality, and Access.

Medicare and Medicaid guidelines that provide incentives for quality outcomes while reducing reimbursements to providers for poor quality outcomes. Improving access to quality care while decreasing overall costs also creates tensions among a variety of interested parties, including state and federal governments, regulatory agencies, legislatures, professional provider organizations, and advocacy groups.

CONTEXT TO NURSING AND HEALTH CARE

Healthcare Delivery

Health policy, as defined previously, is the result of authoritative, public decision making and is negotiated through a political process. The potential is always present that some interests will be disadvantaged compared with other interests as a result of the competition of ideas and values of the American political process. Because health policies, especially at the national level, have the potential to affect large portions of the public, an awareness of social policy, institutional policy, and markets is central to understanding health policy.

Social Policy

Social policy, in its broadest sense, relates to decisions that promote the welfare of the public.[15] Social policy can be directed at a wide variety of social concerns and issues in which the primary policy goal is not necessarily health but the policy still has an impact on health. For example, government policies related to a social policy goal that addresses obesity may result in legislation or regulation that governs the sale of high-fat/high-sugar content foods available in public schools. A state or federal law might govern WIC (women, infants, and children) payments for healthy foods at farmers' markets. A linked health policy goal would be directed at ensuring Medicare/Medicaid payments for exercise and weight loss programs.

Institutional Policy

Social policies are also not always public policies that result from political decision-making. Institutional policies govern the workplace. Nurses are often familiar with the policy and procedure manual of their unit or clinic or home health agency. An organization might have specific institutional policies developed for their workforce that relate to the prevention of obesity, such as providing exercise facilities onsite. Nurses also work with institutional policies that govern nursing practice, such as professional job descriptions. Social policies can take the form of organizational position statements established by professional organizations and advocacy groups. For example, the Student Nurses Association might adopt a resolution supporting exercise classes for student nurses.

Markets

The U.S. healthcare system is situated within an economic system that emphasizes capitalism and markets. In capitalism, markets function to ensure efficient distribution of resources to those goods and services that are the most desirable among many options. A major assumption of market systems is that the exchange of goods and services takes place among knowledgeable participants in a transparent and equitable process. This ideal is not always present in the sophisticated and expensive U.S. healthcare markets. Most Americans are dependent on the expertise of healthcare professionals to help them manage serious health problems. If they also lack adequate health insurance, they might have limited access to necessary health services if they cannot afford to pay for their care on their own.

Market ideals in these circumstances break down as the pursuit of efficient resource allocation results in resources being directed away from important social needs. An example is overallocating healthcare resources to relatively lucrative health markets such as cardiovascular

care in the hospital but limiting resources for childhood immunizations. This creates a need for government interventions to direct resources to goods and services that serve some public interest, provide for equity in market transactions, or subsidize care for vulnerable or neglected populations. In the complex U.S. healthcare system, the marriage of governments and markets is inevitable as policy goals shift between the twin values of efficiency and equity.[16]

Professional Nursing Practice

Within the framework of professional nursing practice, nurses are affected by a variety of policies that establish, regulate, and change their roles within the healthcare systems of the United States. These policies are the result of professional actions that define nursing roles, establish legal nursing authority over practice, and compel nurses to speak out and act on behalf of their patients and their profession.

Scope and Standards of Professional Nursing Practice

The licensing and regulation of health professionals, including nurses, are the responsibility of state governments. States create laws that establish professional practice acts meant to regulate health professionals. A state regulatory agency and a politically appointed board of nursing are tasked with the implementation and administration of nurse practice acts, including issuing licenses to individuals to legally practice nursing. Some state regulatory boards are specifically created for nursing and some boards are tasked with regulation of several healthcare professions, but all of these regulatory boards establish the scope of legally licensed practice and minimum standards for professional performance under that license. Regulatory boards have authority delegated by the state legislature to make rules, and these rules have the force of law. Professional practice errors that violate the provisions of the practice act are subject to disciplinary action by boards and are adjudicated by the regulatory agency through established disciplinary procedures. Boards have the authority to revoke licenses for unsafe practice as defined by the practice act, including actions or behaviors by the nurse that lie outside of the scope and standards of practice established by the license.

The regulatory environment for advanced practice registered nurses (APRNs) highlights the policy and regulatory jurisdictions of the state and federal government. APRNs are licensed by the state, and therefore rules related to their practice are determined by the state legislature. For example, prescriptive authority is variable across states.[17]

Negligence and Malpractice

Related to professional licensing are health policies that govern professional negligence or malpractice. Professional negligence occurs when the actions of the nurse are judged as substandard to what is expected in "reasonable and prudent" standard of practice and that result in harm to others. Whether a nurse is in violation of these standards is dependent on the minimum standards for practice set by the relevant state board of nursing, by practice standards published by professional societies and by standards established through similar cases decided in state courts.

Engagement and Advocacy

Nurses have a profound influence on health policy by becoming engaged in the political process and through their actions in everyday practice. Lipsky introduced the concept of "street-level bureaucracy" to define the impact of frontline workers on public policy.[18] He demonstrated that these frontline workers, such as police officers and social workers, have great influence in implementing policy at the "street level," or where the policy meets its intended beneficiaries. Street-level decision-making translates *policy intent* to *policy as experienced*. Nurses work very closely with patients and families who are the intended recipients and beneficiaries of health policies; therefore nurses are "street-level" workers who have the potential to greatly impact the implementation of policy at the bedside as well as in the community. Nurses deal with policy issues daily while ensuring the confidentiality of patient information, allocating healthcare resources through staffing assignments, or teaching patients about their healthcare rights. All these actions have a health policy impact for patients and their families that can be traced back to an authorized decision-making process. In addition, the clinical expertise of nurses can be used to influence policy at local, state, national, and international levels. Nurses are always engaged in health policy at many different levels, whether as frontline workers or as policy advocates in the regulatory, legislative, judicial, and executive arenas.

Health policies and economic consequences of these policies are everyday realities for most working nurses, regardless of their specialties or their workplace. Access to care is a national health policy issue that is driven, in part, by economics. Americans with health insurance are able to access available healthcare resources with relative ease. Uninsured Americans either do not seek care or they obtain care through federal- and state-sponsored clinical facilities or in the nation's emergency departments. The lack of secured access to primary care or to needed tertiary care results in a chaotic and costly healthcare system in which financial incentives drive health behavior and health outcomes. Nurses encounter a variety of patient care dilemmas caused by economic factors in daily practice. These situations can be the source of frustration and moral distress for many professional nurses, although they can also be the motivation for nurses to engage in political processes that produce health policies.

Nurses are in a unique and pivotal position to impact the cost/quality/access equation through advocacy. The IOM report developed in collaboration with the Robert Wood Johnson Foundation provides a road map for nurses to become active in health policy at the local, state, and national levels.[19] This report calls on all health professionals, regulatory bodies, and policymakers to improve health care by removing scope of practice barriers and increasing education, leadership, and standardized workforce data collection and analysis (Box 56.1). The Future of Nursing Dashboard[20] highlights progress of the Future of Nursing campaign. Progress had been made, but further work is needed in improving data, removing barriers to practice and care, transforming education, collaborating and leading, and promoting diversity. To foster the work needed to successfully implement policy, The Campaign for Action[21] was designed to meet the goals of the Future of Nursing Report.

Nurses can become involved in the campaign and access up-to-date information at the Center to Champion Nursing in America.[22] The campaign and the center provide an example of infrastructure and advocacy needed to ensure that policy is implemented in practice. Advocacy is providing support to others and rallying that support to a cause. Nursing interest groups might unite for the purpose of advancing national health policy reform that expands access to health care for all Americans. In another example, nurses can advocate for nurse-managed centers to be eligible for Federally Qualified Health Clinic (FQHC) status. Nurse practitioners working in an FQHC are eligible to receive a higher rate of reimbursement. Nurse-managed centers have a long history of providing primary health care to underserved patients. By advocating for FQHC status, nurses can support increased access to quality care at an affordable cost.

INTERRELATED CONCEPTS

Health policy is not an isolated concept. Several additional concepts discussed in this book are closely related to health policy (Fig. 56.3). Data and research are used to generate support and interest for a specific health policy agenda. This use of Evidence supports advocacy. Distribution of scarce resources and policy development to enhance the greater good while minimizing harm require the use of ethical decision-making. Balancing the competing values of fairness (Ethics) and efficiency (Health Care Economics) is a major challenge to designing and implementing successful health policy, particularly policies to address Health Disparities. The tension described previously among cost, quality, and access highlights these competing values. Nurses are in a unique position to combine their advocacy role of ensuring patient Safety and Health Care Quality with ethics and health economics values of fairness, access, and cost efficiency. In some contexts, it may be difficult to distinguish health policy from Health Care Law. Health policies are often the result of new laws but health policy can also become the impetus for new laws.

CLINICAL EXEMPLARS

In the United States, nurses can expect to encounter a wide variety of health policies that have a direct impact on their work. A sample of some of the more visible and relevant health policies that shape the environment of nursing is listed in Box 56.2. Although it is beyond the scope of this book to describe each exemplar in detail, a few are featured here with a brief description.

Featured Exemplars
Patient Self-Determination Act
The Patient Self-Determination Act (PDSA) requires healthcare facilities such as hospitals and nursing homes to provide patients with information related to their preferences for end-of-life care. For example, some patients will choose to accept all life-saving measures should their condition deteriorate while hospitalized. Under PDSA, the facility should inform the patients of their right to make their own decisions about their end-of-life care and the facility's policies respecting those decisions. A statement by the patient that informs the family, the provider, and the facility of the patient's wishes is known as an *advance directive* and is covered by the guidelines of this law.[23]

Emergency Medical Treatment and Labor Act of 1986
This act, commonly referred to as EMTLA, was enacted to prevent the denial of emergency services to patients chiefly because they are uninsured and unable to pay for their care. Common practice before this law was to transfer patients to "safety-net" hospitals, usually

---

BOX 56.1 Eight Recommendations From *the Future of Nursing* Report

1. Remove scope-of-practice barriers.
2. Expand opportunities for nurses to lead and diffuse collaborative improvement efforts.
3. Implement nurse residency programs.
4. Increase proportion of nurses with bachelor's degree in nursing to 80% by 2020.
5. Double the number of nurses with a doctorate by 2020.
6. Ensure that nurses engage in lifelong learning.
7. Prepare and enable nurses to lead change to advance health.
8. Build an infrastructure to collect and analyze healthcare workforce data.

Reprinted with permission from Institute of Medicine. (2011). *The future of nursing: Leading change, advancing health*, Washington DC, National Academy of Sciences.

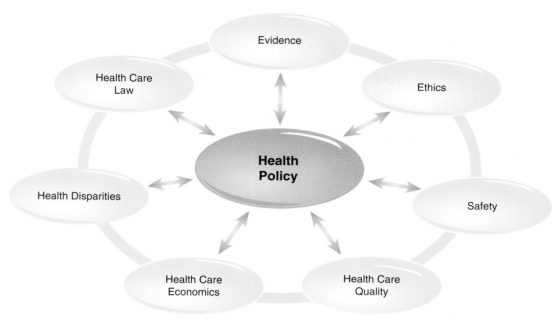

FIGURE 56.3 Health Policy and Interrelated Concepts.

Federal
- Americans with Disabilities Act of 1990
- Emergency Medical Treatment and Labor Act of 1986
- Health Information Technology for Economic and Clinical Health Act of 2009 (electronic health records)
- Health Insurance Portability and Accountability Act of 1996
- Patient Protection and Affordable Care Act of 2010
- Patient Safety and Quality Improvement Act of 2005
- Patient Self-Determination Act of 1998
- Promoting Health/Preventing Disease: Objectives for the Nation, *Healthy People 1990, 2000, 2010, 2020*
- Social Security Act of 1965 (Medicare and Medicaid)
- The Mental Health Parity and Addiction Equity Act of 2008
- U.S. Preventive Services Task Force
- Mandated Health Coverage and Medicaid Expansion 2012[32]

State
- Scope of practice and licensing for nurses as defined by state professional practice acts
- State public health programs and policies related to infectious diseases
- State public health regulations that govern healthcare facilities
- State statutes and case law related to professional negligence and malpractice

Local
- City and county fire codes that govern safe occupancy limits in healthcare facilities
- City and county ordinances that govern facility maintenance, signs, utilities, parking, and/or traffic around hospitals and other health facilities
- City and county tax districts for publicly supported facilities

🌿 **ACCESS EXEMPLAR LINKS IN YOUR GIDDENS EBOOK**

tax-supported public hospitals. EMTLA was meant to stop private hospital facilities from "patient dumping" to public hospitals at taxpayer expense.[24]

Health Information Technology for Economic and Clinical Health Act of 2009

The Health Information Technology for Economic and Clinical Health Act of 2009 (HITECH) amends the Public Health Service Act to establish a nationwide health information technology infrastructure, including the development of health IT standards, interoperability and certification, reports on quality, and reimbursement incentives to improve the quality of health care. A section of the act also addresses privacy and security concerns associated with the electronic transmission of health information through several provisions that strengthen the civil and criminal enforcement of the HIPAA rules.[25,26] As with all federal regulations, rules are updated as new issues arise. These updates are printed in the Federal Register.[27]

2012 Supreme Court Ruling on Mandated Health Coverage and Expansion of Medicaid

The Supreme Court has final authority for determining if congressional laws are congruent with the U.S. Constitution. In the case of *Independent Business v. Sebelius*, the court upheld the constitutionality of mandating health coverage (the *individual mandate*) but ruled that the expansion of Medicaid eligibility outlined in the Affordable Care Act was unconstitutional. This is an example of the interplay of checks and balances between the three branches of government. The legislative branch passed the Affordable Care Act. The judicial branch ruled on a case brought before the Supreme Court upholding one part of the law as constitutional and ruling another part of the law unconstitutional. The administrative branch under the auspices of the U.S. Department of Health and Human Services (USHHS) rewrote regulations to accommodate the ruling that Medicaid expansion cannot be required of states.[28]

Scope of Practice and Licensing for Nurses

The U.S. Constitution is based on federalism—sharing of powers between the national, state, and local governments. The federal government is granted powers explicitly outlined in the Constitution. The 10th Amendment of the Bill of Rights provides that states have powers not outlined in the Constitution and not prohibited by the states.[29] Regulation of healthcare professionals is one of the powers granted to states. Each state issues licenses based on state licensure rules and regulates health professional behavior based on state laws and regulations. For nurses, state licensure is usually regulated through a *nurse practice act*.

CASE STUDY

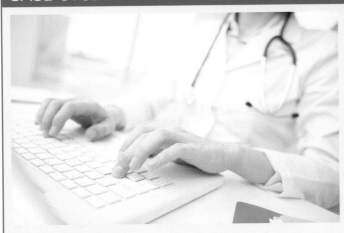

Case Presentation

The confidentiality of medical information became an *agenda* item for Congress when electronic data systems became widely adopted throughout the United States. The increased use of computers in health care had created the capacity for critical healthcare information to be efficiently shared among healthcare providers and among insurance companies. Advocates for patient confidentiality and information privacy argued that the ease of information sharing through electronic transmission of records would result in personal health information becoming available to a wide variety of interested parties. Access to this information could result in a variety of actions, including denial of coverage through employer-sponsored plans to individuals or family members with chronic or debilitating conditions. Other unfavorable outcomes from the unrestricted sharing of private health information could also result, such as the sale of mailing lists of individuals with particular medical conditions to companies with a commercial interest in obtaining those lists.

The intent of the Health Insurance Portability and Accountability Act (HIPAA) of 1996 was to limit the ability of employers to deny health insurance coverage to their employees based on preexisting medical conditions. In the *formulation*

of a policy response, the intervention chosen by Congress was to limit access to healthcare information to only those parties with a legitimate role in the financing and delivery of services, specifically healthcare providers, insurance companies, and third-party contractors.[30] Through HIPAA, Congress directed the USDHHS to *implement* the policy by developing privacy rules that protect electronically transmitted health information. These rules cover any entity that must have access to this information for legitimate purposes and provide guidelines for determining access to and disclosure of protected health information. Criminal and financial penalties are provided for proven HIPAA violations, including federal prison sentences for perpetrators and fines of up to $250,000. Investigations and prosecutions of HIPAA violations are the responsibility of the U.S. Department of Justice.[29]

One of the federal agencies tasked with public review and reporting for federal policies is the U.S. Government Accountability Office (GAO). The GAO has published different reviews of HIPAA at the request of government officials throughout the years since the passage of the statute, and these reports are publicly available on the GAO website. A recent review documents the ongoing issues of implementation of this widespread policy that governs the electronic transmission of healthcare information.[31] HIPAA provides broad guidelines for the protection of patient information that must be interpreted for implementation. Covered entities targeted by the statute are expected to develop HIPAA-compliant policies that govern the treatment of protected health information in their organizations and during transactions with contracted third parties. The GAO report notes that there is still much guidance to be issued by USDHHS to assist these entities in complying with HIPAA guidelines. This guidance will be created through USDHHS rule-making authority and will be publicly available for comment and feedback by affected organizations and the general public during the rule-making process.

Case Analysis Questions

1. In what ways does this case demonstrate components of health policy as a concept?
2. Why was this policy an issue at the federal level as opposed to being managed at the state level?

From shironosov/iStock/Thinkstock/

 ACCESS EXEMPLAR LINKS IN YOUR GIDDENS EBOOK

REFERENCES

1. Knickman, J., & Kovner, A. (2015). The challenge of health care development and health policy. In J. Knickman & A. Kovnor (Eds.), *Jonas and Kovners' health care delivery in the United States* (11th ed., pp. 4–5). New York: Springer Publishing.
2. Peterson, M. (2014). Congress. In J. Morone & D. Elke (Eds.), *Health politics and policy* (5th ed., pp. 30–55). Clifton Park, NY: Delmar.
3. Sparer, M., & Thompson, F. (2015). Government and health insurance: The policy process. In J. Knickman & A. Kovner (Eds.), *Jonas and Kovners' health care delivery in the United States* (11th ed., pp. 29–51). New York: Springer Publishing.
4. Shortell, S., & Kaluzny, A. (2006). Organization theory and health services management. In S. Shortell & A. Kaluzny (Eds.), *Health care management: Organization design and behavior* (5th ed., pp. 5–41). Clifton Park, NY: Delmar.
5. Dye, T. (2016). *Understanding public policy* (15th ed.). Pearson.
6. Mason, D., Leavitt, J., & Chaffee, M. (2013). Policy and politics: A framework for action. In D. Mason, J. Leavitt, & M. Chaffee (Eds.), *Policy and politics in nursing and health care* (6th ed., pp. 1–16). St Louis: Saunders.
7. Longest, B., & Darr, K. (2010). *Managing health services organizations and systems* (5th ed.). Baltimore: Health Professions Press.
8. Keepnews, D., Betts, V., & Gentry, J. (2016). Nursing and the courts. In D. Mason, D. Gardner, F. Outlaw, & E. O'Grady (Eds.), *Policy and politics in nursing and health care* (7th ed., pp. 447–456). St Louis: Elsevier.

9. Anderson, J. E. (2010). *Public policymaking: An introduction* (7th ed.). Boston: Wadsworth Cengage.

10. Thompson, F., & Cantor, J. (2014). Federalism. In J. Morone & D. Elke (Eds.), *Health politics and policy* (5th ed., pp. 94–115). Clifton Park, NY: Delmar.

11. Weil, A. (2013). Promoting cooperative federalism through state shared savings. *Health Affairs, 32*(8), 1493–1500.

12. Stone, D. (2014). Values in health policy: Understanding fairness and efficiency. In J. Morone & D. Elke (Eds.), *Health politics and policy* (5th ed., pp. 2–3). Clifton Park, NY: Delmar.

13. Institute of Medicine. (2000). *To err is human: Building a safer health system*. Washington, DC: National Academies Press.

14. Institute of Medicine. (2001). *Crossing the quality chasm: A new health system for the 21st century*. Washington, DC: National Academies Press.

15. O'Grady, E., Mason, D., Outlaw, F., & Gardner, D. (2016). Frameworks for action in policy and politics. In D. Mason, D. Gardner, F. Outlaw, & E. O'Grady (Eds.), *Policy and politics in nursing and health care* (7th ed., pp. 1–21). St. Louis: Elsevier.

16. Rice, T. (2014). Markets and politics. In J. Morone & D. Elke (Eds.), *Health politics and policy* (5th ed., pp. 14–25). Clifton Park, NY: Delmar.

17. American Association of Nurse Practitioners. *State practice environment 2018*. Retrieved from https://www.aanp.org/legislation-regulation/state-legislation/state-practice-environment.

18. Lipsky, M. (1980). *Street-level bureaucracy: Dilemmas of the individual in public services*. New York: Russell Sage Foundation.

19. Institute of Medicine. (2010). *The future of nursing: Leading change, advancing health*. Washington, DC: National Academies Press.

20. Future of Nursing Campaign for Action Dashboard. (2017). Retrieved from https://campaignforaction.org/wp-content/uploads/2017/07/Dashboard-Indicators_Dec17.pdf.

21. Campaign for Action. (2018). Retrieved from https://campaignforaction.org.

22. Center to Champion Nursing in America. (2018). Retrieved from https://www.aarp.org/ppi/initiatives/.

23. American Bar Association. (2015). *Health care advanced directives*. Retrieved from http://www.americanbar.org/groups/public_education/resources/law_issues_for_consumers/patient_self_determination_act.html.

24. Rosenblum, S., Cartwright-Smith, L., Hirsch, J., et al. (2012). Case studies at Denver Health: "Patient dumping" in the emergency department despite EMTALA, the law that banned it. *Health Affairs, 31*(8), 1749–1756.

25. U.S. Department of Health and Human Services. (2009). *HITECH act enforcement interim final rule*. Retrieved from http://www.hhs.gov/ocr/privacy/hipaa/administrative/enforcementrule/hitechenforcementifr.html.

26. HealthIT.gov. (2015). *Health IT legislation and regulation*. Retrieved from http://www.healthit.gov/policy-researchers-implementers/health-it-legislation.

27. Federal Register. (2013). *Modifications to the HIPPA Privcy, Security, Enforcement, and Breach Notification Rules Under the HITECH Act*. Retrieved from https://www.gpo.gov/fdsys/pkg/FR-2013-01-25/pdf/2013-01073.pdf.

28. Courts, U.S. (n.d.). *About the Supreme Court*. Retrieved from http://www.uscourts.gov/educational-resources/get-informed/supreme-court/about-supreme-court.aspx.

29. The White House. (n.d.). *State & local government*. Retrieved from http://www.whitehouse.gov/our-government/state-and-local-government. see also http://bensguide.gpo.gov/9-12/government/federalism2.html.

30. Flores, J., & Dodier, A. (2005). HIPAA: Past, present and future implications for nurses. *Online Journal of Issues in Nursing, 10*(2), Manuscript 4.

31. Harman, L. (2005). HIPAA: A few years later. *Online Journal of Issues in Nursing, 10*(2), Manuscript 2.

32. Rosenblum, S., & Westmorland, T. (2012). The Supreme Court's surprising decision on the Medicaid expansion: How will the federal government and states proceed? *Health Affairs, 31*(8), 1663–1672.

CONCEPT

57

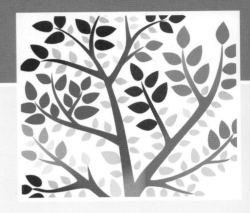

Health Care Law

Kathleen A. Hessler

Ours is a government of liberty, by, through and under the law. No man is above it, and no man is below it.
—**Theodore Roosevelt**

Healthcare delivery in the United States is a complex network of business systems that include healthcare providers, payers, and adaptable organizations. Healthcare businesses must continue to evolve to meet the rapidly changing demands of the legal and regulatory environment. There are numerous explanations for the complexity in today's healthcare systems. Key reasons include the gap in care affordability, disparate geographic locations and delivery systems, an increase in fraudulent billing activity across provider types, and increasing medical specializations in the delivery of care. Additionally, the emphasis on quality of care and the rise of state medical malpractice cases across the country have created greater scrutiny on the importance of the standards of care and evidence-based best practices for all healthcare professionals. Furthermore, these professionals are subject to state statutes and regulations regarding their license to practice under the state law. Nurses must be aware of the various aspects of healthcare law and its applications. More importantly, nurses must understand the impact and consequences of these laws on nursing practice.

DEFINITION

Law is a system of rules that are created by a society or government to promote or regulate specific behaviors and relationships, to manage crime, and to establish business agreements. Laws may either prohibit action or require action on the part of individuals, businesses, or the government. Health law is a specialization in the field of law, which deals with a myriad of aspects of health care, including, but not limited to, the practices of healthcare practitioners and provider entities, the rights of patients, quality of care issues, and requirements of payment for medical and healthcare services. Healthcare professional licensure issues and certification matters are recognized by many as part of the spectrum of healthcare law as are state medical malpractice acts. For the purpose of this concept presentation, healthcare law is defined as "the practice of law involving federal, state, or local law and rules or regulations regarding the delivery of healthcare services. In addition to healthcare provider issues and regulations of providers, health law includes legal issues regarding relationships between and among providers and payors."[1]

SCOPE

The scope of healthcare law involves a collection of laws that have a direct impact on the delivery of health care or on the relationships among those in the business of health care or between the provider, payors, and consumers and patients of health care. The executive, legislative, and judicial branches of federal and state governments hold the authority for the creation, implementation, and enforcement of law. The process for creating healthcare law is through the United States Congress or the state *legislative processes*, *regulatory activities* by government agencies, or through *precedent setting judicial opinions* resulting from court cases. These processes represent an interwoven process that fosters a continuing evolution in healthcare law (Fig. 57.1).

Sources of Law

Healthcare law originates from primary and secondary sources of state and federal law, including, but not limited to, constitutional law, statutory law, administrative law, common law, tort law, contract law, criminal law, and in some instances, employment law (Fig. 57.2).

Federal statutory law is formed under the authority of the Federal United States Constitution and enacted through Congress. Similarly, each state authorizes the creation of law under its constitution, or similar document, and enacts law through the state legislative process. And just as our federal government has an organized judicial branch, so does each state. While federal law preempts state laws, state laws may be more restrictive than federal law; in these cases, the state's more restrictive measures govern. If state law conflicts with federal law, federal law governs. In some situations, like medical marijuana, the federal government has chosen to ignore enforcement measures in the face of state law.

Constitutional Law

Constitutional law deals with the fundamental principles by which a government exercises its authority. The United States Constitution defines the role, powers, and structures of our government—namely, the executive, legislative, and judicial branches. It also describes the basic rights of citizens and relationships between our federal government and the sovereignty of the states. Although the Constitution does not have a direct relationship to health care, the most frequently used grant of power in the Constitution for the enactment of healthcare legislation is found in Article I, Section 8 (last sentence): "To make all Laws, which shall be necessary and proper for carrying into Execution the foregoing

Powers"[2] (commonly known as the taxing and spending power as well as the power to regulate interstate commerce).

While the United States Supreme Court has not interpreted the Constitution as guaranteeing citizens the right to health care, the Supreme Court has held that the Due Process Clause of the Fourteenth Amendment provides protection under the Constitution for certain "liberty rights" related to privacy. Legislation created by federal or state governments that implicates the right to privacy has been reviewed under the strict scrutiny standard of review. Historically, the right to privacy has been upheld to encompass several rights, including, but not limited to, the right to use contraception (*Griswold v. Connecticut*, 1965),[3] to have an abortion (*Roe v. Wade*, 1973),[4] and the right to refuse medical treatment that sustains life as confirmed in the 1990 case of *Cruzan v. Missouri*.[5]

Statutory (Legislative) Law

Federal and state statutory laws are important sources of healthcare law. These are laws that arise from legislative action. Many legislative laws at both the federal and the state level are enacted with the intent to directly impact the businesses or provider relationships in health care or to provide some form of health care for defined groups of people, such as the poor or chronically ill. Other laws may not have been enacted with the intent to directly affect health care, but they may influence the business of health care nonetheless, such as insurance laws. Because each state has an independent legislative body, the laws that are enacted may vary in title and scope, but the underlying authority to legislate for the general health and welfare of the people is the same.

As an example, the Social Security Act Amendments of 1965 are the federal legislation that established the Medicare and Medicaid programs.[6] While the Medicare program is fully administered and funded by the federal government, the Medicaid programs are administered by the states and share the responsibility of financing the programs with the federal government. Some states have several separate Medicaid programs.

Administrative Law and Regulation

Administrative agencies protect public interest and act as agents for the executive branches of the federal and state governments. Government

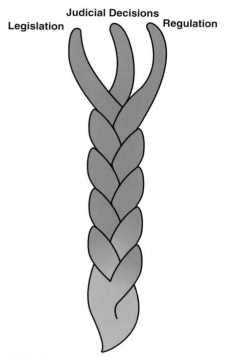

FIGURE 57.1 Scope of Health Care Law.

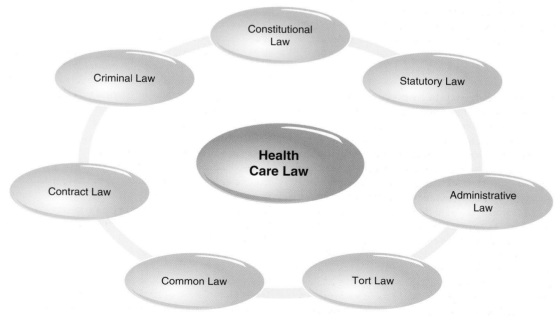

FIGURE 57.2 Sources of Law.

agencies, as part of the executive branch of government, have the power to enact rules and regulations to promote public health and ensure that the intent of legislation passed by the Congress or the state legislature is executed under the authority of the statute. They also have the authority to enforce the law and levy fines and remedies pursuant to regulation. Regulations aim to address healthcare system objectives, such as protecting the public's health by promoting quality services, preventing and controlling communicable disease, protecting the public against bioterrorism, ensuring disaster preparedness of healthcare providers, reducing healthcare costs through oversight of health insurance programs, promoting access to care, and protecting consumers who are in the market for health insurance and other types of coverage.

Examples of a federal administrative Cabinet-level department that has a significant effect on healthcare law is the U.S. Department of Health and Human Services (DHHS or HHS) and its multiple government agencies. The U.S. Department of Veteran Affairs (DVA) is a peer organization to HHS and promotes and provides healthcare services for veterans. Each state has its own Department of Health (DOH) and Department of Human Services (DHS). The states also have the authority to regulate the practice of healthcare practitioners through state licensing boards, which are vested with executive powers to implement regulations through statutory practice acts.

Common Law

Common law, also referred to as judge-made law, case law, or judicial precedent, is a body of law derived from decisions made by appellate or supreme courts. The opinions of appeals court and Supreme Court become precedent to bind judges and litigants in the future in the applicable jurisdiction. Common law can evolve and change with time, depending on the facts and legal issues in a case. Common law stands on equal footing with regulations and statutory law. However, case law decisions may further limit or expand statutory or regulatory law if the legislation or regulations are ambiguous and the court's opinion includes an interpretation of the law that was previously unclear. Sometimes one area of the country may not have addressed a question that another area of the country has already answered in the courts, and it may adopt the ruling of another area without going through the process of litigating the question in the courts.

Tort Law

A tort is a wrongful and unreasonable action or omission to an individual or entity against a person who suffers harm from the act or omission. The individual harmed, also referred to as the *plaintiff* in a lawsuit, suffers a loss, which results in liability by the person responsible for the injury—referred to as the *defendant* in a lawsuit. A tort is customarily defined as a civil wrong under state statute or common law and is the basis for civil lawsuits. The most familiar basis for individual liability of nurses, physicians, and other healthcare providers, including hospitals, is rooted in tort law and is often referred to as medical negligence or medical malpractice. Tort law has been responsible for shaping and defining many quality and safety standards of health care.

The goals of tort law are (1) to provide relief to the harmed party, (2) to impose liability on those responsible for the harm, and (3) to deter others from such harmful acts. There are three categories of tort law: *intentional torts*, such as assault or battery; *negligent or unintentional torts*, such as a slip and fall or a car accident; and *strict liability*, where no degree of care matters, such as ultrahazardous materials or dangerous animals.

Contract Law

Contract law is the body of law that governs mutual agreements between two or more individuals or groups of people or businesses. Contract law is a prominent mechanism under which healthcare services and transactions are conducted. The complex network of healthcare contracts extends but is not limited to healthcare contracts between insurance companies and consumers as well as agreements between insurance carriers and provider hospitals, physicians, durable medical equipment companies, and pharmacies. Healthcare business transactions (the buying and selling of healthcare business) are accomplished through contracts, as are other business relationships between healthcare entities and vendor businesses.

Contracts govern relationships between the Centers for Medicare & Medicaid Services (CMS) and the State Survey Agency's agreement to monitor certified Medicare healthcare providers in that state. Additionally, CMS contracts with companies to pay and audit Medicare claims for compliance with Medicare program and billing requirements. These are called Medicare Administrative Contractors (MACs).[7] Other examples of healthcare government contractors are Recovery Auditor Contractors (RACs), Zone Program Integrity Contractors (ZPICs), United Program Integrity Contractors (UPICs), and Quality Improvement Organizations (QICs).[8]

Admission agreements and patient consent forms of some healthcare services may be construed as a contract between the patient and the healthcare facility or provider. Some healthcare entities require patients to sign arbitration agreements on admission, just as many employers require new employees to sign such contractual agreements. However, the validity of patient arbitration agreements continues to be challenged in the courts; the courts do not always uphold them as valid contracts.

Criminal Law

Criminal law relates to crime and prohibits conduct that threatens or harms others or endangers the property or health or safety of individuals. It is distinguishable from civil law as it authorizes punitive treatment of the offender. The federal government and each state have its own criminal code. Criminal penalties are levied under healthcare laws, including felonies associated with Medicare or insurance reimbursement fraud, abusive billing or referral practices, and misrepresentation of practitioner qualifications.

In particular, the federal Anti-Kickback Statute[9] is a criminal statute that prohibits the exchange, or an offer to exchange, anything of value to induce referrals to federal or state healthcare programs. Convictions for a single violation under this Statute have increased under the Bipartisan Budget Act of 2018 to fines of $25,000 to $100,000 and up to 10 years' imprisonment. Over the past several decades, a staggering number of healthcare providers have been indicted and convicted or have been excluded from providing healthcare services under the Medicare or state Medicaid programs for engaging in behaviors that solicit or pay for referrals of Medicare patients or beneficiaries.

Some states have passed criminal statutes that encourage prosecution of healthcare workers in cases of intentional or neglectful patient care. For instance, in New Mexico, a state statute called Resident Abuse and Neglect[10] empowers the State's Attorney General's Office to prosecute healthcare providers or caregivers who harm residents in a care facility.

ATTRIBUTES AND CRITERIA

Attributes and criteria represent identified characteristics and elements of a concept to enhance consistency in meaning and application of the concept. These include the structural elements of a concept and "rules" that must be present to qualify as a concept. Three major attributes for Health Care Law are as follows:

- Laws are created by Congress or the state legislatures on behalf of healthcare consumers to achieve healthcare policy goals.

- Regulatory agencies are charged with drafting and implementing regulations to ensure the effectiveness, and the intent of the statutes are accomplished without overly burdensome activity.
- Enforcement procedures are associated with subsequent punishment. Examples include fines and settlements, exclusion from government payment sources, auditing and monitoring programs, and jail time (if criminal law is implicated).

In addition to these attributes, there are generally accepted standards or guidelines that can be utilized to judge or determine adherence to the law and to assist providers in interpreting the law. These may include government guidance documents such as Medicare Interpretive Guidelines, advisory opinions, compliance program guidance, work plans, or other government tools. Other measures that have an impact on healthcare law include accreditation standards, evidence-based best practices, codes of conduct, standards of ethics, and social expectations and customs.

Though government guidance, accreditation standards, and codes of conduct are different from healthcare laws (they are not legally binding), if such guidance or standards are followed, a provider is likely to be deemed in compliance with these standards. In addition, a provider's compliance may be used as a defense in mitigating allegations of wrong-doing in litigation, government fraud actions, and alleged regulatory deficiencies. Healthcare law can be distinguished and differentiated from accreditation requirements, social expectations, and customs by considering the major and minor attributes presented in Box 57.1.

THEORETICAL LINKS

Legal theory is also known as *jurisprudence* and is the theoretical study of law, principally by philosophers. However, in the 20th century, social scientists studied the theory of law, striving to gain a deeper under-standing of legal reasoning, legal systems, and institutions as well as the role law plays in our society.[11] There are several theories of juris-prudence, but the one most applicable to healthcare law is *normative jurisprudence*, which "is concerned with 'evaluative' theories of law. It deals with what the goal or purpose of law is or what moral or political theories provide a foundation for the law."[12] In addition to the questions of defining what law is, normative jurisprudence tries to answer what the proper function of law is or what actions should be subject to legal sanctions and what level of punishment should be allowed.

The need for healthcare laws has been determined through social practices, values, and morals, and the evolution of a complex healthcare industry that touches every American. There have been arguments over the course of many decades as to whether all Americans have a right to health care. The healthcare laws have evolved in an effort—albeit not always successful—to distribute health care fairly and equitably and to make it affordable to all. Healthcare laws are also enacted to monitor and punish bad behavior and bad actors who try to profit unlawfully in the healthcare industry.

CONTEXT TO NURSING AND HEALTH CARE

The field of healthcare law is complicated and continues to evolve with the passing of statutory laws and the subsequent implementation of regulations by the applicable federal or state agencies. Many of these laws have a direct or indirect impact on nursing practice and livelihood. This section touches on the most important areas of healthcare law that impact the professional practice of nurses working in health care today. The body of law and its impact on health care is vast and nurses should try to keep abreast of issues that are pertinent to their area of practice as well as to healthcare delivery.

Federal Statutory Laws Impacting Health Care

Federal statutory laws have had sweeping effects on the delivery of health care over the past half-century or more. Some examples include the Social Security Amendments of 1965 and 1983.[13] Others include the Consolidated Omnibus Budget Reconciliation Act (COBRA) of 1986 and the Omnibus Budget Reconciliation Act (OBRA) 1987 (also known as the Federal Nursing Home Reform Act),[14] the Patient Self-Determination Act of 1991,[15] and the Health Insurance Portability and Accountability Act (HIPAA).[16] The most sweeping healthcare law in recent years that has affected all Americans, especially healthcare con-sumers and healthcare providers who participate in the Medicare program, is the Patient Protection and Affordable Care Act 2010,[17] also known as the Affordable Care Act (ACA) or Obamacare. This federal statute requires Centers for Medicare and Medicaid Services (CMS) to draft and implement a vast array of regulations over several years' time. Implementation of regulations continues to require significant effort in the development of policy and in the monitoring of healthcare pro-viders to ensure compliance with new insurance requirements, billing and payment changes, compliance program requirements, and quality of care initiatives. Documentation of nursing care provided to patients should comply with the documentation requirements set forth by CMS for designated service lines, such as hospitals, home health, hospice, and others. Additionally, nurse notes should be accurate, timely, and reflect compliance with standards of care and quality initiatives.

Administration and Regulation
Federal Regulation and Administrative Agencies

The US Department of Health and Human Services (HHS)[18] is a federal Cabinet-level department under which eleven federal agencies operate. (Box 57.2). The agencies administer a variety of health and human services and conduct research while protecting and serving Americans. For example, CMS has a broad authority to draft the Medicare and Medicaid Conditions of Participation (CoPs) regulations for hospitals, skilled nursing facilities, home health agencies, and hospice providers, to name a few. These regulations focus on patient and resident rights,

---

BOX 57.1   Attributes and Criteria of Health Care Law

Attributes
- Created by a government body with appropriate authority, such as a legis-lature, agency, or court (judicial decision)
- Requires or prohibits actions
- Usually has enforceable sanctions such as fines, exclusion for government programs, auditing, and monitoring programs such as Corporate Integrity Agreements or Imprisonment
- Publicly available and accessible by any individual or group
- Consistent with national and state constitutions
- Can be modified, changed, or upheld through authoritative action

Criteria
- Guidance to promote a policy goal and provide steps to achieve compliance
- Interpretive guidelines such as State Operations Manuals (SOM)—Guide to Surveyors
- Standards of practice or best practices
- Reports from government agencies and data analytics
- Law and guidance may be self-limited, expiring after some time-period
- May vary in scope

BOX 57.2 Operating Agencies of the U.S. Department of Health and Human Service

- Administration for Children and Families (ACF)
- Administration for Community Living (ACL)
- Agency for Healthcare Research and Quality (AHRQ)
- Agency for Toxic Substances and Disease Registry (ATSDR)
- Centers for Disease Control and Prevention (CDC)
- Centers for Medicare & Medicaid Services (CMS)
- Food and Drug Administration (FDA)
- Health Resources and Services Administration (HRSA)
- Indian Health Services (IHS)
- National Institutes of Health (NIH)
- Substance Abuse and Mental Health Services Administration (SAMHSA)

health standards that define quality and safety, consents for treatment, coordination of care and care planning, quality assurance and performance improvement programs, and other expectations for healthcare organizations participating in the Medicare and Medicaid programs. Healthcare organizations must be in compliance with the full range of CoPs regulations before they are granted certification to bill the Medicare or Medicaid programs. In addition to the federal agencies, HHS houses other offices and important programs that have healthcare oversight. For example, the Office for Human Research Protections (OHRP) protects the rights of human subjects involved in health research supported by HHS. This office was created in response to findings from the famous 1979 Belmont Report,[19] which exposed abuses and atrocities of subjects involved in research conducted by the federal government.

Licensing and Scope of Nursing Practice

All states and U.S. territories have legislated a Nurse Practice Act (NPA). This act establishes a Board of Nursing (BON) that has the authority to draft regulations or administrative rules to clarify and implement the act. Proposed rules and regulations must be consistent with the NPA and must go through a process of public review before enactment. Once enacted, they have the full force of the law in that state.[20] The goals of a BON are to protect the public's health and welfare through monitoring safe and competent nursing care. In addition to establishing the educational, examination, and competency requirements necessary to obtain a nursing license, practice acts and regulatory agencies also establish and enforce the context and scope of licensure within which regulated professionals must comply to retain their status as licensees in good standing. The scope of practice for professional nursing is the range of permissible activity as defined by the law; it defines what nurses can and cannot do.

Because the scope of nursing practice is defined by state legislation, there is variability from state to state in the range of activities that are legally authorized. It is important that a nurse become familiar with the practice act and the scope of practice in the state or territory where the nurse works. Some states are compact states offering nurses one multistate license; nurses should ensure they understand the scope of their compact license if they plan to work in more than one state. Although there is general consistency for the scope of practice for the professional registered nurse, there is significant variability for the defined scope of practice of a licensed practical or vocational nurse (LPN or LVN). Finally, the range of practice for an advanced practice registered nurse (APRN) varies considerably from state to state.

The BON also investigates and decides cases involving alleged violations of the state practice act and licensure. When a nurse is in violation of the practice act, the state board exercises its power to discipline the nurse to a degree consistent with the board's assessment of the severity of the problem and potential risk to the public. Disciplinary actions can range from censure and penalties, mandatory education, and ethics programs to progressively more undesirable consequences, such as probation, suspension, and revocation or denial of licensure. Boards are required to report disciplinary actions to the National Practitioner Data Bank (NPDB). The NPDB is used by healthcare entities as a workforce tool for licensing, hiring, and credentialing decisions. Unlicensed practice of nursing is a criminal violation, and if a person is convicted, he/she may result in fines and/or imprisonment in most states.[21]

Licensing of Healthcare Organizations

States have the authority to license and regulate healthcare facilities and businesses. Licensure requirements vary in terms of the services provided, the need for the service, physical location, building structure, safety, and staffing requirements. Most states require licensing of hospitals, nursing facilities, home health agencies, and hospices. Assisted living facilities (ALF) are state licensed with no accompanying federal regulations. The State Survey Agency will survey healthcare facilities and providers under the state licensing requirements that often mirror or are more restrictive than the Medicare CoPs. If a facility or business becomes certified under the Medicare program, the provider will be subject to both state and federal monitoring surveys.

Healthcare Fraud

Government oversight for healthcare fraud extends across multiple state and federal agencies and includes a vast network of activity and enforcement. Fraudulent and abusive billing practices have been detected over many years and have resulted in billions of lost dollars to the Medicare program. During 1995–1996, under the Clinton administration, HHS OIG conducted a pilot study called "Operation Restore Trust" in five states. More than 40 million dollars was recovered to the Medicare program with resulting criminal convictions and successful civil settlements.[22] This led to the establishment of the national Health Care Fraud and Abuse Control Program (HCFAC) in 1997.

Every year, the HCFAC provides enormous paybacks to the government from alleged fraudulent or abusive practices. In the fiscal year 2017, federal health fraud recoveries totaled $2.6 billion.[23] Additionally, this program led to an increasing number of civil and criminal convictions as well as provider exclusions from federal government healthcare programs. For example, under the Federal False Claims Act, the Department of Justice (DOJ) opened 967 new criminal healthcare fraud investigations in 2017 and filed criminal charges in 439 cases for healthcare fraud–related crimes.[24]

Medical Negligence and Medical Malpractice

Medical negligence is enforced under state statutory law as well as tort law and is referred to as medical malpractice. In general, there are four elements to a civil medical malpractice lawsuit for which the plaintiff or accusing party must prove to receive compensation. The patient must show evidence that the nurse, physician, or alleged healthcare provider (1) owed the patient a duty/standard of care, (2) breached the duty/standard to provide adequate care, (3) caused injury to the patient (causation), and (4) caused an injury that resulted in damages.

Duty of Care

The evidence presented by the patient plaintiff must establish that the nurse or healthcare provider owed a professional duty to the person harmed beyond the duty to exercise ordinary care. Professional duty arises from a special relationship between healthcare providers and patients. The standard of care for nurses is the degree of care that would be exercised by a "reasonably prudent nurse" acting under the same or similar circumstances. Examples of standards of care may include hospital or provider policies and procedures, the Code of Ethics for Nurses,[25] scope of practice under the state NPA, and accreditation standards such as The Joint Commission. Nurses with different areas of expertise or specialty practice are held accountable to the standard of care applicable to that specialty.

Breach of Duty

The second element that must be satisfied to establish liability is a breach of duty. Healthcare providers breach their duty to patients when they fall below the standard of care or deviate from the standard. It is important to remember that not all deviations from the standard of care will result in tort liability. For example, it is below the standard of care for a nursing professional to administer the wrong dose of medication to a patient. If the medication error does not result in harm or injury to the patient, the nurse will not likely face tort liability. However, the nurse may be terminated from employment or be subject to a disciplinary action by the state BON.

Causation

Causation is the link between breach and injury. If the injury would **not** have occurred "but for" the defendant's actions, there is causation. Causation establishes that the breach of duty legally caused injury to the patient. The breach of duty or violation of standard of care must be the direct or proximate cause of the harm that the patient experienced; in other words, if the breach had not occurred, no harm would have come to the patient. In many instances, causation can be difficult to prove in medical malpractice cases.

Injury or Harm

The final element to be satisfied in a negligence action is proof of injury or harm. The resultant harm may be physical or a combination of physical, mental, emotional, or financial harm. In some states, a patient cannot recover from emotional harm alone without an accompanying physical disability. An injury must be established by a preponderance of the evidence. Damages can be economic or noneconomic. Economic damages such as loss of work and medical care are easier to determine when compared with noneconomic damages, such as pain and suffering, loss of consortium, or others. A jury may award punitive damages if they believed (and were instructed accordingly from the judge) that the action or inaction of the healthcare provider was so egregious that the negligence rose to a level of gross negligence.

Employer/Employee Liability

Professional liability can attach to an employer for the negligent acts of its employee. This is known as vicarious liability, and it arises from the common law doctrine of *respondent superior*, a Latin-derived term that means "let the master answer." Under vicarious liability, an employer can be liable for the acts of its employee if the employee was acting as the agent of the employer and the actions that resulted in injury occurred within the scope of employment. To reduce the risk of liability, nurses should be cognizant of best practice measures and include timely and truthful documentation to accurately support the services that were rendered, including, but not limited to, patient education and training. Nurses should clearly understand and review the clinical policies and procedures where they work and understand the clinical regulatory requirements for the service line in which they are practicing (e.g., hospital, nursing facility, or home health or hospice agency). Additionally, nurses must be up-to-date on nursing procedure and expertise in the areas they practice. A nurse should seek additional training if he/she does not feel qualified to perform a specific task such as wound care or administration of chemotherapy. Nurses should consider options to purchase professional liability insurance. While a hospital or other healthcare provider may cover a nurse in an allegation of medical or nursing malpractice under the entity's insurance coverage, that coverage may be limited and does not usually extend to BON actions or other unforeseen events.

Laws That Affirm Patient Decision-Making
Consent for Treatment

Historically, medical consent laws were largely shaped by common law. The common-law principle of self-determination essentially guarantees an individual's right to privacy and protection against the actions of others that threaten bodily harm. One of the first cases in the United States that established principles of consent for medical treatment was *Schloendorff v. Society of New York Hospital* (1914).[26] The case involved a woman who was admitted to a hospital for a stomach ulcer and the physician ultimately diagnosed a fibroid tumor. Although the patient consented to an examination under ether anesthesia, she refused the offered surgery. After the examination, the surgeon took her into the operating room and removed the tumor without her consent. Ultimately, there were consequences from the surgery and the plaintiff filed suit based on the harm she sustained from complications of the surgery. This case underscores a patient's right to make decisions about their body, especially when an invasive procedure is being performed.

The concept of consent evolved into a process known as *informed consent*. Healthcare practitioners are obligated to disclose and explain procedures and treatment (including the risks and benefits of the procedure and disclosures about alternatives to the proposed procedure) to a patient in language that they understand. Researchers are also obligated to obtain informed consent from individuals who participate as subjects in research. Consent must be given voluntarily in writing by the patient who has the requisite capacity to consent. Prior to receiving healthcare services, it is a normal practice for a patient to sign paperwork consenting to receiving care that is generally provided in a particular setting. Even with this general consent, a nurse should always alert a patient prior to touching; the nurse should explain what she/he is going to do and why. If a patient refuses a specific treatment, the nurse should be respectful of the patient's wishes and communicate with the patient what the risks are in refusing the treatment. The nurse must notify the ordering practitioner of the patient's refusal. Additionally, the nurse should document the refusal (including the conversation with the patient about the risks of refusing the ordered treatment) and notification of the practitioner in the patient's health record.

Competence and Capacity

The application of informed consent assumes that a patient is competent and has the capacity to make reasonable decisions when all the necessary information is provided. Healthcare professionals may confuse competency with capacity or they may use the terms interchangeably.

Competence is a legal term that means a person has sufficient capacity and ability to make reasoned decisions. A person who is competent may make "poor" decisions or use "bad" judgment in making decisions. Such flawed decision-making does not render someone incompetent to make reasoned decisions. The determination of incompetence is a judicial decision; in other words, a judge must make a legal determination of competency. Adults are presumed to be competent unless there is credible evidence revealing an inability to make a reasoned decision. If a person is determined to be legally incompetent, then the court will appoint a guardian over the person to make healthcare decisions and provide safety measures. If a person can make reasoned decisions but is unable to make decisions regarding financial or business matters, a court may appoint a conservator to handle their financial affairs only. Children under 18 years of age are presumed to lack competence unless proven otherwise. However, some state laws allow children of a certain age to make specific healthcare decisions without parental consent. If a guardian or conservator has been appointed by the court, a copy of these documents should be placed in the clinical record. Nurses should read and understand such documents and the extent of powers vested to the guardian.

Capacity refers to an evaluation or assessment of a person's ability to understand, appreciate, and manipulate information to form rational decisions. It is determined by a physician or other healthcare practitioner, not by a judge. Capacity may be affected by drugs or the current/underlying medical condition. For instance, a person with a progressive dementia may be able to decide what they want for breakfast but may not be able to make a reasoned decision on whether to accept chemotherapy treatment for newly diagnosed cancer. Capacity can also change over time. For example, a person who undergoes brain surgery for a tumor may be deemed incapacitated for a period of time after the surgery. Nurses spend more time with a patient and may detect situations where a person is not making reasoned decisions; therefore nursing documentation of objective observations is important to other practitioners in evaluating a patient's changing capacity.

Substituted Judgement and Best Interest Standards

When a patient is unable to give consent directly, a surrogate or agent can give consent on behalf of the patient. If a surrogate is not designated in advance by the patient and the patient was not deemed incompetent and assigned a guardian, the nurse should look to the state advance directive laws. Within the context of these laws, most states list surrogate decision-makers based on their relationship to the patient. Usually, the spouse is designated as the legal decision-maker. Next in line is typically the adult children, or majority thereof. The extent of the list is specific to the state law.

If the surrogate decision-maker has discussed the wishes and desires of treatment or end-of-life care in advance with the patient who is now incapable of making own decisions, the surrogate is ethically bound to abide by the patient's wishes and stand in their shoes. This is called *substituted judgment*. If it is not clear what healthcare treatment or refusal of care an incompetent or incapacitated patient would choose, then the surrogate is ethically obligated to act in the best interest of the patient, known as the *best interest* standard. Surrogates may have a difficult time deciding to withdraw or withhold treatments, despite knowing what the patient would want them to do or what is in their best interest.

Advance Directives

Healthcare entities that receive federal funds are required to provide patients with written information about their rights to make their own healthcare decisions, including the right to execute written healthcare directives in advance, the right to refuse medical treatment, and to appoint a person or agent to speak and make decisions on their behalf if they become incapacitated. The provider must ask patients if they have advance directives and document the patient's response in the medical record. The patient should be encouraged to provide these documents and they should be placed in the patient's medical record. A nurse should become familiar with the contents of a patient's directives. Providers are prohibited from discriminating against patients, based on whether they have advance directive.

All states have laws outlining the specific details of drafting and executing advance directives. These laws encourage compliance with the patient's directive by giving healthcare providers, who act in reliance

on these documents, immunity from civil or criminal liability. Some states impose criminal liability if a patient's advance directives are not followed.

Laws Affecting End of Life

The current discussions on end-of-life issues and the law have far surpassed the age of the right to refuse treatment that would hasten death. The issue of whether mentally competent, but terminally ill patients, should have the right to hasten their death has been a hot topic of discussion and activity since controversial Jack Kevorkian advocated for assisted suicide on behalf of terminally ill patients in the early 1990s.

Oregon enacted the nation's first Death with Dignity Act in 1997,[27] followed by Washington, Montana, Vermont, California, Colorado, Washington, DC, and Hawaii. More than 25 other states have introduced various forms of legislation advocating for these end-of-life options. Although many people liken these acts to state-assisted suicide laws, the language in the statutes distinguish the Death with Dignity Acts from state assisted suicide laws. Nonetheless, these laws are being challenged in state courts by opponents filing lawsuits challenging the legalities of the statute. For instance, on May 15, 2018, a judge in Riverside County overturned California's End-of-Life Options Act. However, on June 15, 2018, a California appeals court reinstated the act while the case proceeds through the court system.

Death with dignity laws allow physicians to write a prescription for a lethal dose of medication that a mentally competent but terminally ill patient can use to end his or her life if the patient has less than 6 months to live. Various safeguards and protocols to be followed by the prescribing physician are included in the laws. For instance, Oregon's Act requires, in part, that the patient make two oral requests at least 15 days apart to the physician followed by a written request signed in the presence of two witnesses, one of whom cannot be a relative of the patient. It also requires two physicians to confirm the patient's diagnosis and prognosis and assess the patient's competency and mental health. Most states with such laws allow provider entities to opt in or out of participating. For instance, the provider who opts out may be required to educate the patient on other options and to provide measures for the patient to be transferred to an entity or provider who will abide by the patient's lawful wishes. It is important to note that because the Veterans Administration Hospitals operate under federal law, it is illegal for the Veterans hospitals, physicians, and clinics to participate in prescribing lethal doses of medicine, regardless of a state's death with dignity law.

Confidentiality Laws

Patients have a right to confidentiality in regard to their health care. The HIPAA laws includes strict requirements about the protection of patient information and distribution thereof; the law is strictly enforced with significant penalties. Likewise, state laws may have confidentiality statutes specific to patient information. This era of electronic medical record systems requires a heightened awareness of these laws. Nurses should learn the pertinent substantive requirements of patient privacy and security laws that are applicable to their practice and always be cognizant of and respectful of a patient's right to confidentiality and privacy.

INTERRELATED CONCEPTS

Four concepts are interrelated to healthcare law: Health Policy, Ethics, Health Care Economics, and Health Care Quality, as shown in Fig. 57.3. At its most basic level, a law is a set of rules that are designed to help meet a specific policy or goal. As such, **Health Policy** encompasses

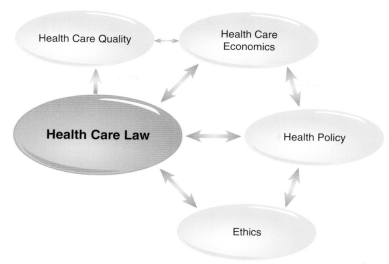

FIGURE 57.3 Health Care Law and Interrelated Concepts.

the goal or expected outcomes, and healthcare laws require interventions or prohibitions that are intended to accomplish the health policy goal or expected outcome. Ethics is a set of values which guide our society and under which many healthcare policies and laws are made. In other words, our society's adherence to an ethical principle may drive a desire to adopt a policy and create laws that promote the policy.

Another concept that is closely interrelated to health care law is Health Care Economics. As previously described, many laws have a financial incentive to compel compliance with the law. There are organizations and departments within healthcare organizations whose job is to ensure compliance with many healthcare laws and regulations. Within a healthcare organization or hospital, this task may be the responsibility of the compliance officer or compliance department. The compliance officer monitors the organization's activities so that the organization can continue to receive payments from the government and is not subject to any fines.

Finally, the concept of Health Care Quality is increasingly more interrelated to healthcare law. For example, as an added incentive to encourage healthcare provider compliance, the government healthcare programs have initiated value-based purchasing initiatives that require healthcare entities to maintain data on specific quality measures at a predetermined level of acceptance in order for the provider to receive the highest level of reimbursement. Additionally, some enforcement agencies have brought actions under the false claims laws for government claims billed and paid under the theory of "worthless services," arguing that the patient did not receive the care as ordered or the quality of services per healthcare standards was not met.

CLINICAL EXEMPLARS

There are a multitude of exemplars of healthcare law, many of which have been highlighted throughout this concept presentation; the most common and important of these are presented in Box 57.3. Some exemplars are listed in more than one category. This illustrates the interrelated nature of the source of laws.

Featured Exemplars
Social Security Act Amendments of 1965 (Medicare and Medicaid)

The Social Security Act Amendments of 1965 created a trust fund for the establishment of the Medicare and Medicaid insurance programs for those who do not have medical insurance through employment (retired individuals and the unemployed).[28] The Medicare program has undergone many changes since it was initially enacted, and the federal government (CMS) can decide what rules healthcare organizations must follow to be eligible for reimbursement. One of the most significant changes was the adoption of payment based on diagnosis-related groups in 1983, which was also eventually adopted by insurance companies to compensate healthcare organizations for the care of those patients. Provider payment structures under CMS continue to evolve.

Emergency Medical Treatment and Active Labor Act of 1986

The Emergency Medical Treatment and Active Labor Act (EMTALA) was a provision of the COBRA of 1986.[29] The policy underlying EMTALA is that hospitals with active emergency departments have a duty to care for those requiring emergency medical services irrespective of a patient's ability to pay. Medicare-participating hospitals that offer emergency services must provide an appropriate medical screening exam to a patient who presents for treatment. The hospital must stabilize any emergency medical condition before transferring the patient to another facility. If the hospital is unable to stabilize the patient's condition, the hospital can arrange for transfer to appropriate level of care.

Health Insurance Portability and Accountability Act of 1996

The HIPAA of 1996 was enacted to provide individuals with preexisting medical conditions access to health insurance if they changed or lost their job. Another element of HIPAA is to prevent healthcare fraud and abuse and promote medical liability reform. The act also included a provision (known as the Privacy Rule) for health information privacy requirements for individually identifiable health information. The Privacy Rule protects the confidentiality of health information relating to the provision or payment of health care for a past, present,

BOX 57.3   EXEMPLARS OF HEALTH CARE LAW

Federal Statutory Laws
- Social Security Act Amendments of 1965
- Social Security Act Amendments of 1983
- Federal False Claims Act of 1986
- Emergency Medical Treatment and Active Labor Act of 1986 (EMTALA)
- Omnibus Budget Reconciliation Act of 1987
- Patient Self-Determination Act of 1991
- Health Insurance Portability and Accountability Act of 1996 (HIPAA)
- Patient Protection and Affordable Care Act of 2010 (also known as the ACA and Obamacare)
- Americans with Disabilities Act of 1990 (ADA)

Federal Regulations
- Centers for Medicare and Medicaid (CMS) CoPs for Hospitals, Nursing Facilities, Home Health and Hospice Agencies (enforced by the States with a contract between CMS and a State Survey Agency)
- HHS/OIG Health Care Provider Self-Disclosures
- Emergency Preparedness Rule (EP)

State Statutory or Regulatory Laws
- Criminal Background Checks
- Immunizations
- Public health and safety: disease surveillance, disaster preparedness
- Consent
- Confidentiality
- Advance Directives/Living Wills/Statutory Surrogates

- Death with Dignity, Aid-In-Dying, or End of Life Options Acts
- Good Samaritan Acts
- State Nurse Practice Acts and Scope of Practice

Torts
- Negligence
- Medical Malpractice
- Patient Abandonment

Contracts
- State contract law
- Health insurance plans: consumers and insurer
- Agreements between the government/insurance payers and providers
- Agreements between providers and healthcare organizations
- Independent Contractor Agreements
- Admission Agreements for nursing facilities, assisted living, and continuing care communities

Criminal Liability
- Federal and State Anti-Kickback Laws
- Medicare and Medicaid Fraud
- Non-Government Health Plan Insurance Fraud
- Patient Criminal Abuse and Neglect
- Assisted suicide laws
- Active euthanasia
- Sexual assault

ACCESS EXEMPLAR LINKS IN YOUR GIDDENS EBOOK

or future physical or mental health condition but does permit the "minimum necessary" use and disclosure of protected health information without patient authorization for purposes of treatment, payment, and healthcare operations.[30]

Health Information Technology for Economic and Clinical Health Act, 2009

The Health Information Technology for Economic and Clinical Health (HITECH) Act was enacted as part of the American Recovery and Reinvestment Act of 2009. HITECH broadened the scope of HIPAA's Privacy Rule and provided for more enforcement of noncompliance by establishing increased levels of culpability and raising penalty amounts for compliance violations.[31] In addition, HITECH includes specific requirements for notifying individuals when their protected health information has been breached or improperly used or disclosed without authorization.

Patient Protection and Affordable Care Act of 2010

The ACA includes provisions to enable Americans with preexisting conditions to more easily afford insurance, the creation of health insurance exchanges to make insurance coverage more accessible and affordable for some individuals and small businesses, and the elimination of insurance copays for preventive care. The law also requires that every American have minimum essential health insurance.[32] This controversial provision of the law (whether or not it is constitutional for the government to compel individuals to purchase insurance) and others has been challenged in the court. Challenges continue under the Trump administration to overturn and or modify portions of the ACA.

Federal False Claims Act of 1986

The Federal False Claims Act is the most effective tool used by the government in combating healthcare fraud and abusive billing practices. A person or entity may be in violation of this law if she/he or the entity (A) knowingly presents or causes to be presented a false or fraudulent claim for payment or approval or (B) knowingly makes, uses, or causes to be made or used a false record or statement material to a false or fraudulent claim.[33] This law also allows for whistleblowers to bring actions against a provider. Evidence to support the government's allegations of false claims usually originates from lack of documentation to show that a patient received the services that were ordered. Additionally, evidence may reveal a lack of clinical documentation to show that the patient needed the services provided. In other words, the terms "medical necessity" or "eligibility" to receive services under the Medicare or Medicare programs must be proven through documentation.

CASE STUDY

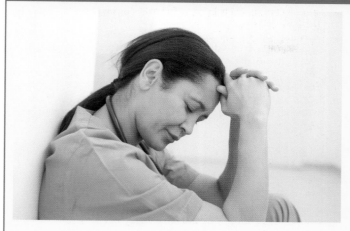

Case Presentation

On July 4, 2006, Julie Thao, RN, an experienced obstetrics nurse with years of expertise worked an extended shift that ended at midnight, and she returned to duty at 7 a.m. on July 5. Shortly before noon on July 5, Thao made a lethal medication error while assigned as the primary nurse to a teenage patient who was admitted to the birthing unit at St. Mary's Hospital for induction of labor.[34]

On July 5, Thao spent almost an hour with the patient on admission explaining the birthing process and answering questions, with much of her focus on alleviating the patient's anxiety. During that time, Thao failed to place an identification wristband on the patient's wrist, in violation of hospital policy. Because the patient tested positive for group B *Streptococcus*, the physician ordered an antibiotic to be administered intravenously (IV) at 11:00 a.m. Anticipating that the patient would need an epidural during labor, Thao gathered epidural medications

(bupivacaine and fentanyl) without a physician's order, took these to the patient's room, and placed them on the counter where the antibiotic was ready and waiting to be administered. At 11:30 a.m., Thao picked up the IV bag that she believed contained the antibiotic and began the infusion intravenously. However, Thao administered the IV bag containing the unordered epidural medication (which is supposed to be administered into the spine).

Almost immediately, the patient appeared to be seizing, and Thao stopped the infusion. Despite efforts to resuscitate the patient, Thao's error resulted in the death of the patient, whose baby was saved by an emergency C-section at 12:20 p.m. Thao was terminated from her position at St. Mary's Hospital, and the patient's family filed a civil lawsuit against the hospital.

The Wisconsin Board of Nursing suspended Thao's license for 9 months, followed by a 2-year practice limitation with terms and conditions, including a requirement to make educational presentations to nurses or nursing students on the topic of preventing medication errors.

A subsequent criminal complaint charged Thao with patient abuse and neglect causing great bodily harm, a felony that carried a penalty of imprisonment and a significant monetary fine.[35] Thao's alleged criminal conduct was characterized as "(1) failing to obtain a doctor's order before introducing medication into the patient's room, (2) not looking at the medication prior to administration, (3) failing to adhere to the 5 'rights' of medication administration, and (4) failing to scan the barcodes on the medication as required."[36] Thao eventually received probation after pleading no contest to two criminal misdemeanors counts related to the unlawful dispensing and possession of the epidural medication.[37]

Case Analysis Questions

1. Consider Fig. 57.2. Which of the sources of law does this case represent?
2. Under what basis did the Wisconsin Board of Nursing have the authority to suspend Ms. Thao's license and impose a 2-year practice limitation?

From Wavebreakmedia Ltd/Wavebreak Media/Thinkstock.

 ACCESS EXEMPLAR LINKS IN YOUR GIDDENS EBOOK

REFERENCES

1. The Florida Bar. (2018). Health Law. Retrieved from https://www.floridabar.org/about/cert/cert-hl/.
2. National Archives. *The Constitution of the United States: A Transcription.* Retrieved from https://www.archives.gov/founding-docs/constitution-transcript.
3. *Griswold v. Connecticut*, 381 U.S. 479 (1965).
4. *Roe v. Wade*, 410 U.S. 113, (1973).
5. *Cruzan v. Missouri Department of Health*, 497 U.S. 261, (1990).
6. Social Security Act Amendments of 1965, Pub. L. No. 89-97, 79 Stat. 285, 1965.
7. Centers for Medicare & Medicaid Services. (2017). What is a MAC. Retrieved from https://www.cms.gov/Medicare/Medicare-Contracting/Medicare-Administrative-Contractors/What-is-a-MAC.html.
8. Centers for Medicare and Medicaid Services. (n.d.). Improving the medicare claims review process. Retrieved from https://www.cms.gov/Research-Statistics-Data-and-Systems/Monitoring-Programs/Medicare-FFS-Compliance-Programs/Medical-Review/Downloads/What_Is_TPE-Infosheet.pdf.
9. Federal Anti-Kickback Statute, 42 U.S.C. § 1320a-b7.
10. New Mexico Statutes, *Resident Abuse and Neglect* Chapter 30: Criminal Offenses Article 47: 30-47-1 through 30-47-10.
11. Wikipedia. *Jurisprudence*. Retrieved from https://en.wikipedia.org/wiki/Jurisprudence.
12. Ibid.
13. Social Security Act Amendments of 1965, Pub. L. No. 89-97, 79 Stat. 285, 1965 and Social Security Amendments of 1983, Pub. L. No. 98-21, 97 Stat. 65, 1983.
14. Consolidated Omnibus Budget Reconciliation Act of 1986, Pub. L. No. 99-272,100 Stat 82, 1986 and the Omnibus Budget Reconciliation Act of 1987 (OBRA), 42 U.S.C. 1396r(b)(4) & 42 U.S.C. 1395i-3(b)(4) also known as the Nursing Home Reform Act and the Federal Regulations: 42 CFR 483.25.
15. Patient Self-Determination Act, 42 U.S.C. § 1395 cc(f), 1991.
16. Health Insurance Portability and Accountability Act, 42 U.S.C. § 1320(d)(6), 1996.
17. Patient Protection and Affordable Care Act, Pub. L. No. 111-148, 124 Stat. 119, 2010, as amended by the Health Care and Education Reconciliation Act of 2010, Pub. L. No. 111-152, 124 Stat. 1029, 2010.
18. U.S. Department of Health & Human Services. (2017). HHS Organizational Chart. Retrieved from https://www.hhs.gov/about/agencies/orgchart/index.html.
19. Wikipedia. (2017). Tuskegee syphilis experiment. Retrieved from https://en.wikipedia.org/wiki/Tuskegee_syphilis_experiment.
20. NCSBN National Council of State Boards Nursing. (2018). *Nurse Practice Act Toolkit.* Retrieved from https://www.ncsbn.org/npa-toolkit.htm.
21. National Practitioner Data Bank. (n.d.). Retrieved from https://www.npdb.hrsa.gov/resources/aboutLegsAndRegs.jsp.
22. Department of Health and Human Services Office of Inspector General. (1995). *Operation Restore Trust Activities.* Retrieved from https://oig.hhs.gov/oei/reports/oei-12-96-00020.pdf.
23. Office of Inspector General, U.S. Department of Health & Human Services. *Health Care Fraud and Abuse Control Program Report-Fiscal Year 2017.* Retrieved from https://oig.hhs.gov/reports-and-publications/hcfac/.

24. Ibid.

25. American Nurses Association. (2015). *Code of Ethics for Nurses*, Nursebooks.org.

26. *Schloendorff v. Society of New York Hospital,* 105 N.E. 92 (N.Y. 1914).

27. Oregon Death with Dignity Act, *Ore Rev Stat* §§ 127.800–127.897:800–995, 1994.

28. Social Security Act Amendments of 1965, Pub. L. No. 89-97, 79 Stat. 285, 1965.

29. Emergency Medical Treatment and Active Labor Act, 42 U.S.C. § 1395dd, 1986.

30. U.S. Department of Health and Human Services. (2003). Office for Civil Rights: *Summary of HIPAA privacy rule.* Washington, DC: Author.

31. Health Information Technology for Economic and Clinical Health Act, 42 U.S.C. § 17921, 2009.

32. Patient Protection and Affordable Care Act, Pub. L. No. 111-148, 124 Stat. 119, 2010, as amended by the Health Care and Education Reconciliation Act of 2010, Pub. L. No. 111-152, 124 Stat. 1029, 2010.

33. 31 U.S. Code § §3729 to 3733 False Claims.

34. In the matter of the disciplinary proceedings against Julie Thao, R.N., Respondent. State of Wisconsin Board of Nursing, December 14, 2006, Final Decision and Order LS0612145NUR.

35. Collins, S. (2007). Criminalization of negligence in nursing: A new trend? *The Florida Nurse, 28.*

36. Ibid. p. 28.

37. Wisconsin Court System. Circuit court access, (n.d.). Retrieved from http://wcca.wicourts.gov.

Page numbers followed by "*f*" indicate figures, "*t*" indicate tables, and "*b*" indicate boxes.